COMPLETE GUIDE TO PRESCRIPTION & NONPRESCRIPTION

DRUGS

By H. WINTER GRIFFITH, M.D.

Technical consultants:
John D. Palmer, M.D., Ph.D.
William N. Jones, B.S., M.S.
Stephen W. Moore, M.D.
Miriam L. Levinson, Pharm.D.

Over 5000 Brand Names
Over 700 Generic Names

A Perigee Book

A Perigee Book
Published by The Berkley Publishing Group
A division of Penguin Putnam Inc.
375 Hudson Street,
New York, New York 10014

Cover photograph by Michael Howell

First edition: October 1999
ISBN: 0-399-52541-6
ISSN: 1082-2585

Published simultaneously in Canada.

The Penguin Putnam Inc. World Wide Web site address is
http://www.penguinputnam.com

Printed in the United States of America

10 9 8 7 6 5 4 3 2 1

CONTENTS

ABOUT THE AUTHOR

H. Winter Griffith, M.D., authored 25 medical books, including the *Complete Guide to Symptoms, Illness & Surgery; Complete Guide to Pediatric Symptoms, Illness & Medications*; and *Complete Guide to Sports Injuries*, each now published by The Body Press/Perigee Books. Others include *Instructions for Patients; Drug Information for Patients; Instructions for Dental Patients; Information and Instructions for Pediatric Patients; Vitamins, Minerals and Supplements*; and *Medical Tests—Doctor Ordered and Do-It-Yourself.* Dr. Griffith received his medical degree from Emory University in 1953. After 20 years in private practice, he established and was the first director of a basic medical science program at Florida State University. He then became an associate professor of family and community medicine at the University of Arizona College of Medicine. Until his death in 1993, Dr. Griffith lived in Tucson, Arizona.

Technical Consultants

John D. Palmer, M.D., Ph.D.
   Associate professor of pharmacology, University of Arizona College of
      Medicine
   Associate professor of medicine (clinical pharmacology), University of Arizona
      College of Medicine

William N. Jones, Pharmacist, B.S., M.S.
   Clinical pharmacy coordinator, Veterans Administration Medical Center,
      Tucson, Arizona
   Adjunct assistant professor, Department of Pharmacy Practice, College of
      Pharmacy, University of Arizona

Stephen W. Moore, M.D.
   Family physician, Tucson, Arizona

Miriam L. Levinson, Pharm.D.
   Clinical specialist for drug information at Meriter Hospital in Madison, Wisconsin

DRUGS AND YOU

A drug cannot "cure." It aids the body's natural defenses to promote recovery. Likewise, a manufacturer or doctor cannot guarantee a drug will be useful for everyone. The complexity of the human body, individual responses in different people and in the same person under different circumstances, past and present health, age and gender influence how well a drug works.

All effective drugs produce desirable changes in the body, but a drug can also cause undesirable adverse reactions or side effects in some people. Despite uncertainties, the drug discoveries of recent years have given us tools to save lives and reduce discomfort. Before you decide whether to take a drug, you or your doctor must ask, "Will the benefits outweigh the risks?"

The purpose of this book is to give you enough information about the most widely used drugs so you can make a wise decision. The information will alert you to potential or preventable problems. You can learn what to do if problems arise.

The information is derived from many authoritative sources and represents the consensus of many experts. Every effort has been made to ensure accuracy and completeness. Where information from different sources conflicts, the majority's opinion is used, coupled with the clinical judgment of the technical consultants. Drug information changes with continuing observations by clinicians and users.

Each year, new drug charts are added and existing charts are updated when appropriate. However, because drug information is constantly changing, you should always talk to your doctor or pharmacist if you have any questions or concerns.

Information in this book applies to generic drugs in both the United States and Canada. Generic names do not vary in these countries, but brand names do.

BE SAFE! TELL YOUR DOCTOR

Some suggestions for wise drug use apply to all drugs. Always give your doctor, dentist, or health-care provider complete information about the drugs you take, including your medical history, your medical plans and your progress while under medication.

MEDICAL HISTORY

Tell the important facts of your medical history including illness and previous experience with drugs. Include allergic or adverse reactions you have had to any medicine or other substance in the past. Describe the allergic symptoms you have, such as hay fever, asthma, eye watering and itching, throat irritation and reactions to food. People who have allergies to common substances are more likely to develop drug allergies.

List all drugs you take. Don't forget vitamin and mineral supplements; skin, rectal or vaginal medicines; eyedrops and eardrops; antacids; antihistamines; cold and cough remedies; inhalants and nasal sprays; aspirin, aspirin combinations or other pain relievers; motion sickness remedies; weight-loss aids; salt and sugar substitutes; caffeine; oral contraceptives; sleeping pills, "tonics" or herbal preparations.

FUTURE MEDICAL PLANS

Discuss plans for elective surgery (including dental surgery), pregnancy and breast-feeding. These conditions may require discontinuing or modifying the dosages of medicines you may be taking.

QUESTIONS

Don't hesitate to ask questions about a drug. Your doctor, nurse or pharmacist will be able to provide more information if they are familiar with you and your medical history.

YOUR ROLE

Learn the generic names and brand names of all your medicines. Write them down to help you remember. If a drug is a combination, learn the names of its generic ingredients.

TAKING A DRUG

Never take medicine in the dark! Recheck the label before each use. You could be taking the *wrong* drug! Tell your doctor about any unexpected new symptoms you have while taking medicine. You may need to change medicines or have a dose adjustment.

STORAGE

Keep all medicines out of children's reach and in childproof containers. Store drugs in a cool, dry place, such as a kitchen cabinet or bedroom. Avoid medicine cabinets in bathrooms. They get too moist and warm at times.

Keep medicine in its original container, tightly closed. Don't remove the label! If directions call for refrigeration, keep the medicine cool, but don't freeze it.

DISCARDING

Don't save leftover medicine to use later. Discard it before the expiration date shown on the container. Dispose safely to protect children and pets.

REFILLS

All refills must be ordered by your doctor or dentist, either in the first prescription or later. The pharmacy that originally filled the prescription can refill it without checking with your doctor or previous pharmacy. If you go to a *new* pharmacy, you must have a new prescription, or the new pharmacist must call your doctor or original pharmacy to see if a refill is authorized.

If you need a refill, call your pharmacist and order your refill by number and name.

Use one pharmacy for the whole family if you can. The pharmacist then has a record of all of your drugs and can communicate effectively with your doctor, you and your family.

ALCOHOL & MEDICATIONS

Alcohol and drugs of abuse defeat the purpose of many medications. For example, alcohol causes depression; if you drink and are depressed, antidepressants will not relieve the depression. If you have a problem with drinking or drugs, discuss it with your doctor. There are many ways to help you conquer such a problem.

ALERTNESS

Many of the medicines used to treat disorders may alter your alertness. If you drive, work around machinery, or must avoid sedation, discuss the problem with your doctor; usually there are ways (e.g., the time of day you take the medicine) to manage the problem.

LEARN ABOUT DRUGS

Study the information in this book's charts regarding your medications. Read each chart completely. Because of space limitations, most information that fits more than one category appears only once. Any time you are prescribed a new medication, read the information on the chart for that drug, then take the time to review the charts on other medications you already take. Read any instruction sheets or printed warnings provided by your doctor or pharmacist.

Take care of yourself. You are the most important member of your health-care team.

DRUG ADVERTISING

Ads can cause confusion. Be sure and get sufficient information about any drug you think may help you. Ask your doctor or pharmacist.

GUIDE TO DRUG CHARTS

The drug information in this book is organized in condensed, easy-to-read charts. Each drug is described in a two-page format, as shown in the sample chart below and opposite. Charts are arranged alphabetically by drug generic names, and in some instances, such as *ADRENOCORTICOIDS, TOPICAL,* by drug class name.

A *generic name* is the official chemical name for a drug. A *brand name* is a drug manufacturer's registered trademark for a generic drug. Brand names listed on the charts include

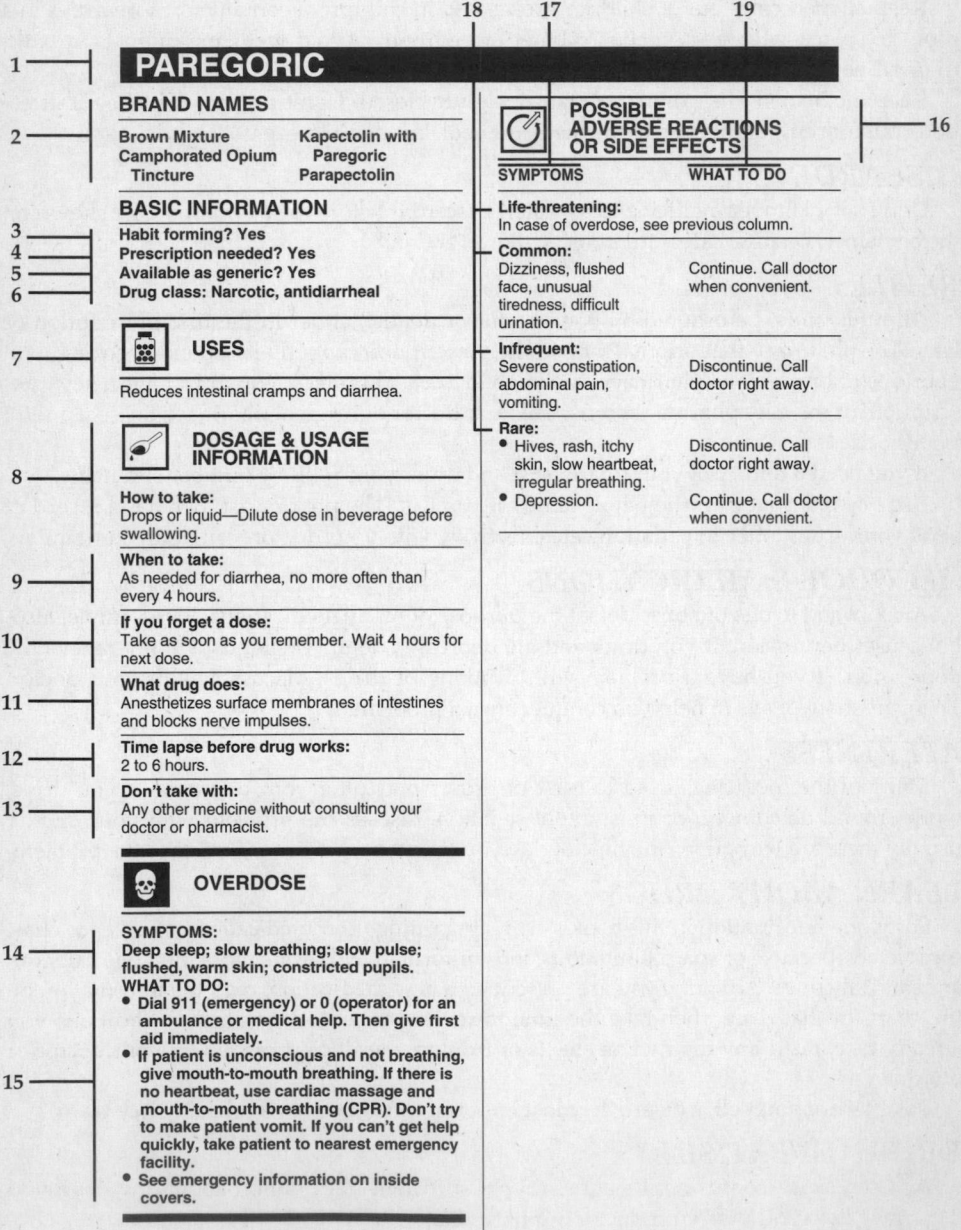

PAREGORIC

BRAND NAMES

Brown Mixture	Kapectolin with
Camphorated Opium	Paregoric
Tincture	Parapectolin

BASIC INFORMATION

Habit forming? Yes
Prescription needed? Yes
Available as generic? Yes
Drug class: Narcotic, antidiarrheal

USES

Reduces intestinal cramps and diarrhea.

DOSAGE & USAGE INFORMATION

How to take:
Drops or liquid—Dilute dose in beverage before swallowing.

When to take:
As needed for diarrhea, no more often than every 4 hours.

If you forget a dose:
Take as soon as you remember. Wait 4 hours for next dose.

What drug does:
Anesthetizes surface membranes of intestines and blocks nerve impulses.

Time lapse before drug works:
2 to 6 hours.

Don't take with:
Any other medicine without consulting your doctor or pharmacist.

OVERDOSE

SYMPTOMS:
Deep sleep; slow breathing; slow pulse; flushed, warm skin; constricted pupils.
WHAT TO DO:
• Dial 911 (emergency) or 0 (operator) for an ambulance or medical help. Then give first aid immediately.
• If patient is unconscious and not breathing, give mouth-to-mouth breathing. If there is no heartbeat, use cardiac massage and mouth-to-mouth breathing (CPR). Don't try to make patient vomit. If you can't get help quickly, take patient to nearest emergency facility.
• See emergency information on inside covers.

POSSIBLE ADVERSE REACTIONS OR SIDE EFFECTS

SYMPTOMS	WHAT TO DO
Life-threatening:	
In case of overdose, see previous column.	
Common:	
Dizziness, flushed face, unusual tiredness, difficult urination.	Continue. Call doctor when convenient.
Infrequent:	
Severe constipation, abdominal pain, vomiting.	Discontinue. Call doctor right away.
Rare:	
• Hives, rash, itchy skin, slow heartbeat, irregular breathing.	Discontinue. Call doctor right away.
• Depression.	Continue. Call doctor when convenient.

those from the United States and Canada. A generic drug may have one or many brand names.

To find information about a generic drug, look it up in the index. To learn about a brand name, check the index, where each brand name is followed by the name(s) of its generic ingredients and their chart page number(s).

The chart design is the same for every drug. When you are familiar with the chart, you can quickly find information you want to know about a drug.

On the next few pages, each of the numbered chart sections below is explained. This information will guide you in reading and understanding the charts that begin on page 2.

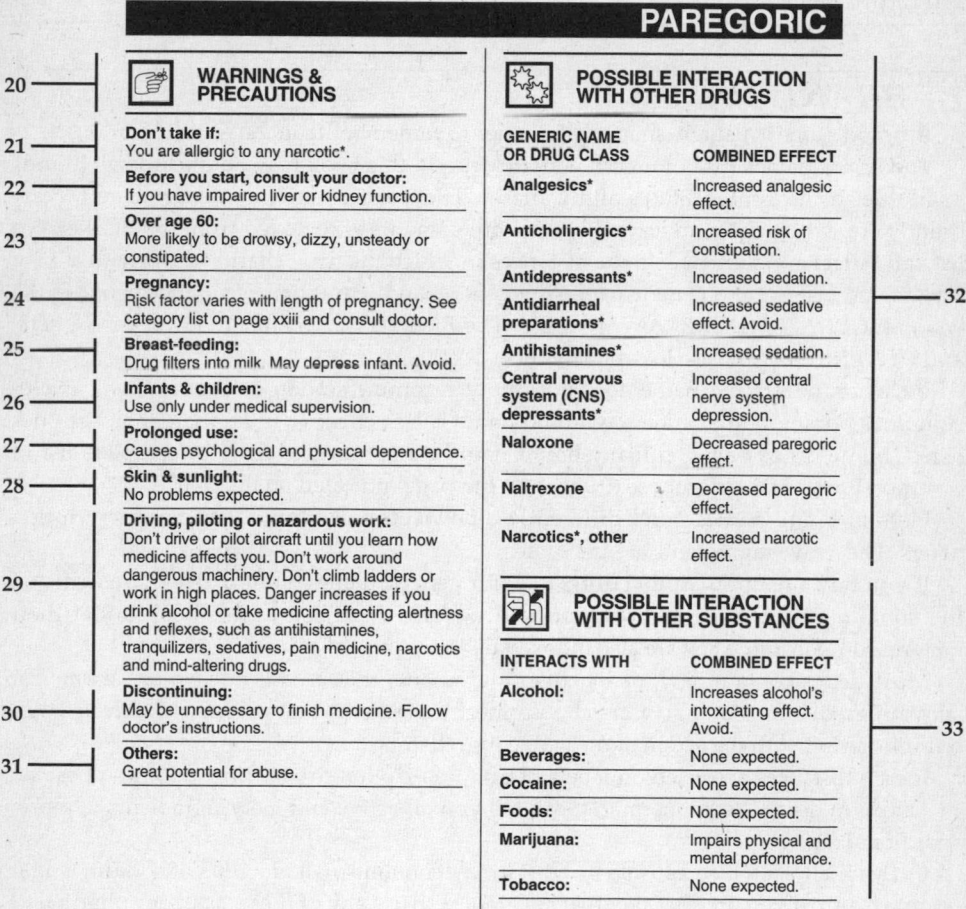

PAREGORIC

20 — **WARNINGS & PRECAUTIONS**

21 — **Don't take if:**
You are allergic to any narcotic*.

22 — **Before you start, consult your doctor:**
If you have impaired liver or kidney function.

23 — **Over age 60:**
More likely to be drowsy, dizzy, unsteady or constipated.

24 — **Pregnancy:**
Risk factor varies with length of pregnancy. See category list on page xxiii and consult doctor.

25 — **Breast-feeding:**
Drug filters into milk. May depress infant. Avoid.

26 — **Infants & children:**
Use only under medical supervision.

27 — **Prolonged use:**
Causes psychological and physical dependence.

28 — **Skin & sunlight:**
No problems expected.

29 — **Driving, piloting or hazardous work:**
Don't drive or pilot aircraft until you learn how medicine affects you. Don't work around dangerous machinery. Don't climb ladders or work in high places. Danger increases if you drink alcohol or take medicine affecting alertness and reflexes, such as antihistamines, tranquilizers, sedatives, pain medicine, narcotics and mind-altering drugs.

30 — **Discontinuing:**
May be unnecessary to finish medicine. Follow doctor's instructions.

31 — **Others:**
Great potential for abuse.

POSSIBLE INTERACTION WITH OTHER DRUGS

GENERIC NAME OR DRUG CLASS	COMBINED EFFECT
Analgesics*	Increased analgesic effect.
Anticholinergics*	Increased risk of constipation.
Antidepressants*	Increased sedation.
Antidiarrheal preparations*	Increased sedative effect. Avoid.
Antihistamines*	Increased sedation.
Central nervous system (CNS) depressants*	Increased central nerve system depression.
Naloxone	Decreased paregoric effect.
Naltrexone	Decreased paregoric effect.
Narcotics*, other	Increased narcotic effect.

— 32

POSSIBLE INTERACTION WITH OTHER SUBSTANCES

INTERACTS WITH	COMBINED EFFECT
Alcohol:	Increases alcohol's intoxicating effect. Avoid.
Beverages:	None expected.
Cocaine:	None expected.
Foods:	None expected.
Marijuana:	Impairs physical and mental performance.
Tobacco:	None expected.

— 33

*See Glossary

1—GENERIC OR CLASS NAME

Each drug chart is titled by generic name or by the name of the drug class, such as *DIGITALIS PREPARATIONS.*

Sometimes a drug is known by more than one generic name. The chart is titled by the most common one. Less common generic names appear in parentheses following the first. For example, vitamin C is also known as ascorbic acid. Its chart title is *VITAMIN C (Ascorbic Acid).* The index will include a reference for each name.

Your drug container may show a generic name, a brand name or both. If you have only a brand name, use the index to find the drug's generic name(s) and chart page number(s).

If your drug container shows no name, ask your doctor or pharmacist for the name and record it on the container.

2—BRAND NAMES

A brand name is usually shorter and easier to remember than the generic name.

The brand names listed for each generic drug in this book may not include all brands available in the United States and Canada. The most common ones are listed. New brands appear on the market, and brands are sometimes removed from the market. No list can reflect every change. In the instances in which the drug chart is titled with a drug class name instead of a generic name, the generic and brand names all appear under the heading *GENERIC AND BRAND NAMES.* The *BRAND NAMES* are in lower-case letters, and *GENERIC NAMES* are in capital letters.

Inclusion of a brand name does not imply recommendation or endorsement. Exclusion does not imply that a missing brand name is less effective or less safe than the ones listed. Some drugs have too many brand names to list on one chart. A complete list of common brand names for those drugs is on the page indicated on the chart.

Lists of brand names don't differentiate between prescription and nonprescription drugs. The active ingredients are the same.

If you buy a nonprescription drug, look for generic names of the active ingredients on the container. Common nonprescription drugs are described in this book under their generic components. They are also indexed by brand name.

Most drugs contain *inert,* or inactive, ingredients that are *fillers, dyes* or *solvents* for active ingredients. Manufacturers choose inert ingredients that preserve the drug without interfering with the action of the active ingredients.

Inert substances are listed on labels of nonprescription drugs. They do not appear on prescription drugs. Your pharmacist can tell you all active and inert ingredients in a prescription drug.

Occasionally, a tablet, capsule or liquid may contain small amounts of sodium, sugar or potassium. If you are on a diet that severely restricts any of these, ask your pharmacist or doctor to suggest another form.

Some liquid medications contain alcohol. Avoid them if you are susceptible to the adverse effects of alcohol consumption.

BASIC INFORMATION

3—HABIT FORMING

A drug habit can be physical or psychological. Either leads to drug dependence. Dependence occurs when there is a strong or compelling desire to continue taking the drug to experience its effects or to avoid the symptoms caused by its withdrawal.

Psychological dependence does not cause dangerous withdrawal effects. It may cause stress and unwanted behavior changes until the habit is broken.

4—PRESCRIPTION NEEDED?

"Yes" means a doctor must prescribe the drug for you. "No" means you can buy the drug without prescription. Sometimes low strengths of a drug are available without prescription, while high strengths require prescription.

The information about the drug applies whether it requires prescription or not. If the generic ingredients are the same, nonprescription drugs have the same dangers, warnings, precautions and interactions as prescription drugs. A nonprescription (over-the-counter) drug has dosing and other instructions printed on the container label. Always read them carefully before you take the drug. The information and warnings on containers for nonprescription drugs may not be as complete as the information in this book. Check both sources.

5—AVAILABLE AS GENERIC?

Some generic drugs have patent restrictions that protect the manufacturer or distributor of that drug. These drugs may be purchased only by brand name.

In recent years, drug manufacturers have marketed more drugs under generic names. Drugs purchased by generic name are usually less expensive than brand names.

Some states allow pharmacists to fill prescriptions by brand names or generic names. This allows patients to buy the least expensive form of a drug.

A doctor may specify a brand name because he or she trusts a known source more than an unknown manufacturer of generic drugs. You and your doctor should decide together whether you should buy a medicine by generic name or brand name.

Generic drugs manufactured in other countries are not subject to regulation by the U.S. Food and Drug Administration. All drugs manufactured in the United States are subject to regulation.

6—DRUG CLASS

Drugs that possess similar chemical structures or similar therapeutic effects are grouped into classes. Most drugs within a class produce similar benefits, side effects, adverse reactions and interactions with other drugs and substances. For example, all the generic drugs in the narcotic drug class will have similar effects on the body.

Some information on the charts applies to all drugs in a class. For example, a reference may be made to narcotics. The index lists the class—narcotics—and lists drugs in that class.

The names for classes of drugs are not standardized, so classes listed in other references may vary from the classes in this book.

7—USES

This section lists the disease or disorder for which a drug is prescribed.

Most uses listed are approved by the U.S. Food and Drug Administration. Some uses are listed if experiments and clinical trials indicate effectiveness and safety. Still, other uses are included that may not be officially sanctioned, but for which doctors commonly prescribe the drug.

The use for which your doctor prescribes the drug may not appear. You and your doctor should discuss the reason for any prescription medicine you take. You alone will probably decide whether to take a nonprescription drug. This section may help you make a wise decision.

DOSAGE & USAGE INFORMATION

8—HOW TO TAKE

Drugs are available in tablets, capsules, liquids, suppositories, injections, transdermal patches (See Glossary), aerosol inhalants and topical forms such as drops, sprays, creams, ointments and lotions. This section gives general instructions for taking or using each form.

This information supplements drug label information. If your doctor's instructions differ from the suggestions, follow your *doctor's* instructions.

Instructions are left out for how *much* to take. Dose amounts can't be generalized. Dosages of prescription drugs must be individualized for you by your doctor. Be sure the dosage instructions are on the label. Advice to "take as directed" is not helpful if you forget the doctor's instructions or didn't understand them. Nonprescription drugs have instructions on the labels regarding how much to take.

9—WHEN TO TAKE

Dose schedules vary for medicines and for patients.

Drugs prescribed on a schedule should usually be taken at approximately the same times each day. Some *must* be taken at regular intervals to maintain a steady level of the drug in the body. If the schedule interferes with your sleep, consult your doctor.

Instructions to take on an empty stomach mean the drug is absorbed best in your body this way. Other drugs must be taken with liquid or food because they irritate the stomach.

Instructions for other dose schedules are usually on the label. Variations in standard dose schedules may apply because some medicines interact with others if you take them at the same time.

10—IF YOU FORGET A DOSE

Suggestions in this section vary from drug to drug. Most tell you when to resume taking the medicine if you forget a scheduled dose.

Establish habits so you won't forget doses. Forgotten doses decrease a drug's therapeutic effect.

11—WHAT DRUG DOES

This is a simple description of the drug's action in the body. The wording is generalized and may not be a complete explanation of the complex chemical process that takes place. For some drugs, the method of action is unknown.

12—TIME LAPSE BEFORE DRUG WORKS

The times given are approximations. Times vary a great deal from person to person, and from time to time in the same person. The figures give you some idea of when to expect improvement or side effects.

13—DON'T TAKE WITH

Some drugs create problems when taken in combination with other substances. Most problems are detailed in the Interaction column of each chart. This section mentions substances that don't appear in the Interaction column.

Occasionally, an interaction is singled out if the combination is particularly harmful.

OVERDOSE

14—SYMPTOMS

The symptoms listed are most likely to develop with accidental or purposeful overdose. Overdosage may not cause all symptoms listed. Sometimes symptoms are identical to ones listed as side effects. The difference is intensity and severity. You will have to judge. Consult a doctor or poison control center if you have any doubt.

15—WHAT TO DO

If you suspect an overdose, whether symptoms are apparent or not, follow instructions in this section. Expanded instructions for emergency treatment for overdose are on the inside back cover.

16—POSSIBLE ADVERSE REACTIONS OR SIDE EFFECTS

Adverse reactions or side effects are symptoms that may occur when you take a drug. They are effects on the body other than the desired therapeutic effect.

The term *side effects* implies expected and usually unavoidable effects of a drug. Side effects have nothing to do with the drug's intended use.

For example, the generic drug paregoric reduces intestinal cramps and vomiting. It also often causes a flushed face. The flushing is a side effect that is harmless and does not affect the drug's therapeutic potential. Many side effects disappear in a short time without treatment.

The term *adverse reaction* is more significant. For example, paregoric can cause a serious adverse allergic reaction in some people. This reaction can include hives, rash and severe itch.

Some adverse reactions can be prevented, which is one reason this information is included in the book. Most adverse reactions are minor and last only a short time. With many drugs, adverse reactions that might occur will frequently diminish in intensity as your body adjusts to the medicine.

The majority of drugs, used properly for valid reasons, offer benefits that outweigh potential hazards.

17—SYMPTOMS

Symptoms of commonly known side effects and adverse reactions are listed. Other drug responses may be listed under "Prolonged use," "Skin & sunlight" or "Others." You may experience a symptom that is not listed. It may be a side effect or adverse reaction to the drug, or it may be an additional symptom of the illness. If you are unsure, call your doctor.

18—FREQUENCY

This is an estimation of how often symptoms occur in persons who take the drug. The four most common categories of frequency can be found under the **SYMPTOMS** heading and are as follows. **Life-threatening** means exactly what it says; seek emergency treatment immediately. **Common** means these symptoms are expected and sometimes inevitable. **Infrequent** means the symptoms occur in approximately 1% to 10% of patients. **Rare** means symptoms occur in fewer than 1%.

19—WHAT TO DO

Follow the guidelines provided opposite the symptoms that apply to you. If you are concerned or confused, call your doctor.

20—WARNINGS & PRECAUTIONS

Read these entries to determine special information that applies to you.

21—DON'T TAKE IF

This section lists circumstances when drug use is not safe. On some drug labels and in formal medical literature, these circumstances are called *contraindications*.

22—BEFORE YOU START, CONSULT YOUR DOCTOR

This section lists conditions, especially disease conditions, under which a drug should be used only with caution and medical supervision.

23—OVER AGE 60

As a person ages, physical changes occur that require special considerations. Liver and kidney functions decrease, metabolism slows and the prostate gland enlarges in men.

Most drugs are metabolized or excreted at a rate dependent on kidney and liver functions. Smaller doses or longer intervals between doses may be necessary to prevent unhealthy concentration of a drug. Toxic effects and adverse reactions occur more frequently and cause more serious problems in older people.

24—PREGNANCY

The best rule to follow during pregnancy is to avoid all drugs, including tobacco and alcohol. Any medicine—prescription or nonprescription—requires medical advice and supervision.

This section will alert you if there is evidence that a drug harms the unborn child. Lack of evidence does not guarantee a drug's safety.

The definitions of the pregnancy risk categories of drugs used by the Food and Drug Administration (FDA) are listed on page xxiii.

25—BREAST-FEEDING

Many drugs filter into a mother's milk. Some drugs have dangerous or unwanted effects on the nursing infant. This section suggests ways to minimize harm to the child.

26—INFANTS & CHILDREN

Many drugs carry special warnings and precautions for children because of a child's size and immaturity. In medical terminology, *newborns* are babies up to 2 weeks old, *infants* are 2 weeks to 1 year, and *children* are 1 to 12 years.

27—PROLONGED USE

With the exception of immediate allergic reactions, most drugs produce no ill effects during short periods of treatment. However, relatively safe drugs taken for long periods may produce unwanted effects. These are listed. Drugs should be taken in the smallest doses and for the shortest time possible. Nevertheless, some diseases and conditions require a prolonged or even lifelong period of treatment. Therefore, follow-up medical examinations and laboratory tests recommended when a drug is used for long periods are listed. Your doctor may want to change drugs occasionally or alter your treatment regimen to minimize problems.

The words "functional dependence" sometimes appear in this section. This does not mean *physical* or *psychological addiction*. Sometimes a body function ceases to work naturally because it has been replaced or interfered with by the drug. The body then becomes dependent on the drug to continue the function.

28—SKIN & SUNLIGHT

Many drugs cause *photosensitivity*, which means increased skin sensitivity to ultraviolet rays from sunlight or artificial rays from a sunlamp. This section will alert you to this potential problem.

29—DRIVING, PILOTING OR HAZARDOUS WORK

Any drug that alters moods or that decreases alertness, muscular coordination or reflexes may make these activities particularly hazardous. The effects may not appear in all people, or they may disappear after a short exposure to the drug. If this section contains a warning, use caution until you determine how a new drug affects you.

30—DISCONTINUING

Some patients stop taking a drug when symptoms begin to go away, although complete recovery may require longer treatment.

Other patients continue taking a drug when it is no longer needed. This section gives warnings about prematurely discontinuing. Some drugs cause symptoms days or weeks after they have been discontinued.

31—OTHERS

Warnings and precautions appear here if they don't fit into the other categories. This section includes special instructions, reminders, storage instructions, warnings to persons with chronic illness and other information.

32—POSSIBLE INTERACTION WITH OTHER DRUGS

People often must take two or more drugs at the same time. Many of these drug combinations have the potential to interact adversely. Fortunately, this adverse reaction occurs in only a small proportion of people who take the interacting combinations. Drugs interact in your body with other drugs, whether prescription or nonprescription. Interactions affect absorption, metabolism, elimination or distribution of either drug. Other factors that can influence drug interactions are the patient's age, state of health and the way the drugs are administered: time taken, how taken, dosage, dosage forms and duration of treatment. The chart lists interactions by generic name, drug class or drug-induced effect. An asterisk (*) beside a drug class name in this column reminds you to "See Glossary" in the back of the book, where that drug class is described and where generic drug names for that class are listed.

If a drug class appears, the drug you are looking up may interact with any drug in that class. Drugs in each class that are included in the book are listed in the index. Occasionally drugs that are not included in this book appear in the Interaction column.

Interactions are sometimes beneficial. You may not be able to determine from the chart which interactions are good and which are bad. Don't guess. Consult your doctor or pharmacist if you take drugs that interact. Some combinations can be fatal.

Some drugs have too many interactions to list on one chart. The additional interactions appear on the continuation page indicated at the bottom of the list.

Testing has not been done on all possible drug combinations. It is important to let your doctor or pharmacist know about any drugs you take, both prescription and nonprescription.

33—POSSIBLE INTERACTION
WITH OTHER SUBSTANCES

The substances listed here are repeated on every drug chart. All people eat food and drink beverages. Many adults consume alcohol. Many people use cocaine and smoke tobacco or marijuana. This section shows possible interactions between these substances and each drug.

INFORMATION ABOUT SUBSTANCES OF ABUSE

Each of the drug charts beginning on page 2 contains a section listing the interactions of alcohol, marijuana and cocaine with the therapeutic drug in the bloodstream. These three drugs are singled out because of their widespread use and abuse. The information is factual, not judgmental.

The long-term effects of alcohol and tobacco abuse are numerous. They have been well publicized, and information is provided here as a reminder of the inherent dangers of these drugs.

Drugs of potential abuse include those that are addictive and harmful. They usually produce a temporary, false sense of well-being. The long-term effects, however, are harmful and can be devastating to the body and psyche of the addict.

Refresh your memory frequently about the potential harm from prolonged use of *any* drugs or substances you take. Avoid unwise use of habit-forming drugs.

These are the most common drugs of abuse:

TOBACCO (NICOTINE)

What it does: Tobacco smoke contains noxious, addictive and cancer-producing ingredients. They include nicotine, carbon monoxide, ammonia, and a variety of harmful tars. Carcinogens in smoke probably come from the tars. Most are present in chewing tobacco and snuff as well as smoke from cigarettes, cigars and pipes. Tobacco smoke interferes with the immune mechanisms of the body.

Short-term effects of average amount: Relaxation of mood if you are a steady smoker. Constriction of blood vessels.

Short-term effects of large amount inhaled: Headache, appetite loss, nausea.

Long-term effects: Greatly enhanced chances of developing lung cancer. Impaired breathing and chronic lung disease (asthma, emphysema, chronic bronchitis, lung abscess and others) much more likely. Heart and blood vessel disease more frequent and more severe when they happen. These include myocardial infarction (heart attack), coronary artery disease, heartbeat irregularities, generalized atherosclerosis (hardening of the arteries, making brain, heart, and kidney more vulnerable to disease), peripheral vascular disease such as intermittent claudication, Buerger's disease and others. Tobacco and nicotine lead to an increased incidence of abortion and significantly reduce the birth weight of children brought to term and delivered of women who smoke during pregnancy. Tobacco smoking not only causes higher frequency of lung cancer, but also increases the likelihood of developing cancer of the throat, larynx, mouth, esophagus, bladder and pancreas.

ALCOHOL

What it does:

• Central Nervous System

Depresses, does not stimulate, the action of all parts of the central nervous system. It depresses normal mental activity and normal muscle function. Short-term effects of an average amount: relaxation, breakdown of inhibitions, euphoria, decreased alertness. Short-term effects of large amounts: nausea, stupor, hangover, unconsciousness, even death. Alcoholism is associated with accidents of all types, marital and family problems, work impairment, legal problems and social problems. Continued abuse of alcohol may result in damage to peripheral nerves and cause various types of brain disorders, including loss of balance and dementia.

• Gastrointestinal System

Increases stomach acid, poisons liver function. Chronic alcoholism frequently leads to permanent damage to the liver.

• Heart and Blood Vessels

Decreased normal function, leading to heart diseases such as cardiomyopathy and disorders of the blood vessels and kidney, such as high blood pressure. Bleeding from the esophagus and stomach frequently accompany liver disease caused by chronic alcoholism.

• Unborn Fetus (teratogenicity)

Alcoholism in the mother carrying a fetus causes *fetal alcohol syndrome (FAS)*, which includes the production of mental deficiency, facial abnormalities, slow growth and other major and minor malformations in the newborn.

Signs of Use:

Early signs: Prominent smell of alcohol on the breath, behavior changes (aggressiveness; passivity; lack of sexual inhibition; poor judgment; outbursts of uncontrolled emotion, such as rage or tearfulness).

Intoxication signs: Unsteady gait, slurred speech, poor performance of any brain or muscle function, stupor or coma in *severe* alcoholic intoxication with slow, noisy breathing, cold and clammy skin, heartbeat faster than usual.

Long-term Effects:

Addiction: Compulsive use of alcohol. Persons addicted to alcohol have severe withdrawal symptoms when alcohol is unavailable. Even with successful treatment, addiction to alcohol (and other drugs that cause addiction) has a high tendency to relapse. (Memories of euphoric feelings plus family, social, emotional, psychological and genetic factors probably are all important factors in producing the addiction.)

Liver disease: Usually cirrhosis; also, deleterious effects on the unborn child of an alcoholic mother.

Loss of sexual function: Impotence, erectile dysfunction, loss of libido.

Increased incidence of cancer: Mouth, pharynx, larynx, esophagus, liver and lung.

Interference with expected or normal actions of many medications: Detailed on every chart in this book, drugs such as sedatives, pain killers, narcotics, antihistamines, anticonvulsants, anticoagulants and others.

Marijuana (cannabis, hashish)

What it does: Heightens perception, causes mood swings, relaxes mind and body.
Signs of use: Red eyes, lethargy, uncoordinated body movements.
Long-term effects: Decreased motivation. Possible brain, heart, lung and reproductive system damage. High dose may initiate symptoms of previously latent schizophrenia.

Amphetamines

What they do: Speed up physical and mental processes to cause a false sense of energy and excitement. The moods are temporary and unreal.
Signs of use: Dilated pupils, insomnia, trembling.
Long-term effects or overdose: Violent behavior, paranoia, inflammation of blood vessels, renal failure, possible death from overdose.

Anabolic Steroids

What they do: Enhance strength, increase muscle mass.
Signs of use: Significant mood swings, aggressiveness.
Long-term effects or overdose: Possible heart problems, paranoid delusions and mania, liver and adrenal gland damage, infertility and impotence in men, male characteristics in women.

Barbiturates

What they do: Produce drowsiness and lethargy.
Signs of use: Confused speech, lack of coordination and balance.
Long-term effects or overdose: Disrupt normal sleep pattern. Possible death from overdose, especially in combination with alcohol.

Cocaine

What it does: Stimulates the nervous system, heightens sensations and may produce hallucinations.
Signs of use: Trembling, intoxication, dilated pupils, constant sniffling.
Long-term effects or overdose: Ulceration of nasal passages where sniffed. Itching all over body, sometimes with open sores. Possible brain damage or heart rhythm disturbance. Possible death from overdose.

Opiates (codeine, heroin, methadone, morphine, opium)

What they do: Relieve pain, create temporary and false sense of well-being.
Signs of use: Constricted pupils, mood swings, slurred speech, sore eyes, lethargy, weight loss, sweating.
Long-term effects or overdose: Malnutrition, extreme susceptibility to infection, the need to increase drug amount to produce the same effects. Possible death from overdose.

PHENCYCLIDINE (PCP, ANGEL DUST)

What they do: Produce euphoria accompanied by a feeling of numbness.
Signs of use: Psychosis or violent behavior, dizziness, loss of motor skills, disorientation.
Long-term effects or overdose: Seizures, high or low blood pressure, rigid muscles. Possible death from overdose.

PSYCHEDELIC DRUGS (LSD, MESCALINE)

What they do: Produce hallucinations, either pleasant or frightening.
Signs of use: Dilated pupils, sweating, trembling, fever, chills.
Long-term effects or overdose: Lack of motivation, unpredictable behavior, narcissism, recurrent hallucinations without drug use ("flashbacks"). Possible death from overdose.

VOLATILE SUBSTANCES (GLUE, SOLVENTS, NITROUS OXIDE, OTHER VOLATILE COMPOUNDS)

What they do: Produce hallucinations, temporary false sense of well-being and possible unconsciousness.
Signs of use: Dilated pupils, flushed face, confusion, respiratory failure, coma.
Long-term effects or overdose: Permanent brain, liver, kidney damage. Possible death from overdose.

CHECKLIST FOR SAFER DRUG USE

- Tell your doctor about *any* drug you take (even aspirin, allergy pills, cough and cold preparations, antacids, laxatives, vitamins, etc.) *before* you take *any* new drug.

- Learn all you can about drugs you may take *before* you take them. Information sources are your doctor, your nurse, your pharmacist, this book, other books in your public library and the Internet.

- Keep an up-to-date list of all the medicines you take in a wallet or purse. Include name, dose and frequency.

- Don't take drugs prescribed for someone else—even if your symptoms are the same.

- Keep your prescription drugs to yourself. Your drugs may be harmful to someone else.

- Tell your doctor about any symptoms you believe are caused by a drug—prescription or nonprescription—that you take.

- Take only medicines that are *necessary*. Avoid taking nonprescription drugs while taking prescription drugs for a medical problem.

- Before your doctor prescribes for you, tell him about your previous experiences with any drug—beneficial results, side effects, adverse reactions or allergies.

- Take medicine in good light after you have identified it. If you wear glasses to read, put them on to check drug labels. It is easy to take the wrong drug at the wrong time.

- Don't keep any drugs that change mood, alertness or judgment—such as sedatives, narcotics or tranquilizers—by your bedside. These cause many accidental deaths by overdose. You may unknowingly repeat a dose when you are half asleep or confused.

- Know the names of your medicines. These include the generic name, the brand name and the generic names of all ingredients in a combination drug. Your doctor, nurse or pharmacist can give you this information.

- Study the labels on all nonprescription drugs. If the information is incomplete or if you have questions, ask the pharmacist for more details.

- If you must deviate from your prescribed dose schedule, tell your doctor.

- Shake liquid medicines before taking (if directed).

- Store all medicines away from moisture and heat. Bathroom medicine cabinets are usually unsuitable.

- If a drug needs refrigeration, don't freeze.

- Obtain a standard measuring spoon from your pharmacy for liquid medicines. Kitchen teaspoons and tablespoons are not accurate enough.

- Follow diet instructions when you take medicines. Some work better on a full stomach, others on an empty stomach. Some drugs are more useful with special diets. For example, medicine for high blood pressure may be more effective if accompanied by a sodium-restricted diet.

- Tell your doctor about any allergies you have to any substance (e.g., food) or adverse reactions to medicines you've had in the past. A previous allergy to a drug may make it dangerous to prescribe again. People with other allergies, such as eczema, hay fever, asthma, bronchitis and food allergies, are more likely to be allergic to drugs.

- Prior to surgery, tell your doctor, anesthesiologist or dentist about any drug you have taken in the past few weeks. Advise them of any cortisone drugs you have taken within two years.

- If you become pregnant while taking any medicine, including birth control pills, tell your doctor immediately.

- Avoid *all* drugs while you are pregnant, if possible. If you must take drugs during pregnancy, record names, amounts, dates and reasons.

- If you see more than one doctor, tell each one about drugs others have prescribed.

- When you use nonprescription drugs, report it so the information is on your medical record.

- Store all drugs away from the reach of children.

- Note the expiration date on each drug label. Discard outdated ones safely. If no expiration date appears and it has been at least one year since taking the medication, it may be best to discard it.

- Pay attention to the information in the drug charts about safety while driving, piloting or working in dangerous places.

- Alcohol, cocaine, marijuana or other mood-altering drugs, as well as tobacco—mixed with some drugs—can cause a life-threatening interaction, prevent your medicine from being effective or delay your return to health. Common sense dictates that you avoid them during illness.

- Some medications are subject to theft. For example, a repair person in your home who is abusing drugs may ask to use your bathroom, and while there "check out" your medicine cabinet. Sedatives, stimulants and analgesics are especially likely to be stolen, but almost any medication is subject to theft.

- If possible, use the same pharmacy for all your medications. Every pharmacy keeps a "drug profile," and if it is complete, the pharmacist may stop medications that are likely to cause serious interactions. Also, having a record of all your medications in one place helps your doctor or an emergency room doctor get a complete picture in case of an emergency.

- If you have a complicated medical history or a condition that might render you unable to communicate (e.g., diabetes or epilepsy), wear a Medic-Alert identification bracelet or neck tag. Call 800-344-3226 for information.

- If you are giving medicine to children, read all instructions carefully. Use the specific dosing device (dropper, cup, etc.) that comes with the product. Don't exceed recommended dose. It does not help and can cause health risks.

COMPLIANCE WITH DOCTORS' RECOMMENDATIONS

For medical purposes, *compliance* is defined as the extent to which a patient follows the instructions of a doctor and includes taking medications on schedule, keeping appointments and following directions for changes in lifestyle, such as changing one's diet or exercise.

Although the cost of obtaining medical advice and medication is one of the largest items in a family budget, many people defeat the health-care process by departing from the doctor's recommendations. This failure to carry out the doctor's instructions is the single most common cause of treatment failure. Perhaps the instructions were not presented clearly, or you may not have understood them or realized their importance and benefits.

FACTORS THAT CAN CAUSE PROBLEMS WITH COMPLIANCE:

- Treatment recommendations that combine two or more actions (such as instructions to take medication, see a therapist and join a support group).
- Recommendations that require lifestyle changes (such as dieting).
- Recommendations that involve long-term regimens (such as taking a medication for life).
- Recommendations for very young patients or for the elderly (another person has to be responsible for following the instructions).

EXAMPLES OF NONCOMPLIANCE:

- Medications are forgotten or discontinued too soon. Forgetting to take a medication is the most common of all shortcomings, especially if a medication must be taken more than once a day. If you need to take a medication several times a day, set out a week's supply in an inexpensive pill box that you can carry with you.
- Side effects of medications are a common problem. Almost all medications have some unpleasant side effects. Often these disappear after a few days, but if they don't, let your doctor know right away. Side effects can often be controlled by changing to a similar medication or by adding medications that control the side effects.
- Not taking a drug because it is unpleasant (e.g., bad tasting). Ask your doctor about options.
- Cost is another reason why there are treatment failures; because of a tight budget, a person may take a medication less frequently than prescribed or just not purchase it. If you can't afford a medication, perhaps a less costly one can be prescribed or your doctor can find other ways to provide it.
- Laboratory tests, x-rays or other recommended medical studies are not obtained, perhaps due to concerns about costs or fear of the tests themselves.
- Recommendations about behavioral changes such as diet or exercise are ignored (old habits are difficult for anyone to change).
- Suggested immunizations are not obtained, sometimes due to fear of needles.
- Follow-up visits to the doctor are not made, or appointments are cancelled, perhaps due to problems finding transportation or long waiting times in the doctor's office.

COMMUNICATING WITH YOUR DOCTOR:

- If you don't understand something, ask.
- If there are reasons why you cannot follow a recommendation, speak up.
- If you have reservations or fears about treatment, discuss them.

Remember, it is your health and your money that are at issue. You and your doctor are—or should be—working together to make you well.

COUGH AND COLD MEDICINES

Coughs and colds are among humans' most common ailments, and the commercial medicines available for treatment are numerous.

There are hundreds of brands of medicines (each with a registered name) designed to relieve symptoms caused by the common cold, influenza and other minor respiratory illnesses. Most of these medications are over-the-counter (OTC) medicines and can be purchased without a prescription. Cold medicines do not cure the infection or hasten the healing process.

Although these drugs may be safe when taken alone, interactions between these medicines and other nonprescription or prescription drugs, when taken together, may produce undesirable or unsafe results. So, for your own safety, you should study the information in this book with regard to the ingredients of each brand-name cough or cold medicine you are taking. Follow these steps to learn about the safety of your drug:

1. Determine the brand name of your drug.

2. Look on the label for the generic ingredients that are used in your brand of medicine.

3. For each generic ingredient, consult the index or look up each generic drug in the alphabetized drug charts. Read the information about how to use the drug safely, especially regarding its use (interaction) with other drugs you may be taking simultaneously.

The generic ingredients of cough and cold medicines fall into several drug classes:

Antihistamines control allergy symptoms. Antihistamines may cause drowsiness, decreased reflexes and decreased ability to concentrate. Therefore, don't drive vehicles or pilot aircraft until you learn how this medicine affects you. Don't work around dangerous machinery. Don't climb ladders or work in high places. The danger increases if you drink alcohol or take other medicines that affect alertness and reflexes, such as other antihistamines, tranquilizers, sedatives, pain medicines, narcotics or mind-altering drugs. They all may cause other side effects or adverse reactions.

Decongestants relieve symptoms of nasal or bronchial congestion. All decongestants may cause nervousness, irregular heartbeats in some people, dizziness, confusion and other side effects. Conduct your daily activities with these effects in mind.

Antitussives reduce frequency and severity of cough. These may be either *narcotic* (codeine and hydrocodone) or *non-narcotic* (dextromethorphan). Narcotic cough suppressants are habit-forming and may cause some of the same mental changes that can take place with antihistamines. The most common non-narcotic antitussive medicine, dextromethorphan, is not habit-forming but has other side effects.

Expectorants loosen secretions to make them easier to cough up. The most common expectorant is guaifenesin, which has very few side effects but doesn't loosen secretions very efficiently.

Analgesics relieve aches and pains. The most common analgesics in cough and cold medicines are aspirin, acetaminophen and ibuprofen.

To learn the details about any cough or cold remedy you may take, look up the brand names in the index of this book. Then consult the generic drug charts listed for each brand name.

PREGNANCY RISK CATEGORY INFORMATION

The pregnancy risk category assigned to a medication identifies the potential risk for that particular drug to cause birth defects or death to an unborn child (fetus). These categories are assigned by applying the definitions of the Food and Drug Administration (FDA) to the available clinical information about the drug. Most drugs are tested only on animals and not on humans for safety during pregnancy, because such testing would subject unborn children to unnecessary risks.

It is best to avoid all drugs during pregnancy, but this rating system can help you and your doctor to assess the risk-to-benefit ratio should drug treatment become necessary. You and your doctor should discuss these benefits and risks carefully before any drug treatment is initiated. You should not take any medications (including nonprescription drugs such as laxatives or cold remedies) without your doctor's approval.

Definitions of the drug categories, labeled A, B, C, D, and X, are listed below:

- A: Adequate studies in pregnant women have failed to show a risk to the fetus in the first trimester of pregnancy, and there is no evidence of risk in later trimesters.

- B: Animal studies have not shown an adverse effect on the fetus, but there are no adequate studies in pregnant women; or animal studies have shown an adverse effect on the fetus, but adequate studies in pregnant women have not shown a risk to the fetus.

- C: Animal studies have shown an adverse effect on the fetus, but there are no adequate studies in humans; or there are no studies in animals or women. The drug may be used by pregnant women because of its benefits and despite its potential risks.

- D: There is evidence of risk to the human fetus, but the potential benefits of use by pregnant women may be acceptable despite the potential risks (e.g., a woman might take such a drug in a life-threatening situation or for a serious disease for which safer drugs cannot be used or are ineffective).

- X: Studies in animals and humans show fetal abnormalities, or reports of adverse reactions indicate evidence of fetal risk. The risks involved clearly outweigh potential benefits, and the drug is contraindicated for pregnant women.

DRUG CHARTS

ACARBOSE

BRAND NAMES

Precose

BASIC INFORMATION

Habit forming? No
Prescription needed? Yes
Available as generic? No
Drug class: Antihyperglycemic, antidiabetic

 ## USES

Treatment for hyperglycemia (excess sugar in the blood) that cannot be controlled by diet alone in patients with type II non-insulin-dependent diabetes mellitus (NIDDM). May be used alone or in combination with other antidiabetic drugs.

 ## DOSAGE & USAGE INFORMATION

How to take:
Tablet—Swallow with liquid. Take at the very beginning of a meal.

When to take:
Usually 3 times a day or as directed by doctor. Dosage may be increased at 4- to 8-week intervals until maximum benefits are achieved.

Continued next column

 ## OVERDOSE

SYMPTOMS:
- **Symptoms of lactic acidosis (acid in the blood)—chills, diarrhea, severe muscle pain, sleepiness, slow heartbeat, breathing difficulty, unusual weakness.**
- **Symptoms of hypoglycemia (not a problem with acarbose used alone)—stomach pain, anxious feeling, cold sweats, chills, confusion, convulsions, cool pale skin, excessive hunger, nausea or vomiting, rapid heartbeat, nervousness, shakiness, unsteady walk, unusual weakness or tiredness, vision changes, unconsciousness.**

WHAT TO DO:
- **For mild low blood sugar symptoms, drink or eat something containing sugar right away.**
- **For more severe symptoms, dial 911 (emergency) or 0 (operator) for an ambulance or medical help. Then give first aid immediately.**
- **See emergency information on inside covers.**

If you forget a dose:
Take as soon as you remember. If it is almost time for the next dose, then skip the missed dose and wait for your next scheduled dose (don't double this dose).

What drug does:
Impedes the digestion and absorption of carbohydrates and their subsequent conversion into glucose, improving control of blood glucose, and may reduce the complications of diabetes. However, acarbose does not cure diabetes.

Time lapse before drug works:
May take several weeks for full effectiveness.

Don't take with:
Any other prescription or nonprescription drug without consulting your doctor or pharmacist.

 ## POSSIBLE ADVERSE REACTIONS OR SIDE EFFECTS

SYMPTOMS	WHAT TO DO
Life-threatening: In case of overdose or low blood sugar, see previous column.	
Common: Diarrhea, stomach cramps, gas, bloating, feeling of fullness in stomach, nausea.	Continue. Call doctor when convenient.
Infrequent: None expected.	
Rare: Lactic acidosis or severe low blood sugar (see symptoms under Overdose).	Discontinue. Call doctor right away or seek emergency help.

WARNINGS & PRECAUTIONS

Don't take if:
You are allergic to acarbose.

Before you start, consult your doctor:
- If you have any kidney or liver disease or any heart or blood vessel disorder.
- If you have any chronic health problem.
- If you have an infection, illness or any condition that can cause low blood sugar.
- If you have a history of acid in the blood (metabolic acidosis or ketoacidosis).
- If you have inflammatory bowel disease or any other intestinal disorder.
- If you are allergic to any medication, food or other substance.

Over age 60:
No special problems expected. A lower starting dosage may be recommended by your doctor.

Pregnancy:
Decide with your doctor if drug benefits justify risks to unborn child. Risk category B (see page xxiii).

Breast-feeding:
It is unknown if drug passes into milk. Avoid drug or discontinue nursing until you finish medicine. Consult doctor for advice on maintaining milk supply.

Infants & children:
Safety and efficacy have not been established. Use only under close medical supervision.

Prolonged use:
- Schedule regular doctor visits to determine if the drug is continuing to be effective in controlling the diabetes and to check for any problems in kidney function.
- You will most likely require an antidiabetic medicine for the rest of your life.
- You will need to test your blood glucose levels several times a day, or for some, once to several times a week.
- Acarbose may reduce absorption of iron, causing anemia. Discuss with your doctor.

Skin & sunlight:
No special problems expected.

Driving, piloting or hazardous work:
No special problems expected.

Discontinuing:
Don't discontinue without consulting your doctor even if you feel well. You can have diabetes without feeling any symptoms. Untreated diabetes can cause serious problems.

Others:
- Advise any doctor or dentist whom you consult that you take this medicine. Drug may interfere with the accuracy of some medical tests.
- Follow any special diet your doctor may prescribe. It can help control diabetes.
- Consult doctor if you become ill with vomiting or diarrhea.
- Use caution when exercising. Ask your doctor about an appropriate exercise program.
- Wear medical identification stating that you have diabetes and take this medication.
- Learn to recognize the symptoms of low blood sugar. You and your family need to know what to do if these symptoms occur.
- Have a glucagon kit and syringe in the event severe low blood sugar occurs.
- High blood sugar (hyperglycemia) may occur with diabetes. Ask your doctor about symptoms to watch for and treatment steps to take.
- Educate yourself about diabetes.

POSSIBLE INTERACTION WITH OTHER DRUGS

GENERIC NAME OR DRUG CLASS	COMBINED EFFECT
Amylase (Pancreatic enzyme)	Decreased acarbose effect.
Charcoal, activated	Decreased acarbose effect.
Hyperglycemia-causing medications*	Increased risk of hyperglycemia.
Metformin	Decreased acarbose effect. Increased risk of side effects.
Pancreatin (Pancreatic enzyme)	Decreased acarbose effect.

POSSIBLE INTERACTION WITH OTHER SUBSTANCES

INTERACTS WITH	COMBINED EFFECT
Alcohol:	May increase effect of acarbose. Avoid excessive amounts.
Beverages:	No special problems.
Cocaine:	No special problems.
Foods:	No special problems.
Marijuana:	No special problems.
Tobacco:	No special problems.

*See Glossary

ACETAMINOPHEN

BRAND NAMES

See complete list of brand names in the *Generic and Brand Name Directory*, page 860.

BASIC INFORMATION

Habit forming? No
Prescription needed? No
Available as generic? Yes
Drug class: Analgesic, fever reducer

USES

Treatment of mild to moderate pain and fever. Acetaminophen does not relieve redness, stiffness or swelling of joints or tissue inflammation. Use aspirin or other drugs for inflammation.

DOSAGE & USAGE INFORMATION

How to take:
- Tablet or capsule—Swallow with liquid.
- Effervescent granules—Dissolve granules in 4 oz. of cool water. Drink all the water.
- Elixir—Swallow with liquid.
- Suppositories—Remove wrapper and moisten suppository with water. Gently insert larger end into rectum. Push well into rectum with finger.
- Powder—Sprinkle over liquid, then swallow.

When to take:
As needed, no more often than every 3 hours.

If you forget a dose:
Take as soon as you remember. Wait 3 hours for next dose.

What drug does:
May affect hypothalamus—part of brain that helps regulate body heat and receives body's pain messages.

Continued next column

OVERDOSE

SYMPTOMS:
Stomach upset, irritability, sweating, diarrhea, loss of appetite, abdominal cramps, convulsions, coma.
WHAT TO DO:
- Call your doctor or poison control center for advice if you suspect overdose, even if not sure. Symptoms may not appear until damage has occurred.
- See emergency information on inside covers.

Time lapse before drug works:
15 to 30 minutes. May last 4 hours.

Don't take with:
- Other drugs with acetaminophen. Too much acetaminophen can damage liver and kidneys.
- Any other medicine without consulting your doctor or pharmacist.

POSSIBLE ADVERSE REACTIONS OR SIDE EFFECTS

SYMPTOMS	WHAT TO DO
Life-threatening: In case of overdose, see previous column.	
Common: None expected.	
Infrequent: None expected.	
Rare: Extreme fatigue; rash, itch, hives; sore throat and fever; unexplained bleeding or bruising; blood in urine; painful, decreased or frequent urination; yellow skin or eyes.	Discontinue. Call doctor right away.

WARNINGS & PRECAUTIONS

Don't take if:
- You are allergic to acetaminophen.
- Your symptoms don't improve after 2 days' use. Call your doctor.

Before you start, consult your doctor:
If you have kidney disease or liver damage.

Over age 60:
Don't exceed recommended dose. You can't eliminate drug as efficiently as younger persons.

Pregnancy:
No proven harm to unborn child. Avoid if possible. Consult doctor. Risk category B (see page xxiii).

Breast-feeding:
No proven harm to nursing infant.

Infants & children:
Use only under medical supervision.

Prolonged use:
- May affect blood system and cause anemia. Limit use to 5 days for children 12 and under, and 10 days for adults.
- Talk to your doctor about the need for follow-up medical examinations or laboratory studies to check liver function, kidney function.

Skin & sunlight:
No problems expected.

Driving, piloting or hazardous work:
Avoid if you feel drowsy. Otherwise, no restrictions.

Discontinuing:
Discontinue in 2 days if symptoms don't improve.

Others:
May interfere with the accuracy of some medical tests.

POSSIBLE INTERACTION WITH OTHER DRUGS

GENERIC NAME OR DRUG CLASS	COMBINED EFFECT
Anticoagulants, oral*	May increase anticoagulant effect. If combined fre-quently, prothrombin time should be monitored.
Aspirin and other salicylates*	Prolonged use of high doses of both drugs may lead to kidney disease.
Isoniazid	Increased risk of liver damage.
Nicotine	Increased effect of acetaminophen.

POSSIBLE INTERACTION WITH OTHER SUBSTANCES

INTERACTS WITH	COMBINED EFFECT
Alcohol:	Drowsiness; long-term use may cause toxic effect in liver.
Beverages:	None expected.
Cocaine:	None expected. However, cocaine may slow body's recovery. Avoid.
Foods:	None expected.
Marijuana:	Increased pain relief. However, marijuana may slow body's recovery. Avoid.
Tobacco:	None expected.

ACETAMINOPHEN & SALICYLATES

GENERIC AND BRAND NAMES

See complete list of generic and brand names in the *Generic and Brand Name Directory*, page 862.

BASIC INFORMATION

Habit forming? No
Prescription needed? No
  High strength: Yes
  Low strength: No
  Yes, for some combinations
Available as generic? No
Drug class: Analgesic, fever reducer, anti-inflammatory (nonsteroidal)

USES

- Treatment of mild pain and fever.
- Salicylates are useful in the treatment of inflammatory conditions such as stiffness, swelling, joint pain of arthritis or rheumatism. For long-term use for inflammatory problems, separate drugs instead of this combination may be safer and more effective.

DOSAGE & USAGE INFORMATION

How to take:
- Tablet or capsule—swallow with liquid.
- Effervescent granules—dissolve granules in 4 oz. of cool water.

When to take:
As needed, no more often than every 3 hours or as prescribed by your doctor.

If you forget a dose:
Take as soon as you remember. Wait 3 hours for next dose.

Continued next column

OVERDOSE

SYMPTOMS:
Ringing in ears; nausea; vomiting; diarrhea; dizziness; fever; deep, rapid breathing; hallucinations; coma; unusual sweating; blood in urine; thirst; vision problems; nervousness.
WHAT TO DO:
- **Dial 911 (emergency) or 0 (operator) for an ambulance or medical help. Then give first aid immediately.**
- **See emergency information on inside covers.**

What drug does:
- May affect hypothalamus, the part of the brain that helps regulate body heat and receives body's pain messages.
- May affect production of prostaglandins to reduce inflammation.

Time lapse before drug works:
15 to 30 minutes. May last 4 hours.

Don't take with:
- Other drugs with acetaminophen or aspirin or other salicylates. Too much can cause damage to liver, kidneys and peripheral nerves.
- Any laxative containing cellulose.
- If medicine you take has a buffering agent added, don't take with tetracyclines.
- Any other medicine without consulting your doctor or pharmacist.

POSSIBLE ADVERSE REACTIONS OR SIDE EFFECTS

SYMPTOMS	WHAT TO DO
Life-threatening:	
In case of overdose, see previous column.	
Common:	
• Jaundice, vomiting blood, black stools, cloudy urine, nausea and vomiting, unexplained tiredness, discomfort on urinating.	Discontinue. Call doctor right away.
• Indigestion or heartburn.	Continue. Call doctor when convenient.
Infrequent:	
Shortness of breath; wheezing (for medicines containing aspirin); decreased urine volume; feet swelling; black or tarry stools; pain on urinating; nausea and vomiting; skin rash, hives; sore throat, fever; easy bruising.	Discontinue. Call doctor right away.
Rare:	
• While taking medicine: Sudden decrease in urine volume.	Discontinue. Call doctor right away.
• After discontinuing medicine: Swelling of feet; rapid weight gain; bloating or puffiness; any urinary problems, such as painful, cloudy or bloody urine.	Check with doctor immediately.

WARNINGS & PRECAUTIONS

Don't take if:
- You are allergic to acetaminophen or any salicylates.*
- Your symptoms don't improve after 3 days use.
- You take a buffered form and need to restrict sodium in your diet.
- You have a peptic ulcer.
- You have a bleeding disorder.

Before you start, consult your doctor:
- If you have ever had peptic ulcers.
- If you have had gout.
- If you have asthma or nasal polyps.
- If you have kidney disease or liver damage.

Over age 60:
Don't exceed recommended dose. More likely to be harmful to kidney and liver or cause hidden bleeding in stomach or intestines. Watch for black stools or decreased urine output.

Pregnancy:
Risk factors vary for drugs in this group. See category list on page xxiii and consult doctor.

Breast-feeding:
Drug passes into milk. Avoid drug or discontinue nursing until you finish medicine. Consult doctor on maintaining milk supply.

Infants & children:
Overdose frequent and severe. Keep containers out of children's reach. Do not give to persons under age 18 who have fever and discomfort of viral illness, especially chicken pox and influenza. Probably increases risk of Reye's syndrome*.

Prolonged use:
- High doses for severe inflammatory conditions taken for long periods may increase likelihood of kidney damage.
- Talk to your doctor about the need for follow-up medical examinations or laboratory studies to check liver function, kidney function.

Skin & sunlight:
No special problems expected.

Driving, piloting or hazardous work:
No problems expected unless you feel drowsy.

Discontinuing:
No problems expected.

Others:
- Children up to 12 years—Don't take more than 5 doses per day for more than 5 consecutive days.
- Adults—Don't take for more than 10 consecutive days.
- Urine test for sugar may be inaccurate.
- Don't take if container has a strong vinegar-like odor.
- May interfere with the accuracy of some medical tests.

POSSIBLE INTERACTION WITH OTHER DRUGS

GENERIC NAME OR DRUG CLASS	COMBINED EFFECT
Adrenocorticoids, systemic	Increased risk of ulcers. Increased adrenocorticoid effect.
Antacids*	Decreased acetaminophen and salicylates effect.
Anticoagulants*	Increased anticoagulant effect. Abnormal bleeding.
Antidiabetic agents*, oral	Low blood sugar.
Anti-inflammatory drugs nonsteroidal (NSAIDs)*	Risk of stomach bleeding and ulcers.
Aspirin and other salicylates*	Likely toxicity.
Barbiturates*	Increased liver toxicity.
Carbamazepine	Increased liver toxicity.
Carteolol	Decreased antihypertensive effect of carteolol.

Continued on page 896

POSSIBLE INTERACTION WITH OTHER SUBSTANCES

INTERACTS WITH	COMBINED EFFECT
Alcohol:	Increased chance of stomach irritation and bleeding.
Beverages:	None expected.
Cocaine:	None expected. However, cocaine may deter body's recovery. Avoid.
Foods:	None expected.
Marijuana:	Possible increased pain relief, but marijuana may deter body's recovery. Avoid.
Tobacco:	None expected.

*See Glossary

ACETOHYDROXAMIC ACID (AHA)

BRAND NAMES

Lithostat

BASIC INFORMATION

Habit forming? No
Prescription needed? Yes
Available as generic? No
Drug class: Antibacterial (antibiotic),
antiurolithic

USES

- Treatment for chronic urinary tract infections.
- Prevents formation of urinary tract stones. Will not dissolve stones already present.

DOSAGE & USAGE INFORMATION

How to take:
Tablet—Swallow with liquid. If you can't swallow whole, crumble tablet and take with liquid or food.

When to take:
At the same time each day, according to instructions on prescription label.

If you forget a dose:
Take as soon as you remember up to 2 hours late. If more than 2 hours, wait for next scheduled dose (don't double this dose).

What drug does:
Stops enzyme action that makes urine too alkaline. Alkaline urine favors bacterial growth and stone formation and growth.

Time lapse before drug works:
1 to 3 weeks.

Don't take with:
- Alcohol or iron.
- Any other medicine without consulting your doctor or pharmacist.

OVERDOSE

SYMPTOMS:
Loss of appetite, tremor, nausea, vomiting.
WHAT TO DO:
Overdose unlikely to threaten life. If person takes much larger amount than prescribed, call doctor, poison control center or hospital emergency room for instructions.

POSSIBLE ADVERSE REACTIONS OR SIDE EFFECTS

SYMPTOMS	WHAT TO DO
Life-threatening:	
In case of overdose, see previous column.	
Common:	
Appetite loss, nausea, vomiting, anxiety, depression, mild headache, unusual tiredness.	Continue. Call doctor when convenient.
Infrequent:	
• Loss of coordination, slurred speech, severe headache, sudden change in vision, shortness of breath, clot or pain over a blood vessel, sudden chest pain, leg pain in calf (deep vein blood clot).	Discontinue. Seek emergency treatment.
• Rash on arms and face.	Continue. Call doctor when convenient.
Rare:	
• Sore throat, fever, unusual bleeding, bruising.	Discontinue. Call right away.
• Hair loss.	Continue. Call doctor when convenient.

WARNINGS & PRECAUTIONS

Don't take if:
You have severe chronic kidney disease.

Before you start, consult your doctor:
- If you are anemic.
- If you have or have had phlebitis or thrombophlebitis.

Over age 60:
Adverse reactions and side effects may be more frequent and severe than in younger persons.

Pregnancy:
Studies inconclusive on harm to unborn child. Animal studies show fetal abnormalities. Don't use. Risk category X (see page xxiii).

Breast-feeding:
Studies inconclusive. May have a potential for adverse reactions in nursing children. Avoid drug or discontinue nursing until you finish medicine. Consult doctor on maintaining milk supply.

Infants & children:
Not recommended. Safety and dosage have not been established.

Prolonged use:
Talk to your doctor about the need for follow-up medical examinations or laboratory studies to check blood pressure, liver function, kidney function, urinary pH.

Skin & sunlight:
No problems expected.

Driving, piloting or hazardous work:
Don't drive or pilot aircraft until you learn how medicine affects you. Don't work around dangerous machinery. Don't climb ladders or work in high places. Danger increases if you drink alcohol or take medicine affecting alertness and reflexes, such as antihistamines, tranquilizers, sedatives, pain medicines, narcotics and mind-altering drugs.

Discontinuing:
Don't discontinue without consulting doctor. Dose may require gradual reduction if you have taken drug for a long time. Doses of other drugs may also require adjustment.

Others:
No problems expected.

POSSIBLE INTERACTION WITH OTHER DRUGS

GENERIC NAME OR DRUG CLASS	COMBINED EFFECT
Iron	Decreased effects of both drugs.

POSSIBLE INTERACTION WITH OTHER SUBSTANCES

INTERACTS WITH	COMBINED EFFECT
Alcohol:	Severe skin rash common in many patients within 30 to 45 minutes after drinking alcohol.
Beverages:	None expected.
Cocaine:	None expected.
Foods:	None expected.
Marijuana:	None expected.
Tobacco:	None expected.

*See Glossary

ADRENOCORTICOIDS (Nasal Inhalation)

GENERIC AND BRAND NAMES

BECLOMETHASONE
(nasal)
Beconase
Beconase AQ
Vancenase
Vancenase AQ
BUDESONIDE
(nasal)
Rhinocort Aqua
Rhinocort Nasal
Inhaler
Rhinocort Turbuhaler
DEXAMETHASONE
(nasal)
Dexacort Turbinaire

FLUNISOLIDE
(Nasal)
Nasalide
Nasarel
Rhinalar
FLUTICASONE
(nasal)
Flonase
MOMETASONE
Nasonex
TRIAMCINOLONE
(nasal)
Nasacort
Nasacort AQ

BASIC INFORMATION

Habit forming? No
Prescription needed? Yes
Available as generic? Yes, for some
Drug class: Adrenocorticoid (nasal); anti-inflammatory (steroidal), nasal

USES

- Treats nasal allergy.
- Treats nasal polyps.
- Treats noninfectious inflammatory nasal conditions.

DOSAGE & USAGE INFORMATION

How to take:
- Read patient instruction sheet supplied with your prescription. Usually 1 or 2 sprays into each nostril every 12 hours.
- Save container for possible refills.

When to take:
At the same time each day, according to instructions on prescription label.

Continued next column

OVERDOSE

SYMPTOMS:
None expected.
WHAT TO DO:
Overdose unlikely to threaten life. If person takes much larger amount than prescribed, call doctor, poison control center or hospital emergency room for instructions.

If you forget a dose:
Use as soon as you remember up to an hour late. If you remember more than an hour late, skip this dose. Don't double the next dose.

What drug does:
- Subdues inflammation by decreasing secretion of prostaglandins in cells of the lining of the nose and by inhibiting release of histamine.
- Very little, if any, of the nasal adrenocorticoid gets absorbed into the bloodstream.

Time lapse before drug works:
Usually 5 to 7 days, but may be as long as 2 to 3 weeks.

Don't take with:
Any other medicine without consulting your doctor or pharmacist.

POSSIBLE ADVERSE REACTIONS OR SIDE EFFECTS

SYMPTOMS	WHAT TO DO
Life-threatening: None expected.	
Common: Burning or dryness of nose, sneezing.	Continue. Call doctor when convenient.
Infrequent: Crusting inside the nose, nosebleed, sore throat, ulcers in nose, cough, dizziness, headache, hoarseness, nausea, runny nose, bloody mucus.	Discontinue. Call doctor right away.
Rare: • White patches in nose or throat. • Eye pain, wheezing respiration.	Discontinue. Call doctor right away. Discontinue. Seek emergency treatment.

WARNINGS & PRECAUTIONS

Don't take if:
You are allergic to cortisone or any cortisone-like medication.

Before you start, consult your doctor:
If you know you are allergic to any of the propellants in the spray. These include benzalkonium chloride, disodium acetate, phenylethanol, fluorocarbons, propylene glycol.

Over age 60:
No special problems expected.

Pregnancy:
Risk factors vary for drugs in this group. See category list on page xxiii and consult doctor.

Breast-feeding:
Drug may pass into milk. Avoid drug or discontinue nursing until you finish medicine. Consult doctor on maintaining milk supply.

Infants & children:
Use only under medical supervision.

Prolonged use:
Not recommended.

Skin & sunlight:
No special problems expected.

Driving, piloting or hazardous work:
Don't drive or pilot aircraft until you learn how medicine affects you. Don't work around dangerous machinery. Don't climb ladders or work in high places. Danger increases if you drink alcohol or take medicine affecting alertness and reflexes.

Discontinuing:
No special problems expected.

Others:
No special problems expected.

 ## POSSIBLE INTERACTION WITH OTHER DRUGS

GENERIC NAME OR DRUG CLASS	COMBINED EFFECT
None expected.	

 ## POSSIBLE INTERACTION WITH OTHER SUBSTANCES

INTERACTS WITH	COMBINED EFFECT
Alcohol:	None expected.
Beverages:	None expected.
Cocaine:	None expected.
Foods:	None expected.
Marijuana:	None expected.
Tobacco:	None expected.

ADRENOCORTICOIDS (Oral Inhalation)

GENERIC AND BRAND NAMES

BECLOMETHASONE
  (oral inhalation)
  Beclodisk
  Becloforte
  Beclovent
  Beclovent Rotacaps
  Vanceril
BUDESONIDE
  (oral inhalation)
  Pulmicort Nebuamp
  Pulmicort Turbuhaler
DEXAMETHASONE
  (oral inhalation)
  Decadron Respihaler

FLUNISOLIDE
  (oral inhalation)
  Aerobid
  Aerobid-M
  Bronalide
FLUTICASONE
  (oral inhalation)
  Flovent
TRIAMCINOLONE
  (oral inhalation)
  Azmacort

BASIC INFORMATION

Habit forming? No
Prescription needed? Yes
Available as generic? No
**Drug class: Anti-inflammatory (inhalation),
  antiasthmatic**

USES

Treatment for prevention of symptoms in patients with chronic bronchial asthma. Does not relieve the symptoms of an acute asthma attack.

DOSAGE & USAGE INFORMATION

How to take:
Oral inhaler—Follow instructions that come with your prescription or take as directed by your doctor. If you don't understand the instructions or have any questions, consult your doctor or pharmacist. Most effective if taken regularly. More effective if taken with a spacer. Talk with your doctor or pharmacist.

Continued next column

OVERDOSE

SYMPTOMS:
None expected.
WHAT TO DO:
Overdose unlikely to threaten life. If person takes much larger amount than prescribed, call doctor, poison control center or hospital emergency room for instructions.

When to take:
Your doctor will determine the dosage amount and schedule that will help control the asthma symptoms and lessen risks of side effects. Usually 1 to 2 inhaled puffs 3 to 4 times a day is sufficient.

If you forget a dose:
Take as soon as you remember. Then spread out the remaining doses for that day at regularly spaced intervals.

What drug does:
Helps prevent inflammation in the lungs and breathing passages. May decrease progression of severe disease.

Time lapse before drug works:
1 to 4 weeks for the initial response and up to several months for full benefits.

Don't take with:
Any other medicine without consulting your doctor or pharmacist.

POSSIBLE ADVERSE REACTIONS OR SIDE EFFECTS

SYMPTOMS	WHAT TO DO
Life-threatening: None expected.	
Common: Dry mouth, cough, throat irritation, hoarseness or other voice changes.	Continue. Call doctor when convenient.
Infrequent: Dry throat, headache, nausea, skin bruising, unpleasant taste, white curd-like patches in mouth or throat, pain when eating or swallowing (thrush).	Continue. Call doctor when convenient.
Rare: Increased wheezing; difficulty in breathing; pain, tightness or burning in chest; behavior changes (restlessness, nervousness, depression) with budesonide.	Continue, but call doctor right away

WARNINGS & PRECAUTIONS

Don't use if:
You are allergic to any corticosteroids*.

Before you start, consult your doctor:
- If you have osteoporosis.
- If you have or have had tuberculosis.
- If you are taking oral corticosteroid drugs.

Over age 60:
No special problems expected.

Pregnancy:
Decide with your doctor if drug benefits justify any possible risk to unborn child. Risk category C (see page xxiii).

Breast-feeding:
Unknown effect. Decide with your doctor if you should continue breast-feeding while using this drug.

Infants & children:
- Should be safe with regular low-dosage regimen. There have been a few reports that long-term use or higher doses may decrease growth rate or cause reduced adrenal gland function. Be sure you and your child's doctor discuss all benefits and risks of the drug.
- Children using large doses of this drug are more susceptible to infectious disease (chicken pox, measles). Avoid exposure to infected people and keep all immunizations up to date.

Prolonged use:
- Talk to your doctor about the need for follow-up medical examinations or laboratory studies to check adrenal function, growth and development in children, pulmonary function, and inhalation technique.
- The drug may lose its effectiveness. If this occurs, consult your doctor.

Skin & sunlight:
No special problems expected.

Driving, piloting or hazardous work:
No special problems expected.

Discontinuing:
Don't discontinue this drug after prolonged use without consulting doctor. Dosage may require a gradual reduction before stopping to avoid any withdrawal symptoms.

Others:
- Advise any doctor or dentist whom you consult that you use this medicine.
- Carry or wear identification to state that you use this medicine.
- Call your doctor if you have any injury, infection or other stress to your body.
- Take medicine only as directed. Do not increase or reduce dosage without doctor's approval.

POSSIBLE INTERACTION WITH OTHER DRUGS

GENERIC NAME OR DRUG CLASS	COMBINED EFFECT
None significant.	

POSSIBLE INTERACTION WITH OTHER SUBSTANCES

INTERACTS WITH	COMBINED EFFECT
Alcohol:	None expected.
Beverages:	None expected.
Cocaine:	Effects not known. Best to avoid.
Foods:	None expected.
Marijuana:	Effects not known. Best to avoid.
Tobacco:	Asthma patients should avoid.

ADRENOCORTICOIDS (Systemic)

GENERIC AND BRAND NAMES

See complete list of generic and brand names in the *Generic and Brand Name Directory*, page 862.

BASIC INFORMATION

Habit forming? No
Prescription needed? Yes
Available as generic? Yes
Drug class: Corticosteroid, anti-inflammatory (steroidal), immunosuppressant

USES

- Used for their anti-inflammatory and immuno-suppressive effect in the treatment of many different medical problems including some cancers.
- Treatment for some allergic diseases, blood disorders, kidney diseases, asthma and emphysema.
- Replaces corticosteroid lost due to adrenal deficiencies.

DOSAGE & USAGE INFORMATION

How to take:
- Tablet, capsules or liquid—Swallow with liquid or food to lessen stomach irritation. If you can't swallow whole, crumble tablet or open capsules.
- Enema—Follow package instructions.

When to take:
At the same times each day. Take once-a-day or once-every-other-day doses in mornings.

If you forget a dose:
- Several-doses-per-day prescription—Take as soon as you remember up to 2 hours late. If more than 2 hours, wait for next scheduled dose (don't double this dose).

Continued next column

OVERDOSE

SYMPTOMS:
Severe headache or retained fluids, convulsions, heart failure.
WHAT TO DO:
- **Dial 911 (emergency) or 0 (operator) for an ambulance or medical help. Then give first aid immediately.**
- **See emergency information on inside covers.**

- Once-a-day dose or less—Wait for next dose. Double this dose.

What drug does:
Decreases inflammatory responses. Suppresses immune response. Stimulates bone marrow.

Time lapse before drug works:
2 to 4 days.

Don't take with:
Any other prescription or nonpescription drug without consulting your doctor or pharmacist.

POSSIBLE ADVERSE REACTIONS OR SIDE EFFECTS

SYMPTOMS	WHAT TO DO
Life-threatening:	
Hives, rash, intense itching, faintness, swelling soon after a dose (anaphylaxis).	Seek emergency treatment immediately.
Common:	
Acne, indigestion, nausea, vomiting, gaseousness, headache, insomnia, dizziness, appetite increased, weight gain, poor wound healing, swollen legs or feet.	Continue. Call doctor when convenient.
Infrequent:	
• Black, bloody or tarry stool; various infections; decreased or blurred vision; fever.	Discontinue. Call doctor right away.
• Mood or emotional changes, insomnia, restlessness, frequent urination, round face, irregular menstrual periods, euphoria, muscle cramps or weakness, stomach or hip or shoulder pain, thirstiness, fatigue, loss of appetite (with triamcinolone).	Continue. Call doctor when convenient.
Rare:	
• Irregular heartbeat, convulsions, leg or thigh pain.	Discontinue. Call doctor right away.
• Skin rash, joint pain, unusual hair growth on face or body, hallucinations, confusion, excitement, darkened or lightened skin color, rectal problems with use of rectal products (irritation, blisters, bleeding).	

WARNINGS & PRECAUTIONS

Don't take if:
- You are allergic to any cortisone drug*.
- You have active case of tuberculosis, systemic fungal infection, herpes infection of eyes or peptic ulcer disease.

Before you start, consult your doctor:
If you have, or have had, heart disease, congestive heart failure, diabetes, AIDS, HIV infection, glaucoma, underactive or overactive thyroid, high blood pressure, myasthenia gravis, blood clots in legs or lungs, peptic ulcer disease, tuberculosis, recent or current chickenpox or measles, kidney or liver disease, esophagitis, cold sores, osteoporosis, systemic lupus erythematosus or hyperlipidemia.

Over age 60:
Adverse reactions and side effects may be more frequent and severe than in younger persons. Likely to aggravate edema, diabetes or ulcers. Likely to cause cataracts and osteoporosis (softening of the bones) with long term use.

Pregnancy:
Decide with your doctor if drug benefits justify risk to unborn child. Risk category C (see page xxiii).

Breast-feeding:
Drug passes into milk. Avoid drug or discontinue nursing until you finish medicine. Consult doctor for advice on maintaining milk supply.

Infants & children:
Use only under close medical supervision.

Prolonged use:
- May lead to glaucoma, cataracts, diabetes, fragile bones and thin skin, growth retardation in children, functional dependence*.
- Talk to your doctor about the need for follow-up medical examinations or laboratory studies to check progress, blood pressure, serum electrolytes, stools for blood, other blood studies, eyes, growth in children.

Skin & sunlight:
No problems expected.

Driving, piloting or hazardous work:
No problems expected.

Discontinuing:
- Don't discontinue without doctor's advice until you complete prescribed dose, even though symptoms diminish or disappear.
- Drug dose needs to be gradually reduced after long-term therapy. Don't stop drug suddenly.
- Drug can affect your response to surgery, illness, injury or stress for 2 years after discontinuing. Tell anyone who takes medical care of you within 2 years about use of this drug.

Others:
- Avoid immunizations if possible.

*See Glossary

- Resistance to infection is less while taking this medicine. Consult doctor if infection occurs.
- Consult doctor about sudden weight gain or swelling.
- Advise any doctor or dentist whom you consult that you take this medicine.
- May cause recurrence of tuberculosis.
- Can interfere with the accuracy of some medical tests.
- Wear or carry medical identification that indicates use of this drug.

POSSIBLE INTERACTION WITH OTHER DRUGS

GENERIC NAME OR DRUG CLASS	COMBINED EFFECT
Antacids*	Decreased effect of prednisone and dexamethasone.
Anticholinergics*	Possible glaucoma.
Anticoagulants*, oral	Decreased anti-coagulant effect.
Anticonvulsants, hydantoin*	Decreased adreno-corticoid effect.
Antidepressants, tricyclic*	Increased risk of mental side effects.
Antidiabetics*, oral	Decreased anti-diabetic effect.
Antihistamines*	Decreased adreno-corticoid effect.
Anti-inflammatory drugs, nonsteroidal (NSAIDs)*	Increased risk of ulcers. Increased adrenocorticoid effect.
Aspirin	Increased adreno-corticoid effect.

Continued on page 896

POSSIBLE INTERACTION WITH OTHER SUBSTANCES

INTERACTS WITH	COMBINED EFFECT
Alcohol:	Risk of stomach ulcers.
Beverages:	No proven problems.
Cocaine:	Overstimulation. Avoid.
Foods:	No proven problems.
Marijuana:	Decreased immunity.
Tobacco:	Increased adreno-corticoid effect.

ADRENOCORTICOIDS (Topical)

GENERIC AND BRAND NAMES

See complete list of generic and brand names in the *Generic and Brand Name Directory*, page 862.

BASIC INFORMATION

Habit forming? No
Prescription needed? For some
Available as generic? Yes
Drug class: Adrenocorticoid (topical)

 USES

Relieves redness, swelling, itching, skin discomfort of hemorrhoids; insect bites; poison ivy, oak, sumac; soaps, cosmetics; jewelry; burns; sunburn; numerous skin rashes; eczema; discoid lupus erythematosus; swimmers' ear; sun poisoning; hair loss; scars; penphigus; psoriasis; pityriasis rosea.

 DOSAGE & USAGE INFORMATION

How to use:
- Cream, lotion, ointment, gel—Apply small amount and rub in gently.
- Topical aerosol—Follow directions on container. Don't breathe vapors.
- Other forms—Follow directions on container.

When to use:
When needed or as directed. Don't use more often than directions allow.

If you forget an application:
Use as soon as you remember.

What drug does:
Reduces inflammation by affecting enzymes that produce inflammation.

Time lapse before drug works:
15 to 20 minutes.

Don't use with:
Any other medicine without consulting your doctor or pharmacist.

 OVERDOSE

SYMPTOMS:
None expected.
WHAT TO DO:
If person swallows or inhales drug, call doctor, poison control center or hospital emergency room for instructions.

 POSSIBLE ADVERSE REACTIONS OR SIDE EFFECTS

SYMPTOMS   WHAT TO DO

Life-threatening:
None expected.

Common:
None expected.

Infrequent:
Infection on skin with pain, redness, blisters, pus; skin irritation with burning, itching, blistering or peeling; acne-like skin eruptions. | Continue. Call doctor when convenient.

Rare:
None expected.

Note: Side effects are unlikely if topical adrenocorticoids are used in low doses for short periods of time. High doses for long periods can possibly cause the adverse reactions of cortisone (see CORTISONE).

WARNINGS & PRECAUTIONS

Don't take if:
You are allergic to any topical adrenocorticoid (cortisone) preparation.

Before you start, consult your doctor:
- If you plan pregnancy within medication period.
- If you have diabetes.
- If you have infection at treatment site.
- If you have stomach ulcer.
- If you have tuberculosis.

Over age 60:
Adverse reactions and side effects may be more frequent and severe than in younger persons, especially thinning of the skin.

Pregnancy:
Decide with your doctor whether drug benefits justify risk to unborn child. Risk category C (see page xxiii).

Breast-feeding:
No problems expected.

Infants & children:
- Use only under medical supervision. Too much for too long can be absorbed into blood stream through skin and retard growth.
- For infants in diapers, avoid plastic pants or tight diapers.

Prolonged use:
- Increases chance of absorption into blood stream to cause side effects of oral cortisone drugs.
- May thin skin where used.
- Talk to your doctor about the need for follow-up medical examinations or laboratory studies to check complete blood counts (white blood cell count, platelet count, red blood cell count, hemoglobin, hematocrit), adrenal function.

Skin & sunlight:
Desoximetasone may cause rash or intensify sunburn in areas exposed to sun or ultraviolet light (photosensitivity reaction). Avoid over-exposure. Notify doctor if reaction occurs.

Driving, piloting or hazardous work:
No problems expected.

Discontinuing:
May be unnecessary to finish medicine. Follow doctor's instructions.

Others:
- Don't use a plastic dressing longer than 2 weeks.
- Aerosol spray—Store in cool place. Don't use near heat or open flame or while smoking. Don't puncture, break or burn container.
- Don't use for acne or gingivitis.

 ## POSSIBLE INTERACTION WITH OTHER DRUGS

GENERIC NAME OR DRUG CLASS	COMBINED EFFECT
Antibacterials* (topical)	Decreased antibiotic effects.
Antifungals* (topical)	Decreased antifungal effect.

 ## POSSIBLE INTERACTION WITH OTHER SUBSTANCES

INTERACTS WITH	COMBINED EFFECT
Alcohol:	None expected.
Beverages:	None expected.
Cocaine:	None expected.
Foods:	None expected.
Marijuana:	None expected.
Tobacco:	None expected.

*See Glossary

ALENDRONATE

BRAND NAMES

Fosamax

BASIC INFORMATION

Habit forming? No
Prescription needed? Yes
Available as generic? No
Drug class: Osteoporosis therapy,
  bisphosphonate

 ## USES

- Prevention and treatment of postmenopausal osteoporosis (thinning of bones) in females. Osteoporosis is a major cause of bone fractures.
- Treatment for Paget's disease of bone.

 ## DOSAGE & USAGE INFORMATION

How to take:
Tablet—Swallow with a full glass of water (6 to 8 oz.). To help the medicine reach your stomach faster and to prevent throat irritation, don't lie down for 30 minutes after you take it.

When to take:
At the same time each day. Take in the morning at least 30 to 60 minutes before eating, drinking or taking any other medications.

If you forget a dose:
Skip the missed dose entirely, then resume schedule the next morning. Do not double this dose.

What drug does:
Slows down the loss of bone tissue and increases bone mass in women with osteo-porosis. Osteoporosis is a progressive disease in which bone breakdown increases faster than bone formation.

Time lapse before drug works:
Up to 6 months or longer.

Continued next column

 ## OVERDOSE

SYMPTOMS:
Increased severity of heartburn, stomach cramps, throat irritation.
WHAT TO DO:
Overdose unlikely to threaten life. If person takes much larger amount than prescribed, call doctor, poison control center or hospital emergency room for instructions.

Don't take with:
- Any other prescription or nonprescription drug without consulting your doctor or pharmacist.
- Any other medication at the same time as alendronate. Wait 30 minutes.

 ## POSSIBLE ADVERSE REACTIONS OR SIDE EFFECTS

SYMPTOMS	WHAT TO DO
Life-threatening: None expected.	
Common: Stomach pain.	Continue. Call doctor when convenient.
Infrequent: Bone or muscle pain, nausea, constipation or diarrhea, gas, bloated feeling, heartburn, throat pain or irritation, swallowing difficulty, headache.	Continue. Call doctor when convenient.
Rare: Skin rash.	Continue. Call doctor when convenient.

WARNINGS & PRECAUTIONS

Don't take if:
You are allergic to alendronate or etidronate.

Before you start, consult your doctor:
- If you are allergic to any medication, food or other substance.
- If you currently have a gastrointestinal problem.
- If you have low blood levels of calcium (hypocalcemia) or vitamin D deficiency.
- If you have kidney problems.

Over age 60:
No special problems expected.

Pregnancy:
Normally not used in premenopausal women. Risk category C (see page xxiii).

Breast-feeding:
Unknown if drug passes into milk. Avoid drug or discontinue nursing until you finish medicine. Consult doctor for advice on maintaining milk supply.

Infants & children:
Not recommended for this age group.

Prolonged use:
- No special problems expected. Long-term safety has not been established, and medical studies are continuing.
- Visit your doctor regularly to determine if the drug is continuing to control bone loss and to monitor your calcium levels.

Skin & sunlight:
No special problems expected.

Driving, piloting or hazardous work:
No special problems expected.

Discontinuing:
Don't discontinue without your doctor's approval.

Others:
- In addition to taking the drug, weight-bearing exercise and adequate dietary intake of calcium and vitamin D are essential in preventing bone loss. Dietary supplements of 1000 mg elemental calcium and 400 I.U. vitamin D daily may be recommended by your doctor.
- Advise any doctor or dentist whom you consult that you take this medicine.
- May affect the results of some medical tests.
- Smoking and alcohol consumption are risk factors for osteoporosis and should be discontinued.

POSSIBLE INTERACTION WITH OTHER DRUGS

GENERIC NAME OR DRUG CLASS	COMBINED EFFECT
Antacids*	Decreased effect of alendronate. Take 30 minutes after alendronate.
Aspirin-containing products	Increased risk of stomach irritation.
Calcium supplements*	Decreased effect of alendronate. Take 30 minutes after alendronate.
Hormone replacement therapy*	Unknown effect. Not recommended.
Vitamin supplements	Decreased effect of alendronate. Take 30 minutes after alendronate.

POSSIBLE INTERACTION WITH OTHER SUBSTANCES

INTERACTS WITH	COMBINED EFFECT
Alcohol:	No special problems expected, but alcohol is a risk factor for osteoporosis.
Beverages: Any beverage other than plain water.	Decreased effect of alendronate. Wait 30 minutes after taking alendronate.
Cocaine:	No special problems expected.
Foods: Any food.	Decreased effect of alendronate. Wait 30 minutes after taking alendronate.
Marijuana:	No special problems expected.
Tobacco:	No special problems expected, but smoking is a risk factor for osteoporosis.

ALLOPURINOL

BRAND NAMES

Alloprin	Novopural
Apo-Allopurinol	Purinol
Lopurin	Zyloprim

BASIC INFORMATION

Habit forming? No
Prescription needed? Yes
Available as generic? Yes
Drug class: Antigout

USES

- Treatment for chronic gout.
- Prevention of kidney stones caused by uric acid.

DOSAGE & USAGE INFORMATION

How to take:
Tablet—Swallow with liquid or food to lessen stomach irritation.

When to take:
At the same times each day.

If you forget a dose:
- 1 dose per day—Take as soon as you remember up to 6 hours late. If more than 6 hours, wait for next scheduled dose (don't double this dose).
- More than 1 dose per day—Take as soon as you remember up to 3 hours late. If more than 3 hours, wait for next scheduled dose (don't double this dose).

What drug does:
Slows formation of uric acid by inhibiting enzyme (xanthine oxidase) activity.

Time lapse before drug works:
Reduces blood uric acid in 1 to 3 weeks. May require 6 months to prevent acute gout attacks.

Don't take with:
Any other medicine without consulting your doctor or pharmacist.

OVERDOSE

SYMPTOMS:
None expected.
WHAT TO DO:
Overdose unlikely to threaten life. If person takes much larger amount than prescribed, call doctor, poison control center or hospital emergency room for instructions.

POSSIBLE ADVERSE REACTIONS OR SIDE EFFECTS

SYMPTOMS	WHAT TO DO
Life-threatening: None expected.	
Common: Rash, hives, itch.	Discontinue. Call doctor right away.
Infrequent: • Jaundice (yellow skin or eyes.)	Discontinue. Call doctor right away.
• Drowsiness, diarrhea, stomach pain, nausea or vomiting without other symptoms, headache.	Continue. Call doctor when convenient.
Rare: • Sore throat, fever, unusual bleeding or bruising.	Discontinue. Call doctor right away.
• Numbness, tingling, pain in hands or feet.	Continue. Call doctor when convenient.

WARNINGS & PRECAUTIONS

Don't take if:
You are allergic to allopurinol.

Before you start, consult your doctor:
If you have had liver or kidney problems.

Over age 60:
Adverse reactions and side effects may be more frequent and severe than in younger persons.

Pregnancy:
Decide with your doctor whether drug benefits justify risk to unborn child. Risk category C (see page xxiii).

Breast-feeding:
Drug passes into milk. Avoid drug or discontinue nursing. Consult doctor for advice on maintaining milk supply.

Infants & children:
Not recommended.

Prolonged use:
Talk to your doctor about the need for follow-up medical examinations or laboratory studies to check liver function, kidney function, complete blood counts (white blood cell count, platelet count, red blood cell count, hemoglobin, hematocrit), and serum uric-acid determinations.

Skin & sunlight:
No problems expected.

Driving, piloting or hazardous work:
Avoid if you feel drowsy. Use may disqualify you for piloting aircraft.

Discontinuing:
Don't discontinue without doctor's advice until you complete prescribed dose, even though symptoms diminish or disappear.

Others:
Acute gout attacks may increase during first weeks of use. If so, consult doctor about additional medicine.

POSSIBLE INTERACTION WITH OTHER DRUGS

GENERIC NAME OR DRUG CLASS	COMBINED EFFECT
Amoxicillin	Likely skin rash.
Ampicillin	Likely skin rash.
Anticoagulants, oral*	May increase anticoagulant effect.
Antidiabetics, oral*	Increased uric acid elimination.
Azathioprine	Greatly increased azathioprine effect.
Chlorpropamide	May increase chlorpropamide effect.
Chlorthalidone	Decreased all opurinol effect.
Cyclophosphamide	Increased cyclophosphamide toxicity.
Diuretics, thiazide*	Decreased allopurinol effect.
Ethacrynic acid	Decreased allopurinol effect.
Furosemide	Decreased allopurinol effect.
Indapamide	Decreased allopurinol effect.
Iron supplements*	Excessive accumulation of iron in tissues.
Mercaptopurine	Increased mercaptopurine effect.
Metolazone	Decreased allopurinol effect.
Probenecid	Increased allopurinol effect.
Theophylline	May increase theophylline effect.

POSSIBLE INTERACTION WITH OTHER SUBSTANCES

INTERACTS WITH	COMBINED EFFECT
Alcohol:	None expected, but may impair management of gout.
Beverages:	Caffeine drinks. Decreased allopurinol effect.
Cocaine:	Decreased allopurinol effect. Avoid.
Foods:	None expected. Low-purine diet* recommended.
Marijuana:	Occasional use— None expected. Daily use—Possible increase in uric acid level.
Tobacco:	None expected.

*See Glossary

ALPHA ADRENERGIC RECEPTOR BLOCKERS

GENERIC AND BRAND NAMES

DOXAZOSIN
  Cardura
PRAZOSIN
  Minipress
  Minizide

TAMSULOSIN
  Flomax
TERAZOSIN
  Hytrin

BASIC INFORMATION

Habit forming? No
Prescription needed? Yes
Available as generic? Yes, for some
Drug class: Antihypertensive

USES

- Treatment for high blood pressure.
- May improve congestive heart failure.
- Treatment for Raynaud's disease.
- Treatment for benign prostatic hyperplasia.

DOSAGE & USAGE INFORMATION

How to take:
Tablet or capsule—Swallow with liquid. If you can't swallow whole, crumble tablet or open capsule and take with liquid or food.

When to take:
At the same times each day.

If you forget a dose:
Take as soon as you remember up to 2 hours late. If more than 2 hours, wait for next scheduled dose (don't double this dose).

Continued next column

OVERDOSE

SYMPTOMS:
Extreme weakness; rapid or irregular heartbeat; loss of consciousness; cold, sweaty skin; weak, rapid pulse; coma.
WHAT TO DO:
- Dial 911 (emergency) or 0 (operator) for an ambulance or medical help. Then give first aid immediately.
- If patient is unconscious and not breathing, give mouth-to-mouth breathing. If there is no heartbeat, use cardiac massage and mouth-to-mouth breathing (CPR). Don't try to make patient vomit. If you can't get help quickly, take patient to nearest emergency facility.
- See emergency information on inside covers.

What drug does:
Expands and relaxes blood vessel walls to lower blood pressure.

Time lapse before drug works:
30 minutes.

Don't take with:
Any other medicine without consulting your doctor or pharmacist.

POSSIBLE ADVERSE REACTIONS OR SIDE EFFECTS

SYMPTOMS	WHAT TO DO
Life-threatening: In case of overdose, see previous column.	
Common: Headache, dizziness.	Continue. Call doctor when convenient.
Infrequent: • Rash or itchy skin, blurred vision, shortness of breath, difficulty breathing, chest pain, rapid heartbeat.	Discontinue. Call doctor right away.
• Appetite loss, constipation or diarrhea, abdominal pain, nausea, vomiting, fluid retention, joint or muscle aches, tiredness, weakness and faintness when arising from bed or chair.	Continue. Call doctor when convenient.
• Headache, irritability, depression, dry mouth, stuffy nose, increased urination, drowsiness.	Continue. Tell doctor at next visit.
Rare: Decreased sexual function, numbness or tingling in hands or feet.	Continue. Call doctor when convenient.

WARNINGS & PRECAUTIONS

Don't take if:
You are allergic to alpha adrenergic receptor blockers.

Before you start, consult your doctor:
- If you experience lightheadedness or fainting with other antihypertensive drugs.
- If you are easily depressed.
- If you have impaired brain circulation or have had a stroke.
- You will have surgery within 2 months, including dental surgery, requiring general or spinal anesthesia.
- If you have coronary heart disease (with or without angina).
- If you have kidney disease or impaired liver function.

Over age 60:
Begin with no more than 1 mg. per day for first 3 days. Increases should be gradual and supervised by your doctor. Don't stand while taking. Sudden changes in position may cause falls. Sit or lie down promptly if you feel dizzy. If you have impaired brain circulation or coronary heart disease, excessive lowering of blood pressure should be avoided. Report problems to your doctor immediately.

Pregnancy:
Risk factors vary for drugs in this group. See category page xxiii and consult doctor.

Breast-feeding:
No proven problems. Consult doctor.

Infants & children:
Not recommended.

Prolonged use:
Talk to your doctor about the need for follow-up medical examinations or laboratory studies.

Skin & sunlight:
No problems expected.

Driving, piloting or hazardous work:
Don't drive or pilot aircraft until you learn how medicine affects you. Don't work around dangerous machinery. Don't climb ladders or work in high places.

Discontinuing:
Don't discontinue without doctor's advice until you complete prescribed dose, even though symptoms diminish or disappear.

Others:
- First dose likely to cause dizziness or light-headedness. Take drug at night and get out of bed slowly next morning.
- Advise any doctor or dentist whom you consult that you take this medicine.
- May affect the results in some medical tests.

POSSIBLE INTERACTION WITH OTHER DRUGS

GENERIC NAME OR DRUG CLASS	COMBINED EFFECT
Amphetamines*	Decreased alpha adrenergic blocker effect.
Antihypertensives, other*	Increased anti-hypertensive effect. Dosages may require adjustments.
Anti-inflammatory drugs, nonsteroidal (NSAIDs)*	Decreased effect of alpha adrenergic blocker.
Estrogen	Decreased effect of alpha adrenergic blocker.
Sympathomimetics*	Decreased effect of alpha adrenergic blocker.

POSSIBLE INTERACTION WITH OTHER SUBSTANCES

INTERACTS WITH	COMBINED EFFECT
Alcohol:	Excessive blood pressure drop.
Beverages:	None expected.
Cocaine:	Increased risk of heart block and high blood pressure.
Foods:	None expected.
Marijuana:	Possible fainting. Avoid.
Tobacco:	Possible spasm of coronary arteries. Avoid.

*See Glossary

ALPROSTADIL

BRAND NAMES

Caverject   Muse

BASIC INFORMATION

Habit forming? No
Prescription needed? Yes
Available as generic? No
Drug class: Impotence therapy

USES

Treatment for impotence in some men who have erectile dysfunction due to neurologic, vascular, psychological or mixed causes.

DOSAGE & USAGE INFORMATION

How to use:
- Injection—The first injection will be given in the doctor's office to determine proper dosage and to train you in preparing and self-injecting the drug. When using it at home, follow the instructions provided with the prescription or use as directed by your doctor to inject drug into the penis.
- Intraurethral—Use as a single dose suppository 10 to 30 minutes prior to intercourse.

When to take:
Usually 10 to 30 minutes prior to sexual intercourse. Do not use injection more than 3 times in one week, and do not use more than once in a 24-hour period. Do not use more than 2 suppositories in one 24 hour period.

If you forget a dose:
Not used on a scheduled basis.

What drug does:
Increases the blood flow into the penis and decreases the blood flow from the penis. The change in blood flow causes the penis to swell and elongate.

Continued next column

OVERDOSE

SYMPTOMS:
Prolonged penile erection.
WHAT TO DO:
Overdose unlikely to threaten life. If someone uses larger amount than prescribed, call doctor, poison control center or hospital emergency room for instructions.

Time lapse before drug works:
5 to 20 minutes. Erections may last up to 60 minutes.

Don't take with:
Any other medication without consulting your doctor or pharmacist.

POSSIBLE ADVERSE REACTIONS OR SIDE EFFECTS

SYMPTOMS	WHAT TO DO
Life-threatening: None expected.	
Common:	
• Pain at site of injection, aching or burning pain during erection.	Discontinue. Call doctor when convenient.
• Pinching sensation at injection site.	Continue. Tell doctor at next visit.
Infrequent: None expected.	
Rare:	
• Erection lasting more than 4 hours is not priapism; (priapism is defined as an erection lasting more than 6 hours). Could cause permanent damage to the penis.	Call doctor right away or seek emergency care.
• Bruising or bleeding at site of injection; redness, swelling, tenderness, lumpiness, itching, rash, irritation, strange feeling, numbness or curving of the erect penis; slight bleeding from urethra, swelling of leg veins, dizziness, fainting, rapid pulse. Female partners may have mild vaginal itching or burning.	Discontinue. Call doctor when convenient.

WARNINGS & PRECAUTIONS

Don't use if:
You are allergic to alprostadil or you have been advised not to have sex.

Before you start, consult your doctor:
- If you have liver disease.
- If you have sickle cell anemia or trait.
- If you have multiple myeloma or leukemia.
- If you have a penile implant or any type of penile malformation.
- If you are allergic to any other medications.
- If you have a history of priapism (prolonged penile erection).

Over age 60:
Effects on this age group are variable. Consult doctor.

Pregnancy:
Not used by females. Men should not use the product to have sexual intercourse with a pregnant woman unless the couple uses a condom barrier.

Breast-feeding:
Not used by females.

Infants & children:
Not used in this age group.

Prolonged use:
Have regular checkups with your doctor while using this drug to determine the effectiveness of the treatment and to check for any penile problems.

Skin & sunlight:
No special problems expected.

Driving, piloting or hazardous work:
No special problems expected.

Discontinuing:
No special problems expected.

Others:
- Don't increase dosage or frequency of use without your doctor's approval.
- Follow label instructions, and dispose of all needles properly after use. Do not reuse or share needles.
- The injection of this drug provides no protection from sexually transmitted diseases. Other protective measures, such as condoms, should be used when necessary to prevent the spread of sexually transmitted diseases.
- Slight bleeding may occur at injection site. Apply pressure if this occurs. If bleeding persists, consult doctor.

POSSIBLE INTERACTION WITH OTHER DRUGS

GENERIC NAME OR DRUG CLASS	COMBINED EFFECT
None significant.	

POSSIBLE INTERACTION WITH OTHER SUBSTANCES

INTERACTS WITH	COMBINED EFFECT
Alcohol:	No special problems expected.
Beverages:	No special problems expected.
Cocaine:	No special problems expected.
Foods:	No special problems expected.
Marijuana:	No special problems expected.
Tobacco:	No special problems expected.

AMINOBENZOATE POTASSIUM

BRAND NAMES

KPAB
Potaba
Potaba Envules
Potaba Powder

Potassium
Aminobenzoate
Potassium
Para-
aminobenzoate

BASIC INFORMATION

Habit forming? No
Prescription needed? Yes
Available as generic? No
Drug class: Antifibrosis

USES

Reduces inflammation and relieves contractions in tissues lying under the skin that have become tight from such disorders as dermatomyositis, Peyronie's disease, scleroderma, pemphigus, morphea.

DOSAGE & USAGE INFORMATION

How to take:
- Tablets—Dissolve in liquid or take with food to prevent stomach upset.
- Capsules—Take with full glass of liquid.
- Oral solution—Swallow with liquid to lessen stomach upset.
- Powder—Mix with liquid.

When to take:
At the same times each day, according to instructions on prescription label. Usually taken with meals and at bedtime with a snack.

If you forget a dose:
Take as soon as you remember up to 2 hours late. If more than 2 hours, wait for next scheduled dose (don't double this dose).

What drug does:
May increase ability of diseased tissues to use oxygen.

Continued next column

OVERDOSE

SYMPTOMS:
Nausea, vomiting.
WHAT TO DO:
Overdose unlikely to threaten life. If person takes much larger amount than prescribed, call doctor, poison control center or hospital emergency room for instructions.

Time lapse before drug works:
May require 3 to 10 months for improvement to begin.

Don't take with:
Any other medicine without consulting your doctor or pharmacist.

POSSIBLE ADVERSE REACTIONS OR SIDE EFFECTS

SYMPTOMS	WHAT TO DO
Life-threatening: None expected.	
Common: Appetite loss, nausea, rash, fever.	Continue. Call doctor when convenient.
Infrequent:	
• Low blood sugar (hunger, anxiety, cold sweats, rapid pulse). on the way to emergency room.)	Discontinue. Seek emergency treatment. (Note: Take sugar or honey
• Sore throat with fever and chills.	Discontinue. Call doctor right away.
Rare: None expected.	

26

AMINOBENZOATE POTASSIUM

WARNINGS & PRECAUTIONS

Don't take if:
You are allergic to aminobenzoate potassium or para-aminobenzoic acid (PABA).

Before you start, consult your doctor:
- If you have low blood sugar.
- If you have diabetes mellitus.
- If you have kidney disease.

Over age 60:
Adverse reactions and side effects may be more frequent and severe than in younger persons, particularly low blood sugar.

Pregnancy:
Risk factor not designated. See category list on page xxiii and consult doctor.

Breast-feeding:
Unknown effect. Consult doctor.

Infants & children:
Not recommended. Safety and dosage have not been established.

Prolonged use:
Talk to your doctor about the need for follow-up medical examinations or laboratory studies to check complete blood counts (white blood cell count, platelet count, red blood cell count, hemoglobin, hematocrit).

Skin & sunlight:
No problems expected.

Driving, piloting or hazardous work:
No problems expected.

Discontinuing:
No problems expected.

Others:
If you become acutely ill and cannot eat well for even a short while, tell your doctor. These circumstances can lead to low blood sugar, and dosage may need adjustment.

POSSIBLE INTERACTION WITH OTHER DRUGS

GENERIC NAME OR DRUG CLASS	COMBINED EFFECT
Dapsone	Decreased dapsone effect.
Salicylates*	May increase salicylate blood level.
Sulfa drugs* (sulfonamides)	Decreased sulfa effect.

POSSIBLE INTERACTION WITH OTHER SUBSTANCES

INTERACTS WITH	COMBINED EFFECT
Alcohol:	None expected.
Beverages:	None expected.
Cocaine:	None expected.
Foods:	None expected.
Marijuana:	None expected.
Tobacco:	None expected.

*See Glossary

AMINOGLUTETHIMIDE

BRAND NAMES

Cytadren

BASIC INFORMATION

Habit forming? No
Prescription needed? Yes
Available as generic? No
Drug class: Antiadrenal, antineoplastic

USES

- Treats Cushing's syndrome.
- Treats breast malignancies.

DOSAGE & USAGE INFORMATION

How to take:
Tablets—Swallow with liquid. If you can't swallow whole, crumble tablet and take with liquid or food. Instructions to take on empty stomach mean 1 hour before or 2 hours after eating.

When to take:
Follow doctor's instructions exactly.

If you forget a dose:
Take as soon as you remember up to 2 hours late. If more than 2 hours, wait for next scheduled dose (don't double this dose).

What drug does:
Suppresses adrenal cortex.

Time lapse before drug works:
1 to 2 hours.

Don't take with:
Any other medicines (including over-the-counter drugs such as cough and cold medicines, laxatives, antacids, diet pills, caffeine, nose drops or vitamins) without consulting your doctor.

OVERDOSE

SYMPTOMS:
None expected.
WHAT TO DO:
Overdose unlikely to threaten life. If person takes much larger amount than prescribed, call doctor, poison control center or hospital emergency room for instructions.

POSSIBLE ADVERSE REACTIONS OR SIDE EFFECTS

SYMPTOMS	WHAT TO DO
Life-threatening: None expected.	
Common: Skin rash on face and hands.	Continue. Tell doctor at next visit.
Infrequent: • Dizziness, drowsiness, unexplained fatigue, low back pain, pain on urinating, clumsiness, unusual eye movements, appetite loss.	Discontinue. Call doctor right away.
• Vomiting, skin darkening, depression, headache, muscle pain.	Continue. Call doctor when convenient.
Rare: Unusual bleeding or bruising	Discontinue. Call doctor right away.

WARNINGS & PRECAUTIONS

Don't take if:
• You have recently been exposed to chicken pox.
• You have shingles (herpes zoster).

Before you start, consult your doctor:
• If you have decreased thyroid function (hypothyroidism).
• If you have any form of infection.

Over age 60:
Adverse reactions and side effects may be more frequent and severe than in younger persons. You may need smaller doses for shorter periods of time.

Pregnancy:
Risk category D (see page xxiii).

Breast-feeding:
Effect not documented. Consult your doctor.

Infants & children:
Effect not documented. Consult your doctor.

Prolonged use:
Talk to your doctor about the need for follow-up medical examinations or laboratory studies to check thyroid function, liver function, serum electrolytes (sodium potassium, chloride) and blood pressure.

Skin & sunlight:
No problems expected.

Driving, piloting or hazardous work:
No problems expected.

Discontinuing:
No special problems expected.

Others:
• Advise any doctor or dentist whom you consult that you take this medicine.
• May affect results in some medical tests.
• May cause decreased thyroid function.

POSSIBLE INTERACTION WITH OTHER DRUGS

GENERIC NAME OR DRUG CLASS	COMBINED EFFECT
Anticoagulants*	Decreased anti-coagulant effect.
Clozapine	Toxic effect on the central nervous system.
Cortisone-like drugs*	Decreased cortisone effects.
Dexamethasone	Dexamethasone effect decreased by half.
Trilostane	Too much decrease in adrenal function.

POSSIBLE INTERACTION WITH OTHER SUBSTANCES

INTERACTS WITH	COMBINED EFFECT
Alcohol:	Increased stomach irritation.
Beverages: Coffee, tea, cocoa.	Increased stomach irritation.
Cocaine:	No proven problems.
Foods:	No proven problems.
Marijuana:	No proven problems.
Tobacco:	No proven problems.

AMIODARONE

BRAND NAMES

Cordarone

BASIC INFORMATION

Habit forming? No
Prescription needed? Yes
Available as generic? No
Drug class: Antiarrhythmic

USES

Prevents and treats life-threatening heartbeat irregularities involving both the large chambers of the heart (auricles and ventricles).

DOSAGE & USAGE INFORMATION

How to take:
Tablets—Swallow whole with liquid or food to lessen stomach irritation. If you can't swallow whole, crumble tablet and take with liquid or food.

When to take:
According to prescription instructions.

If you forget a dose:
Skip this dose and resume regular schedule. Do not double the next dose. If you forget 2 doses or more, consult your doctor.

What drug does:
- Slows nerve impulses in the heart.
- Makes heart muscle fibers less responsive to abnormal electrical impulses arising in the electrical regulatory system of the heart.

Continued next column

OVERDOSE

SYMPTOMS:
Irregular heartbeat, loss of consciousness, seizures.
WHAT TO DO:
- **Dial 911 (emergency) or 0 (operator) for an ambulance or medical help. Then give first aid immediately.**
- **If patient is unconscious and not breathing, give mouth-to-mouth breathing. If there is no heartbeat, use cardiac massage and mouth-to-mouth breathing (CPR). Don't try to make patient vomit. If you can't get help quickly, take patient to nearest emergency facility.**
- **See emergency information on inside covers.**

Time lapse before drug works:
2 to 3 days to 2 to 3 months.

Don't take with:
Any other medicine without consulting your doctor or pharmacist.

POSSIBLE ADVERSE REACTIONS OR SIDE EFFECTS

SYMPTOMS	WHAT TO DO
Life-threatening:	
Shortness of breath, difficulty breathing, cough.	Discontinue. Seek emergency treatment.
Common:	
• Walking difficulty, fever, numbness or tingling in hands or feet, shakiness, weakness in arms and legs.	Discontinue. Call doctor right away.
• Constipation, headache, appetite loss, nausea, vomiting.	Continue. Call doctor when convenient.
Infrequent:	
• Skin color change to blue-gray, blurred vision, cold feeling, dry eyes, nervousness, scrotum swelling or pain, insomnia, swollen feet and ankles, fast or slow heartbeat, eyes hurt in light, weight gain or loss, sweating.	Discontinue. Call doctor right away.
• Bitter or metallic taste, diminished sex drive, dizziness, flushed face, coldness and unusual tiredness.	Continue. Call doctor when convenient.
Rare:	
Jaundice, skin rash.	Discontinue. Call doctor right away.

WARNINGS & PRECAUTIONS

Don't take if:
You are allergic to amiodarone.

Before you start, consult your doctor:
- If you have liver, kidney or thyroid disease.
- If you have heart disease other than coronary artery disease.

Over age 60:
- Adverse reactions and side effects may be more frequent and severe than in younger persons. Ask about smaller doses.
- Pain in legs (while walking) considerably more likely.

Pregnancy:
Risk category D (see page xxiii).

Breast-feeding:
Drug passes into milk. Avoid drug or discontinue nursing until you finish medicine. Consult doctor for advice on maintaining milk supply.

Infants & children:
Safety not established. Use only under close medical supervision.

Prolonged use:
- Blue-gray discoloration of skin may appear.
- Don't discontinue without consulting doctor. Dose may require gradual reduction if you have taken drug for a long time. Doses of other drugs may also require adjustment.
- Talk to your doctor about the need for follow-up medical examinations or laboratory studies to check ECG*, SGPT*, serum alkaline phosphatase, SGOT*, thyroid function.

Skin & sunlight:
May cause rash or intensify sunburn in areas exposed to sun or ultraviolet light (photosensitivity reaction). Avoid overexposure. Notify doctor if reaction occurs.

Driving, piloting or hazardous work:
Avoid if you feel dizzy or lightheaded. Otherwise, no problems expected.

Discontinuing:
- Don't discontinue without consulting doctor. Dose may require gradual reduction if you have taken drug for a long time. Doses of other drugs may also require adjustment.
- Notify doctor if cough, fever, breathing difficulty or shortness of breath occur after discontinuing medicine.

Others:
- Learn to check your own pulse. If it drops to lower than 50 or rises to higher than 100 beats per minute, don't take amiodarone until you consult your doctor.
- May interfere with the accuracy of some medical tests.

POSSIBLE INTERACTION WITH OTHER DRUGS

GENERIC NAME OR DRUG CLASS	COMBINED EFFECT
Antiarrhythmics, other*	Increased likelihood of heartbeat irregularity.
Anticoagulants*	Increased anticoagulant effect.
Beta-adrenergic blocking agents*	Increased likelihood of slow heartbeat.
Calcium channel blockers*	Possible heart block.
Cholestyramine	May decrease amiodarone blood levels.
Digitalis	Increased digitalis effect.
Diltiazem	Increased likelihood of slow heartbeat.
Diuretics*	Increased risk of heartbeat irregularity due to low potassium level.
Encainide	Increased effect of toxicity on the heart muscle.
Flecainide	Increased flecainide effect.
Isoniazid	Increased risk of liver damage.
Nicardipine	Possible increased effect and toxicity of each drug.
Nifedipine	Increased likelihood of slow heartbeat.
Phenytoin	Increased effect of phenytoin.
Procainamide	Increased procainamide effect.
Propafenone	Increased effect of both drugs and increased risk of toxicity.
Quinidine	Increased quinidine effect.
Verapamil	Increased likelihood of slow heartbeat.

POSSIBLE INTERACTION WITH OTHER SUBSTANCES

INTERACTS WITH	COMBINED EFFECT
Alcohol:	Increased risk of heartbeat irregularity. Avoid.
Beverages:	None expected.
Cocaine:	Increased risk of heartbeat irregularity. Avoid.
Foods:	None expected.
Marijuana:	Possible irregular heartbeat. Avoid.
Tobacco:	Possible irregular heartbeat. Avoid.

AMLEXANOX

BRAND NAMES

Aphthasol

BASIC INFORMATION

Habit forming? No
Prescription needed? Yes
Available as generic? No
Drug class: Antiaphthous ulcer agent

 ## USES

Treatment for severe canker sores (aphthous ulcers) in the mouth.

 ## DOSAGE & USAGE INFORMATION

How to use:
Oral paste—Use fingertips to apply paste directly to each canker sore following oral hygiene.

When to use:
Use as soon as symptoms of a canker sore appear. Apply four times a day—after meals and before bedtime. Wash hands after application.

If you forget a dose:
Use as soon as you remember. If it is almost time for the next dose, wait for the next dose (don't double this dose).

What drug does:
Exact healing mechanism is unknown. Appears to stop the inflammatory process and hypersensitivity reaction.

Time lapse before drug works:
Pain relief may occur within hours or up to 24 hours. Complete healing time will take several days.

Don't use with:
Any other medicine without consulting your doctor or pharmacist.

 ## OVERDOSE

SYMPTOMS:
None expected.
WHAT TO DO:
- If person accidentally swallows drug, call doctor, poison control center or hospital emergency room for instructions.
- See emergency information on inside covers.

 ## POSSIBLE ADVERSE REACTIONS OR SIDE EFFECTS

SYMPTOMS	WHAT TO DO
Life-threatening: None expected.	
Common: None expected.	
Infrequent: Slight pain or stinging or burning at site of application.	No action necessary.
Rare: Diarrhea, nausea, rash.	Discontinue. Call doctor when convenient.

WARNINGS & PRECAUTIONS

Don't take if:
You are allergic to amlexanox.

Before you start, consult your doctor:
If you are allergic to any medication, food or other substance.

Over age 60:
No problems expected.

Pregnancy:
Decide with your doctor if drug benefits outweigh risks to unborn child. Risk category B (see page xxiii).

Breast-feeding:
It is unknown if drug passes into milk. Absorption into the body has occurred with this drug. Avoid drug or discontinue nursing until you finish medicine. Consult doctor for advice on maintaining milk supply.

Infants & children:
Safety and efficacy have not been established. Use only under close medical supervision.

Prolonged use:
Normally only used for up to10 days of treatment.

Skin & sunlight:
No problems expected.

Driving, piloting or hazardous work:
No problems expected.

Discontinuing:
May be unnecessary to finish medicine. Discontinue when canker sores heal.

Others:
- If canker sores do not heal after 10 days, consult your dentist or health-care provider.
- Advise any doctor or dentist whom you consult that you take this medicine.
- Has not been studied in people with weakened immune systems.

POSSIBLE INTERACTION WITH OTHER DRUGS

GENERIC NAME OR DRUG CLASS	COMBINED EFFECT
None expected.	

POSSIBLE INTERACTION WITH OTHER SUBSTANCES

INTERACTS WITH	COMBINED EFFECT
Alcohol:	None expected.
Beverages:	None expected.
Cocaine:	None expected.
Foods:	None expected.
Marijuana:	None expected.
Tobacco:	None expected.

AMPHETAMINES

GENERIC AND BRAND NAMES

AMPHETAMINE &
DEXTROAMPHET-
AMINE
Adderall
DEXTROAMPHETAMINE
Dexedrine
Dexedrine Spansule
Oxydess
Spancap

METHAMPHETAMINE
Desoxyn
Desoxyn Gradumet

BASIC INFORMATION

Habit forming? Yes
Prescription needed? Yes
Available as generic? Yes
Drug class: Central nervous system
  stimulant

USES

- Prevents narcolepsy (attacks of uncontrollable sleepiness).
- Controls hyperactivity in children under special circumstances.

DOSAGE & USAGE INFORMATION

How to take:
- Tablet—Swallow with liquid.
- Extended-release capsules and tablets—Swallow each dose whole with liquid; do not crush.

When to take:
- At the same times each day.
- Short-acting form—Don't take later than 6 hours before bedtime.
- Long-acting form—Take on awakening.

If you forget a dose:
- Short-acting form—Take up to 2 hours late. If more than 2 hours, wait for next dose (don't double this dose).

Continued next column

OVERDOSE

SYMPTOMS:
Rapid heartbeat, hyperactivity, high fever, hallucinations, suicidal or homicidal feelings, convulsions, coma.
WHAT TO DO:
- **Dial 911 (emergency) or 0 (operator) for an ambulance or medical help. Then give first aid immediately.**
- **See emergency information at end of book**

- Long-acting form—Take as soon as you remember. Wait 20 hours for next dose.

What drug does:
- Hyperactivity—Decreases motor restlessness and increases ability to pay attention.
- Narcolepsy—Increases motor activity and mental alertness; diminishes drowsiness.

Time lapse before drug works:
15 to 30 minutes (short-acting).

Don't take with:
Any other medicine without consulting your doctor or pharmacist.

POSSIBLE ADVERSE REACTIONS OR SIDE EFFECTS

SYMPTOMS	WHAT TO DO
Life-threatening:	
In case of overdose, see previous column.	
Common:	
• Irritability, nervousness, insomnia, euphoria. signs of addiction*.	Continue. Call doctor when convenient.
• Dry mouth.	Continue. Tell doctor at next visit.
• Fast, pounding heartbeat.	Discontinue. Call doctor right away.
Infrequent:	
• Dizziness, reduced alertness, blurred vision, unusual sweating.	Discontinue. Call doctor right away.
• Headache, diarrhea or constipation, appetite loss, stomach pain, nausea, vomiting, weight loss, diminished sex drive, impotence.	Continue. Call doctor when convenient.
Rare:	
• Rash; hives; chest pain or irregular heartbeat; uncontrollable movements of head, neck, arms, legs.	Discontinue. Call doctor right away.
• Mood changes, swollen breasts.	Continue. Call doctor when convenient.

WARNINGS & PRECAUTIONS

Don't take if:
- You are allergic to any amphetamine.
- You will have surgery within 2 months, including dental surgery, requiring general or spinal anesthesia.

Before you start, consult your doctor:
- If you plan to become pregnant within medication period.
- If you have glaucoma.
- If you have diabetes.
- If you have a history of substance abuse.
- If you have heart or blood vessel disease or high blood pressure.
- If you have overactive thyroid, anxiety or tension.
- If you have a severe mental illness (especially children).

Over age 60:
Adverse reactions and side effects may be more frequent and severe than in younger persons.

Pregnancy:
Decide with your doctor if drug benefits justify risk to unborn child. Consult doctor. Risk category C (see page xxiii).

Breast-feeding:
Drug passes into milk.

Infants & children:
Not recommended for children under 12.

Prolonged use:
- Habit forming.
- Talk to your doctor about the need for follow-up medical examinations or laboratory studies to check blood pressure, growth charts in children, reassessment of need for continued treatment.

Skin & sunlight:
No problems expected.

Driving, piloting or hazardous work:
Don't drive or pilot aircraft until you learn how medicine affects you. Don't work around dangerous machinery. Don't climb ladders or work in high places. Danger increases if you drink alcohol or take medicine affecting alertness and reflexes.

Discontinuing:
May be unnecessary to finish medicine, but don't suddenly stop. Follow doctor's instructions.

Others:
- This is a dangerous drug and must be closely supervised. Don't use for appetite control or depression. Potential for damage and abuse.
- During withdrawal phase, may cause prolonged sleep of several days.
- Don't use for fatigue or to replace rest.

POSSIBLE INTERACTION WITH OTHER DRUGS

GENERIC NAME OR DRUG CLASS	COMBINED EFFECT
Antidepressants, tricyclic*	Decreased amphetamine effect.
Antihypertensives*	Decreased anti-hypertensive effect.
Beta-adrenergic blocking agents*	High blood pressure, slow heartbeat.
Carbonic anhydrase inhibitors*	Increased amphetamine effect.
Central nervous system (CNS) stimulants*, other	Excessive CNS stimulation.
Doxazosin	Decreased doxazosin effect.
Furazolidine	Sudden and severe high blood pressure.
Haloperidol	Decreased amphetamine effect.
Monoamine oxidase (MAO) inhibitors*	May severely increase blood pressure.
Phenothiazines*	Decreased amphetamine effect.
Prazosin	Decreased prazosin effect.
Sodium bicarbonate	Increased amphetamine effect.
Sympathomimetics*	Seizures.
Thyroid hormones*	Heartbeat irregularities.

POSSIBLE INTERACTION WITH OTHER SUBSTANCES

INTERACTS WITH	COMBINED EFFECT
Alcohol:	Decreased amphetamine effect. Avoid.
Beverages: Caffeine drinks.	Overstimulation. Avoid.
Cocaine:	Dangerous stimulation of nervous system. Avoid.
Foods:	None expected.
Marijuana:	Frequent use—Severely impaired mental function.
Tobacco:	None expected.

ANAGRELIDE

BRAND NAMES

Agrylin

BASIC INFORMATION

Habit forming? No
Prescription needed? Yes
Available as generic? No
Drug class: Platelet count–reducing agent, antithrombocythemia

USES

Reduces elevated platelet counts and the risk of thrombosis (formation of a blood clot); also makes symptoms more tolerable in patients with essential thrombocythemia.

DOSAGE & USAGE INFORMATION

How to take:
Capsule—Swallow with liquid. Take with or without food.

When to take:
At the same time each day. Dose may be adjusted to maintain proper platelet count.

If you forget a dose:
Take as soon as you remember. If it is almost time for the next dose, then skip the missed dose and wait for your next scheduled dose (don't double this dose).

What drug does:
Exact mechanism is unknown.

Time lapse before drug works:
One to two weeks.

Don't take with:
Any other prescription or nonprescription drug without consulting your doctor or pharmacist.

OVERDOSE

SYMPTOMS:
None expected immediately. May lower platelet count, leading to increased bleeding.
WHAT TO DO:
Overdose unlikely to threaten life. If person takes much larger amount than prescribed, call doctor, poison control center or hospital emergency room for instructions.

POSSIBLE ADVERSE REACTIONS OR SIDE EFFECTS

SYMPTOMS	WHAT TO DO
Life-threatening: Severe headache or weakness; pain or pressure in chest, jaw, neck, back or arms; swelling of feet or legs; severe tiredness or weakness; increased heart rate; difficulty breathing or shortness of breath.	Seek emergency treatment immediately.
Common: • Abdominal pain, weakness, dizziness palpitations, shortness of breath.	Continue. Call doctor right away.
• Diarrhea, heartburn, gas, bloating, headache, loss of appetite, general feeling of discomfort or illness, nausea, pain.	Continue. Call doctor if symptoms persist.
Infrequent: • Blurred or double vision, painful or difficult urination, blood in urine, tingling in hands or feet, unusual bruising or bleeding, flushing, faintness.	Discontinue. Call doctor right away.
• Canker sore, joint pain, back pain, confusion, constipation, fever or chills, insomnia, leg cramps, depression, nervousness, runny nose, ringing in ears, skin rash, itching, sleepiness, sensitivity to light, vomiting.	Continue. Call doctor if symptoms persist.
Rare: Hair loss.	Tell doctor at next visit.

WARNINGS & PRECAUTIONS

Don't take if:
You are allergic to anagrelide.

Before you start, consult your doctor:
- If you have any kidney or liver disease or any heart or blood vessel disorder.
- If you have any chronic health problem.
- If you are pregnant or nursing.

Over age 60:
No problems expected.

Pregnancy:
Decide with your doctor if drug benefits justify risk to unborn child. Risk category C (see page xxiii).

Breast-feeding:
It is unknown if drug passes into milk. Avoid drug or discontinue nursing until you finish medicine. Consult doctor for advice on maintaining milk supply.

Infants & children:
Safety and efficacy have not been established in patients under 16. Use only under close medical supervision.

Prolonged use:
Schedule regular visits with your doctor for laboratory examinations to monitor the continued effectiveness of the medication.

Skin & sunlight:
No problems expected.

Driving, piloting or hazardous work:
No problems expected.

Discontinuing:
Don't discontinue without consulting your doctor even if you feel well.

Others:
- Close medical supervision, including frequent platelet counts, required at start of therapy with this drug.
- Advise any doctor or dentist whom you consult that you are using this medicine.

POSSIBLE INTERACTION WITH OTHER DRUGS

GENERIC NAME OR DRUG CLASS	COMBINED EFFECT
Sulcrafate	May interfere with anagrelide absorption. Don't take at the same time.

POSSIBLE INTERACTION WITH OTHER SUBSTANCES

INTERACTS WITH	COMBINED EFFECT
Alcohol:	None expected.
Beverages:	None expected.
Cocaine:	Effects unknown. Avoid.
Foods:	None expected.
Marijuana:	Effects unknown. Avoid.
Tobacco:	None expected.

ANDROGENS

GENERIC AND BRAND NAMES

See complete list of generic and brand names in the *Generic and Brand Name Directory*, page 863.

BASIC INFORMATION

Habit forming? No
Prescription needed? Yes
Available as generic? Yes
Drug class: Androgen

 USES

- Corrects male hormone deficiency.
- Reduces "male menopause" symptoms (loss of sex drive, depression, anxiety).
- Decreases calcium loss of osteoporosis (softened bones).
- Blocks growth of breast cancer cells in females.
- Corrects undescended testicles in male children.
- Reduces breast pain and fullness following childbirth.
- Augments treatment of aplastic anemia.
- Stimulates weight gain after illness, injury or for chronically underweight persons.
- Stimulates growth in treatment of dwarfism.

 DOSAGE & USAGE INFORMATION

How to take:
- Tablets or capsules—With food to lessen stomach irritation.
- Injection—Once or twice a month.
- Transdermal—Follow instructions provided with prescription.

When to take:
At the same time each day.

If you forget a dose:
Take as soon as you remember up to 2 hours late. If more than 2 hours, wait for next scheduled dose (don't double this dose).

 OVERDOSE

SYMPTOMS:
None expected.
WHAT TO DO:
Overdose unlikely to threaten life. If person takes much larger amount than prescribed, call doctor, poison control center or hospital emergency room for instructions.

What drug does:
- Stimulates cells that produce male sex characteristics.
- Replaces hormone deficiencies.
- Stimulates red-blood-cell production.
- Suppresses production of estrogen (female sex hormone).

Time lapse before drug works:
Varies with problems treated. May require 2 or 3 months of regular use for desired effects.

Don't take with:
Any other medicine without consulting your doctor or pharmacist.

 POSSIBLE ADVERSE REACTIONS OR SIDE EFFECTS

SYMPTOMS	WHAT TO DO
Life-threatening: Intense itching, weakness, loss of consciousness.	Seek emergency treatment immediately.
Common:	
• Acne or oily skin, deep voice, enlarged clitoris in females; frequent erections, swollen breasts in men; mild to moderate redness or itching at site of patch.	Continue. Call doctor when convenient.
• Sore mouth; higher sex drive, decreased testicle size, impotence in men.	Continue. Tell doctor at next visit.
Infrequent:	
• Yellow skin or eyes.	Discontinue. Seek emergency treatment.
• Depression or confusion, flushed face, rash or itch, nausea, vomiting, diarrhea, swollen feet or legs, headache, shortness of breath, rapid weight gain, chills, difficult urination; vaginal bleeding in women; scrotum pain in men.	Discontinue. Call doctor right away.
Rare:	
• Hives, black stool.	Discontinue. Seek emergency treatment.
• Sore throat, fever, abdominal pain.	Discontinue. Call doctor right away.
• Appetite loss, halitosis.	Continue. Call doctor when convenient.

WARNINGS & PRECAUTIONS

Don't take if:
You are allergic to any male hormone.

Before you start, consult your doctor:
- If you might be pregnant.
- If you have cancer of prostate.
- If you have heart disease or arteriosclerosis.
- If you have kidney or liver disease.
- If you have breast cancer (males).
- If you have high blood pressure.
- If you have migraine attacks.
- If you have high level of blood calcium.
- If you have epilepsy.

Over age 60:
- May stimulate sexual activity.
- Can make high blood pressure or heart disease worse.
- Can enlarge prostate and cause urinary retention.

Pregnancy:
Risk to unborn child outweighs drug benefits. Don't use. Risk category X (see page xxiii).

Breast-feeding:
Drug passes into milk. Avoid drug or discontinue nursing until you finish medicine. Consult doctor for advice on maintaining milk supply.

Infants & children:
Don't give to children younger than 2. Use with older children only under medical supervision.

Prolonged use:
- Reduces sperm count and volume of semen.
- Possible kidney stones.
- Unnatural hair growth and deep voice in women.
- Talk to your doctor about the need for follow-up medical examinations or laboratory studies to check complete blood counts (white blood cell count, platelet count, red blood cell count, hemoglobin, hematocrit).

Skin & sunlight:
No problems expected.

Driving, piloting or hazardous work:
No problems expected.

Discontinuing:
No problems expected.

Others:
- May cause atrophy of testicles.
- Will not increase strength in athletes.
- May cause liver cancer.
- In women, may cause male-like changes such as deepened voice, increased hair growth.

POSSIBLE INTERACTION WITH OTHER DRUGS

GENERIC NAME OR DRUG CLASS	COMBINED EFFECT
Anticoagulants*	Increased anticoagulant effect.
Antidiabetic agents*	Increased antidiabetic effect.
Chlorzoxazone	Decreased androgen effect.
Cyclosporine	Increased cyclosporine effect.
Hepatotoxic drugs* (other)	Increased liver toxicity.
Insulin	Increased antidiabetic effect.
Oxyphenbutazone	Decreased androgen effect.
Phenobarbital	Decreased androgen effect.
Phenylbutazone	Decreased androgen effect.

POSSIBLE INTERACTION WITH OTHER SUBSTANCES

INTERACTS WITH	COMBINED EFFECT
Alcohol:	None expected.
Beverages:	None expected.
Cocaine:	No proven problems.
Foods: Salt.	Excessive fluid retention (edema). Decrease salt intake while taking male hormones.
Marijuana:	Decreased blood levels of androgens.
Tobacco:	No proven problems.

ANDROGENS & ESTROGENS

GENERIC AND BRAND NAMES

See complete list of generic and brand names in the *Generic and Brand Name Directory*, page 864.

BASIC INFORMATION

Habit forming? No
Prescription needed? Yes
Available as generic? Yes
Drug class: Androgens-estrogens

 USES

- Prevents breast fullness in new mothers after childbirth.
- Relieves menopause symptoms such as unnecessary sweating, hot flashes, chills, faintness and dizziness.

 DOSAGE & USAGE INFORMATION

How to take:
- Injection—Given deeply intramuscular.
- Tablets—Swallow with liquid or food to lessen stomach irritation.

When to take:
When directed.

If you forget a dose:
Check with your doctor.

What drug does:
- Restores normal estrogen level in tissues.
- Stimulates cells that produce male sex characteristics.
- Replaces hormones lost due to deficiencies.
- Stimulates red blood cell production.
- Suppresses production of estrogen.

Time lapse before drug works:
10 to 20 days.

Don't take with:
Any other medicine without consulting your doctor or pharmacist.

 OVERDOSE

SYMPTOMS:
Headache (severe), coordination loss, vision changes, chest pain, shortness of breath (sudden), speech slurring.
WHAT TO DO:
Overdose unlikely to threaten life. If person takes much larger amount than prescribed, call doctor, poison control center or hospital emergency room for instructions.

 POSSIBLE ADVERSE REACTIONS OR SIDE EFFECTS

SYMPTOMS	WHAT TO DO
Life-threatening:	
In case of overdose, see previous column.	
Hives, black stool, black or bloody vomit, intense itching, weakness, loss of consciousness.	Discontinue. Seek emergency treatment.
Common:	
Red or flushed face; rash; swollen, tender breasts.	Discontinue. Call doctor right away.
Depression, irritability, dizziness, confusion, acne or oily skin, enlarged clitoris, deepened voice, appetite loss, increased sex drive, unnatural hair growth, headache, constipation.	Continue. Call doctor when convenient.
Infrequent:	
Nausea, vomiting, diarrhea, unusual vaginal bleeding or discharge, uncontrolled muscle movements.	Discontinue. Call doctor right away.
Swollen feet and ankles, migraine headache.	Continue. Call doctor when convenient.
Rare:	
Jaundice, abdominal pain.	Discontinue. Call doctor right away.
Brown blotches on skin; hair loss; sore throat, fever, mouth sores.	Continue. Call doctor when convenient.

 WARNINGS & PRECAUTIONS

Don't take if:
- You are allergic to any male hormone or any estrogen-containing drugs.
- You have impaired liver function.
- You have had blood clots, stroke or heart attack.
- You have unexplained vaginal bleeding.

Before you start, consult your doctor:
- If you might be pregnant or plan to become pregnant within 3 months.
- If you have heart disease, arteriosclerosis, diabetes, liver disease, high blood pressure, asthma, congestive heart failure, kidney disease or gallstones.

- If you have a high level of blood calcium.
- If you have had migraine headaches, epilepsy or porphyria.
- If you have had cancer of breast or reproductive organs, fibrocystic breast disease, fibroid tumors of the uterus or endometriosis.

Over age 60:
- May stimulate sexual activity.
- Can make high blood pressure or heart disease worse.
- Controversial. You and your doctor must decide if drug risks outweigh benefits.

Pregnancy:
Risk to unborn child outweighs drug benefits. Don't use. Risk category X (see page xxiii).

Breast-feeding:
Drug passes into milk. Avoid drug or discontinue nursing until you finish medicine. Consult doctor for advice on maintaining milk supply.

Infants & children:
Not recommended.

Prolonged use:
- Increased growth of fibroid tumors of uterus.
- Possible kidney stones.
- Unnatural hair growth and deep voice in women.
- Talk to your doctor about the need for follow-up medical examinations or laboratory studies to check pap smear, liver function, mammogram, complete blood counts (white blood cell count, platelet count, red blood cell count, hemoglobin, hematocrit).
- Possible breast lumps, jaundice, sore throat, fever. If any of these occur, call your doctor.

Skin & sunlight:
One or more drugs in this group may cause rash or intensify sunburn in areas exposed to sun or utltraviolet light (photosensitivity reaction). Avoid overexposure. Notify doctor if reaction occurs.

Driving, piloting or hazardous work:
No problems expected.

Discontinuing:
You may need to discontinue estrogens periodically. Consult your doctor.

Others:
- In rare instances, may cause blood clot in lung, brain or leg. Symptoms are *sudden* severe headache, coordination loss, vision change, chest pain, breathing difficulty, slurred speech, pain in legs or groin. Seek emergency treatment immediately.
- Will not increase strength in athletes.
- Carefully read the paper delivered with your prescription called "Information for the Patient."
- Don't smoke.

POSSIBLE INTERACTION WITH OTHER DRUGS

GENERIC NAME OR DRUG CLASS	COMBINED EFFECT
Anticoagulants*, oral	Increased effect of anticoagulant.
Anticonvulsants*, hydantoin	Increased seizures.
Antidiabetics*, oral	Unpredictable increase or decrease in blood sugar.
Antifibrinolytic agents*	Increased possibility of blood clotting.
Carbamazepine	Increased seizures.
Chlorzoxazone	Decreased androgen effect.
Cholestyramine	Decreased cholestyramine effect.
Clofibrate	Decreased clofibrate effect.
Colestipol	Decreased colestipol effect.

Continued on page 897

POSSIBLE INTERACTION WITH OTHER SUBSTANCES

INTERACTS WITH	COMBINED EFFECT
Alcohol:	None expected.
Beverages:	None expected.
Cocaine:	No proven problems.
Foods: Salt.	Excessive fluid retention (edema). Decrease salt intake while taking male hormones.
Marijuana:	Decreased blood levels of androgens. Possible menstrual irregularities and bleeding between periods.
Tobacco:	Increased risk of blood clots leading to stroke or heart attack.

ANESTHETICS (Mucosal-Local)

GENERIC AND BRAND NAMES

BENZOCAINE
  Anbesol Baby Gel
  Anbesol Maximum
    Strength Gel
  Anbesol Maximum
    Strength Liquid
  Baby Anbesol
  Baby Orabase
  Baby Oragel
  Baby Oragel
    Nighttime Formula
  Benzodent
  Children's
    Cloraseptic
    Lozenges
  Dentapaine
  Dentocaine
  Dent-Zel-Ite
  Hurricaine
  Numzident
  Num-Zit Gel
  Num-Zit Lotion
  Orabase-B with
    Benzocaine
  Orajel Extra
    Strength
  Orajel Liquid
  Orajel Maximum
    Strength
  Oratect Gel
  Rid-A-Pain
  SensoGARD Canker
    Sore Relief
  Spec-T Sore Throat
    Anesthetic
  Topicaine

BENZOCAINE &
  MENTHOL
  Chloraseptic
    Lozenges
    Cherry Flavor
BENZOCAINE &
  PHENOL
  Anbesol Gel
  Anbesol Liquid
  Anbesol Regular
    Strength Gel
  Anbesol Regular
    Strength Liquid
DYCLONINE
  Children's Sucrets
  Sucrets Maximum
    Strength
  Sucrets Regular
    Strength
LIDOCAINE
  Xylocaine
  Xylocaine Viscous
  Zilactin-L
TETRACAINE
  Supracaine

BASIC INFORMATION

Habit forming? No
Prescription needed? Yes, for some
Available as generic? Yes, for some
Drug class: Anesthetic (topical)

 ## OVERDOSE

SYMPTOMS:
Overabsorption by body—Dizziness, blurred vision, seizures, drowsiness.
WHAT TO DO:
- **Dial 911 (emergency) or 0 (operator) for an ambulance or medical help. Then give first aid immediately.**
- **Not for internal use. If child accidentally swallows, call poison control center.**
- **See emergency information on inside covers.**

 ## USES

Relieves pain or irritation in mouth caused by toothache, teething, mouth sores, dentures, braces, dental appliances. Also relieves pain of sore throat for short periods of time.

 ## DOSAGE & USAGE INFORMATION

How to use:
- For mouth problems—Apply to sore places with cotton-tipped applicator. Don't swallow.
- For throat—Gargle, but don't swallow.
- For aerosol spray—Don't inhale.

When to use:
As directed by physician or label on package.

If you forget a dose:
Use as soon as you remember.

What drug does:
Blocks pain impulses to the brain.

Time lapse before drug works:
Immediately.

Don't use with:
Any other medicine without consulting your doctor or pharmacist.

POSSIBLE ADVERSE REACTIONS OR SIDE EFFECTS

SYMPTOMS	WHAT TO DO
Life-threatening: Unusual anxiety, excitement, nervousness, irregular or slow heartbeat.	Discontinue. Seek emergency treatment.
Common: None expected.	
Infrequent: Redness, irritation, sores not present before treatment, rash, itchy skin, hives.	Discontinue. Call doctor right away.
Rare: None expected.	

WARNINGS & PRECAUTIONS

Don't use if:
You are allergic to any of the products listed.

Before you start, consult your doctor:
- If you are allergic to anything.
- If you have infection, canker sores or other sores in your mouth.
- If you take medicine for myasthenia gravis, eye drops for glaucoma or any sulfa medicine.

Over age 60:
Adverse reactions and side effects may be more frequent and severe than in younger persons. Ask doctor about smaller doses.

Pregnancy:
Risk factors vary for drugs in this group. See category list on page xxiii and consult doctor.

Breast-feeding:
No problems expected, but check with doctor.

Infants & children:
No problems expected, but check with doctor.

Prolonged use:
Not intended for prolonged use.

Skin & sunlight:
No problems expected.

Driving, piloting or hazardous work:
Wait to see if causes dizziness, sweating, drowsiness or blurred vision. If not, no problems expected.

Discontinuing:
No problems expected.

Others:
- Keep cool, but don't freeze.
- Don't puncture, break or burn aerosol containers.
- Don't eat, drink or chew gum for 1 hour after use.
- Heat and moisture in bathroom medicine cabinet can cause breakdown of medicine. Store someplace else.
- Before anesthesia, tell dentist about any medicines you take or use.

POSSIBLE INTERACTION WITH OTHER DRUGS

GENERIC NAME OR DRUG CLASS	COMBINED EFFECT
So remote, they are not considered clinically significant.	

POSSIBLE INTERACTION WITH OTHER SUBSTANCE

INTERACTS WITH	COMBINED EFFECT
Alcohol:	Adverse reactions more common.
Beverages:	None expected.
Cocaine:	May cause too much nervousness and trembling. Avoid.
Foods:	None expected.
Marijuana:	None expected.
Tobacco:	Avoid. Tobacco makes mouth problems worse.

ANESTHETICS (Rectal)

GENERIC AND BRAND NAMES

BENZOCAINE
  Americaine
    Hemorrhoidal
  Ethyl
    Aminobenzoate
DIBUCAINE
  Nupercainal
PRAMOXINE
  Fleet Relief
  Proctofoam
  Tronolane
  Tronothane

TETRACAINE
  Pontocaine Cream
**TETRACAINE &
  MENTHOL**
  Pontocaine
    Ointment

BASIC INFORMATION

Habit forming? No
Prescription needed? Yes, for some
Available as generic? Yes, Dibucaine.
  No others, but most brands are available
  without prescription.
Drug class: Anesthetic (rectal)

 ## USES

- Relieves pain, itching and swelling of hemorrhoids (piles).
- Relieves pain of rectal fissures (breaks in lining membrane of the anus).

 ## DOSAGE & USAGE INFORMATION

How to use:
- Rectal cream or ointment—Apply to surface of rectum with fingers. Insert applicator into rectum no farther than 1/2 and apply inside. Wash applicator with warm soapy water or discard.
- Aerosol foam—Read patient instructions. Don't insert into rectum. Use the special applicator and wash carefully after using.

Continued next column

 ## OVERDOSE

SYMPTOMS:
None expected.
WHAT TO DO:
Not intended for internal use. If child accidentally swallows, call poison control center.

- Suppository—Remove wrapper and moisten with water. Lie on side. Push blunt end of suppository into rectum with finger. If suppository is too soft, run cold water over wrapper or put in refrigerator for 15 to 45 minutes before using.
- Pads—For external use only. Follow instructions on label. Do not use for more than 1 week without doctor's approval.

When to use:
As directed.

If you forget a dose:
Use as soon as you remember.

What drug does:
Deadens nerve endings to pain and touch.

Time lapse before drug works:
5 to 15 minutes.

Don't use with:
Any other medicine without consulting your doctor or pharmacist.

 ## POSSIBLE ADVERSE REACTIONS OR SIDE EFFECTS

SYMPTOMS	WHAT TO DO
Life-threatening: None expected.	
Common: None expected.	
Infrequent:	
• Nervousness, trembling, hives, rash, itch, inflammation or tenderness not present before application, slow heartbeat.	Discontinue. Call doctor right away.
• Dizziness, blurred vision, swollen feet.	Continue. Call doctor when convenient.
Rare:	
• Blood in urine.	Discontinue. Call doctor right away.
• Increased or painful urination.	Continue. Call doctor when convenient.

WARNINGS & PRECAUTIONS

Don't use if:
You are allergic to any topical anesthetic.

Before you start, consult your doctor:
- If you have skin infection at site of treatment.
- If you have had severe or extensive skin disorders such as eczema or psoriasis.
- If you have bleeding hemorrhoids.

Over age 60:
Adverse reactions and side effects may be more frequent and severe than in younger persons.

Pregnancy:
Risk factors vary for drugs in this group. See category list on page xxiii and consult doctor.

Breast-feeding:
No problems expected. Consult doctor.

Infants & children:
Use caution. More likely to be absorbed through skin and cause adverse reactions.

Prolonged use:
Possible excess absorption. Don't use longer than 3 days for any one problem.

Skin & sunlight:
No problems expected.

Driving, piloting or hazardous work:
No problems expected.

Discontinuing:
May be unnecessary to finish medicine. Follow doctor's instructions.

Others:
- Report any rectal bleeding to your doctor.
- Keep cool, but don't freeze.

POSSIBLE INTERACTION WITH OTHER DRUGS

GENERIC NAME OR DRUG CLASS	COMBINED EFFECT
Sulfa drugs*	Decreased anti-infective effect of sulfa drugs.

POSSIBLE INTERACTION WITH OTHER SUBSTANCE

INTERACTS WITH	COMBINED EFFECT
Alcohol:	None expected.
Beverages:	None expected.
Cocaine:	Possible nervous system toxicity. Avoid.
Foods:	None expected.
Marijuana:	None expected.
Tobacco:	None expected.

ANESTHETICS (Topical)

GENERIC AND BRAND NAMES

See complete list of generic and brand names in the *Generic and Brand Name Directory*, page 864.

BASIC INFORMATION

Habit forming? No
Prescription needed?
  High strength: Yes
  Low strength: No
Available as generic? Yes
Drug class: Anesthetic (topical)

USES

Relieves pain and itch of sunburn, insect bites, scratches and other minor skin irritations.

DOSAGE & USAGE INFORMATION

How to use:
All forms—Use only enough to cover irritated area. Follow instructions on label or use as directed by doctor. Avoid using on large areas of skin.

When to use:
When needed for discomfort, no more often than every hour.

If you forget an application:
Use as needed.

What drug does:
Blocks pain impulses from skin to brain.

Time lapse before drug works:
3 to 15 minutes.

Don't take with:
Any other medicine without consulting your doctor or pharmacist.

OVERDOSE

SYMPTOMS:
If swallowed or inhaled—Dizziness, nervousness, trembling, seizures.
WHAT TO DO:
- **Dial 911 (emergency) or 0 (operator) for an ambulance or medical help. Then give first aid immediately.**
- **See emergency information on inside covers.**

POSSIBLE ADVERSE REACTIONS OR SIDE EFFECTS

SYMPTOMS	WHAT TO DO
Life-threatening: None expected.	
Common: None expected.	
Infrequent: Hives-like swellings on skin or in mouth or throat; skin problems not present before treatment (rash, burning, stinging, tenderness, redness).	Discontinue. Call doctor right away.
Rare: If too much of drug absorbed into body (very rare)—Nervousness, slow heartbeat, dizziness, blurred or double vision, confusion, convulsions, noises in ears, feeling hot or cold, numbness, trembling, anxiety, paleness, tiredness or weakness.	Discontinue. Call doctor right away.

WARNINGS & PRECAUTIONS

Don't use if:
You are allergic to any topical anesthetic.

Before you start, consult your doctor:
- If you have skin infection at site of treatment.
- If you have had severe or extensive skin disorders such as eczema or psoriasis.
- If you have bleeding hemorrhoids.

Over age 60:
Adverse reactions and side effects may be more frequent and severe than in younger persons.

Pregnancy:
Risk factors vary for drugs in this group. See category list on page xxiii and consult doctor.

Breast-feeding:
No problems expected. Consult doctor.

Infants & children:
Use caution. More likely to be absorbed through skin and cause adverse reactions.

Prolonged use:
Possible excess absorption. Don't use longer than 3 days for any one problem.

Skin & sunlight:
May cause rash or intensify sunburn in areas exposed to sun or ultraviolet light (photosensitivity reaction). Avoid overexposure. Notify doctor if reaction occurs.

Driving, piloting or hazardous work:
No problems expected.

Discontinuing:
May be unnecessary to finish medicine. Follow doctor's instructions.

Others:
- Contact doctor if condition being treated doesn't improve within a week. Call sooner if new symptoms develop or pain worsens.
- Wash hands carefully after use.

POSSIBLE INTERACTION WITH OTHER DRUGS

GENERIC NAME OR DRUG CLASS	COMBINED EFFECT
Sulfa drugs*	Decreased effect of sulfa drugs for infection.

POSSIBLE INTERACTION WITH OTHER SUBSTANCE

INTERACTS WITH	COMBINED EFFECT
Alcohol:	None expected.
Beverages:	None expected.
Cocaine:	Possible nervous system toxicity. Avoid.
Foods:	None expected.
Marijuana:	None expected.
Tobacco:	None expected.

GENERIC AND BRAND NAMES

APROSARTAN	**LOSARTAN**
Trovan	Cozaar
CANDESARTAN	Hyzaar
Atacand	**TELMISARTAN**
EPROSARTAN	Micandis
Teveten	**VALSARTAN**
IRBESARTAN	Diovan
Avapro	Diovan HCT

BASIC INFORMATION

Habit forming? No
Prescription needed? Yes
Available as generic? No
Drug class: Antihypertensive, angiotensin II receptor antagonist

USES

Treatment for hypertension (high blood pressure). May be used alone or in combination with other antihypertensive medications.

DOSAGE & USAGE INFORMATION

How to take:
Tablet—Swallow with liquid. May be taken with or without food.

When to take:
Once or twice daily as directed.

If you forget a dose:
Take as soon as you remember. If it is almost time for the next dose, then skip the missed dose and wait for your next scheduled dose (don't double this dose).

What drug does:
Lowers blood pressure by relaxing the blood vessels to allow improved blood flow in the body.

Time lapse before drug works:
May take several weeks for full effectiveness.

Continued next column

OVERDOSE

SYMPTOMS:
Slow or irregular heartbeat, faintness, dizziness, lightheadedness.
WHAT TO DO:
Overdose unlikely to threaten life. If person takes much larger amount than prescribed, call doctor, poison control center or hospital emergency room for instructions.

Don't take with:
Any other prescription or nonprescription drug without consulting your doctor or pharmacist.

POSSIBLE ADVERSE REACTIONS OR SIDE EFFECTS

SYMPTOMS	WHAT TO DO
Life-threatening: None expected.	
Common: Headache.	Continue. Call doctor when convenient.
Infrequent:	
• Dizziness, fever or sore throat (upper respiratory infection).	Continue, but call doctor right away.
• Diarrhea, back pain, cough, fatigue, stuffy nose.	Continue. Call doctor when convenient.
Rare: Dry cough, trouble sleeping, muscle cramps, leg pain.	Continue. Call doctor when convenient.

WARNINGS & PRECAUTIONS

Don't take if:
You are allergic to losartan.

Before you start, consult your doctor:
- If you have any kidney or liver disease.
- If you are allergic to any medication, food or other substance.

Over age 60:
No special problems expected.

Pregnancy:
Decide with your doctor if drug benefits justify risks to unborn child. Risk category C for first trimester and category D for second and third trimesters (see page xxiii).

Breast-feeding:
One or more of these drugs pass into milk in laboratory animals. Avoid drug or discontinue nursing until you finish medicine. Consult doctor for advice on maintaining milk supply.

Infants & children:
Not recommended for children under age 18.

Prolonged use:
- No special problems expected. Hypertension usually requires life-long treatment.
- Schedule regular doctor visits to determine if drug is continuing to be effective in controlling the hypertension and to check for any kidney problems.

Skin & sunlight:
No special problems expected.

Driving, piloting or hazardous work:
Don't drive or pilot aircraft until you learn how medicine affects you. Don't work around dangerous machinery. Don't climb ladders or work in high places. Danger increases if you drink alcohol or take other medicines affecting alertness and reflexes.

Discontinuing:
Don't discontinue without consulting your doctor, even if you feel well. You can have hypertension without feeling any symptoms. Untreated high blood pressure can cause serious problems.

Others:
- Advise any doctor or dentist whom you consult that you take this medicine. May interfere with the accuracy of some medical tests.
- Follow any special diet your doctor may prescribe. It can help control hypertension.
- Consult doctor if you become ill with vomiting or diarrhea.
- Use caution when exercising or performing activities in hot weather and with excessive sweating. You may experience dizziness, lightheadedness or faintness.

POSSIBLE INTERACTION WITH OTHER DRUGS

GENERIC NAME OR DRUG CLASS	COMBINED EFFECT
Anti-inflammatory drugs, nonsteroidal (NSAIDs)*	Decreased anti-hypertensive effect.
Cyclosporine	Excess potassium levels in the body.
Diuretics*	Increased anti-hypertensive effect.
Diuretics, potassium-sparing*	Excess potassium levels in the body.
Hypotension-causing drugs*, other	Increased anti-hypertensive effect.
Indomethacin	Decreased anti-hypertensive effect.
Potassium-containing medications	Excess potassium levels in the body.
Potassium supplements*	Excess potassium levels in the body.
Sympathomimetics*	Decreased anti-hypertensive effect.

POSSIBLE INTERACTION WITH OTHER SUBSTANCES

INTERACTS WITH	COMBINED EFFECT
Alcohol:	Unknown effect. Consult doctor.
Beverages: Low-salt milk.	Excess potassium in the body.
Cocaine:	Unknown effect. Consult doctor.
Foods: Salt substitutes containing potassium.	Excess potassium in the body.
Marijuana:	Increased sedation. Avoid.
Tobacco:	No special problems expected.

*See Glossary

ANGIOTENSIN-CONVERTING ENZYME (ACE) INHIBITORS

GENERIC AND BRAND NAMES

See complete list of generic and brand names in the *Generic and Brand Name Directory*, page 864.

BASIC INFORMATION

Habit forming? No
Prescription needed? Yes
Available as generic? Yes, for some
Drug class: Antihypertensive, ACE inhibitor

 USES

- Treatment for high blood pressure and congestive heart failure.
- Treatment for kidney disease in diabetic patients.
- Treatment for acute myocardial infarction within 24 hours of occurrence.

 DOSAGE & USAGE INFORMATION

How to take:
Tablet—Swallow with liquid. Instructions to take on empty stomach mean 1 hour before or 2 hours after eating.

When to take:
At the same times each day, usually 2-3 times daily. Take first dose at bedtime and lie down immediately.

If you forget a dose:
Take as soon as you remember up to 2 hours late. If more than 2 hours, wait for next scheduled dose (don't double this dose).

What drug does:
- Reduces resistance in arteries.
- Strengthens heartbeat.

Time lapse before drug works:
60 to 90 minutes.

Don't take with:
Any other medicine without consulting your doctor or pharmacist.

 OVERDOSE

SYMPTOMS:
Low blood pressure, fever, chills, sore throat, fainting, convulsions, coma.
WHAT TO DO:
- **Dial 911 (emergency) or 0 (operator) for an ambulance or medical help. Then give first aid immediately.**
- **See emergency information on inside covers.**

 POSSIBLE ADVERSE REACTIONS OR SIDE EFFECTS

SYMPTOMS	WHAT TO DO
Life-threatening: Hives, rash, intense itching, faintness soon after a dose (anaphylaxis); difficulty breathing.	Seek emergency treatment immediately.
Common: Rash, loss of taste.	Discontinue. Call doctor right away.
Infrequent: • Swelling of mouth, face, hands or feet.	Discontinue. Seek emergency treatment.
• Dizziness, fainting, chest pain, fast or irregular heartbeat, confusion, nervousness, numbness and tingling in hands or feet.	Discontinue. Call doctor right away.
• Diarrhea, headache, tiredness, cough.	Continue. Call doctor when convenient.
Rare: • Sore throat, cloudy urine, fever, chills.	Discontinue. Call doctor right away.
• Nausea, vomiting, indigestion, abdominal pain.	Continue. Call doctor when convenient.

 WARNINGS & PRECAUTIONS

Don't take if:
- You are allergic to any ACE inhibitor*.
- You are receiving blood from a blood bank.
- You will have surgery within 2 months, including dental surgery, requiring general or spinal anesthesia.

Before you start, consult your doctor:
- If you have had a stroke.
- If you have angina or heart or blood vessel disease.
- If you have any autoimmune disease, including AIDS or lupus.
- If you have high level of potassium in blood.
- If you have kidney or liver disease.
- If you are on severe salt-restricted diet.
- If you have a bone marrow disorder.

Over age 60:
Adverse reactions and side effects may be more frequent and severe than in younger persons.

ANGIOTENSIN-CONVERTING ENZYME (ACE) INHIBITORS

Pregnancy:
Risk factors vary for drugs in this group. See category list on page xxiii and consult doctor.

Breast-feeding:
Drug passes into milk. Avoid drug or discontinue nursing until you finish medicine. Consult doctor for advice on maintaining milk supply.

Infants & children:
Under close medical supervision only.

Prolonged use:
- May decrease white cells in blood or cause protein loss in urine.
- Request periodic laboratory blood counts and urine tests.

Skin & sunlight:
One or more drugs in this group may cause rash or intensify sunburn in areas exposed to sun or utltraviolet light (photosensitivity reaction). Avoid overexposure. Notify doctor if reaction occurs.

Driving, piloting or hazardous work:
Avoid if you become dizzy or faint. Otherwise, no problems expected.

Discontinuing:
Don't discontinue without consulting doctor. Dose may require gradual reduction if you have taken drug for a long time. Doses of other drugs may also require adjustment.

Others:
- Stop taking diuretics or increase salt intake 1 week before starting any ACE inhibitor.
- Avoid exercising in hot weather.
- May affect results in some medical tests.
- Advise any doctor or dentist whom you consult that you take this medicine.

POSSIBLE INTERACTION WITH OTHER DRUGS

GENERIC NAME OR DRUG CLASS	COMBINED EFFECT
Amiloride	Possible excessive potassium in blood.
Antihypertensives, other*	Increased anti-hypertensive effect. Dosage of each may require adjustment.
Beta-adrenergic blocking agents*	Increased anti-hypertensive effect. Dosage of each may require adjustment.
Carteolol	Increased anti-hypertensive effects of both drugs. Dosages may require adjustment.

Chloramphenicol	Possible blood disorders.
Diuretics*	Possible severe blood pressure drop with first dose.
Diclofenac	May decrease ACE inhibitor effect.
Guanfacine	Increased effect of both drugs.
Nicardipine	Possible excessive potassium in blood. Dosages may require adjustment.
Nimodipine	Possible excessive potassium in blood. Dangerous blood pressure drop.
Nitrates*	Possible excessive blood pressure drop.
Nonsteroidal anti-inflammatory drugs (NSAIDs)*	Decreased ACE inhibitor effect.
Pentamidine	May increase bone marrow depression or make kidney damage more likely.
Pentoxifylline	Increased anti-hypertensive effect.
Potassium	May raise potassium levels in blood to toxic levels.

Continued on page 897

POSSIBLE INTERACTION WITH OTHER SUBSTANCES

INTERACTS WITH	COMBINED EFFECT
Alcohol:	Possible excessive blood pressure drop.
Beverages: Low-salt milk.	Possible excessive potassium in blood.
Cocaine	Increased risk of heart block and high blood pressure.
Foods: Salt substitutes.	Possible excessive potassium.
Marijuana:	Increased dizziness.
Tobacco:	May decrease ACE inhibitor effect.

*See Glossary

ANGIOTENSIN-CONVERTING ENZYME (ACE) INHIBITORS & HYDROCHLOROTHIAZIDE

GENERIC AND BRAND NAMES

See complete list of generic and brand names in the *Generic and Brand Names Directory*, page 864.

BASIC INFORMATION

Habit forming? No
Prescription needed? Yes
Available as generic? No
Drug class: Antihypertensive, diuretic (thiazide), ACE inhibitor

USES

* Treatment for high blood pressure and congestive heart failure.
* Reduces fluid retention.

DOSAGE & USAGE INFORMATION

How to take:
Tablet—Swallow with liquid. Instructions to take on empty stomach mean 1 hour before or 2 hours after eating.

When to take:
At the same times each day, usually 2 to 3 times daily. Take first dose at bedtime and lie down immediately.

If you forget a dose:
Take as soon as you remember up to 2 hours late. If more than 2 hours, wait for next scheduled dose (don't double this dose).

What drug does:
* Forces sodium and water excretion, reducing body fluid.
* Relaxes muscle cells of small arteries.
* Reduced body fluid and relaxed arteries lower blood pressure.
* Reduces resistance in arteries.
* Strengthens heartbeat.

Continued next column

OVERDOSE

SYMPTOMS:
Cramps, weakness, drowsiness, weak pulse, low blood pressure.
WHAT TO DO:
* **Dial 911 (emergency) or 0 (operator) for an ambulance or medical help. Then give first aid immediately.**
* **See emergency information on inside covers.**

Time lapse before drug works:
4 to 6 hours. May require several weeks to lower blood pressure.

Don't take with:
Nonprescription drugs without consulting doctor.

POSSIBLE ADVERSE REACTIONS OR SIDE EFFECTS

SYMPTOMS	WHAT TO DO
Life-threatening:	
Irregular heartbeat (fast or uneven); hives, rash, intense itching, faintness soon after a dose (anaphylaxis).	Discontinue. Seek emergency treatment.
Common:	
• Dry mouth, thirst, tiredness, weakness, muscle cramps, vomiting, chest pain, skin rash, coughing, weak pulse.	Discontinue. Call doctor right away.
• Taste loss, dizziness.	Continue. Call doctor when convenient.
Infrequent:	
• Face, mouth, hands swell.	Discontinue. Call doctor right away.
• Nausea, diarrhea.	Continue. Call doctor when convenient.
Rare:	
Jaundice (yellow eyes and skin), bruising, back pain.	Discontinue. Call doctor right away.

WARNINGS & PRECAUTIONS

Don't take if:
* You are allergic to any ACE inhibitor or any thiazide diuretic drug.
* You are receiving blood from a blood bank.
* If you will have surgery within 2 months, including dental surgery, requiring general or spinal anesthesia.

Before you start, consult your doctor:
* If you have had a stroke.
* If you have angina, heart or blood vessel disease, a high level of potassium in blood, lupus, gout, liver, pancreas or kidney disorder.
* If you have any autoimmune disease, including AIDS or lupus.
* If you are on severe salt-restricted diet.
* If you are allergic to any sulfa drug.
* If you have a bone marrow disorder.

ANGIOTENSIN-CONVERTING ENZYME (ACE) INHIBITORS & HYDROCHLOROTHIAZIDE

Over age 60:
Adverse reactions and side effects may be more frequent and severe than in younger persons, especially dizziness and excessive potassium loss.

Pregnancy:
Risk factors vary for drugs in this group. See category list on page xxiii and consult doctor.

Breast-feeding:
Drug passes into milk. Avoid drug or discontinue nursing until you finish medicine. Consult doctor for advice on maintaining milk supply.

Infants & children:
Not recommended.

Prolonged use:
Talk to your doctor about the need for follow-up medical examinations or laboratory studies to check blood pressure, ECG*, liver function, kidney function.

Skin & sunlight:
One or more drugs in this group may cause rash or intensify sunburn in areas exposed to sun or utltraviolet light (photosensitivity reaction). Avoid overexposure. Notify doctor if reaction occurs.

Driving, piloting or hazardous work:
Don't drive or pilot aircraft until you learn how medicine affects you. Don't work around dangerous machinery. Don't climb ladders or work in high places. Danger increases if you drink alcohol or take medicine affecting alertness and reflexes, such as antihistamines, tranquilizers, sedatives, pain medicine, narcotics and mind-altering drugs.

Discontinuing:
Don't discontinue without consulting doctor. Dose may require gradual reduction if you have taken drug for a long time. Doses of other drugs may also require adjustment.

Others:
- Hot weather and fever may cause dehydration and drop in blood pressure. Dose may require temporary adjustment. Weigh daily and report any unexpected weight decreases to your doctor.
- May cause rise in uric acid, leading to gout.
- May cause blood-sugar rise in diabetics.

POSSIBLE INTERACTION WITH OTHER DRUGS

GENERIC NAME OR DRUG CLASS	COMBINED EFFECT
Allopurinol	Decreased allopurinol effect.
Amiloride	Possible excessive potassium in blood.
Antidepressants, tricyclic*	Dangerous drop in blood pressure. Avoid combination unless under medical supervision.
Antihypertensives, other*	Increased antihypertensive effect. Dosage of each may require adjustment.
Anti-inflammatory drugs nonsteroidal (NSAIDs)*	Decreased captopril effect.
Barbiturates*	Increased hydrochlorothiazide effect.
Beta-adrenergic blocking agents*	Increased antihypertensive effect. Dosage of each may require adjustments.
Carteolol	Increased antihypertensive effects of both drugs. Dosages may require adjustment.
Chloramphenicol	Possible blood disorders.
Cholestyramine	Decreased hydrochlorothiazide effect.
Digitalis preparations*	Excessive potassium loss that causes dangerous heart rhythms.

Continued on page 898

POSSIBLE INTERACTION WITH OTHER SUBSTANCES

INTERACTS WITH	COMBINED EFFECT
Alcohol:	Dangerous blood pressure drop. Avoid.
Beverages: Low-salt milk.	Possible excessive potassium in blood.
Cocaine	Increased risk of heart block and high blood pressure.
Foods: Salt substitutes.	Possible excessive potassium.
Marijuana:	Increased dizziness; may increase blood-pressure.
Tobacco:	May decrease blood pressure lowering effect.

ANTACIDS

GENERIC AND BRAND NAMES

See complete list of generic and brand names in the *Generic and Brand Name Directory*, page 864.

BASIC INFORMATION

Habit forming? No
Prescription needed? No
Available as generic? Yes, for some.
Drug class: Antacid

USES

Treatment for hyperacidity in upper gastrointestinal tract, including stomach and esophagus. Symptoms may be heartburn or acid indigestion. Diseases include peptic ulcer, gastritis, esophagitis, hiatal hernia.

DOSAGE & USAGE INFORMATION

How to take:
Follow package instructions.

When to take:
1 to 3 hours after meals unless directed otherwise by your doctor.

If you forget a dose:
Take as soon as you remember, but not simultaneously with any other medicine.

What drug does:
- Neutralizes some of the hydrochloric acid in the stomach.
- Reduces action of pepsin, a digestive enzyme.

Continued next column

OVERDOSE

SYMPTOMS:
Dry mouth, shallow breathing, diarrhea or constipation, headache, mental confusion, weakness, fatigue, stupor, bone pain.
WHAT TO DO:
- **Overdose unlikely to threaten life. Depending on severity of symptoms and amount taken, call doctor, poison control center or hospital emergency room for instructions.**
- **Dial 911 (emergency) or 0 (operator) for an ambulance or medical help. Then give first aid immediately.**
- **See emergency information on inside covers.**

Time lapse before drug works:
15 minutes for antacid effect.

Don't take with:
Other medicines at the same time. Decreases absorption of other drugs. Wait 2 hours between doses.

POSSIBLE ADVERSE REACTIONS OR SIDE EFFECTS

SYMPTOMS	WHAT TO DO
Life-threatening: None expected.	
Common: Chalky taste.	Continue. Tell doctor at next visit.
Infrequent: Mild constipation, increased thirst, laxative effect, unpleasant taste in mouth, stomach cramps, stool color changes (whitish or speckling).	Continue. Call doctor when convenient.
Rare: Bone pain, frequent or urgent urination, muscle weakness or pain, nausea, weight gain, severe constipation, dizziness, headache, appetite loss, mood changes, vomiting, nervousness, swollen feet and ankles, tiredness or weakness.	Discontinue. Call doctor right away.

Note: Side effects are rare unless too much medicine is taken for a long time.

WARNINGS & PRECAUTIONS

Don't take if:
- You are allergic to any antacid.
- You have a high blood-calcium level.

Before you start, consult your doctor:
If you have kidney disease, chronic constipation, colitis, diarrhea, symptoms of appendicitis, stomach or intestinal bleeding, irregular heartbeat.

Over age 60:
Adverse reactions and side effects may be more frequent and severe than in younger persons. Diarrhea or constipation particularly likely.

Pregnancy:
Risk factors vary for drugs in this group. See category list on page xxiii and consult doctor.

Breast-feeding:
Drug passes into milk. Consult doctor.

Infants & children:
Use only under medical supervision.

Prolonged use:
- High blood level of calcium (if your antacid contains calcium) which disturbs electrolyte balance.
- Kidney stones, impaired kidney function.
- Talk to your doctor about the need for follow-up medical examinations or laboratory studies to check kidney function, serum calcium, serum potassium.

Skin & sunlight:
No problems expected.

Driving, piloting or hazardous work:
No problems expected.

Discontinuing:
May be unnecessary to finish medicine. Follow doctor's instructions.

Others:
- Don't take longer than 2 weeks unless under medical supervision.
- May affect results in some medical tests.

POSSIBLE INTERACTION WITH OTHER DRUGS

GENERIC NAME OR DRUG CLASS	COMBINED EFFECT
Alendronate	Decreased alendronate effect. Take antacid 30 minutes after alendronate.
Capecitabine	Increased risk of capecitabine toxicity.
Chlorpromazine	Decreased chlorpromazine effect.
Ciprofloxacin	May cause kidney dysfunction.
Dexamethasone	Decreased dexamethasone effect.
Digitalis preparations*	Decreased digitalis effect.
Iron supplements*	Decreased iron effect.
Isoniazid	Decreased isoniazid effect.
Ketoconazole	Reduced ketoconazole effect.
Levodopa	Increased levodopa effect.

Mecamylamine	Increased mecamylamine effect.
Meperidine	Increased meperidine effect.
Methenamine	Reduced methenamine effect.
Nalidixic acid	Decreased nalidixic acid effect.
Nicardipine	Possible decreased nicardipine effect.
Nizatidine	Decreased nizatidine absorption.
Ofloxacin	Decreased ofloxacin effect.
Oxyphenbutazone	Decreased oxyphenbutazone effect.
Para-aminosalicylic acid (PAS)	Decreased PAS effect.
Penicillins*	Decreased penicillin effect.
Prednisone	Decreased prednisone effect.
Pseudoephedrine	Increased pseudoephedrine effect.
Salicylates*	Increased salicylate effect.
Tetracyclines	Decreased tetracycline effect.
Ticlopidine	Decreased ticlopidine effect.

POSSIBLE INTERACTION WITH OTHER SUBSTANCES

INTERACTS WITH	COMBINED EFFECT
Alcohol:	Decreased antacid effect.
Beverages: Milk.	May cause bone discomfort.
Cocaine:	No proven problems.
Foods:	Decreased antacid effect. Wait 1 hour after eating.
Marijuana:	Decreased antacid effect.
Tobacco:	Decreased antacid effect.

*See Glossary

GENERIC AND BRAND NAMES

ALBENDAZOLE
  Albenza
IVERMECTIN
  Stromectol
MEBENDAZOLE
  Mebendacin
  Mebutar
  Nemasole
  Vermox
PYRANTEL
  Antiminth
  Aut
  Cobantril
  Helmex

Lombriareu
Reese's Pinworm
  Medicine
  Trilombrin
PYRVINIUM
  Vanquin
  Viprynium
THIABENDAZOLE
  Foldan
  Mintezol
  Mintezol Topical
  Minzolum
  Triasox

BASIC INFORMATION

Habit forming? No
Prescription needed? Yes
Available as generic? Yes
Drug class: Anthelmintics, antiparasitic

USES

- Treatment of roundworms, pinworms, whipworms, hookworms and other intestinal parasites.
- Treatment of hydatid disease and neurocysticercosis; stronglyoidiasis and onchocerciasis.

DOSAGE & USAGE INFORMATION

How to take or apply:
- Tablet—Swallow with liquid or food to lessen stomach irritation.
- Topical suspension—Apply to end of each tunnel or burrow made by worm.
- Chewable tablets—Chew thoroughly before swallowing.
- Oral suspension—Follow package instructions.

Continued next column

OVERDOSE

SYMPTOMS:
Increased severity of adverse reactions and side effects.
WHAT TO DO:
Overdose unlikely to threaten life. If person takes much larger amount than prescribed, call doctor, poison control center or hospital emergency room for instructions.

When to take:
Morning and evening with food to increase uptake.

If you forget a dose:
Skip dose and begin treatment again. Often only one or two doses are needed to complete treatment.

What drug does:
Kills or paralyzes the parasites. They then pass out of the body in the feces. Usually the type of worm parasite must be identified so the appropriate drug can be prescribed.

Time lapse before drug works:
Some take only hours, others, 1-3 days.

Don't take with:
Any other medicine without consulting your doctor or pharmacist.

POSSIBLE ADVERSE REACTIONS OR SIDE EFFECTS

SYMPTOMS	WHAT TO DO
Life-threatening: None expected.	
Common: None expected.	
Infrequent: • Abdominal pain, diarrhea, dizziness, fever, nausea, rectal itching.	Continue. Call doctor when convenient.
• Red stools, asparagus-like urine smell, bad taste in mouth.	No action necessary.
Rare: Skin rash, itching, sore throat and fever, weakness (severe), hair loss, headache, blurred vision, seizures.	Discontinue. Call doctor right away.

WARNINGS & PRECAUTIONS

Don't take if:
You are allergic to any anthelmintics.

Before you start, consult your doctor:
- If you have liver disease.
- If you have Crohn's disease.
- If you have ulcerative colitis.

Over age 60:
Adverse reactions and side effects may be more frequent and severe than in younger persons. You may need smaller doses for shorter periods of time.

Pregnancy:
Risk factors vary for drugs in this group. See category list on page xxiii and consult doctor.

Breast-feeding:
Unknown effect. Consult your doctor.

Infants & children:
No problems expected. Don't give to a child under age 2 without doctor's approval.

Prolonged use:
- Not intended for long-term use.
- Talk to your doctor about the need for follow-up medical examinations or laboratory studies to check stools, cellophane tape swabs pressed against rectal area to check for parasite eggs, complete blood counts (white blood cell count, platelet count, red blood cell count, hemoglobin, hematocrit).

Skin & sunlight:
Thiabendazole may cause rash or intensify sunburn in areas exposed to sun or ultraviolet light (photosensitivity reaction). Avoid overexposure. Notify doctor if reaction occurs.

Driving, piloting or hazardous work:
Use caution if the medicine causes you to feel dizzy or weak. Otherwise, no problems expected.

Discontinuing:
No problems expected.

Others:
- Take full course of treatment. Repeat course may be necessary if follow-up examinations reveal persistent infection.
- Wash all bedding after treatment to prevent re-infection.

POSSIBLE INTERACTION WITH OTHER DRUGS

GENERIC NAME OR DRUG CLASS	COMBINED EFFECT
Carbamazepine	Decreased effect of mebendazole.
Phenytoin	Decreased effect of mebendazole.
Piperazine	Decreased effect of each drug.
Theophylline	Increased effect of theophylline (with thiabendazole use.)

POSSIBLE INTERACTION WITH OTHER SUBSTANCES

INTERACTS WITH	COMBINED EFFECT
Alcohol:	Decreased mebendazole effect. Avoid.
Beverages:	None expected.
Cocaine:	None expected.
Foods:	None expected.
Marijuana:	None expected.
Tobacco:	None expected.

*See Glossary

ANTHRALIN (Topical)

BRAND NAMES

Anthra-Derm
Anthraforte
Anthranol
Anthrascalp
Dithranol
Drithocreme
Drithocreme HP

Dritho-Scalp
Lasan
Lasan HP
Lasan Pomade
Lasan Unguent
Micanol

BASIC INFORMATION

Habit forming? No
Prescription needed? Yes
Available as generic? No
Drug class: Antipsoriasis, hair growth stimulant

USES

- Treats quiescent or chronic psoriasis.
- Stimulates hair growth in some people (not an approved use by the FDA).

DOSAGE & USAGE INFORMATION

How to use:
- Wear plastic gloves for all applications.
- If directed, apply at night.
- Cream, lotion, ointment—Bathe and dry area before use. Apply small amount and rub gently.
- If for short contact, same as above for cream.
- Leave on 20 to 30 minutes. Then remove medicine by bathing or shampooing.
- If for scalp overnight—Shampoo before use to remove scales or medicine. Dry hair. Part hair several times and apply to scalp. Wear plastic cap on head. Clean off next morning with petroleum jelly, then shampoo.

When to use:
As directed.

If you forget a dose:
Use as soon as you remember.

What drug does:
Reduces growth activity within abnormal cells by inhibiting enzymes.

Continued next column

OVERDOSE

SYMPTOMS:
None expected.
WHAT TO DO:
Not for internal use. If child accidentally swallows, call poison control center.

Time lapse before drug works:
May require several weeks or more.

Don't use with:
Any other medicine without consulting your doctor or pharmacist.

POSSIBLE ADVERSE REACTIONS OR SIDE EFFECTS

SYMPTOMS	WHAT TO DO
Life-threatening: None expected.	
Common: None expected.	
Infrequent: Redness or irritation of skin not present before application, rash.	Discontinue. Call doctor when convenient.
Rare: None expected.	

WARNINGS & PRECAUTIONS

Don't use if:
- You are allergic to anthralin.
- You have infected skin.

Before you start, consult your doctor:
- If you have chronic kidney disease.
- If you are allergic to anything.

Over age 60:
No problems expected, but check with doctor.

Pregnancy:
Studies in animals and humans have not been done. Consult doctor. Risk category C (see page xxiii).

Breast-feeding:
No problems expected, but check with doctor.

Infants & children:
No problems expected, but check with doctor.

Prolonged use:
No problems expected, but check with doctor.

Skin & sunlight:
May cause rash or intensify sunburn in areas exposed to sun or ultraviolet light (photosensitivity reaction). Avoid overexposure. Notify doctor if reaction occurs.

Driving, piloting or hazardous work:
No problems expected.

Discontinuing:
No problems expected.

Others:
- Keep cool, but don't freeze.
- Apply petroleum jelly to normal skin or scalp to protect areas not being treated.
- Will stain hair, clothing, shower, bathtub or sheets. Wash as soon as possible.
- Heat and moisture in bathroom medicine cabinet can cause breakdown of medicine. Store someplace else.

POSSIBLE INTERACTION WITH OTHER DRUGS

GENERIC NAME OR DRUG CLASS	COMBINED EFFECT
Antidiabetic agents*	Increased sensitivity to sun exposure.
Coal tar preparations*	Increased sensitivity to sun exposure.
Diuretics, thiazide*	Increased sensitivity to sun exposure.
Griseofulvin	Increased sensitivity to sun exposure.
Methosalen	Increased sensitivity to sun exposure.
Nalidixic acid	Increased sensitivity to sun exposure.
Phenothiazines*	Increased sensitivity to sun exposure.
Sulfa drugs*	Increased sensitivity to sun exposure.
Tetracyclines*	Increased sensitivity to sun exposure.
Trioxsalen	Increased sensitivity to sun exposure.

POSSIBLE INTERACTION WITH OTHER SUBSTANCES

INTERACTS WITH	COMBINED EFFECT
Alcohol:	None expected.
Beverages:	None expected.
Cocaine:	None expected.
Foods:	None expected.
Marijuana:	None expected.
Tobacco:	None expected.

ANTIACNE, CLEANSING (Topical)

GENERIC AND BRAND NAMES

ALCOHOL &
  ACETONE
Seba-Nil
ALCOHOL &
  SULFUR
Liquimat
Postacne

SULFURATED
  LIME
Vlemasque
Vlemickxs Solution

BASIC INFORMATION

Habit forming? No
Prescription needed? No
Available as generic? Yes
Drug class: Anti-acne agent, cleansing agent

USES

Treats acne or oily skin.

DOSAGE & USAGE INFORMATION

How to use:
* Lotion, gel or pledget—Start with small amount and wipe over face to remove dirt and surface oil. Don't apply to wounds or burns. Don't rinse with water and avoid contact with eyes. Skin may be more sensitive in dry or cold climates.
* Plaster—Follow package instructions.

When to use:
As directed. May increase frequency up to 3 or more times daily as tolerated. Warm, humid weather may allow more frequent use.

If you forget a dose:
Use as soon as you remember and then go back to regular schedule.

Continued next column

OVERDOSE

SYMPTOMS:
None expected.
WHAT TO DO:
* Not for internal use. If child accidentally swallows, call poison control center.
* Dial 911 (emergency) or 0 (operator) for an ambulance or medical help. Then give first aid immediately.
* See emergency information on inside covers.

What drug does:
Helps remove oil from skin's surface.

Time lapse before drug works:
Works immediately.

Don't use with:
Other topical acne treatments unless directed by doctor.

POSSIBLE ADVERSE REACTIONS OR SIDE EFFECTS

SYMPTOMS	WHAT TO DO
Life-threatening: None expected.	
Common: None expected.	
Infrequent: • Skin infection, pustules or rash; unusual pain, swelling or redness of treated skin.	Discontinue. Call doctor right away.
• Burning, dryness, stinging, peeling of skin.	Continue. Call doctor when convenient.
Rare: None expected.	

WARNINGS & PRECAUTIONS

Don't use if:
You have to apply over a wounded or burned area.

Before you start, consult your doctor:
If you use benzoyl peroxide, resorcinol, salicylic acid, sulfur or tretinoin (vitamin A acid).

Over age 60:
No problems expected.

Pregnancy:
Risk category not assigned to this drug group. Consult doctor about use.

Breast-feeding:
No problems expected, but check with doctor.

Infants & children:
No problems expected, but check with doctor. Use only under close medical supervision.

Prolonged use:
Excessive drying of skin.

Skin & sunlight:
No special problems expected.

Driving, piloting or hazardous work:
No problems expected, but check with doctor.

Discontinuing:
No problems expected, but check with doctor.

Others:
Some anti-acne agents are flammable. Don't use near fire or while smoking.

POSSIBLE INTERACTION WITH OTHER DRUGS

GENERIC NAME OR DRUG CLASS	COMBINED EFFECT
Abrasive or medicated soaps	Irritation or too much drying.
After-shave lotions	Irritation or too much drying.
Antiacne topical preparations (other)	Irritation or too much drying.
"Cover-up" cosmetics	Irritation or too much drying.
Drying cosmetic soaps	Irritation or too much drying.
Isotretinoin	Irritation or too much drying.
Mercury compounds	May stain skin black and smell bad.
Perfumed toilet water	Irritation or too much drying.
Preparations containing skin-peeling agents such as benzoyl peroxide, resorcinol, salicylic acid, sulfur, tretinoin	Irritation or too much drying.

POSSIBLE INTERACTION WITH OTHER SUBSTANCES

INTERACTS WITH	COMBINED EFFECT
Alcohol:	None expected.
Beverages:	None expected.
Cocaine:	None expected.
Foods:	None expected.
Marijuana:	None expected.
Tobacco:	None expected.

ANTIALLERGIC AGENTS (Ophthalmic)

GENERIC AND BRAND NAMES

EMEDASTINE
 Emadine
LEVOCABASTINE
 Livostin

LODOXAMIDE
 Alomide
OLOPATADINE
 Patanol

BASIC INFORMATION

Habit forming? No
Prescription needed? Yes
Available as generic? No
Drug class: Ophthalmic antiallergic agents,
 antihistaminic

 ## USES

Prevention and treatment of seasonal allergic
(hay fever) eye disorders. May be referred to as
seasonal conjunctivitis, vernal conjunctivitis,
vernal keratitis and vernal keratoconjunctivitis.

 ## DOSAGE & USAGE INFORMATION

How to use:
Eye solution
• Wash hands.
• Apply pressure to inside corner of eye with
 middle finger.
• Continue pressure for 1 minute after placing
 medicine in eye.
• Tilt head backward. Pull lower lid away from
 eye with index finger of the same hand.
• Drop eye drops into pouch and close eye.
 Don't blink.
• Keep eyes closed for 1 to 2 minutes.

When to use:
1 to 2 drops 4 times a day or as directed by
doctor.

If you forget a dose:
Use as soon as you remember, then return to
regular schedule.

Continued next column

 ## OVERDOSE

SYMPTOMS:
None expected.
WHAT TO DO:
**Not intended for internal use. If child
accidentally swallows, call poison control
center.**

Time lapse before drug works:
Levocabastine—7 days, with confirmed
improvement.
Lodoxamide—3 days.
Olopatadine—8 hours.

What drug does:
• Lodoxamide acts as a mast cell* stabilizer to
 prevent a hypersensitivity reaction to certain
 allergens such as pollen.
• Levocabastine and olopatadine are histamine
 H_1 receptor antagonists that block
 hypersensitivity responses to allergens.

Time lapse before drug works:
Relief of symptoms may begin immediately, but
full benefit might take a few days.

Don't use with:
Any other medications without first consulting
doctor or pharmacist.

 ## POSSIBLE ADVERSE REACTIONS OR SIDE EFFECTS

SYMPTOMS	WHAT TO DO
Life-threatening: None expected.	
Common: Brief and mild burning or stinging when drops are administered.	No action necessary.
Infrequent: Blurred vision, feeling that something is in the the eye, redness of eye, eye irritation not present before, eye tearing or discharge.	Discontinue. Call doctor right away.
Rare: • Aching in eye, crusting in corner of eye or eyelid, dryness of eyes or nose, drowsiness or sleepiness, feeling of heat in eye or body, nausea, stomach discomfort, sneezing, sticky or tired feeling of eye.	Continue. Call doctor when convenient.
• Redness or irritation of eyelid, swelling of eye, pain in eye, sensitivity to light, headache, dizziness, skin rash.	Discontinue. Call doctor right away.

WARNINGS & PRECAUTIONS

Don't use if:
You are allergic to levocabastine or lodoxamide.

Before you start, consult your doctor:
- If you wear soft contact lenses.
- You are allergic to any other medications, foods or other substances.

Over age 60:
No special problems expected.

Pregnancy:
Risk category C for levocabastine and olopatadine and B for lodoxamide (see page xxiii). Consult doctor.

Breast-feeding:
lodoxamide passes into breast milk after administration into the eye. It is unknown if levocabastine or olopatadine pass into breast milk. Consult doctor.

Infants & children:
No information available on safety or effectiveness for children under age 2 for lodoxamide and under age 12 for levocabastine. Consult doctor.

Prolonged use:
No special problems expected.

Skin & sunlight:
No special problems expected.

Driving, piloting or hazardous work:
Avoid if you feel dizzy or side effects cause vision problems.

Discontinuing:
No special problems expected.

Others:
- Don't use leftover medicine for other eye problems without your doctor's approval.
- If symptoms don't improve after a few days of use, call your doctor.

POSSIBLE INTERACTION WITH OTHER DRUGS

GENERIC NAME OR DRUG CLASS	COMBINED EFFECT
None significant.	

POSSIBLE INTERACTION WITH OTHER SUBSTANCES

INTERACTS WITH	COMBINED EFFECT
Alcohol:	None expected.
Beverages:	None expected.
Cocaine	None expected.
Foods:	None expected.
Marijuana:	None expected.
Tobacco:	None expected.

ANTIBACTERIALS, ANTIFUNGALS (Topical)

GENERIC AND BRAND NAMES

CLIOQUINOL &
  HYDROCORTISONE
  Vioform Hydro-
    cortisone Cream
  Vioform Hydro-
    cortisone Lotion
  Vioform Hydro-
    cortisone Mild
    Cream
  Vioform Hydro-
    cortisone Mild
    Ointment
  Vioform Hydro-
    cortisone Ointment

SULFADIAZINE
  Flamazine
  Flint SSD
  Sildamac
  Silvadene
  SSD
  SSD AF
  Thermazine

BASIC INFORMATION

Habit forming? No
Prescription needed? Yes
Available as generic? Yes, some are
Drug class: Antibacterial (topical),
  antifungal (topical)

 ## USES

Treats eczema, other inflammatory skin
conditions, athlete's foot, skin infections.

 ## DOSAGE & USAGE INFORMATION

How to use:
- Cream, lotion, ointment—Bathe and dry area
  before use. Apply small amount and rub
  gently.
- Keep away from eyes.

When to use:
2 to 4 times a day.

If you forget a dose:
Use as soon as you remember.

Continued next column

 ## OVERDOSE

SYMPTOMS:
Severe nausea, vomiting, diarrhea.
WHAT TO DO:
- Not for internal use. If child accidentally
  swallows, call poison control center.
- Dial 911 (emergency) or 0 (operator) for an
  ambulance or medical help. Then give first
  aid immediately.
- See emergency information on inside
  covers.

What drug does:
Kills some types of fungus and bacteria on
contact.

Time lapse before drug works:
2 to 4 weeks, sometimes longer.

Don't use with:
Other ointments, creams or lotions without
consulting doctor.

 ## POSSIBLE ADVERSE REACTIONS OR SIDE EFFECTS

SYMPTOMS	WHAT TO DO
Life-threatening: None expected.	
Common: May stain skin around nails.	Continue. Tell doctor at next visit.
Infrequent: Stomach cramps; hives; itching, burning, peeling, red, stinging, swelling skin.	Discontinue. Call doctor right away.
Rare: None expected.	

WARNINGS & PRECAUTIONS

Don't use if:
You are allergic to clioquinol, iodine or any iodine-containing preparation.

Before you start, consult your doctor:
If you are allergic to anything that touches your skin.

Over age 60:
No problems expected.

Pregnancy:
Risk factors vary for drugs in this group. See category list on page xxiii and consult doctor.

Breast-feeding:
No problems expected, but check with doctor.

Infants & children:
No problems expected, but check with doctor.

Prolonged use:
No problems expected, but check with doctor.

Skin & sunlight:
No special problems expected.

Driving, piloting or hazardous work:
No problems expected, but check with doctor.

Discontinuing:
No problems expected, but check with doctor.

Others:
- If not improved in 2 weeks, check with doctor.
- May stain clothing or bed linens.
- May stain hair, skin and nails yellow.
- If accidentally gets into eyes, flush with clear water immediately.
- Tests of thyroid function may yield inaccurate results if you use clioquinol within 1 month before testing.

POSSIBLE INTERACTION WITH OTHER DRUGS

GENERIC NAME OR DRUG CLASS	COMBINED EFFECT
None expected.	

POSSIBLE INTERACTION WITH OTHER SUBSTANCES

INTERACTS WITH	COMBINED EFFECT
Alcohol:	None expected.
Beverages:	None expected.
Cocaine:	None expected.
Foods:	None expected.
Marijuana:	None expected.
Tobacco:	None expected.

*See Glossary

ANTIBACTERIALS FOR ACNE (Topical)

GENERIC AND BRAND NAMES

CHLORTETRACYCLINE
(topical)
  Aureomycin
CLINDAMYCIN
(topical)
  Cleocin T Gel
  Cleocin T Lotion
  Cleocin T Topical
    Solution
  Clinda-Derm
  Dalacin T Topical
    Solution

ERYTHROMYCIN
(topical)
  Akne-Mycin
  A/T/S
  Benzamycin
  Erycette
  EryDerm
  EryGel
  EryMax
  ErySol
  Erythro-statin
  ETS
  Sans-Acne
  Staticin
  Theramycin Z
  T-Stat
TETRACYCLINE
(topical)
  Achromycin
  Topicycline

BASIC INFORMATION

Habit forming? No
Prescription needed? Yes
Available as generic? Yes
Drug class: Antibacterial (topical)

USES

Treats acne by killing skin bacteria that may be part of the cause of acne.

DOSAGE & USAGE INFORMATION

How to use:
- Pledgets and solutions are flammable. Use away from flame or heat.
- Apply medication to entire area, not just to pimples.
- If you use other acne medicines on skin, wait an hour after using erythromycin before applying other medicine.

Continued next column

OVERDOSE

SYMPTOMS:
None expected.
WHAT TO DO:
Not for internal use. If child accidentally swallows, call poison control center.

- Cream, lotion, ointment—Bathe and dry area before use. Apply small amount and rub gently.

When to use:
2 times a day, morning and evening, or as directed by your doctor.

If you forget a dose:
Use as soon as you remember.

What drug does:
Kills bacteria on skin, skin glands or in hair follicles.

Time lapse before drug works:
3 to 4 weeks to begin improvement.

Don't use with:
Other skin medicine without telling your doctor.

POSSIBLE ADVERSE REACTIONS OR SIDE EFFECTS

SYMPTOMS	WHAT TO DO
Life-threatening: None expected.	
Common: Stinging or burning of skin for a few minutes after application; faint yellow skin color, especially around hair roots (with chlortetracycline, meclocycline or tetracycline).	Continue. Tell doctor at next visit.
Infrequent: Red, peeling, itching, irritated or dry skin.	Continue. Call doctor when convenient.
Rare (extremely): Symptoms of excess medicine absorbed by body—Abdominal pain, diarrhea, fever, nausea, vomiting, bloating, thirst, weakness, weight loss.	Discontinue. Call doctor right away.

WARNINGS & PRECAUTIONS

Don't use if:
You are allergic to erythromycins, clindamycins or tetracyclines.

Before you start, consult your doctor:
- If you are allergic to any substance that touches your skin.
- If you use benzoyl peroxide, resorcinol, salicylic acid, sulfur or tretinoin (vitamin A acid).

Over age 60:
No problems expected.

Pregnancy:
Risk factors vary for drugs in this group. See category list on page xxiii and consult doctor.

Breast-feeding:
No problems expected, but check with doctor.

Infants & children:
No problems expected, but check with doctor.

Prolonged use:
Excess irritation to skin.

Skin & sunlight:
No special problems expected.

Driving, piloting or hazardous work:
No problems expected, but check with doctor.

Discontinuing:
No problems expected, but check with doctor.

Others:
- Use water-base cosmetics.
- Keep medicine away from mouth or eyes.
- If accidentally gets into eyes, flush immediately with clear water.
- Keep away from heat or flame.
- Keep cool, but don't freeze.

POSSIBLE INTERACTION WITH OTHER DRUGS

GENERIC NAME OR DRUG CLASS	COMBINED EFFECT
Abrasive or medicated soaps	Irritation or too much drying.
After-shave lotions	Irritation or too much drying.
Anti-acne topical preparations (other)	Irritation or too much drying.
"Cover-up" cosmetics	Irritation or too much drying.
Drying cosmetic soaps	Irritation or too much drying.
Isotretinoin	Irritation or too much drying.
Mercury compounds	May stain skin black and smell bad.
Perfumed toilet water	Irritation or too much drying.
Preparations containing skin peeling agents such as benzoyl peroxide, resorcinol, salicylic acid, sulfur, tretinoin	Irritation or too much drying.

POSSIBLE INTERACTION WITH OTHER SUBSTANCES

INTERACTS WITH	COMBINED EFFECT
Alcohol:	None expected.
Beverages:	None expected.
Cocaine:	None expected.
Foods:	None expected.
Marijuana:	None expected.
Tobacco:	None expected.

ANTIBACTERIALS (Ophthalmic)

GENERIC AND BRAND NAMES

See complete list of generic and brand names in the *Generic and Brand Name Directory*, page 865.

BASIC INFORMATION

Habit forming? No
Prescription needed? Yes
Available as generic? Yes, for some
Drug class: Antibacterial (ophthalmic)

USES

- Helps body overcome eye infections on surface tissues of the eye.
- Treatment for corneal ulcers, bacterial.

DOSAGE & USAGE INFORMATION

How to use:
Eye drops
- Wash hands.
- Apply pressure to inside corner of eye with middle finger.
- Continue pressure for 1 minute after placing medicine in eye.
- Tilt head backward. Pull lower lid away from eye with index finger of the same hand.
- Drop eye drops into pouch and close eye. Don't blink.
- Keep eyes closed for 1 to 2 minutes.

Eye ointment
- Wash hands.
- Pull lower lid down from eye to form a pouch.
- Squeeze tube to apply thin strip of ointment into pouch.
- Close eye for 1 to 2 minutes.
- Don't touch applicator tip to any surface (including the eye). If you accidentally touch tip, clean with warm soap and water.
- Keep container tightly closed.
- Keep cool, but don't freeze.
- Wash hands immediately after using.

Continued next column

OVERDOSE

SYMPTOMS:
None expected.
WHAT TO DO:
Not intended for internal use. If child accidentally swallows, call poison control center.

When to use:
As directed. Don't miss doses.

If you forget a dose:
Use as soon as you remember.

What drug does:
Penetrates bacterial cell membrane and prevents cells from multiplying.

Time lapse before drug works:
Begins in 1 hour. May require 7 to 10 days to control infection.

Don't use with:
Any other eye drops or ointment without checking with your ophthalmologist.

POSSIBLE ADVERSE REACTIONS OR SIDE EFFECTS

SYMPTOMS	WHAT TO DO
Life-threatening: None expected.	
Common: Ointments cause blurred vision for a few minutes.	Continue. Tell doctor at next visit.
Infrequent:	
• Signs of irritation not present before drug use.	Discontinue. Call doctor right away.
• Burning or stinging of the eye.	Continue. Call doctor when convenient.
Rare (with chloramphenicol): Sore throat, pale skin, fever, unusual bleeding or bruising.	Discontinue. Call doctor right away.

WARNINGS & PRECAUTIONS

Don't use if:
You are allergic to any antibiotic used on skin, ears, vagina or rectum.

Before you start, consult your doctor:
If you have had an allergic reaction to any medicine, food or other substances.

Over age 60:
No problems expected.

Pregnancy:
Risk factors vary for drugs in this group. See category list on page xxiii and consult doctor.

Breast-feeding:
No problems expected, but check with doctor.

Infants & children:
No problems expected. Use only under medical supervision.

Prolonged use:
Sensitivity reaction may develop.

Skin & sunlight:
No problems expected.

Driving, piloting or hazardous work:
No problems expected.

Discontinuing:
Possible rare adverse reaction of bone marrow depression that leads to aplastic anemia may occur after discontinuing chloramphenicol.

Others:
* Notify doctor if symptoms fail to improve in 2 to 4 days.
* Keep medicine cool, but don't freeze.

POSSIBLE INTERACTION WITH OTHER DRUGS

GENERIC NAME OR DRUG CLASS	COMBINED EFFECT
Clinically significant interactions with oral or injected medicines unlikely.	

POSSIBLE INTERACTION WITH OTHER SUBSTANCES

INTERACTS WITH	COMBINED EFFECT
Alcohol:	None expected.
Beverages:	None expected.
Cocaine:	None expected.
Foods:	None expected.
Marijuana:	None expected.
Tobacco:	None expected.

GENERIC AND BRAND NAMES

CHLORAMPHENICOL
  Chloromycetin
  Sopamycetin
COLISTIN, NEOMYCIN
  & HYDRO-
  CORTISONE
  Coly-Mycin S
GENTAMICIN (Otic)
  Garamycin Otic
  Solution
HYDROCORTISONE
  & ACETIC ACID
  Acetasol HC
  Otic Tridesilon
  Solution
  Otomycet-HC
  VasotateHC
  Vosol HC

NEOMYCIN,
POLYMIXIN B &
HYDROCORTI-
SONE
  Antibiotic Ear
  Cortarigen Modified
  Ear Drops
  Cort-Biotic
  Cortisporin
  Drotic
  Ear-Eze
  LazerSporin
  Masporin Otic
  Octigen
  Ortega Otic-M
  Oticair
  Otimar
  Otobione
  Otocidin
  Otocort
  Pediotic

BASIC INFORMATION

Habit forming? No
Prescription needed? Yes
Available as generic? Yes
Drug class: Antibacterial (otic)

 USES

Ear infections in external ear canal (not middle ear) caused by susceptible germs (bacteria, virus, fungus).

 OVERDOSE

SYMPTOMS:
None expected.
WHAT TO DO:
Not intended for internal use. If child accidentally swallows, call poison control center.

 DOSAGE & USAGE INFORMATION

How to use:
Ear drops
- Warm ear drops under running water around the unopened bottle.
- Lie down with affected ear up.
- Adults—Pull ear lobe back and up.
- Children—Pull ear lobe down and back.
- Drop medicine into ear canal until canal is full.
- Stay lying down for 2 minutes.
- Gently insert cotton plug into ear to prevent leaking.

Ear ointment
- Apply small amount to skin just inside the ear canal.
- Use finger or piece of sterile gauze.
- Don't use cotton-tipped applicators.

When to use:
As directed on label.

If you forget a dose:
Use as soon as you remember.

What drug does:
Kills germs that infect the skin of the external ear canal.

Time lapse before drug works:
15 minutes.

Don't use with:
Other ear medications unless directed by your doctor.

 POSSIBLE ADVERSE REACTIONS OR SIDE EFFECTS

SYMPTOMS	WHAT TO DO
Life-threatening: None expected.	
Common: None expected.	
Infrequent:	
• Itching, burning, redness, swelling.	Discontinue. Call doctor right away.
• Burning or stinging of the ear.	Continue. Call doctor when convenient.
Rare (with chloramphenicol): Pale skin, sore throat, fever, unusual bleeding or bruising, unusual tiredness or weakness.	Discontinue. Call doctor right away.

WARNINGS & PRECAUTIONS

Don't use if:
You are allergic to any of the medicines listed.

Before you start, consult your doctor:
If eardrum is punctured.

Over age 60:
No problems expected.

Pregnancy:
Risk factors vary for drugs in this group. See category list on page xxiii and consult doctor.

Breast-feeding:
No problems expected. Consult doctor.

Infants & children:
No problems expected.

Prolonged use:
Not intended for prolonged use. Don't use longer than 7 to 10 days for any one problem.

Skin & sunlight:
No special problems expected.

Driving, piloting or hazardous work:
No problems expected.

Discontinuing:
Possible rare adverse reaction of bone marrow depression that leads to aplastic anemia after discontinuing chloramphenicol.

Others:
Keep cool, but don't freeze.

POSSIBLE INTERACTION WITH OTHER DRUGS

GENERIC NAME OR DRUG CLASS	COMBINED EFFECT
None expected.	

POSSIBLE INTERACTION WITH OTHER SUBSTANCES

INTERACTS WITH	COMBINED EFFECT
Alcohol:	None expected.
Beverages:	None expected.
Cocaine:	None expected.
Foods:	None expected.
Marijuana:	None expected.
Tobacco:	None expected.

ANTIBACTERIALS (Topical)

GENERIC AND BRAND NAMES

CHLORAMPHENICOL
 (topical)
 Chloromycetin
GENTAMICIN
 Garamycin
 Gentamar
 G-Myticin
  Antibiotic
MUPIROCIN
 Bactroban
 Bactroban Nasal
NEOMYCIN &
 POLYMIXIN B
 Neosporin

NEOMYCIN,
 POLYMIXIN B &
 BACITRACIN
 Bactine First Aid
 Foille
 Mycitracin
 Neo-Polycin
 Neosporin
 Maximum
 Strength
 Ointment
 Neosporin
 Ointment
 Topisporin
 Triple Antibiotic

BASIC INFORMATION

Habit forming? No
Prescription needed? Yes
Available as generic? Yes
Drug class: Antibacterial (topical)

USES

Treats skin infections that may accompany burns, superficial boils, insect bites or stings, skin ulcers, minor surgical wounds.

DOSAGE & USAGE INFORMATION

How to use:
- Cream, lotion, ointment—Bathe and dry area before use. Apply small amount and rub gently. May cover with gauze or bandage if desired.
- Nasal ointment—Follow instructions provided with prescription.

When to use:
3 or 4 times daily, or as directed by doctor.

Continued next column

OVERDOSE

SYMPTOMS:
None expected.
WHAT TO DO:
Not for internal use. If child accidentally swallows, call poison control center.
- **Dial 911 (emergency) or 0 (operator) for an ambulance or medical help. Then give first aid immediately.**
- **See emergency information on inside covers.**

If you forget a dose:
Use as soon as you remember.

What drug does:
Kills susceptible bacteria by interfering with bacterial DNA and RNA.

Time lapse before drug works:
Begins first day. May require treatment for a week or longer to cure infection.

Don't use with:
Any other medicine without consulting your doctor or pharmacist.

POSSIBLE ADVERSE REACTIONS OR SIDE EFFECTS

SYMPTOMS	WHAT TO DO
Life-threatening: None expected.	
Common: None expected.	
Infrequent: Itching, swollen or red skin; rash.	Discontinue. Call doctor right away.
Rare: Any sort of hearing loss (with neomycin products); pale skin, sore throat, fever, unusual bleeding or bruising, unusual tiredness or weakness (with chloramphenicol).	Discontinue. Call doctor right away.

WARNINGS & PRECAUTIONS

Don't use if:
You are allergic to chloramphenicol, gentamicin or related antibiotics (name usually ends with "mycin" or "micin"), mupirocin, neomycin, polymyxins.

Before you start, consult your doctor:
If any of the lesions on the skin are open sores.

Over age 60:
No problems expected.

Pregnancy:
Risk factors vary for drugs in this group. See category list on page xxiii and consult doctor.

Breast-feeding:
No problems expected, but check with doctor.

Infants & children:
No problems expected, but check with doctor.

Prolonged use:
No problems expected, but check with doctor.

Skin & sunlight:
No special problems expected.

Driving, piloting or hazardous work:
No problems expected, but check with doctor.

Discontinuing:
No problems expected, but check with doctor.

Others:
* Heat and moisture in bathroom medicine cabinet can cause breakdown of medicine. Store someplace else.
* Keep cool, but don't freeze.

POSSIBLE INTERACTION WITH OTHER DRUGS

GENERIC NAME OR DRUG CLASS	COMBINED EFFECT
Any other topical medication	Hypersensitivity* reactions more likely to occur.

POSSIBLE INTERACTION WITH OTHER SUBSTANCES

INTERACTS WITH	COMBINED EFFECT
Alcohol:	None expected.
Beverages:	None expected.
Cocaine:	None expected.
Foods:	None expected.
Marijuana:	None expected.
Tobacco:	None expected.

*See Glossary

ANTICHOLINERGICS

GENERIC AND BRAND NAMES

See complete list of generic and brand names in the *Generic and Brand Name Directory*, page 866.

BASIC INFORMATION

Habit forming? No
Prescription needed?
  Low strength: No
  High strength: Yes
Available as generic? Yes
Drug class: Antispasmodic, anticholinergic

USES

- Reduces spasms of digestive system, bladder and urethra.
- Treatment of bronchial spasms.
- Used as a component in some cough and cold preparations.
- Treatment of peptic ulcers.

DOSAGE & USAGE INFORMATION

How to take:
- Tablet—Swallow with liquid or food to lessen stomach irritation.
- Aerosol—Dilute in saline and inhale as nebulizer.

When to take:
30 minutes before meals (unless directed otherwise by doctor).

If you forget a dose:
Take as soon as you remember up to 2 hours late. If more than 2 hours, wait for next scheduled dose (don't double this dose).

What drug does:
Blocks nerve impulses at parasympathetic nerve endings, preventing muscle contractions and gland secretions of organs involved.

Continued next column

OVERDOSE

SYMPTOMS:
Dilated pupils, rapid pulse and breathing, dizziness, fever, hallucinations, confusion, slurred speech, agitation, flushed face, convulsions, coma.
WHAT TO DO:
- **Dial 911 (emergency) or 0 (operator) for an ambulance or medical help. Then give first aid immediately.**
- **See emergency information on inside covers.**

Time lapse before drug works:
15 to 30 minutes.

Don't take with:
- Antacids* or antidiarrheals*.
- Any other medicine without consulting your doctor or pharmacist.

POSSIBLE ADVERSE REACTIONS OR SIDE EFFECTS

SYMPTOMS	WHAT TO DO
Life-threatening:	
In case of overdose, see previous column.	
Common:	
• Confusion, delirium, rapid heartbeat.	Discontinue. Call doctor right away.
• Nausea, vomiting, decreased sweating.	Continue. Call doctor when convenient.
• Constipation.	Continue. Tell doctor at next visit.
• Dryness in ears, nose, throat, mouth.	No action necessary.
Infrequent:	
• Headache, difficult or painful urination, nasal congestion, altered taste, increased sensitivity to light.	Continue. Call doctor when convenient.
• Lightheadedness.	Discontinue. Call doctor right away.
Rare:	
Rash or hives, eye pain, blurred vision, fever.	Discontinue. Call doctor right away.

WARNINGS & PRECAUTIONS

Don't take if:
- You are allergic to any anticholinergic.
- You have trouble with stomach bloating.
- You have difficulty emptying your bladder completely.
- You have narrow-angle glaucoma.
- You have severe ulcerative colitis.

Before you start, consult your doctor:
- If you have open-angle glaucoma.
- If you have angina or any heart disease or heart rhythm problem.
- If you have chronic bronchitis or asthma.
- If you have liver, kidney or thyroid disease.
- If you have hiatal hernia or esophagitis.
- If you have enlarged prostate or urinary retention.
- If you have myasthenia gravis.
- If you have peptic ulcer.
- If you will have surgery within 2 months, including dental surgery, requiring general or spinal anesthesia.

Over age 60:
Adverse reactions and side effects may be more frequent and severe than in younger persons.

Pregnancy:
Risk factors vary for drugs in this group. See category list on page xxiii and consult doctor.

Breast-feeding:
Drug may pass into milk and could affect milk flow. Avoid drug or discontinue nursing until you finish medicine. Consult doctor for advice on maintaining milk supply.

Infants & children:
Use only under medical supervision.

Prolonged use:
Chronic constipation, possible fecal impaction. Consult doctor immediately.

Skin & sunlight:
No special problems expected.

Driving, piloting or hazardous work:
Use disqualifies you for piloting aircraft. Otherwise, no problems expected.

Discontinuing:
May be unnecessary to finish medicine. Follow doctor's instructions.

Others:
Advise any doctor or dentist whom you consult that you take this medicine.

POSSIBLE INTERACTION WITH OTHER DRUGS

GENERIC NAME OR DRUG CLASS	COMBINED EFFECT
Adrenocorticoids, systemic	Possible glaucoma.
Amantadine	Increased anti-cholinergic effect.
Antacids*	Space doses of the drugs 2 to 3 hours apart.
Anticholinergics, other*	Increased anti-cholinergic effect.
Antidepressants, tricyclic*	Increased anti-cholinergic effect. Increased sedation.
Antihistamines*	Increased anti-cholinergic effect.
Attapulgite	Decreased anti-cholinergic effect.
Haloperidol	Increased internal eye pressure.
Ketoconazole	Decreased ketoconazole effect.
Methylphenidate	Increased anti-cholinergic effect.
Molindone	Increased anti-cholinergic effect.
Monoamine oxidase (MAO) inhibitors*	Increased anti-cholinergic effect.
Narcotics*	Increased risk of severe constipation.
Orphenadrine	Increased anti-cholinergic effect.
Phenothiazines*	Increased anti-cholinergic effect.
Potassium supplements*	Possible intestinal ulcers with oral potassium tablets.
Quinidine	Increased anti-cholinergic effect.

POSSIBLE INTERACTION WITH OTHER SUBSTANCES

INTERACTS WITH	COMBINED EFFECT
Alcohol:	None expected.
Beverages:	None expected.
Cocaine:	Excessively rapid heartbeat. Avoid.
Foods:	None expected.
Marijuana:	Drowsiness and dry mouth.
Tobacco:	None expected.

ANTICOAGULANTS (Oral)

GENERIC AND BRAND NAMES

ANISINDIONE
  Miradon

WARFARIN SODIUM
  Coumadin
  Panwarfarin
  Sofarin
  Warfilone

BASIC INFORMATION

Habit forming? No
Prescription needed? Yes
Available as generic? Yes
Drug class: Anticoagulant

 ## USES

Reduces blood clots. Used for abnormal clotting inside blood vessels.

 ## DOSAGE & USAGE INFORMATION

How to take:
Tablet—Swallow with liquid. If you can't swallow whole, crumble tablet and take with liquid or food.

When to take:
At the same time each day.

If you forget a dose:
Take as soon as you remember up to 12 hours late. If more than 12 hours, wait for next scheduled dose (don't double this dose). Inform your doctor of any missed doses.

What drug does:
Blocks action of vitamin K necessary for blood clotting.

Time lapse before drug works:
36 to 48 hours.

Don't take with:
Any other medicine without consulting your doctor or pharmacist.

 ## OVERDOSE

SYMPTOMS:
Bloody vomit, coughing blood, bloody or black stools, red urine.
WHAT TO DO:
- **Dial 911 (emergency) or 0 (operator) for an ambulance or medical help. Then give first aid immediately.**
- **See emergency information on inside covers.**

 ## POSSIBLE ADVERSE REACTIONS OR SIDE EFFECTS

SYMPTOMS	WHAT TO DO
Life-threatening:	
In case of overdose, see previous column.	
Common:	
Bloating, gas.	Continue. Tell doctor at next visit.
Infrequent:	
• Black stools or bloody vomit, coughing up blood.	Discontinue. Seek emergency treatment.
• Rash, hives, itch, blurred vision, sore throat, easy bruising, bleeding, cloudy or red urine, back pain, jaundice, fever, chills, fatigue, weakness, painful urination, decreased amount of urine, heavy menstruation, bleeding gums.	Discontinue. Call doctor right away.
• Diarrhea, cramps, nausea, vomiting, swollen feet or legs, hair loss.	Continue. Call doctor when convenient.
Rare:	
• Bleeding into and under skin.	Discontinue. Seek emergency treatment.
• Dizziness, headache, mouth sores.	Discontinue. Call doctor right away.

 ## WARNINGS & PRECAUTIONS

Don't take if:
- You have been allergic to any oral anticoagulant.
- You have a bleeding disorder.
- You have an active peptic ulcer.
- You have ulcerative colitis.

Before you start, consult your doctor:
- If you take any other drugs, including nonprescription drugs.
- If you have high blood pressure.
- If you have heavy or prolonged menstrual periods.
- If you have diabetes.
- If you have a bladder catheter.
- If you have serious liver or kidney disease.
- If you will have surgery within 2 months, including dental surgery, requiring general or spinal anesthesia.

Over age 60:
Adverse reactions and side effects may be more frequent and severe than in younger persons.

Pregnancy:
Risk factors vary for drugs in this group. See category list on page xxiii and consult doctor.

Breast-feeding:
Drug filters into milk. May harm child. Avoid.

Infants & children:
Use only under doctor's supervision.

Prolonged use:
Talk to your doctor about the need for follow-up medical examinations or laboratory studies to check prothorombin time, stool and urine for blood.

Skin & sunlight:
No problems expected.

Driving, piloting or hazardous work:
- Avoid hazardous activities that could cause injury.
- Don't drive if you feel dizzy or have blurred vision.

Discontinuing:
Don't discontinue without consulting doctor. Dose may require gradual reduction if you have taken drug for a long time. Doses of other drugs may also require adjustment.

Others:
- Carry identification to state that you take anticoagulants.
- Advise any doctor or dentist whom you consult that you take this medicine.

 ## POSSIBLE INTERACTION WITH OTHER DRUGS

GENERIC NAME OR DRUG CLASS	COMBINED EFFECT
Acetaminophen	Increased effect of anticoagulant.
Adrenocorticoids, systemic	Decreased anticoagulant effect.
Allopurinol	Increased effect of anticoagulant.
Aminoglutethmide	Decreased effect of anticoagulant.
Amiodarone	Increased effect of anticoagulant.
Androgens*	Increased effect of anticoagulant.
Antacids* (large doses)	Decreased effect of anticoagulant.
Antibiotics*	Increased effect of anticoagulant.
Antidiabetic agents*	Increased effect of anticoagulant.

Antihistamines*	Unpredictable increased or decreased effect of anticoagulant.
Anti-inflammatory drugs, nonsteroidal (NSAIDs)*	Increased risk of bleeding.
Anti-inflammatory drugs, nonsteroidal (ophthalmic)*	May increase bleeding tendency.
Aspirin	Possible spontaneous bleeding.
Barbiturates*	Decreased effect of anticoagulant.
Benzodiazepines*	Unpredictable increased or decreased effect of anticoagulant.
Bismuth subsalicylate	Increased risk of bleeding.
Calcium supplements*	Decreased effect of anticoagulant.
Carbamazepine	Decreased effect of anticoagulant.
Cefixime	Increased effect of anticoagulant.
Chloramphenicol	Increased effect of anticoagulant.
Cholestyramine	Decreased effect of anticoagulant.

Continued on page 898

 ## POSSIBLE INTERACTION WITH OTHER SUBSTANCES

INTERACTS WITH	COMBINED EFFECT
Alcohol:	Can increase or decrease effect of anticoagulant. Use with caution.
Beverages:	None expected.
Cocaine:	None expected.
Foods: High in vitamin K such as fish, liver, spinach, cabbage, cauliflower, Brussels sprouts.	May decrease anticoagulant effect.
Marijuana:	None expected.
Tobacco:	Decreased effect of anticoagulant.

ANTICONVULSANTS, HYDANTOIN

GENERIC AND BRAND NAMES

ETHOTOIN
  Peganone
MEPHENYTOIN
  Mesantoin

PHENYTOIN
  Dilantin
  Dilantin 30
  Dilantin 125
  Dilantin Infatabs
  Dilantin Kapseals
  Diphenylan

BASIC INFORMATION

Habit forming? No
Prescription needed? Yes
Available as generic? Yes
Drug class: Anticonvulsant (hydantoin)

 USES

- Prevents some forms of epileptic seizures.
- Stabilizes irregular heartbeat.

 DOSAGE & USAGE INFORMATION

How to take:
- Tablet—Swallow with liquid.
- Chewable tablets—Chew well before swallowing.
- Suspension—Shake well before taking with liquid.

When to take:
At the same time each day.

If you forget a dose:
- If drug taken 1 time per day—Take as soon as you remember up to 12 hours late. If more than 12 hours, wait for next scheduled dose (don't double this dose).
- If taken several times per day—Take as soon as possible, then return to regular schedule.

Continued next column

 OVERDOSE

SYMPTOMS:
Jerky eye movements; stagger; slurred speech; imbalance; drowsiness; blood pressure drop; slow, shallow breathing; coma.
WHAT TO DO:
- Dial 911 (emergency) or 0 (operator) for an ambulance or medical help. Then give first aid immediately.
- See emergency information on inside covers.

What drug does:
Promotes sodium loss from nerve fibers. This lessens excitability and inhibits spread of nerve impulses.

Time lapse before drug works:
7 to 10 days continual use.

Don't take with:
Any other medicine without consulting your doctor or pharmacist.

 POSSIBLE ADVERSE REACTIONS OR SIDE EFFECTS

SYMPTOMS	WHAT TO DO
Life-threatening:	
Severe allergic reaction (rash, fever, swollen glands, kidney failure).	Seek emergency help.
Common:	
• Bleeding, swollen or tender gums.	Continue, but call doctor right away.
• Mild dizziness or drowsiness, constipation.	Continue. Call doctor when convenient.
Infrequent:	
• Hallucinations, confusion, stagger, fever, uncontrolled eye movements, increase in seizures, rash, change in vision, agitation, sore throat, diarrhea, slurred speech, muscle twitching.	Continue, but call doctor right away.
• Increased body and facial hair, breast swelling, insomnia, enlargement of facial features.	Continue. Call doctor when convenient.
Rare:	
Nausea; vomiting; unusual bleeding or bruising; swollen lymph nodes; stomach pain; yellow skin or eyes; joint pain; light gray stools; loss of appetite; weight loss; trouble breathing; uncontrolled movements of arms, legs, hands, lips, tongue or cheeks; slowed growth; learning problems.	Continue, but call doctor right away.

 WARNINGS & PRECAUTIONS

Don't take if:
You are allergic to any hydantoin anticonvulsant.

Before you start, consult your doctor:
- If you have had impaired liver function or disease.
- If you will have surgery within 2 months, including dental surgery, requiring general or spinal anesthesia.
- If you have diabetes.
- If you have a blood disorder.

Over age 60:
Adverse reactions and side effects may be more frequent and severe than in younger persons.

Pregnancy:
Decide with your doctor if drug benefits justify risk to unborn child. Risk category C (see page xxiii).

Breast-feeding:
Drug passes into milk. Avoid drug or discontinue nursing until you finish medicine. Consult doctor for advice on maintaining milk supply.

Infants & children:
Use only under medical supervision.

Prolonged use:
- Weakened bones.
- Lymph gland enlargement.
- Possible liver damage.
- Numbness and tingling of hands and feet.
- Continual back-and-forth eye movements.
- Talk to your doctor about the need for follow-up medical examinations or laboratory studies to check complete blood counts (white blood cell count, platelet count, red blood cell count, hemoglobin, hematocrit), liver function, EEG*.

Skin & sunlight:
One or more drugs in this group may cause rash or intensify sunburn in areas exposed to sun or ultraviolet light (photosensitivity reaction). Avoid overexposure. Notify doctor if reaction occurs.

Driving, piloting or hazardous work:
Don't drive or pilot aircraft until you learn how medicine affects you. Don't work around dangerous machinery. Don't climb ladders or work in high places. Danger increases if you drink alcohol or take medicine affecting alertness and reflexes.

Discontinuing:
Don't discontinue without consulting doctor. Dose may require gradual reduction if you have taken drug for a long time. Doses of other drugs may also require adjustment.

Others:
- May cause learning disability.
- Good dental care is important while using this medicine.
- Advise any doctor or dentist whom you consult about the use of this drug.

POSSIBLE INTERACTION WITH OTHER DRUGS

GENERIC NAME OR DRUG CLASS	COMBINED EFFECT
Adrenocorticoids, systemic	Decreased adrenocorticoid effect.
Amiodarone	Increased anticonvulsant effect.
Antacids*	Decreased anticonvulsant effect.
Anticoagulants*	Increased effect of both drugs.
Antidepressants, tricyclic*	May need to adjust anticonvulsant dose.
Antivirals, HIV/AIDS*	Increased risk of peripheral neuropathy with phenytoin.
Barbiturates*	Changed seizure pattern.
Calcium	Decreased effects of both drugs.
Carbamazepine	Possible increased anticonvulsant metabolism.
Carbonic anhydrase inhibitors*	Increased chance of bone disease.
Central nervous system (CNS) depressants*	Oversedation.
Chloramphenicol	Increased anticonvulsant effect.

Continued on page 899

POSSIBLE INTERACTION WITH OTHER SUBSTANCES

INTERACTS WITH	COMBINED EFFECT
Alcohol:	Possible decreased anticonvulsant effect. Use with caution.
Beverages:	None expected.
Cocaine:	Possible seizures.
Foods:	None expected.
Marijuana:	Drowsiness, unsteadiness, decreased anticonvulsant effect.
Tobacco:	None expected.

*See Glossary

ANTICONVULSANTS, SUCCINIMIDE

GENERIC AND BRAND NAMES

ETHOSUXIMIDE
Zarontin

METHOSUXIMIDE
Celontin

BASIC INFORMATION

Habit forming? No
Prescription needed? Yes
Available as generic? Yes, for some
Drug class: Anticonvulsant (succinimide)

USES

Controls seizures in treatment of some forms of epilepsy.

DOSAGE & USAGE INFORMATION

How to take:
Capsule or syrup—Swallow with liquid or food to lessen stomach irritation.

When to take:
Every day in regularly spaced doses, according to prescription.

If you forget a dose:
Take as soon as you remember up to 2 hours late. If more than 2 hours, wait for next scheduled dose (don't double this dose).

What drug does:
Depresses nerve transmissions in part of brain that controls muscles.

Time lapse before drug works:
3 hours.

Continued next column

OVERDOSE

SYMPTOMS:
Severe drowsiness, slow or irregular breathing, coma.
WHAT TO DO:
- **Dial 911 (emergency) or 0 (operator) for an ambulance or medical help. Then give first aid immediately.**
- **If patient is unconscious and not breathing, give mouth-to-mouth breathing. If there is no heartbeat, use cardiac massage and mouth-to-mouth breathing (CPR). Don't try to make patient vomit. If you can't get help quickly, take patient to nearest emergency facility.**
- **See emergency information on inside covers.**

Don't take with:
Any other medicine without consulting your doctor or pharmacist.

POSSIBLE ADVERSE REACTIONS OR SIDE EFFECTS

SYMPTOMS	WHAT TO DO
Life-threatening:	
In case of overdose, see previous column.	
Common:	
• Nausea, vomiting, appetite loss, dizziness, drowsiness, hiccups, stomach pain, headache, loss of appetite.	Continue. Call doctor when convenient.
• Muscle pain, skin rash or itching, swollen glands, sore throat, fever.	Continue, but call doctor right away.
• Change in urine color (pink, red, red-brown).	No action necessary.
Infrequent:	
Nightmares, irritability, mood changes, tiredness, difficulty concentrating.	Continue, but call doctor right away.
Rare:	
Unusual bleeding or bruising, depression, swollen glands, chills, increased seizures, shortness of breath, wheezing, chest pain, sores in mouth or on lips.	Continue, but call doctor right away.

WARNINGS & PRECAUTIONS

Don't take if:
You are allergic to any succinimide anticonvulsant.

Before you start, consult your doctor:
- If you plan to become pregnant within medication period.
- If you take other anticonvulsants.
- If you have blood disease.
- If you have kidney or liver disease.

Over age 60:
Adverse reactions and side effects may be more frequent and severe than in younger persons.

Pregnancy:
Risk factors vary for drugs in this group. See category list on page xxiii and consult doctor.

Breast-feeding:
Drug passes into milk. Avoid drug or discontinue nursing. Consult your doctor about maintaining milk supply.

Infants & children:
Use only under medical supervision.

Prolonged use:
Talk to your doctor about the need for follow-up medical examinations or laboratory studies to check complete blood counts (white blood cell count, platelet count, red blood cell count, hemoglobin, hematocrit), liver function, kidney function, urine.

Skin & sunlight:
No problems expected.

Driving, piloting or hazardous work:
Don't drive or pilot aircraft until you learn how medicine affects you. Don't work around dangerous machinery. Don't climb ladders or work in high places. Danger increases if you drink alcohol or take medicine affecting alertness and reflexes, such as antihistamines, tranquilizers, sedatives, pain medicine, narcotics and mind-altering drugs.

Discontinuing:
Don't discontinue without doctor's advice until you complete prescribed dose, even though symptoms diminish or disappear.

Others:
- Your response to medicine should be checked regularly by your doctor. Dose and schedule may have to be altered frequently to fit individual needs.
- Periodic blood cell counts, kidney and liver function studies recommended.
- May discolor urine pink to red-brown. No action necessary.
- Advise any doctor or dentist whom you consult about the use of this medicine.

POSSIBLE INTERACTION WITH OTHER DRUGS

GENERIC NAME OR DRUG CLASS	COMBINED EFFECT
Anticonvulsants, other*	Increased effect of both drugs.
Antidepressants, tricyclic*	May provoke seizures.
Antipsychotics*	May provoke seizures.
Central nervous system (CNS) depressants*	Decreased anticonvulsant effect.
Haloperidol	Decreased haloperidol effect; changed seizure pattern.
Phenytoin	Increased phenytoin effect.

POSSIBLE INTERACTION WITH OTHER SUBSTANCES

INTERACTS WITH	COMBINED EFFECT
Alcohol:	May provoke seizures.
Beverages:	None expected.
Cocaine:	May provoke seizures.
Foods:	None expected.
Marijuana:	May provoke seizures.
Tobacco:	None expected.

GENERIC AND BRAND NAMES

See complete list of generic and brand names in the *Generic and Brand Name Directory*, page 866.

BASIC INFORMATION

Habit forming? No
Prescription needed? Yes
Available as generic? Yes
Drug class: Antidepressant (tricyclic)

 ## USES

- Gradually relieves symptoms of depression.
- Used to decrease bedwetting in children.
- Pain relief (sometimes).
- Clomipramine is used to treat obsessive-compulsive disorder.
- Protriptyline may be used to treat attention-deficit disorder.
- Treatment for narcolepsy, bulimia, panic attacks, cocaine withdrawal, attention-deficit disorder.
- May be useful for restless leg syndrome.

 ## DOSAGE & USAGE INFORMATION

How to take:
Tablet, capsule or syrup—Swallow with liquid.

When to take:
At the same time each day, usually at bedtime.

Continued next column

 ## OVERDOSE

SYMPTOMS:
Hallucinations, drowsiness, enlarged pupils, respiratory failure, fever, cardiac arrhythmias, convulsions, coma.
WHAT TO DO:
- **Dial 911 (emergency) or 0 (operator) for an ambulance or medical help. Then give first aid immediately.**
- **If patient is unconscious and not breathing, give mouth-to-mouth breathing. If there is no heartbeat, use cardiac massage and mouth-to-mouth breathing (CPR). Don't try to make patient vomit. If you can't get help quickly, take patient to nearest emergency facility.**
- **See emergency information at end of book.**

If you forget a dose:
Bedtime dose—If you forget your once-a-day bedtime dose, don't take it more than 3 hours late. If more than 3 hours, wait for next scheduled dose. Don't double this dose.

What drug does:
Probably affects part of brain that controls messages between nerve cells.

Time lapse before drug works:
2 to 4 weeks. May require 4 to 6 weeks for maximum benefit.

Don't take with:
Any prescription or nonprescription drugs without consulting your doctor or pharmacist.

 ## POSSIBLE ADVERSE REACTIONS OR SIDE EFFECTS

SYMPTOMS	WHAT TO DO
Life-threatening:	
In case of overdose, see previous column.	
Common:	
• Tremor.	Discontinue. Call doctor right away.
• Headache, dry mouth or unpleasant taste, constipation or diarrhea, nausea, indigestion, fatigue, weakness, drowsiness, nervousness, anxiety, excessive sweating.	Continue. Call doctor when convenient.
• Insomnia, "sweet tooth."	Continue. Tell doctor at next visit.
Infrequent:	
• Convulsions.	Discontinue. Seek emergency treatment.
• Hallucinations, shakiness, dizziness, fainting, blurred vision, eye pain, vomiting, irregular heartbeat or slow pulse, inflamed tongue, abdominal pain, jaundice, hair loss, rash, fever, chills, joint pain, palpitations, hiccups, visual changes.	Discontinue. Call doctor right away.
• Difficult or frequent urination; decreased sex drive; muscle aches; abnormal dreams; nasal congestion; weakness and faintness when arising from bed or chair; back pain.	Continue. Call doctor when convenient.

Rare:

Itchy skin; sore throat; involuntary movements of jaw, lips and tongue; nightmares; confusion; swollen breasts; swollen testicles.	Discontinue. Call doctor right away.

WARNINGS & PRECAUTIONS

Don't take if:
- You are allergic to any tricyclic antidepressant.
- You drink alcohol in excess.
- You have had a heart attack within 6 weeks.
- You have glaucoma.
- You have taken MAO inhibitors* within 2 weeks.
- Patient is younger than 12.

Before you start, consult your doctor:
- If you will have surgery within 2 months, including dental surgery, requiring general or spinal anesthesia.
- If you have an enlarged prostate or glaucoma.
- If you have heart disease or high blood pressure.
- If you have stomach or intestinal problems.
- If you have an overactive thyroid.
- If you have asthma.
- If you have liver disease.

Over age 60:
More likely to develop urination difficulty and serious side effects such as seizures, hallucinations, shaking, dizziness, fainting, headache, insomnia.

Pregnancy:
Risk factors vary for drugs in this group. See category list on page xxiii and consult doctor.

Breast-feeding:
Drug may pass into milk. Avoid drug or discontinue nursing until you finish medicine. Consult doctor about maintaining milk supply.

Infants & children:
Don't give to children younger than 12 except under medical supervision.

Prolonged use:
Talk to your doctor about the need for follow-up medical examinations or laboratory studies to check complete blood counts (white blood cell count, platelet count, red blood cell count, hemoglobin, hematocrit), blood pressure, eyes, teeth.

Skin & sunlight:
One or more drugs in this group may cause rash or intensify sunburn in areas exposed to sun or ultraviolet light (photosensitivity reaction). Avoid overexposure and use sunscreen. Notify doctor if reaction occurs.

Driving, piloting or hazardous work:
Don't drive or pilot aircraft until you learn how medicine affects you. Don't work around dangerous machinery. Don't climb ladders or work in high places. Danger increases if you drink alcohol or take medicine affecting alertness and reflexes.

Discontinuing:
- Don't discontinue without consulting doctor. Dose may require gradual reduction if you have taken drug for a long time. Doses of other drugs may also require adjustment.
- Withdrawal symptoms such as convulsions, muscle cramps, nightmares, insomnia, abdominal pain. Call your physician right away if any of these occur.

Others:
- May affect results in some medical tests.
- Advise any doctor or dentist whom you consult that you take this medicine.

POSSIBLE INTERACTION WITH OTHER DRUGS

GENERIC NAME OR DRUG CLASS	COMBINED EFFECT
Adrenocorticoids, systemic	Increased risk of mental side effects.
Anticoagulants*, oral	Possible increased anticoagulant effect.
Anticholinerglcs*	Increased anticholinergic effect.
Antihistamines*	Increased antihistamine effect.
Barbiturates*	Decreased antidepressant effect. Increased sedation.

Continued on page 901

POSSIBLE INTERACTION WITH OTHER SUBSTANCES

Alcohol: Beverages or medicines with alcohol.	Excessive intoxication. Avoid.
Beverages:	None expected.
Cocaine:	Increased risk of heartbeat irregularity.
Foods:	None expected.
Marijuana:	Excessive drowsiness. Increased risk of side effects. Avoid.
Tobacco:	Possible decreased tricyclic antidepressant effect.

ANTIDIABETIC AGENTS, SULFONYLUREA

GENERIC AND BRAND NAMES

See complete list of generic and brand names in the *Generic and Brand Name Directory*, page 866.

BASIC INFORMATION

Habit forming? No
Prescription needed? Yes
Available as generic? Yes, for some.
Drug class: Antidiabetic (oral), sulfonylurea

 USES

- Treatment for diabetes in adults who can't control blood sugar by diet, weight loss and exercise.
- Treatment for diabetes insipidus (chlorpropamide).

 DOSAGE & USAGE INFORMATION

How to take:
- Tablet—Swallow with liquid or food to lessen stomach irritation. If you can't swallow whole, crumble tablet and take with liquid or food.
- Extended-release tablet—Swallow whole with liquid. Do not crush or chew tablet.

When to take:
At the same times each day.

If you forget a dose:
Take as soon as you remember up to 2 hours late. If more than 2 hours, wait for next scheduled dose (don't double this dose).

What drug does:
Stimulates pancreas to produce more insulin. Insulin in blood forces cells to use sugar in blood.

Time lapse before drug works:
3 to 4 hours. May require 2 weeks for maximum benefit.

Don't take with:
Any other medicine without consulting your doctor or pharmacist.

 OVERDOSE

SYMPTOMS:
Excessive hunger, nausea, anxiety, cool skin, cold sweats, drowsiness, rapid heartbeat, weakness, unconsciousness, coma.
WHAT TO DO:
- **Dial 911 (emergency) or 0 (operator) for an ambulance or medical help. Then give first aid immediately.**
- **See emergency information on inside covers.**

 POSSIBLE ADVERSE REACTIONS OR SIDE EFFECTS

SYMPTOMS	WHAT TO DO
Life-threatening: In case of overdose, see previous column.	
Common:	
• Dizziness.	Discontinue. Call doctor right away.
• Diarrhea, appetite loss, nausea, stomach pain, heartburn, constipation.	Continue. Call doctor when convenient.
Infrequent:	
• Low blood sugar (hunger, anxiety, cold sweats, rapid pulse), shortness of breath.	Discontinue. Seek emergency treatment.
• Headache.	Discontinue. Call doctor right away.
Rare: Fatigue, itchy skin or rash, sore throat, fever, ringing in ears, unusual bleeding or bruising, jaundice, edema, weakness, confusion.	Discontinue. Call doctor right away.

 WARNINGS & PRECAUTIONS

Don't take if:
- You are allergic to any sulfonurea.
- You have impaired kidney or liver function.

Before you start, consult your doctor:
- If you have a severe infection.
- If you have thyroid disease.
- If you take insulin.
- If you have heart disease.

Over age 60:
Dose usually smaller than for younger adults. Avoid episodes of low blood sugar because repeated ones can damage brain permanently.

Pregnancy:
Discuss any use of these drugs with your doctor. Risk factors vary for drugs in this group. See category list on page xxiii and consult doctor.

Breast-feeding:
Drug filters into milk. May lower baby's blood sugar. Avoid.

Infants & children:
Don't give to infants or children.

Prolonged use:
- Adverse effects more likely.

- Talk to your doctor about the need for follow-up medical examinations or laboratory studies to check blood sugar, complete blood counts (white blood cell count, platelet count, redblood cell count, hemoglobin, hematocrit), eyes.

Skin and sunlight:
One or more drugs in this group may cause rash or intensify sunburn in areas exposed to sun or ultraviolet light (photosensitivity reaction). Avoid overexposure. Notify doctor if reaction occurs.

Driving, piloting or hazardous work:
No problems expected unless you develop hypoglycemia (low blood sugar). If so, avoid driving or hazardous activity.

Discontinuing:
Don't discontinue without consulting doctor. Dose may require gradual reduction if you have taken drug for a long time. Doses of other drugs may also require adjustment.

Others:
- Don't exceed recommended dose. Hypoglycemia (low blood sugar) may occur, even with proper dose schedule. You must balance medicine, diet and exercise.
- May affect results in some medical tests.
- Advise any doctor or dentist whom you consult that you take this medicine.

POSSIBLE INTERACTION WITH OTHER DRUGS

GENERIC NAME OR DRUG CLASS	COMBINED EFFECT
Adrenocorticoids, systemic	Decreased anti-diabetic effect.
Androgens*	Increased blood sugar lowering.
Anticoagulants*	Unpredictable prothrombin times.
Anticonvulsants, hydantoin*	Decreased blood sugar lowering.
Anti-inflammatory nonsteriodal drugs (NSAIDs)*	Increased blood-sugar lowering.
Aspirin	Increased blood sugar lowering.
Beta-adrenergic blocking agents*	Increased blood sugar lowering. Possible increased difficulty in regulating blood sugar levels.
Bismuth subsalicylate	Increased insulin effect. May require dosage adjustment.

Chloramphenicol	Increased blood sugar lowering.
Cimetidine	Increased blood sugar lowering.
Clofibrate	Increased blood sugar lowering.
Contraceptives, oral*	Decreased blood sugar lowering.
Dapsone	Increased risk of adverse effect on blood cells.
Desmopressin	May increase desmopressin effect.
Dexfenfluramine	May require dosage change as weight loss occurs.
Dextrothyroxine	Antidiabetic may require adjustment.
Digoxin	Possible decreased digoxin effect.
Diuretics* (loop, thiazide)	Decreased blood sugar lowering.
Epinephrine	Increased blood sugar lowering.
Estrogens*	Increased blood sugar lowering.
Fluconazole	Greater than expected drop in blood sugar. If any oral antidiabetic drug is taken with fluconazole, blood sugars must be monitored carefully.
Guanethidine	Unpredictable blood sugar lowering effect.

Continued on page 902

POSSIBLE INTERACTION WITH OTHER SUBSTANCES

INTERACTS WITH	COMBINED EFFECT
Alcohol:	Disulfiram reaction.* Avoid.
Beverages:	None expected.
Cocaine:	No proven problems.
Foods:	None expected.
Marijuana:	Decreased blood sugar lowering. Avoid.
Tobacco:	None expected.

*See Glossary

GENERIC AND BRAND NAMES

See complete list of generic and brand names in the *Generic and Brand Name Directory*, page 866.

BASIC INFORMATION

Habit forming? No
Prescription needed? Yes
Available as generic? Yes
Drug class: Antidyskinetic, antiparkinson, dopamine agonists

USES

- Treatment of Parkinson's disease.
- Treatment of adverse effects of certain central nervous system drugs.
- Treatment for Tourette's syndrome.

DOSAGE & USAGE INFORMATION

How to take:
- Tablets—Swallow with liquid. If you can't swallow whole, crumble tablet and take with liquid or food to lessen stomach irritation.
- Extended-release capsule or elixir—Take with food to lessen stomach irritation.

When to take:
At the same times each day.

If you forget a dose:
Take as soon as you remember up to 2 hours late. If more than 2 hours, wait for next scheduled dose (don't double this dose).

Continued next column

OVERDOSE

SYMPTOMS:
Agitation, dilated pupils, hallucinations, dry mouth, rapid heartbeat, sleepiness.
WHAT TO DO:
- **Dial 911 (emergency) or 0 (operator) for an ambulance or medical help. Then give first aid immediately.**
- **If patient is unconscious and not breathing, give mouth-to-mouth breathing. If there is no heartbeat, use cardiac massage and mouth-to-mouth breathing (CPR). Don't try to make patient vomit. If you can't get help quickly, take patient to nearest emergency facility.**
- **See emergency information on inside covers.**

What drug does:
- Balances chemical reactions necessary to send nerve impulses within base of brain.
- Improves muscle control and reduces stiffness.

Time lapse before drug works:
1 to 2 hours. Full effect may take 2 to 3 days.

Don't take with:
Any other medication without consulting your doctor or pharmacist.

POSSIBLE ADVERSE REACTIONS OR SIDE EFFECTS

SYMPTOMS	WHAT TO DO
Life-threatening: In case of overdose, see previous column.	
Common: • Blurred vision, light sensitivity, unusual body movements, painful or difficult or frequent urination, vomiting, hallucinations.	Continue, but call doctor right away.
• Dry mouth, tiredness, weakness feeling, drowsiness or insomnia, constipation, nausea, lightheadedness.	Continue. Call doctor when convenient.
Infrequent: Headache, memory loss, abdominal pain, weakness and faintness when arising from bed or chair, nervousness, impotence, sore throat, cough or wheezing, viral infection, appetite loss, restlessness.	Continue. Call doctor when convenient.
Rare: • Rash, hives, eye pain, delusions, amnesia, paranoia, fever, swollen neck glands, vision changes, chest pain, swallowing or breathing difficulty, numbness or tingling or swelling in hands or feet, urine bloody or cloudy, ear buzzing, irregular heartbeat.	Continue. Call doctor right away.
• Confusion, dizziness, sore mouth or tongue, muscle cramps or weakness, depression.	Continue. Call doctor when convenient.

Note: Most symptoms representing side effects either disappear or decrease when dose is reduced. Consult doctor.

WARNINGS & PRECAUTIONS

Don't take if:
You are allergic to any antidyskinetic.

Before you start, consult your doctor:
- If you have glaucoma or retinal problems.
- If you have had high blood pressure, heart disease, impaired liver function.
- If you have hypotension or orthostatic hypotension*.
- If you have had tardive dyskinesia*.
- If you have had kidney disease, urination difficulty, prostatic hypertrophy or intestinal obstruction.
- If you have had myasthenia gravis.

Over age 60:
More sensitive to drug. Aggravates symptoms of enlarged prostate. Causes impaired thinking, hallucinations, nightmares. Consult doctor about any of these.

Pregnancy:
Decide with your doctor whether drug benefits justify risk to unborn child. Risk category C (see page xxiii).

Breast-feeding:
Effects unknown. May inhibit lactation. Consult doctor.

Infants & children:
Use only under doctor's supervision.

Prolonged use:
- Possible glaucoma.
- Talk to your doctor about the need for follow-up medical examinations to assess drug's effectiveness and examination to check eye pressure.

Skin & sunlight:
No special problems expected.

Driving, piloting or hazardous work:
Don't drive or pilot aircraft until you learn how medicine affects you. Don't work around dangerous machinery. Don't climb ladders or work in high places. Danger increases if you drink alcohol or take medicine affecting alertness and reflexes, such as antihistamines, tranquilizers, sedatives, pain medicine, narcotics and mind-altering drugs.

Discontinuing:
- Don't discontinue without consulting doctor. Dose may require gradual reduction if you have taken drug for a long time. Doses of other drugs may also require adjustment.
- After discontinuing, if you experience extrapyramidal reaction* recurrence or worsening, orthostatic hypotension, fast heartbeat, trouble in sleeping, consult doctor.

Others:
- Internal eye pressure should be measured regularly.
- Avoid becoming overheated.
- Use caution when arising from a sitting or lying position.
- Advise any doctor or dentist whom you consult that you take this medicine.

POSSIBLE INTERACTION WITH OTHER DRUGS

GENERIC NAME OR DRUG CLASS	COMBINED EFFECT
Antacids*	Possible decreased absorption.
Anticholinergics, others*	Increased anticholinergic effect.
Antidepressants, tricyclic*	Increased antidyskinetic effect.
Antihistamines*	Increased antidyskinetic effect.
Carbidopa	Increased effect of carbidopa.
Chlorpromazine	Decreased effect of chlorpromazine.
Ciprofloxacin	Increased effect of ropinirole.
Central nervous system (CNS) depressants*	May add to any sedative effect.
Dopamine antagonists*	Decreased effect of pramipexole and ropinirole.
Estrogens	Increased effect of ropinirole.

Continued on page 902

POSSIBLE INTERACTION WITH OTHER SUBSTANCES

INTERACTS WITH	COMBINED EFFECT
Alcohol:	Oversedation. Avoid.
Beverages:	None expected.
Cocaine:	Decreased antidyskinetic effect. Avoid.
Foods:	None expected.
Marijuana:	None expected.
Tobacco:	Decreased effect of ropinirole.

ANTIFIBRINOLYTIC AGENTS

GENERIC AND BRAND NAMES

AMINOCAPROIC ACID **TRANEXAMIC ACID**
  Amicar   Cyclokapron

BASIC INFORMATION

Habit forming? No
Prescription needed? Yes
Available as generic? Yes
Drug class: Antifibrinolytic, antihemorrhagic

USES

- Treats serious bleeding, especially occurring after surgery, dental or otherwise.
- Sometimes used before surgery in hopes of preventing excessive bleeding in patients with disorders that increase the chance of serious bleeding.

DOSAGE & USAGE INFORMATION

How to take:
- Tablet—Swallow with liquid or food to lessen stomach irritation. If you can't swallow whole, crumble tablet and take with liquid or food.
- Syrup—Take as directed on label.

When to take:
As directed by your doctor.

If you forget a dose:
Take as soon as you remember. Don't double this dose.

What drug does:
Inhibits activation of plasminogen to cause blood clots to disintegrate.

Time lapse before drug works:
Within 2 hours.

Don't take with:
- Thrombolytic chemicals such as streptokinase, urokinase.
- Any other medicine without consulting your doctor or pharmacist.

OVERDOSE

SYMPTOMS:
None expected for oral forms. Injectable forms may cause drop in blood pressure or slow heartbeat.
WHAT TO DO:
Follow doctor's instructions.

POSSIBLE ADVERSE REACTIONS OR SIDE EFFECTS

SYMPTOMS	WHAT TO DO
Life-threatening: Shortness of breath, slurred speech, leg or arm numbness.	Seek emergency treatment.
Common: Diarrhea, nausea, vomiting, severe menstrual cramps.	Continue. Call doctor when convenient.
Infrequent: Dizziness; headache; muscular pain and weakness; red eyes; ringing in ears; skin rash; abdominal pain; stuffy nose; decreased urine; swelling of feet, face, legs; rapid weight gain.	Continue. Call doctor when convenient.
Rare: • Unusual tiredness, blurred vision, clotting of menstrual flow.	Continue. Call doctor when convenient.
• Signs of thrombosis (sudden, severe headache; pains in chest, groin or legs; loss of coordination; shortness of breath; slurred speech; vision changes; weakness or numbness in arms or leg).	Seek emergency treatment.

WARNINGS & PRECAUTIONS

Don't take if:
- You are allergic to aminocaproic acid or tranexamic acid.
- You have a diagnosis of disseminated intravascular coagulation (DIC).

Before you start, consult your doctor:
- If you have heart disease.
- If you have bleeding from the kidney.
- If you have had impaired liver function.
- If you have had kidney disease or urination difficulty.
- If you have blood clots in parts of the body.

Over age 60:
No changes from other age groups expected.

Pregnancy:
Risk factors vary for drugs in this group. See category list on page xxiii and consult doctor.

Breast-feeding:
No problems documented. Consult doctor.

Infants & children:
Use for children only under doctor's supervision.

Prolonged use:
Talk to your doctor about the need for follow-up medical examinations or laboratory studies to check eyes.

Skin & sunlight:
No problems expected.

Driving, piloting or hazardous work:
Don't drive or pilot aircraft until you learn how medicine affects you. Don't work around dangerous machinery. Don't climb ladders or work in high places. Danger increases if you drink alcohol or take medicine affecting alertness and reflexes, such as antihistamines, tranquilizers, sedatives, pain medicine, narcotics and mind-altering drugs.

Discontinuing:
Don't discontinue without consulting doctor. Dose may require gradual reduction if you have taken drug for a long time. Doses of other drugs may also require adjustment.

Others:
- Should not be used in patients with disseminated intravascular coagulation.
- Have eyes checked frequently.

POSSIBLE INTERACTION WITH OTHER DRUGS

GENERIC NAME OR DRUG CLASS	COMBINED EFFECT
Contraceptives, oral*	Increased possibility of blood clotting.
Estrogens*	Increased possibility of blood clotting.
Thrombolytic agents* (alteplase, streptokinase, urokinase)	Decreased effects of both drugs.

POSSIBLE INTERACTION WITH OTHER SUBSTANCES

INTERACTS WITH	COMBINED EFFECT
Alcohol:	Decreases effectiveness. Avoid.
Beverages:	No problems expected.
Cocaine:	Combined effect unknown. Avoid.
Foods:	No problems expected.
Marijuana:	Combined effect unknown. Avoid.
Tobacco:	Combined effect unknown. Avoid.

ANTIFUNGALS (Topical)

GENERIC AND BRAND NAMES

See complete list of generic and brand names in the *Generic and Brand Name Directory*, page 866.

BASIC INFORMATION

Habit forming? No
Prescription needed? Yes, for some
Available as generic? Yes, for some
Drug class: Antifungal (topical)

USES

Fights fungus infections such as ringworm of the scalp, athlete's foot, jockey itch, "sun fungus," nail fungus and others.

DOSAGE & USAGE INFORMATION

How to use:
- Solution—Apply to affected area once daily for one week.
- Cream, lotion, ointment, gel—Bathe and dry area before use. Apply small amount and rub gently.
- Powder—Apply lightly to skin.
- Shampoo—Follow package instructions.
- Don't bandage or cover treated areas with plastic wrap.
- Follow other instructions from manufacturer listed on label.

When to use:
Twice a day, morning and evening, unless otherwise directed by your doctor.

If you forget a dose:
Use as soon as you remember.

What drug does:
Kills fungi by damaging the fungal cell wall.

Continued next column

OVERDOSE

SYMPTOMS:
None expected.
WHAT TO DO:
- Not for internal use. If child accidentally swallows, call poison control center.
- Dial 911 (emergency) or 0 (operator) for an ambulance or medical help. Then give first aid immediately.
- See emergency information on inside covers.

Time lapse before drug works:
May require 6 to 8 weeks for cure.

Don't use with:
Other skin medicines without telling your doctor.

POSSIBLE ADVERSE REACTIONS OR SIDE EFFECTS

SYMPTOMS	WHAT TO DO
Life-threatening: None expected.	
Common: None expected.	
Infrequent: Itching, redness, swelling of treated skin not present before treatment.	Discontinue. Call doctor right away.
Rare: None expected.	

WARNINGS & PRECAUTIONS

Don't use if:
You are allergic to any topical antifungal medicine listed.

Before you start, consult your doctor:
If you are allergic to anything that touches your skin.

Over age 60:
No problems expected.

Pregnancy:
Risk factors vary for drugs in this group. See category list on page xxiii and consult doctor.

Breast-feeding:
No problems expected, but check with doctor.

Infants & children:
No problems expected, but check with doctor. Some drugs in this group have not been studied in children under 12.

Prolonged use:
No problems expected, but check with doctor.

Skin & sunlight:
No special problems expected.

Driving, piloting or hazardous work:
No problems expected, but check with doctor.

Discontinuing:
No problems expected, but check with doctor.

Others:
- Avoid contact with eyes.
- Heat and moisture in bathroom medicine cabinet can cause breakdown of medicine. Store someplace else.
- Keep medicine cool, but don't freeze.
- Store away from heat or sunlight.
- Don't use on other members of the family without consulting your doctor.
- If using for jock itch, avoid wearing tight underwear.
- If using for athlete's foot, dry feet carefully after bathing, wear clean cotton socks with sandals or well-ventilated shoes.

POSSIBLE INTERACTION WITH OTHER DRUGS

GENERIC NAME OR DRUG CLASS	COMBINED EFFECT
None expected.	

POSSIBLE INTERACTION WITH OTHER SUBSTANCES

INTERACTS WITH	COMBINED EFFECT
Alcohol:	None expected.
Beverages:	None expected.
Cocaine:	None expected.
Foods:	None expected.
Marijuana:	None expected.
Tobacco:	None expected.

ANTIFUNGALS (Vaginal)

GENERIC AND BRAND NAMES

See complete list of generic and brand names in the *Generic and Brand Name Directory*, page 867.

BASIC INFORMATION

Habit forming? No
Prescription needed? Yes, for some
Available as generic? Yes, some
Drug class: Antifungal (vaginal)

USES

Treats fungus infections of the vagina.

DOSAGE & USAGE INFORMATION

How to use:
- Vaginal creams—Insert into vagina with applicator as illustrated in patient instructions that comes with prescription.
- Vaginal tablets—Insert with applicator as illustrated in instructions.
- Vaginal suppositories—Insert as illustrated in instructions.

When to use:
According to instructions. Usually once or twice daily.

If you forget a dose:
Use as soon as you remember.

What drug does:
Destroys fungus cells membrane causing loss of essential elements to sustain fungus cell life.

Time lapse before drug works:
Begins immediately. May require 2 weeks of treatment to cure vaginal fungus infections. Recurrence common.

Don't use with:
Other vaginal preparations or douches unless otherwise instructed by your doctor.

OVERDOSE

SYMPTOMS:
None expected.
WHAT TO DO:
Overdose unlikely to threaten life.

POSSIBLE ADVERSE REACTIONS OR SIDE EFFECTS

SYMPTOMS	WHAT TO DO
Life-threatening: None expected.	
Common: None expected.	
Infrequent: Vaginal burning, itching, irriation, swelling of labia, redness, increased discharge (not present before starting medicine).	Discontinue. Call doctor right away.
Rare: Skin rash, hives, irritation of sex partner's penis.	Discontinue. Call doctor right away.

WARNINGS & PRECAUTIONS

Don't use if:
- You are allergic to any of the products listed.
- You have pre-existing liver disease.

Before you start, consult your doctor:
If you are pregnant.

Over age 60:
No problems expected.

Pregnancy:
Risk factors vary for drugs in this group. See category list on page xxiii and consult doctor.

Breast-feeding:
No problems expected. Consult doctor.

Infants & children:
Use only under close medical supervision.

Prolonged use:
No problems expected.

Skin & sunlight:
No problems expected.

Driving, piloting or hazardous work:
No problems expected.

Discontinuing:
Recurrence likely if you stop before time suggested.

Others:
- Gentian Violet and some of the other products can stain clothing. Sanitary napkins may protect against staining.
- Keep the genital area clean. Use plain unscented soap.
- Take showers rather than tub baths.
- Wear cotton underpants or pantyhose with a cotton crotch. Avoid underpants made from non-ventilating materials. Wear freshly laundered underpants.
- Don't sit around in wet clothing—especially a wet bathing suit.
- If you will take antibiotics in the future, ask your doctor about eating yogurt, sour cream, buttermilk or taking acidophilus tablets.
- After urination or bowel movements, cleanse by wiping or washing from front to back (vagina to anus).
- Don't douche unless your doctor recommends it.
- If urinating causes burning, urinate through a tubular device, such as a toilet-paper roll or plastic cup with the end cut out.

POSSIBLE INTERACTION WITH OTHER DRUGS

GENERIC NAME OR DRUG CLASS	COMBINED EFFECT
Clinically significant interactions with oral or injected medicines unlikely.	

POSSIBLE INTERACTION WITH OTHER SUBSTANCES

INTERACTS WITH	COMBINED EFFECT
Alcohol:	None expected.
Beverages:	None expected.
Cocaine:	None expected.
Foods:	None expected.
Marijuana:	None expected.
Tobacco:	None expected.

*See Glossary

ANTIGLAUCOMA, LONG-ACTING (Ophthalmic)

GENERIC AND BRAND NAMES

DEMECARIUM
  Humorsol
ECHOTHIOPHATE
  Phospholine Iodide
ISOFLUROPHATE
  Floropryl

BASIC INFORMATION

Habit forming? No
Prescription needed? Yes
Available as generic? No
Drug class: Antiglaucoma (ophthalmic)

 USES

- Treats glaucoma (open-angle type).
- Treats glaucoma after some forms of eye surgery and a few other eye disorders.

 DOSAGE & USAGE INFORMATION

How to use:
Eye drops
- Wash hands.
- Apply pressure to inside corner of eye with middle finger.
- Continue pressure for 1 minute after placing medicine in eye.
- Tilt head backward. Pull lower lid away from eye with index finger of the same hand.
- Drop eye drops into pouch and close eye. Don't blink.
- Keep eyes closed for 1 to 2 minutes.
- Press finger to tear duct in corner of eye for 2 minutes to prevent possible absorption by body.

Eye ointment
- Wash hands.
- Pull lower lid down from eye to form a pouch.
- Squeeze tube to apply thin strip of ointment into pouch.
- Close eye for 1 to 2 minutes.
- Don't touch applicator tip to any surface (including the eye). If you accidentally touch tip, clean with warm soap and water.

Continued next column

 OVERDOSE

SYMPTOMS:
None expected.
WHAT TO DO:
Not intended for internal use. If child accidentally swallows, call poison control center.

- Keep container tightly closed.
- Keep cool, but don't freeze.
- Wash hands immediately after using.
- Press finger to tear duct in corner of eye for 2 minutes to prevent possible absorption by body.

When to use:
As directed on label.

If you forget a dose:
Use as soon as you remember.

What drug does:
Inactivates an enzyme to reduce pressure inside the eye.

Time lapse before drug works:
5 to 60 minutes.

Don't use with:
Any other eye medicine without consulting your doctor.

 POSSIBLE ADVERSE REACTIONS OR SIDE EFFECTS

SYMPTOMS	WHAT TO DO
Life-threatening: None expected.	
Common: Pupils become small.	No action necessary.
Infrequent: Blurred vision, change in vision, eye pain, eyelids twitch, headache, watery eyes.	Discontinue. Call doctor right away.
Rare: Decreased vision with veil or curtain appearing, loss of bladder control, slow heartbeat, increased sweating, weakness, difficult breathing, vomiting, nausea, diarrhea.	Discontinue. Call doctor right away.

ANTIGLAUCOMA, LONG-ACTING (Ophthalmic)

WARNINGS & PRECAUTIONS

Don't use if:
You are allergic to demecarium, echothiophate, isoflurophate

Before you start, consult your doctor:
- If you have a history of retinal detachment.
- If you plan surgery under general or local anesthesia.
- If you have asthma, epilepsy, Down syndrome, eye infection or other eye disease, heart disease, Parkinson's disease, ulcer in stomach or duodenum.

Over age 60:
No problems expected.

Pregnancy:
Risk factors vary for drugs in this group. See category list on page xxiii and consult doctor.

Breast-feeding:
Unknown effect. Consult doctor.

Infants & children:
Use under medical supervision only.

Prolonged use:
No problems expected.

Skin & sunlight:
No problems expected.

Driving, piloting or hazardous work:
Don't drive or pilot aircraft until you learn how medicine affects you. Don't work around dangerous machinery. Don't climb ladders or work in high places. Danger increases if you drink alcohol or take medicine affecting alertness and reflexes, such as antihistamines, tranquilizers, sedatives, pain medicine, narcotics and mind-altering drugs.

Discontinuing:
- Discontinue 2 to 3 weeks prior to eye surgery.
- Otherwise, don't discontinue without consulting your doctor. Dose may require gradual reduction if you have used drug for a long time. Doses of other drugs may also require adjustment.

Others:
- Keep appointments for regular eye examinations to measure pressure in the eye.
- Keep cool, but don't freeze.
- Eyeglass prescription may need changing.

POSSIBLE INTERACTION WITH OTHER DRUGS

GENERIC NAME OR DRUG CLASS	COMBINED EFFECT
Anticholinergics*	Increased risk of toxicity.
Atropine (ophthalmic)	May not be safe. Check with doctor.
Cholinesterase inhibitors*	Increased risk of toxicity.
Cyclopentolate (ophthalmic)	Reduces effect of antiglaucoma eye medicines.
Fibuprofen (ophthalmic)	May decrease antiglaucoma effect.
Insecticides or pesticides with organic phosphates	Increased toxic absorption of pesticides.
Medicines to treat myasthenia gravis	Additive toxicity.
Physostigmine (ophthalmic)	Shortens action of antiglaucoma medicines.
Topical anesthetics	Increased risk of toxic effects of antiglaucoma eye medicines.

POSSIBLE INTERACTION WITH OTHER SUBSTANCES

INTERACTS WITH	COMBINED EFFECT
Alcohol:	None expected.
Beverages:	None expected.
Cocaine:	None expected.
Foods:	None expected.
Marijuana:	None expected.
Tobacco:	None expected.

ANTIGLAUCOMA, SHORT-ACTING (Ophthalmic)

GENERIC AND BRAND NAMES

CARBACHOL
  Carbastat
  Carboptic
  Isopto Carbachol
  Miostat
DIPIVEFRIN
  AKPro
  Ophtho-Dipivefrin
  Propine C Cap

EPINEPHRINE
  Epifrin
  Epinal
  Eppy/N
  Glaucon
PHYSOSTIGMINE
  Eserine
  Isopto Eserine

BASIC INFORMATION

Habit forming? No
Prescription needed? Yes
Available as generic? Yes, some are
Drug class: Antiglaucoma (ophthalmic)

 ## USES

Treats glaucoma (open-angle, secondary, angle-closure during or after eye surgery).

 ## DOSAGE & USAGE INFORMATION

How to use:
Eye drops
- Wash hands.
- Apply pressure to inside corner of eye with middle finger.
- Continue pressure for 1 minute after placing medicine in eye.
- Tilt head backward. Pull lower lid away from eye with index finger of the same hand.
- Drop eye drops into pouch and close eye. Don't blink.
- Keep eyes closed for 1 to 2 minutes.

Eye ointment
- Wash hands.
- Pull lower lid down from eye to form a pouch.
- Squeeze tube to apply thin strip of ointment into pouch.

Continued next column

 ## OVERDOSE

SYMPTOMS:
None expected.
WHAT TO DO:
Not intended for internal use. If child accidentally swallows, call poison control center.

- Close eye for 1 to 2 minutes.
- Don't touch applicator tip to any surface (including the eye). If you accidentally touch tip, clean with warm soap and water.
- Keep container tightly closed.
- Keep cool, but don't freeze.
- Wash hands immediately after using.

When to use:
As directed on label.

If you forget a dose:
Use as soon as you remember.

What drug does:
Inactivates enzyme and facilitates movement of fluid (aquemous humor) into and out of the eye.

Time lapse before drug works:
10-30 minutes.

Don't use with:
Any other medicine without consulting your doctor.

 ## POSSIBLE ADVERSE REACTIONS OR SIDE EFFECTS

SYMPTOMS	WHAT TO DO
Life-threatening: None expected.	
Common: Headache; stinging, burning, watery eyes.	Continue. Call doctor when convenient.
Infrequent: Eye pain, changes in vision, blurred vision.	Discontinue. Call doctor right away.
Rare: Faintness, increased sweating, irregular or fast heartbeat, paleness.	Discontinue. Call doctor right away.

WARNINGS & PRECAUTIONS

Don't use if:
You are allergic to any eye medicine for glaucoma.

Before you start, consult your doctor:
- If you plan to have eye or dental surgery.
- If you have any eye disease.
- If you have heart problems or high blood pressure.
- If you have diabetes.

Over age 60:
Adverse reactions and side effects may be more frequent and severe than in younger persons. Ask doctor about smaller doses.

Pregnancy:
Risk factors vary for drugs in this group. See category list on page xxiii and consult doctor.

Breast-feeding:
Safety unestablished. Avoid if possible. Consult doctor.

Infants & children:
Use only under close medical supervision.

Prolonged use:
May be necessary.

Skin & sunlight:
No problems expected.

Driving, piloting or hazardous work:
Don't drive or pilot aircraft until you learn how medicine affects you. Don't work around dangerous machinery. Don't climb ladders or work in high places. Danger increases if you drink alcohol or take medicine affecting alertness and reflexes, such as antihistamines, tranquilizers, sedatives, pain medicine, narcotics and mind-altering drugs.

Discontinuing:
Don't discontinue without consulting your doctor. Dose may require gradual reduction if you have used drug for a long time. Doses of other drugs may also require adjustment.

Others:
- Most normal physical activities, including swimming or other exercise, are okay while you use this medicine.
- Keep cool, but don't freeze.
- Keep appointments for regular eye examinations to measure pressure in the eye.

POSSIBLE INTERACTION WITH OTHER DRUGS

GENERIC NAME OR DRUG CLASS	COMBINED EFFECT
Other eye drugs	May decrease antiglaucoma effect.

POSSIBLE INTERACTION WITH OTHER SUBSTANCES

INTERACTS WITH	COMBINED EFFECT
Alcohol:	None expected.
Beverages:	None expected.
Cocaine:	None expected.
Foods:	None expected.
Marijuana:	None expected.
Tobacco:	None expected.

ANTIHISTAMINES

GENERIC AND BRAND NAMES

See complete list of generic and brand names in the *Generic and Brand Name Directory*, page 867.

BASIC INFORMATION

Habit forming? No
Prescription needed?
 High strength: Yes
 Low strength: No
Available as generic? Yes
Drug class: Antihistamine

USES

- Reduces allergic symptoms such as hay fever, hives, rash or itching.
- Prevents motion sickness, nausea, vomiting.
- Relieves symptoms associated with the common cold.
- Induces sleep.
- Reduces stiffness and tremors of Parkinson's disease.

DOSAGE & USAGE INFORMATION

How to take:
Follow label directions.

When to take:
Varies with form. Follow label directions.

If you forget a dose:
Take as soon as you remember up to 2 hours late. If more than 2 hours, wait for next scheduled dose (don't double this dose).

What drug does:
- Blocks action of histamine after an allergic response triggers histamine release in sensitive cells. Histamines cause itching, sneezing, runny nose and eyes and other symptoms.
- Appears to work in the vomiting center of the brain to control nausea and vomiting and help prevent motion sickness.

Time lapse before drug works:
15 minutes to 1 hour.

Continued next column

OVERDOSE

SYMPTOMS:
Convulsions, red face, hallucinations, coma.
WHAT TO DO:
- **Dial 911 (emergency) or 0 (operator)for an ambulance or medical help. Then give first aid immediately.**
- **See emergency information on inside covers.**

Don't take with:
Any other medicine without consulting your doctor or pharmacist.

POSSIBLE ADVERSE REACTIONS OR SIDE EFFECTS

SYMPTOMS	WHAT TO DO
Life-threatening: In case of overdose, see previous column.	
Common: Drowsiness (less likely with cetirizine, loratadine or astemizole); dizziness; dryness of mouth, nose or throat.	Continue. Tell doctor at next visit.
Infrequent:	
• Change in vision, clumsiness, rash.	Discontinue. Call doctor right away.
• Less tolerance for contact lenses, painful or difficult urination.	Continue. Call doctor when convenient.
• Appetite loss.	Continue. Tell doctor at next visit.
Rare: Nightmares, agitation, irritability, sore throat, fever, rapid heartbeat, unusual bleeding or bruising, fatigue, weakness, confusion, fainting, seizures.	Discontinue. Call doctor right away.

WARNINGS & PRECAUTIONS

Don't take if:
You are allergic to any antihistamine.

Before you start, consult your doctor:
- If you have glaucoma.
- If you have enlarged prostate.
- If you have asthma.
- If you have kidney disease.
- If you have peptic ulcer.
- If you will have surgery within 2 months, including dental surgery, requiring general or spinal anesthesia.

Over age 60:
Don't exceed recommended dose. Adverse reactions and side effects may be more frequent and severe than in younger persons, especially urination difficulty, diminished alertness and other brain and nervous-system symptoms.

Pregnancy:
Risk factors vary for drugs in this group. See category list on page xxiii and consult doctor.

Breast-feeding:
Drug passes into milk. Avoid drug or discontinue nursing until you finish medicine. Consult doctor for advice on maintaining milk supply.

Infants & children:
Not recommended for premature or newborn infants. Otherwise, no problems expected.

Prolonged use:
Avoid. May damage bone marrow and nerve cells.

Skin & sunlight:
May cause rash or intensify sunburn in areas exposed to sun or sunlamp.

Driving, piloting or hazardous work:
Don't drive or pilot aircraft until you learn how medicine affects you. Don't work around dangerous machinery. Don't climb ladders or work in high places. Danger increases if you drink alcohol or take medicine affecting alertness and reflexes, such as antihistamines, tranquilizers, sedatives, pain medicine, narcotics and mind-altering drugs.

Discontinuing:
No problems expected.

Others:
- May mask symptoms of hearing damage from aspirin, other salicylates, cisplatin, paromomycin, vancomycin or anticonvulsants. Consult doctor if you use these.
- Advise any doctor or dentist whom you consult that you take this medicine.

POSSIBLE INTERACTION WITH OTHER DRUGS

GENERIC NAME OR DRUG CLASS	COMBINED EFFECT
Adrenocorticoids, systemic	Decreased adrenocorticoid effect.
Anticholinergics*	Increased anticholinergic effect.
Anticoagulants, oral*	Decreased antihistamine effect.
Antidepressants*	Excess sedation. Avoid.
Antihistamines, other*	Excess sedation. Avoid.
Carteolol	Decreased antihistamine effect.
Central nervous system (CNS) depressants*	May increase sedation.
Clozapine	Toxic effect on the central nervous system.
Dirithromycin	Serious heart rhythm problems with astemizole. Avoid.
Dronabinol	Increased effects of both drugs. Avoid.
Erythromycins*	Increased risk of cardiac toxicity with astemizole.
Fluvoxamine	Serious heart rhythm problems with astemizole. Avoid.
Hypnotics*	Excess sedation. Avoid.
Itraconazole	Increased risk of cardiac toxicity and death with astemizole.
Ketocanazole	Increased risk of cardiac toxicity and death with astemizole.
Mind-altering drugs*	Excess sedation. Avoid.
Molindone	Increased sedative and antihistamine effect.
Monoamine oxidase (MAO) inhibitors*	Increased antihistamine effect.
Nabilone	Greater depression of central nervous system.
Narcotics*	Excess sedation. Avoid.
Nefazodone	Serious heart rhythm problems with astemizole. Avoid.

Continued on page 902

POSSIBLE INTERACTION WITH OTHER SUBSTANCES

INTERACTS WITH	COMBINED EFFECT
Alcohol:	Excess sedation. Avoid.
Beverages: Caffeine drinks.	Less antihistamine sedation.
Cocaine:	Decreased antihistamine effect. Avoid.
Foods:	None expected.
Marijuana:	Excess sedation. Avoid.
Tobacco:	None expected.

ANTIHISTAMINES, NONSEDATING

GENERIC AND BRAND NAMES

ASTEMIZOLE
  Hismanal
CETIRIZINE
  Reactine
  Zyrtec
FEXOFENADINE
  Allegra
  Allegra-D

LORATADINE
  Claritin
  Claritin Extra
  Claritin RediTabs
  Claritin-D
  Claritin-D 12 Hour
  Claritin-D 24 Hour

BASIC INFORMATION

Habit forming? No
Prescription needed? Yes, for some
Available as generic? Yes, for some
Drug class: Antihistamine

USES

- Reduces allergic symptoms caused by hay fever (seasonal allergic rhinitis), such as sneezing, runny nose, itchy nose or throat, itchy and watery eyes.
- Treatment for chronic idiopathic urticaria (hives).
- Used to help relieve some asthma symptoms.
- Other uses as recommended by your doctor.

DOSAGE & USAGE INFORMATION

How to take:
Capsule, tablet, suspension, syrup—Swallow with liquid. Most may be taken with food or milk to lessen stomach irritation. Astemizole needs to be taken on an empty stomach, 1 hour before or 2 hours after eating.

When to take:
Varies with form. Follow label directions.

If you forget a dose:
Take as soon as you remember up to 2 hours late. If more than 2 hours, wait for next scheduled dose (don't double this dose).

Continued next column

OVERDOSE

SYMPTOMS:
Serious irregular heartbeat, convulsions, severe headache, nausea.
WHAT TO DO:
- Dial 911 (emergency) or 0 (operator) for an ambulance or medical help. Then give first aid immediately.
- See emergency information on inside covers.

What drug does:
Blocks action of histamine after an allergic response triggers histamine release in sensitive cells. Histamines cause itching, sneezing, runny nose and eyes and other symptoms.

Time lapse before drug works:
1 to 2 hours.

Don't take with:
Any other medicine without consulting your doctor or pharmacist.

POSSIBLE ADVERSE REACTIONS OR SIDE EFFECTS

SYMPTOMS	WHAT TO DO
Life-threatening: In case of overdose, see previous column.	
Common: Dryness of mouth, nose or throat.	Continue. Tell doctor at next visit.
Infrequent: Increased appetite, weight gain, mild stomach or intestinal problems, cold or flu-like symptoms.	Continue. Call doctor when convenient.
Rare: • Heart rhythm disturbances, fainting.	Discontinue. Call doctor right away or get emergency care.
• Allergic reaction such as mild skin rash, headache, nausea, dizziness, nervousness, fatigue, muscle aches. Drowsiness may occur even though these drugs are nonsedating.	Discontinue. Call doctor when. convenient.

WARNINGS & PRECAUTIONS

Don't take if:
You are allergic to any antihistamine.

Before you start, consult your doctor:
- If you have any type of heart disorder.
- If you have glaucoma.
- If you have enlarged prostate or urinary retention problems.
- If you have asthma or a respiratory disease.
- If you have liver or kidney disease.
- If you have peptic ulcer.
- If you have electrolyte abnormality, such as low potassium (hypokalemia).

Over age 60:
Adverse reactions and side effects may be more frequent and severe than in younger persons.

Pregnancy:
Risk factors vary for drugs in this group. See category list on page xxiii and consult doctor.

Breast-feeding:
Drug may pass into milk. Avoid drug or discontinue nursing until you finish medicine. Consult doctor for advice on maintaining milk supply.

Infants & children:
- Use cetirizine only under close medical supervision.
- All others are not recommended for children under age 12.

Prolonged use:
Antihistamines are normally taken during the hay fever season. They are not intended for long-term uninterrupted use.

Skin & sunlight:
Rarely, may cause rash or intensify sunburn in areas exposed to sun or ultraviolet light (photosensitivity reaction). Avoid overexposure. Notify doctor if reaction occurs.

Driving, piloting or hazardous work:
No problems expected.

Discontinuing:
No problems expected.

Others:
- Claritin-D 24 Hour Extended Release round-shaped tablets have been replaced by oval-shaped tablets due to reports of throat obstruction. You should replace the old round-shaped tablets with the new oval-shaped tablets and be sure to swallow them with a full glass of water.
- Don't exceed recommended dose. This can increase the risk of adverse reactions.
- Advise any doctor or dentist whom you consult that you take this medicine.

POSSIBLE INTERACTION WITH OTHER DRUGS

GENERIC NAME OR DRUG CLASS	COMBINED EFFECT
Anticholinergics	Increased anti-cholinergic effect.
Central nervous system (CNS) depressants*	May add to any sedative effect.
Erythromycins*	Heart rhythm problems. Avoid.
Fluvoxamine	Increased antihistamine effect.

Itraconazole	Heart rhythm problems with astemizole. Avoid.
Ketocanazole	Heart rhythm problems with astemizole. Avoid.
Leukotriene modifiers	Effects unknown. Consult doctor.
Macrolide antibiotics	Increased risk of adverse reactions.
Metronidazole	Heart rhythm problems with astemizole. Avoid.
Monoamine oxidase (MAO) inhibitors	Increased sedation. Avoid.
Nefazodone	Heart rhythm problems with astemizole. Avoid.
QT interval prolongation-causing drugs*	Heart rhythm problems. Avoid.
Zafirlukast	May increase effect of astemizole.

POSSIBLE INTERACTION WITH OTHER SUBSTANCES

INTERACTS WITH	COMBINED EFFECT
Alcohol:	May cause sedation. Avoid.
Beverages:	None expected.
Cocaine:	Decreased antihista-mine effect. Avoid.
Foods:	None expected.
Marijuana:	May cause sedation. Avoid.
Tobacco:	None expected.

ANTIHISTAMINES, PHENOTHIAZINE-DERIVATIVE

GENERIC AND BRAND NAMES

See complete list of generic and brand names in the *Generic and Brand Name Directory*, page 871.

BASIC INFORMATION

Habit forming? No
Prescription needed? Yes
Available as generic? Yes
Drug class: Tranquilizer (phenothiazine), antihistamine

USES

- Relieves itching of hives, skin allergies, chickenpox.
- Treatment for hay fever, motion sickness, vertigo.
- Treatment for nausea and vomiting.

DOSAGE & USAGE INFORMATION

How to take:
- Tablet or syrup—Swallow with liquid or food to lessen stomach irritation.
- Extended-release capsules—Swallow each dose whole. If you take regular tablets, you may chew or crush them.

When to take:
At the same times each day.

If you forget a dose:
Take as soon as you remember up to 2 hours late. If more than 2 hours, wait for next scheduled dose (don't double this dose).

Continued next column

OVERDOSE

SYMPTOMS:
Fast heartbeat, flushed face, shortness of breath, clumsiness, drowsiness, muscle spasms, jerking movements of head and face.
WHAT TO DO:
- **Dial 911 (emergency) or 0 (operator) for an ambulance or medical help. Then give first aid immediately.**
- **See emergency information on inside covers.**

What drug does:
- Blocks action of histamine after an allergic response triggers histamine release in sensitive cells. Histamines cause itching, sneezing, runny nose and eyes and other symptoms.
- Appears to work in the vomiting center of the brain to control nausea and vomiting and help prevent motion sickness.

Time lapse before drug works:
15 minutes to 1 hour.

Don't take with:
- Antacid or medicine for diarrhea.
- Nonprescription drug for cough, cold or allergy.
- Any other medicine without consulting your doctor or pharmacist.

POSSIBLE ADVERSE REACTIONS OR SIDE EFFECTS

SYMPTOMS	WHAT TO DO
Life-threatening:	
In case of overdose, see previous column.	
Common:	
Drowsiness; dryness of mouth, nose or throat; nasal congestion.	Continue. Call doctor when convenient.
Infrequent:	
• Nightmares, unusual excitement, nervousness, irritability, loss of appetite, sweating.	Continue. Call doctor when convenient.
• Difficult urination; blurred or changed vision; dizziness; ringing in ears; skin rash; uncontrolled, jerky movements (with high doses); slow, snakelike movement of arms; spasm of neck muscles; stiffening of tongue; eyes rolling upward.	Discontinue. Call doctor right away.
Rare:	
Sore throat, fever, confusion, yellow skin or eyes, fast heartbeat, feeling faint, unusual tiredness or weakness, unusual bleeding or bruising.	Discontinue. Call doctor right away.

ANTIHISTAMINES, PHENOTHIAZINE-DERIVATIVE

 WARNINGS & PRECAUTIONS

Don't take if:
- You are allergic to any phenothiazine.
- You have a blood or bone marrow disease.

Before you start, consult your doctor:
- If you will have surgery within 2 months, including dental surgery, requiring general or spinal anesthesia.
- If you have asthma, emphysema or other lung disorder.
- If you take nonprescription ulcer medicine, asthma medicine or amphetamines.

Over age 60:
Adverse reactions and side effects may be more frequent and severe than in younger persons. More likely to develop tardive dyskinesia (involuntary movement of jaws, lips, tongue, chewing). Report this to your doctor immediately. Early treatment can help.

Pregnancy:
Decide with your doctor if drug benefits justify risk to unborn child. Risk category C (see page xxiii).

Breast-feeding:
Drug passes into milk. Avoid drug or discontinue nursing until you finish medicine. Consult doctor for advice on maintaining milk supply.

Infants & children:
Don't give to children younger than 2.

Prolonged use:
- May lead to tardive dyskinesia (involuntary movement of jaws, lips, tongue; chewing).
- Talk to your doctor about the need for follow-up medical examinations or laboratory studies to check complete blood counts (white blood cell count, platelet count, red blood cell count, hemoglobin, hematocrit), liver function, eyes.

Skin & sunlight:
One or more drugs in this group may cause rash or intensify sunburn in areas exposed to sun or ultraviolet light (photosensitivity reaction). Avoid overexposure. Notify doctor if reaction occurs.

Driving, piloting or hazardous work:
Don't drive or pilot aircraft until you learn how medicine affects you. Don't work around dangerous machinery. Don't climb ladders or work in high places. Danger increases if you drink alcohol or take medicine affecting alertness and reflexes.

Discontinuing:
May be unnecessary to finish medicine. Follow doctor's instructions.

Others:
May affect results in some medical tests.

 POSSIBLE INTERACTION WITH OTHER DRUGS

GENERIC NAME OR DRUG CLASS	COMBINED EFFECT
Antacids*	Decreased antihistamine effect.
Anticholinergics*	Increased anticholinergic effect.
Anticonvulsants, hydantoin*	Increased anticonvulsant effect.
Antidepressants, tricyclic*	Increased antihistamine effect.
Antihistamines*, other	Increased antihistamine effect.
Antithyroid drugs*	Increased risk of bone marrow depression.
Appetite suppressants*	Decreased appetite suppressant effect.
Barbiturates*	Oversedation.
Carteolol	Decreased antihistamine effect.
Central nervous system (CNS) depressants*	Dangerous degree of sedation.
Cisapride	Decreased antihistamine effect.
Clozapine	Toxic effect on the central nervous system.

Continued on page 903

POSSIBLE INTERACTION WITH OTHER SUBSTANCES

INTERACTS WITH	COMBINED EFFECT
Alcohol:	Dangerous oversedation.
Beverages:	None expected.
Cocaine:	Decreased trimeprazine effect. Avoid.
Foods:	None expected.
Marijuana:	Drowsiness.
Tobacco:	None expected.

ANTI-INFLAMMATORY DRUGS, NONSTEROIDAL (NSAIDs)

GENERIC AND BRAND NAMES

See complete list of generic and brand names in the *Generic and Brand Name Directory*, page 871.

BASIC INFORMATION

Habit forming? No
Prescription needed? Yes, for some.
Available as generic? Yes, for some.
Drug class: Anti-inflammatory (nonsteroidal), analgesic, antigout agent, fever-reducer

USES

- Treatment for joint pain, stiffness, inflammation and swelling of arthritis and gout.
- Treatment for pain, fever and inflammation.
- Treatment for dysmenorrhea (painful or difficult menstruation).
- Treats juvenile rheumatoid arthritis.

DOSAGE & USAGE INFORMATION

How to take:
- Tablet or capsule—Swallow with liquid or food to lessen stomach irritation. If you can't swallow whole, crumble tablet and take with liquid or food. Don't crumble delayed release tablet.
- Liquid—Take as directed on bottle. Don't freeze.
- Rectal suppositories—Remove wrapper and moisten suppository with water. Gently insert into rectum, large end first. If suppository is too soft, chill in refrigerator or cool water before removing wrapper.

When to take:
At the same times each day.

If you forget a dose:
Take as soon as you remember up to 2 hours late. If more than 2 hours, wait for next scheduled dose (don't double this dose).

Continued next column

OVERDOSE

SYMPTOMS:
Confusion, agitation, severe headache, incoherence, convulsions, possible hemorrhage from stomach or intestine, coma.
WHAT TO DO:
- **Dial 911 (emergency) or 0 (operator)for an ambulance or medical help. Then give first aid immediately.**
- **See emergency information on inside covers.**

What drug does:
Reduces tissue concentration of prostaglandins (hormones which produce inflammation and pain).

Time lapse before drug works:
Begins in 4 to 24 hours. May require 3 weeks regular use for maximum benefit.

Don't take with:
Any other medicine without consulting your doctor or pharmacist.

POSSIBLE ADVERSE REACTIONS OR SIDE EFFECTS

SYMPTOMS	WHAT TO DO
Life-threatening:	
Hives, rash, intense itching, faintness soon after a dose (anaphylaxis in aspirin-sensitive persons).	Seek emergency treatment immediately.
Common:	
• Dizziness, nausea, stomach cramps, headache.	Continue. Call doctor when convenient.
• Diarrhea, skin rash, bleeding from rectum (with suppositories).	Discontinue. Call doctor right away.
Infrequent:	
• Depression; drowsiness; ringing in ears; swollen feet, face or legs; constipation or diarrhea; vomiting; gaseousness; dry mouth; tremors; insomnia.	Continue. Call doctor when convenient.
• Muscle cramps, numbness or tingling in hands or feet, mouth ulcers, rapid weight gain.	Discontinue. Call doctor right away.
Rare:	
• Convulsions; confusion; rash, hives or itch; blurred vision; black, bloody, tarry stool; difficult breathing; tightness in chest; rapid heartbeat; unusual bleeding or bruising; blood in urine; jaundice; psychosis; frequent, painful urination; fainting; sore throat; fever; chills; diminished hearing; eye pain; nose bleeds; severe abdominal pain.	Discontinue. Call doctor right away.
• Fatigue, weakness, menstrual irregularities.	Continue. Call doctor when convenient.

WARNINGS & PRECAUTIONS

Don't take if:
- You are allergic to aspirin or any nonsteroidal, anti-inflammatory drug.
- You have gastritis, peptic ulcer, enteritis, ileitis, ulcerative colitis, asthma, heart failure, high blood pressure or bleeding problems.
- Patient is younger than 15.

Before you start, consult your doctor:
- If you have epilepsy.
- If you have Parkinson's disease.
- If you have been mentally ill.
- If you have impaired kidney or liver function.

Over age 60:
Adverse reactions and side effects may be more frequent and severe than in younger persons.

Pregnancy:
Risk factors vary for drugs in this group. See category list on page xxiii and consult doctor.

Breast-feeding:
May harm child. Avoid.

Infants & children:
Not recommended for anyone younger than 15. Use only under medical supervision.

Prolonged use:
- Eye damage.
- Reduced hearing.
- Sore throat, fever.
- Weight gain.
- Talk to your doctor about the need for follow-up medical examinations or laboratory studies to check complete blood counts (white blood cell count, platelet count, red blood cell count, hemoglobin, hematocrit), liver function, stools for blood, eyes.

Skin & sunlight:
One or more drugs in this group may cause rash or intensify sunburn in areas exposed to sun or ultraviolet light (photosensitivity reaction). Avoid overexposure. Notify doctor if reaction occurs.

Driving, piloting or hazardous work:
Don't drive or pilot aircraft until you learn how medicine affects you. Don't work around dangerous machinery. Don't climb ladders or work in high places. Danger increases if you drink alcohol or take medicine affecting alertness and reflexes, such as antihistamines, tranquilizers, sedatives, pain medicine, narcotics and mind-altering drugs.

Discontinuing:
No problems expected. If drug has been taken for a long time, consult doctor before discontinuing.

Others:
Advise any doctor or dentist whom you consult that you take this medicine

POSSIBLE INTERACTION WITH OTHER DRUGS

GENERIC NAME OR DRUG CLASS	COMBINED EFFECT
Adrenocorticoids, systemic	Increased risk of ulcers. Increased adrenocorticoid effect.
Angiotensin-converting enzyme (ACE) inhibitors*	May decrease ACE inhibitor effect.
Antacids*	Decreased pain relief.
Anticoagulants, oral*	Increased risk of bleeding.
Anticonvulsants, hydantoin*	Increased anti-convulsant effect.
Anti-inflammatory pain relievers (any combination of)	Danger of increased side effects such as stomach bleeding.
Aspirin	Increased risk of stomach ulcer.
Beta-adrenergic blocking agents*	Decreased anti-hypertensive effect.
Carteolol	Decreased anti-hypertensive effect.
Cephalosporins*	Increased risk of bleeding.
Didanosine	Increased risk of pancreatitis (sulindac only).

Continued on page 903

POSSIBLE INTERACTION WITH OTHER SUBSTANCES

INTERACTS WITH	COMBINED EFFECT
Alcohol:	Possible stomach ulcer or bleeding.
Beverages:	None expected.
Cocaine:	None expected.
Foods:	None expected.
Marijuana:	Increased pain relief from NSAIDs.
Tobacco:	None expected.

*See Glossary

ANTI-INFLAMMATORY DRUGS, NONSTEROIDAL (NSAIDs) (Ophthalmic)

GENERIC AND BRAND NAMES

DICLOFENAC
  Voltaren Ophtha
  Voltaren
  Ophthalmic
FLURBIPROFEN
  Ocufen

INDOMETHACIN
  Indocid
KETOROLAC
  Acular
SUPROFEN
  Profenal

BASIC INFORMATION

Habit forming? No
Prescription needed? Yes
Available as generic? Yes, for some
Drug class: Ophthalmic anti-inflammatory agents, nonsteroidal

USES

- Used to prevent problems during and following eye surgery, such as cataract removal.
- Treatment for eye itching caused by seasonal allergic conjunctivitis.

DOSAGE & USAGE INFORMATION

How to use:
Eye solution
- Wash hands.
- Apply pressure to inside corner of eye with middle finger.
- Continue pressure for 1 minute after placing medicine in eye.
- Tilt head backward. Pull lower lid away from eye with index finger of the same hand.
- Drop eye drops into pouch and close eye. Don't blink.
- Keep eyes closed for 1 to 2 minutes.

When to use:
As directed by your doctor or on the label. Your doctor or nurse may instill the drug before an eye operation.

If you forget a dose:
Use as soon as you remember.

Continued next column

OVERDOSE

SYMPTOMS:
None expected.
WHAT TO DO:
Not intended for internal use. If child accidentally swallows, call poison control center.

What drug does:
Blocks prostaglandin production. Prostaglandins cause inflammatory responses and constriction of the pupil.

Time lapse before drug works:
Immediately.

Don't use with:
Any other medications without first consulting doctor or pharmacist.

POSSIBLE ADVERSE REACTIONS OR SIDE EFFECTS

SYMPTOMS	WHAT TO DO
Life-threatening: None expected.	
Common: Brief and mild burning or stinging when drops are administered.	No action necessary.
Infrequent: None expected.	
Rare: Allergic reaction (itching, tearing); redness, swelling or bleeding in eye not present before; eye pain; sensitivity to light.	Discontinue. Call doctor right away.

ANTI-INFLAMMATORY DRUGS, NONSTEROIDAL (NSAIDs) (Ophthalmic)

WARNINGS & PRECAUTIONS

Don't use if:
- You are allergic to any eye medication.
- You are allergic to any nonsteroidal anti-inflammatory drugs taken orally, e.g., aspirin.

Before you start, consult your doctor:
- If you have any bleeding disorder such as hemophilia.
- If you have or have had herpes simplex keratitis (an inflammation of the cornea).
- If you have allergies to any medications, foods or other substances.

Over age 60:
No special problems expected.

Pregnancy:
Risk category C (see page xxiii). Decide with your doctor whether drug benefit justifies risk to unborn child.

Breast-feeding:
Unknown if drug passes into breast milk after administration into the eye. Consult doctor.

Infants & children:
No information available on safety or effectiveness. Consult doctor.

Prolonged use:
Not intended for long-term use.

Skin & sunlight:
No special problems expected.

Driving, piloting or hazardous work:
No special problems expected.

Discontinuing:
No special problems expected.

Others:
Don't use leftover medicine for other eye problems without your doctor's approval. Some eye infections could be made worse.

POSSIBLE INTERACTION WITH OTHER DRUGS

GENERIC NAME OR DRUG CLASS	COMBINED EFFECT
Anticoagulants*, oral	May increase bleeding tendency.
Antiglaucoma drugs*	May decrease antiglaucoma effect (with flubiprofen).
Carbachol	Decreased carbachol effect.

POSSIBLE INTERACTION WITH OTHER SUBSTANCES

INTERACTS WITH	COMBINED EFFECT
Alcohol:	None expected.
Beverages:	None expected.
Cocaine	None expected.
Foods:	None expected.
Marijuana:	None expected.
Tobacco:	None expected.

ANTI-INFLAMMATORY DRUGS, STEROIDAL (Ophthalmic)

GENERIC AND BRAND NAMES

See complete list of generic and brand names in the *Generic and Brand Name Directory*, page 872.

BASIC INFORMATION

Habit forming? No
Prescription needed? Yes
Available as generic? Yes
Drug class: Adrenocorticoid (ophthalmic); anti-inflammatory, steroidal (ophthalmic)

USES

- Relieves redness and irritation due to allergies or other irritants.
- Prevents damage to eye.
- Treatment for anterior uveitis (a type of eye infection).

DOSAGE & USAGE INFORMATION

How to use:
Eye drops
- Wash hands.
- Apply pressure to inside corner of eye with middle finger.
- Continue pressure for 1 minute after placing medicine in eye.
- Tilt head backward. Pull lower lid away from eye with index finger of the same hand.
- Drop eye drops into pouch and close eye. Don't blink.
- Keep eyes closed for 1 to 2 minutes.

Eye ointment
- Wash hands.
- Pull lower lid down from eye to form a pouch.
- Squeeze tube to apply thin strip of ointment into pouch.
- Close eye for 1 to 2 minutes.
- Don't touch applicator tip to any surface (including the eye). If you accidentally touch tip, clean with warm soap and water.
- Keep container tightly closed.

Continued next column

OVERDOSE

SYMPTOMS:
None expected.
WHAT TO DO:
Not intended for internal use. If child accidentally swallows, call poison control center.

- Keep cool, but don't freeze.
- Wash hands immediately after using.

When to use:
As directed.

If you forget a dose:
Use as soon as you remember.

What drug does:
Affects cell membranes and decreases response to irritating substances.

Time lapse before drug works:
Immediately.

Don't use with:
Medicines for abdominal cramps or glaucoma without first consulting doctor.

POSSIBLE ADVERSE REACTIONS OR SIDE EFFECTS

SYMPTOMS	WHAT TO DO
Life-threatening: None expected.	
Common: None expected.	
Infrequent: Watery, stinging, burning eyes.	Continue. Call doctor when convenient.
Rare:	
• Eye pain, blurred vision, drooping eyelid, halos around lights, enlarged pupils, flashes of light.	Discontinue. Call doctor right away.
• Eye symptoms (discharge, dryness, irritation, tearing, sensation of foreign body); sore throat; runny or stuffy nose.	Continue. Call doctor when convenient.

ANTI-INFLAMMATORY DRUGS, STEROIDAL (Ophthalmic)

WARNINGS & PRECAUTIONS

Don't use if:
You are allergic to any cortisone medicine.

Before you start, consult your doctor:
- If you have or ever have had any eye infection, glaucoma, virus (herpes) or fungus infection of the eye, tuberculosis of the eye.
- If you wear contact lenses (may need to discontinue wearing temporarily).

Over age 60:
No problems expected.

Pregnancy:
Risk factors vary for drugs in this group. See category list on page xxiii and consult doctor.

Breast-feeding:
Safety unestablished. Avoid if possible. Consult doctor.

Infants & children:
Use for short periods of time only.

Prolonged use:
- Recheck with eye doctor at regular intervals.
- May develop glaucoma, hypertension of the eye, damage to optic nerve, vision changes, cataracts or infections due to suppressive effects of drug.

Skin & sunlight:
No problems expected.

Driving, piloting or hazardous work:
No problems expected.

Discontinuing:
No problems expected.

Others:
- Cortisone eye medicines should not be used for bacterial, viral, fungal or tubercular infections.
- Keep cool, but don't freeze.
- Notify doctor if condition doesn't improve within 3 days.
- Contact lens wearers have increased risk of infection.

POSSIBLE INTERACTION WITH OTHER DRUGS

GENERIC NAME OR DRUG CLASS	COMBINED EFFECT
Antiglaucoma drugs*, long- and short-acting	Decreased antiglaucoma effect.

POSSIBLE INTERACTION WITH OTHER SUBSTANCES

INTERACTS WITH	COMBINED EFFECT
Alcohol:	None expected.
Beverages:	None expected.
Cocaine:	None expected.
Foods:	None expected.
Marijuana:	None expected.
Tobacco:	None expected.

ANTI-INFLAMMATORY DRUGS, STEROIDAL (Otic)

GENERIC AND BRAND NAMES

BETAMETHASONE (otic)
Betnesol
DEXAMETHASONE (otic)
Ak-Dex
Decadron
I-Methasone

HYDROCORTISONE (otic)
Cortamed
Cortisol

BASIC INFORMATION

Habit forming? No
Prescription needed? Yes
Available as generic? No
Drug class: Anti-inflammatory, steroidal (otic); adrenocorticoid (otic)

 ## USES

- Treats allergic conditions involving external ear.
- Used together with antibiotics to treat ear infections.
- Treats seborrheic and eczematoid dermatitis involving the ear.

 ## DOSAGE & USAGE INFORMATION

How to use:
Ear drops
- Warm ear drops under running water around the unopened bottle.
- Lie down with affected ear up.
- Adults—Pull ear lobe back and up.
- Children—Pull ear lobe down and back.
- Drop medicine into ear canal until canal is full.
- Stay lying down for 2 minutes.
- Gently insert cotton plug into ear to prevent leaking.

Continued next column

 ## OVERDOSE

SYMPTOMS:
None expected.
WHAT TO DO:
Not intended for internal use. If child accidentally swallows, call poison control center.

Ear ointment
- Apply small amount to skin just inside the ear canal.
- Use finger or piece of sterile gauze.
- Don't use cotton-tipped applicators.

When to use:
As directed by your doctor.

If you forget a dose:
Use as soon as you remember.

What drug does:
Decreases tissue inflammation, decreases scarring.

Time lapse before drug works:
15 minutes.

Don't use with:
Other ear medications unless directed by your doctor.

 ## POSSIBLE ADVERSE REACTIONS OR SIDE EFFECTS

SYMPTOMS	WHAT TO DO
Life-threatening: None expected.	
Common: None expected.	
Infrequent: Itching, burning, redness, swelling.	Discontinue. Call doctor right away.
Rare: None expected.	

ANTI-INFLAMMATORY DRUGS, STEROIDAL
(Otic)

 WARNINGS & PRECAUTIONS

Don't use if:
You are allergic to any of the medications listed under Brand and Generic Names.

Before you start, consult your doctor:
• If eardrum is punctured.
• If you have a viral infection.
• If you have a fungal ear infection.

Over age 60:
No problems expected.

Pregnancy:
Risk factors vary for drugs in this group. See category list on page xxiii and consult doctor.

Breast-feeding:
No problems expected. Consult doctor.

Infants & children:
Use small amounts only.

Prolonged use:
Not intended for prolonged use.

Skin & sunlight:
No problems expected.

Driving, piloting or hazardous work:
No problems expected.

Discontinuing:
No problems expected.

Others:
Keep cool, but don't freeze.

 POSSIBLE INTERACTION WITH OTHER DRUGS

GENERIC NAME OR DRUG CLASS	COMBINED EFFECT
None expected.	

 POSSIBLE INTERACTION WITH OTHER SUBSTANCES

INTERACTS WITH	COMBINED EFFECT
Alcohol:	None expected.
Beverages:	None expected.
Cocaine:	None expected.
Foods:	None expected.
Marijuana:	None expected.
Tobacco:	None expected.

ANTIMALARIAL

GENERIC AND BRAND NAMES

HALOFANTRINE　　**MEFLOQUINE**
　Halfan　　　　　　Lariam

BASIC INFORMATION

Habit forming? No
Prescription needed? Yes
Available as generic? No
Drug class: Antiprotozoal, antimalarial, antiparasitic

USES

- Treats malaria caused by *plasmodium falciparum* (either chloroquine-sensitive or chloroquine-resistant).
- Treats malaria caused by *plasmodium vivax*.
- Mefloquine helps prevent malaria in people traveling into areas where malaria is prevalent.

DOSAGE & USAGE INFORMATION

How to take:
- Mefloquine tablet—Swallow with food, milk or water to lessen stomach irritation.
- Halofantrine tablet—Take on an empty stomach.
- Halofantrine suspension—Varies by age and weight; follow physician's directions.

When to take:
- Mefloquine treatment is usually given as 5 tablets in a single dose, while prevention with mefloquine should start a week prior to travel.
- Halofantrine tablets and suspension are taken every 6 hours, 3 times a day for one day on an empty stomach, 1 hour before or 2 hours after a meal.

Continued next column

OVERDOSE

SYMPTOMS:
Seizures, heart rhythm disturbances.
WHAT TO DO:
- **Dial 911 (emergency) or 0 (operator) for an ambulance or medical help. Then give first aid immediately.**
- **Induce vomiting and see a doctor immediately because of the potential cardiotoxic effect. Treat vomiting or diarrhea with standard fluid therapy.**
- **See emergency information on inside covers.**

If you forget a dose:
Take as soon as you remember, then return to regular dosing schedule.

What drug does:
Exact mechanism unknown. Mefloquine kills parasite in one of its developmental stages, while halofantrine treats malaria in its acute stage.

Time lapse before drug works:
6 to 24 hours.

Don't take with:
- Sulfadoxine and pyrimethamine combination (Fansidar).
- Any other medicines (including over-the-counter drugs such as cough and cold medicines, laxatives, antacids, diet pills, caffeine, nose drops or vitamins) without consulting your doctor or pharmacist.

POSSIBLE ADVERSE REACTIONS OR SIDE EFFECTS

SYMPTOMS	WHAT TO DO
Life-threatening: Seizures.	Seek emergency treatment immediately.
Common:	
• Dizziness, headache, lightheadedness, abdominal pain, diarrhea, nausea or vomiting, rash, visual disturbances.	Discontinue. Call doctor right away.
• Insomnia, appetite loss.	Continue. Call doctor when convenient.
Infrequent: None expected.	
Rare: Change in heart rate, confusion, anxiety, depression, hallucinations, psychosis, black urine or decrease in urine amount, chest or lower back pain, rapid breathing.	Discontinue. Call doctor right away.

WARNINGS & PRECAUTIONS

Don't take if:
You are allergic to mefloquine, halofantrine, quinine, quinidine or related medications.

Before you start, consult your doctor:
- It you plan to become pregnant within the medication period or 2 months after.
- If you have heart trouble, especially heart block.
- If you have depression or other emotional problems.
- If you are giving this to a child under 40 pounds of body weight.
- If you have epilepsy or a seizure disorder.

Over age 60:
Adverse reactions and side effects may be more frequent and severe than in younger persons.

Pregnancy:
Not recommended. If traveling to an area where malaria is endemic, consult your doctor about prophylaxis. Risk category C (see page xxiii).

Breast-feeding:
One or more of these drugs may pass into mother's milk. Avoid drug or discontinue nursing.

Infants & children:
- For halofantrine pediatric use, consult your doctor.
- Mefloquine is not recommended for children under 2.

Prolonged use:
Not recommended.

Skin & sunlight:
No problems expected.

Driving, piloting or hazardous work:
Don't drive or pilot aircraft until you learn how medicine affects you. Don't work around dangerous machinery. Don't climb ladders or work in high places. Danger increases if you drink alcohol or take medicine affecting alertness and reflexes.

Discontinuing:
Don't discontinue without doctor's advice until you complete the prescribed dosage.

Others:
- Periodic physical (including eye) examinations and blood studies recommended.
- Resistance to one or more of these drugs by some strains of malaria has been reported, so prevention and treatment of malaria may not be uniformly effective.

POSSIBLE INTERACTION WITH OTHER DRUGS

GENERIC NAME OR DRUG CLASS	COMBINED EFFECT
Antiseizure medications	Possible lowered seizure control.
Beta-adrenergic blocking agents*	Heartbeat irregularities or cardiac arrest. Avoid.
Calcium channel blockers*	Heartbeat irregularities.
Chloroquine	Increased chance of seizures. Avoid.
Divalproex	Increased risk of seizures.
Propranolol	Heartbeat irregularities.
Quinidine	Increased chance of seizures and heart rhythm disturbances.
Quinine	Increased chance of seizures and heart rhythm disturbances.
Typhoid vaccine (oral)	Concurrent use may decrease effectiveness of vaccine.
Valproic acid	Decreased valproic acid effect.

POSSIBLE INTERACTION WITH OTHER SUBSTANCES

INTERACTS WITH	COMBINED EFFECT
Alcohol:	Possible liver toxicity. Avoid.
Beverages: Any alcoholic beverage.	Possible liver toxicity. Avoid.
Cocaine:	No problems expected.
Foods:	No problems expected.
Marijuana:	No problems expected.
Tobacco:	No problems expected.

ANTIMYASTHENICS

GENERIC AND BRAND NAMES

AMBENONIUM
  Mytelase Caplets
NEOSTIGMINE
  Prostigmin

PYRIDOSTIGMINE
  Mestinon
  Mestinon Timespans
  Regonol

BASIC INFORMATION

Habit forming? No
Prescription needed? Yes
Available as generic? No
Drug class: Cholinergic, antimyasthenic

USES

- Diagnosis and treatment of myasthenia gravis.
- Treatment of urinary retention and abdominal distention.
- Antidote to adverse effects of muscle relaxants used in surgery.

DOSAGE & USAGE INFORMATION

How to take:
- Tablet or syrup—Swallow with liquid or food to lessen stomach irritation.
- Extended-release tablets—Swallow each dose whole. If you take regular tablets, you may chew or crush them.

When to take:
As directed, usually 3 or 4 times a day.

Continued next column

OVERDOSE

SYMPTOMS:
Muscle weakness or paralysis, cramps, twitching or clumsiness; severe diarrhea, nausea, vomiting, stomach cramps or pain; breathing difficulty; confusion, irritability, nervousness, restlessness, fear; unusually slow heartbeat; seizures; blurred vision; extreme fatigue.
WHAT TO DO:
- **Dial 911 (emergency) or 0 (operator) for an ambulance or medical help. Then give first aid immediately.**
- **See emergency information on inside covers.**

If you forget a dose:
Take as soon as you remember up to 2 hours late. If more than 2 hours, wait for next scheduled dose (don't double this dose).

What drug does:
Inhibits the chemical activity of an enzyme (cholinesterase) so nerve impulses can cross the junction of nerves and muscles.

Time lapse before drug works:
Usually takes 10 to 14 days to determine if drug helps relieve symptoms.

Don't take with:
Any other medicine without consulting your doctor or pharmacist.

POSSIBLE ADVERSE REACTIONS OR SIDE EFFECTS

SYMPTOMS	WHAT TO DO
Life-threatening: In case of overdose, see previous column.	
Common: Excess saliva, unusual sweating. mild diarrhea, nausea, vomiting, stomach cramps or pain.	Continue. Call doctor when convenient.
Infrequent: Constricted pupils, watery eyes, lung congestion, frequent urge to urinate, confusion, slurred speech.	Continue. But call doctor right away.
Rare: Other symptoms.	Continue. Call doctor when convenient.

WARNINGS & PRECAUTIONS

Don't take if:
You are allergic to any cholinergic* or bromide.

Before you start, consult your doctor:
- If you plan to become pregnant within medication period.
- If you have bronchial asthma.
- If you have heartbeat irregularities.
- If you have urinary obstruction or urinary tract infection.

Over age 60:
Adverse reactions and side effects may be more frequent and severe than in younger persons.

Pregnancy:
Decide with your doctor if drug benefits justify risk to unborn child. Risk category C (see page xxiii).

Breast-feeding:
Pyridostigmine passes into milk. It is unknown if others pass into milk. Avoid drug or discontinue nursing until you finish medicine. Consult doctor for advice on maintaining milk supply.

Infants & children:
Use only under close medical supervision.

Prolonged use:
Medication may lose effectiveness. Ask your doctor about discontinuing drug for a few days to possibly help restore effect.

Skin & sunlight:
No problems expected.

Driving, piloting or hazardous work:
Don't drive or pilot aircraft until you learn how medicine affects you. Don't work around dangerous machinery. Don't climb ladders or work in high places. Danger increases if you drink alcohol or take medicine affecting alertness and reflexes, such as antihistamines, tranquilizers, sedatives, pain medicine, narcotics and mind-altering drugs.

Discontinuing:
Don't discontinue without doctor's advice until you complete prescribed dose, even though symptoms diminish or disappear.

Others:
- Advise any doctor or dentist whom you consult that you take this medicine.
- Be cautious about participating in hot weather activities since drug may cause excessive sweating.

POSSIBLE INTERACTION WITH OTHER DRUGS

GENERIC NAME OR DRUG CLASS	COMBINED EFFECT
Anesthetics, local or general*	Decreased effect of antimyasthenic.
Antiarrhythmics*	Decreased effect of antimyasthenic.
Anticholinergics*	May mask severe side effects.
Cholinergics*, other	Possible brain and nervous system toxicity.
Guanadrel	Decreased effect of antimyasthenic.
Guanethidine	Decreased effect of antimyasthenic.
Mecamylamine	Decreased effect of antimyasthenic.
Procainamide	Decreased effect of antimyasthenic.
Quinidine	Decreased effect of antimyasthenic.

POSSIBLE INTERACTION WITH OTHER SUBSTANCES

INTERACTS WITH	COMBINED EFFECT
Alcohol:	No proven problems with small doses.
Beverages:	None expected.
Cocaine:	Decreased antimyasthenic effect. Avoid.
Foods:	None expected.
Marijuana:	No proven problems.
Tobacco:	No proven problems.

ANTIPYRINE & BENZOCAINE (Topical-Otic)

BRAND NAMES

A/B Otic	Aurodex
Allergen	Dolotic
Analgesic Ear	Earache Drops
Drops	Earocol
Antiben	Otiprin
Aurafair	Oto
Auralgan	Otocalm

BASIC INFORMATION

Habit forming? No
Prescription needed? Yes
Available as generic? Yes
Drug class: Analgesic (otic), anesthetic

USES

- Relieves pain of middle ear infections (otitis media). It does not treat the infection itself.
- Used to soften earwax so it can be removed.

DOSAGE & USAGE INFORMATION

How to use:
- Warm ear drops under running water around the unopened bottle.
- Lie down with affected ear up.
- Adults—Pull ear lobe back and up.
- Children—Pull ear lobe down and back.
- Drop medicine into ear canal until canal is full.
- Stay lying down for 2 minutes.
- Gently insert cotton plug into ear to prevent leaking.

When to use:
Every 1 to 2 hours for 4 hours, then 4 times a day when needed for pain.

If you forget a dose:
Use as soon as you remember.

What drug does:
Functions as a topical anesthetic/analgesic on the eardrum.

Time lapse before drug works:
10 minutes.

Continued next column

OVERDOSE

SYMPTOMS:
None expected.
WHAT TO DO:
Not intended for internal use. If child accidentally swallows, call poison control center.

Don't use with:
Any other medicine without consulting your doctor or pharmacist.

POSSIBLE ADVERSE REACTIONS OR SIDE EFFECTS

SYMPTOMS	WHAT TO DO
Life-threatening: None expected.	
Common: None expected.	
Infrequent: Itching or burning in ear (probably represents allergic reaction).	Discontinue. Call doctor right away.
Rare: None expected.	

ANTIPYRINE & BENZOCAINE (Topical-Otic)

WARNINGS & PRECAUTIONS

Don't use if:
You are allergic to any local anesthetic (name usually ends with "caine").

Before you start, consult your doctor:
If eardrum is ruptured.

Over age 60:
No problems expected.

Pregnancy:
Consult doctor. Risk category C (see page xxiii).

Breast-feeding:
No problems expected. Consult doctor.

Infants & children:
No problems expected.

Prolonged use:
Not intended for prolonged use.

Skin & sunlight:
No problems expected.

Driving, piloting or hazardous work:
No problems expected.

Discontinuing:
No problems expected.

Others:
- Keep cool, but don't freeze.
- Don't touch tip of dropper to any other surface.
- Don't rinse the dropper. Wipe with clean cloth and close tightly.

POSSIBLE INTERACTION WITH OTHER DRUGS

GENERIC NAME OR DRUG CLASS	COMBINED EFFECT
None expected.	

POSSIBLE INTERACTION WITH OTHER SUBSTANCES

INTERACTS WITH	COMBINED EFFECT
Alcohol:	None expected.
Beverages:	None expected.
Cocaine:	None expected.
Foods:	None expected.
Marijuana:	None expected.
Tobacco:	None expected.

ANTISEBORRHEICS (Topical)

GENERIC AND BRAND NAMES

See complete list of generic and brand names in the *Generic and Brand Name Directory*, page 872.

BASIC INFORMATION

Habit forming? No
Prescription needed? Yes
Available as generic? Yes
Drug class: Antiseborrheic

USES

Treats dandruff or seborrheic dermatitis of scalp.

DOSAGE & USAGE INFORMATION

How to use:
- Wet hair and scalp.
- Apply enough medicine to form lather.
- Rub in well. Keep away from eyes.
- Allow to remain on scalp 3 to 5 minutes then rinse.
- Repeat above steps once.

Continued next column

OVERDOSE

SYMPTOMS:
None expected.
WHAT TO DO:
- Not for internal use. If child accidentally swallows, call poison control center.
- Dial 911 (emergency) or 0 (operator) for an ambulance or medical help. Then give first aid immediately.
- See emergency information on inside covers.

When to use:
As directed by doctor. Twice a week for shampoo is average.

If you forget a dose:
Use as soon as you remember.

What drug does:
Slows cell growth in scales on scalp.

Time lapse before drug works:
Varies a great deal. If no improvement in 2 weeks, notify doctor.

Don't use with:
- Other scalp preparations without notifying doctor.
- Any other medicine without consulting your doctor or pharmacist.

POSSIBLE ADVERSE REACTIONS OR SIDE EFFECTS

SYMPTOMS	WHAT TO DO
Life-threatening: None expected.	
Common: None expected.	
Infrequent:	
• Irritation not present before using, rash.	Discontinue. Call doctor when convenient.
• Dryness or itching scalp.	Continue. Call doctor when convenient.
Rare: None expected.	

WARNINGS & PRECAUTIONS

Don't use if:
- You have had an allergic reaction to chloroxine, clioquinol (iodochlorhydroxyquin), iodoquinol (diiodohydroxyquin) or edate sodium.
- Scalp is blistered or infected with oozing or raw areas.

Before you start, consult your doctor:
If you are allergic to anything.

Over age 60:
No problems expected.

Pregnancy:
Risk factors vary for drugs in this group. See category list on page xxiii and consult doctor.

Breast-feeding:
No problems expected, but check with doctor.

Infants & children:
No problems expected, but check with doctor.

Prolonged use:
No problems expected, but check with doctor.

Skin & sunlight:
No special problems expected.

Driving, piloting or hazardous work:
No problems expected, but check with doctor.

Discontinuing:
No problems expected, but check with doctor.

Others:
- If medicine accidentally gets into eyes, flush them immediately with cool water.
- Heat and moisture in bathroom medicine cabinet can cause breakdown of medicine. Store someplace else.
- Keep cool, but don't freeze.

POSSIBLE INTERACTION WITH OTHER DRUGS

GENERIC NAME OR DRUG CLASS	COMBINED EFFECT
Other medical shampoos	May accentuate adverse reactions of each medicine.

POSSIBLE INTERACTION WITH OTHER SUBSTANCES

INTERACTS WITH	COMBINED EFFECT
Alcohol:	None expected.
Beverages:	None expected.
Cocaine:	None expected.
Foods:	None expected.
Marijuana:	None expected.
Tobacco:	None expected.

ANTITHYROID DRUGS

GENERIC AND BRAND NAMES

METHIMAZOLE	PROPYLTHIOURACIL
Tapazole	Propyl-Thyracil
Thiamazole	

BASIC INFORMATION

Habit forming? No
Prescription needed? Yes
Available as generic? Yes
Drug class: Antihyperthyroid

USES

- Treatment of overactive thyroid (hyperthyroidism).
- Treatment of angina in patients who have overactive thyroid.

DOSAGE & USAGE INFORMATION

How to take:
Tablet—Swallow with liquid or food to lessen stomach irritation. If you can't swallow whole, crumble tablet and take with liquid or food.

When to take:
At the same times each day.

If you forget a dose:
Take as soon as you remember up to 2 hours late. If more than 2 hours, wait for next scheduled dose (don't double this dose).

What drug does:
Prevents thyroid gland from producing excess thyroid hormone.

Time lapse before drug works:
10 to 20 days.

Don't take with:
- Anticoagulants
- Any other medicine without consulting your doctor or pharmacist.

OVERDOSE

SYMPTOMS:
Bleeding, spots on skin, jaundice (yellow eyes and skin), loss of consciousness.
WHAT TO DO:
Overdose unlikely to threaten life. If person takes much larger amount than prescribed, call doctor, poison control center or hospital emergency room for instructions.

POSSIBLE ADVERSE REACTIONS OR SIDE EFFECTS

SYMPTOMS	WHAT TO DO
Life-threatening:	
In case of overdose, see previous column.	
Common:	
Skin rash, itching, dryness.	Continue. Call doctor right away.
Infrequent:	
• Dizziness, sore throat with chills and fever, abdominal pain.	Continue. Call doctor right away.
• Taste loss, constipation, diarrhea.	Continue. Call doctor when convenient.
Rare:	
Headache; enlarged lymph glands; irregular or rapid heartbeat; unusual bruising or bleeding; backache; numbness or tingling in toes, fingers or face; joint pain; muscle aches; menstrual irregularities; jaundice; tired, weak, sleepy, listless; swollen eyes or feet; black stools; excessive cold feeling; puffy skin; irritability.	Continue. Call doctor right away.

WARNINGS & PRECAUTIONS

Don't take if:
You are allergic to antithyroid medicines.

Before you start, consult your doctor:
- If you have liver disease.
- If you have blood disease.
- If you have an infection.
- If you take anticoagulants.

Over age 60:
Adverse reactions and side effects may be more frequent and severe than in younger persons.

Pregnancy:
Consult doctor. Risk category D (see page xxiii).

Breast-feeding:
Drug filters into milk. Consult doctor.

Infants & children:
Use only under special medical supervision by experienced clinician.

Prolonged use:
- Adverse reactions and side effects more common.
- Talk to your doctor about the need for follow-up medical examinations or laboratory studies to check thyroid function, complete blood counts (white blood cell count, platelet count, red blood cell count, hemoglobin, hematocrit).

Skin & sunlight:
No problems expected.

Driving, piloting or hazardous work:
Don't drive or pilot aircraft until you learn how medicine affects you. Don't work around dangerous machinery. Don't climb ladders or work in high places. Danger increases if you drink alcohol or take medicine affecting alertness and reflexes, such as antihistamines, tranquilizers, sedatives, pain medicine, narcotics and mind-altering drugs.

Discontinuing:
Don't discontinue without consulting doctor. Dose may require gradual reduction if you have taken drug for a long time. Doses of other drugs may also require adjustment.

Others:
- Advise any doctor or dentist whom you consult that you take this medicine.
- Ask your doctor about the symptoms of over-active or underactive thyroid and what to do if they occur.

POSSIBLE INTERACTION WITH OTHER DRUGS

GENERIC NAME OR DRUG CLASS	COMBINED EFFECT
Amiodarone	Decreased anti-thyroid effect.
Anticoagulants*	Increased effect of anticoagulants.
Antineoplastic drugs*	Increased chance to suppress bone marrow.
Chloramphenicol	Increased chance to suppress bone marrow.
Clozapine	Toxic effect on bone marrow.
Digitalis preparations*	Increased digitalis effect.
Iodine	Decreased anti-thyroid effect.
Levamisole	Increased risk of bone marrow depression.
Lithium	Decreased thyroid activity.
Potassium iodide	Decreased anti-thyroid effect.
Tiopronin	Increased risk of toxicity to bone marrow.

POSSIBLE INTERACTION WITH OTHER SUBSTANCES

INTERACTS WITH	COMBINED EFFECT
Alcohol:	Increased possibility of liver toxicity. Avoid.
Beverages:	No problems expected.
Cocaine:	Increased toxicity potential of medicines. Avoid.
Foods:	No problems expected.
Marijuana:	Increased rapid or irregular heartbeat. Avoid.
Tobacco:	Increased chance of rapid heartbeat. Avoid.

ANTIVIRALS FOR HERPES VIRUS

GENERIC AND BRAND NAMES

ACYCLOVIR
  Avirax
  Zovirax
FAMCICLOVIR
  Famvir

GANCICLOVIR
  Cytovene
VALACYCLOVIR
  Valtrex

BASIC INFORMATION

Habit forming? No
Prescription needed? Yes
Available as generic? Yes, for some
Drug class: Antiviral

USES

- Treatment for symptoms of herpes virus infections (does not cure the disorders). These infections include herpes simplex, genital herpes and herpes zoster (also known as shingles). Herpes infections may occur on the lips and mouth, genitals, skin and the brain.
- May be used to treat chickenpox and other viral infections as prescribed by your doctor.
- Ganciclovir is used for treatment of cytomegalovirus (CMV) eye infection in persons whose immune system is impaired.

DOSAGE & USAGE INFORMATION

How to take:
Tablet, capsule or oral suspension—Swallow with liquid. If you can't swallow whole, open capsule or crumble tablet and take with liquid or food. Take ganciclovir with food and do not open capsule. Other drugs may be taken with or without food. Measure oral suspension with specially marked measuring device.

When to take:
At the same times each day and night. Drugs work best if started within 48 hours of diagnosis (or when symptoms first appear).

Continued next column

OVERDOSE

SYMPTOMS:
None expected.
WHAT TO DO:
Overdose unlikely to threaten life. If person takes much larger amount than prescribed or accidentally swallows topical form of drug, call doctor, poison control center or hospital emergency room for instructions.

If you forget a dose:
Take as soon as you remember up to 2 hours late. If more than 2 hours, wait for next dose (don't double this dose).

What drug does:
Inhibits the growth and spread of the virus thereby decreasing length of infection and lessening the severity of the symptoms.

Time lapse before drug works:
Begins the first day, but may take several days for symptoms (pain, burning and blisters) to improve.

Don't take with:
Any other medicine without consulting your doctor or pharmacist.

POSSIBLE ADVERSE REACTIONS OR SIDE EFFECTS

SYMPTOMS	WHAT TO DO
Life-threatening: None expected.	
Common: None expected.	
Infrequent: Headache, nausea, diarrhea, vomiting, tiredness, dizziness; with ganciclovir—sore throat and fever, unusual bleeding or bruising, mood changes.	Continue. Call doctor when convenient.
Rare: None expected.	

WARNINGS & PRECAUTIONS

Don't take if:
You are allergic to antiviral agents.

Before you start, consult your doctor:
- If you have kidney disease.
- If you are allergic to any medication, food or other substance.

Over age 60:
No special problems expected.

Pregnancy:
Risk factors vary for drugs in this group. See category page xxiii and consult doctor.

Breast-feeding:
Drugs may pass into milk. Avoid nursing until you finish medicine. Consult doctor for advice on maintaining milk supply.

Infants & children:
Use only under medical supervision.

Prolonged use:
Not intended for long-term use.

Skin & sunlight:
No special problems expected.

Driving, piloting or hazardous work:
Avoid if you experience dizziness after taking drug, otherwise no problems expected.

Discontinuing:
Don't discontinue without doctor's advice until you complete prescribed dose, even though symptoms diminish or disappear.

Others:
- Advise any doctor or dentist whom you consult that you take this medicine.
- If symptoms don't improve within a few days, or if they worsen, consult doctor.
- If drug is prescribed for genital herpes, be sure you use proper precautions to prevent spreading the disorder to your sexual partner. If unsure, ask your doctor for information.
- Keep affected skin area clean and dry.
- Decrease blister irritation by wearing loose-fitting clothing.

POSSIBLE INTERACTION WITH OTHER DRUGS

GENERIC NAME OR DRUG CLASS	COMBINED EFFECT
Bone marrow depressants*	Increased risk of bone marrow depression with ganciclovir.
Cimetidine	Increased antiviral effect.
Nephrotoxic medications*	Increased risk of nephrotoxicity.
Zidovudine	Increased effect of zidovudine. Use with caution.

POSSIBLE INTERACTION WITH OTHER SUBSTANCES

INTERACTS WITH	COMBINED EFFECT
Alcohol:	None expected.
Beverages:	None expected.
Cocaine:	None expected.
Foods:	None expected.
Marijuana:	None expected.
Tobacco:	None expected.

*See Glossary

ANTIVIRALS FOR INFLUENZA

GENERIC AND BRAND NAMES

AMANTIDINE	**RIMANTIDINE**
Symadine	Flumadine
Symmetrel	

BASIC INFORMATION

Habit forming? No
Prescription needed? Yes
Available as generic? Yes
Drug class: Antiviral, antiparkinsonism

USES

- Prevention and treatment for Type-A flu infections.
- Relief for symptoms of Parkinson's disease (amantidine).

DOSAGE & USAGE INFORMATION

How to take:
- Capsule—Swallow with liquid or food to lessen stomach irritation.
- Syrup—Dilute dose in beverage before swallowing.

When to take:
At the same times each day. For Type-A flu it is especially important to take regular doses as prescribed.

If you forget a dose:
Take as soon as you remember. Wait 4 hours for next dose. Return to schedule.

What drug does:
- Type-A flu—May block penetration of tissue cells by infectious material from virus cells.
- Parkinson's disease and drug-induced extrapyramidal* reactions—Improves muscular condition and coordination.

Continued next column

OVERDOSE

SYMPTOMS:
Heart rhythm disturbances, blood pressure drop, convulsions, hallucinations, violent behavior, confusion, slurred speech, rolling eyes.
WHAT TO DO:
- Dial 911 (emergency) or 0 (operator) for an ambulance or medical help. Then give first aid immediately.
- See emergency information on inside covers.

Time lapse before drug works:
- Type-A flu—48 hours.
- Parkinson's disease—2 days to 2 weeks.

Don't take with:
- Alcohol
- Any other medicine without consulting your doctor or pharmacist.

POSSIBLE ADVERSE REACTIONS OR SIDE EFFECTS

SYMPTOMS	WHAT TO DO
Life-threatening: In case of overdose, see previous column.	
Common: Headache, difficulty in concentrating, dizziness or lightheadedness, insomnia, irritability, nervousness, nightmares (these side effects infrequent with rimantadine).	Continue. Call doctor when convenient.
Infrequent:	
• With amantadine— Blurred or changed vision, confusion, difficult urination, hallucinations, fainting.	Discontinue. Call doctor right away.
• Constipation; dry mouth, nose or throat; vomiting, appetite loss, nausea.	Continue. Call doctor when convenient.
Rare:	
• With amantadine— Swelling or irritated eyes; depression; swelling of hands, legs or feet; skin rash.	Discontinue. Call doctor right away.
• Seizures (may occur in persons with a history of seizures).	Discontinue. Seek emergency help.

WARNINGS & PRECAUTIONS

Don't take if:
You are allergic to amantadine or rimantadine.

Before you start, consult your doctor:
- If you have had epilepsy or other seizures.
- If you have had heart disease or heart failure.
- If you have had liver or kidney disease.
- If you have had peptic ulcers.
- If you have had eczema or skin rashes.
- If you have had emotional or mental disorders or taken drugs for them.

Over age 60:
Adverse reactions and side effects may be more frequent and severe than in younger persons.

Pregnancy:
Decide with your doctor whether benefits justify risk to unborn child. Risk category C (see page xxiii).

Breast-feeding:
Drug may pass into milk. Avoid drug or discontinue nursing until you finish medicine. Consult doctor for advice on maintaining milk supply.

Infants & children:
Use only under medical supervision.

Prolonged use:
Skin splotches, feet swelling, rapid weight gain, shortness of breath. Consult doctor.

Skin & sunlight:
One or more drugs in this group may cause rash or intensify sunburn in areas exposed to sun or ultraviolet light (photosensitivity reaction). Avoid overexposure. Notify doctor if reaction occurs.

Driving, piloting or hazardous work:
Don't drive or pilot aircraft until you learn how medicine affects you. Don't work around dangerous machinery. Don't climb ladders or work in high places. Danger increases if you drink alcohol or take medicine affecting alertness and reflexes.

Discontinuing:
- Parkinson's disease—Don't discontinue without doctor's advice until you complete prescribed dose, even though symptoms diminish or disappear.
- Type-A flu—Discontinue 48 hours after symptoms disappear.

Others:
- Parkinson's disease—May lose effectiveness in 3 to 6 months. Consult doctor.
- These drugs are not effective for influenza-B virus.
- Drug-resistant strains of the virus may occur within the same household.

 ## POSSIBLE INTERACTION WITH OTHER DRUGS

GENERIC NAME OR DRUG CLASS	COMBINED EFFECT
Acetaminophen	With rimantadine—Decreased antiviral effect.
Anticholinergics*	With amantadine—Increased benefit, but excessive anticholinergic dose produces mental confusion, hallucinations, delirium.
Antidepressants, tricyclic*	With amantadine—Increased risk of confusion, hallucinations, nightmares.
Antidyskinetics*	With amantadine—Increased risk of confusion, hallucinations, nightmares.
Antihistamines*	With amantadine—Increased risk of confusion, hallucinations, nightmares.
Aspirin	With rimantadine—Decreased antiviral effect.
Central nervous system (CNS) stimulants*	With amantadine—Increased risk of adverse reactions.
Levodopa	With amantadine—Increased benefit of levodopa. Can cause agitation.

 ## POSSIBLE INTERACTION WITH OTHER SUBSTANCES

INTERACTS WITH	COMBINED EFFECT
Alcohol:	Increased alcohol effect. Possible fainting.
Beverages:	None expected.
Cocaine:	Dangerous overstimulation.
Foods:	None expected.
Marijuana:	None expected.
Tobacco:	None expected.

*See Glossary

ANTIVIRALS (Ophthalmic)

GENERIC AND BRAND NAMES

IDOXURIDINE
Herplex Eye Drops
Stoxil Eye Ointment

TRIFLURIDINE
Trifluorothymidine
Viroptic

BASIC INFORMATION

Habit forming? No
Prescription needed? Yes
Available as generic? No
Drug class: Antiviral (ophthalmic)

 USES

Treats virus infections of the eye (usually herpes simplex virus).

 DOSAGE & USAGE INFORMATION

How to use:
Eye drops
- Wash hands.
- Apply pressure to inside corner of eye with middle finger.
- Continue pressure for 1 minute after placing medicine in eye.
- Tilt head backward. Pull lower lid away from eye with index finger of the same hand.
- Drop eye drops into pouch and close eye. Don't blink.
- Keep eyes closed for 1 to 2 minutes.

Eye ointment
- Wash hands.
- Pull lower lid down from eye to form a pouch.
- Squeeze tube to apply thin strip of ointment into pouch.
- Close eye for 1 to 2 minutes.
- Don't touch applicator tip to any surface (including the eye). If you accidentally touch tip, clean with warm soap and water.
- Keep container tightly closed.
- Keep cool, but don't freeze.
- Wash hands immediately after using.

Continued next column

 OVERDOSE

SYMPTOMS:
None expected.
WHAT TO DO:
Not intended for internal use. If child accidentally swallows, call poison control center.

When to use:
As directed. Usually 1 drop every 2 hours up to maximum of 9 drops daily.

If you forget a dose:
Use as soon as you remember.

What drug does:
Destroys reproductive capacity of virus.

Time lapse before drug works:
Begins work immediately. Usual course of treatment is 7 days.

Don't use with:
Other eye drops, boric acid or ointment without consulting doctor.

 POSSIBLE ADVERSE REACTIONS OR SIDE EFFECTS

SYMPTOMS	WHAT TO DO
Life-threatening None expected.	
Common Stinging or burning eyes.	Continue. Tell doctor at next visit.
Infrequent Blurred vision for a few minutes (with ointment).	No action necessary.
Rare Itchy, red eyes; swollen eyelid or eye; excess flow of tears; dimming or haziness of vision.	Discontinue. Call doctor right away.

WARNINGS & PRECAUTIONS

Don't use if:
You are allergic to trifluridine or idoxuridine.

Before you start, consult your doctor:
- If you have had any other eye problems.
- If you use eye drops for glaucoma.

Over age 60:
No problems expected.

Pregnancy:
Risk factors vary for drugs in this group. See category list on page xxiii and consult doctor.

Breast-feeding:
No problems expected, but safety not established. Consult doctor.

Infants & children:
Use only under close medical supervision.

Prolonged use:
Avoid unless directed by your eye doctor.

Skin & sunlight:
No problems expected.

Driving, piloting or hazardous work:
No problems expected.

Discontinuing:
Don't discontinue without consulting doctor.

Others:
- Don't use more often or longer than prescribed.
- Keep cool, but don't freeze.
- If problem doesn't improve within a week, notify your doctor.

POSSIBLE INTERACTION WITH OTHER DRUGS

GENERIC NAME OR DRUG CLASS	COMBINED EFFECT
Eye products containing boric acid	Increased risk of toxicity to eye.

POSSIBLE INTERACTION WITH OTHER SUBSTANCES

INTERACTS WITH	COMBINED EFFECT
Alcohol:	None expected.
Beverages:	None expected.
Cocaine:	None expected.
Foods:	None expected.
Marijuana:	None expected.
Tobacco:	None expected.

ANTIVIRALS (Topical)

GENERIC AND BRAND NAMES

ACYCLOVIR
Zovirax Ointment

PENCICLOVIR
Denavir

BASIC INFORMATION

Habit forming? No
Prescription needed? Yes
Available as generic? No
Drug class: Antiviral

 ## USES

- Treatment of symptoms of herpes infections of the skin, mucous membranes, lips, mouth and genitals.
- May be used for other skin disorders as prescribed by your doctor.

 ## DOSAGE & USAGE INFORMATION

How to take:
- Acyclovir ointment—Apply to skin and mucous membranes every 3 hours (6 times a day) for 7 days. Use rubber glove when applying. Apply 1/2-inch strip to each sore or blister. Wash before using.
- Penciclovir cream—Use only on lips and face. Avoid eye area. Use every 2 hours, while awake, for 4 days.

When to use:
Use as soon as symptoms begin to appear (burning, pain or blisters).

If you forget a dose:
Apply as soon as you remember, then continue with regular schedule.

What drug does:
- Inhibits reproduction of virus in cells without killing normal cells.
- Does not cure. Herpes breakout often recurs.

Time lapse before drug works:
2 hours.

Don't take with:
Any other topical medicine without consulting your doctor or pharmacist.

 ## OVERDOSE

SYMPTOMS:
None expected.
WHAT TO DO:
If person accidentally swallows topical form of drug, call doctor, poison control center or hospital emergency room for instructions.

 ## POSSIBLE ADVERSE REACTIONS OR SIDE EFFECTS

SYMPTOMS	WHAT TO DO
Life-threatening: None expected.	
Common: May cause mild pain, burning, itching or stinging.	Continue. Call doctor when convenient.
Infrequent: None expected.	
Rare: Skin rash.	Continue. Call doctor when convenient.

WARNINGS & PRECAUTIONS

Don't take if:
You are allergic to topical acyclovir or penciclovir.

Before you start, consult your doctor:
If you are allergic to any medication, food or other substance.

Over age 60:
Adverse reactions and side effects may be more frequent and severe than in younger persons.

Pregnancy:
Decide with your doctor whether drug benefits justify risk to unborn child. Risk category C (see page xxiii).

Breast-feeding:
Is is unknown if topical antivirals are absorbed and then pass into breast milk. Consult doctor.

Infants & children:
Use only under special medical supervision.

Prolonged use:
Don't use longer than prescribed time.

Skin & sunlight:
No problems expected.

Driving, piloting or hazardous work:
No problems expected.

Discontinuing:
May be unnecessary to finish medicine. Follow doctor's instructions.

Others:
- Women: Get pap smear every 6 months because those with herpes infections are possibly at increased risk to develop cancer of the cervix. Avoid sexual activity until all blisters or sores heal.
- Don't get topical medicine in eyes.
- Check with doctor if no improvement in 1 week.

POSSIBLE INTERACTION WITH OTHER DRUGS

GENERIC NAME OR DRUG CLASS	COMBINED EFFECT
None expected.	

POSSIBLE INTERACTION WITH OTHER SUBSTANCES

INTERACTS WITH	COMBINED EFFECT
Alcohol:	No problems expected.
Beverages:	No problems expected.
Cocaine:	No problems expected.
Foods:	No problems expected.
Marijuana:	No problems expected.
Tobacco:	No problems expected.

APPETITE SUPPRESSANTS

GENERIC AND BRAND NAMES

See complete list of generic and brand names in the *Generic and Brand Name Directory*, page 872.

BASIC INFORMATION

Habit forming? Yes
Prescription needed? Yes
Available as generic? Yes
Drug class: Appetite suppressant

USES

Suppresses appetite. Temporary treatment for obesity.

DOSAGE & USAGE INFORMATION

How to take:
- Tablet or capsule—Swallow with liquid. You may chew or crush tablet.
- Extended-release tablets or capsules—Swallow each dose whole with liquid; do not crush.
- Elixir—Swallow with liquid.

When to take:
- Long-acting forms—10 to 14 hours before bedtime.
- Short-acting forms—1 hour before meals. Last dose no later than 4 to 6 hours before bedtime.

If you forget a dose:
- Long-acting form—Take as soon as you remember up to 2 hours late. If more than 2 hours, wait for next scheduled dose (don't double this dose).
- Short-acting form—Wait for next scheduled dose. Don't double this dose.

Continued next column

OVERDOSE

SYMPTOMS:
Irritability, overactivity, trembling, insomnia, mood changes, fever, rapid heartbeat, confusion, disorientation, hallucinations, convulsions, coma.
WHAT TO DO:
- **Dial 911 (emergency) or 0 (operator) for an ambulance or medical help. Then give first aid immediately.**
- **See emergency information on inside covers.**

What drug does:
Apparently stimulates brain's appetite control center.

Time lapse before drug works:
Begins in 1 hour. Short-acting form lasts 4 hours. Long-acting form lasts 14 hours.

Don't take with:
Nonprescription drugs without consulting doctor.

POSSIBLE ADVERSE REACTIONS OR SIDE EFFECTS

SYMPTOMS	WHAT TO DO
Life-threatening: In case of overdose, see previous column.	
Common: Irritability, nervousness, insomnia, false sense of well-being.	Continue. Call doctor when convenient.
Infrequent:	
• Irregular or pounding heartbeat, urgent or difficult urination.	Discontinue. Call doctor right away.
• Blurred vision, unpleasant taste or dry mouth, constipation or diarrhea, nausea, vomiting, cramps, changes in sex drive, increased sweating, headache, nightmares, weakness.	Continue. Call doctor when convenient.
Rare:	
• Rash or hives, breathing difficulty.	Discontinue. Call doctor right away.
• Hair loss.	Continue. Call doctor when convenient.

WARNINGS & PRECAUTIONS

Don't take if:
- You are allergic to any sympathomimetic or phenylpropanolamine.
- You have glaucoma.
- You have taken MAO inhibitors within 2 weeks.
- You plan to become pregnant within medication period.
- You have a history of drug or alcohol abuse.
- You have irregular or rapid heartbeat.

Before you start, consult your doctor:
- If you have high blood pressure or heart disease.
- If you have an overactive thyroid, nervous tension or anxiety.
- If you have epilepsy.
- If you will have surgery within 2 months, including dental surgery, requiring general or spinal anesthesia.
- If you take any other nonprescription medicine.

Over age 60:
Adverse reactions and side effects may be more frequent and severe than in younger persons.

Pregnancy:
Risk factors vary for drugs in this group. See category list on page xxiii and consult doctor.

Breast-feeding:
Safety not established. Consult doctor.

Infants & children:
Don't give to children younger than 12.

Prolonged use:
- Loses effectiveness. Avoid.
- Talk to your doctor about the need for follow-up medical examinations or laboratory studies.

Skin & sunlight:
No problems expected.

Driving, piloting or hazardous work:
Don't drive or pilot aircraft until you learn how medicine affects you. Don't work around dangerous machinery. Don't climb ladders or work in high places. Danger increases if you drink alcohol or take medicine affecting alertness and reflexes, such as antihistamines, tranquilizers, sedatives, pain medicine, narcotics and mind-altering drugs.

Discontinuing:
- Don't discontinue without consulting doctor. Dose may require gradual reduction if you have taken drug for a long time. Doses of other drugs may also require adjustment.
- Consult doctor if following symptoms occur after stopping the drug—depression, nausea and vomiting, stomach cramps, insomnia, nightmares, extreme tiredness or weakness.

Others:
- Don't increase dose without doctor's approval.
- Advise any doctor or dentist whom you consult that you take this medicine.

POSSIBLE INTERACTION WITH OTHER DRUGS

GENERIC NAME OR DRUG CLASS	COMBINED EFFECT
Antidiabetic agents*, oral or insulin	May require dosage adjustment of anti-diabetic agent.
Antihypertensives*	Decreased anti-hypertensive effect.
Appetite suppressants, other*	Dangerous overstimulation.
Caffeine	Increased stimulant effect.
Central nervous system (CNS) depressants*	Increased depressive effects of both drugs.
Central nervous system (CNS) stimulants*	Increased stimulant effects of both drugs.
Guanethidine	Decreased guanethidine effect.
Methyldopa	Decreased methyldopa effect.
Monoamine oxidase (MAO) inhibitors*	Dangerous blood pressure rise.
Phenothiazines*	Decreased appetite suppressant effect.
Rauwolfia alkaloids*	Decreased effect of rauwolfia alkaloids.

POSSIBLE INTERACTION WITH OTHER SUBSTANCES

INTERACTS WITH	COMBINED EFFECT
Alcohol:	Increased sedation.
Beverages: Caffeine drinks.	Excessive stimulation.
Cocaine:	Convulsions or excessive nervousness.
Foods:	None expected.
Marijuana:	Frequent use— Irregular heartbeat.
Tobacco:	None expected.

ASPIRIN

BRAND NAMES

See complete list of brand names in the *Generic and Brand Name Directory*, page 873.

BASIC INFORMATION

Habit forming? No
Prescription needed? No
Available as generic? Yes
Drug class: Analgesic, anti-inflammatory (nonsteroidal)

USES

- Reduces pain, fever, inflammation.
- Relieves swelling, stiffness, joint pain of arthritis or rheumatism.
- Antiplatelet effect to reduce chances of heart attack and/or stroke.

DOSAGE & USAGE INFORMATION

How to take:

- Tablet or capsule—Swallow with liquid or food to lessen stomach irritation.
- Extended-release tablets or capsules—Swallow each dose whole.
- Effervescent tablets—Dissolve in water.
- Chewing gum tablets—Chew completely. Don't swallow whole.
- Dispersible tablets—Dissolve in the mouth before swallowing.
- Chewable tablets—Chew before swallowing or dissolve in small amount of liquid before swallowing.

Continued next column

OVERDOSE

SYMPTOMS:

- **Mild overdose—Confusion, severe diarrhea, stomach pain, increased thirst, vision problems, ringing or buzzing in ears, dizziness, lightheadedness, severe headache.**
- **Severe overdose—Bloody urine; hallucinations; severe nervousness, excitement or confusion; shortness of breath; trouble breathing; convulsions.**
- **In some children—The only symptoms may be behavior changes, severe drowsiness or tiredness, fast or deep breathing.**

WHAT TO DO:

- **Dial 911 (emergency) or 0 (operator) for an ambulance or medical help. Then give first aid immediately.**
- **See emergency information on inside covers.**

- Suppositories—Remove wrapper and moisten suppository with water. Gently insert into rectum, large end first.

When to take:
Pain, fever, inflammation—As needed, no more often than every 4 hours.

If you forget a dose:
- Pain, fever—Take as soon as you remember. Wait 4 hours for next dose.
- Arthritis—Take as soon as you remember up to 2 hours late. Return to regular schedule.

What drug does:
- Affects hypothalamus, the part of the brain which regulates temperature by dilating small blood vessels in skin.
- Prevents clumping of platelets (small blood cells) so blood vessels remain open.
- Decreases prostaglandin effect.
- Suppresses body's pain messages.

Time lapse before drug works:
30 minutes for pain, fever, arthritis.

Don't take with:
- Tetracyclines. Space doses 1 hour apart.
- Any other medicine without consulting your doctor or pharmacist.

POSSIBLE ADVERSE REACTIONS OR SIDE EFFECTS

SYMPTOMS	WHAT TO DO
Life-threatening: Black or bloody vomit; blood in urine; difficulty breathing; hives, rash, intense itching, faintness soon after a dose (anaphylaxis).	Seek emergency treatment immediately.
Common: Heartburn, indigestion, mild nausea or vomiting.	Continue. Call doctor when convenient.
Infrequent: Trouble sleeping; rectal irritation (with suppository).	Continue. Call doctor when convenient.
Rare: Severe headache, convulsions, extreme drowsiness, flushing or other change in skin color, any loss of hearing, severe vomiting, swelling of face, vision problems, bloody or black stools, ringing in ears, severe stomach cramps or pain (all symptoms more likely with repeated doses for long periods since aspirin can build up in the body).	Discontinue. Call doctor right away or seek emergency treatment

WARNINGS & PRECAUTIONS

Don't take if:
- You need to restrict sodium in your diet. Buffered effervescent tablets and sodium salicylate are high in sodium.
- You are sensitive to aspirin or aspirin has a strong vinegar-like odor, which means it has decomposed.
- You have a peptic ulcer of stomach or duodenum or a bleeding disorder.

Before you start, consult your doctor:
- If you have had stomach or duodenal ulcers.
- If you have had gout.
- If you have asthma or nasal polyps.
- If you have kidney or liver disease.

Over age 60:
More likely to cause hidden bleeding in stomach or intestines. Watch for dark stools.

Pregnancy:
Risk category C; D in third trimester (see page xxiii). Consult doctor.

Breast-feeding:
Drug passes into milk. Avoid drug or discontinue nursing until you finish medicine. Consult doctor for advice on maintaining milk supply.

Infants & children:
- Overdose frequent and severe. Keep bottles out of children's reach.
- Do not give to persons under age 18 who have fever and discomfort of viral illness, especially chicken pox and influenza. Probably increases risk of Reye's syndrome.

Prolonged use:
- Talk to your doctor about the need for follow-up medical examinations or laboratory studies to check liver function, complete blood counts (white blood cell count, platelet count, red blood cell count, hemoglobin, hematocrit).
- Kidney damage may result. Periodic kidney function tests recommended.

Skin & sunlight:
No special problems expected.

Driving, piloting or hazardous work:
No restrictions unless you feel drowsy.

Discontinuing:
For chronic illness—Don't discontinue without doctor's advice until you complete prescribed dose, even though symptoms diminish or disappear.

Others:
- Aspirin can complicate surgery, pregnancy, labor and delivery, and illness.
- For arthritis—Don't change dose without consulting doctor.
- Urine tests for blood sugar may be inaccurate.
- Don't take if pills have vinegar-like odor.

POSSIBLE INTERACTION WITH OTHER DRUGS

GENERIC NAME OR DRUG CLASS	COMBINED EFFECT
Acebutolol	Decreased anti-hypertensive effect of acebutolol.
Adrenocorticoids, systemic	Increased adreno-corticoid effect.
Alendronate	Increased risk of stomach irritation.
Allopurinol	Decreased allopurinol effect.
Angiotensin-converting enzyme (ACE) inhibitors*	Decreased ACE inhibitor effect.
Antacids*	Decreased aspirin effect.
Anticoagulants*	Increased anti-coagulant effect. Abnormal bleeding.
Antidiabetic agents, oral*	Low blood sugar.
Anti-inflammatory drugs nonsteroidal (NSAIDs)*	Risk of stomach bleeding and ulcers.
Bumetanide	Possible aspirin toxicity.
Carteolol	Decreased anti-hypertensive effect of carteolol.

Continued on page 904

POSSIBLE INTERACTION WITH OTHER SUBSTANCES

INTERACTS WITH	COMBINED EFFECT
Alcohol:	Possible stomach irritation and bleeding. Avoid.
Beverages:	None expected.
Cocaine:	None expected.
Foods:	None expected.
Marijuana:	Possible increased pain relief, but marijuana may slow body's recovery. Avoid.
Tobacco:	None expected.

*See Glossary

ATOVAQUONE

BRAND NAMES

Mepron

BASIC INFORMATION

Habit forming? No
Prescription needed? Yes
Available as generic? No
Drug class: Antiprotozoal

USES

- Treats mild to moderate pneumocystis carinii pneumonia.
- May be effective for other parasitic infections such as toxoplasmosis and malaria.

DOSAGE & USAGE INFORMATION

How to take:
Tablet—Swallow with liquid. If you cannot swallow whole, crumble tablet and take with liquid or food.

When to take:
At the same times each day. Take with meals that are high in fat (eggs, cheese, butter, milk, meat, pizza, nuts) to increase absorption.

If you forget a dose:
Take as soon as you remember up to 2 hours late. If more than 2 hours, wait for next scheduled dose (don't double this dose).

What drug does:
Stops harmful growth of susceptible organisms.

Time lapse before drug works:
3 weeks.

Don't take with:
Any other prescription or nonprescription drug without consulting your doctor or pharmacist.

OVERDOSE

SYMPTOMS:
None expected.
WHAT TO DO:
Overdose unlikely to threaten life. If person takes much larger amount than prescribed, call doctor, poison control center or hospital emergency room for instructions.

POSSIBLE ADVERSE REACTIONS OR SIDE EFFECTS

SYMPTOMS	WHAT TO DO
Life-threatening: None expected.	
Common:	
• Fever, skin rash.	Discontinue. Call doctor right away.
• Nausea or vomiting, diarrhea, headache, cough, trouble sleeping.	Continue. Call doctor when convenient.
Infrequent: None expected.	
Rare: None expected	

WARNINGS & PRECAUTIONS

Don't take if:
You are allergic to atovaquone.

Before you start, consult your doctor:
If you have any gastrointestinal disorder.

Over age 60:
No problems expected.

Pregnancy:
Discuss with your doctor whether drug benefits justify risk to unborn child. Risk category C (see page xxiii).

Breast-feeding:
Not known if drug passes into breast milk. Avoid drug or discontinue nursing until you finish medicine. Consult doctor for advice on maintaining milk supply.

Infants & children:
Give only under close medical supervision.

Prolonged use:
Not intended for long-term use.

Skin & sunlight:
No problems expected.

Driving, piloting or hazardous work:
No problems expected.

Discontinuing:
No problems expected.

Others:
- Advise any doctor or dentist whom you consult that you take this medicine.
- May affect the results in some medical tests.
- Talk to your doctor about the need for follow-up medical examinations or laboratory studies to check blood counts and liver function.

POSSIBLE INTERACTION WITH OTHER DRUGS

GENERIC NAME OR DRUG CLASS	COMBINED EFFECT
None significant.	

POSSIBLE INTERACTION WITH OTHER SUBSTANCES

INTERACTS WITH	COMBINED EFFECT
Alcohol:	None expected.
Beverages:	None expected.
Cocaine:	None expected.
Foods:	None expected.
Marijuana:	None expected.
Tobacco:	None expected.

ATROPINE, HYOSCYAMINE, METHENAMINE, METHYLENE BLUE, PHENYLSALICYLATE & BENZOIC ACID

BRAND NAMES

Atrosept
Dolsed
Hexalol
Prosed/DS
Trac Tabs 2X
UAA
Uridon Modified
Urimed

Urinary
  Antiseptic No. 2
Urised
Uriseptic
Uritab
Uritin
Uro-Ves
U-Tract

BASIC INFORMATION

Habit forming? No
Prescription needed? Yes
Available as generic? No
Drug class: Analgesic (urinary), anti-spasmodic, anti-infective (urinary)

USES

A combination medicine to control infection, spasms and pain caused by urinary tract infections.

DOSAGE & USAGE INFORMATION

How to take:
Tablet—Swallow with liquid or food to lessen stomach irritation.

When to take:
30 minutes before meals (unless directed otherwise by doctor).

Continued next column

OVERDOSE

SYMPTOMS:
Dilated pupils, rapid pulse and breathing, dizziness, fever, hallucinations, confusion, slurred speech, agitation, flushed face, convulsions, coma.
WHAT TO DO:
- Dial 911 (emergency) or 0 (operator) for an ambulance or medical help. Then give first aid immediately.
- See emergency information on inside covers.

If you forget a dose:
Take as soon as you remember up to 2 hours late. If more than 2 hours, wait for next scheduled dose (don't double this dose).

What drug does:
Makes urine acid. Blocks nerve impulses at parasympathetic nerve endings, preventing muscle contractions and gland secretions of organs involved. Methenamine destroys some germs.

Time lapse before drug works:
15 to 30 minutes.

Don't take with:
- Antacids* or antidiarrheals*.
- Any other medicine without consulting your doctor or pharmacist.

POSSIBLE ADVERSE REACTIONS OR SIDE EFFECTS

SYMPTOMS	WHAT TO DO
Life-threatening: Heartbeat irregularity, shortness of breath or difficulty breathing.	Seek emergency treatment immediately.
Common: Dry mouth, throat, ears, nose.	Continue. Call doctor when convenient.
Infrequent: • Flushed, red face; drowsiness; difficult urination; nausea and vomiting; abdominal pain; ringing or buzzing in ears; severe drowsiness; back pain; lightheadedness.	Discontinue. Call doctor right away.
• Headache, nasal congestion, altered taste.	Continue. Call doctor when convenient.
Rare: Blurred vision; pain in eyes; skin rash, hives.	Discontinue. Seek emergency treatment.

WARNINGS & PRECAUTIONS

Don't take if:
- You are allergic to any of the ingredients or aspirin.
- Brain damage in child.
- You have glaucoma.

ATROPINE, HYOSCYAMINE, METHENAMINE, METHYLENE BLUE, PHENYLSALICYLATE & BENZOIC ACID

Before you start, consult your doctor:
- If you are on any special diet such as low-sodium.
- If you have had a hiatal hernia, bronchitis, asthma, liver disease, stomach or duodenal ulcers.
- If you have asthma, nasal polyps, bleeding disorder, glaucoma or enlarged prostate.
- If you will have any surgery within 2 months.
- If you have heart disease.

Over age 60:
- Adverse reactions and side effects may be more frequent and severe than in younger persons.
- More likely to cause hidden bleeding in stomach or intestines. Watch for dark stools.

Pregnancy:
Risk factors vary for drugs in this group. See category list on page xxiii and consult doctor.

Breast-feeding:
Drug passes into milk. Avoid or discontinue nursing until you finish medicine.

Infants & children:
Side effects more likely. Not recommended in children under 12.

Prolonged use:
May lead to constipation or kidney damage. Request lab studies to monitor effects of prolonged use.

Skin & sunlight:
No problems expected.

Driving, piloting or hazardous work:
May disqualify for piloting aircraft during time you take medicine.

Discontinuing:
May be unnecessary to finish medicine. Follow your symptoms and doctor's advice.

Others:
- Salicylates can complicate surgery, pregnancy, labor and delivery, and illness.
- Urine tests for blood sugar may be inaccurate.
- Drink cranberry juice or eat prunes or plums to help make urine more acid.

POSSIBLE INTERACTION WITH OTHER DRUGS

GENERIC NAME OR DRUG CLASS	COMBINED EFFECT
Allopurinol	Decreased allopurinol effect.
Amantadine	Increased atropine and belladonna effect.
Antacids*	Decreased salicylate and methenamine effect.
Anticoagulants*	Increased anticoagulant effect. Abnormal bleeding.
Anticholinergics, other*	Increased atropine and belladonna effect.
Antidepressants, other*	Increased sedation.
Antidiabetics, oral*	Low blood sugar.
Antihistamines*	Increased atropine and hyoscyamine effect.
Anti-inflammatory drugs, nonsteroidal (NSAIDs)*	Risk of stomach bleeding and ulcers.
Aspirin	Likely salicylate toxicity.
Beta-adrenergic blocking agents*	Decreased antihypertensive effect.
Carbonic anhydrase inhibitors*	Decreased methenamine effect.
Cortisone drugs*	Increased internal eye pressure, increased cortisone effect. Risk of ulcers and stomach bleeding.

Continued on page 904

POSSIBLE INTERACTION WITH OTHER SUBSTANCES

INTERACTS WITH	COMBINED EFFECT
Alcohol:	Excessive sedation. Possible stomach irritation and bleeding. Avoid.
Beverages:	None expected.
Cocaine:	Excessively rapid heartbeat. Avoid.
Foods:	None expected.
Marijuana:	Drowsiness and dry mouth. May slow body's recovery.
Tobacco:	Dry mouth.

*See Glossary

137

ATTAPULGITE

BRAND NAMES

Diar-Aid
Diasorb
Fowlers Diarrhea
    Tablets
Kaopectate
Kaopectate Advanced
    Formula
Kaopectate
    Maximum Strength
Rheaban
St. Joseph
    Antidiarrheal

BASIC INFORMATION

Habit forming? No
Prescription needed? No
Available as generic? Yes
Drug class: Antidiarrheal

USES

Treats diarrhea. Used in conjunction with fluids, appropriate diet and rest. Treats symptoms only. Does not cure any disorder that causes diarrhea.

DOSAGE & USAGE INFORMATION

How to take:
- Tablets—Swallow with liquid. If you can't swallow whole, crumble tablet and take with liquid or food. Instructions to take on empty stomach mean 1 hour before or 2 hours after eating.
- Chewable tablets—Chew well before swallowing.
- Oral suspension—Follow label instructions.

When to take:
2 hours before or 3 hours after taking any other oral medications. Outside of this restriction, take a dose after each loose bowel movement until diarrhea is controlled.

If you forget a dose:
Take as soon as you remember, then resume regular schedule.

Continued next column

OVERDOSE

SYMPTOMS:
None expected.
WHAT TO DO:
Overdose unlikely to threaten life. If person takes much larger amount than prescribed, call doctor, poison control center or hospital emergency room for instructions.

What drug does:
Absorbs bacteria and toxins and reduces water loss. Attapulgite does not get absorbed into the body.

Time lapse before drug works:
5 to 8 hours.

Don't take with:
Any other medicine without consulting your doctor or pharmacist.

POSSIBLE ADVERSE REACTIONS OR SIDE EFFECTS

SYMPTOMS	WHAT TO DO
Life-threatening: None expected.	
Common: None expected.	
Infrequent: Constipation (usually mild and of short duration).	Continue. Call doctor when convenient.
Rare: None expected.	

WARNINGS & PRECAUTIONS

Don't take if:
- You are allergic to attapulgite.
- You or your doctor suspects intestinal obstruction.

Before you start, consult your doctor:
If you are dehydrated (signs are a dry mouth, loose skin, sunken eyes and parched lips).

Over age 60:
- Dehydration is more likely in this age group.
- Side effects of constipation are more likely.

Pregnancy:
Risk category not designated. See list on page xxiii and consult doctor.

Breast-feeding:
No problems expected, but consult doctor.

Infants & children:
Use only under close medical supervision for children up to 3 years of age. This age group is quite susceptible to fluid and electrolyte loss.

Prolonged use:
Not intended for prolonged use.

Skin & sunlight:
No special problems expected.

Driving, piloting or hazardous work:
No special problems expected.

Discontinuing:
May be unnecessary to finish medicine. Follow doctor's instructions.

Others:
No special problems expected.

POSSIBLE INTERACTION WITH OTHER DRUGS

GENERIC NAME OR DRUG CLASS	COMBINED EFFECT
Digitalis	May decrease effectiveness of digitalis.
Lincomycin*	May decrease effectiveness of lincomycins.
Any other medicine taken by mouth	When taken at the same time, neither drug may be as effective. Take other medicines 2 hours before or 3 hours after attapulgite.

POSSIBLE INTERACTION WITH OTHER SUBSTANCES

INTERACTS WITH	COMBINED EFFECT
Alcohol:	No proven problems.
Beverages:	No proven problems.
Cocaine:	No proven problems.
Foods: Prunes, prune juice and other fruits or foods that may cause diarrhea.	Decreased effect of attapulgite.
Marijuana:	No proven problems.
Tobacco:	No proven problems.

AZATHIOPRINE

BRAND NAMES

Imuran

BASIC INFORMATION

Habit forming? No
Prescription needed? Yes
Available as generic? Yes
Drug class: Immunosuppressant, antirheumatic

 USES

- Protects against rejection of transplanted organs (e.g., kidney, heart).
- Treats severe active rheumatoid arthritis and other immunologic diseases if simpler treatment plans have been ineffective.

 DOSAGE & USAGE INFORMATION

How to take:
Tablets—Swallow with liquid. If you can't swallow whole, crumble tablet and take with liquid or food. Instructions to take on empty stomach mean 1 hour before or 2 hours after eating.

When to take:
Follow your doctor's instructions. Usually once a day.

If you forget a dose:
Take as soon as you remember up to 2 hours late. If more than 2 hours, wait for next scheduled dose (don't double this dose).

What drug does:
Unknown; probably inhibits synthesis of DNA and RNA.

Time lapse before drug works:
6 to 8 weeks.

Don't take with:
Any other medicines (including over-the-counter drugs such as cough and cold medicines, laxatives, antacids, diet pills, caffeine, nose drops or vitamins) without consulting your doctor.

 OVERDOSE

SYMPTOMS:
None expected.
WHAT TO DO:
Overdose unlikely to threaten life. If person takes much larger amount than prescribed, call doctor, poison control center or hospital emergency room for instructions.

 POSSIBLE ADVERSE REACTIONS OR SIDE EFFECTS

SYMPTOMS	WHAT TO DO
Life-threatening: Rapid heart rate, sudden fever, muscle or joint pain, cough, shortness of breath.	Seek emergency treatment immediately.
Common: • Infection or low blood count causing fever and chills, back pain cough, painful urination; anemia (tiredness or weakness); nausea; vomiting.	Discontinue. Call doctor right away.
• Appetite loss.	Continue. Call doctor when convenient.
Infrequent: Jaundice (yellow eyes, skin), skin rash.	Discontinue. Call doctor right away.
Rare: Low platelet count causing bleeding or bruising, tarry or black stools, bloody urine, red spots under skin; severe abdominal pain; mouth sores.	Discontinue. Call doctor right away.

WARNINGS & PRECAUTIONS

Don't take if:
- You are allergic to azathioprine
- You have chicken pox.
- You have shingles (herpes zoster).

Before you start, consult your doctor:
- If you have gout.
- If you have liver or kidney disease.
- If you have an infection.

Over age 60:
Adverse reactions and side effects may be more frequent and severe than in younger persons. You may need smaller doses for shorter periods of time.

Pregnancy:
Risk to unborn child outweighs drug benefits. Don't use. Risk category D (see page xxiii).

Breast-feeding:
Drug passes into milk. Avoid drug or discontinue nursing until you finish medicine. Consult doctor for advice on maintaining milk supply.

Infants & children:
No special problems expected.

Prolonged use:
- May increase likelihood of problems upon discontinuing.
- Talk to your doctor about the need for follow-up medical examinations or laboratory studies to check thyroid function, liver function, electrolytes (sodium potassium, chloride), blood pressure and complete blood counts (white blood count, platelet count, red blood cell count, hemoglobin, hematocrit) every week during first two months, then once a month.

Skin & sunlight:
No special problems expected.

Driving, piloting or hazardous work:
Avoid if you feel confused, drowsy or dizzy.

Discontinuing:
May still experience symptoms of bone marrow depression, such as: blood in stools, fever or chills, blood spots under the skin, back pain, hoarseness, bloody urine. If any of these occur, call your doctor right away.

Others:
- Advise any doctor or dentist whom you consult that you take this medicine.
- May affect results in some medical tests.

POSSIBLE INTERACTION WITH OTHER DRUGS

GENERIC NAME OR DRUG CLASS	COMBINED EFFECT
Allopurinol	Greatly increased azathioprine activity.
Antivirals, HIV/AIDS*	Increased risk of pancreatitis.
Clozapine	Toxic effect on bone marrow.
Tiopronin	Increased risk of toxicity to bone marrow.
Immunosuppressants, other*	Higher risk of developing infection or malignancies.
Levamisole	Increased risk of bone marrow depression.
Vaccines	May decrease effectiveness or cause disease itself.

POSSIBLE INTERACTION WITH OTHER SUBSTANCES

INTERACTS WITH	COMBINED EFFECT
Alcohol:	No special problems expected.
Beverages:	No special problems expected.
Cocaine:	Increased likelihood of adverse reactions. Avoid.
Foods:	No special problems expected.
Marijuana:	Increased likelihood of adverse reactions. Avoid.
Tobacco:	No special problems expected.

AZELAIC ACID

BRAND NAMES

Azelex

BASIC INFORMATION

Habit forming? No
Prescription needed? Yes
Available as generic? No
Drug class: Antiacne agent,
  hypopigmentation agent

 ## USES

- Topical treatment for mild to moderate acne vulgaris.
- May be used for treatment of melasma (chloasma), a skin condition in which brownish patches of pigmentation appear on the face.

 ## DOSAGE & USAGE INFORMATION

How to use:
Cream—Wash the affected skin area and then apply the prescribed amount of cream and rub it into the skin. Rub it in thoroughly, but gently, to avoid irritation. Wash hands after applying.

When to use:
Usually twice a day (morning and evening).

If you forget a dose:
Use as soon as you remember.

What drug does:
The drug helps prevents the development of new acne lesions (whiteheads), but the exact mechanism is unknown. It appears to have some antibacterial and anti-inflammatory effect, and also helps in skin renewal.

Time lapse before drug works:
Results should be visible in about 4 weeks, but full benefits may take months.

Don't use with:
Other topical medications without consulting your doctor or pharmacist.

 ## OVERDOSE

SYMPTOMS:
None expected.
WHAT TO DO:
If person accidently swallows drug, call doctor, poison control center or hospital emergency room for instructions.

 ## POSSIBLE ADVERSE REACTIONS OR SIDE EFFECTS

SYMPTOMS	WHAT TO DO
Life-threatening:	
None expected.	
Common:	
Peeling, itching, redness or dryness of skin; tingling, burning or stinging may occur when medicine first used.	Continue. Call doctor when convenient.
Infrequent:	
None expected.	
Rare:	
Lightening of skin or white spots in persons with darker complexions.	Discontinue. Call doctor when. convenient.

WARNINGS & PRECAUTIONS

Don't use if:
You are sensitive to azelaic acid.

Before you start, consult your doctor:
- If you are allergic to any medicine, food or other substance, or have a family history of allergies.
- If you have a dark complexion.

Over age 60:
No special problems expected, however the drug has not been tested extensively in this age group.

Pregnancy:
Consult doctor. Risk category B (see page xxiii).

Breast-Feeding:
No special problems expected. Consult doctor.

Infants & children:
Normally not used in this age group. Safety and effectiveness in children under age 12 has not been established.

Prolonged use:
No problems expected.

Skin & sunlight:
No problems expected.

Driving, piloting or hazardous work:
No problems expected.

Discontinuing:
No problems expected.

Others:
- Use as directed. Don't increase or decrease dosage without doctor's approval. Using more of the cream or using it more frequently than prescribed won't improve results and may cause excessive skin irritation.
- The side effects involving skin irritation usually go away with continued use. If they continue beyond 4 weeks, or are severe, consult doctor about reducing the dosage to once a day.
- You may use water-based cosmetics while undergoing treatment with this drug.

POSSIBLE INTERACTION WITH OTHER DRUGS

GENERIC NAME OR DRUG CLASS	COMBINED EFFECT
None expected.	

POSSIBLE INTERACTION WITH OTHER SUBSTANCES

INTERACTS WITH	COMBINED EFFECT
Alcohol:	None expected.
Beverages:	None expected.
Cocaine:	None expected.
Foods:	None expected.
Marijuana:	None expected.
Tobacco:	None expected.

AZELASTINE

BRAND NAMES

Astelin

BASIC INFORMATION

Habit forming? No
Prescription needed? Yes
Available as generic? No
Drug class: Antihistamine (H_1 receptor)

 ## USES

Reduces allergic symptoms caused by hay fever (seasonal allergic rhinitis), such as sneezing, runny nose, stuffy nose, itchy and watery eyes.

 ## DOSAGE & USAGE INFORMATION

How to use:
Nasal spray—Blow nose before using. Prime the pump per package instructions. Spray in nostrils (2 sprays per nostril).

When to take:
Usually once or twice a day according to doctor's instructions.

If you forget a dose:
Take as soon as you remember. If it is almost time for next dose, wait for next scheduled dose (don't double this dose).

What drug does:
Blocks action of histamine after an allergic response triggers histamine release in sensitive cells. Histamines cause itching, sneezing, runny nose and eyes and other symptoms.

Time lapse before drug works:
1 to 3 hours.

Don't take with:
Any other medicine or herbal remedy without consulting your doctor or pharmacist.

 ## OVERDOSE

SYMPTOMS:
May increase sleepiness, but an overdose with this dosage form is unlikely to occur.
WHAT TO DO:
If person uses much larger amount than prescribed, call doctor, poison control center or hospital emergency room for instructions.

 ## POSSIBLE ADVERSE REACTIONS OR SIDE EFFECTS

SYMPTOMS	WHAT TO DO
Life-threatening: None expected.	
Common: Sleepiness, bitter taste.	Usually no action needed. If symptoms continue, call doctor.
Infrequent: Dry mouth, weight gain, headache, sore throat, mild burning in the nose, nausea, sneezing, muscle aches, small amount of bloody mucus from nose.	Continue. Call doctor when convenient.
Rare: Allergic reaction, skin rash, shortness of breath, changes in vision, eye pain, bloody urine, mouth or lip sores, fast heartbeat, wheezing.	Discontinue. Call doctor right away.

WARNINGS & PRECAUTIONS

Don't take if:
You are allergic to azelastine.

Before you start, consult your doctor:
- If you have kidney problems.
- If you are allergic to any medication, food or other substance.

Over age 60:
No problems expected.

Pregnancy:
Decide with your doctor if drug benefits justify risks to unborn child. Risk category C (see page xxiii).

Breast-feeding:
It is not known if drugs pass into milk. Avoid drug or discontinue nursing until you finish medicine. Consult doctor for advice on maintaining milk supply.

Infants & children:
Not recommended for children under age 12.

Prolonged use:
Antihistamines are normally taken during the hay fever season. They are not intended for long-term uninterrupted use.

Skin & sunlight:
No problems expected.

Driving, piloting or hazardous work:
Don't drive or pilot aircraft until you learn how medicine affects you. Don't work around dangerous machinery. Don't climb ladders or work in high places. Danger increases if you drink alcohol or take other medicines affecting alertness and reflexes such as antihistamines, tranquilizers, sedatives, pain medicine, narcotics and mind-altering drugs.

Discontinuing:
No problems expected.

Others:
- Don't exceed recommended dose. It could increase the risk of adverse reactions.
- Advise any doctor or dentist whom you consult that you take this medicine.
- Avoid getting the spray in your eyes.
- Pump must be "primed" before first use if unused 3-4 days before. To prime pump, activate for 3-4 sprays or until a fine mist appears.

POSSIBLE INTERACTION WITH OTHER DRUGS

GENERIC NAME OR DRUG CLASS	COMBINED EFFECT
Central nervous system (CNS) depressants*	May add to any sedative effect.
Cimetidine	Increased azelastine effect. May see increased sedation.

POSSIBLE INTERACTION WITH OTHER SUBSTANCES

INTERACTS WITH	COMBINED EFFECT
Alcohol:	May cause excessive sedation. Avoid.
Beverages:	None expected.
Cocaine:	Decreased antihistamine effect. Avoid.
Foods:	None expected.
Marijuana:	May cause sedation. Avoid.
Tobacco:	None expected.

*See Glossary

BACLOFEN

BRAND NAMES

Lioresal

BASIC INFORMATION

Habit forming? No
Prescription needed? Yes
Available as generic? Yes
Drug class: Muscle relaxant for multiple
  sclerosis

USES

- Relieves spasms, cramps and spasticity of muscles caused by medical problems, including multiple sclerosis and spine injuries.
- Reduces number and severity of trigeminal neuralgia attacks.

DOSAGE & USAGE INFORMATION

How to take:
Tablet—Swallow with liquid or food to lessen stomach irritation.

When to take:
3 or 4 times daily as directed.

If you forget a dose:
Take as soon as you remember up to 2 hours late. If more than 2 hours, wait for next scheduled dose (don't double this dose).

What drug does:
Blocks body's pain and reflex messages to brain.

Time lapse before drug works:
Variable. Few hours to weeks.

Continued next column

OVERDOSE

SYMPTOMS:
Blurred vision, blindness, difficult breathing, vomiting, drowsiness, muscle weakness, convulsive seizures.
WHAT TO DO:
- **Dial 911 (emergency) or 0 (operator) for an ambulance or medical help. Then give first aid immediately.**
- **If patient is unconscious and not breathing, give mouth-to-mouth breathing. If there is no heartbeat, use cardiac massage and mouth-to-mouth breathing (CPR). Don't try to make patient vomit. If you can't get help quickly, take patient to nearest emergency facility.**
- **See emergency information on inside covers.**

Don't take with:
Any other medicine without consulting your doctor or pharmacist.

POSSIBLE ADVERSE REACTIONS OR SIDE EFFECTS

SYMPTOMS	WHAT TO DO
Life-threatening: In case of overdose, see previous column.	
Common: Dizziness, lightheadedness, confusion, drowsiness, nausea.	Continue. Call doctor when convenient.
Infrequent:	
• Rash with itching, numbness or tingling in hands or feet.	Discontinue. Call doctor right away.
• Headache, abdominal pain, diarrhea or constipation, appetite loss, muscle weakness, difficult or painful urination, male sex problems, nasal congestion, clumsiness, slurred speech, insomnia.	Continue. Call doctor when convenient.
Rare:	
• Fainting, weakness, hallucinations, depression, chest pain, muscle pain, pounding heatbeat.	Discontinue. Call doctor right away.
• Ringing in ears, lowered blood pressure, dry mouth, taste disturbance, euphoria, weight gain.	Continue. Call doctor when convenient.

WARNINGS & PRECAUTIONS

Don't take if:
- You are allergic to any muscle relaxant.
- Muscle spasm due to strain or sprain.

Before you start, consult your doctor:
- If you have Parkinson's disease.
- If you have cerebral palsy.
- If you have had a recent stroke.
- If you have had a recent head injury.
- If you have arthritis.
- If you have diabetes.
- If you have epilepsy.
- If you have psychosis.
- If you have kidney disease.
- If you will have surgery within 2 months, including dental surgery, requiring general or spinal anesthesia.

Over age 60:
Adverse reactions and side effects may be more frequent and severe than in younger persons.

Pregnancy:
Decide with your doctor if drug benefits justify risk to unborn child. Risk category C (see page xxiii).

Breast-feeding:
Avoid nursing or discontinue until you finish medicine. Consult doctor about maintaining milk supply.

Infants & children:
Not recommended.

Prolonged use:
Epileptic patients should be monitored with EEGs. Diabetics should more closely monitor blood sugar levels. Obtain periodic liver function tests.

Skin & sunlight:
No problems expected.

Driving, piloting or hazardous work:
Don't drive or pilot aircraft until you learn how medicine affects you. Don't work around dangerous machinery. Don't climb ladders or work in high places. Danger increases if you drink alcohol or take medicine affecting alertness and reflexes, such as antihistamines, tranquilizers, sedatives, pain medicine, narcotics and mind-altering drugs.

Discontinuing:
Don't discontinue without consulting doctor. Dose may require gradual reduction if you have taken drug for a long time. Doses of other drugs may also require adjustment.

Others:
No problems expected.

POSSIBLE INTERACTION WITH OTHER DRUGS

GENERIC NAME OR DRUG CLASS	COMBINED EFFECT
Anesthetics, general*	Increased sedation. Low blood pressure. Avoid.
Antidiabetic drugs*, insulin or oral	Need to adjust diabetes medicine dosage.
Central nervous system (CNS) depressants* (antidepressants,* antihistamines,* narcotics,* other muscle relaxants,* sedatives,* sleeping pills,* tranquilizers*)	Increased sedation Low blood pressure. Avoid.

Clozapine	Toxic effect on the central nervous system.
Ethinamate	Dangerous increased effects of ethinamate. Avoid combining.
Fluoxetine	Increased depressant effects of both drugs.
Guanfacine	May increase depressant effects of either drug.
Leucovorin	High alcohol content of leucovorin may cause adverse effects.
Methyprylon	Increased sedative effect, perhaps to dangerous level. Avoid.
Nabilone	Greater depression of the central nervous system.
Sertraline	Increased depressive effects of both drugs.

POSSIBLE INTERACTION WITH OTHER SUBSTANCES

INTERACTS WITH	COMBINED EFFECT
Alcohol:	Increased sedation. Low blood pressure. Avoid.
Beverages:	No problems expected.
Cocaine:	Increased spasticity. Avoid.
Foods:	No problems expected.
Marijuana:	Increased spasticity. Avoid.
Tobacco:	May interfere with absorption of medicine.

BARBITURATES

GENERIC AND BRAND NAMES

See complete list of generic and brand names in the *Generic and Brand Name Directory*, page 873.

BASIC INFORMATION

Habit forming? Yes
Prescription needed? Yes
Available as generic? Yes, for some
Drug class: Sedative-hypnotic agent, anticonvulsant

 ## USES

- Reduces likelihood of seizures (tonic-clonic seizure pattern and simple partial) in epilepsy.
- Preventive treatment for febrile seizures.
- Reduces anxiety or nervous tension.
- As an ingredient in combination drugs to treat gastrointestinal disorders, headaches and asthma.
- Aids sleep at night (on a short-term basis).

 ## DOSAGE & USAGE INFORMATION

How to take:
- Capsule—Swallow with liquid. If you can't swallow whole, open capsule and take with liquid or food. Instructions to take on empty stomach mean 1 hour before or 2 hours after eating.
- Elixir—Swallow with liquid.
- Rectal suppositories—Remove wrapper and moisten suppository with water. Gently insert into rectum, pointed end first. If suppository is too soft, chill in refrigerator or cool water before removing wrapper.
- Tablet—Swallow with liquid or food to lessen stomach irritation. If you can't swallow whole, crumble tablet and take with liquid or food.

Continued next column

 ## OVERDOSE

SYMPTOMS:
Deep sleep, trouble breathing, weak pulse, coma.
WHAT TO DO:
- **Dial 911 (emergency) or 0 (operator) for an ambulance or medical help. Then give first aid immediately.**
- **If patient is unconscious and not breathing, give mouth-to-mouth breathing. If there is no heartbeat use cardiac massage and mouth-to-mouth breathing (CPR). Don't try to make patient vomit. If you can't get help quickly, take patient to emergency facility. See emergency facts at end of book.**

When to take:
At the same times each day.

If you forget a dose:
Take as soon as you remember up to 2 hours late. If more than 2 hours, wait for next scheduled dose (don't double this dose).

What drug does:
May partially block nerve impulses at nerve-cell connections.

Time lapse before drug works:
60 minutes; will take several weeks for maximum antiepilepsy effect.

Don't take with:
Nonprescription drugs without consulting doctor or pharmacist.

 ## POSSIBLE ADVERSE REACTIONS OR SIDE EFFECTS

SYMPTOMS	WHAT TO DO
Life-threatening: In case of overdose, see previous column.	
Common: Dizziness, drowsiness, clumsiness, unsteadiness. signs of addiction*.	Continue. Call doctor when convenient.
Infrequent: Confusion, headache, irritability, feeling faint, nausea, vomiting, depression, nightmares, trouble sleeping.	Continue, but call doctor right away.
Rare: Agitation, slow heartbeat, difficult breathing, bleeding sores on lips, fever, chest pain, unexplained bleeding or bruising, muscle or joint pain, skin rash or hives, thickened or scaly skin, white spots in mouth, tightness in chest, face swelling, sore throat, yellow eyes or skin, hallucinations, unusual tiredness or weakness	Continue, but call doctor right away.

 ## WARNINGS & PRECAUTIONS

Don't take if:
- You are allergic to any barbiturate.
- You have porphyria.

Before you start, consult your doctor:
- If you have epilepsy.
- If you have kidney or liver damage.
- If you have asthma.
- If you have anemia.
- If you have chronic pain.
- If you will have surgery within 2 months, including dental surgery, requiring general or spinal anesthesia.

Over age 60:
Adverse reactions and side effects may be more frequent and severe than in younger persons. Use small doses.

Pregnancy:
Risk to unborn child outweighs drug benefits. Don't use. Risk category D (see page xxiii).

Breast-feeding:
Drug passes into milk. Avoid drug or discontinue nursing until you finish medicine. Consult doctor for advice on maintaining milk supply.

Infants & children:
Use only under doctor's supervision.

Prolonged use:
- May cause addiction, anemia, chronic intoxication. Unlikely to occur with the usual anticonvulsant or sedative dosage levels.
- May lower body temperature, making exposure to cold temperatures hazardous.
- Talk to your doctor about the need for follow-up medical examinations or laboratory studies to check blood sugar, kidney function.

Skin and sunlight:
No problems expected.

Driving, piloting or hazardous work:
Don't drive or pilot aircraft until you learn how medicine affects you. Don't work around dangerous machinery. Don't climb ladders or work in high places. Danger increases if you drink alcohol or take medicine affecting alertness and reflexes.

Discontinuing:
If you become addicted, don't stop taking barbiturates suddenly. Seek medical help for safe withdrawal.

Others:
- May affect results in some medical tests.
- Barbiturate addiction is common. Withdrawal effects may be fatal.
- Advise any doctor or dentist whom you consult that you take this medicine.

POSSIBLE INTERACTION WITH OTHER DRUGS

GENERIC NAME OR DRUG CLASS	COMBINED EFFECT
Adrenocorticoids, systemic	Decreased prednisone effect. Oversedation.
Anticoagulants, oral*	Decreased effect of anticoagulant.
Anticonvulsants*	Changed seizure patterns.
Antidepressants, tricyclic*	Decreased antidepressant effect. Possible dangerous oversedation.
Antidiabetic, agents, oral*	Increased effect of barbiturate.
Antihistamines*	Dangerous sedation. Avoid.
Aspirin	Decreased aspirin effect.
Beta-adrenergic blocking agents*	Decreased effect of beta-adrenergic blocker.
Carbamazepine	Decreased carbamazepine effect.
Carteolol	Increased barbiturate effect. Dangerous sedation.
Clozapine	Toxic effect on the central nervous system.
Contraceptives, oral*	Decreased contraceptive effect.
Dextrothyroxine	Decreased barbiturate effect.
Divalproex	Dangerous sedation. Avoid.
Doxycycline	Decreased doxycycline effect.
Griseofulvin	Decreased griseofulvin effect.

Continued on page 905

POSSIBLE INTERACTION WITH OTHER SUBSTANCES

INTERACTS WITH	COMBINED EFFECT
Alcohol:	Possible fatal oversedation. Avoid.
Beverages:	None expected.
Cocaine:	Decreased barbiturate effect.
Foods:	None expected.
Marijuana:	Excessive sedation. Avoid.
Tobacco:	None expected.

BARBITURATES, ASPIRIN & CODEINE
(Also contains caffeine)

GENERIC AND BRAND NAMES

See complete list of generic and brand names in the *Generic and Brand Name Directory*, page 873.

BASIC INFORMATION

Habit forming? Yes
Prescription needed? Yes
Available as generic? Yes
Drug class: Narcotic, analgesic

 USES

- Reduces anxiety or nervous tension (low dose).
- Reduces pain, fever, inflammation.

 DOSAGE & USAGE INFORMATION

How to take:
- Tablet or capsule—Swallow with liquid or food to lessen stomach irritation. If you can't swallow whole, crumble tablet or open capsule and take with liquid or food.
- Extended-release tablets or capsules— Swallow each dose whole.

When to take:
When needed. No more often than every 4 hours.

If you forget a dose:
Take as soon as you remember. Wait 4 hours for next dose.

Continued next column

 OVERDOSE

SYMPTOMS:
Deep sleep, slow and weak pulse, ringing in ears, nausea, vomiting, dizziness, fever, deep and rapid breathing, hallucinations, convulsions, coma.
WHAT TO DO:
- **Dial 911 (emergency) or 0 (operator) for an ambulance or medical help. Then give first aid immediately.**
- **If patient is unconscious and not breathing, give mouth-to-mouth breathing. If there is no heartbeat, use cardiac massage and mouth-to-mouth breathing (CPR). Don't try to make patient vomit. If you can't get help quickly, take patient to nearest emergency facility.**
- **See emergency information on inside covers.**

What drug does:
- May partially block nerve impulses at nerve-cell connections.
- Affects hypothalamus, the part of the brain which regulates temperature by dilating small blood vessels in skin.
- Prevents clumping of platelets (small blood cells) so blood vessels remain open.
- Decreases prostaglandin effect.
- Blocks pain messages to brain and spinal cord.
- Reduces sensitivity of brain's cough-control center.

Time lapse before drug works:
30 minutes.

Don't take with:
Nonprescription drugs without consulting doctor.

 POSSIBLE ADVERSE REACTIONS OR SIDE EFFECTS

SYMPTOMS	WHAT TO DO
Life-threatening: Wheezing, tightness in chest, pinpoint pupils.	Seek emergency treatment immediately.
Common: Dizziness, drowsiness, heartburn, flushed face, depression, false sense of well-being, increased urination.	Continue. Call doctor when convenient.
Infrequent: Jaundice; vomiting blood; easy bruising; skin rash, hives; confusion; depression; sore throat, fever, mouth sores; difficult urination; hearing loss; slurred speech; blood in urine; decreased vision.	Discontinue. Call doctor right away.
Rare: Insomnia, nightmares, constipation, headache, nervousness, flushed face, increased sweating, unusual tiredness.	Continue. Call doctor when convenient.

BARBITURATES, ASPIRIN & CODEINE
(Also contains caffeine)

 WARNINGS & PRECAUTIONS

Don't take if:
- You are allergic to any barbiturate or narcotic.
- You have a peptic ulcer of stomach or duodenum, bleeding disorder, porphyria.

Before you start, consult your doctor:
- If you have had stomach or duodenal ulcers.
- If you have asthma, epilepsy, kidney or liver damage, anemia, chronic pain, gout.
- If you will have surgery within 2 months, including dental surgery, requiring general or spinal anesthesia.

Over age 60:
- Adverse reactions and side effects may be more frequent and severe than in younger persons.
- More likely to cause hidden bleeding in stomach or intestines. Watch for dark stools.
- More likely to be drowsy, dizzy, unsteady or constipated. Use only if absolutely necessary.

Pregnancy:
Risk factors vary for drugs in this group. See category list on page xxiii and consult doctor.

Breast-feeding:
Drug passes into milk. Avoid drug or discontinue nursing until you finish medicine. Consult doctor for advice on maintaining milk supply.

Infants & children:
- Overdose frequent and severe. Keep bottles out of children's reach.
- Use only under doctor's supervision.
- Do not give to persons under age 18 who have fever and discomfort of viral illness, especially chicken pox and influenza. Probably increases risk of Reye's syndrome*.

Prolonged use:
- Kidney damage. Periodic kidney function test recommended.
- May cause addiction, anemia, chronic intoxication.
- May lower body temperature, making exposure to cold temperatures hazardous.

Skin & sunlight:
One or more drugs in this group may cause rash or intensity sunburn in areas exposed to sun or ultraviolet light (photosensitivity reaction). Avoid overexposure. Notify doctor if reaction occurs.

Driving, piloting or hazardous work:
Don't drive or pilot aircraft until you learn how medicine effects you. Don't work around dangerous machinery. Don't climb ladders or work in high places. Danger increases if you drink alcohol or take medicine affecting alertness and reflexes, such as antihistamines, tranquilizers, sedatives, pain medicine, narcotics and mind-altering drugs.

Discontinuing:
May be unnecessary to finish medicine. Follow doctor's instructions. If you develop withdrawal symptoms of hallucinations, agitation or sleeplessness after discontinuing, call doctor right away.

Others:
- Aspirin can complicate surgery; illness; pregnancy, labor and delivery.
- For arthritis—Don't change dose without consulting doctor.
- Urine tests for blood sugar may be inaccurate.
- Great potential for abuse.

 POSSIBLE INTERACTION WITH OTHER DRUGS

GENERIC NAME OR DRUG CLASS	COMBINED EFFECT
Adrenocorticoids, systemic	Increased risk of ulcers.
Allopurinol	Decreased allopurinol effect.
Analgesics, other*	Increased analgesic effect.
Antacids*	Decreased aspirin effect.
Anticoagulants, oral*	Increased anticoagulant effect. Abnormal bleeding.

Continued on page 905

 POSSIBLE INTERACTION WITH OTHER SUBSTANCES

INTERACTS WITH	COMBINED EFFECT
Alcohol:	Possible stomach irritation and bleeding, possible fatal oversedation. Avoid.
Beverages:	None expected.
Cocaine:	Increased cocaine toxic effects. Avoid.
Foods:	None expected.
Marijuana:	Possible increased pain relief, but marijuana may slow body's recovery. Impairs physical and mental performance. Avoid.
Tobacco:	None expected.

*See Glossary

BECAPLERMIN

BRAND NAMES

Regranex

BASIC INFORMATION

Habit forming? No
Prescription needed? Yes
Available as generic? No
Drug class: Platelet-derived growth factor.

USES

Treatment of skin ulcers in patients with diabetes mellitus.

DOSAGE & USAGE INFORMATION

How to use:
Gel—Apply to the affected area. Follow all instructions provided with the prescription. Dosage may change as wound heals.

When to use:
At the same time each day. Change the wound dressing between applications of the medication.

If you forget a dose:
Apply it as soon as possible. If it is almost time for your next dose, skip the missed dose and go back to your regular dosing schedule. Do not double doses.

What drug does:
Stimulates growth of cells involved in wound repair.

Time lapse before drug works:
Up to six months.

Don't use with:
Any other prescription or nonprescription drug without consulting your doctor.

OVERDOSE

SYMPTOMS:
None expected.
WHAT TO DO:
Overdose unlikely to threaten life. If person uses much larger amount than prescribed, call doctor, poison control center or hospital emergency room for instructions.

POSSIBLE ADVERSE REACTIONS OR SIDE EFFECTS

SYMPTOMS	WHAT TO DO
Life-threatening: None expected.	
Common: None expected.	
Infrequent: Rash in area of skin ulcer.	Discontinue. Call doctor right away.
Rare: None expected.	

WARNINGS & PRECAUTIONS

Don't take if:
- You are allergic to becaplermin, parabens or metacresol.
- You have any new growths or wounds in the application area.

Before you start, consult your doctor:
- If you have any other medical problem.
- If you are allergic to any other substances, such as food preservatives or dyes.

Over age 60:
No problems expected.

Pregnancy:
Decide with your doctor if drug benefits justify risk to unborn child. Risk category C (see page xxiii).

Breast-feeding:
It is not known if drug passes into milk. Avoid drugs or discontinue nursing until you finish medicine. Consult doctor for advice on maintaining milk supply.

Infants & children:
Safety and efficacy in children under age 16 has not been established.

Prolonged use:
No problems expected. Your doctor should periodically evaluate your response to the drug and adjust the dose according to the rate of change in the width and length of the diabetic ulcer.

Skin & sunlight:
No problems expected.

Driving, piloting or hazardous work:
No problems expected.

Discontinuing:
Don't discontinue without consulting doctor.

Others:
- Do not place tip of tube onto ulcer or any other object; it may contaminate the medication.
- Be sure you follow application instructions carefully.
- Avoid bearing weight on the affected extremity.
- Wash hands carefully before preparing your dose.
- Keep this medication in refrigerator; do not freeze.

POSSIBLE INTERACTION WITH OTHER DRUGS

GENERIC NAME OR DRUG CLASS	COMBINED EFFECT
None expected.	

POSSIBLE INTERACTION WITH OTHER SUBSTANCES

INTERACTS WITH	COMBINED EFFECT
Alcohol:	None expected.
Beverages:	None expected.
Cocaine:	Effects unknown. Avoid.
Foods:	None expected.
Marijuana:	Effects unknown. Avoid.
Tobacco:	None expected.

BELLADONNA ALKALOIDS & BARBITURATES

GENERIC AND BRAND NAMES

See complete list of generic and brand names in the *Generic and Brand Name Directory*, page 874.

BASIC INFORMATION

Habit forming? Yes
Prescription needed? Yes
Available as generic? Some yes, some no
Drug class: Antispasmodic, anticholinergic, sedative

 ## USES

- Reduces spasms of digestive system, bladder and urethra.
- Reduces anxiety or nervous tension (low dose).
- Relieves insomnia (higher bedtime dose).

 ## DOSAGE & USAGE INFORMATION

How to take:
- Tablet, liquid or capsule—Swallow with liquid or food to lessen stomach irritation. If you can't swallow whole, crumble tablet or open capsule and take with liquid or food.
- Extended-release tablets or capsules— Swallow each dose whole.
- Chewable tablets—Chew well before swallowing.
- Drops—Dilute dose in beverage before swallowing.

When to take:
At the same times each day.

If you forget a dose:
Take as soon as you remember up to 2 hours late. If more than 2 hours, wait for next scheduled dose (don't double this dose).

Continued next column

 ## OVERDOSE

SYMPTOMS:
Blurred vision, confusion, convulsions, irregular heartbeat, hallucinations, coma.
WHAT TO DO:
- **Dial 911 (emergency) or 0 (operator) for an ambulance or medical help. Then give first aid immediately.**
- **See emergency information on inside covers.**

What drug does:
- May partially block nerve impulses at nerve cell connections.
- Blocks nerve impulses at parasympathetic nerve endings, preventing muscle contractions and gland secretions of organs involved.

Time lapse before drug works:
15 to 30 minutes.

Don't take with:
- Antacids* or antidiarrheals*.
- Any other medicine without consulting your doctor or pharmacist.

 ## POSSIBLE ADVERSE REACTIONS OR SIDE EFFECTS

SYMPTOMS	WHAT TO DO
Life-threatening: Unusual excitement, restlessness, fast heartbeat, breathing difficulty.	Seek emergency treatment immediately.
Common: • Dry mouth, throat, nose; drowsiness; constipation; dizziness; nausea; vomiting; "hangover" effect; depression; confusion.	Discontinue. Call doctor right away.
• Reduced sweating, slurred speech, agitation, nasal congestion, altered taste.	Continue. Call doctor when convenient.
Infrequent: Difficult urination; difficult swallowing; rash or hives; face, lip or eyelid swelling; joint or muscle pain; lightheadedness.	Discontinue. Call doctor right away.
Rare: Jaundice; unusual bruising or bleeding; hives, skin rash; pain in eyes; blurred vision; sore throat, fever, mouth sores; unexplained bleeding or bruising.	Discontinue. Call doctor right away.

WARNINGS & PRECAUTIONS

Don't take if:
- You are allergic to any barbiturate or any anticholinergic.
- You have prophyria, trouble with stomach bloating, difficulty emptying your bladder completely, narrow-angle glaucoma, severe ulcerative colitis.

Before you start, consult your doctor:
- If you have open-angle glaucoma, angina, chronic bronchitis or asthma, hiatal hernia, liver disease, enlarged prostate, myasthenia gravis, peptic ulcer, epilepsy, kidney or liver damage, anemia, chronic pain, thyroid disease.
- If you will have surgery within 2 months, including dental surgery, requiring general or spinal anesthesia.

Over age 60:
Adverse reactions and side effects may be more frequent and severe than in younger persons. Ask your doctor about small doses.

Pregnancy:
Risk factors vary for drugs in this group. See category list on page xxiii and consult doctor.

Breast-feeding:
Drug passes into milk. Avoid drug or discontinue nursing until you finish medicine.

Infants & children:
Use only under doctor's supervision.

Prolonged use:
- May cause addiction, anemia, chronic intoxication.
- May lower body temperature, making exposure to cold temperatures hazardous.

Skin & sunlight:
One or more drugs in this group may cause rash or intensity sunburn in areas exposed to sun or ultraviolet light (photosensitivity reaction). Avoid overexposure. Notify doctor if reaction occurs.

Driving, piloting or hazardous work:
Don't drive or pilot aircraft until you learn how medicine affects you. Don't work around dangerous machinery. Don't climb ladders or work in high places. Danger increases if you drink alcohol or take medicine affecting alertness and reflexes.

Discontinuing:
May be unnecessary to finish medicine. Follow doctor's instructions. If you develop withdrawal symptoms of hallucinations, agitation or sleeplessness after discontinuing, call doctor right away.

Others:
- Great potential for abuse.
- Advise any doctor or dentist whom you consult that you take this medicine.

POSSIBLE INTERACTION WITH OTHER DRUGS

GENERIC NAME OR DRUG CLASS	COMBINED EFFECT
Acetaminophen	Possible decreased barbiturate effect.
Adrenocorticoids, systemic	Possible glaucoma.
Amantadine	Increased belladonna effect.
Antacids*	Decreased belladonna effect.
Anticoagulants, oral*	Decreased anti-coagulant effect.
Anticholinergics, other*	Increased belladonna effect.
Anticonvulsants*	Changed seizure patterns.
Antidepressants, tricyclic*	Possible dangerous oversedation. Avoid.
Antidiabetics, oral*	Increased barbiturate effect.
Antihistamines*	Dangerous sedation. Avoid.
Anti-inflammatory drugs nonsteroidal (NSAIDs)*	Decreased anti-inflammatory effect.
Aspirin	Decreased aspirin effect.

Continued on page 906

POSSIBLE INTERACTION WITH OTHER SUBSTANCES

INTERACTS WITH	COMBINED EFFECT
Alcohol:	Possible fatal oversedation. Avoid.
Beverages:	None expected.
Cocaine:	Excessively rapid heartbeat. Avoid.
Foods:	None expected.
Marijuana:	Drowsiness and dry mouth. Avoid.
Tobacco:	Decreased effectiveness of acid reduction in stomach.

*See Glossary

BENZODIAZEPINES

GENERIC AND BRAND NAMES

See complete list of generic and brand names in the *Generic and Brand Name Directory*, page 874.

BASIC INFORMATION

Habit forming? Yes
Prescription needed? Yes
Available as generic? Yes, for most
Drug class: Tranquilizer (benzodiazepine), anticonvulsant

 USE

- Treatment for anxiety disorders and panic disorders.
- Treatment for muscle spasm.
- Treatment for seizure disorders.
- Treatment for alcohol withdrawal.
- Treatment for insomnia (short-term).

 DOSAGE & USAGE INFORMATION

How to take:
- Tablet or capsule—Swallow with liquid. If you can't swallow whole, crumble tablet or open capsule and take with liquid or small amount of food.
- Extended-release capsule—Swallow capsule whole. Do not open or chew.
- Oral suspension—Dilute dose in water, soda or sodalike beverage or small amount of food such as applesauce or pudding.
- Sublingual tablet—Do not chew or swallow. Place under tongue until dissolved.
- Rectal gel—Follow instructions provided with prescription or as directed by the doctor.

Continued next column

 OVERDOSE

SYMPTOMS:
Drowsiness, weakness, tremor, stupor, coma.
WHAT TO DO:
- **Dial 911 (emergency) or 0 (operator) for an ambulance or medical help. Then give first aid immediately.**
- **If patient is unconscious and not breathing, give mouth-to-mouth breathing. If there is no heartbeat, use cardiac massage and mouth-to-mouth breathing (CPR). Don't try to make patient vomit. If you can't get help quickly, take patient to nearest emergency facility.**
- **See emergency information at end of book.**

When to take:
At the same time each day, according to instructions on prescription label.

If you forget a dose:
Take as soon as you remember up to 2 hours late. If more than 2 hours, wait for next scheduled dose (don't double this dose).

What drug does:
Affects limbic system of brain, the part that controls emotions.

Time lapse before drug works:
May take 6 weeks for full benefit; depends on drug when treating anxiety.

Don't take with:
Any other medicine without consulting your doctor or pharmacist.

 POSSIBLE ADVERSE REACTIONS OR SIDE EFFECTS

SYMPTOMS	WHAT TO DO
Life-threatening:	
In case of overdose, see previous column.	
Common:	
Clumsiness, drowsiness, dizziness. signs of addiction*.	Continue. Call doctor when convenient.
Infrequent:	
• Hallucinations, confusion, depression, irritability, rash, itch, vision changes, sore throat, fever, chills.	Discontinue. Call doctor right away.
• Constipation or diarrhea, nausea, vomiting, difficult urination, vivid dreams, behavior changes, abdominal pain, headache, dry mouth.	Continue. Call doctor when convenient.
Rare:	
• Slow heartbeat, breathing difficulty.	Discontinue. Seek emergency treatment.
• Mouth, throat ulcers; jaundice.	Discontinue. Call doctor right away.
• Decreased sex drive.	Continue. Call doctor when convenient.

 WARNINGS & PRECAUTIONS

Don't take if:
- You are allergic to any benzodiazepine.
- You have myasthenia gravis.
- You are an active or recovering alcoholic.
- Patient is younger than 6 months.

Before you start, consult your doctor:
- If you have liver, kidney or lung disease.
- If you have diabetes, epilepsy or porphyria.
- If you have glaucoma.

Over age 60:
Adverse reactions and side effects may be more frequent and severe than in younger persons. You may need smaller doses for shorter periods of time. You may develop increased sedation or agitation or difficulty walking.

Pregnancy:
Risk factors vary for drugs in this group. See category list on page xxiii and consult doctor.

Breast-feeding:
Drug passes into milk. Avoid drug or discontinue nursing until you finish medicine. Consult doctor for advice on maintaining milk supply.

Infants & children:
Use only under medical supervision.

Prolonged use:
May impair liver function.

Skin & sunlight:
- One or more drugs in this group may cause rash or intensify sunburn in areas exposed to sun or ultraviolet light (photosensitivity reaction). Avoid overexposure and use sunscreen. Notify doctor if reaction occurs.
- Hot weather, heavy exercise and sweating may reduce excretion and cause overdose in some people with one or more of these drugs.

Driving, piloting or hazardous work:
Don't drive or pilot aircraft until you learn how medicine affects you. Don't work around dangerous machinery. Don't climb ladders or work in high places. Danger increases if you drink alcohol or take medicine affecting alertness and reflexes.

Discontinuing:
Don't discontinue without consulting doctor. Dose may require gradual reduction if you have taken drug for a long time. Doses of other drugs may also require adjustment.

Others:
- Blood sugar may rise in diabetics, requiring insulin adjustment.
- Don't use for insomnia more than 4-7 days.
- Caution—Keep in safe secure place to avoid theft.
- Advise any doctor or dentist whom you consult that you take this medicine.

POSSIBLE INTERACTION WITH OTHER DRUGS

GENERIC NAME OR DRUG CLASS	COMBINED EFFECT
Anticonvulsants*	Change in seizure pattern.
Antidepressants, tricyclic*	Increased sedative effect of both drugs.
Antihistamines*	Increased sedative effect of both drugs.
Central nervous system (CNS) depressants*	Increased sedative effect.
Cimetidine	Increased benzo-diazepine effect.
Clozapine	Toxic effect on the central nervous system.
Contraceptives, oral*	Increased benzo-diazepine effect.
Disulfiram	Increased benzo-diazepine effect.
Erythromycins*	Increased benzo-diazepine effect.
Fluoxetine	Increased sedative effect.
Fluvoxamine	Increased sedative effect.
Ketoconazole	Increased benzo-diazepine effect.
Levodopa	Possible decreased levodopa effect.
Mirtazapine	Increased sedative effect. Avoid.
Molindone	Increased tranquilizer effect.
Monoamine oxidase (MAO) inhibitors*	Convulsions, deep sedation, rage.

Continued on page 907

POSSIBLE INTERACTION WITH OTHER SUBSTANCES

INTERACTS WITH	COMBINED EFFECT
Alcohol:	Heavy sedation. Avoid.
Beverages:	None expected.
Cocaine:	Decreased benzo-diazepine effect.
Foods:	None expected.
Marijuana:	Heavy sedation. Avoid.
Tobacco:	Decreased benzo-diazepine effect.

BENZOYL PEROXIDE

BRAND NAMES

See complete list of brand names in the *Generic and Brand Name Directory*, page 874.

BASIC INFORMATION

Habit forming? No
Prescription needed? No
Available as generic? Yes
Drug class: Anti-acne (topical)

USES

- Treatment for acne.
- Treats pressure sores.

DOSAGE & USAGE INFORMATION

How to use:
Cream, gel, pads, sticks, lotion, cleansing bar or facial mask—Wash affected area with plain soap and water. Dry gently with towel. Rub medicine into affected areas. Keep away from eyes, nose, mouth. Wash hands after using.

When to use:
Apply 1 or more times daily. If you have a fair complexion, start with single application at bedtime.

If you forget an application:
Use as soon as you remember.

What drug does:
Slowly releases oxygen from skin, which controls some skin bacteria. Also causes peeling and drying, helping control blackheads and whiteheads.

Time lapse before drug works:
1 to 2 weeks.

Don't use with:
Any other medicine without consulting your doctor or pharmacist.

OVERDOSE

SYMPTOMS:
None expected.
WHAT TO DO:
- **If person swallows drug, call doctor, poison control center or hospital emergency room for instructions.**
- **See emergency information on inside covers.**

POSSIBLE ADVERSE REACTIONS OR SIDE EFFECTS

SYMPTOMS	WHAT TO DO
Life-threatening: None expected.	
Common: Mild redness and chapping of skin during first few weeks of use.	No action necessary.
Infrequent: • Rash, excessive dryness, peeling skin. • Painful skin irritation.	Discontinue. Call doctor right away. Continue. Call doctor when convenient.
Rare: None expected.	

WARNINGS & PRECAUTIONS

Don't take if:
You are allergic to benzoyl peroxide.

Before you start, consult your doctor:
• If you plan to become pregnant within medication period.
• If you take oral contraceptives.
• If you are using any other prescription or nonprescription medicine for acne.
• If you are using abrasive skin cleansers or medicated cosmetics.

Over age 60:
No problems expected.

Pregnancy:
Consult doctor. Risk category C (see page xxiii).

Breast-feeding:
No proven problems. Consult doctor.

Infants & children:
Not recommended.

Prolonged use:
Permanent rash or scarring.

Skin & sunlight:
May cause rash or intensify sunburn in areas exposed to sun or ultraviolet light (photosensitivity reaction). Avoid overexposure. Notify doctor if reaction occurs.

Driving, piloting or hazardous work:
No problems expected.

Discontinuing:
• May be unnecessary to finish medicine. Discontinue when acne improves.
• If acne doesn't improve in 2 weeks, call doctor.

Others:
• Drug may bleach hair or dyed fabrics, including clothing or carpet.
• Store away from heat in cool, dry place.
• Avoid contact with eyes, lips, nose and sensitive areas of the neck.

POSSIBLE INTERACTION WITH OTHER DRUGS

GENERIC NAME OR DRUG CLASS	COMBINED EFFECT
Antiacne topical preparations, other	Excessive skin irritation.
Skin-peeling agents (salicylic acid, sulfur, resorcinol, tretinoin)	Excessive skin irritation.

POSSIBLE INTERACTION WITH OTHER SUBSTANCES

INTERACTS WITH	COMBINED EFFECT
Alcohol:	None expected.
Beverages:	None expected.
Cocaine:	None expected.
Foods: Cinnamon, foods with benzoic acid.	Skin rash.
Marijuana:	None expected.
Tobacco:	None expected.

BETA CAROTENE

BRAND NAMES

Solatene
Numerous multiple vitamin and mineral
supplements. Check labels.

BASIC INFORMATION

Habit forming? No
Prescription needed? No
Available as generic? Yes
Drug class: Nutritional supplement

USES

- Used as a nutritional supplement.
- Prevents night blindness.
- Used as an adjunct to the treatment of
  steatorrhea, chronic fever, obstructive
  jaundice, pancreatic insufficiency, protein
  deficiency, total parenteral nutrition and photosensitivity in photo porphyria.

DOSAGE & USAGE INFORMATION

How to take:
Tablet or capsule—Swallow with liquid. If you
can't swallow whole, crumble tablet or open
capsule and take with liquid or food.

When to take:
At the same time each day, according to
directions on package or prescription label.

If you forget a dose:
Take as soon as you remember (don't double
this dose).

What drug does:
Enables the body to manufacture vitamin A,
which is essential for the normal functioning of
the retina, normal growth and development and
normal testicular and ovarian function.

Time lapse before drug works:
Total effect may take several weeks.

Don't take with:
No restrictions.

OVERDOSE

SYMPTOMS:
Yellow skin
WHAT TO DO:
**Overdose unlikely to threaten life. If person
takes much larger amount than prescribed,
call doctor, poison control center or hospital
emergency room for instructions.**

POSSIBLE ADVERSE REACTIONS OR SIDE EFFECTS

SYMPTOMS	WHAT TO DO
Life-threatening: None expected.	
Common: Yellow palms, hands, soles of feet.	Continue. Call doctor when convenient.
Infrequent: None expected.	
Rare:	
• Joint pain, unusual bleeding or bruising.	Discontinue. Call doctor right away.
• Diarrhea, dizziness.	Continue. Call doctor when convenient.

WARNINGS & PRECAUTIONS

Don't take if:
You are hypersensitive to beta carotene

Before you start, consult your doctor:
- If you have liver or kidney disease.
- If you have hypervitaminosis*.

Over age 60:
No problems expected.

Pregnancy:
Consult doctor. Risk category C (see page xxiii).

Breast-feeding:
No problems expected.

Infants & children:
No problems expected.

Prolonged use:
No problems expected.

Skin & sunlight:
No special problems expected.

Driving, piloting or hazardous work:
No special problems expected.

Discontinuing:
No special problems expected.

Others:
- Some researchers claim that beta carotene may reduce the occurrence of some cancers. There is insufficient data to substantiate this claim.
- May affect results of some medical tests.

POSSIBLE INTERACTION WITH OTHER DRUGS

GENERIC NAME OR DRUG CLASS	COMBINED EFFECT
Cholestyramine	Decreased absorption of beta carotene.
Colestipol	Decreased absorption of beta carotene.
Mineral oil	Decreased absorption of beta carotene.
Neomycin	Decreased absorption of beta carotene.

POSSIBLE INTERACTION WITH OTHER SUBSTANCES

INTERACTS WITH	COMBINED EFFECT
Alcohol:	None expected.
Beverages:	None expected.
Cocaine:	None expected.
Foods:	None expected.
Marijuana:	None expected.
Tobacco:	None expected.

BETA-ADRENERGIC BLOCKING AGENTS

GENERIC AND BRAND NAMES

See complete list of generic and brand names in the *Generic and Brand Name Directory*, page 875.

BASIC INFORMATION

Habit forming? No
Prescription needed? Yes
Available as generic? Yes, for some.
Drug class: Antiadrenergic, antianginal, antiarrhythmic, antihypertensive

USES

- Treats high blood pressure (hypertension).
- Some beta-blockers are used to relieve angina (chest pain).
- May be used to treat irregular heartbeat.
- May be used to treat anxiety disorders and other conditions as determined by your doctor.
- Treats tremors (some types).
- Reduces frequency of vascular headaches (does not relieve headache pain).

DOSAGE & USAGE INFORMATION

How to take:
Tablet, liquid or extended-release capsule—Swallow with liquid. If you can't swallow whole, crumble tablet or open capsule and take with liquid or food. Don't crush capsule or extended-release tablet.

When to take:
With meals or immediately after.

If you forget a dose:
Take as soon as you remember. Return to regular schedule, but allow 3 hours between doses.

Continued next column

OVERDOSE

SYMPTOMS:
Weakness, slow or weak pulse, blood pressure drop, fainting, difficulty breathing, convulsions, cold and sweaty skin.
WHAT TO DO:
- **Dial 911 (emergency) or 0 (operator) for an ambulance or medical help. Then give first aid immediately.**
- **See emergency information at end of book.**

What drug does:
- Blocks certain actions of sympathetic nervous system.
- Lowers heart's oxygen requirements.
- Slows nerve impulses through heart.
- Reduces blood vessel contraction in heart, scalp and other body parts.

Time lapse before drug works:
1 to 4 hours.

Don't take with:
Nonprescription drugs or drugs in Interaction column without consulting doctor or pharmacist.

POSSIBLE ADVERSE REACTIONS OR SIDE EFFECTS

SYMPTOMS	WHAT TO DO
Life-threatening:	
Congestive heart failure (severe shortness of breath, rapid heartbeat); severe asthma.	Discontinue. Seek emergency treatment.
Common:	
• Pulse slower than 50 beats per minute.	Discontinue. Call doctor right away.
• Drowsiness, fatigue, numbness or tingling of fingers or toes, dizziness, diarrhea, nausea, weakness.	Continue. Call doctor when convenient.
• Cold hands or feet; dry mouth, eyes and skin.	Continue. Tell doctor at next visit.
Infrequent:	
• Hallucinations, nightmares, insomnia, headache, difficult breathing, joint pain, anxiety, chest pain.	Discontinue. Call doctor right away.
• Confusion, reduced alertness, depression, impotence, abdominal pain.	Continue. Call doctor when convenient.
• Constipation.	Continue. Tell doctor at next visit.
Rare:	
• Rash, sore throat, fever.	Discontinue. Call doctor right away.
• Unusual bleeding and bruising; dry, burning eyes.	Continue. Call doctor when convenient.

WARNINGS & PRECAUTIONS

Don't take if:
- You are allergic to any beta-adrenergic blocker.
- You have asthma.
- You have hay fever symptoms.
- You have taken a monoamine oxidase (MAO) inhibitor* in the past 2 weeks.

Before you start, consult your doctor:
- If you have heart disease or poor circulation to the extremities.
- If you have hay fever, asthma, chronic bronchitis, emphysema.
- If you have overactive thyroid function.
- If you have impaired liver or kidney function.
- If you will have surgery within 2 months, including dental surgery, requiring general or spinal anesthesia.
- If you have diabetes or hypoglycemia.

Over age 60:
Adverse reactions and side effects may be more frequent and severe than in younger persons.

Pregnancy:
Risk factors vary for drugs in this group. See category list on page xxiii and consult doctor.

Breast-feeding:
Drug passes into milk. Avoid drug or discontinue nursing until you finish medicine. Consult doctor for advice on maintaining milk supply.

Infants & children:
Not recommended.

Prolonged use:
Talk to your doctor about the need for follow-up medical examinations or laboratory studies to check blood pressure, ECG*, kidney function, blood sugar.

Skin & sunlight:
No problems expected.

Driving, piloting or hazardous work:
Don't drive or pilot aircraft until you learn how medicine affects you. Don't work around dangerous machinery. Don't climb ladders or work in high places. Danger increases if you drink alcohol or take medicine affecting alertness and reflexes.

Discontinuing
Don't discontinue without consulting doctor. Dose may require gradual reduction if you have taken drug for a long time. Doses of other drugs may also require adjustment. Angina may result from abrupt discontinuing.

Others:
- May mask diabetic hypoglycemia symptoms.
- May affect results in some medical tests.
- Advise any doctor or dentist whom you consult that you take this medicine.

POSSIBLE INTERACTION WITH OTHER DRUGS

GENERIC NAME OR DRUG CLASS	COMBINED EFFECT
Angiotensin-converting (ACE) inhibitors*	Increased anti-hypertensive effects of both drugs. Dosages may require adjustment.
Antidiabetics*	Increased anti-diabetic effect.
Antihistamines*	Decreased antihistamine effect.
Antihypertensives*	Increased anti-hypertensive effect.
Anti-inflammatory drugs, nonsteroidal (NSAIDs)*	Decreased anti-hypertensive effect of beta blocker.
Betaxolol eyedrops	Possible increased beta blocker effect.
Calcium channel blockers*	Additional blood pressure drop.
Clonidine	Additional blood pressure drop. High blood pressure if clonidine stopped abruptly.
Dextrothyroxine	Possible decreased beta blocker effect.

Continued on page 908

POSSIBLE INTERACTION WITH OTHER SUBSTANCES

INTERACTS WITH	COMBINED EFFECT
Alcohol:	Excessive blood pressure drop. Avoid.
Beverages:	None expected.
Cocaine:	Irregular heartbeat; decreased beta-adrenergic effect. Avoid.
Foods:	None expected.
Marijuana:	Daily use—Impaired circulation to hands and feet.
Tobacco:	Possible irregular heartbeat.

*See Glossary

BETA-ADRENERGIC BLOCKING AGENTS & THIAZIDE DIURETICS

GENERIC AND BRAND NAMES

See complete list of generic and brand names in the *Generic and Brand Name Directory*, page 875.

BASIC INFORMATION

Habit forming? No
Prescription needed? Yes
Available as generic? Yes
Drug class: Beta-adrenergic blocker, diuretic (thiazide)

USES

- Controls, but doesn't cure, high blood pressure.
- Reduces fluid retention (edema).
- Reduces angina attacks.
- Stabilizes irregular heartbeat.
- Lowers blood pressure.
- Reduces frequency of migraine headaches. (Does not relieve headache pain.)
- Other uses prescribed by your doctor.

DOSAGE & USAGE INFORMATION

How to take:
Extended-release capsules—Swallow with liquid. If you can't swallow whole, open capsule and take with liquid or food.

When to take:
At the same time each day.

If you forget a dose:
Take as soon as you remember up to 4 hours late. If more than 4 hours, wait for next scheduled dose (don't double this dose).

What drug does:
- Forces sodium and water excretion, reducing body fluid.
- Relaxes muscle cells of small arteries.

Continued next column

OVERDOSE

SYMPTOMS:
Irregular heartbeat (usually too slow), seizures, confusion, fainting, convulsions, coma.
WHAT TO DO:
- **Dial 911 (emergency) or 0 (operator) for an ambulance or medical help. Then give first aid immediately.**
- **See emergency information on inside covers.**

- Reduced body fluid and relaxed arteries lower blood pressure.
- Blocks some of the actions of sympathetic nervous system.
- Lowers heart's oxygen requirements.
- Slows nerve impulses through heart.
- Reduces blood vessel contraction in heart, scalp and other body parts.

Time lapse before drug works:
- 1 to 4 hours for beta-blocker effect.
- May require several weeks to lower blood pressure.

Don't take with:
Any other medicines, even over-the-counter drugs such as cough/cold medicines, diet pills, nose drops, caffeine, without consulting your doctor.

POSSIBLE ADVERSE REACTIONS OR SIDE EFFECTS

SYMPTOMS	WHAT TO DO
Life-threatening:	
Wheezing, chest pain, seizures, irregular heartbeat.	Seek emergency treatment immediately.
Common:	
• Dry mouth, weak pulse, vomiting, muscle cramps, increased thirst, mood changes, nausea.	Discontinue. Call doctor right away.
• Weakness, tiredness, dizziness, mental depression, diminished sex drive, constipation, nightmares, insomnia.	Continue. Call doctor when convenient.
Infrequent:	
• Cold feet and hands, chest pain, breathing difficulty, anxiety, nervousness, headache, appetite loss, abdominal pain, numbness and tingling in fingers and toes, slow heartbeat.	Discontinue. Call doctor right away.
• Confusion, diarrhea.	Continue. Call doctor when convenient.
Rare:	
• Hives, skin rash; joint pain; jaundice; fever, sore throat, mouth ulcers.	Discontinue. Call doctor right away.
• Impotence, back pain.	Continue. Call doctor when convenient.

BETA-ADRENERGIC BLOCKING AGENTS & THIAZIDE DIURETICS

 WARNINGS & PRECAUTIONS

Don't take if:
- You are allergic to any beta-adrenergic blocker or any thiazide diuretic drug.
- You have asthma or hay fever symptoms.
- You have taken MAO Inhibitors in past two weeks.

Before you start, consult your doctor:
- If you have heart disease or poor circulation to the extremities.
- If you have hay fever, asthma, chronic bronchitis, emphysema, overactive thyroid function, impaired liver or kidney function, gout, diabetes, hypoglycemia, pancreas disorder, systemic lupus erythematosus.
- If you are allergic to any sulfa drug or tartrazine dye.
- If you will have surgery within 2 months, including dental surgery, requiring general or spinal anesthesia.

Over age 60:
Adverse reactions and side effects may be more frequent and severe than in younger persons, especially dizziness and excessive potassium loss.

Pregnancy:
Risk factors vary for drugs in this group. See category list on page xxiii and consult doctor.

Breast-feeding:
Drug passes into milk. Avoid drug or discontinue nursing until you finish medicine. Consult doctor for advice on maintaining milk supply.

Infants & children:
Not recommended.

Prolonged use:
- Weakens heart muscle contractions.
- You may need medicine to treat high blood pressure for the rest of your life.
- Talk to your doctor about the need for follow-up medical examinations or laboratory studies.

Skin & sunlight:
One or more drugs in this group may cause rash or intensity sunburn in areas exposed to sun or ultraviolet light (photosensitivity reaction). Avoid overexposure. Notify doctor if reaction occurs.

Driving, piloting or hazardous work:
Don't drive or pilot aircraft until you learn how medicine affects you. Don't work around dangerous machinery. Don't climb ladders or work in high places. Danger increases if you drink alcohol or take medicine affecting alertness and reflexes, such as antihistamines, tranquilizers, sedatives, pain medicine, narcotics and mind-altering drugs.

Discontinuing:
Don't discontinue without consulting doctor. Dose may require gradual reduction if you have taken drug for a long time. Doses of other drugs may also require adjustment.

Others:
- May mask hypoglycemia symptoms.
- Hot weather and fever may cause dehydration and drop in blood pressure. Dose may require temporary adjustment. Weigh daily and report any unexpected weight decreases to your doctor.
- May cause rise in uric acid, leading to gout.
- May cause blood sugar rise in diabetics.

 POSSIBLE INTERACTION WITH OTHER DRUGS

GENERIC NAME OR DRUG CLASS	COMBINED EFFECT
Allopurinol	Decreased allopurinol effect.
Aminophylline	Decreased effectiveness of both.
Antidepressants, tricyclic*	Dangerous drop in blood pressure. Avoid combination unless under medical supervision.

Continued on page 908

 POSSIBLE INTERACTION WITH OTHER SUBSTANCES

INTERACTS WITH	COMBINED EFFECT
Alcohol:	Dangerous blood pressure drop. Avoid.
Beverages:	None expected.
Cocaine:	Irregular heartbeat, decreased beta blocker effect. Avoid.
Foods: Licorice.	Excessive potassium loss that causes dangerous heart rhythms.
Marijuana:	May increase blood pressure.
Tobacco:	May increase blood pressure and make heart work harder. Avoid.

BETA-ADRENERGIC BLOCKING AGENTS (Ophthalmic)

GENERIC AND BRAND NAMES

BETAXOLOL
  (ophthalmic)
  Betoptic
  Betoptic S
CARTEOLOL
  (ophthalmic)
  Ocupress
LEVOBUNOLOL
  (ophthalmic)
  AKBeta
  Betagen C Cap B.I.D.
  Betagen C Cap Q.D.
  Betagen Standard
   Cap
METIPRANOLOL
  (ophthalmic)
  OptiPranolol

TIMOLOL
  (ophthalmic)
  Apo-Timop
  Beta-Tim
  Betimol
  Cosopt
  Gen-Timolol
  Med Timolol
  Novo-Timol
  Nu-Timolol
  Timodal
  Timoptic
  Timoptic in
   Ocudose
  Timoptic-XE

BASIC INFORMATION

Habit forming? No
Prescription needed? Yes
Available as generic? Yes, for some
Drug class: Antiglaucoma

USES

Treatment for glaucoma and ocular hypertension.

DOSAGE & USAGE INFORMATION

How to take:
Eye drops—Follow directions on prescription.

Continued next column

OVERDOSE

SYMPTOMS:
Slow heartbeat, low blood pressure, broncho-spasm, heart failure (these symptoms are what might be expected if similar drugs were taken orally).
WHAT TO DO:
* **For overdose in the eye, flush with warm tap water and call doctor immediately.**
* **For accidentally ingested overdose or signs of system toxicity, dial 911 (emergency) or 0 (operator) for an ambulance or medical help. Then give first aid immediately.**
* **See emergency information on inside covers.**

When to take:
At the same time each day according to doctor's instructions.

If you forget a dose—
* Once-a-day dose—Apply as soon as you remember. If almost time for next dose, wait and apply at regular time (don't double this dose).
* More than once-a-day dose—Apply as soon as you remember. If close to time for next dose, wait and apply at regular time (don't double this dose).

What drug does:
Appears to reduce production of aqueous humor (fluid inside eye), thereby reducing pressure inside eye.

Time lapse before drug works:
1 to 6 hours.

Don't take with:
Any other prescription or nonprescription drug without consulting your doctor.

POSSIBLE ADVERSE REACTIONS OR SIDE EFFECTS

SYMPTOMS	WHAT TO DO
Life-threatening: In case of overdose, see previous column.	
Common: Redness of eye or inside of eyelid, decreased night vision, stinging or irritation of eye when medicine applied.	Continue. Call doctor when convenient.
Infrequent: None expected.	
Rare:	
• Changes in vision; blurred vision; sensation of foreign body in eye; dryness, inflammation, discharge or pain in eye; crusty eyelids; increased sensitivity to light.	Continue. Call doctor when convenient.
• Symptoms of system absorption may occur.	See information for Possible Adverse Reactions or Side Effects under Beta-Adrenergic Blocking Agents.

BETA-ADRENERGIC BLOCKING AGENTS
(Ophthalmic)

 WARNINGS & PRECAUTIONS

Don't take if:
You are allergic to any beta-adrenergic blocking agent taken orally or used in the eye.

Before you start, consult your doctor:
- If you have asthma, a bronchial disorder or pulmonary disease.
- If you have any heart disease or heart problem.
- If you have diabetes, low blood pressure, over-active thyroid or myasthenia gravis.

Over age 60:
Adverse reactions and side effects may be more frequent and severe than in younger persons.

Pregnancy:
Decide with your doctor whether drug benefits justify risk to unborn child. Risk category C (see page xxiii).

Breast-feeding:
Drug passes into milk. Avoid drug or discontinue nursing until you finish medicine. Consult doctor for advice on maintaining milk supply.

Infants & children:
Give only under close medical supervision. Children may be more sensitive to drug and side effects.

Prolonged use:
Talk to your doctor about the need for follow-up medical examinations to check pressure inside eye.

Skin & sunlight:
No special problems expected.

Driving, piloting or hazardous work:
Don't drive or pilot aircraft until you learn how medicine affects you. Don't work around dangerous machinery. Don't climb ladders or work in high places.

Discontinuing:
- Don't discontinue without doctor's approval.
- May need to discontinue drug temporarily before major surgery. Your doctor will provide instructions.

Others:
Advise any doctor or dentist whom you consult that you take this medicine.

 POSSIBLE INTERACTION WITH OTHER DRUGS

GENERIC NAME OR DRUG CLASS	COMBINED EFFECT

Drug interactions are unlikely unless a significant amount of the eye medication is absorbed into the system. Potential interactions that may occur are similar to those listed in Possible Drug Interactions With Other Drugs under Beta-Adrenergic Blocking Agents.

 POSSIBLE INTERACTION WITH OTHER SUBSTANCES

INTERACTS WITH	COMBINED EFFECT
Alcohol:	None expected.
Beverages:	None expected.
Cocaine:	None expected.
Foods:	None expected.
Marijuana:	None expected.
Tobacco:	None expected.

BETHANECHOL

BRAND NAMES

Duvoid   Urecholine
Urabeth

BASIC INFORMATION

Habit forming? No
Prescription needed? Yes
Available as generic? Yes
Drug class: Cholinergic

 USES

- Helps initiate urination following surgery, or for persons with urinary infections or enlarged prostate.
- Treats reflux esophagitis.

 DOSAGE & USAGE INFORMATION

How to take:
Tablet—Swallow with liquid, 1 hour before or 2 hours after eating.

When to take:
At the same times each day.

If you forget a dose:
Take as soon as you remember up to 2 hours late. If more than 2 hours, wait for next scheduled dose (don't double this dose).

What drug does:
Affects chemical reactions in the body that strengthen bladder muscles.

Continued next column

 OVERDOSE

SYMPTOMS:
Shortness of breath, wheezing or chest tightness, unconsciousness, coma.
WHAT TO DO:
- Dial 911 (emergency) or 0 (operator) for an ambulance or medical help. Then give first aid immediately.
- If patient is unconscious and not breathing, give mouth-to-mouth breathing. If there is no heartbeat, use cardiac massage and mouth-to-mouth breathing (CPR). Don't try to make patient vomit. If you can't get help quickly, take patient to nearest emergency facility.
- See emergency information on inside covers.

Time lapse before drug works:
30 to 90 minutes.

Don't take with:
Any other medicine without consulting your doctor or pharmacist.

 POSSIBLE ADVERSE REACTIONS OR SIDE EFFECTS

SYMPTOMS	WHAT TO DO
Life-threatening: In case of overdose, see previous column.	
Common: None expected.	
Infrequent: Dizziness, headache, faintness, blurred or changed vision, diarrhea, nausea, vomiting, stomach discomfort, belching, excessive urge to urinate.	Continue. Call doctor when convenient.
Rare: Shortness of breath, wheezing, tightness in chest.	Discontinue. Call doctor right away.

WARNINGS & PRECAUTIONS

Don't take if:
You are allergic to any cholinergic.

Before you start, consult your doctor:
- If you plan to become pregnant within medication period.
- If you have asthma.
- If you have epilepsy.
- If you have heart or blood vessel disease.
- If you have high or low blood pressure.
- If you have overactive thyroid.
- If you have intestinal blockage.
- If you have Parkinson's disease.
- If you have stomach problems (including ulcer).
- If you have had bladder or intestinal surgery within 1 month.

Over age 60:
Adverse reactions and side effects may be more frequent and severe than in younger persons.

Pregnancy:
Decide with your doctor if drug benefits justify risk to unborn child. Risk category C (see page xxiii).

Breast-feeding:
Unknown effect. Consult doctor.

Infants & children:
Use only under medical supervision.

Prolonged use:
No problems expected.

Skin & sunlight:
No problems expected.

Driving, piloting or hazardous work:
Don't drive or pilot aircraft until you learn how medicine effects you. Don't work around dangerous machinery. Don't climb ladders or work in high places. Danger increases if you drink alcohol or take medicine affecting alertness and reflexes, such as antihistamines, tranquilizers, sedatives, pain medicine, narcotics and mind-altering drugs.

Discontinuing:
May be unnecessary to finish medicine. Follow doctor's instructions.

Others:
- Be cautious about standing up suddenly.
- Interferes with laboratory studies of liver and pancreas function.
- Side effects more likely with injections.

POSSIBLE INTERACTION WITH OTHER DRUGS

GENERIC NAME OR DRUG CLASS	COMBINED EFFECT
Cholinergics, other*	Increased effect of both drugs. Possible toxicity.
Ganglionic blockers*	Decreased blood pressure.
Nitrates*	Decreased bethanechol effect.
Procainamide	Decreased bethanechol effect.
Quinidine	Decreased bethanechol effect.

POSSIBLE INTERACTION WITH OTHER SUBSTANCES

INTERACTS WITH	COMBINED EFFECT
Alcohol:	None expected.
Beverages:	None expected.
Cocaine:	None expected.
Foods:	None expected.
Marijuana:	None expected.
Tobacco:	None expected.

BISMUTH SUBSALICYLATE

BRAND NAMES

Helidac   Pepto-Bismol

BASIC INFORMATION

Habit forming? No
Prescription needed? No
Available as generic? Yes
Drug class: Antidiarrheal, antacid

USES

- Treats symptoms of diarrhea, heartburn, nausea, acid indigestion.
- Helps prevent traveler's diarrhea.
- Treats ulcers.
- Used with other medications to treat a stomach infected by the bacteria H. Pylori.

DOSAGE & USAGE INFORMATION

How to take:
- Tablets—Swallow with water.
- Chewable tablets—Chew well before swallowing.
- Liquid—Take as directed on label.

When to take:
As directed on label or by your doctor.

If you forget a dose:
Take as soon as you remember. Don't double this dose.

What drug does:
- Binds toxin of some bacteria.
- Stimulates absorption of fluid and electrolytes across the intestinal wall.
- Decreases inflammation and increased motility of the intestinal muscles and lining.

Time lapse before drug works:
30 minutes to 1 hour.

Continued next column

OVERDOSE

SYMPTOMS:
Hearing loss, ringing or buzzing in the ears, severe drowsiness or tiredness, severe excitement or nervousness, fast or deep breathing.
WHAT TO DO:
- **Dial 911 (emergency) or 0 (operator) for an ambulance or medical help. Then give first aid immediately.**
- **See emergency information on inside covers.**

Don't take with:
Any other medicine without consulting your doctor or pharmacist.

POSSIBLE ADVERSE REACTIONS OR SIDE EFFECTS

SYMPTOMS	WHAT TO DO
Life-threatening: In case of overdose, see previous column.	
Common: Black stools, dark tongue. (These symptoms are normal and medically insignificant.)	No action necessary.
Infrequent: None expected.	
Rare: Abdominal pain, increased sweating, muscle weakness, drowsiness, anxiety, trembling, hearing loss, ringing or buzzing in ears, confusion, dizziness, headache, increased thirst, vision problems, severe constipation, continuing diarrhea, trouble breathing (all more likely to occur with high doses or chronic use).	Discontinue. Call doctor right away.

WARNINGS & PRECAUTIONS

Don't take if:
- You are allergic to aspirin, salicylates or other nonsteroidal anti-inflammatory drugs.
- You have stomach ulcers that have ever bled.
- The patient is a child with fever.

Before you start, consult your doctor:
- If you are on a low-sodium, low-sugar or other special diet.
- If you have had diarrhea for more than 24 hours. This is especially applicable to infants, children and those over 60.
- If you have had kidney disease.

Over age 60:
- Consult doctor before using.
- May cause severe constipation.

Pregnancy:
Decide with your doctor if drug benefits justify risk to unborn child. Risk category C; D in third trimester (see page xxiii).

Breast-feeding:
- Drug passes into milk. Avoid or discontinue nursing until you finish medicine.
- May harm baby if mother takes large amounts.

Infants & children:
Not recommended for children 3 and younger. May cause constipation.

Prolonged use:
May cause constipation.

Skin & sunlight:
No problems expected.

Driving, piloting or hazardous work:
Don't drive or pilot aircraft if you take high or prolonged dose until you learn how medicine affects you. Don't work around dangerous machinery. Don't climb ladders or work in high places. Danger increases if you drink alcohol or take medicine affecting alertness and reflexes, such as antihistamines, tranquilizers, sedatives, pain medicine, narcotics and mind-altering drugs.

Discontinuing:
No problems expected.

Others:
- Pepto-Bismol contains salicylates. When given to children with flu or chicken pox, salicylates may cause a serious illness called Reye's syndrome*. An overdose in children can cause the same problems as aspirin poisoning.
- May cause false urine sugar tests.
- Dehydration can develop if too much body fluid has been lost. Consult doctor if any of the following symptoms occur: decreased urination, dizziness or lightheadedness, dryness of mouth, increased thirst, wrinkled skin.

- Don't store tablet form of drug in bathroom or near kitchen sink. Heat and moisture can cause it to break down.
- Consult doctor if diarrhea doesn't improve within 2 days.
- Read labels of any other drugs being used, such as for pain or inflammation. They may contain salicylates* and can lead to increased risk of side effects and overdose.

POSSIBLE INTERACTION WITH OTHER DRUGS

GENERIC NAME OR DRUG CLASS	COMBINED EFFECT
Anticoagulants*	Increased risk of bleeding.
Insulin or oral antidiabetic drugs*	Increased insulin effect. May require dosage adjustment.
Probenecid	Decreased effect of probenecid.
Salicylates*, other	Increased risk of salicylate toxicity.
Sulfinpyrazone	Decreased effect of sulfinpyrazone.
Tetracylines*	Decreased absorption of tetracycline.
Thrombolytic agents*	Increased risk of bleeding.

POSSIBLE INTERACTION WITH OTHER SUBSTANCES

INTERACTS WITH	COMBINED EFFECT
Alcohol:	None expected.
Beverages:	None expected.
Cocaine:	Decreased Pepto-Bismol effect. Avoid.
Foods:	None expected.
Marijuana:	None expected.
Tobacco:	None expected.

BROMOCRIPTINE

BRAND NAMES

Alti-Bromocriptine	Parlodel
Apo-Bromocriptine	Parlodel Snaptabs

BASIC INFORMATION

Habit forming? No
Prescription needed? Yes
Available as generic? Yes
Drug class: Antiparkinsonism

 ## USES

- Controls Parkinson's disease symptoms such as rigidity, tremors and unsteady gait.
- Treats male and female infertility.
- Treats acromegaly (an overproduction of growth hormone).
- Treats some pituitary tumors.

 ## DOSAGE & USAGE INFORMATION

How to take:
Tablet or capsule—Swallow with liquid or food to lessen stomach irritation. If you can't swallow whole, crumble tablet or open capsule and take with liquid or food.

When to take:
At the same times each day.

If you forget a dose:
Take as soon as you remember up to 2 hours late. If more than 2 hours, wait for next scheduled dose (don't double this dose).

Continued next column

 ## OVERDOSE

SYMPTOMS:
Muscle twitch, spastic eyelid closure, nausea, vomiting, diarrhea, irregular and rapid pulse, weakness, fainting, confusion, agitation, hallucination, coma.
WHAT TO DO:
- **Dial 911 (emergency) or 0 (operator) for an ambulance or medical help. Then give first aid immediately.**
- **If patient is unconscious and not breathing, give mouth-to-mouth breathing. If there is no heartbeat, use cardiac massage and mouth-to-mouth breathing (CPR). Don't try to make patient vomit. If you can't get help quickly, take patient to nearest emergency facility.**
- **See emergency information on inside covers.**

What drug does:
Restores chemical balance necessary for normal nerve impulses.

Time lapse before drug works:
2 to 3 weeks to improve; several months or longer for maximum benefit.

Don't take with:
Any other medicine without consulting your doctor or pharmacist.

 ## POSSIBLE ADVERSE REACTIONS OR SIDE EFFECTS

SYMPTOMS	WHAT TO DO
Life-threatening:	
In case of overdose, see previous column.	
Common:	
Dizziness, mild nausea, lightheadedness when getting up, headache.	Continue. Call doctor when convenient.
Infrequent:	
Constipation, diarrhea, tiredness, drowsiness, dry mouth, depression, tingling and numbness of hands and feet.	Continue. Call doctor when convenient.
Rare:	
• Severe nausea and vomiting (may be bloody), vision changes, nervousness, sudden weakness, unusual headache, excess sweating, seizures, fainting, chest pain, black or tarry stools, uncontrollable body movements.	Discontinue. Call doctor right away.
• Stomach or back pain, runny nose, urinary frequency.	Continue. Call doctor when convenient.

WARNINGS & PRECAUTIONS

Don't take if:
- You are allergic to bromocriptine or ergotamine.
- You have taken a monoamine oxidase (MAO) inhibitor* in the past 2 weeks.
- You have glaucoma (narrow-angle type).

Before you start, consult your doctor:
- If you have diabetes or epilepsy.
- If you have had high blood pressure, heart or lung disease.
- If you have had liver or kidney disease.
- If you have a peptic ulcer.
- If you have a history of mental problems.
- If you will have surgery within 2 months, requiring general or spinal anesthesia.

Over age 60:
Adverse reactions and side effects may be more frequent and severe than in younger persons.

Pregnancy:
Decide with your doctor if drug benefits justify risk to unborn child. Risk category B (see page xxiii).

Breast-feeding:
Drug inhibits milk production. Avoid.

Infants & children:
Not recommended if under 15 years old.

Prolonged use:
- May lead to uncontrolled movements of head, face, mouth, tongue, arms or legs.
- Changes in lung tissue and excess fluid in chest cavity may occur.
- Talk to your doctor about the need for follow-up medical examinations or laboratory studies to check blood pressure, x-rays, growth hormone levels.

Skin & sunlight:
No problems expected.

Driving, piloting or hazardous work:
Don't drive or pilot aircraft until you learn how medicine effects you. Don't work around dangerous machinery. Don't climb ladders or work in high places. Danger increases if you drink alcohol or take medicine affecting alertness and reflexes, such as antihistamines, tranquilizers, sedatives, pain medicine, narcotics and mind-altering drugs.

Discontinuing:
Don't discontinue without doctor's advice until you complete prescribed dose, even though symptoms diminish or disappear.

Others:
- Expect to start with small doses and increase gradually to lessen frequency and severity of adverse reactions.
- Advise any doctor or dentist whom you consult that you take this medicine.

POSSIBLE INTERACTION WITH OTHER DRUGS

GENERIC NAME OR DRUG CLASS	COMBINED EFFECT
Antihypertensives*	May decrease blood pressure.
Antiparkinsonism drugs, other*	Increased bromocriptine effect.
Ergot alkaloids, other	Increased risk of high blood pressure.
Erythromycin	Increased bromocriptine effect.
Haloperidol	Decreased bromocriptine effect.
Levodopa	Decreased antiparkinson effect.
Methyldopa	Decreased bromocriptine effect.
Papaverine	Decreased bromocriptine effect.
Phenothiazines*	Decreased bromocriptine effect.
Risperidone	Increased bromocriptine effect.
Ritonavir	Increased bromocriptine effect.

POSSIBLE INTERACTION WITH OTHER SUBSTANCES

INTERACTS WITH	COMBINED EFFECT
Alcohol:	Decreased alcohol tolerance. Avoid
Beverages:	None expected.
Cocaine:	Decreased bromocriptine effect. Avoid.
Foods:	None expected.
Marijuana:	Increased fatigue, lethargy, fainting. Avoid.
Tobacco:	Interferes with absorption. Avoid.

BRONCHODILATORS, ADRENERGIC

GENERIC AND BRAND NAMES

See complete list of generic and brand names in the *Generic and Brand Name Directory*, page 875.

BASIC INFORMATION

Habit forming? No
Prescription needed? Yes, for most
Available as generic? Yes, for some
Drug class: Sympathomimetic

USES

- Relieves bronchial asthma.
- Decreases congestion of breathing passages.
- Suppresses allergic reactions.
- Relieves exercise-induced bronchospasm.

DOSAGE & USAGE INFORMATION

How to take:
- Tablet or capsule—Swallow with liquid. You may chew or crush tablet.
- Extended-release tablets—Swallow each dose whole.
- Syrup—Take as directed on bottle.
- Drops—Dilute dose in beverage.
- Aerosol inhalor—Follow directions in package.

When to take:
As needed, no more often than every 4 hours.

If you forget a dose:
Take up to 2 hours late. If more than 2 hours, wait for next dose (don't double this dose).

What drug does:
- Prevents cells from releasing allergy-causing chemicals (histamines).
- Relaxes muscles of bronchial tubes.
- Decreases blood-vessel size and blood flow, thus causing decongestion.

Time lapse before drug works:
30 to 60 minutes.

Continued next column

OVERDOSE

SYMPTOMS:
Severe anxiety, confusion, delirium, muscle tremors, rapid and irregular pulse, severe weakness.
WHAT TO DO:
- **Dial 911 (emergency) or 0 (operator) for an ambulance or medical help. Then give first aid immediately.**
- **See emergency information on inside covers.**

Don't take with:
- Nonprescription drugs with ephedrine, pseudoephedrine or epinephrine.
- Nonprescription drugs for cough, cold, allergy or asthma without consulting doctor.
- Any other medicine without consulting your doctor or pharmacist.

POSSIBLE ADVERSE REACTIONS OR SIDE EFFECTS

SYMPTOMS	WHAT TO DO
Life-threatening:	
In case of overdose, see previous column.	
Common:	
• Nervousness, restlessness, trembling.	Continue. Call doctor when convenient.
• Dry mouth or throat.	Continue. Tell doctor at next visit.
Infrequent:	
• Fast heartbeat, nausea, vomiting, headache, dizziness, lightheadedness.	Discontinue. Call doctor right away.
• Trouble sleeping, appetite loss, coughing.	Continue. Call doctor when convenient.
Rare:	
• Increased wheezing, difficulty breathing, chest discomfort or pain, irregular heartbeat, painful or difficult urination, allergic reaction (bluish, reddish or flushed skin; rash; itching; hives; swelling of face area; wheezing).	Discontinue. Call doctor right away.
• Smell or taste changes.	No action necessary

WARNINGS & PRECAUTIONS

Don't take if:
You are allergic to ephedrine, any bronchodilator* drug or sulfites used in some preparations.

Before you start, consult your doctor:
- If you have high blood pressure.
- If you have diabetes.
- If you have cardiovascular disease.
- If you have overactive thyroid gland.
- If you have difficulty urinating.
- If you have taken any monoamine oxidase(MAO) inhibitor* in past 2 weeks.
- If you have taken digitalis preparations* in the last 7 days.

- If you will have surgery within 2 months, including dental surgery, requiring general or spinal anesthesia.
- If you have pheochromocytoma.

Over age 60:
More likely to develop high blood pressure, heart rhythm disturbances, angina and to feel drug's stimulant effects.

Pregnancy:
Risk factors vary for drugs in this group. See category list on page xxiii and consult doctor.

Breast-feeding:
Drug passes into milk. Avoid drug or discontinue nursing until you finish medicine. Consult doctor for advice on maintaining milk supply.

Infants & children:
No problems expected for most. Use only under close medical supervision.

Prolonged use:
- Excessive doses—Rare toxic psychosis.
- Men with enlarged prostate gland may have more urination difficulty.
- Talk to your doctor about the need for follow-up medical examinations or laboratory studies to check ECG*, blood pressure.

Skin & sunlight:
No problems expected.

Driving, piloting or hazardous work:
Avoid if you feel dizzy. Otherwise, no problems expected.

Discontinuing:
May be unnecessary to finish medicine. Follow doctor's instructions.

Others:
- May affect results in some medical tests.
- Complications increase if you use more than prescribed. If you need to use more frequently, consult your doctor.

POSSIBLE INTERACTION WITH OTHER DRUGS

GENERIC NAME OR DRUG CLASS	COMBINED EFFECT
Antidepressants, tricyclic*	Increased effect of bronchodilator. Excessive stimulation of heart and blood pressure.
Antihypertensives*	Decreased antihypertensive effect.
Beta-adrenergic blocking agents*	Decreased effects of both drugs.
Digitalis preparations*	Serious heart rhythm disturbances.

Epinephrine	Increased bronchodilator effect.
Ergot preparations*	Serious blood-pressure rise.
Finasteride	Decreased finasteride effect.
Furazolidine	Sudden severe increase in blood pressure.
Guanadrel	Decreased effect of both drugs.
Guanethidine	Decreased effect of both drugs.
Maprotiline	Increased heart stimulation.
Methyldopa	Possible increased blood pressure.
Monoamine oxidase (MAO) inhibitors*	Increased bronchodilator effect. Dangerous blood pressure rise.
Nicotine	Decreased effect of isoproterenol.
Nitrates*	Possible decreased effects of both drugs.
Phenothiazines*	Possible increased bronchodilator toxicity. Possible decreased bronchodilator effect.
Pseudoephedrine	Increased bronchodilator effect.

Continued on page 909

POSSIBLE INTERACTION WITH OTHER SUBSTANCES

INTERACTS WITH	COMBINED EFFECT
Alcohol:	None expected.
Beverages: Caffeine drinks.	Nervousness or insomnia.
Cocaine:	High risk of heartbeat irregularities and high blood pressure.
Foods:	None expected.
Marijuana:	Rapid heartbeat, possible heart rhythm disturbance.
Tobacco:	None expected.

*See Glossary

BRONCHODILATORS, XANTHINE

GENERIC AND BRAND NAMES

See complete list of generic and brand names in the *Generic and Brand Name Directory*, page 876.

BASIC INFORMATION

Habit forming? No
Prescription needed? Yes
Available as generic? Yes
Drug class: Bronchodilator (xanthine)

USES

- Treatment for bronchial asthma symptoms.
- Treatment for chronic bronchitis, emphysema and other pulmonary diseases.

DOSAGE & USAGE INFORMATION

How to take:
- Tablet or capsule—Swallow with liquid.
- Extended-release tablets or capsules— Swallow each dose whole. If you take regular tablets, you may chew or crush them.
- Suppositories—Remove wrapper and moisten suppository with water. Gently insert larger end into rectum. Push well into rectum with finger.
- Syrup, elixir or oral solution—Take as directed on bottle.
- Enema—Use as directed on label.

When to take:
Most effective taken on empty stomach 1 hour before or 2 hours after eating. However, may take with food to lessen stomach upset.

If you forget a dose:
Take as soon as you remember up to 2 hours late. If more than 2 hours, wait for next scheduled dose (don't double this dose).

What drug does:
Relaxes and expands bronchial tubes.

Continued next column

OVERDOSE

SYMPTOMS:
Restlessness, irritability, confusion, black or tarry stool, breathing difficulty, pounding and irregular heartbeat, vomiting blood, delirium, convulsions, rapid pulse, coma.
WHAT TO DO:
- **Dial 911 (emergency) or 0 (operator) for an ambulance or medical help. Then give first aid immediately.**
- **See emergency information on inside covers.**

Time lapse before drug works:
15 to 30 minutes.

Don't take with:
Any other medicine without consulting your doctor or pharmacist.

POSSIBLE ADVERSE REACTIONS OR SIDE EFFECTS

SYMPTOMS	WHAT TO DO
Life-threatening: In case of overdose, see previous column.	
Common: Headache, irritability, nervousness, nausea, restlessness, insomnia, vomiting, stomach pain.	Continue. Call doctor when convenient.
Infrequent: • Rash or hives, flushed face, diarrhea, rapid breathing, irregular heartbeat.	Discontinue. Call doctor right away.
• Dizziness or light-headedness, appetite loss, trembling, fatigue, weakness.	Continue. Call doctor when convenient.
Rare: Frequent urination.	Continue. Call doctor when convenient.

WARNINGS & PRECAUTIONS

Don't take if:
- You are allergic to any bronchodilator.
- You have an active peptic ulcer.

Before you start, consult your doctor:
- If you have had impaired kidney or liver function.
- If you have gastritis.
- If you have a peptic ulcer.
- If you have high blood pressure or heart disease.
- If you take medication for gout.

Over age 60:
Adverse reactions and side effects may be more frequent and severe than in younger persons.

Pregnancy:
Decide with your doctor if drug benefits justify risk to unborn child. Risk category C (see page xxiii).

Breast-feeding:
Drug passes into milk. Avoid drug or discontinue nursing until you finish medicine. Consult doctor for advice on maintaining milk supply.

Infants & children:
Use only under medical supervision.

Prolonged use:
Stomach irritation may occur.

Skin & sunlight:
No problems expected.

Driving, piloting or hazardous work:
Avoid if lightheaded or dizzy. Otherwise, no problems expected.

Discontinuing:
May be unnecessary to finish medicine. Follow doctor's instructions.

Others:
No problems expected.

POSSIBLE INTERACTION WITH OTHER DRUGS

GENERIC NAME OR DRUG CLASS	COMBINED EFFECT
Allopurinol	Increased theophylline effect.
Aminoglutethimide	Possible decreased bronchodilator effect.
Beta-agonists*	Increased effect of both drugs.
Beta-adrenergic blocking agents*	Decreased bronchodilator effect.
Cimetidine	Increased bronchodilator effect.
Ciprofloxin	Increased xanthine bronchodilator in blood. Dosage adjustments necessary.
Clarithromycin	Increased concentration of theophylline.
Clindamycin	May increase bronchodilator effect.
Corticosteroids*	Possible increased bronchodilator effect.
Erythromycin	Increased bronchodilator effect.
Finasteride	Decreased finasteride effect.
Fluvoxamine	Increased theophylline effect.
Furosemide	Increased furosemide effect.
Lansoprazole	May require dosage adjustment of theophylline.
Leukotriene modifiers	Unknown effects. Consult doctor.

Lincomycins*	May increase bronchodilator effect.
Lithium	Decreased lithium effect.
Moricizine	Decreased bronchodilator effect.
Nicotine	Possible increased bronchodilator effect.
Norfloxacin	Increased xanthine bronchodilator in blood. Dosage adjustments necessary.
Phenobarbital	Decreased bronchodilator effect.
Phenytoin	Decreased effect of both drugs.
Probenecid	Increased effect of dyphylline.
Ranitidine	Possible increased bronchodilator effect and toxicity.
Rauwolfia alkaloids*	Rapid heartbeat.
Rifampin	Decreased bronchodilator effect.
Sulfinpyrazone	Increased effect of dyphylline.
Sympathomimetics*	Possible increased bronchodilator effect.
Tacrine	Increased bronchodilator effect.

Continued on page 910

POSSIBLE INTERACTION WITH OTHER SUBSTANCES

INTERACTS WITH	COMBINED EFFECT
Alcohol:	None expected.
Beverages: Caffeine drinks.	Nervousness and insomnia.
Cocaine:	Excess stimulation. Avoid.
Foods:	None expected.
Marijuana:	Slightly increased antiasthmatic effect of bronchodilator. Decreased effect with chronic use.
Tobacco:	Decreased bronchodilator effect.

*See Glossary

BUPROPION

BRAND NAMES

Wellbutrin

Wellbutrin SR
Zyban

BASIC INFORMATION

Habit forming? No
Prescription needed? Yes
Available as generic? No
Drug class: Antidepressant

 USES

- Relieves severe depression. (Has less effect on sexual functioning than some other antide-pressants and may be more acceptable to some patients.)
- May be used in combination with other therapy for smoking cessation.

 DOSAGE & USAGE INFORMATION

How to take:
- Tablets—Swallow with liquid. If you can't swallow whole, crumble tablet and take with liquid or food (but drug does have a bitter taste). May take with food to lessen stomach irritation.
- Sustained-release tablets—Swallow with liquid. Do not crumble sustained release tablet.

When to take:
At the same times each day, according to instructions on prescription label.

If you forget a dose:
Take as soon as you remember up to 4 hours late. If more than 4 hours, wait for next scheduled dose (don't double this dose). Do not take more often than every 6 hours.

What drug does:
Blocks certain chemicals that are necessary for nerve transmission in the brain. Boosts dopamine and norepinephrine (two brain chemicals) that are also boosted by nicotine.

Continued next column

 OVERDOSE

SYMPTOMS:
Confusion, agitation, seizures, coma.
WHAT TO DO:
- Dial 911 (emergency) or 0 (operator) for an ambulance or medical help. Then give first aid immediately. Do not induce vomiting.
- See emergency information at end of book.

Time lapse before drug works:
3 to 4 weeks.

Don't take with:
Any other medicine without consulting your doctor or pharmacist.

 POSSIBLE ADVERSE REACTIONS OR SIDE EFFECTS

SYMPTOMS	WHAT TO DO
Life-threatening:	
In case of overdose, see previous column.	
Common:	
• Excitement, anxiety, insomnia, restlessness. constipation, loss of appetite, dry mouth, dizziness, nausea or vomiting, unusual weight loss.	Continue. Call doctor when convenient.
• Confusion, heart-beat irregularity, severe headache.	Discontinue. Call doctor right away.
Infrequent:	
Rash, blurred vision, drowsiness, chills, fever, hallucinations, fatigue, nightmares.	Discontinue. Call doctor right away
Rare:	
Fainting, seizures.	Discontinue. Call doctor right away.

WARNINGS & PRECAUTIONS

Don't take if:
- You are allergic to bupropion.
- You have anorexia nervosa or bulimia.
- You have had recent head injury.
- You have a brain or spinal cord tumor.

Before you start, consult your doctor:
- If you have manic phases to your illness.
- If you abuse drugs.
- If you have seizures.
- If you have liver, kidney or heart disease.

Over age 60:
No problems expected.

Pregnancy:
No proven harm to unborn child, but avoid if possible. Risk category B (see page xxiii).

Breast-feeding:
Drug passes into milk. May cause adverse reactions. Avoid drug or discontinue breast-feeding. Consult doctor about maintaining milk supply.

Infants & children:
Effect not documented. Consult your doctor.

Prolonged use:
Talk to your doctor about the need for follow-up medical examinations or laboratory studies to check kidney function, liver function and serum bupropion levels in blood.

Skin & sunlight:
No problems expected.

Driving, piloting or hazardous work:
Don't drive or pilot aircraft until you learn how medicine affects you. Don't work around dangerous machinery. Don't climb ladders or work in high places. Danger increases if you drink alcohol or take medicine affecting alertness and reflexes.

Discontinuing:
Don't discontinue without doctor's approval. Dose may require gradual reduction to avoid adverse effects.

Others:
- May affect results in some medical tests.
- Advise any doctor or dentist whom you consult that you take this medicine.

POSSIBLE INTERACTION WITH OTHER DRUGS

GENERIC NAME OR DRUG CLASS	COMBINED EFFECT
Antidepressants, tricyclic*	Increased risk of seizures.
Carbamazepine	Decreased carbamazepine effect. Risk of seizures.
Cimetidine	Increased bupropion effect.
Clozapine	Increased risk of seizures.
Fluoxetine	Increased risk of seizures.
Haloperidol	Increased risk of seizures.
Levodopa	Increased levodopa effect.
Lithium	Increased risk of seizures.
Loxapine	Increased risk of seizures.
Maprotiline	Increased risk of seizures.
Molindone	Increased risk of seizures.
Monoamine oxidase (MAO) inhibitors*	Increased risk of side effects.
Phenothiazines*	Increased risk of seizures.
Phenytoin	Increased phenytoin effect and risk of seizures.
Thioxanthenes*	Increased risk of seizures.
Trazodone	Increased risk of seizures.

POSSIBLE INTERACTION WITH OTHER SUBSTANCES

INTERACTS WITH	COMBINED EFFECT
Alcohol:	Increased risk of seizures. Avoid.
Beverages: Coffee, tea, cocoa.	Increased side effects such as restlessness, insomnia.
Cocaine:	Increased risk of seizures. Avoid.
Foods:	No special problems expected.
Marijuana:	Increased risk of seizures. Avoid.
Tobacco:	No special problems expected.

*See Glossary

BUSPIRONE

BRAND NAMES

BuSpar

BASIC INFORMATION

Habit forming? Probably not
Prescription needed? Yes
Available as generic? No
Drug class: Antianxiety agent

 ## USES

- Treats chronic anxiety disorders with nervousness or tension. Not intended for treatment of ordinary stress of daily living. Causes less sedation than some anti-anxiety drugs. Not useful for acute anxiety.
- Useful in agitation associated with dementia.
- Reduces agggression and irritability in patients with dementia, brain injury, mental retardation.
- Used for anxiety in alcoholics or substance abusers (buspirone has low abuse potential).
- Reduces frequency of vascular headaches (does not relieve headache pain).
- Not useful in withdrawal from sedatives.

 ## DOSAGE & USAGE INFORMATION

How to take:
Tablets—Take with food.

When to take:
As directed. Usually 3 times daily. Food increases absorption.

If you forget a dose:
Take as soon as you remember, but skip this dose and don't double the next dose if it is almost time for the next dose.

What drug does:
Chemical family azaspirodecanedione; *not* a benzodiazepine. Probably has an effect on neurotransmitter systems.

Continued next column

 ## OVERDOSE

SYMPTOMS:
Severe drowsiness or nausea, vomiting, small pupils, unconsciousness.
WHAT TO DO:
- **Dial 911 (emergency) or 0 (operator) for an ambulance or medical help. Then give first aid immediately.**
- **See emergency information at end of book.**

Time lapse before drug works:
2 or 4 weeks before beneficial effects may be observed.

Don't take with:
Alcohol, other tranquilizers, antihistamines, muscle relaxants, sedatives or narcotics.

 ## POSSIBLE ADVERSE REACTIONS OR SIDE EFFECTS

SYMPTOMS	WHAT TO DO
Life-threatening: Chest pain; pounding, fast heartbeat (rare).	Discontinue. Seek emergency treatment.
Common: Lightheadedness, headache, nausea, restlessness, dizziness (if these side effects continue).	Discontinue. Call doctor right away.
Infrequent: Drowsiness, dry mouth, ringing in ears, nightmares or vivid dreams, unusual fatigue.	Continue. Call doctor when convenient.
Rare: Numbness or tingling in feet or hands; sore throat; fever; depression or confusion; uncontrollable movements of tongue, lips, arms and legs; slurred speech; psychosis; blurred vision.	Discontinue. Call doctor right away.

WARNINGS & PRECAUTIONS

Don't take if:
You are allergic to buspirone.

Before you start, consult your doctor:
- If you have ever been addicted to any substance.
- If you have chronic kidney or liver disease.
- If you are already taking *any* medicine.

Over age 60:
Adverse reactions and side effects may be more frequent and severe than in younger persons.

Pregnancy:
No problems expected, but better to avoid if possible. Consult doctor. Risk category B (see page xxiii)

Breast-feeding:
Unknown if drug passes into milk. Avoid nursing until you finish medicine. Consult doctor for advice on maintaining milk supply.

Infants & children:
Safety and efficacy not established for under 18 years old.

Prolonged use:
- Not recommended for prolonged use. Adverse side effects more likely.
- Request follow-up studies to check kidney function, blood counts, and platelet counts.

Skin & sunlight:
No problems expected.

Driving, piloting or hazardous work:
Don't drive or pilot aircraft until you learn how medicine affects you. Don't work around dangerous machinery. Don't climb ladders or work in high places. Danger increases if you drink alcohol or take medicine affecting alertness and reflexes, such as antihistamines, tranquilizers, sedatives, pain medicine, narcotics and mind-altering drugs.

Discontinuing:
No problems expected.

Others:
- Before elective surgery requiring local or general anesthesia, tell your dentist, surgeon or anesthesiologist that you take buspirone.
- Advise any doctor or dentist whom you consult that you take this medicine.
- This medication is expensive and is not available in a generic form.

 ## POSSIBLE INTERACTION WITH OTHER DRUGS

GENERIC NAME OR DRUG CLASS	COMBINED EFFECT
Antihistamines*	Increased sedative effect of both drugs.
Barbiturates*	Excessive sedation. Sedative effect of both drugs may be increased.
Benzodiazepines*	Recent use of benzodiazepines may lessen effect of buspirone.
Central nervous system (CNS) depressants*	Increased sedative effect.
Monoamine oxidase MAO inhibitors*	May increase blood pressure.
Narcotics*	Excessive sedation. Sedative effect of both drugs may be increased.

 ## POSSIBLE INTERACTION WITH OTHER SUBSTANCES

INTERACTS WITH	COMBINED EFFECT
Alcohol:	Excess sedation. Use caution.
Beverages: Caffeine-containing drinks.	Avoid. Decreased anti-anxiety effect of buspirone.
Cocaine:	Avoid. Decreased anti-anxiety effect of buspirone.
Foods:	None expected.
Marijuana:	Avoid. Decreased anti-anxiety effect of buspirone.
Tobacco:	Avoid. Decreased anti-anxiety effect of buspirone.

*See Glossary

BUSULFAN

BRAND NAMES

Myleran

BASIC INFORMATION

Habit forming? No
Prescription needed? Yes
Available as generic? No
Drug class: Antineoplastic,
   immunosuppressant

 ## USES

- Treatment for some kinds of cancer.
- Suppresses immune response after transplant and in immune disorders.

 ## DOSAGE & USAGE INFORMATION

How to take:
Tablet—Swallow with liquid after light meal. Don't drink fluids with meals. Drink extra fluids between meals. Avoid sweet or fatty foods.

When to take:
At the same time each day.

If you forget a dose:
Take as soon as you remember. Don't ever double dose.

What drug does:
Inhibits abnormal cell reproduction. May suppress immune system.

Time lapse before drug works:
Up to 6 weeks for full effect.

Don't take with:
Any other medicine without consulting your doctor or pharmacist.

 ## OVERDOSE

SYMPTOMS:
Bleeding, chills, fever, collapse, stupor, seizure.
WHAT TO DO:
- Dial 911 (emergency) or 0 (operator) for an ambulance or medical help. Then give first aid immediately.
- If patient is unconscious and not breathing, give mouth-to-mouth breathing. If there is no heartbeat, use cardiac massage and mouth-to-mouth breathing (CPR). Don't try to make patient vomit. If you can't get help quickly, take patient to nearest emergency facility.
- See emergency information on inside covers.

 ## POSSIBLE ADVERSE REACTIONS OR SIDE EFFECTS

SYMPTOMS	WHAT TO DO
Life-threatening:	
In case of overdose, see previous column.	
Common:	
• Unusual bleeding or bruising, mouth sores with sore throat, chills and fever, black stools, lip sores, menstrual irregularities.	Discontinue. Call doctor right away.
• Hair loss.	Continue. Call doctor when convenient.
• Nausea, vomiting, diarrhea (almost always occurs), tiredness, weakness.	Continue. Tell doctor at next visit.
Infrequent:	
• Mental confusion, shortness of breath.	Continue. Call doctor when convenient.
• Cough, joint pain, dizziness, appetite loss.	Continue. Tell doctor at next visit.
Rare:	
• Jaundice, cataracts, symptoms of myasthenia gravis.*	Discontinue. Call doctor right away.
• Swollen breasts.	Continue. Call doctor when convenient.

WARNINGS & PRECAUTIONS

Don't take if:
- You have had hypersensitivity to alkylating antineoplastic drugs.
- Your physician has not explained the serious nature of your medical problem and risks of taking this medicine.

Before you start, consult your doctor:
- If you have gout.
- If you have had kidney stones.
- If you have active infection.
- If you have impaired kidney or liver function.
- If you have taken other antineoplastic drugs or had radiation treatment in last 3 weeks.

Over age 60:
Adverse reactions and side effects may be more frequent and severe than in younger persons.

Pregnancy:
Consult doctor. Risk to child is significant. Risk category D (see page xxiii).

Breast-feeding:
Drug passes into milk. Don't nurse.

Infants & children:
Use only under care of medical supervisors who are experienced in anticancer drugs.

Prolonged use:
- Adverse reactions more likely the longer drug is required.
- Talk to your doctor about the need for follow-up medical examinations or laboratory studies to check complete blood counts (white blood cell count, platelet count, red blood cell count, hemoglobin, hematocrit), serum uricacid.

Skin & sunlight:
No problems expected.

Driving, piloting or hazardous work:
No problems expected.

Discontinuing:
Don't discontinue without doctor's advice until you complete prescribed dose, even though symptoms diminish or disappear. Some side effects may follow discontinuing. Report to doctor blurred vision, convulsions, confusion, persistent headache.

Others:
- May cause sterility.
- May increase chance of developing leukemia.

POSSIBLE INTERACTION WITH OTHER DRUGS

GENERIC NAME OR DRUG CLASS	COMBINED EFFECT
Antigout drugs*	Decreased antigout effect.
Antineoplastic drugs, other*	Increased effect of all drugs (may be beneficial).
Chloramphenicol	Increased likelihood of toxic effects of both drugs.
Clozapine	Toxic effect on bone marrow.
Lovastatin	Increased heart and kidney damage.
Tiopronin	Increased risk of toxicity to bone marrow.
Vaccines, live or killed	Increased risk of toxicity or reduced effectiveness of vaccine.

POSSIBLE INTERACTION WITH OTHER SUBSTANCES

INTERACTS WITH	COMBINED EFFECT
Alcohol:	May increase chance of intestinal bleeding.
Beverages:	No problems expected.
Cocaine:	Increases chance of toxicity.
Foods:	Reduces irritation in stomach.
Marijuana:	No problems expected.
Tobacco:	Increases lung toxicity.

*See Glossary

BUTORPHANOL

BRAND NAMES

Stadol NS

BASIC INFORMATION

Habit forming? Yes
Prescription needed? Yes
Available as generic? No
Drug class: Narcotic analgesic

USES

- Treatment for migraine headache pain and postoperative pain.
- Treatment for other types of pain for which a narcotic analgesic is appropriate.

DOSAGE & USAGE INFORMATION

How to take:
Nasal spray—Spray in one nostril using the metered-dose pump.

When to take:
For pain as directed by your doctor. Usual treatment consists of one dose in one nostril followed by a second dose in 60 to 90 minutes if pain persists. Your doctor may direct that the initial 2-dose sequence may be repeated in 3 to 4 hours as needed.

If you forget a dose:
Unlikely to be a problem since the drug is taken for pain and not routinely.

What drug does:
Blocks the pain impulses at specific sites in the brain and spinal cord.

Time lapse before drug works:
Within 15 minutes of the first dose.

Don't take with:
Any other medicine without consulting your doctor or pharmacist.

OVERDOSE

SYMPTOMS:
Heartbeat irregularities, breathing difficulty, coma.
WHAT TO DO:
- **Dial 911 (emergency) or 0 (operator) for an ambulance or medical help. Then give first aid immediately.**
- **See emergency information on inside covers.**

POSSIBLE ADVERSE REACTIONS OR SIDE EFFECTS

SYMPTOMS	WHAT TO DO
Life-threatening: In case of overdose, see previous column.	
Common: Drowsiness, dizziness, nausea or vomiting, nasal congestion or irritation.	Discontinue. Call doctor when convenient.
Infrequent: Constipation (with continued use), faintness, high or low blood pressure.	Discontinue. Call doctor when convenient.
Rare: • Taste changes, ear ringing, dry mouth.	No action necessary.
• Difficult breathing, heart palpitations.	Discontinue. Call doctor right away.

BUTORPHANOL

 ## WARNINGS & PRECAUTIONS

Don't take if:
You are allergic to butorphanol or the preservative benzethonium chloride*, which is used in the manufacture of the drug.

Before you start, consult your doctor:
- If you have a respiratory disorder or a central nervous system disease.
- If you have had adverse reactions to other narcotics*.
- If you have a history of emotional problems.
- If you have heart, kidney or liver disease.

Over age 60:
Adverse reactions and side effects (particularly dizziness) may be more frequent and severe than in younger persons.

Pregnancy:
Risk category C (see page xxiii). Decide with your doctor if drug benefits justify any possible risk to unborn child.

Breast-feeding:
Drug may pass into milk. Decide with your doctor if you should continue breast-feeding while taking this drug.

Infants & children:
Not recommended for children under age 18. Safety and effectiveness have not been established.

Prolonged use:
Long-term use effects are unknown. Probably habit forming. Consult with your doctor on a regular basis while using this drug.

Skin & sunlight:
No special problems expected.

Driving, piloting or hazardous work:
Don't drive or pilot aircraft until you learn how medicine affects you. Don't work around dangerous machinery. Don't climb ladders or work in high places. Danger increases if you drink alcohol or take medicine affecting alertness and reflexes.

Discontinuing:
Don't discontinue this drug after prolonged use without consulting doctor. Dosage may require a gradual reduction before stopping to avoid any withdrawal symptoms.

Others:
- When first using this drug, get up slowly from a sitting or lying position to avoid any dizziness, faintness or lightheadedness.
- Advise any doctor or dentist whom you consult that you take this medicine.
- Take medicine only as directed. Do not increase or reduce dosage without doctor's approval.

 ## POSSIBLE INTERACTION WITH OTHER DRUGS

GENERIC NAME OR DRUG CLASS	COMBINED EFFECT
Central nervous system (CNS) depressants*, other	Increased sedative effect.
Oxymetazoline	Delays start of butorphanol effect.

POSSIBLE INTERACTION WITH OTHER SUBSTANCES

INTERACTS WITH	COMBINED EFFECT
Alcohol:	Increased sedative affect. Avoid.
Beverages:	None expected.
Cocaine:	Effect not known. Best to avoid.
Foods:	None expected.
Marijuana:	Effect not known. Best to avoid.
Tobacco:	None expected.

*See Glossary

CAFFEINE

BRAND NAMES

See complete list of brand names in the *Generic and Brand Name Directory*, page 876.

BASIC INFORMATION

Habit forming? Yes
Prescription needed? No
Available as generic? Yes
Drug class: Stimulant (xanthine), vasoconstrictor

 USES

- Treatment for drowsiness and fatigue (occasional use only).
- Treatment for migraine and other vascular headaches in combination with ergot.

 DOSAGE & USAGE INFORMATION

How to take:
- Tablet or liquid—Swallow with liquid or food to lessen stomach irritation. If you can't swallow whole, crumble tablet and take with liquid or food.
- Extended-release capsules—Swallow whole with liquid.
- Powder—Stir powder into water or other liquid. The powder may also be placed on the tongue and then followed by liquid.

When to take:
At the same times each day.

If you forget a dose:
Take as soon as you remember up to 2 hours late. If more than 2 hours, wait for next scheduled dose (don't double this dose).

What drug does:
- Constricts blood vessel walls.
- Stimulates central nervous system.

Continued next column

 OVERDOSE

SYMPTOMS:
Excitement, insomnia, rapid heartbeat (infants can have slow heartbeat), confusion, fever, hallucinations, convulsions, coma.
WHAT TO DO:
- Dial 911 (emergency) or 0 (operator) for an ambulance or medical help. Then give first aid immediately.
- See emergency information at end of book.

Time lapse before drug works:
30 minutes.

Don't take with:
Nonprescription drugs without consulting your doctor or pharmacist.

 POSSIBLE ADVERSE REACTIONS OR SIDE EFFECTS

SYMPTOMS	WHAT TO DO
Life-threatening:	
In case of overdose, see previous column.	
Common:	
• Rapid heartbeat, low blood sugar (hunger, anxiety, cold sweats, rapid pulse) with tremor, irritability (mild).	Discontinue. Call doctor right away.
• Nervousness, insomnia.	Continue. Tell doctor at next visit.
• Increased urination.	No action necessary.
Infrequent:	
• Confusion, irritability (severe).	Discontinue. Call doctor right away.
• Nausea, indigestion, burning feeling in stomach.	Continue. Call doctor when convenient.
Rare:	
None expected.	

WARNINGS & PRECAUTIONS

Don't take if:
- You are allergic to any stimulant.
- You have heart disease.
- You have active peptic ulcer of stomach or duodenum.

Before you start, consult your doctor:
- If you have irregular heartbeat.
- If you have hypoglycemia (low blood sugar).
- If you have epilepsy.
- If you have a seizure disorder.
- If you have high blood pressure.
- If you have insomnia.

Over age 60:
Adverse reactions and side effects may be more frequent and severe than in younger persons.

Pregnancy:
Decide with your doctor if drug benefits justify risk to unborn child. Risk category C (see page xxiii).

Breast-feeding:
Drug passes into milk. Avoid drug or discontinue nursing until you finish medicine. Consult doctor for advice on maintaining milk supply.

Infants & children:
Not recommended.

Prolonged use:
Stomach ulcers.

Skin & sunlight:
No problems expected.

Driving, piloting or hazardous work:
No problems expected.

Discontinuing:
Will cause withdrawal symptoms of headache, irritability, drowsiness. Discontinue gradually if you use caffeine for a month or more.

Others:
Consult your doctor if drowsiness or fatigue continues, recurs or is not relieved by caffeine.

 ## POSSIBLE INTERACTION WITH OTHER DRUGS

GENERIC NAME OR DRUG CLASS	COMBINED EFFECT
Caffeine-containing drugs, other	Increased risk of overstimulation.
Central nervous system (CNS) stimulants*	Increased risk of overstimulation.
Cimetidine	Increased caffeine effect.
Contraceptives, oral*	Increased caffeine effect.
Isoniazid	Increased caffeine effect.
Monoamine oxidase (MAO) inhibitors*	Dangerous blood pressure rise.
Sympathomimetics*	Overstimulation.
Xanthines*	Increased risk of overstimulation.

 ## POSSIBLE INTERACTION WITH OTHER SUBSTANCES

INTERACTS WITH	COMBINED EFFECT
Alcohol:	Decreased alcohol effect.
Beverages: Caffeine drinks (coffee, tea or soft drinks).	Increased caffeine effect. Use caution.
Cocaine	Convulsions or excessive nervousness.
Foods:	No proven problems.
Marijuana:	Increased effect of both drugs. May lead to dangerous, rapid heartbeat. Avoid.
Tobacco:	Increased heartbeat. Avoid. Decreased caffeine effect.

*See Glossary

CALCIPOTRIENE

BRAND NAMES

Dovonex

BASIC INFORMATION

Habit forming? No
Prescription needed? Yes
Available as generic? No
Drug class: Antipsoriatic

 ## USES

Treats discoid or "plaque" psoriasis, the most common form of the disorder.

 ## DOSAGE & USAGE INFORMATION

How to use:
Cream, ointment or topical solution—Apply a thin layer to the affected skin. Rub in gently and completely. It should not be used on the face.

When to use:
Twice a day.

If you forget a dose:
Apply ointment as soon as you remember, then return to regular schedule.

What drug does:
Calcipotriene is a vitamin D product that helps regulate skin cell production and development.

Time lapse before drug works:
2 weeks. May take up to 8 weeks for maximum benefits that can include marked improvement in symptoms for most patients or complete clearing for others.

Don't use with:
Other topical or systemic drugs without consulting with your doctor or pharmacist.

 ## OVERDOSE

SYMPTOMS:
May be absorbed into the system through excessive topical application and increase the levels of calcium, which could cause muscle weakness, excess fatigue, depression, loss of appetite and nausea.
WHAT TO DO:
Overdose unlikely to threaten life. If symptoms occur, call doctor for instructions. If child accidentally swallows, call poison control center.

 ## POSSIBLE ADVERSE REACTIONS OR SIDE EFFECTS

SYMPTOMS	WHAT TO DO
Life-threatening: None expected.	
Common: Irritation, burning, itching of the skin.	Discontinue. Call doctor when convenient.
Infrequent: Redness, dryness, peeling or skin rash, worsening of psoriasis.	Discontinue. Call doctor when convenient.
Rare: None expected.	

WARNINGS & PRECAUTIONS

Don't use if:
- You are allergic to calcipotriene or any of its components.
- You have hypercalcemia (excess of calcium in the system).

Before you start, consult your doctor:
If you have had allergic reactions to other topical drugs.

Over age 60:
Adverse reactions and side effects may be more frequent and severe than in younger persons.

Pregnancy:
Decide with your doctor if drug benefits justify any possible risk to unborn child. Risk category C (see page xxiii).

Breast-feeding:
Unknown if drug passes into milk. Avoid nursing until you finish medicine. Consult doctor for advice on maintaining milk supply.

Infants & children:
Safety in children has not been established. Use only under close medical supervision. Adverse reactions and side effects may be more frequent and severe.

Prolonged use:
Not intended for long-term use. Usual length of treatment is 8 weeks. If your doctor recommends continued treatment with calcipotriene, discuss the need for follow-up laboratory studies to check calcium levels

Skin & sunlight:
No special problems expected.

Driving, piloting or hazardous work:
No special problems expected.

Discontinuing:
No special problems expected.

Others:
Wash hands after applying the drug.

POSSIBLE INTERACTION WITH OTHER DRUGS

GENERIC NAME OR DRUG CLASS	COMBINED EFFECT
None expected.	

POSSIBLE INTERACTION WITH OTHER SUBSTANCES

INTERACTS WITH	COMBINED EFFECT
Alcohol:	None expected.
Beverages:	None expected.
Cocaine:	None expected.
Foods:	None expected.
Marijuana:	None expected.
Tobacco:	None expected.

CALCITONIN

BRAND NAMES

Miacalcin

BASIC INFORMATION

Habit forming? No
Prescription needed? Yes
Available as generic? No
Drug class: Osteoporosis therapy

 ## USES

Treatment for postmenopausal osteoporosis (thinning of bones) in females. Osteoporosis is a major cause of bone fractures.

 ## DOSAGE & USAGE INFORMATION

How to take:
Nasal spray—One spray per day in a nostril, alternating nostrils daily. Follow directions on label about activating and using the pump supplied with the medication.

When to take:
At the same time each day.

If you forget a dose:
Take as soon as you remember up to 12 hours late. If more than 12 hours, wait for next scheduled dose (don't double this dose).

What drug does:
The exact mechanism is not fully understood. It slows down the loss of bone tissue and increases bone mass in women with osteoporosis.

Time lapse before drug works:
Up to 6 months or longer.

Don't take with:
Any other prescription or nonprescription drug without consulting your doctor or pharmacist.

 ## OVERDOSE

SYMPTOMS:
None reported.
WHAT TO DO:
Overdose unlikely to threaten life. If person takes much larger amount than prescribed, call doctor, poison control center or hospital emergency room for instructions.

 ## POSSIBLE ADVERSE REACTIONS OR SIDE EFFECTS

SYMPTOMS	WHAT TO DO
Life-threatening:	
Rare allergic reaction—Breathing difficulty; swelling of hands, feet, face, mouth, neck; skin rash.	Discontinue. Seek emergency treatment.
Common:	
Nasal inflammation, dryness, crusting, sores, irritation, itching, redness; swollen, runny, stuffy nose; small amount of nasal bleeding, discomfort, tenderness.	Continue. Call doctor when convenient.
Infrequent:	
Back pain, joint pain, headache, mild bloody nose, flushing, nausea, sinus infection.	Continue. Call doctor when convenient.
Rare:	
None expected.	

WARNINGS & PRECAUTIONS

Don't take if:
You are allergic to calcitonin.

Before you start, consult your doctor:
If you are allergic to any medication, food or other substance. A skin test may be performed before beginning treatment with calcitonin.

Over age 60:
No special problems expected.

Pregnancy:
Not normally used in premenopausal women. Risk category C (see page xxiii).

Breast-feeding:
Not normally used in premenopausal women.

Infants & children:
Not recommended for this age group.

Prolonged use:
• No special problems expected.
• Visit your doctor regularly to determine if the drug is continuing to control bone loss and to have periodic nasal examinations to check for ulceration or irritation.

Skin & sunlight:
No special problems expected.

Driving, piloting or hazardous work:
No special problems expected.

Discontinuing:
Don't discontinue without your doctor's approval.

Others:
• In addition to taking the drug, weight-bearing exercise and adequate dietary intake of calcium and vitamin D are essential in preventing bone loss. Dietary supplements of 1000 mg elemental calcium and 400 I.U. vitamin D daily may be recommended by your doctor.
• Advise any doctor or dentist whom you consult that you take this medicine.
• May affect the results of some medical tests.

POSSIBLE INTERACTION WITH OTHER DRUGS

GENERIC NAME OR DRUG CLASS	COMBINED EFFECT
None significant.	

POSSIBLE INTERACTION WITH OTHER SUBSTANCES

INTERACTS WITH	COMBINED EFFECT
Alcohol:	No special problems expected.
Beverages:	No special problems expected.
Cocaine:	No special problems expected.
Foods:	No special problems expected.
Marijuana:	No special problems expected.
Tobacco:	No special problems expected.

*See Glossary

GENERIC AND BRAND NAMES

See complete list of generic and brand names in *Generic and Brand Name Directory*, page 876.

BASIC INFORMATION

Habit forming? No
Prescription needed? Yes
Available as generic? Yes
Drug class: Calcium channel blocker, antiarrhythmic, antianginal

USES

- Used for angina attacks, irregular heartbeat, high blood pressure.
- Treats migraine.

DOSAGE & USAGE INFORMATION

How to take:
- Tablet or capsule—Swallow with liquid. You may chew or crush tablet.
- Extended-release tablets or capsules— Swallow each dose whole with liquid; do not crush tablet or open capsule.

When to take:
At the same times each day. Take verapamil with food.

If you forget a dose:
Take as soon as you remember up to 2 hours late. If more than 2 hours, wait for next scheduled dose (don't double this dose).

Continued next column

OVERDOSE

SYMPTOMS:
Unusually fast or unusually slow heartbeat, loss of consciousness, cardiac arrest.
WHAT TO DO:
- **Dial 911 (emergency) or 0 (operator) for an ambulance or medical help. Then give first aid immediately.**
- **If patient is unconscious and not breathing, give mouth-to-mouth breathing. If there is no heartbeat, use cardiac massage and mouth-to-mouth breathing (CPR). Don't try to make patient vomit. If you can't get help quickly, take patient to nearest emergency facility.**
- **See emergency information at end of book.**

What drug does:
- Reduces work that heart must perform.
- Reduces normal artery pressure.
- Increases oxygen to heart muscle.

Time lapse before drug works:
1 to 2 hours.

Don't take with:
Any other medicine without consulting your doctor or pharmacist.

POSSIBLE ADVERSE REACTIONS OR SIDE EFFECTS

SYMPTOMS	WHAT TO DO
Life-threatening:	
In case of overdose, see previous column.	
Common:	
Tiredness.	Continue. Tell doctor at next visit.
Infrequent:	
• Unusually fast or unusually slow heart-beat, wheezing, cough, shortness of breath.	Discontinue. Call doctor right away.
• Dizziness; numbness or tingling in hands and feet; swollen feet, ankles or legs; difficult urination.	Continue. Call doctor when convenient.
• Nausea, constipation.	Continue. Tell doctor at next visit.
Rare:	
• Fainting, depression, psychosis, rash, jaundice.	Discontinue. Call doctor right away.
• Headache, insomnia, vivid dreams, hair loss.	Continue. Tell doctor at next visit.

WARNINGS & PRECAUTIONS

Don't take if:
- You are allergic to calcium channel blockers.
- You have very low blood pressure.

Before you start, consult your doctor:
- If you have kidney or liver disease.
- If you have high blood pressure.
- If you have heart disease other than coronary artery disease.

Over age 60:
Adverse reactions and side effects may be more frequent and severe than in younger persons.

Pregnancy:
Decide with your doctor if drug benefits justify risk to unborn child. Risk category C (see page xxiii).

Breast-feeding:
Safety not established. Avoid if possible. Consult doctor.

Infants & children:
Not recommended.

Prolonged use:
Talk to your doctor about the need for follow-up medical examinations or laboratory studies to check blood pressure, liver function, kidney function, ECG*.

Skin & sunlight:
One or more drugs in this group may cause rash or intensify sunburn in areas exposed to sun or ultraviolet light (photosensitivity reaction). Avoid overexposure. Notify doctor if reaction occurs.

Driving, piloting or hazardous work:
Avoid if you feel dizzy. Otherwise, no problems expected.

Discontinuing:
Don't discontinue without doctor's advice until you complete prescribed dose, even though symptoms diminish or disappear.

Others:
- Learn to check your own pulse rate. If it drops to 50 beats per minute or lower, don't take drug until your consult your doctor.
- Advise any doctor or dentist whom you consult that you take this medicine.

 POSSIBLE INTERACTION WITH OTHER DRUGS

GENERIC NAME OR DRUG CLASS	COMBINED EFFECT
Angiotensin-converting enzyme (ACE) inhibitors*	Possible excessive potassium in blood. Dosages may require adjustment.
Antiarrhythmics*	Possible increased effect and toxicity of each drug.
Anticoagulants, oral*	Possible increased anticoagulant effect.
Anticonvulsants, hydantoin*	Increased anticonvulsant effect.
Antihypertensives*	Blood pressure drop. Dosages may require adjustment.
Beta-adrenergic blocking agents*	Possible irregular heartbeat and congestive heart failure.
Calcium (large doses)	Possible decreased effect of calcium channel blocker.

Carbamazepine	May increase carbamazepine effect and toxicity.
Cimetidine	Possible increased effect of calcium channel blocker.
Cyclosporine	Increased cyclosporine toxicity.
Digitalis preparations*	Increased digitalis effect. May need to reduce dose.
Disopyramide	May cause dangerously slow, fast or irregular heartbeat.
Diuretics*	Dangerous blood pressure drop. Dosages may require adjustment.
Encainide	Increased effect of toxicity on heart muscle.
Fluvoxamine	Slow heartbeat (with diltiazem).
HMG-CoA reductase inhibitors	Increased effect of HMG-CoA reductase inhibitor.
Hypokalemia-causing medications*	Increased antihypertensive effect.
Leukotriene modifiers	Increased effect of calcium channel blocker.
Lithium	Possible decreased lithium effect.

Continued on page 910

 POSSIBLE INTERACTION WITH OTHER SUBSTANCES

INTERACTS WITH	COMBINED EFFECT
Alcohol:	Dangerously low blood pressure. Avoid.
Beverages: Grapefruit juice.	Possible increased drug effect.
Cocaine:	Possible irregular heartbeat. Avoid.
Foods:	None expected.
Marijuana:	Possible irregular heartbeat. Avoid.
Tobacco:	Possible rapid heartbeat. Avoid.

CALCIUM SUPPLEMENTS

GENERIC AND BRAND NAMES

See complete list of generic and brand names in the *Generic and Brand Name Directory*, page 877.

BASIC INFORMATION

Habit forming? No
Prescription needed? For some
Available as generic? Yes
Drug class: Antihypocalcemic, dietary replacement

 ## USES

- Treats or prevents osteoporosis (thin, porous, easily fractured bones). Frequently prescribed with estrogen beginning at menopause.
- Helps heart, muscle and nervous system to work properly.
- Dietary supplement when calcium ingestion is insufficient or there is a deficiency such as osteomalacia or rickets.

 ## DOSAGE & USAGE INFORMATION

How to take:
- Take in addition to foods high in calcium (milk, yogurt, sardines, cheese, canned salmon, turnip greens, broccoli, shrimp, tofu).
- Tablet—Swallow with liquid or food to lessen stomach irritation. If you can't swallow whole, crumble tablet and take with food or liquid.
- Syrup—Take before meals.
- Suspension—Swallow with liquid or food to lessen stomach irritation.

When to take:
As directed. Don't take within 2 hours of any other medicine you take by mouth.

If you forget a dose:
Use as soon as you remember.

Continued next column

 ## OVERDOSE

SYMPTOMS:
Confusion, irregular heartbeat, depression, bone pain, coma.
WHAT TO DO:
- Dial 911 (emergency) or 0 (operator) for an ambulance or medical help. Then give first aid immediately.
- See emergency information on inside covers.

What drug does:
- Participates in metabolism of all activities essential for normal life and function of cells.
- Provides calcium necessary for bone, nerve function.

Time lapse before drug works:
15 to 30 minutes.

Don't take with:
- Any other medicine until 2 hours have passed since taking calcium.
- Any other medicine without consulting your doctor or pharmacist.

 ## POSSIBLE ADVERSE REACTIONS OR SIDE EFFECTS

SYMPTOMS	WHAT TO DO
Life-threatening: Irregular or very slow heart rate.	Discontinue. Seek emergency treatment.
Common: None expected.	
Infrequent: Constipation, diarrhea, drowsiness, headache, appetite loss, dry mouth, weakness.	Discontinue. Call doctor right away.
Rare: Frequent, painful or difficult urination; increased thirst; nausea, vomiting; rash; urine frequency increased and volume larger; confusion; high blood pressure; eyes sensitive to light.	Discontinue. Call doctor right away.

 ## WARNINGS & PRECAUTIONS

Don't take if:
- You are allergic to calcium.
- You have a high blood calcium level.

Before you start, consult your doctor:
If you have diarrhea, heart disease, kidney stones, kidney disease, sarcoidosis, malabsorption.

Over age 60:
No problems expected.

Pregnancy:
Consult doctor. Risk category C (see page xxiii).

Breast-feeding:
No problems expected. Consult doctor.

Infants & children:
Use only under close medical supervision.

Prolonged use:
- Side effects more likely.
- Talk to your doctor about the need for follow-up medical examinations or laboratory studies to check serum calcium determinations, blood pressure, urine.

Skin & sunlight:
No problems expected.

Driving, piloting or hazardous work:
No problems expected.

Discontinuing:
No problems expected.

Others:
- Exercise, along with vitamin D from sunshine and calcium, helps prevent osteoporosis.
- Don't use bone meal or dolomite as a source for calcium supplement (they may contain lead).

 POSSIBLE INTERACTION WITH OTHER DRUGS

GENERIC NAME OR DRUG CLASS	COMBINED EFFECT
Alendronate	Decreased alendronate effect. Take calcium 30 minutes after alendronate.
Anticoagulants, oral*	Decreased anticoagulant effect.
Calcitonin	Decreased calcitonin effect.
Calcium-containing medicines, other	Increased calcium effect.
Chlorpromazine	Decreased chlorpromazine effect.
Contraceptives, oral*	May increase absorption of calcium—frequently a desirable combined effect.
Corticosteroids*	Decreased calcium absorption and effect.
Digitalis preparations*	Decreased digitalis effect.
Diuretics, thiazide*	Increased calcium in blood.
Estrogens*	May increase absorption of calcium—frequently a desirable combined effect.
Etidronate	Decreased etidronate absorption. Take drugs 2 hours apart.
Iron supplements*	Decreased iron effect.
Meperidine	Increased meperidine effect.
Mexiletine	May slow elimination of mexiletine and cause need to adjust dosage.
Nalidixic acid	Decreased effect of nalidixic acid.
Nicardipine	Possible decreased nicardipine effect.
Nimodipine	Possible decreased nimodipine effect.
Oxyphenbutazone	Decreased oxyphenbutazone effect.
Para-aminosalicylic acid (PAS)	Decreased PAS effect.
Penicillins*	Decreased penicillin effect.
Pentobarbital	Decreased pentobarbital effect.
Phenylbutazone	Decreased phenylbutazone effect.
Phenytoin	Decreased phenytoin absorption.
Pseudoephedrine	Increased pseudoephedrine effect.
Quinidine	Increased quinidine effect.
Salicylates*	Increased salicylate effect.

Continued on page 910

POSSIBLE INTERACTION WITH OTHER SUBSTANCES

INTERACTS WITH	COMBINED EFFECT
Alcohol:	Decreased absorption of calcium.
Beverages:	No problems expected.
Cocaine:	No proven problems.
Foods: Don't take within 1 or 2 hours of eating.	Decreased absorption of calcium.
Marijuana:	Decreased absorption of calcium.
Tobacco:	Decreased absorption of calcium.

*See Glossary

CAPECITABINE

BRAND NAMES

Xeloda

BASIC INFORMATION

Habit forming? No
Prescription needed? Yes
Available as generic? No
Drug class: Antineoplastic

 ## USES

Treats metastatic breast cancer in patients resistant to both paclitaxel and an anthracycline containing chemotherapy regimen.

 ## DOSAGE & USAGE INFORMATION

How to take:
Tablets—Swallow with water. If you can't swallow whole, crumble tablet and take with liquid or food.

When to take:
Take in two divided doses every 12 hours after a meal and with water.

If you forget a dose:
Do not take missed dose or double next dose. Continue your regular dosing schedule and consult your doctor.

What drug does:
Capecitabine is converted in the body to the substance 5-fluorouracil. In some patients, this substance kills cancer cells and decreases the size of the tumor.

Time lapse before drug works:
Results may not show for several months.

Don't take with:
Any other prescription or nonprescription drug without consulting your doctor.

 ## OVERDOSE

SYMPTOMS:
Nausea, vomiting, diarrhea, gastrointestinal irritation and bleeding, and bone marrow depression.
WHAT TO DO:
Overdose unlikely to threaten life. If person takes much larger amount than prescribed, call doctor, poison control center or hospital emergency room for instructions.

 ## POSSIBLE ADVERSE REACTIONS OR SIDE EFFECTS

SYMPTOMS	WHAT TO DO
Life-threatening: None expected.	
Common:	
• Diarrhea (if you have more than 4 bowel movements in a day or any diarrhea at night); vomiting (more than once a day); nausea; loss of appetite; stomatitis (pain, redness or swelling in mouth); hand and foot syndrome (pain, redness or swelling in hands or feet); fever (100.5 or higher).	Discontinue. Call doctor right away.
• Diarrhea, nausea and vomiting, rash, dry or itchy skin, tiredness, weakness, dizziness, headache.	Continue. Call doctor when convenient.
Infrequent: Jaundice.	Continue. Call doctor right away.
Rare: None expected.	

WARNINGS & PRECAUTIONS

Don't take if:
You are allergic to 5-fluorouracil.

Before you start, consult your doctor:
- If you have an infection or any other medical problem.
- If you have heart problems.
- If you are taking the vitamin folic acid.
- If you are pregnant or if you plan to become pregnant.
- If you have had liver problems.

Over age 60:
Adverse reactions and side effects, especially gastrointestinal, may be more severe and frequent than in younger patients.

Pregnancy:
Animal studies show fetal abnormalities and increased risk of abortion. Discuss with your doctor whether drug benefits justify risk to unborn child. Risk category D (see page xxiii).

Breast-feeding:
Not known if drug passes into milk. Avoid drug or discontinue nursing until you finish medicine. Consult doctor for advice on maintaining milk supply.

Infants & children:
Safety and effectiveness of use in children not established.

Prolonged use:
Talk to your doctor about the need for follow-up medical examinations or laboratory studies.

Skin & sunlight:
No problems expected.

Driving, piloting or hazardous work:
Avoid if you feel side effects such as nausea and vomiting.

Discontinuing:
Your doctor will determine the schedule.

Others:
Advise any doctor or dentist whom you consult that you take this medicine.

 POSSIBLE INTERACTION WITH OTHER DRUGS

GENERIC NAME OR DRUG CLASS	COMBINED EFFECT
Antacids	Increased risk of capecitabine toxicity.
Leucovorin	Increased risk of capecitabine toxicity.

 POSSIBLE INTERACTION WITH OTHER SUBSTANCES

INTERACTS WITH	COMBINED EFFECT
Alcohol:	None expected.
Beverages:	None expected.
Cocaine:	Effects unknown. Avoid.
Foods:	None expected.
Marijuana:	Effects unknown. Avoid.
Tobacco:	None expected.

CAPSAICIN

BRAND NAMES

ArthriCare	Methacin
ARTH-RX	Zotrix
Axsain	Zotrix-HP
Capsagel	

BASIC INFORMATION

Habit forming? No
Prescription needed? No
Available as generic? Yes
Drug class: Analgesic (topical)

 ## USES

- Treats neuralgias, such as pain that occurs following shingles (herpes zoster) or neuropathy of the feet, ankles and fingers (common in diabetes).
- Treats discomfort caused by arthritis.

 ## DOSAGE & USAGE INFORMATION

How to use:
Cream—Apply a small amount and rub carefully on the affected areas. Use every day. Wash hands after applying. Don't apply to irritated skin. Don't bandage over treated areas.

When to use:
Apply 3 or 4 times a day.

If you forget a dose:
Use as soon as you remember.

What drug does:
Depletes the nerves of the substance that triggers pain sensation.

Time lapse before drug works:
Begins to work immediately. Frequently takes 2 to 3 weeks for full benefit, but may take up to 6 or 8 weeks.

Don't use with:
No problems expected.

 ## OVERDOSE

SYMPTOMS:
None expected.
WHAT TO DO:
Not intended for internal use. If child accidentally swallows, call poison control center.

 ## POSSIBLE ADVERSE REACTIONS OR SIDE EFFECTS

SYMPTOMS	WHAT TO DO
Life-threatening: None expected.	
Common: Stinging or burning sensation at application site.	Nothing. It usually improves in 2 to 3 days or becomes less severe the longer you use the drug.
Infrequent: None expected.	
Rare: None expected.	

WARNINGS & PRECAUTIONS

Don't use if:
You are allergic to capsaicin or to the fruit of capsaicin plants (for example, hot peppers).

Before you start, consult your doctor:
If you have any allergies.

Over age 60:
No problems expected.

Pregnancy:
Consult doctor. Risk category C (see page xxiii).

Breast-feeding:
No problems expected. Consult doctor.

Infants & children:
Not recommended for children under age 2.

Prolonged use:
No problems expected.

Skin & sunlight:
No problems expected.

Driving, piloting or hazardous work:
No problems expected.

Discontinuing:
Discontinue if there are no signs of improvement within a month.

Others:
- Capsaicin is not a local anesthetic*.
- Although capsaicin may help relieve the pain of neuropathy, it does not cure any disorder.
- If you accidently get some capsaicin in your eye, flush with water.

POSSIBLE INTERACTION WITH OTHER DRUGS

GENERIC NAME OR DRUG CLASS	COMBINED EFFECT
None expected.	

POSSIBLE INTERACTION WITH OTHER SUBSTANCES

INTERACTS WITH	COMBINED EFFECT
Alcohol:	No proven problems.
Beverages:	No proven problems.
Cocaine:	No proven problems.
Foods:	No proven problems.
Marijuana:	No proven problems.
Tobacco:	No proven problems.

CARBAMAZEPINE

BRAND NAMES

Apo-Carbamazepine
Epitol
Mazepine
Novocarbamaz
PMS Carbamazepine

Taro-Carbamazepine
Tegretol
Tegretol Chewtabs
Tegretol CR

BASIC INFORMATION

Habit forming? No
Prescription needed? Yes
Available as generic? Yes
Drug class: Analgesic, anticonvulsant, antimanic agent

USES

- Decreases frequency, severity and duration of attacks of tic douloureux*.
- Treats bipolar (manic-depressive) disorder.
- Prevents seizures.
- Used for pain relief, alcohol withdrawal.

DOSAGE & USAGE INFORMATION

How to take:
Regular or chewable tablet—Swallow with liquid or food to lessen stomach irritation.

When to take:
At the same times each day.

If you forget a dose:
Take as soon as you remember up to 2 hours late. If more than 2 hours, wait for next scheduled dose (don't double this dose).

Continued next column

OVERDOSE

SYMPTOMS:
Involuntary movements, drowsiness, irregular heartbeat, irregular bleeding, decreased urination, decreased blood pressure, dilated pupils, flushed skin, stupor, coma.
WHAT TO DO:
- Dial 911 (emergency) or 0 (operator) for an ambulance or medical help. Then give first aid immediately.
- If patient is unconscious and not breathing, give mouth-to-mouth breathing. If there is no heartbeat, use cardiac massage and mouth-to-mouth breathing (CPR). Don't try to make patient vomit. If you can't get help quickly, take patient to nearest emergency facility.
- See emergency information at end of book.

What drug does:
Reduces excitability of nerve fibers in brain, thus inhibiting repetitive spread of nerve impulses. Reduces transmission of pain messages at certain nerve terminals.

Time lapse before drug works:
- Tic douloureux—24 to 72 hours.
- Bipolar disorder—Unknown.
- Seizures—1 to 2 weeks.

Don't take with:
Any other medicine without consulting your doctor or pharmacist. May inactiviate other medications, such as birth control pills.

POSSIBLE ADVERSE REACTIONS OR SIDE EFFECTS

SYMPTOMS	WHAT TO DO
Life-threatening:	
In case of overdose, see previous column.	
Common:	
• Blurred vision.	Continue. Call doctor when convenient.
• Back-and-forth eye movements.	Discontinue. Call doctor right away.
Infrequent:	
• Confusion, slurred speech, fainting, depression, headache, hallucinations, hives, rash, mouth sores, sore throat, fever, unusual bleeding or bruising, unusual fatigue, jaundice.	Discontinue. Call doctor right away.
• Diarrhea, nausea, vomiting, constipation, dry mouth, impotence.	Continue. Call doctor when convenient.
Rare:	
• Breathing difficulty; irregular, pounding or slow heartbeat; chest pain; uncontrollable body jerks; numbness, weakness or tingling in hands and feet; tender, bluish legs or feet; less urine; swollen lymph glands, blood disorder (symptoms of anemia, bleeding, frequent infections).	Discontinue. Call doctor right away.
• Frequent urination, muscle pains, joint aches.	Continue. Call doctor when convenient.

WARNINGS & PRECAUTIONS

Don't take if:
- You are allergic to carbamazepine or any tricyclic antidepressant*.
- You have had liver or bone marrow disease.
- You have taken a monoamine oxidase (MAO) inhibitor* in the past 2 weeks.

Before you start, consult your doctor:
- If you have high blood pressure, thrombophlebitis or heart disease.
- If you have glaucoma.
- If you have emotional or mental problems.
- If you have liver or kidney disease.
- If you have a history of blood disorders.
- If you are taking any other medications.
- If you drink more than 2 alcoholic drinks per day.

Over age 60:
Adverse reactions and side effects may be more frequent and severe than in younger persons.

Pregnancy:
Decide with your doctor whether drug benefits justify risk to unborn child. Risk category C (see page xxiii).

Breast-feeding:
Drug passes into milk. Avoid drug or discontinue nursing until you finish medicine. Consult doctor for advice on maintaining milk supply.

Infants & children:
Approved for children under age 6 with epilepsy for treatment of seizures and for trigeminal neuralgia.

Prolonged use:
- Lowers sex drive.
- Talk to your doctor about the need for follow-up medical examinations or laboratory studies to check complete blood counts (white blood cell count, platelet count, red blood cell count, hemoglobin, hematocrit), serum iron and serum levels.

Skin & sunlight:
May cause rash or intensity sunburn in areas exposed to sun or ultraviolet light (photosensitivity reaction). Avoid overexposure and use sunscreen. Notify doctor if reaction occurs.

Driving, piloting or hazardous work:
Don't drive or pilot aircraft until you learn how medicine effects you. Don't work around dangerous machinery. Don't climb ladders or work in high places. Danger increases if you drink alcohol or take medicine affecting alertness and reflexes.

Discontinuing:
Don't discontinue without doctor's advice until you complete prescribed dose, even though symptoms diminish or disappear.

Others:
- Use only if less hazardous drugs are not effective. Stay under medical supervision.
- Periodic blood tests are needed.
- Advise any doctor or dentist whom you consult that you take this medicine.

POSSIBLE INTERACTION WITH OTHER DRUGS

GENERIC NAME OR DRUG CLASS	COMBINED EFFECT
Adrenocorticoids, systemic	Decreased adrenocorticoid effect.
Anticoagulants, oral*	Decreased anticoagulant effect.
Anticonvulsants, hydantoin* or succinimide*	Decreased effect of both drugs.
Antidepressants, tricyclic*	Confusion. Possible psychosis.
Barbiturates*	Possible increased barbiturate metabolism.
Bupropion	Decreased carbamazepine effect. Seizure risk.
Cimetidine	Increased carbamazepine effect.
Cisapride	Decreased carbamazepine effect.
Citalopram	May lessen effect of citalopram.

Continued on page 910

POSSIBLE INTERACTION WITH OTHER SUBSTANCES

INTERACTS WITH	COMBINED EFFECT
Alcohol:	Increased sedative effect of alcohol. Avoid.
Beverages:	None expected.
Cocaine:	Increased adverse effects of carbamazepine. Avoid.
Foods:	None expected.
Marijuana:	Increased adverse effects of carbamazepine. Avoid.
Tobacco:	None expected.

*See Glossary

CARBIDOPA & LEVODOPA

BRAND NAMES

Sinemet   Sinemet CR

BASIC INFORMATION

Habit forming? No
Prescription needed? Yes
Available as generic? Yes
Drug class: Antiparkinsonism

USES

Controls Parkinson's disease symptoms such as rigidity, tremor and unsteady gait.

DOSAGE & USAGE INFORMATION

How to take:
- Tablet—Swallow with liquid or food to lessen stomach irritation. If you can't swallow whole, crumble tablet and take with liquid or food.
- Extended-release tablet—Swallow each dose whole; do not crumble.

When to take:
At the same times each day.

If you forget a dose:
Take as soon as you remember up to 2 hours late. If more than 2 hours, wait for next scheduled dose (don't double this dose).

What drug does:
Restores chemical balance necessary for normal nerve impulses.

Continued next column

OVERDOSE

SYMPTOMS:
Muscle twitch, spastic eyelid closure, nausea, vomiting, diarrhea, irregular and rapid pulse, weakness, fainting, confusion, agitation, hallucination, coma.
WHAT TO DO:
- **Dial 911 (emergency) or 0 (operator) for an ambulance or medical help. Then give first aid immediately.**
- **If patient is unconscious and not breathing, give mouth-to-mouth breathing. If there is no heartbeat, use cardiac massage and mouth-to-mouth breathing (CPR). Don't try to make patient vomit. If you can't get help quickly, take patient to nearest emergency facility.**
- **See emergency information on inside covers.**

Time lapse before drug works:
2 to 3 weeks to improve; 6 weeks or longer for maximum benefit.

Don't take with:
Any other medicine without consulting your doctor or pharmacist.

POSSIBLE ADVERSE REACTIONS OR SIDE EFFECTS

SYMPTOMS	WHAT TO DO
Life-threatening:	
In case of overdose, see previous column.	
Common:	
• Mood changes, uncontrollable body movements, diarrhea.	Continue. Call doctor when convenient.
• Dry mouth, body odor.	No action necessary.
Infrequent:	
• Fainting, severe dizziness, headache, insomnia, nightmares, rash, itch, nausea, vomiting, irregular heartbeat.	Discontinue. Call doctor right away.
• Flushed face, blurred vision, muscle twitching, discolored or dark urine, difficult urination.	Continue. Call doctor when convenient.
• Constipation, tiredness.	Continue. Tell doctor at next visit.
Rare:	
• High blood pressure.	Discontinue. Call doctor right away.
• Upper abdominal pain, anemia.	Continue. Call doctor when convenient.

WARNINGS & PRECAUTIONS

Don't take if:
- You are allergic to levodopa or carbidopa.
- You have taken MAO inhibitors in past 2 weeks.
- You have glaucoma (narrow-angle type).

Before you start, consult your doctor:
- You have diabetes or epilepsy.
- If you have had high blood pressure, heart or lung disease.
- If you have had liver or kidney disease.
- If you have a peptic ulcer.
- If you have malignant melanoma.
- If you will have surgery within 2 months, including dental surgery, requiring general or spinal anesthesia.

Over age 60:
Adverse reactions and side effects may be more frequent and severe than in younger persons.

Pregnancy:
Decide with your doctor whether drug benefits justify risk to unborn child. Risk category C (see page xxiii).

Breast-feeding:
Drug filters into milk. May harm child. Avoid.

Infants & children:
Not recommended.

Prolonged use:
- May lead to uncontrolled movements of head, face, mouth, tongue, arms or legs.
- Talk to your doctor about the need for follow-up medical examinations or laboratory studies to check complete blood counts (white blood cell count, platelet count, red blood cell count, hemoglobin, hematocrit), liver function, eyes, kidney function.

Skin & sunlight:
No problems expected.

Driving, piloting or hazardous work:
Don't drive or pilot aircraft until you learn how medicine affects you. Don't work around dangerous machinery. Don't climb ladders or work in high places. Danger increases if you drink alcohol or take medicine affecting alertness and reflexes, such as antihistamines, tranquilizers, sedatives, pain medicine, narcotics and mind-altering drugs.

Discontinuing:
Don't discontinue without doctor's advice until you complete prescribed dose, even though symptoms diminish or disappear.

Others:
Expect to start with small dose and increase gradually to lessen frequency and severity of adverse reactions.

 POSSIBLE INTERACTION WITH OTHER DRUGS

GENERIC NAME OR DRUG CLASS	COMBINED EFFECT
Anticonvulsants*, hydantoin	Decreased effect of carbidopa and levodopa.
Antidepressants*	Weakness or faintness when arising from bed or chair.
Antihypertensives*	Decreased blood pressure and effect of carbidopa and levodopa.
Antiparkinsonism drugs, other*	Increased effect of carbidopa and levodopa.
Bupropion	Increased levodopa effect.
Haloperidol	Decreased effect of carbidopa and levodopa.
Methyldopa	Decreased effect of carbidopa and levodopa.
Monoamine oxidase (MAO) inhibitors*	Dangerous rise in blood pressure.
Papaverine	Decreased effect of carbidopa and levodopa.
Phenothiazines*	Decreased effect of carbidopa and levodopa.
Phenytoin	Decreased effect of carbidopa and levodopa.
Pyridoxine (Vitamin B-6)	Decreased effect of carbidopa and levodopa.
Rauwolfia alkaloids*	Decreased effect of carbidopa and levodopa.
Selegiline	May require adjustment in dosage of carbidopa and levodopa.

 POSSIBLE INTERACTION WITH OTHER SUBSTANCES

INTERACTS WITH	COMBINED EFFECT
Alcohol:	None expected.
Beverages:	None expected.
Cocaine:	Decreased cabidopa and levodopa effect. High rise of hearbeat irregularities. Avoid.
Foods:	None expected.
Marijuana:	Increased fatigue, lethargy, fainting.
Tobacco:	None expected.

CARBOHYDRATES & ELECTROLYTES

BRAND NAMES

Gastrolyte
Kao Lectrolyte
Lytren RHS
Oral rehydration salts
ORS-bicarbonate
ORS-citrate
Pedialyte

Pedialyte Freezer
  Pops
Rapolyte
Rehydralyte
Resol
Ricelyte

BASIC INFORMATION

Habit forming? No
Prescription needed? Not for all
Available as generic? Yes
Drug class: Electrolyte replenisher

USES

Replenishes fluids and electrolytes (salts) in dehydrated people.

DOSAGE & USAGE INFORMATION

How to take:
- Powder form—Follow package instructions for mixing solution. Mix new solution each day of use. If thirsty between doses of solution, drink plain water (except nursing babies).
- Oral solution—Follow instructions on container. Avoid other electrolyte-containing foods or liquids such as fruits, fruit juices or foods with added salt while taking solution.

When to take:
According to doctor's instructions. Frequency of need varies greatly.

If you forget a dose:
Take as soon as you remember up to 2 hours late. If more than 2 hours, wait for next scheduled dose (don't double this dose).

What drug does:
Prevents and treats electrolyte imbalance due to severe diarrhea..

Continued next column

OVERDOSE

SYMPTOMS:
Seizures.
WHAT TO DO:
- Dial 911 (emergency) or 0 (operator) for an ambulance or medical help. Then give first aid immediately.
- See emergency information on inside covers.

Time lapse before drug works:
8 to 12 hours.

Don't take with:
Any other medicines (including over-the-counter drugs such as cough and cold medicines, laxatives, antacids, diet pills, caffeine, nose drops or vitamins) without consulting your doctor

POSSIBLE ADVERSE REACTIONS OR SIDE EFFECTS

SYMPTOMS	WHAT TO DO
Life-threatening:	
In case of overdose, see previous column.	
Common:	
Mild vomiting.	Continue treatment. Slowly and frequently take small amounts of the solution.
Infrequent:	
None expected.	
Rare:	
• Too-high blood sodium level, causing convulsions, muscle twitching, swelling of feet or legs.	Discontinue. Seek emergency treatment.
• Overhydration (puffy eyes).	Discontinue. Call doctor right away.

WARNINGS & PRECAUTIONS

Don't take if:
- Kidneys are not functioning.
- Patient is unable to drink.
- There is severe and sustained vomiting.

Before you start, consult your doctor:
If patient is younger than 6 months.

Over age 60:
No problems expected; well tolerated by older patients.

Pregnancy:
Risk category not designated. See page xxiii and consult doctor.

Breast-feeding:
No problems expected. Consult doctor.

Infants & children:
Safe and effective in young; not yet evaluated in premature infants.

Prolonged use:
Talk to your doctor about the need for follow-up medical examinations or laboratory studies to check body weight, blood pressure, serum electrolytes and serum pH.

Skin & sunlight:
No problems expected.

Driving, piloting or hazardous work:
No problems expected.

Discontinuing:
No special problems expected.

Others:
- Contact doctor if diarrhea does not improve after 2 days.
- May affect results in some medical tests.

POSSIBLE INTERACTION WITH OTHER DRUGS

GENERIC NAME OR DRUG CLASS	COMBINED EFFECT
None expected.	

POSSIBLE INTERACTION WITH OTHER SUBSTANCES

INTERACTS WITH	COMBINED EFFECT
Alcohol:	Dangerous. Avoid.
Beverages:	Continuing milk all right. Others as tolerated.
Cocaine:	Dangerous. Avoid.
Foods: Rice, cereal, bananas, cooked potatoes or other carbohydrate-rich foods as tolerated.	Helps maintain nutrition.
Marijuana:	Dangerous. Avoid.
Tobacco:	May increase diarrhea. Avoid.

CARBONIC ANHYDRASE INHIBITORS

GENERIC AND BRAND NAMES

ACETAZOLAMIDE
  Acetazolam
  Ak-Zol
  Apo Acetazolamide
  Dazamide
  Diamox
  Storzolamide

BRINZOLAMIDE
  Azopt
DICHLORPHENAMIDE
  Daranide
METHAZOLAMIDE
  MZM
  Neptazane

BASIC INFORMATION

Habit forming? No
Prescription needed? Yes
Available as generic? Yes
Drug class: Carbonic anhydrase inhibitor

 ## USES

- Treatment of glaucoma.
- Treatment of epileptic seizures.
- Treatment of body fluid retention.
- Treatment for shortness of breath, insomnia and fatigue at high altitudes.
- Treatment for prevention of altitude illness.

 ## DOSAGE & USAGE INFORMATION

How to take:
- Sustained-release tablets—Swallow whole with liquid or food to lessen stomach irritation.
- Extended-release capsules—Swallow whole with liquid.
- Topical—1 drop in the affected eye 3 times a day.

When to take:
- 1 dose per day—At the same time each morning.
- More than 1 dose per day—Take last dose several hours before bedtime.

Continued next column

 ## OVERDOSE

SYMPTOMS:
Drowsiness, confusion, excitement, nausea, vomiting, numbness in hands and feet, coma.
WHAT TO DO:
- **Call your doctor or poison control center for advice if you suspect overdose, even if not sure. Symptoms may not appear until damage has occurred.**
- **See emergency information on inside covers.**

If you forget a dose:
Take as soon as you remember. Continue regular schedule.

What drug does:
- Inhibits action of carbonic anhydrase, an enzyme. This lowers the internal eye pressure by decreasing fluid formation in the eye.
- Forces sodium and water excretion, reducing body fluid.

Time lapse before drug works:
2 hours.

Don't take with:
Nonprescription drugs without consulting doctor.

 ## POSSIBLE ADVERSE REACTIONS OR SIDE EFFECTS

SYMPTOMS	WHAT TO DO
Life-threatening: Convulsions.	Seek emergency treatment immediately.
Common: None expected.	
Infrequent: Back pain, sedation, fatigue, weakness, tingling or burning in feet or hands.	Continue. Call doctor when convenient.
Rare: • Headache; mood changes; nervousness; clumsiness; trembling; confusion; hives, itch, rash; sores; ringing in ears; hoarseness; dry mouth; thirst; sore throat; fever; appetite change; nausea; vomiting; black, tarry stool; breathing difficulty; irregular or weak heartbeat; easy bleeding or bruising; muscle cramps; painful or frequent urination; blood in urine.	Continue. Call doctor right away.
• Depression, loss of libido.	Continue. Call doctor when convenient.

WARNINGS & PRECAUTIONS

Don't take if:
- You are allergic to any carbonic anhydrase inhibitor.
- You have liver or kidney disease.
- You have Addison's disease (adrenal gland failure).
- You have diabetes.

Before you start, consult your doctor:
- If you have gout or lupus.
- If you are allergic to any sulfa drug.
- If you will have surgery within 2 months, including dental surgery, requiring general or spinal anesthesia.

Over age 60:
- Don't exceed recommended dose.
- If you take a digitalis preparation, eat foods high in potassium content or take a potassium supplement.

Pregnancy:
Avoid if possible, especially first 3 months. Consult doctor. Risk category C (see page xxiii).

Breast-feeding:
Avoid drug or don't nurse your infant. Consult doctor about maintaining milk supply.

Infants & children:
Not recommended for children younger than 12.

Prolonged use:
May cause kidney stones, vision change, loss of taste and smell, jaundice or weight loss.

Skin & sunlight:
One or more drugs in this group may cause rash or intensity sunburn in areas exposed to sun or ultraviolet light (photosensitivity reaction). Avoid overexposure. Notify doctor if reaction occurs.

Driving, piloting or hazardous work:
Avoid if you feel drowsy or dizzy. Otherwise, no problems expected.

Discontinuing:
Don't discontinue without medical advice.

Others:
Medicine may increase sugar levels in blood and urine. Diabetics may need insulin adjustment.

POSSIBLE INTERACTION WITH OTHER DRUGS

GENERIC NAME OR DRUG CLASS	COMBINED EFFECT
Adrenocorticoids, systemic	Increased loss of calcium.
Amphetamines*	Increased amphetamine effect.
Anticonvulsants*	Increased loss of bone minerals.
Antidepressants, tricyclic*	Increased anti-depressant effect.
Antidiabetics, oral*	Increased potassium loss.
Aspirin	Decreased aspirin effect.
Ciprofloxacin	May cause kidney dysfunction.
Digitalis preparations*	Possible digitalis toxicity.
Diuretics*	Increased potassium loss.
Lithium	Decreased lithium effect.
Mecamylamine	Increased mecamylamine effect.
Methenamine	Decreased methenamine effect.
Mexiletene	May slow elimination of mexiletine and cause need to adjust dosage.
Quinidine	Increased quinidine effect.
Salicylates*	Salicylate toxicity.
Sympathomimetics*	Increased sympathomimetic effect.

POSSIBLE INTERACTION WITH OTHER SUBSTANCES

INTERACTS WITH	COMBINED EFFECT
Alcohol:	None expected.
Beverages:	None expected.
Cocaine:	Avoid. Decreased carbonic anhydrase inhibitor effect.
Foods: Potassium-rich foods.*	Eat these to decrease potassium loss.
Marijuana:	Avoid. Increased carbonic anhydrase inhibitor effect.
Tobacco:	May decrease absorption of carbonic anhydrase inhibitors.

CELLULOSE SODIUM PHOSPHATE

BRAND NAMES

Calcibind

BASIC INFORMATION

Habit forming? No
Prescription needed? Yes
Available as generic? No
Drug class: Antiurolithic

 ## USES

Prevents formation of calcium kidney stones.

 ## DOSAGE & USAGE INFORMATION

How to take:
Oral suspension—Dissolve in full glass of liquid and swallow. Note: Drink 8 ounces of water or other liquid every hour while you are awake.

When to take:
- According to instructions on prescription label. Usually 3 times a day with meals.
- Don't take within 1-1/2 hours of taking any laxative or antacid containing magnesium.

If you forget a dose:
Take as soon as you remember up to 2 hours late. If more than 2 hours, wait for next scheduled dose (don't double this dose).

What drug does:
Combines with calcium in food to prevent absorption into the bloodstream.

Time lapse before drug works:
None. Works right away.

Don't take with:
Any other medicines (including over-the-counter drugs such as cough and cold medicines, laxatives, antacids, diet pills, caffeine, nose drops or vitamins) without consulting your doctor.

 ## OVERDOSE

SYMPTOMS:
Drowsiness, mental changes, muscle spasms, seizures.
WHAT TO DO:
- Dial 911 (emergency) or 0 (operator) for an ambulance or medical help. Then give first aid immediately.
- See emergency information on inside covers.

 ## POSSIBLE ADVERSE REACTIONS OR SIDE EFFECTS

SYMPTOMS	WHAT TO DO
Life-threatening:	
In case of overdose, see previous column.	
Common:	
Loose bowel movements.	Continue. Call doctor when convenient.
Infrequent:	
Abdominal pain.	Discontinue. Call doctor right away.
Rare:	
None expected.	

CELLULOSE SODIUM PHOSPHATE

WARNINGS & PRECAUTIONS

Don't take if:
- You have bone disease.
- You have hyperparathyroidism.
- You have too little calcium in your blood.

Before you start, consult your doctor:
- If you have heart disease.
- If you have kidney disease.

Over age 60:
No special problems expected.

Pregnancy:
Decide with your doctor if drug benefits justify risk to unborn child. Risk category C (see page xxiii).

Breast-feeding:
No special problems expected. Consult doctor.

Infants & children:
Not recommended up to age 16.

Prolonged use:
Talk to your doctor about the need for follow-up medical examinations or laboratory studies to check serum calcium and magnesium concentrations (every 6 months), serum parathyroid hormone, urinary calcium and urinary oxalate levels (occasionally).

Skin & sunlight:
No problems expected.

Driving, piloting or hazardous work:
Avoid if you feel confused, drowsy or dizzy.

Discontinuing:
No special problems expected.

Others:
Advise any doctor or dentist whom you consult that you take this medicine.

POSSIBLE INTERACTION WITH OTHER DRUGS

GENERIC NAME OR DRUG CLASS	COMBINED EFFECT
Calcium-containing medications	Decreased effect of cellulose sodium phosphate.
Magnesium-containing medicines (includes many laxatives* and antacids*)	Decreased magnesium effect.
Vitamin C (ascorbic acid)	Decreased vitamin C effect.

POSSIBLE INTERACTION WITH OTHER SUBSTANCES

INTERACTS WITH	COMBINED EFFECT
Alcohol:	No special problems expected.
Beverages: Milk or other dairy products or tea.	Decreases effectiveness of cellulose sodium phosphate.
Cocaine:	No special problems expected.
Foods: Spinach, broccoli, rhubarb.	Decreases effectiveness of cellulose sodium phosphate.
Marijuana:	No special problems expected.
Tobacco:	No special problems expected.

*See Glossary

209

CEPHALOSPORINS

GENERIC AND BRAND NAMES

CEFACLOR
  Ceclor
CEFADROXIL
  Duricef
  Ultracef
CEFDINIR
  Omnicef
CEFIXIME
  Suprax
CEFOTETAN
  Cefotan
CEFPODOXIME
  Vantin
CEFPROZIL
  Cefzil

CEFUROXIME
  Ceftin
CEPHALEXIN
  Apo-Cephalex
  Cefanex
  Ceporex
  C-Lexin
  Keflet
  Keflex
  Keftab
  Novolexin
  Nu-Cephalex
CEPHRADINE
  Anspor
  Velosef

BASIC INFORMATION

Habit forming? No
Prescription needed? Yes
Available as generic? Yes
Drug class: Antibacterial

USES

Treatment of bacterial infections. Will not cure viral infections such as cold and flu.

DOSAGE & USAGE INFORMATION

How to take:
- Tablet or capsule—Swallow with liquid. If you can't swallow whole, crumble tablet or open capsule and take with liquid or food.
- Extended-release tablet—Swallow with liquid. Do not open capsule.
- Liquid—Use measuring spoon. Mix according to package instructions.

Continued next column

OVERDOSE

SYMPTOMS:
Abdominal cramps, nausea, vomiting, severe diarrhea with mucus or blood in stool, convulsions.
WHAT TO DO:
Overdose unlikely to threaten life. If person takes much larger amount than prescribed, call doctor, poison control center or hospital emergency room for instructions.

When to take:
- At same times each day, 1 hour before or 2 hours after eating.
- Take until gone or as directed.

If you forget a dose:
Take as soon as you remember or double next dose. Return to regular schedule.

What drug does:
Kills susceptible bacteria.

Time lapse before drug works:
May require several days to affect infection.

Don't take with:
Any other medicine without consulting your doctor or pharmacist.

POSSIBLE ADVERSE REACTIONS OR SIDE EFFECTS

SYMPTOMS	WHAT TO DO
Life-threatening: Hives, rash, intense itching, faintness soon after a dose (anaphylaxis); difficulty breathing.	Seek emergency treatment immediately.
Common: Mild diarrhea, nausea, vomiting, sore mouth or tongue, mild stomach cramps (all less common with some cephalosporins).	Continue. Call doctor when convenient.
Infrequent: None expected.	
Rare: • Severe stomach cramps, severe diarrhea with mucus or blood in stool, fever, unusual weakness or tiredness, weight loss, bleeding or bruising, increased thirst, decreased urine, dizziness, joint pain, appetite loss, skin symptoms (rash, itching, redness, swelling), yellow skin or eyes.	Discontinue. Call doctor right away.
• Genital itching or vaginal discharge.	Continue. Call doctor when convenient.

WARNINGS & PRECAUTIONS

Don't take if:
You are allergic to any cephalosporin antibiotic.

Before you start, consult your doctor:
- If you are allergic to any penicillin antibiotic.
- If you have a kidney disorder.
- If you have colitis or enteritis.

Over age 60:
Adverse reactions and side effects may be more frequent and severe than in younger persons. More likely to itch around rectum and genitals.

Pregnancy:
No proven harm to unborn child. Avoid if possible. Consult doctor. Risk category B (see page xxiii).

Breast-feeding:
Drug passes into milk. Avoid drug or discontinue nursing until you finish medicine. Consult doctor for advice on maintaining milk supply.

Infants & children:
No special warnings.

Prolonged use:
- Kills beneficial bacteria that protect body against other germs. Unchecked germs may cause secondary infections.
- Talk to your doctor about the need for follow-up medical examinations or laboratory studies to check prothrombin time.

Skin & sunlight:
No problems expected.

Driving, piloting or hazardous work:
No problems expected.

Discontinuing:
Don't discontinue without doctor's advice until you complete prescribed dose, even though symptoms diminish or disappear.

Others:
- Don't use drug for other medical problems without doctor's approval.
- If diarrhea occurs, consult doctor.

POSSIBLE INTERACTION WITH OTHER DRUGS

GENERIC NAME OR DRUG CLASS	COMBINED EFFECT
Anticoagulants*	Increased anticoagulant effect.
Anti-inflammatory drugs, nonsteroidal (NSAIDs)*	Increased risk of peptic ulcer.
Erythromycins*	Decreased antibiotic effect of cephalosporin.
Chloramphenicol	Decreased antibiotic effect of cephalosporin.
Probenecid	Increased cephalosporin effect.
Tetracyclines*	Decreased antibiotic effect of cephalosporin.

POSSIBLE INTERACTION WITH OTHER SUBSTANCES

INTERACTS WITH	COMBINED EFFECT
Alcohol:	Increased kidney toxicity, likelihood of disulfiram-like* effect.
Beverages:	None expected.
Cocaine:	None expected, but cocaine may slow body's recovery. Avoid.
Foods:	Slow absorption. Take with liquid 1 hour before or 2 hours after eating.
Marijuana:	None expected, but marijuana may slow body's recovery. Avoid.
Tobacco:	None expected.

CHARCOAL, ACTIVATED

BRAND NAMES

Acta-Char
Acta-Char Liquid
Actidose-Aqua
Actidose with Sorbitol
Aqueous Charcodote
Charac-50
Charac-tol 50
Charcoaid
Charcocaps

Charcodote
Charcodote TFS
Insta-Char
Liqui-Char
Pediatric Aqueous
  Charcodote
Pediatric Charcodote
SuperChar

BASIC INFORMATION

Habit forming? No
Prescription needed? No
Available as generic? Yes
Drug class: Antidote (adsorbent)

 ## USES

- Treatment of poisonings from medication.
- Treatment (infrequent) for diarrhea or excessive gaseousness.

 ## DOSAGE & USAGE INFORMATION

How to take:
- Tablet or capsule—Swallow with liquid. If you can't swallow whole, crumble tablet or open capsule and take with liquid or food.
- Liquid—Take as directed on label. Don't mix with chocolate syrup, ice cream or sherbet.

When to take:
- For poisoning—Take immediately after poisoning. If your doctor or emergency poison control center has also recommended syrup of ipecac, don't take charcoal for 30 minutes or until vomiting from ipecac stops.
- For diarrhea or gas—Take at same times each day.
- Take 2 or more hours after taking other medicines.

Continued next column

 ## OVERDOSE

SYMPTOMS:
None expected.
WHAT TO DO:
Overdose unlikely to threaten life. If person takes much larger amount than prescribed, call doctor, poison control center or hospital emergency room for instructions.

If you forget a dose:
- For poisonings—Not applicable.
- For diarrhea or gas—Take as soon as you remember up to 2 hours late. If more than 2 hours, wait for next scheduled dose (don't double this dose).

What drug does:
- Helps prevent poison from being absorbed from stomach and intestines.
- Helps absorb gas in intestinal tract.

Time lapse before drug works:
Begins immediately.

Don't take with:
Ice cream or sherbet.

 ## POSSIBLE ADVERSE REACTIONS OR SIDE EFFECTS

SYMPTOMS	WHAT TO DO
Life-threatening: None expected.	
Always: Black bowel movements.	No action necessary.
Infrequent: None expected.	
Rare: Unless taken with cathartic, can cause constipation when taken for overdose of other medicine.	Take a laxative after crisis is over.

212

WARNINGS & PRECAUTIONS

Don't take if:
The poison was lye or other strong alkali, strong acids (such as sulfuric acid), cyanide, iron, ethyl alcohol or methyl alcohol. Charcoal will not prevent these poisons from causing ill effects.

Before you start, consult your doctor:
If you are taking it as an antidote for poison.

Over age 60:
No problems expected.

Pregnancy:
Consult doctor. Risk category C (see page xxiii).

Breast-feeding:
No problems expected. Consult doctor.

Infants & children:
Don't give to children for more than 3 or 4 days for diarrhea. Continuing for longer periods can interfere with normal nutrition.

Prolonged use:
No problems expected.

Skin & sunlight:
No problems expected.

Driving, piloting or hazardous work:
No problems expected.

Discontinuing:
No problems expected.

Others:
No problems expected.

POSSIBLE INTERACTION WITH OTHER DRUGS

GENERIC NAME OR DRUG CLASS	COMBINED EFFECT
Any medicine taken at the same time	May decrease absorption of medicine. Take drugs 2 hours apart.

POSSIBLE INTERACTION WITH OTHER SUBSTANCES

INTERACTS WITH	COMBINED EFFECT
Alcohol:	None expected
Beverages:	None expected.
Cocaine:	None expected.
Foods: Chocolate syrup, ice cream or sherbet.	Decreased charcoal effect.
Marijuana:	None expected.
Tobacco:	None expected.

*See Glossary

CHLOPHEDIANOL

BRAND NAMES

Ulone

BASIC INFORMATION

Habit forming? No
Prescription needed? Yes
Available as generic? No
Drug class: Cough suppressant

USES

Reduces nonproductive cough due to bronchial irritation.

DOSAGE & USAGE INFORMATION

How to take:
Take syrup without diluting. Don't drink fluids immediately after medicine.

When to take:
3 or 4 times a day when needed. No more often than every 3 hours.

If you forget a dose:
Take as soon as you remember up to 2 hours late. If more than 2 hours, wait for next scheduled dose (don't double this dose).

What drug does:
Reduces cough reflex by direct effect on cough center in brain, and by local anesthetic action.

Time lapse before drug works:
30 minutes to 1 hour.

Don't take with:
- Alcohol or brain depressant or stimulant drugs.
- Any other medicine without consulting your doctor or pharmacist.

OVERDOSE

SYMPTOMS:
Blurred vision, hallucinations, coma.
WHAT TO DO:
- **Dial 911 (emergency) or 0 (operator) for an ambulance or medical help. Then give first aid immediately.**
- **If patient is unconscious and not breathing, give mouth-to-mouth breathing. If there is no heartbeat, use cardiac massage and mouth-to-mouth breathing (CPR). Don't try to make patient vomit. If you can't get help quickly, take patient to nearest emergency facility.**
- **See emergency information on inside covers.**

POSSIBLE ADVERSE REACTIONS OR SIDE EFFECTS

SYMPTOMS	WHAT TO DO
Life-threatening: In case of overdose, see previous column.	
Common: Difficult urination in older men with enlarged prostate.	Continue. Call doctor when convenient.
Infrequent: None expected.	
Rare:	
• Hallucinations, drowsiness, rash or hives, nausea, vomiting, irregular heartbeat.	Discontinue. Call doctor right away.
• Nightmares, excitement or irritability, blurred vision, dry mouth.	Continue. Call doctor when convenient.

CHLOPHEDIANOL

WARNINGS & PRECAUTIONS

Don't take if:
You are allergic to chlophedianol.

Before you start, consult your doctor:
- If medicine is for hyperactive child who takes medicine for treatment.
- If your cough brings up sputum (phlegm).
- If you have heart disease.
- If you will have surgery within 2 months, including dental surgery, requiring general or spinal anesthesia.

Over age 60:
Adverse reactions and side effects may be more frequent and severe than in younger persons.

Pregnancy:
Pregnancy risk not designated. See category list on page xxiii and consult doctor.

Breast-feeding:
Unknown whether medicine filters into milk. Consult doctor.

Infants & children:
Not recommended for children under age 2.

Prolonged use:
Not recommended. If cough persists despite medicine, consult doctor.

Skin & sunlight:
No problems expected.

Driving, piloting or hazardous work:
Don't drive or pilot aircraft until you learn how medicine affects you. Don't work around dangerous machinery. Don't climb ladders or work in high places. Danger increases if you drink alcohol or take medicine affecting alertness and reflexes, such as antihistamines, tranquilizers, sedatives, pain medicine, narcotics and mind-altering drugs.

Discontinuing:
May be unnecessary to finish medicine. Follow doctor's instructions.

Others:
Consult doctor if cough persists despite medication for 7 days or if fever, skin rash or headache accompany cough.

POSSIBLE INTERACTION WITH OTHER DRUGS

GENERIC NAME OR DRUG CLASS	COMBINED EFFECT
Anticonvulsants*	Interferes with actions of both.
Antidepressants, tricyclic*	Excess sedation.
Appetite suppressants*	Excess stimulation.
Central nervous system (CNS) depressants*	Excess sedation.
Monoamine oxidase (MAO) inhibitors*	Excess sedation.
Sympathomimetics*	Excess stimulation.

POSSIBLE INTERACTION WITH OTHER SUBSTANCES

INTERACTS WITH	COMBINED EFFECT
Alcohol:	Excess sedation. Avoid.
Beverages: Coffee, tea, cocoa, cola.	Excess stimulation. Avoid.
Cocaine:	Increased chance of toxic stimulation. Avoid.
Foods:	None expected.
Marijuana:	Increased chance of toxic stimulation. Avoid.
Tobacco:	Decreased effect of chlophedianol.

*See Glossary

CHLORAL HYDRATE

BRAND NAMES

Aquachloral   Novochlorhydrate
Noctec

BASIC INFORMATION

Habit forming? Yes
Prescription needed? Yes
Available as generic? Yes
Drug class: Sedative-hypnotic agent

USES

Short term treatment to relieve insomnia.

DOSAGE & USAGE INFORMATION

How to take:
* Syrup or capsule—Swallow with liquid or food to lessen stomach irritation.
* Suppositories—Remove wrapper and moisten suppository with water. Gently insert smaller end into rectum. Push well into rectum with finger.

When to take:
At the same time each day.

If you forget a dose:
Take as soon as you remember up to 2 hours late. If more than 2 hours, wait for next scheduled dose (don't double this dose).

Continued next column

OVERDOSE

SYMPTOMS:
Confusion, weakness, breathing difficulty, throat irritation, jaundice, stagger, slow or irregular heartbeat, unconsciousness, convulsions, coma.
WHAT TO DO:
* Dial 911 (emergency) or 0 (operator) for an ambulance or medical help. Then give first aid immediately.
* If patient is unconscious and not breathing, give mouth-to-mouth breathing. If there is no heartbeat, use cardiac massage and mouth-to-mouth breathing (CPR). Don't try to make patient vomit. If you can't get help quickly, take patient to nearest emergency facility.
* See emergency information at end of book.

What drug does:
Affects brain centers that control wakefulness and alertness.

Time lapse before drug works:
30 to 60 minutes.

Don't take with:
Any other medicine without consulting your doctor or pharmacist.

POSSIBLE ADVERSE REACTIONS OR SIDE EFFECTS

SYMPTOMS	WHAT TO DO
Life-threatening: In case of overdose, see previous column.	
Common: Nausea, stomach pain, vomiting.	Discontinue. Call doctor right away.
Infrequent: "Hangover" effect, clumsiness or unsteadiness, drowsiness, dizziness, lightheadedness, diarrhea.	Continue. Call doctor when convenient.
Rare: • Hallucinations, agitation, confusion. leukopenia (white blood cells causing sore throat and fever).	Discontinue. Call doctor right away.
• Hives, rash.	Continue. Call doctor when convenient.

WARNINGS & PRECAUTIONS

Don't take if:
You are allergic to chloral hydrate or you have porphyria.

Before you start, consult your doctor:
* If you have had liver, kidney or heart trouble.
* If you are prone to stomach upsets (if medicine is in oral form).
* If you are allergic to tartrazine dye.
* If you have colitis or a rectal inflammation (if medicine is in suppository form).

Over age 60:
Adverse reactions and side effects may be more frequent and severe than in younger persons. More likely to have "hangover" effect.

Pregnancy:
Decide with your doctor if drug benefits justify risk to unborn child. Risk category C (see page xxiii).

Breast-feeding:
Small amounts may filter into breast milk. Best to avoid.

Infants & children:
Use only under medical supervision.

Prolonged use:
- Drug loses its effectiveness as an antianxiety agent or sleep aid after about 2 weeks. Not recommended for longer use.
- Addiction and possible kidney damage may result if used long-term.

Skin & sunlight:
No problems expected.

Driving, piloting or hazardous work:
Don't drive or pilot aircraft until you learn how medicine affects you. Don't work around dangerous machinery. Don't climb ladders or work in high places. Danger increases if you drink alcohol or take medicine affecting alertness and reflexes, such as antihistamines, tranquilizers, sedatives, pain medicine, narcotics and mind-altering drugs.

Discontinuing:
Don't discontinue without consulting doctor. Dose may require gradual reduction if you have taken drug for a long time. Doses of other drugs may also require adjustment.

Others:
- Frequent kidney function tests recommended when drug is used for long time.
- Advise any doctor or dentist whom you consult that you take this medicine.

POSSIBLE INTERACTION WITH OTHER DRUGS

GENERIC NAME OR DRUG CLASS	COMBINED EFFECT
Anticoagulants, oral*	Possible hemorrhaging.
Antidepressants*	Increased chloral hydrate effect.
Antihistamines*	Increased chloral hydrate effect.
Central nervous system (CNS) depressants*	Increased sedative effect.
Clozapine	Toxic effect on the central nervous system.
Fluoxetine	Increased depressant effects of both drugs.
Guanfacine	May increase depressant effects of either drug.
Leucovorin	High alcohol content of leucovorin may cause adverse effects.
Mind-altering drugs*	Increased chloral hydrate effect.
Molindone	Increased tranquilizer effect.
Monoamine oxidase (MAO) inhibitors*	Increased chloral hydrate effect.
Narcotics*	Increased chloral hydrate effect.
Phenothiazines*	Increased chloral hydrate effect.
Sertraline	Increased depressive effects of both drugs.

POSSIBLE INTERACTION WITH OTHER SUBSTANCES

INTERACTS WITH	COMBINED EFFECT
Alcohol:	Increased sedative effects of both. Avoid.
Beverages:	None expected.
Cocaine:	Decreased chloral hydrate effect. Avoid.
Foods:	None expected.
Marijuana:	May severely impair mental and physical functioning. Avoid.
Tobacco:	None expected.

CHLORAMBUCIL

BRAND NAMES

Leukeran

BASIC INFORMATION

Habit forming? No
Prescription needed? Yes
Available as generic? No
Drug class: Antineoplastic, immuno-
suppressant

 USES

- Treatment for some kinds of cancer.
- Suppresses immune response after transplant and in immune disorders.

 DOSAGE & USAGE INFORMATION

How to take:
Tablet—Swallow with liquid after light meal. Don't drink fluids with meals. Drink extra fluids between meals. Avoid sweet or fatty foods.

When to take:
At the same time each day.

If you forget a dose:
Take as soon as you remember. Don't ever double dose.

What drug does:
Inhibits abnormal cell reproduction. May suppress immune system.

Time lapse before drug works:
Up to 6 weeks for full effect.

Don't take with:
Any other medicine without consulting your doctor or pharmacist.

 OVERDOSE

SYMPTOMS:
Bleeding, chills, fever, vomiting, abdominal pain, ataxia, collapse, stupor, seizure.
WHAT TO DO:
- Dial 911 (emergency) or 0 (operator) for an ambulance or medical help. Then give first aid immediately.
- If patient is unconscious and not breathing, give mouth-to-mouth breathing. If there is no heartbeat, use cardiac massage and mouth-to-mouth breathing (CPR). Don't try to make patient vomit. If you can't get help quickly, take patient to nearest emergency facility.
- See emergency information on inside covers.

 POSSIBLE ADVERSE REACTIONS OR SIDE EFFECTS

SYMPTOMS	WHAT TO DO
Life-threatening:	
In case of overdose, see previous column.	
Common:	
• Unusual bleeding or bruising, mouth sores with sore throat, chills and fever, black stools, mouth and lip sores, menstrual irregularities, back pain.	Discontinue. Call doctor right away.
• Hair loss, joint pain.	Continue. Call doctor when convenient.
• Nausea, vomiting, diarrhea, tiredness, weakness.	Continue. Tell doctor at next visit.
Infrequent:	
• Mental confusion, shortness of breath.	Continue. Call doctor when convenient.
• Cough, rash, foot swelling.	Continue. Tell doctor at next visit.
Rare:	
Jaundice, convulsions, hallucinations, muscle twitching.	Discontinue. Call doctor right away.

WARNINGS & PRECAUTIONS

Don't take if:
- You have had hypersensitivity to alkylating antineoplastic drugs.
- Your physician has not explained serious nature of your medical problem and risks of taking this medicine.

Before you start, consult your doctor:
- If you have gout.
- If you have had kidney stones.
- If you have active infection.
- If you have impaired kidney or liver function.
- If you have taken other antineoplastic drugs or had radiation treatment in last 3 weeks.

Over age 60:
Adverse reactions and side effects may be more frequent and severe than in younger persons.

Pregnancy:
Consult doctor. Risk to unborn child is significant. Risk category D (see page xxiii).

Breast-feeding:
Safety not established. Consult doctor.

Infants & children:
Use only under care of medical supervisors who are experienced in anticancer drugs.

Prolonged use:
- Adverse reactions more likely the longer drug is required.
- Talk to your doctor about the need for follow-up medical examinations or laboratory studies to check complete blood counts (white blood cell count, platelet count, red blood cell count, hemoglobin, hematocrit).

Skin & sunlight:
No problems expected.

Driving, piloting or hazardous work:
No problems expected.

Discontinuing:
Don't discontinue without doctor's advice until you complete prescribed dose, even though symptoms diminish or disappear. Some side effects may follow discontinuing. Report to doctor blurred vision, convulsions, confusion, persistent headache.

Others:
- May cause sterility.
- May increase chance of developing leukemia.
- Consult your doctor before you or a household member gets any immunization.

POSSIBLE INTERACTION WITH OTHER DRUGS

GENERIC NAME OR DRUG CLASS	COMBINED EFFECT
Antigout drugs*	Decreased antigout effect.
Antineoplastic drugs, other*	Increased effect of all drugs (may be beneficial).
Chloramphenicol	Increased likelihood of toxic effects of both drugs.
Clozapine	Toxic effect on bone marrow.
Cyclosporine	May increase risk of infection.
Immuno-suppressants*	Increased chance of infection.
Lovastatin	Increased heart and kidney damage.
Tiopronin	Increased risk of toxicity to bone marrow.

POSSIBLE INTERACTION WITH OTHER SUBSTANCES

INTERACTS WITH	COMBINED EFFECT
Alcohol:	May increase chance of intestinal bleeding.
Beverages:	No problems expected.
Cocaine:	Increases chance of toxicity.
Foods:	Reduces irritation in stomach.
Marijuana:	No problems expected.
Tobacco:	Increases lung toxicity.

CHLORAMPHENICOL

BRAND NAMES

Chloromycetin   Novochlorocap

BASIC INFORMATION

Habit forming? No
Prescription needed? Yes
Available as generic? Yes
Drug class: Antibacterial

 ## USES

Treatment of infections susceptible to chloramphenicol. Will not treat viral infections such as cold or flu.

 ## DOSAGE & USAGE INFORMATION

How to take:
Suspension or capsule—Take with a full glass of water.

When to take:
Capsule or suspension—1 hour before or 2 hours after eating.

If you forget a dose:
Take as soon as you remember up to 2 hours late. If more than 2 hours, wait for next scheduled dose (don't double this dose).

What drug does:
Prevents bacteria from growing and reproducing. Will not kill viruses.

Time lapse before drug works:
2 to 5 days, depending on type and severity of infection.

Don't take with:
Any other medicine without consulting your doctor or pharmacist.

 ## OVERDOSE

SYMPTOMS:
Nausea, vomiting, diarrhea.
WHAT TO DO:
Overdose unlikely to threaten life. If person takes much larger amount than prescribed, call doctor, poison control center or hospital emergency room for instructions.

 ## POSSIBLE ADVERSE REACTIONS OR SIDE EFFECTS

SYMPTOMS	WHAT TO DO
Life-threatening: Hives, rash, intense itching, faintness soon after a dose (anaphylaxis).	Seek emergency treatment immediately.
Common: None expected.	
Infrequent: • Swollen face or extremities; diarrhea; nausea; vomiting; numbness, tingling, burning pain or weakness in hands and feet; pale skin; unusual bleeding or bruising.	Discontinue. Call doctor right away.
• Headache, confusion.	Continue. Call doctor when convenient.
Rare: • Pain, blurred vision, possible vision loss, delirium, rash, sore throat, fever, jaundice, anemia.	Discontinue. Call doctor right away.
• In babies: Bloated stomach, uneven breathing, drowsiness, low temperature, gray skin.	Discontinue. Call doctor right away.

 ## WARNINGS & PRECAUTIONS

Don't take if:
• You are allergic to chloramphenicol.
• It is prescribed for a minor disorder such as flu, cold or mild sore throat.

Before you start, consult your doctor:
• If you have had a blood disorder or bone-marrow disease.
• If you have had kidney or liver disease.
• If you have diabetes.

Over age 60:
Adverse reactions and side effects may be more frequent and severe than in younger persons, particularly skin irritation around rectum.

Pregnancy:
Decide with your doctor if drug benefits justify risk to unborn child. Risk category C (see page xxiii).

Breast-feeding:
Drug passes into milk. Avoid drug or discontinue nursing until you finish medicine. Consult doctor for advice on maintaining milk supply.

Infants & children:
Use only under close medical supervision, especially in infants younger than 2.

Prolonged use:
* You may become more susceptible to infections caused by germs not responsive to chloramphenicol.
* Talk to your doctor about the need for follow-up medical examinations or laboratory studies to check complete blood counts (white blood cell count, platelet count, red blood cell count, hemoglobin, hematocrit), chloramphenicol serum levels.

Skin & sunlight:
No problems expected.

Driving, piloting or hazardous work:
Don't drive or pilot aircraft until you learn how medicine affects you. Don't work around dangerous machinery. Don't climb ladders or work in high places. Danger increases if you drink alcohol or take medicine affecting alertness and reflexes.

Discontinuing:
Don't discontinue without doctor's advice until you complete prescribed dose, even though symptoms diminish or disappear.

Others:
* Chloramphenicol can cause serious anemia. Frequent laboratory blood studies, liver and kidney tests recommended.
* Second medical opinion recommended before starting.

POSSIBLE INTERACTION WITH OTHER DRUGS

GENERIC NAME OR DRUG CLASS	COMBINED EFFECT
Anticoagulants*	Increased anticoagulant effect.
Antidiabetics, oral*	Increased antidiabetic effect.
Anticonvulsants*	Increased chance of toxicity to bone marrow.
Antivirals, HIV/AIDS*	Increased risk of peripheral neuropathy.
Cefiximine	Decreased antibiotic effect of cefiximine.
Cephalosporins*	Decreased chloramphenicol effect.

Clindamycin	Decreased clindamycin effect.
Clozapine	Toxic effect on bone marrow.
Cyclophosphamide	Increased cyclophosphamide effect.
Erythromycins	Decreased erythromycin effect.
Flecainide	Possible decreased blood cell production in bone marrow.
Levamisole	Increased risk of bone marrow depression.
Lincomycin	Decreased lincomycin effect.
Lisinopril	Possible blood disorders.
Penicillins*	Decreased penicillin effect.
Phenobarbital	Increased phenobarbital effect.
Phenytoin	Increased phenytoin effect.
Rifampin	Decreased chloramphenicol effect.
Thioguanine	More likelihood of toxicity of both drugs.
Tiopronin	Increased risk of toxicity to bone marrow.
Tocainide	Possible decreased blood cell production in bone marrow.

POSSIBLE INTERACTION WITH OTHER SUBSTANCES

INTERACTS WITH	COMBINED EFFECT
Alcohol:	Possible liver problems. May cause disulfiram reaction.*
Beverages:	None expected.
Cocaine:	No proven problems.
Foods:	None expected.
Marijuana:	None expected.
Tobacco:	None expected.

CHLORHEXIDINE

BRAND NAMES

Peridex   Periogard
Periochip

BASIC INFORMATION

Habit forming? No
Prescription needed? Yes
Available as generic? Yes
Drug class: Antibacterial (dental)

 ## USES

Treatment for gingivitis (inflammation of the gums), periodontal disease and other infections of the mouth.

 ## DOSAGE & USAGE INFORMATION

How to use:
- Oral rinse—Swish in mouth for 30 seconds, then spit out. Do not swallow the solution, and do not rinse mouth with water after using. Use product at full strength; do not dilute.
- Implants—Inserted by dentist.

When to use:
Twice a day after brushing and flossing teeth.

If you forget a dose:
Use as soon as you remember, then return to regular schedule.

What drug does:
Kills or prevents growth of susceptible bacteria.

Time lapse before drug works:
Antibacterial action begins within an hour, but full benefit may take several weeks.

Don't use with:
Other mouthwashes without consulting your dentist or pharmacist.

 ## OVERDOSE

SYMPTOMS:
None expected. If a child swallows several ounces of the solution, may have slurred speech, staggering or stumbling walk, sleepiness.
WHAT TO DO:
If symptoms occur, call doctor for instructions. If child weighing under 22 pounds accidentally swallows more than 4 ounces, seek emergency help. Dial 911 (emergency) or 0 (operator) for an ambulance or medical help. Then give first aid immediately.

 ## POSSIBLE ADVERSE REACTIONS OR SIDE EFFECTS

SYMPTOMS	WHAT TO DO
Life-threatening: None expected.	
Common: Staining of teeth and other oral surfaces, increased tartar, taste changes, minor mouth irritation.	Continue. Call dentist when convenient.
Infrequent: None expected.	
Rare: Allergic reaction (stuffy nose, shortness of breath, skin rash, hives, itching, face swelling); swollen glands on side of face or neck.	Discontinue. Call doctor right away.

WARNINGS & PRECAUTIONS

Don't take if:
You are allergic to chlorhexidine or skin cleaners that contain chlorhexidine.

Before you start, consult your dentist:
- If you have front tooth fillings (may become discolored).
- If you have periodontitis.

Over age 60:
No special problems expected.

Pregnancy:
Consult doctor. Risk category B (see page xxiii).

Breast-feeding:
It is unknown if drug passes into milk. Consult doctor.

Infants & children:
Safety in children under age 18 has not been established.

Prolonged use:
See your dentist every 6 months.

Skin & sunlight:
No special problems expected.

Driving, piloting or hazardous work:
No special problems expected.

Discontinuing:
No special problems expected.

Others:
Brush teeth with a tartar-control toothpaste, and floss daily to help reduce tartar buildup.

POSSIBLE INTERACTION WITH OTHER DRUGS

GENERIC NAME OR DRUG CLASS	COMBINED EFFECT
None expected.	

POSSIBLE INTERACTION WITH OTHER SUBSTANCES

INTERACTS WITH	COMBINED EFFECT
Alcohol:	None expected.
Beverages:	Avoid drinking any fluids for several hours after using mouthwash.
Cocaine:	None expected.
Foods:	Avoid eating any foods for several hours after using mouthwash.
Marijuana:	None expected.
Tobacco:	None expected.

CHLOROQUINE

BRAND NAMES

Aralen

BASIC INFORMATION

Habit forming? No
Prescription needed? Yes
Available as generic? Yes
Drug class: Antiprotozoal, antirheumatic

 ## USES

- Treatment for protozoal infections, such as malaria and amebiasis.
- Treatment for some forms of arthritis and lupus.

 ## DOSAGE & USAGE INFORMATION

How to take:
Tablet—Swallow with food or milk to lessen stomach irritation.

When to take:
- Depends on condition. Is adjusted during treatment.
- Malaria prevention—Begin taking medicine 2 weeks before traveling to areas where malaria is present and until 8 weeks after return.

If you forget a dose:
- 1 or more doses a day—Take as soon as you remember up to 2 hours late. If more than 2 hours, wait for next scheduled dose (don't double this dose).
- 1 dose weekly—Take as soon as possible, then return to regular dosing schedule.

What drug does:
- Inhibits parasite multiplication.
- Decreases inflammatory response in diseased joint.

Continued next column

 ## OVERDOSE

SYMPTOMS:
Severe breathing difficulty, drowsiness, faintness, headache, seizures.
WHAT TO DO:
- **Dial 911 (emergency) or 0 (operator) for an ambulance or medical help. Then give first aid immediately.**
- **See emergency information on inside covers.**

Time lapse before drug works:
1 to 2 hours. For treatment of arthritis symptoms, may take up to 6 months for maximum effectiveness.

Don't take with:
Any other medicine without consulting your doctor or pharmacist.

 ## POSSIBLE ADVERSE REACTIONS OR SIDE EFFECTS

SYMPTOMS	WHAT TO DO
Life-threatening:	
In case of overdose, see previous column.	
Common:	
Headache, appetite loss, abdominal pain.	Continue. Tell doctor at next visit.
Infrequent:	
• Blurred or changed vision.	Discontinue. Call doctor right away.
• Rash or itch, diarrhea, nausea, vomiting, decreased blood pressure, hair loss, blue-black skin or mouth, dizziness, nervousness.	Continue. Call doctor when convenient.
Rare:	
• Mood or mental changes, seizures, sore throat, fever, unusual bleeding or bruising, muscle weakness, convulsions.	Discontinue. Call doctor right away.
• Ringing or buzzing in ears, hearing loss.	Continue. Call doctor when convenient.

WARNINGS & PRECAUTIONS

Don't take if:
You are allergic to chloroquine or hydroxychloroquine.

Before you start, consult your doctor:
- If you plan to become pregnant within the medication period.
- If you have blood disease.
- If you have eye or vision problems.
- If you have a G6PD deficiency.
- If you have liver disease.
- If you have nerve or brain disease (including seizure disorders).
- If you have porphyria.
- If you have psoriasis.
- If you have stomach or intestinal disease.
- If you drink more than 3 oz. of alcohol daily.

Over age 60:
Adverse reactions and side effects may be more frequent and severe than in younger persons.

Pregnancy:
Decide with your doctor if drug benefits justify risk to unborn child. Risk category C (see page xxiii).

Breast-feeding:
Drug passes into milk. Avoid drug or discontinue nursing. Consult doctor about maintaining milk supply.

Infants & children:
Not recommended. Dangerous.

Prolonged use:
- Permanent damage to the retina (back part of the eye) or nerve deafness.
- Talk to your doctor about the need for follow-up medical examinations or laboratory studies to check complete blood counts (white blood cell count, platelet count, red blood cell count, hemoglobin, hematocrit), eyes.

Skin & sunlight:
May cause rash or intensify sunburn in areas exposed to sun or ultraviolet light (photosensitivity reaction). Avoid overexposure. Notify doctor if reaction occurs.

Driving, piloting or hazardous work:
Don't drive or pilot aircraft until you learn how medicine affects you. Don't work around dangerous machinery. Don't climb ladders or work in high places. Danger increases if you drink alcohol or take medicine affecting alertness and reflexes.

Discontinuing:
Don't discontinue without doctor's advice until you complete prescribed dose, even though symptoms diminish or disappear.

Others:
- Periodic physical and blood examinations recommended.
- If you are in a malaria area for a long time, you may need to change to another preventive drug every 2 years.

POSSIBLE INTERACTION WITH OTHER DRUGS

GENERIC NAME OR DRUG CLASS	COMBINED EFFECT
Penicillamine	Possible blood or kidney toxicity.

POSSIBLE INTERACTION WITH OTHER SUBSTANCES

INTERACTS WITH	COMBINED EFFECT
Alcohol:	Possible liver toxicity. Avoid.
Beverages:	None expected.
Cocaine:	None expected.
Foods:	None expected.
Marijuana:	None expected.
Tobacco:	None expected.

CHLORPROTHIXENE

BRAND NAMES

Tarasan

BASIC INFORMATION

Habit forming? No
Prescription needed? Yes
Available as generic? No
Drug class: Tranquilizer (thioxanthene), antiemetic

 USES

- Reduces anxiety, agitation, psychosis.
- Stops vomiting, hiccups.

 DOSAGE & USAGE INFORMATION

How to take:
- Tablet—Swallow with liquid. If you can't swallow whole, crumble tablet and take with liquid or food.
- Oral suspension—Dilute dose in beverage before swallowing.

When to take:
At the same time each day.

If you forget a dose:
Take as soon as you remember up to 2 hours late. If more than 2 hours, wait for next scheduled dose (don't double this dose).

What drug does:
Corrects imbalance of nerve impulses.

Continued next column

 OVERDOSE

SYMPTOMS:
Drowsiness, dizziness, weakness, muscle rigidity, twitching, tremors, confusion, dry mouth, blurred vision, rapid pulse, shallow breathing, low blood pressure, convulsions, coma.
WHAT TO DO:
- **Dial 911 (emergency) or 0 (operator) for an ambulance or medical help. Then give first aid immediately.**
- **If patient is unconscious and not breathing, give mouth-to-mouth breathing. If there is no heartbeat, use cardiac massage and mouth-to-mouth breathing (CPR). Don't try to make patient vomit. If you can't get help quickly, take patient to nearest emergency facility.**
- **See emergency information on inside covers.**

Time lapse before drug works:
3 weeks.

Don't take with:
Any other medicine without consulting your doctor or pharmacist.

 POSSIBLE ADVERSE REACTIONS OR SIDE EFFECTS

SYMPTOMS	WHAT TO DO
Life-threatening:	
Uncontrollable movements of head, neck, arms, legs (rarely).	Discontinue. Seek emergency treatment.
Common:	
• Fainting; jerky, involuntary movements; restlessness; blurred vision; rapid heartbeat.	Discontinue. Call doctor right away.
• Dizziness, drowsiness, constipation, muscle spasms, shuffling walk, decreased sweating, increased appetite, weight gain, sensitivity to light.	Continue. Call doctor when convenient.
• Dry mouth, stuffy nose.	Continue. Tell doctor at next visit.
Infrequent:	
• Rash.	Discontinue. Call doctor right away.
• Less sexual ability, difficult urination.	Continue. Call doctor when convenient.
• Menstrual irregularities, swollen breasts, breast milk secretion.	Continue. Tell doctor at next visit.
Rare:	
Sore throat, fever, jaundice, abdominal pain, lip smacking, cheek puffing, chewing movements of mouth, heatstroke, unusual bleeding or bruising.	Discontinue. Call doctor right away.

 WARNINGS & PRECAUTIONS

Don't take if:
- You are allergic to any thioxanthine or phenothiazine tranquilizer.
- You have serious blood disorder.
- You have Parkinson's disease.
- Patient is younger than 12.

Before you start, consult your doctor:
- If you have had liver or kidney disease.
- If you have epilepsy, glaucoma or prostate trouble.
- If you have high blood pressure or heart disease (especially angina).

- If you use alcohol daily.
- If you will have surgery within 2 months, including dental surgery, requiring general or spinal anesthesia.

Over age 60:
Adverse reactions and side effects may be more frequent and severe than in younger persons.

Pregnancy:
Safety not established. Avoid if possible. Consult doctor. Risk category C (see page xxiii).

Breast-feeding:
Studies inconclusive. Consult your doctor.

Infants & children:
Not recommended.

Prolonged use:
- Pigment deposits in lens and retina of eye.
- Involuntary movements of jaws, lips, tongue (tardive dyskinesia).
- Talk to your doctor about the need for follow-up medical examinations or laboratory studies to check complete blood counts (white blood cell count, platelet count, red blood cell count, hemoglobin, hematocrit), liver function, eyes.

Skin & sunlight:
May cause rash or intensify sunburn in areas exposed to sun or ultraviolet light photosensitivity reaction). Avoid overexposure. Notify doctor if reaction occurs.

Driving, piloting or hazardous work:
Don't drive or pilot aircraft until you learn how medicine affects you. Don't work around dangerous machinery. Don't climb ladders or work in high places. Danger increases if you drink alcohol or take medicine affecting alertness and reflexes.

Discontinuing:
Don't discontinue without consulting doctor. Dose may require gradual reduction if you have taken drug for a long time. Doses of other drugs may also require adjustment.

Others:
Hot temperatures increase chance of heat stroke.

POSSIBLE INTERACTION WITH OTHER DRUGS

GENERIC NAME OR DRUG CLASS	COMBINED EFFECT
Anticholinergics*	Increased anticholinergic effect.
Anticonvulsants*	Change in seizure pattern.
Antidepressants, tricyclic*	Increased chlorprothixene effect. Excessive sedation.
Antihistamines*	Increased chlorprothixene effect. Excessive sedation.
Antihypertensives*	Excessively low blood pressure.
Barbiturates*	Increased chlorprothixene effect Excessive sedation.
Bethanechol	Decreased bethanechol effect.
Bupropion	Increased risk of major seizures.
Dronabinol	Increased effects of both drugs. Avoid.
Epinephrine	Low blood pressure and rapid heartbeat.
Guanethidine	Decreased guanethidine effect.
Levodopa	Decreased levodopa effect.
Mind-altering drugs*	Increased chlorprothixene effect. Excessive sedation.
Monoamine oxidase (MAO) inhibitors*	Excessive sedation.
Narcotics*	Increased chlorprothixene effect. Excessive sedation.
Pergolide	Decreased pergolide effect.
Procarbazine	Increased sedation.
Sedatives*	Increased chlorprothixene effect. Excessive sedation.

Continued on page 911

POSSIBLE INTERACTION WITH OTHER SUBSTANCES

INTERACTS WITH	COMBINED EFFECT
Alcohol:	Excessive brain depression. Avoid.
Beverages:	None expected.
Cocaine:	Decreased chlorprothixene effect. Avoid.
Foods:	None expected.
Marijuana:	Daily use—Fainting likely, possible psychosis.
Tobacco:	None expected.

CHLORZOXAZONE & ACETAMINOPHEN

BRAND NAMES

Parafon Forte

BASIC INFORMATION

Habit forming? Possibly
Prescription needed? Yes
Available as generic? Yes
Drug class: Muscle relaxant, analgesic, fever-reducer

 ## USES

- Adjunctive treatment to rest, analgesics and physical therapy for muscle spasms.
- Treatment of mild to moderate pain and fever.

 ## DOSAGE & USAGE INFORMATION

How to take:
Tablet—Swallow with liquid.

When to take:
As needed, no more often than every 3 hours.

If you forget a dose:
Take as soon as you remember. Wait 3 hours for next dose.

What drug does:
- Blocks body's pain messages to brain. Also causes sedation.
- May affect hypothalamus, the part of the brain that helps regulate body heat and receives body's pain messages.

Time lapse before drug works:
15 to 30 minutes. May last 4 hours.

Continued next column

 ## OVERDOSE

SYMPTOMS:
Nausea, vomiting, diarrhea, anorexia, headache, severe weakness, unusual increase in sweating, fainting, breathing difficulty, irritability, convulsions, sensation of paralysis, coma.
WHAT TO DO:
- **Overdose unlikely to threaten life. Depending on severity of symptoms and amount taken, call doctor, poison control center or hospital emergency room for instructions.**
- **Dial 911 (emergency) or 0 (operator) for an ambulance or medical help. Then give first aid immediately.**
- **See emergency information on inside covers.**

Don't take with:
- Other drugs with acetaminophen. Too much acetaminophen can damage liver and kidneys.
- Any other medicine without consulting your doctor or pharmacist.

 ## POSSIBLE ADVERSE REACTIONS OR SIDE EFFECTS

SYMPTOMS	WHAT TO DO
Life-threatening: Hives, rash, intense itching, faintness soon after a dose (anaphylaxis); extreme weakness, transient paralysis, temporary loss of vision.	Seek emergency treatment immediately.
Common: Dizziness, lightheadedness, drowsiness.	Discontinue. Call doctor right away.
Infrequent: • Difficult or frequent urination, severe back pain, cloudy urine.	Discontinue. Call doctor right away.
• Nervousness, restlessness, irritability, headache, indigestion, depression, agitation, constipation, tiredness, weakness.	Continue. Call doctor when convenient.
Rare: • Sudden decrease in urine output; swelling of lips, face or tongue.	Discontinue. Seek emergency treatment.
• Bloody or black stools, jaundice, unusual bleeding or bruising, sore mouth or throat, fever, hiccups, skin rash, hives.	Discontinue. Call doctor right away.

 ## WARNINGS & PRECAUTIONS

Don't take if:
- You are allergic to any skeletal muscle relaxant or acetaminophen.
- Your symptoms don't improve after 2 days use. Call your doctor.

Before you start, consult your doctor:
- If you have had liver disease.
- If you have kidney disease or liver damage.
- If you plan pregnancy within medication period.
- If you are allergic to tartrazine dye*.

CHLORZOXAZONE & ACETAMINOPHEN

Over age 60:
- Adverse reactions and side effects may be more frequent and severe than in younger persons.
- Don't exceed recommended dose. You can't eliminate drug as efficiently as younger persons.

Pregnancy:
Safety not proven. Avoid if possible. Consult doctor. Risk category C (see page xxiii).

Breast-feeding:
Drug passes into milk. Avoid drug or discontinue nursing until you finish medicine. Consult doctor for advice on maintaining milk supply.

Infants & children:
Not recommended.

Prolonged use:
- May affect blood system and cause anemia. Limit use to 5 days for children 12 and under, and 10 days for adults.
- Talk to your doctor about the need for follow-up medical examinations or laboratory studies to check complete blood counts (white blood cell count, platelet count, red blood cell count, hemoglobin, hematocrit), liver function.

Skin & sunlight:
No problems expected.

Driving, piloting or hazardous work:
Don't drive or pilot aircraft until you learn how medicine affects you. Don't work around dangerous machinery. Don't climb ladders or work in high places. Danger increases if you drink alcohol or take medicine affecting alertness and reflexes, such as antihistamines, tranquilizers, sedatives, pain medicine, narcotics and mind-altering drugs.

Discontinuing:
Don't discontinue without consulting your doctor. Dose may require gradual reduction if you have taken drug for a long time. Doses of other drugs may also require adjustment.

Others:
Periodic liver-function tests recommended if you use this drug for a long time.

 POSSIBLE INTERACTION WITH OTHER DRUGS

GENERIC NAME OR DRUG CLASS	COMBINED EFFECT
Anticoagulants, oral*	May increase anti-coagulant effect. If combined frequently, prothrombin time should be monitored.
Antidepressants*	Increased sedation.
Antihistamines*	Increased sedation.
Clozapine	Toxic effect on the central nervous system.
Dronabinol	Increased effect of dronabinol on central nervous system. Avoid combination.
Mind-altering drugs*	Increased sedation.
Monoamine oxidase (MAO) inhibitors*	Increased effect of both drugs (but safety not established).
Muscle relaxants, others*	Increased sedation.
Narcotics*	Increased sedation.
Phenobarbital	Quicker elimination and decreased effects of acetaminophen.
Sedatives*	Increased sedation.
Sertraline	Increased depressive effects of both drugs.
Sleep inducers*	Increased sedation.
Tetracyclines* (effervescent granules or tablets)	May slow tetracycline absorption. Space doses 2 hours apart.

Continued on page 911

 POSSIBLE INTERACTION WITH OTHER SUBSTANCES

INTERACTS WITH	COMBINED EFFECT
Alcohol:	Drowsiness, increased sedation. Long-term use may cause toxic effect in liver.
Beverages:	No problems expected.
Cocaine:	Lack of coordination. May slow body's recovery. Avoid.
Foods:	No problems expected.
Marijuana:	Increased pain relief, lack of coordination, drowsiness, fainting. May slow body's recovery. Avoid.
Tobacco:	No problems expected.

*See Glossary

CHOLESTYRAMINE

BRAND NAMES

Cholybar   Questran Light
Questran

BASIC INFORMATION

Habit forming? No
Prescription needed? Yes
Available as generic? Yes
Drug class: Antihyperlipidemic, antipruritic

USES

- Removes excess bile acids that occur with some liver problems. Reduces persistent itch caused by bile acids.
- Lowers cholesterol level.
- Treatment of one form of colitis (rare).

DOSAGE & USAGE INFORMATION

How to take:
Powder, granules—Sprinkle into 8 oz. liquid. Let stand for 2 minutes, then mix with liquid before swallowing. Or mix with cereal, soup or pulpy fruit. Don't swallow dry.

When to take:
- 3 or 4 times a day on an empty stomach, 1 hour before or 2 hours after eating.
- If taking other medicines, take 1 hour before or 4 to 6 hours after taking cholestyramine.

If you forget a dose:
Take as soon as you remember up to 2 hours late. If more than 2 hours, wait for next scheduled dose (don't double this dose).

What drug does:
Binds with bile acids to prevent their absorption.

Time lapse before drug works:
- Cholesterol reduction—1 day.
- Bile-acid reduction—3 to 4 weeks.

Continued next column

OVERDOSE

SYMPTOMS:
Increased side effects and adverse reactions.
WHAT TO DO:
Overdose unlikely to threaten life. Depending on severity of symptoms and amount taken, call doctor, poison control center or hospital emergency room for instructions.

Don't take with:
- Any drug or vitamin simultaneously. Space doses 2 hours apart.
- Any other medicine without consulting your doctor or pharmacist.

POSSIBLE ADVERSE REACTIONS OR SIDE EFFECTS

SYMPTOMS	WHAT TO DO
Life-threatening: In case of overdose, see previous column.	
Common: Constipation.	Continue. Call doctor when convenient.
Infrequent: • Belching, bloating, diarrhea, mild nausea, vomiting, stomach pain, rapid weight gain.	Discontinue. Call doctor when convenient.
• Heartburn (mild).	Continue. Call doctor when convenient.
Rare: • Severe stomach pain; black, tarry stool.	Discontinue. Seek emergency treatment.
• Rash, hives, hiccups.	Discontinue. Call doctor right away.
• Sore tongue.	Continue. Call doctor when convenient.

WARNINGS & PRECAUTIONS

Don't take if:
You are allergic to cholestyramine.

Before you start, consult your doctor:
- If you plan to become pregnant within medication period.
- If you have angina, heart or blood-vessel disease.
- If you have stomach problems (including ulcer).
- If you have tartrazine sensitivity.
- If you have constipation or hemorrhoids.
- If you have kidney disease.

Over age 60:
Adverse reactions and side effects may be more frequent and severe than in younger persons.

Pregnancy:
Decide with your doctor whether drug benefits justify risk to unborn child. Risk category C (see page xxiii).

Breast-feeding:
No problems expected, but consult doctor.

Infants & children:
Not recommended.

Prolonged use:
- May decrease absorption of folic acid.
- Talk to your doctor about the need for follow-up medical examinations or laboratory studies to check serum cholesterol and triglycerides.

Skin & sunlight:
No problems expected.

Driving, piloting or hazardous work:
No problems expected.

Discontinuing:
Don't discontinue without doctor's advice until you complete prescribed dose, even though symptoms diminish or disappear.

Others:
No problems expected.

POSSIBLE INTERACTION WITH OTHER DRUGS

GENERIC NAME OR DRUG CLASS	COMBINED EFFECT
Adrenocorticoids, systemic	Decreased adreno-corticoid effect.
Anticoagulants, oral*	Increased anti-coagulant effect.
Beta carotene	Decreased absorption of beta carotene.
Dexfenfluramine	May require dosage change as weight loss occurs.
Dextrothyroxine	Decreased dextro-thyroxine effect.
Digitalis preparations*	Decreased digitalis effect.
Indapamide	Decreased indapamide effect.
Penicillins*	May decrease penicillin effect.
Raloxifene	Decreased effect of raloxifene.
Thiazides*	Decreased absorption of cholestyramine.
Thyroid hormones*	Decreased thyroid effect.
Trimethoprim	Decreased absorption of cholestyramine.
Troglitazone	Decreased effect of troglitazone. Avoid.

Ursodiol	Decreased absorption of ursodiol.
Vancomycin	Increased chance of hearing loss or kidney damage. Decreased therapeutic effect of vancomycin.
Vitamins	Decreased absorption of fat-soluble vitamins (A,D,E,K).
All other medicines	Decreased absorption, so dosages or dosage intervals may require adjustment.

POSSIBLE INTERACTION WITH OTHER SUBSTANCES

INTERACTS WITH	COMBINED EFFECT
Alcohol:	None expected.
Beverages:	None expected.
Cocaine:	None expected.
Foods:	Absorption of vitamins in foods decreased. Take vitamin supplements, particularly A, D, E & K.
Marijuana:	None expected.
Tobacco:	None expected.

CINOXACIN

BRAND NAMES

Cinobac

BASIC INFORMATION

Habit forming? No
Prescription needed? Yes
Available as generic? No
Drug class: Anti-infective (urinary)

 USES

Treatment for urinary tract infections.

 DOSAGE & USAGE INFORMATION

How to take:
Capsules—Swallow with food or milk to lessen stomach irritation. If you can't swallow whole, open capsule and take with liquid or food.

When to take:
At the same times each day.

If you forget a dose:
Take as soon as you remember up to 2 hours late. If more than 2 hours, wait for next scheduled dose (don't double this dose).

What drug does:
Destroys bacteria susceptible to cinoxacin.

Time lapse before drug works:
1 to 2 weeks.

Don't take with:
Any other medicine without consulting your doctor or pharmacist.

 OVERDOSE

SYMPTOMS:
Lethargy, stomach upset, behavioral changes, convulsions and stupor.
WHAT TO DO:
* Dial 911 (emergency) or 0 (operator) for an ambulance or medical help. Then give first aid immediately.
* If patient is unconscious and not breathing, give mouth-to-mouth breathing. If there is no heartbeat, use cardiac massage and mouth-to-mouth breathing (CPR). Don't try to make patient vomit. If you can't get help quickly, take patient to nearest emergency facility.
* See emergency information on inside covers.

 POSSIBLE ADVERSE REACTIONS OR SIDE EFFECTS

SYMPTOMS	WHAT TO DO
Life-threatening: Hives, rash, intense itching, faintness soon after a dose (anaphylaxis).	Seek emergency treatment immediately.
Common: Rash, itch; decreased, blurred or double vision; halos around lights or excess brightness; changes in color vision; nausea, vomiting, diarrhea.	Discontinue. Call doctor right away.
Infrequent: Dizziness, drowsiness, headache, ringing in ears, insomnia, appetite loss.	Continue. Call doctor when convenient.
Rare: Severe stomach pain, seizures, psychosis, joint pain, numbness or tingling in hands or feet (infants and children).	Discontinue. Call doctor right away.

CINOXACIN

WARNINGS & PRECAUTIONS

Don't take if:
- You are allergic to cinoxacin or nalidixic acid.
- You have a seizure disorder (epilepsy, convulsions).

Before you start, consult your doctor:
- If you plan to become pregnant during medication period.
- If you have or have had kidney or liver disease.
- If you have impaired circulation to the brain (hardened arteries).

Over age 60:
Adverse reactions and side effects may be more frequent and severe than in younger persons.

Pregnancy:
Decide with your doctor if drug benefits justify risk to unborn child. Risk category C (see page xxiii).

Breast-feeding:
Unknown effect. Avoid drug or discontinue nursing until you finish medicine. Consult doctor for advice on maintaining milk supply.

Infants & children:
Give only under close medical supervision.

Prolonged use:
Talk to your doctor about the need for follow-up medical examinations or laboratory studies to check kidney function, liver function.

Skin & sunlight:
No special problems expected.

Driving, piloting or hazardous work:
Avoid if you feel drowsy, dizzy or have vision problems. Otherwise, no problems expected.

Discontinuing:
Don't discontinue without consulting doctor. Dose may require gradual reduction if you have taken drug for a long time. Doses of other drugs may also require adjustment.

Others:
May interfere with the accuracy of some medical tests.

POSSIBLE INTERACTION WITH OTHER DRUGS

GENERIC NAME OR DRUG CLASS	COMBINED EFFECT
Probenecid	Decreased cinoxacin effect.

POSSIBLE INTERACTION WITH OTHER SUBSTANCES

INTERACTS WITH	COMBINED EFFECT
Alcohol:	Impaired alertness, judgment and coordination.
Beverages:	None expected.
Cocaine:	Impaired judgment and coordination.
Foods:	None expected.
Marijuana:	Impaired alertness, judgment and coordination.
Tobacco:	None expected.

CISAPRIDE

BRAND NAMES

Propulsid

BASIC INFORMATION

Habit forming? No
Prescription needed? Yes
Available as generic? No
Drug class: Cholinergic

 ## USES

- Treatment and prevention of gastro-esophageal reflux or heartburn.
- Treatment for gastroparesis (a stomach disorder).

 ## DOSAGE & USAGE INFORMATION

How to take:
- Tablet–Swallow with liquid.
- Oral suspension–Take as directed on label.

When to take:
At the same times each day. Take 15 minutes before meals and at bedtime.

If you forget a dose:
Take as soon as you remember up to 2 hours late. If more than 2 hours, wait for next scheduled dose (don't double this dose).

What drug does:
Restores the normal anti-reflux mechanism of the esophagus, helping prevent reflux of gastric contents into the esophagus.

Time lapse before drug works:
30 to 60 minutes.

Don't take with:
Any other prescription or nonprescription drug without consulting your doctor.

 ## OVERDOSE

SYMPTOMS:
None expected.
WHAT TO DO:
Overdose unlikely to threaten life. If person takes much larger amount than prescribed, call doctor, poison control center or hospital emergency room for instructions.

 ## POSSIBLE ADVERSE REACTIONS OR SIDE EFFECTS

SYMPTOMS	WHAT TO DO
Life-threatening: None expected.	
Common: None expected.	
Infrequent: Stomach cramps, diarrhea, constipation, unusual tiredness or weakness, headache, nausea, drowsiness.	Continue. Call doctor when convenient.
Rare: Seizures (in patients with a history of seizures).	Discontinue. Call doctor right away.

WARNINGS & PRECAUTIONS

Don't take if:
You are allergic to cisapride.

Before you start, consult your doctor:
- If you have bleeding from the stomach or abdomen.
- If you have epilepsy or a history of seizures.
- If you have kidney or liver disease.

Over age 60:
Adverse reactions and side effects may be more frequent and severe than in younger persons.

Pregnancy:
Discuss with your doctor whether drug benefits justify risk to unborn child. Risk category C (see page xxiii).

Breast-feeding:
Drug passes into milk. Avoid drug or discontinue nursing until you finish medicine. Consult doctor for advice on maintaining milk supply.

Infants & children:
No problems expected. Use only under close medical supervision.

Prolonged use:
Your body may develop a tolerance* to the drug, which can decrease its effectiveness.

Skin & sunlight:
No problems expected.

Driving, piloting or hazardous work:
Don't drive or pilot aircraft until you learn how medicine affects you. Don't work around dangerous machinery. Don't climb ladders or work in high places. Danger increases if you drink alcohol or take other medicines affecting alertness and reflexes.

Discontinuing:
No problems expected.

Others:
Advise any doctor or dentist whom you consult that you take this medicine.

POSSIBLE INTERACTION WITH OTHER DRUGS

GENERIC NAME OR DRUG CLASS	COMBINED EFFECT
Amantadine	Decreased amantadine effect.
Anticholinergics*	Decreased anticholinergic effect.
Antidepressants*	Decreased antidepressant effect.
Antidyskinetics*	Decreased antidyskinetic effect.
Antihistamines*	Decreased antihistamine effect.
Antipsychotics*	Decreased antipsychotic effect.
Buclizine	Decreased buclizine effect.
Carbamazepine	Decreased carbamazepine effect.
Cimetidine	Increased cimetidine effect.
Cyclobenzaprine	Decreased cyclobenzaprine effect.
Disopyramide	Decreased disopyramide effect.
Enzyme inhibitors*	Serious heart rhythm problems.
Flavoxate	Decreased flavoxate effect.
Itraconazole	Heartbeat irregularities. Avoid.
Ketoconazole	Heartbeat irregularities. Avoid.
Leukotriene modifiers	Increased effect of cisapride.
Meclizine	Decreased meclizine effect.

Methylphenidate	Decreased methylphenidate effect.
Orphenadrine	Decreased orphenadrine effect.
Procainamide	Decreased procainamide effect.
Quinidine	Decreased quinidine effect.
Ranitidine	Increased ranitidine effect.
Trimeprazine	Decreased trimeprazine effect.

POSSIBLE INTERACTION WITH OTHER SUBSTANCES

INTERACTS WITH	COMBINED EFFECT
Alcohol:	Increased absorption of alcohol. Avoid.
Beverages:	None expected.
Cocaine:	None expected.
Foods:	None expected.
Marijuana:	None expected.
Tobacco:	None expected.

*See Glossary

CITALOPRAM

BRAND NAMES

Celexa

BASIC INFORMATION

Habit forming? No
Prescription needed? Yes
Available as generic? No
Drug class: Antidepressant (selective serotonin reuptake inhibitor)

 USES

Treats depression.

 DOSAGE & USAGE INFORMATION

How to take:
Tablets—Swallow with water, with or without food. If you can't swallow whole, crumble tablet and take with liquid or food.

When to take:
At the same time each day.

If you forget a dose:
Take as soon as you remember. If it is near the time of your next dose, skip the missed dose and resume normal schedule. Don't double this dose.

What drug does:
Increases serotonin, one of the chemicals in the brain called neurotransmitters, that plays a role in emotions and psychological disturbances.

Time lapse before drug works:
One to four weeks.

Don't take with:
Any other prescription or nonprescription drug without consulting your doctor or pharmacist.

 OVERDOSE

SYMPTOMS:
Dizziness, sweating, nausea, vomiting, tremor, somnolence, heart rhythm disturbances. In rare cases, amnesia, confusion, coma and convulsions have occurred.
WHAT TO DO:
• **Dial 911 (emergency) or O (operator) for an ambulance or medical help. Then give first aid immediately.**
• **See emergency information at end of book.**

 POSSIBLE ADVERSE REACTIONS OR SIDE EFFECTS

SYMPTOMS	WHAT TO DO
Life-threatening: None expected.	
Common: Drowsiness, dry mouth, insomnia, nausea, changes in sexual desire or function.	Continue. Call doctor if symptoms persist.
Infrequent: • Blurred vision, amnesia, apathy (lack of emotion), breathing difficulty, fever, menstrual changes, increase in urine amount, skin rash, itching.	Discontinue. Call doctor right away.
• Abdominal pain, loss of appetite, anxiety, muscle or joint pain, unusual tiredness or weakness, diarrhea, heartburn, gas, increased salivation or sweating, increased yawning, tingling, burning or prickly feeling on skin, headaches, stuffy or runny nose, change in sense of taste, tooth grinding, trembling, unusual increase or decrease in weight, vomiting.	Continue. Call doctor when convenient.
Rare: Abnormal bleeding (nose bleed or red spots on skin); breast tenderness or enlargement; irregular heartbeat; red, itching, burning or peeling skin; red or irritated eyes; sore throat with fever and chills; sudden body or facial spasms; confusion; drowsiness; lack of energy; painful urination; unusual mood or mental changes; dizziness; fainting; serotonin syndrome.*	Discontinue. Call doctor right away.

WARNINGS & PRECAUTIONS

Don't take if:
- You are allergic to citalopram.
- You currently take (or have taken in the last two weeks) a monoamine oxidase (MAO) inhibitor.

Before you start, consult your doctor:
- If you have any other medical problem.
- If you have had kidney or liver problems.
- If you have a history of seizure disorders.
- If you have a history of drug abuse or dependence.
- If you have a history of mood disorders, such as mania, or thoughts of suicide.
- If you are allergic to any medication, food or other substances.

Over age 60:
Adverse reactions and side effects may be more severe and frequent than in younger patients; dosage may need to be adjusted.

Pregnancy:
Decide with your doctor if drug benefits justify risk to unborn child. Risk category C (see page xxiii).

Breast-feeding:
Drug passes into milk. Avoid drug or discontinue nursing until you finish medicine. Consult doctor for advice on maintaining milk supply.

Infants & children:
Safety and effectiveness in children has not been established.

Prolonged use:
No problems expected. Your doctor should periodically evaluate your response to the drug and adjust the dose if necessary.

Skin & sunlight:
No problems expected.

Driving, piloting or hazardous work:
Don't drive or pilot aircraft until you learn how medicine affects you. Don't work around dangerous machinery. Don't climb ladders or work in high places. Danger increases if you drink alcohol or take medicine affecting alertness and reflexes.

Discontinuing:
Don't discontinue without consulting doctor.

Others:
- Advise any doctor or dentist whom you consult that you take this medicine.
- Take medicine only as directed. Do not increase or reduce dosage without doctor's approval.

POSSIBLE INTERACTION WITH OTHER DRUGS

GENERIC NAME OR DRUG CLASS	COMBINED EFFECT
Antidepressants, tricyclic	Increases levels of tricyclic antidepressant.
Carbamazepine	May lessen effect of citalopram.
Cimetidine	Increased effect of citalopram.
Metoprolol	Increased effect of metoprolol.
Monoamine oxidase (MAO) inhibitors	Can cause a life-threatening reaction. Avoid.
Serotonergics	Serotonin syndrome.*
Warfarin	May increase the effect of warfarin.

POSSIBLE INTERACTION WITH OTHER SUBSTANCES

INTERACTS WITH	COMBINED EFFECT
Alcohol:	Contributes to depression. Avoid.
Beverages:	None expected.
Cocaine:	Effects unknown. Avoid.
Foods:	None expected.
Marijuana:	Effects unknown. Avoid.
Tobacco:	None expected.

CITRATES

BRAND AND GENERIC NAMES

POTASSIUM CITRATE
  Citra Forte
  Urocit-K
POTASSIUM CITRATE
  & CITRIC ACID
  Phanadex
  Polycitra-K
POTASSIUM CITRATE
  & SODIUM CITRATE
  Citrolith

SODIUM CITRATE &
  CITRIC ACID
  Albright's Solution
  Bicitra
  Lanatuss
    Expectorant
  Modified Shohl's
    Solution
  Oracit
  Tussirex with
    Codeine Liquid
TRICITRATES
  Polycitra
  Polycitra LC

BASIC INFORMATION

Habit forming? No
Prescription needed? Yes
Available as generic? No
Drug class: Urinary alkalizer, antiurolithic

USES

- To make urine more alkaline (less acid).
- To treat or prevent recurrence of some types of kidney stones.

DOSAGE & USAGE INFORMATION

How to take:
Tablets or liquid—Take right after a meal or with a bedtime snack.

When to take:
On full stomach, usually after meals or with food.

If you forget a dose:
Take as soon as you remember up to 2 hours late. If more than 2 hours, wait for next scheduled dose (don't double this dose).

Continued next column

OVERDOSE

SYMPTOMS:
Convulsions, coma.
WHAT TO DO:
- Dial 911 (emergency) or 0 (operator) for an ambulance or medical help. Then give first aid immediately.
- See emergency information on inside covers.

What drug does:
Increases urinary alkalinity by excretion of bicarbonate ions.

Time lapse before drug works:
1 hour.

Don't take with:
Any medicine that will decrease mental alertness or reflexes, such as alcohol, other mind-altering drugs, cough/cold medicines, antihistamines, allergy medicine, sedatives, tranquilizers (sleeping pills or "downers"), barbiturates, seizure medicine, narcotics, other prescription medicine for pain, muscle relaxants, anesthetics.

POSSIBLE ADVERSE REACTIONS OR SIDE EFFECTS

SYMPTOMS	WHAT TO DO
Life-threatening: Black, tarry stools; vomiting blood; severe abdominal cramps; irregular heartbeat; shortness of breath.	Discontinue. Seek emergency treatment.
Common: Nausea or vomiting.	Continue. Call doctor when convenient.
Infrequent: Confusion, dizziness, swollen feet and ankles, irritability, depression, muscle pain, nervousness, numbness or tingling in hands or feet, unpleasant taste, weakness.	Discontinue. Call doctor right away.
Rare: Slow breathing, tiredness.	Discontinue. Call doctor right away.

WARNINGS & PRECAUTIONS

Don't take if:
You are allergic to any citrate.

Before you start, consult your doctor:
* If you have any disease involving the adrenal glands, diabetes, chronic diarrhea, heart problems, hypertension, kidney disease, stomach ulcer or gastritis, urinary tract infection, toxemia of pregnancy.
* If you plan strenuous exercise.

Over age 60:
Adverse reactions and side effects may be more frequent and severe than in younger persons. Ask doctor about smaller doses.

Pregnancy:
Avoid if possible. Consult doctor. Risk category C (see page xxiii).

Breast-feeding:
Safety during lactation not established. Consult doctor.

Infants & children:
Use only under close medical supervision.

Prolonged use:
* Adverse reactions more likely.
* Talk to your doctor about the need for follow-up medical examinations or laboratory studies to check complete blood counts (white blood cell count, platelet count, red blood cell count, hemoglobin, hematocrit), serum electrolytes, urine.

Skin & sunlight:
No problems expected.

Driving, piloting or hazardous work:
Don't drive or pilot aircraft until you learn how medicine affects you. Don't work around dangerous machinery. Don't climb ladders or work in high places. Danger increases if you drink alcohol or take medicine affecting alertness and reflexes, such as antihistamines, tranquilizers, sedatives, pain medicine, narcotics and mind-altering drugs.

Discontinuing:
Don't discontinue without consulting doctor. Dose may require gradual reduction if you have taken drug for a long time. Doses of other drugs may also require adjustment.

Others:
* Drink at least 8 ounces of water or other liquid (except milk) every hour while awake.
* Liquid may be chilled (don't freeze) to improve taste.
* Monitor potassium in blood with frequent laboratory studies.

POSSIBLE INTERACTION WITH OTHER DRUGS

GENERIC NAME OR DRUG CLASS	COMBINED EFFECT
Amphetamines*	Increased amphetamine effect.
Antacids*	Toxic effect of citrates (alkalosis).
Calcium supplements*	Increased risk of kidney stones.
Digitalis preparations*	Increased risk of too much potassium in blood.
Methenamine	Decreased effects of methenamine.
Mexiletine	May slow elimination of mexiletine and cause need to adjust dosage.
Quinidine	Prolonged quinidine effect.

POSSIBLE INTERACTION WITH OTHER SUBSTANCES

INTERACTS WITH	COMBINED EFFECT
Alcohol:	Decreased mental alertness.
Beverages: Salt-free milk.	May cause potassium toxicity.
Cocaine:	No proven problems.
Foods: Milk, cheese, ice cream, yogurt, buttermilk, salty foods, salt, salt substitutes.	May increase likelihood of kidney stones.
Marijuana:	No proven problems.
Tobacco:	Increased likelihood of stomach irritation.

CLIDINIUM

BRAND NAMES

Apo-Chlorax
Clindex
Clinoxide
Corium
Librax

Lidox
Lodoxide
Quarzan
Zebrax

BASIC INFORMATION

Habit forming? No
Prescription needed?
  Low strength: No
  High strength: Yes
Available as generic? No
Drug class: Antispasmodic, anticholinergic

USES

Reduces spasms of digestive system, bladder and urethra.

DOSAGE & USAGE INFORMATION

How to take:
Capsule—Swallow with liquid or food to lessen stomach irritation.

When to take:
30 minutes before meals (unless directed otherwise by doctor).

If you forget a dose:
Take as soon as you remember up to 2 hours late. If more than 2 hours, wait for next scheduled dose (don't double this dose).

What drug does:
Blocks nerve impulses at parasympathetic nerve endings, preventing muscle contractions and gland secretions of organs involved.

Time lapse before drug works:
15 to 30 minutes.

Continued next column

OVERDOSE

SYMPTOMS:
Dilated pupils, rapid pulse and breathing, dizziness, fever, hallucinations, confusion, slurred speech, agitation, flushed face, convulsions, coma.
WHAT TO DO:
- Dial 911 (emergency) or 0 (operator) for an ambulance or medical help. Then give first aid immediately.
- See emergency information on inside covers.

Don't take with:
Any other medicine without consulting your doctor or pharmacist.

POSSIBLE ADVERSE REACTIONS OR SIDE EFFECTS

SYMPTOMS	WHAT TO DO
Life-threatening:	
In case of overdose, see previous column.	
Common:	
• Confusion, delirium, rapid heartbeat.	Discontinue. Call doctor right away.
• Nausea, vomiting, decreased sweating.	Continue. Call doctor when convenient.
• Constipation.	Continue. Tell doctor at next visit.
• Dryness in ears, nose, throat, mouth.	No action necessary.
Infrequent:	
• Nasal congestion, altered taste, difficult urination, headache, impotence.	Continue. Call doctor when convenient.
• Lightheadedness.	Discontinue. Call doctor right away.
Rare:	
Rash or hives, eye pain, blurred vision.	Discontinue. Call doctor right away.

WARNINGS & PRECAUTIONS

Don't take if:
- You are allergic to any anticholinergic.
- You have trouble with stomach bloating.
- You have difficulty emptying your bladder completely (enlarged prostate).
- You have narrow-angle glaucoma.
- You have severe ulcerative colitis.

Before you start, consult your doctor:
- If you have open-angle glaucoma.
- If you have angina, chronic bronchitis or asthma, kidney or thyroid disease, hiatal hernia, liver disease, enlarged prostate, myasthenia gravis, peptic ulcer.
- If you will have surgery within 2 months, including dental surgery, requiring general or spinal anesthesia.

Over age 60:
Adverse reactions and side effects may be more frequent and severe than in younger persons.

Pregnancy:
Decide with your doctor whether drug benefits justify risk to unborn child. Risk category C (see page xxiii).

Breast-feeding:
Drug passes into milk and decreases milk flow. Avoid drug or discontinue nursing until you finish medicine. Consult doctor for advice on maintaining milk supply.

Infants & children:
Use only under medical supervision.

Prolonged use:
Chronic constipation, possible fecal impaction. Consult doctor immediately.

Skin & sunlight:
No problems expected.

Driving, piloting or hazardous work:
Don't drive or pilot aircraft until you learn how medicine affects you. Don't work around dangerous machinery. Don't climb ladders or work in high places. Danger increases if you drink alcohol or take medicine affecting alertness and reflexes, such as antihistamines, tranquilizers, sedatives, pain medicine, narcotics, or mind-altering drugs.

Discontinuing:
May be unnecessary to finish medicine. Follow doctor's instructions.

Others:
Advise any doctor or dentist whom you consult that you take this medicine.

POSSIBLE INTERACTION WITH OTHER DRUGS

GENERIC NAME OR DRUG CLASS	COMBINED EFFECT
Amantadine	Increased clidinium effect.
Antacids*	Decreased clidinium effect.
Anticholinergics, other*	Increased clidinium effect.
Antidepressants, tricyclic*	Increased clidinium effect. Increased sedation.
Antidiarrheals*	Increased clidinium effect.
Antihistamines*	Increased clidinium effect.
Attapulgite	Decreased clidinium effect.
Haloperidol	Increased internal eye pressure.
Ketoconazole	Decreased ketoconazole effect.

Meperidine	Increased clidinium effect.
Methylphenidate	Increased clidinium effect.
Molindone	Increased anti-cholinergic effect.
Monoamine oxidase (MAO) inhibitors*	Increased clidinium effect.
Nitrates*	Increased internal eye pressure.
Nizatidine	Increased nizatidine effect.
Orphenadrine	Increased clidinium effect.
Pilocarpine	Loss of pilocarpine effect in glaucoma treatment.
Potassium supplements*	Possible intestinal ulcers with oral potassium tablets.
Tranquilizers*	Increased clidinium effect.
Vitamin C	Decreased clidinium effect. Avoid large doses of vitamin C.

POSSIBLE INTERACTION WITH OTHER SUBSTANCES

INTERACTS WITH	COMBINED EFFECT
Alcohol:	None expected.
Beverages:	None expected.
Cocaine:	Excessively rapid heartbeat. Avoid.
Foods:	None expected.
Marijuana:	Drowsiness and dry mouth.
Tobacco:	None expected.

CLINDAMYCIN

BRAND NAMES

Cleocin

Cleocin Pediatric

Cleocin (Vaginal)

Dalacin C

Dalacin C Palmitate

Dalacin C Phosphate

BASIC INFORMATION

Habit forming? No

Prescription needed? Yes

Available as generic? Yes

Drug class: Antibacterial

 USES

Treatment of bacterial infections that are susceptible to clindamycin.

 DOSAGE & USAGE INFORMATION

How to take:
- Capsule or liquid—Swallow with liquid. Take with a full glass of water or a meal to avoid gastric irritation.
- Vaginal cream—Use applicator supplied with product to insert cream into vagina. Wash hands immediately after using.

When to take:
- Oral—At the same times each day.
- Vaginal cream—Apply at bedtime unless directed differently by your doctor.

If you forget a dose:
Take as soon as you remember up to 2 hours late. If more than 2 hours, wait for next scheduled dose (don't double this dose).

What drug does:
Destroys susceptible bacteria. Does not kill viruses.

Time lapse before drug works:
3 to 5 days.

Don't take with:
Any other medicine without consulting your doctor or pharmacist.

 OVERDOSE

SYMPTOMS:
Severe nausea, vomiting, diarrhea.
WHAT TO DO:
Overdose unlikely to threaten life. If person takes much larger amount than prescribed, call doctor, poison control center or hospital emergency room for instructions.

 POSSIBLE ADVERSE REACTIONS OR SIDE EFFECTS

SYMPTOMS	WHAT TO DO
Life-threatening: Hives, wheezing, faintness, itching, coma.	Seek emergency treatment immediately.
Common: Bloating.	Discontinue. Call doctor right away.
Infrequent: • Unusual thirst; vomiting; stomach cramps; severe and watery diarrhea with blood or mucus; painful, swollen joints; fever; jaundice; tiredness; weakness.	Discontinue. Call doctor right away.
• White patches in mouth; rash, itch around groin, rectum or armpits; vaginal discharge, itching; dizziness; nausea; mild diarrhea; pain during intercourse.	Continue. Call doctor when convenient.
Rare: None expected.	

WARNINGS & PRECAUTIONS

Don't take if:
- You are allergic to lincomycins, clindamycin or doxorubicin.
- You have had ulcerative colitis.

Before you start, consult your doctor:
- If you have had yeast infections of mouth, skin or vagina.
- If you will have surgery within 2 months, including dental surgery, requiring general or spinal anesthesia.
- If you have kidney or liver disease.
- If you have allergies of any kind.
- If you have a history of gastrointestinal disorders.

Over age 60:
Adverse reactions and side effects may be more frequent and severe than in younger persons.

Pregnancy:
Decide with your doctor if drug benefits justify risk to unborn child. Risk category B (see page xxiii).

Breast-feeding:
Drug passes into milk. Avoid drug or discontinue nursing until you finish medicine. Consult doctor for advice on maintaining milk supply.

Infants & children:
Don't give to infants younger than 1 month. Use for children only under medical supervision.

Prolonged use:
- Severe colitis with diarrhea and bleeding.
- You may become more susceptible to infections caused by germs not responsive to clindamycin.
- Talk to your doctor about the need for follow-up medical examinations or laboratory studies to check stool exams and perform proctosigmoidoscopy.

Skin & sunlight:
No problems expected.

Driving, piloting or hazardous work:
No problems expected.

Discontinuing:
- Don't discontinue without doctor's advice until you complete prescribed dose, even though symptoms diminish or disappear.
- If vaginal discharge, itching or pain occurs after discontinuing medicine, consult doctor.

Others:
- May interfere with the accuracy of some medical tests.
- Vaginal cream product may decrease the effectiveness of condoms, cervical caps or diaphragms. Wait 72 hours after treatment to use any of these devices.

POSSIBLE INTERACTION WITH OTHER DRUGS

GENERIC NAME OR DRUG CLASS	COMBINED EFFECT
Antidiarrheal preparations*	Decreased clindamycin effect.
Antimyasthenics*	Decreased anti-myasthenic effect.
Chloramphenicol	Decreased clindamycin effect.
Erythromycins*	Decreased clindamycin effect.
Muscle blockers*	Increased actions of muscle blockers to unsafe degree. Avoid.
Narcotics*	Increased risk of respiratory problems.

POSSIBLE INTERACTION WITH OTHER SUBSTANCES

INTERACTS WITH	COMBINED EFFECT
Alcohol:	None expected.
Beverages:	None expected.
Cocaine:	None expected.
Foods:	None expected.
Marijuana:	None expected.
Tobacco:	None expected.

CLOMIPHENE

BRAND NAMES

Clomid   Serophene
Milophene

BASIC INFORMATION

Habit forming? No
Prescription needed? Yes
Available as generic? Yes
Drug class: Gonad stimulant

 USES

- Treatment for men with low sperm counts.
- Treatment for ovulatory failure in women who wish to become pregnant.

 DOSAGE & USAGE INFORMATION

How to take:
Tablet—Swallow with liquid.

When to take:
- Men—Take at the same time each day.
- Women—Follow physician's instructions carefully.

If you forget a dose:
Take as soon as you remember. If you forget a day, double next dose. If you miss 2 or more doses, consult doctor.

What drug does:
Antiestrogen effect stimulates ovulation and sperm production.

Time lapse before drug works:
Usually 3 to 6 months. Ovulation may occur 6 to 10 days after last day of treatment in any cycle.

Don't take with:
No restrictions.

 OVERDOSE

SYMPTOMS:
Increased severity of adverse reactions and side effects.
WHAT TO DO:
Overdose unlikely to threaten life. If person takes much larger amount than prescribed, call doctor, poison control center or hospital emergency room for instructions.

 POSSIBLE ADVERSE REACTIONS OR SIDE EFFECTS

SYMPTOMS	WHAT TO DO
Life-threatening:	
Sudden shortness of breath.	Seek emergency treatment.
Common:	
• Bloating, abdominal pain, pelvic pain.	Discontinue. Call doctor right away.
• Hot flashes.	Continue. Tell doctor at next visit.
Infrequent:	
• Rash, itch, vomiting, jaundice.	Discontinue. Call doctor right away.
• Constipation, diarrhea, increased appetite, heavy menstrual flow, frequent urination, breast discomfort, weight change, hair loss, nausea, eyes sensitive to light.	Continue. Call doctor when convenient.
Rare:	
• Vision changes.	Discontinue. Call doctor right away.
• Dizziness, headache, tiredness, depression, nervousness.	Continue. Call doctor when convenient.

WARNINGS & PRECAUTIONS

Don't take if:
You are allergic to clomiphene.

Before you start, consult your doctor:
- If you have an ovarian cyst, fibroid uterine tumors or unusual vaginal bleeding.
- If you have inflamed veins caused by blood clots.
- If you have liver disease.
- If you are depressed.

Over age 60:
Not recommended.

Pregnancy:
Stop taking at first sign of pregnancy. Consult doctor. Risk category C (see page xxiii).

Breast-feeding:
Not used.

Infants & children:
Not used.

Prolonged use:
- Not recommended.
- Talk to your doctor about the need for follow-up medical examinations or laboratory studies to check basal body temperature, endometrial biopsy, kidney function, eyes.

Skin & sunlight:
No special problems expected.

Driving, piloting or hazardous work:
- Avoid if you feel dizzy.
- May cause blurred vision.

Discontinuing:
May be unnecessary to finish medicine. Follow doctor's instructions.

Others:
- Have a complete pelvic examination before treatment.
- If you become pregnant, twins or triplets are possible.

 ## POSSIBLE INTERACTION WITH OTHER DRUGS

GENERIC NAME OR DRUG CLASS	COMBINED EFFECT
Thyroglobulin	May increase serum thyroglobulin.
Thyroxine (T-4)	May increase serum thyroxine.

 ## POSSIBLE INTERACTION WITH OTHER SUBSTANCES

INTERACTS WITH	COMBINED EFFECT
Alcohol:	None expected.
Beverages:	None expected.
Cocaine:	None expected.
Foods:	None expected.
Marijuana:	None expected.
Tobacco:	None expected.

CLONIDINE

BRAND NAMES

Catapres   Dixarit
Catapres-TTS

BASIC INFORMATION

Habit forming? No
Prescription needed? Yes
Available as generic? Yes
Drug class: Antihypertensive

USES

- Treatment of narcotic withdrawal syndrome.
- May be used for nicotine withdrawal.
- Prevention of migraine headaches.
- Control of overactivity and tics in children.
- Treatment of high blood pressure.

DOSAGE & USAGE INFORMATION

How to take:
- Tablet—Swallow with liquid.
- Transdermal patch (attaches to skin)—Apply to clean, dry, hairless skin on arm or trunk. Follow all prescription instructions carefully.

When to take:
- Tablet—Once or twice a day as directed.
- Transdermal patch—Replace as directed, usually once a week.

Continued next column

OVERDOSE

SYMPTOMS:
Vomiting, fainting, slow heartbeat, feeling cold, coma, diminished reflexes, shortness of breath, dizziness, extreme tiredness.
WHAT TO DO:
- **Dial 911 (emergency) or 0 (operator) for an ambulance or medical help. Then give first aid immediately.**
- **If patient is unconscious and not breathing, give mouth-to-mouth breathing. If there is no heartbeat, use cardiac massage and mouth-to-mouth breathing (CPR). Don't try to make patient vomit. If you can't get help quickly, take patient to nearest emergency facility.**
- **See emergency information at end of book.**

If you forget a dose:
- Take tablet as soon as you remember. If it is almost time for the next dose, wait for the next scheduled dose (don't double this dose). If you miss more than 2 doses in a row, call your doctor.
- If the once-a-week patch change is 3 days late, call your doctor.

What drug does:
- Reduces nervous system overactivity.
- Relaxes and allows expansion of blood vessel walls.

Time lapse before drug works:
2 to 3 weeks for full benefit.

Don't take with:
- Medicines containing alcohol; read labels carefully.
- Any other medicine without consulting your doctor or pharmacist.

POSSIBLE ADVERSE REACTIONS OR SIDE EFFECTS

SYMPTOMS	WHAT TO DO
Life-threatening:	
In case of overdose, see previous column.	
Common:	
Dizziness, constipation drowsiness, irritated skin (with skin patch), dry mouth, tiredness, headache.	Continue. Call doctor when convenient.
Infrequent:	
• Depression, swollen hands or feet.	Discontinue. Call doctor right away.
• Darkened skin (with skin patch), light-headedness upon rising from sitting or lying, nausea, vomiting, dry or burning eyes, diminished sex drive or ability, appetite loss, nervousness.	Continue. Call doctor when convenient.
Rare:	
Cold fingers and toes, nightmares, slow heart rate.	Discontinue. Call doctor right away.

WARNINGS & PRECAUTIONS

Don't take if:
You are allergic to clonidine.

Before you start, consult your doctor:
- If you will have surgery within 2 months, including dental surgery, requiring general or spinal anesthesia.
- If you have heart disease or kidney disease.
- If you have a peripheral circulation disorder (intermittent claudication, Raynaud's syndrome, Buerger's disease).
- If you have history of depression.
- If you have a disorder affecting the skin or any skin irritation (with use of transdermal patch).

Over age 60:
Adverse reactions and side effects may be more frequent and severe than in younger persons.

Pregnancy:
Decide with your doctor whether drug benefits justify risk to unborn child. Risk category C (see page xxiii).

Breast-feeding:
Unknown whether safe or not. Consult doctor.

Infants & children:
Useful for controlling overactivity or tics.

Prolonged use:
- Don't discontinue without consulting doctor. Dose may require gradual reduction if you have taken drug for a long time. Doses of other drugs may also require adjustment.
- Request yearly eye examinations.
- Talk to your doctor about the need for follow-up medical examinations or laboratory studies.

Skin & sunlight:
Use with caution in hot weather.

Driving, piloting or hazardous work:
Don't drive or pilot aircraft until you learn how medicine affects you. Don't work around dangerous machinery. Don't climb ladders or work in high places. Danger increases if you drink alcohol or take medicine affecting alertness and reflexes.

Discontinuing:
Don't discontinue abruptly. May cause a withdrawal syndrome including anxiety, chest pain, insomnia, headache, nausea, irregular heartbeat, flushed face, sweating. Consult doctor if any symptoms occur after discontinuing the medication.

Others:
- Advise any doctor or dentist whom you consult that you take this medicine.
- For dry mouth, suck sugarless hard candy or chew sugarless gum. If dry mouth continues, consult your dentist.

POSSIBLE INTERACTION WITH OTHER DRUGS

GENERIC NAME OR DRUG CLASS	COMBINED EFFECT
Antidepressants, tricyclic*	Decreased clonidine effect.
Antihypertensives*, other	Excessive blood pressure drop.
Appetite suppressants*	Decreased clonidine effect.
Beta-adrenergic blocking agents*	Possible precipitous change in blood pressure.
Central nervous system (CNS) depressants*	Increased depressive effects of both drugs.

POSSIBLE INTERACTION WITH OTHER SUBSTANCES

INTERACTS WITH	COMBINED EFFECT
Alcohol:	Increased sensitivity to sedative effect of alcohol and very low blood pressure. Avoid.
Beverages:	No problems expected.
Cocaine:	Increased risk of heart block and high blood pressure.
Foods:	No problems expected.
Marijuana:	Weakness on standing.
Tobacco:	No problems expected

*See Glossary

CLONIDINE & CHLORTHALIDONE

BRAND NAMES

Combipres

BASIC INFORMATION

Habit forming? No
Prescription needed? Yes
Available as generic? Yes
Drug class: Antihypertensive, diuretic

USES

- Treatment of high blood pressure.
- Reduces fluid retention (edema) caused by conditions such as heart disorders and liver disease.

DOSAGE & USAGE INFORMATION

How to take:
Tablet—Swallow with liquid. If you can't swallow whole, crumble tablet and take with liquid or food. Don't exceed dose.

When to take:
At the same time each day.

If you forget a dose:
Take as soon as you remember up to 2 hours late. If more than 2 hours, wait for next scheduled dose (don't double this dose).

What drug does:
- Relaxes and allows expansion of blood vessel walls.
- Forces sodium and water excretion, reducing body fluid.

Continued next column

OVERDOSE

SYMPTOMS:
Vomiting; fainting; rapid, irregular, slow heartbeat; diminished reflexes; cramps; shortness of breath; weakness; drowsiness; weak pulse; coma.
WHAT TO DO:
- **Dial 911 (emergency) or 0 (operator) for an ambulance or medical help. Then give first aid immediately.**
- **If patient is unconscious and not breathing, give mouth-to-mouth breathing. If there is no heartbeat, use cardiac massage and mouth-to-mouth breathing (CPR). Don't try to make patient vomit. If you can't get help quickly, take patient to nearest emergency facility.**
- **See emergency information at end of book.**

- Reduced body fluid and relaxed arteries lower blood pressure.

Time lapse before drug works:
4 to 6 hours. May require several weeks to lower blood pressure.

Don't take with:
Any medicine that will decrease mental alertness such as alcohol, antihistamines, cold/cough medicines, sedatives, tranquilizers, narcotics, prescription pain medicine, barbiturates, seizure medicine, anesthetics.

POSSIBLE ADVERSE REACTIONS OR SIDE EFFECTS

SYMPTOMS	WHAT TO DO
Life-threatening: Irregular heartbeat, weak pulse.	Discontinue. Seek emergency treatment.
Common: Dry mouth, increased thirst, muscle cramps, nausea or vomiting, mood changes, drowsiness.	Discontinue. Call doctor right away.
Infrequent: Vomiting, diminished sex desire and performance, insomnia, dizziness, diarrhea, constipation, appetite loss.	Continue. Call doctor when convenient.
Rare: • Jaundice; easy bruising or bleeding; sore throat, fever, mouth ulcers; rash or hives; joint pain; flank pain; abdominal pain.	Discontinue. Call doctor right away.
• Cold fingers and toes, nightmares.	Continue. Call doctor when convenient.

WARNINGS & PRECAUTIONS

Don't take if:
- You are allergic to any thiazide diuretic drug or alpha-adrenergic blocker.
- You are under age 12.

Before you start, consult your doctor:
- If you are allergic to any sulfa drug.
- If you have gout, liver, pancreas or kidney disorder, a peripheral circulation disorder (intermittent claudication, Buerger's disease), history of depression, heart disease.
- If you will have surgery within 2 months, including dental surgery, requiring general or spinal anesthesia.

Over age 60:
Adverse reactions and side effects may be more frequent and severe than in younger persons, especially dizziness and excessive potassium loss.

Pregnancy:
Decide with your doctor if drug benefits justify risk to unborn child. Risk category C (see page xxiii).

Breast-feeding:
Drug passes into milk. Avoid drug or discontinue nursing until you finish medicine. Consult doctor for advice on maintaining milk supply.

Infants & children:
Use only after careful medical supervision after age 12. Avoid before age 12.

Prolonged use:
- Don't discontinue without consulting doctor. Dose may require gradual reduction if you have taken drug for a long time. Doses of other drugs may also require adjustment.
- Request yearly eye examinations.
- Talk to your doctor about the need for follow-up medical examinations or laboratory studies.

Skin & sunlight:
No special problems expected.

Driving, piloting or hazardous work:
Don't drive or pilot aircraft until you learn how medicine affects you. Don't work around dangerous machinery. Don't climb ladders or work in high places. Danger increases if you drink alcohol or take medicine affecting alertness and reflexes, such as antihistamines, tranquilizers, sedatives, pain medicine, narcotics and mind-altering drugs.

Discontinuing:
Don't discontinue abruptly. May cause rebound high blood pressure, anxiety, chest pain, insomnia, headache, nausea, irregular heartbeat, flushed face, sweating.

Others:
- Hot weather and fever may cause dehydration and drop in blood pressure. Dose may require temporary adjustment. Weigh daily and report any unexpected weight decreases to your doctor.
- May cause rise in uric acid, leading to gout.
- May cause blood-sugar rise in diabetics.

POSSIBLE INTERACTION WITH OTHER DRUGS

GENERIC NAME OR DRUG CLASS	COMBINED EFFECT
Allopurinol	Decreased allopurinol effect.
Angiotensin-converting enzyme (ACE) inhibitors*	Possible excessive potassium in blood.

Antidepressants, tricyclic*	Dangerous drop in blood pressure. Avoid combination unless under medical supervision.
Antihypertensives, other*	Excessive blood pressure drop.
Appetite suppressants*	Decreased clonidine effect.
Barbiturates*	Increased chlorthalidone effect.
Beta-adrenergic blocking agents*	Possible precipitous change in blood pressure.
Carteolol	Increased anti-hypertensive effect.
Central nervous system (CNS) depressants*	Increased sedative effect.
Cholestyramine	Decreased chlorthalidone effect.
Digitalis preparations*	Excessive potassium loss that causes dangerous heart rhythms.
Diuretics*	Excessive blood pressure drop.

Continued on page 911

POSSIBLE INTERACTION WITH OTHER SUBSTANCES

INTERACTS WITH	COMBINED EFFECT
Alcohol:	Increased sensitivity to sedative effect of alcohol and very low blood pressure. Avoid.
Beverages: Caffeine-containing drinks.	Decreased clonidine effect.
Cocaine:	Increased risk of heart block and high blood pressure.
Foods: Licorice.	Excessive potassium loss that causes dangerous heart rhythm.
Marijuana:	Weakness on standing. May increase blood pressure.
Tobacco:	None expected.

CLOTRIMAZOLE (Oral-Local)

BRAND NAMES

Mycelex Troches

BASIC INFORMATION

Habit forming? No
Prescription needed? Yes
Available as generic? No
Drug class: Antifungal

 ## USES

- Treats thrush, white mouth (candidiasis).
- Used primarily in immunosuppressed patients to treat and prevent mouth infection.

 ## DOSAGE & USAGE INFORMATION

How to take:
Lozenges—Dissolve slowly and completely in the mouth, 5 times a day. Swallow saliva during this time. Don't swallow lozenge whole and don't chew.

When to take:
14 days or longer.

If you forget a dose:
Take as soon as you remember up to 2 hours late. If more than 2 hours, wait for next scheduled dose (don't double this dose).

What drug does:
Kills fungus by interfering with cell wall membrane and its permeability.

Time lapse before drug works:
1 to 3 hours.

Don't take with:
Any other medicine without consulting your doctor or pharmacist.

 ## OVERDOSE

SYMPTOMS:
None expected, but if large dose has been taken, follow instructions below.
WHAT TO DO:
- Dial 911 (emergency) or 0 (operator) for an ambulance or medical help. Then give first aid immediately.
- See emergency information on inside covers.

 ## POSSIBLE ADVERSE REACTIONS OR SIDE EFFECTS

SYMPTOMS	WHAT TO DO
Life-threatening: None expected.	
Common: None expected.	
Infrequent: Abdominal pain, diarrhea, nausea, vomiting.	Discontinue. Call doctor right away.
Rare: None expected.	

CLOTRIMAZOLE (Oral-Local)

WARNINGS & PRECAUTIONS

Don't take if:
You have severe liver disease.

Before you start, consult your doctor:
If you have had a recent organ transplant.

Over age 60:
Adverse reactions and side effects may be more frequent and severe than in younger persons. You may need smaller doses for shorter periods of time.

Pregnancy:
Decide with your doctor if drug benefits justify risk to unborn child. Risk category C (see page xxiii)

Breast-feeding:
Unknown effect. Consult doctor.

Infants & children:
Use only under medical supervision for children younger than 4 or 5 years.

Prolonged use:
No problems expected.

Skin & sunlight:
No problems expected.

Driving, piloting or hazardous work:
Don't drive or pilot aircraft until you learn how medicine affects you. Don't work around dangerous machinery. Don't climb ladders or work in high places. Danger increases if you drink alcohol or take medicine affecting alertness and reflexes.

Discontinuing:
Don't discontinue without consulting doctor. Dose may require gradual reduction if you have taken drug for a long time. Doses of other drugs may also require adjustment.

Others:
- Continue for full term of treatment. May require several months.
- Check with physician if not improved in 1 week.

POSSIBLE INTERACTION WITH OTHER DRUGS

GENERIC NAME OR DRUG CLASS	COMBINED EFFECT
None expected.	

POSSIBLE INTERACTION WITH OTHER SUBSTANCES

INTERACTS WITH	COMBINED EFFECT
Alcohol:	Decreased effects of clotrimazole.
Beverages:	None expected.
Cocaine:	Decreased effects of clotrimazole.
Foods:	None expected.
Marijuana:	Decreased effects of clotrimazole.
Tobacco:	Decreased effects of clotrimazole.

CLOZAPINE

BRAND NAMES

Clozaril   Leponex

BASIC INFORMATION

Habit forming? No
Prescription needed? Yes. Prescribed only
  through a special program.
Available as generic? Yes
Drug class: Antipsychotic

 USES

Treats severe schizophrenia in patients not
helped by other medicines.

 DOSAGE & USAGE INFORMATION

How to take:
Tablet—Swallow with liquid. If you can't swallow
whole, crumble tablet and take with liquid or
food.

When to take:
Once or twice daily as directed.

If you forget a dose:
Take as soon as you remember up to 2 hours
late. If more than 2 hours, wait for next
scheduled dose (don't double this dose).

What drug does:
Interferes with binding of dopamine. May
produce significant improvement, but may at
times also make schizophrenia worse.

Time lapse before drug works:
Weeks to months before improvement is
evident. Your doctor may increase the dosage to
obtain optimal effectiveness..

Don't take with:
Any other prescription drug, nonprescription
drug or alcohol without first checking with your
doctor or pharmacist.

 OVERDOSE

SYMPTOMS:
Heartbeat fast, slow, irregular;
hallucinations; restlessness; excitement;
drowsiness; breathing difficulty.
WHAT TO DO:
- Dial 911 (emergency) or 0 (operator) for an
  ambulance or medical help. Then give first
  aid immediately.
- See emergency information at end of book.

 POSSIBLE ADVERSE REACTIONS OR SIDE EFFECTS

SYMPTOMS	WHAT TO DO
Life-threatening: High fever, rapid pulse, profuse sweating, muscle rigidity, confusion and irritability, seizures; fever, chills, mouth sores.	Discontinue. Seek emergency treatment.
Common: Dry mouth, blurred vision, constipation, difficulty urinating; sedation, low blood pressure, dizziness.	Continue. Call doctor when convenient.
Infrequent: None expected.	
Rare: • Jerky or involuntary movements, especially of the face, lips, jaw, tongue; slow-frequency tremor of head or limbs, especially while moving; muscle rigidity, lack of facial expression and slow inflexible movements; seizures.	Discontinue. Call doctor right away.
• Pacing or restlessness; (akathisia); intermittent spasms of muscles of face, eyes, tongue, jaw, neck, body or limbs.	Continue. Call doctor when convenient.

WARNINGS & PRECAUTIONS

Don't take if:
- You are significantly mentally depressed.
- You have bone marrow depression from other drugs.
- You have an enlarged prostate.
- You have glaucoma.

Before you start, consult your doctor:
- If you have ever had seizures from any cause.
- If you have liver, heart or gastrointestinal disease or any type of blood disorder.

Over age 60:
Possible greater risk of weakness or dizziness upon standing after sitting or lying down. Greater risk of excitement, confusion. Great risk of difficulty in urination.

Pregnancy:
Risk category B (see page xxiii).

Breast-feeding:
May cause sedation, restlessness or irritability in the nursing infant. Avoid.

Infants & children:
Safety not established. Consult doctor.

Prolonged use:
Effects unknown.

Skin & sunlight:
No problems expected.

Driving, piloting or hazardous work:
Don't drive or pilot aircraft until you learn how medicine affects you. Don't work around dangerous machinery. Don't climb ladders or work in high places. Danger increases if you drink alcohol or take medicine affecting alertness and reflexes.

Discontinuing:
Don't discontinue without consulting doctor. Dose may require gradual reduction if you have taken drug for a long time. Doses of other drugs may also require adjustment.

Others:
- This medicine is available only through a special management program for monitoring and distributing this drug.
- You will need laboratory studies each week for white blood cell and differential counts.

POSSIBLE INTERACTION WITH OTHER DRUGS

GENERIC NAME OR DRUG CLASS	COMBINED EFFECT
Antihypertensives*	Lower than expected blood pressure.
Bone marrow depressants*	Toxic bone marrow depression.
Bupropion	Increased risk of seizures.
Carbamazepine	Decreased clozapine effect.
Central nervous system (CNS) depressants*	Toxic effects on the central nervous system.
Fluoxetine	Increased risk of adverse reactions.
Fluvoxamine	Increased risk of adverse reactions.
Haloperidol	Increased risk of seizures.
Lithium	Increased risk of seizures.
Phenytoin	Decreased clozapine effect.
Risperidone	Increased risperidone effect.
Valproic acid	Increased clozapine effect.

POSSIBLE INTERACTION WITH OTHER SUBSTANCES

INTERACTS WITH	COMBINED EFFECT
Alcohol:	Avoid. Increases toxic effect on the central nervous system.
Beverages: Caffeine drinks.	Excess (more than 3 cups of coffee or equivalent) increases risk of heartbeat irregularities.
Cocaine:	Increased risk of heartbeat irregularities.
Foods:	No special problems expected.
Marijuana:	Increased risk of heartbeat irregularities.
Tobacco:	Decreased serum concentration of clozapine. Avoid.

COAL TAR (Topical)

BRAND NAMES

See complete list of brand names in the *Generic and Brand Name Directory*, page 877.

BASIC INFORMATION

Habit forming? No
Prescription needed? No (for most)
Available as generic? Yes
Drug class: Antiseborrheic, antipsoriatic, keratolytic

 ## USES

Applied to the skin to treat dandruff, seborrhea, dermatitis, eczema and other skin diseases.

 ## DOSAGE & USAGE INFORMATION

How to use:
- Follow package instructions.
- Don't apply to blistered, oozing, infected or raw skin.
- Keep away from eyes.
- Protect treated area from sunshine for 72 hours.

When to use:
According to package instructions.

If you forget a dose:
Use as soon as you remember.

What drug does:
- Kills bacteria and fungus organisms on contact.
- Suppresses overproduction of skin cells.

Time lapse before drug works:
None. Works immediately. May take several days before maximum effect.

Don't take with:
Any other medicine without consulting your doctor or pharmacist.

 ## OVERDOSE

SYMPTOMS:
None expected.
WHAT TO DO:
Overdose unlikely to threaten life. If person takes much larger amount than prescribed, call doctor, poison control center or hospital emergency room for instructions.

 ## POSSIBLE ADVERSE REACTIONS OR SIDE EFFECTS

SYMPTOMS	WHAT TO DO
Life-threatening: None expected.	
Common: Skin stinging.	Continue. Call doctor when convenient.
Infrequent: Skin more irritated.	Continue. Call doctor when convenient.
Rare: Pus forms in lesions on skin.	Continue. Call doctor when convenient.

WARNINGS & PRECAUTIONS

Don't use if:
You have intolerance to coal tar.

Before you start, consult your doctor:
If you have infected skin or open wounds.

Over age 60:
No special problems expected.

Pregnancy:
Consult doctor. Risk category C (see page xxiii).

Breast-feeding:
No special problems expected. Consult doctor.

Infants & children:
Don't use on infants.

Prolonged use:
No special problems expected.

Skin & sunlight:
One or more drugs in this group may cause rash or intensify sunburn in areas exposed to sun or ultraviolet light (photosensitivity reaction). Avoid overexposure. Notify doctor if reaction occurs.

Driving, piloting or hazardous work:
No problems expected.

Discontinuing:
No special problems expected.

Others:
- May affect results in some medical tests.
- Protect treated area from direct sunlight for 72 hours.

POSSIBLE INTERACTION WITH OTHER DRUGS

GENERIC NAME OR DRUG CLASS	COMBINED EFFECT
Psoralens (methoxsalen, trioxsalen)	Excess sensitivity to sun.

POSSIBLE INTERACTION WITH OTHER SUBSTANCES

INTERACTS WITH	COMBINED EFFECT
Alcohol:	No special problems expected.
Beverages:	No special problems expected.
Cocaine:	No special problems expected.
Foods:	No special problems expected.
Marijuana:	No special problems expected.
Tobacco:	No special problems expected.

COLCHICINE

GENERIC NAMES

COLCHICINE

BASIC INFORMATION

Habit forming? No
Prescription needed? Yes
Available as generic? Yes
Drug class: Antigout

 USES

- Relieves joint pain, inflammation, swelling of gout.
- Also used for familial Mediterranean fever, dermatitis herpetiformis, calcium pyrophosphate deposition disease, amyloidosis, Paget's disease of bone, recurrent pericarditis, Behcet's syndrome.

 DOSAGE & USAGE INFORMATION

How to take:
Tablet—Swallow with liquid or food to lessen stomach irritation.

When to take:
- As prescribed. Stop taking when pain stops or at first sign of digestive upset. Wait at least 3 days between treatments.
- Don't take more than 8 doses.

If you forget a dose:
Don't double next dose. Consult doctor.

What drug does:
Decreases acidity of joint tissues and prevents deposits of uric-acid crystals.

Time lapse before drug works:
12 to 48 hours.

Don't take with:
Any other medicine without consulting your doctor or pharmacist.

 OVERDOSE

SYMPTOMS:
Bloody urine; diarrhea; burning feeling in the throat, skin or stomach; nausea or vomiting; muscle weakness; fever; shortness of breath; stupor; convulsions; coma.
WHAT TO DO:
- **Dial 911 (emergency) or 0 (operator) for an ambulance or medical help. Then give first aid immediately.**
- **See emergency information on inside covers.**

 POSSIBLE ADVERSE REACTIONS OR SIDE EFFECTS

SYMPTOMS	WHAT TO DO
Life-threatening:	
In case of overdose, see previous column.	
Common:	
Diarrhea, nausea, vomiting, abdominal pain.	Discontinue. Call doctor right away.
Infrequent:	
Hair loss with long-term use.	Continue. Call doctor when convenient.
Rare:	
Jaundice, black or tarry stool, blood in urine, breathing difficulty, fever, chills, headache, hives, mouth or lip sores, sore throat, unusual bruising or bleeding, unusual tiredness or weakness.	Discontinue. Call doctor right away.

WARNINGS & PRECAUTIONS

Don't take if:
You are allergic to colchicine.

Before you start, consult your doctor:
- If you have had peptic ulcers or ulcerative colitis.
- If you have heart, liver or kidney disease.
- If you will have surgery within 2 months, including dental surgery, requiring general or spinal anesthesia.
- If you have a gastrointestinal disorder.
- If you drink large amounts of alcohol.

Over age 60:
Adverse reactions and side effects may be more frequent and severe than in younger persons. Colchicine has a narrow margin of safety for people in this age group.

Pregnancy:
Consult doctor. Risk category D (see page xxiii).

Breast-feeding:
Drug passes into breast milk. Effect unknown. Consult doctor.

Infants & children:
Not recommended.

Prolonged use:
- Hair loss.
- Numbness or tingling in hands and feet.
- Talk to your doctor about the need for follow-up medical examinations or laboratory studies to check complete blood counts (white blood cell count, platelet count, red blood cell count, hemoglobin, hematocrit).

Skin & sunlight:
No problems expected.

Driving, piloting or hazardous work:
Don't drive or pilot aircraft until you learn how medicine affects you. Don't work around dangerous machinery. Don't climb ladders or work in high places. Danger increases if you drink alcohol or take medicine affecting alertness and reflexes, such as antihistamines, tranquilizers, sedatives, pain medicine, narcotics and mind-altering drugs.

Discontinuing:
- May be unnecessary to finish medicine. Follow doctor's instructions.
- Stop taking if digestive upsets occur before symptoms are relieved.

Others:
- Limit each course of treatment to 8 mg. Don't exceed 3 mg. per 24 hours.
- May cause decreased sperm production in males.
- May interfere with the accuracy of some medical tests.

POSSIBLE INTERACTION WITH OTHER DRUGS

GENERIC NAME OR DRUG CLASS	COMBINED EFFECT
Anticoagulants*	Increased anticoagulant effect.
Anti-inflammatory drugs, nonsteroidal (NSAIDs)*	Increased risk of gastrointestinal problems.
Blood dyscrasia-causing medications*	Increased bone marrow depressant effect.
Bone marrow depressants,* other	Increased bone marrow depressant effect.
Phenylbutazone	Increased chance of ulcers in gastrointestinal tract.
Thioguanine	May need increased dosage of colchicine.
Vitamin B-12	Decreased absorption of vitamin B-12.

POSSIBLE INTERACTION WITH OTHER SUBSTANCES

INTERACTS WITH	COMBINED EFFECT
Alcohol:	Increased risk of gastrointestinal toxicity.
Beverages: Herbal teas.	Increased colchicine effect. Avoid.
Cocaine:	Overstimulation Avoid.
Foods:	No proven problems.
Marijuana:	Decreased colchicine effect.
Tobacco:	No proven problems.

*See Glossary

COLESTIPOL

BRAND NAMES

Colestid

BASIC INFORMATION

Habit forming? No
Prescription needed? Yes
Available as generic? No
Drug class: Antihyperlipidemic

USES

- Reduces cholesterol level in blood in patients with type IIa hyperlipidemia.
- Treats overdose of digitalis.
- Reduces skin itching associated with some forms of liver disease.
- Treats diarrhea after some surgical operations.
- Treatment of one form of colitis (rare).

DOSAGE & USAGE INFORMATION

How to take:
Oral suspension—Mix well with 6 ounces or more or water or liquid, or in soups, pulpy fruits, with milk or in cereals. Will not dissolve.

When to take:
- Before meals.
- If taking other medicine, take it 1 hour before or 4 to 6 hours after taking colestipol.

If you forget a dose:
Take as soon as you remember up to 2 hours late. If more than 2 hours, wait for next scheduled dose (don't double this dose).

What drug does:
Binds with bile acids in intestines, preventing reabsorption.

Time lapse before drug works:
3 to 12 months.

Don't take with:
Any other medicine without consulting your doctor or pharmacist.

OVERDOSE

SYMPTOMS:
Fecal impaction.
WHAT TO DO:
Overdose unlikely to threaten life. If person takes much larger amount than prescribed, call doctor, poison control center or hospital emergency room for instructions.

POSSIBLE ADVERSE REACTIONS OR SIDE EFFECTS

SYMPTOMS	WHAT TO DO
Life-threatening: None expected.	
Common: None expected.	
Infrequent:	
• Black, tarry stools from gastrointestinal bleeding.	Discontinue. Seek emergency treatment.
• Severe abdominal pain.	Discontinue. Call doctor right away.
• Constipation, belching, diarrhea, nausea, unexpected weight loss.	Continue. Call doctor when convenient.
Rare: Hives, skin rash, hiccups.	Discontinue. Call doctor right away.

WARNINGS & PRECAUTIONS

Don't take if:
You are allergic to colestipol.

Before you start, consult your doctor:
- If you have liver disease such as cirrhosis.
- If you are jaundiced.
- If you will have surgery within 2 months, including dental surgery, requiring general or spinal anesthesia.
- If you are constipated.
- If you have peptic ulcer.
- If you have coronary artery disease.

Over age 60:
Constipation more likely. Other adverse effects more likely.

Pregnancy:
Safety not established. Consult doctor. Risk category C (see page xxiii).

Breast-feeding:
No proven harm to child. Consult doctor.

Infants & children:
Only under expert medical supervision.

Prolonged use:
- Request lab studies to determine serum cholesterol and serum triglycerides.
- May decrease absorption of folic acid.

Skin & sunlight:
No problems expected.

Driving, piloting or hazardous work:
No problems expected.

Discontinuing:
Don't discontinue without consulting doctor. Dose may require gradual reduction if you have taken drug for a long time. Doses of other drugs may also require adjustment, particularly digitalis.

Others:
- This medicine does not cure disorders, but helps to control them.
- May interfere with the accuracy of some medical tests.

 ## POSSIBLE INTERACTION WITH OTHER DRUGS

GENERIC NAME OR DRUG CLASS	COMBINED EFFECT
Anticoagulants, oral*	Decreased anti-coagulant effect.
Beta carotene	Decreased absorption of beta carotene.
Dexfenfluramine	May require dosage change as weight loss occurs.
Dextrothyroxine	Decreased dextrothyroxine effect.
Digitalis preparations*	Decreased absorption of digitalis preparations.
Diuretics, thiazide*	Decreased absorption of thiazide diuretics.
Penicillins*	Decreased absorption of penicillins.
Tetracyclines*	Decreased absorption of tetracyclines.
Thiazides*	Decreased absorption of colestipol.
Thyroid hormones*	Decreased thyroid effect.
Trimethoprim	Decreased absorption of colestipol.
Ursodiol	Decreased absorption of ursodiol.

Vancomycin	Increased chance of hearing loss or kidney damage. Decreased therapeutic effect of vancomycin.
Vitamins	Decreased absorption of fat-soluble vitamins (A,D,E,K).
Other medicines	May delay or reduce absorption.

 ## POSSIBLE INTERACTION WITH OTHER SUBSTANCES

INTERACTS WITH	COMBINED EFFECT
Alcohol:	None expected.
Beverages:	None expected.
Cocaine:	None expected.
Foods:	Interferes with absorption of vitamins. Take supplements.
Marijuana:	None expected.
Tobacco:	None expected.

CONDYLOMA ACUMINATUM AGENTS

GENERIC AND BRAND NAMES

IMIQUIMOD
  Aldara
PODOFILOX
  Condylox

PODOPHYLLUM
  Podofin

BASIC INFORMATION

Habit forming? No
Prescription needed? Yes
Available as generic? No
Drug class: Cytotoxic (topical)

USES

- Treatment for *condylomata acuminata*—external genital and perianal warts.
- May be used for other skin disorders as prescribed by your doctor.

DOSAGE & USAGE INFORMATION

How to use:
For all treatments—Always follow instructions provided with prescription. Wash hands before and after applying medicine. Let the solution dry before allowing other skin surfaces to touch the treated area.
- Imiquimod—Apply a thin film of cream to the wart and rub in well. Leave cream on the treated skin 6 to 10 hours, then wash with soap and water.

Continued next column

OVERDOSE

SYMPTOMS:
- Imiquimod: Overdose unlikely. It may increase adverse skin reactions.
- Podofilox or podophyllum: The following symptoms may occur when the body absorbs too much—painful urination, breathing difficulty, dizziness, severe nausea or vomiting, fever, heartbeat irregularity, numbness and tingling of hands and feet, abdominal pain, excitement, irritability, seizures, coma.

WHAT TO DO:
- Dial 911 (emergency) or 0 (operator) for an ambulance or medical help. Then give first aid immediately.
- See emergency information on inside covers.

- Podofilox—Apply drug to warts with cotton applicator (supplied with drug). Allow drug to remain on warts for 1 to 6 hours, then remove with soap and water.
- Podophyllum—Apply petroleum jelly on normal skin surrounding warts. With a glass applicator or cotton swab, carefully apply podophyllum to the warts. Allow drug to remain on warts for 1 to 6 hours after application, then remove with soap and water.

When to use:
- Imiquimod cream—Once every other day 3 times a week. Apply at bedtime for up to 16 weeks.
- Podofilox topical solution—Apply twice a day (12 hours apart) for 3 consecutive days, then discontinue use for 4 consecutive days. May repeat this cycle of treatment 4 times (4 weeks).
- Podophyllum topical solution—Once at 1 week intervals for up to 6 weeks.

If you forget a dose:
Apply it as soon as you remember, then return to regular schedule.

What drug does:
Kills cells and erodes tissue.

Time lapse before drug works:
Several weeks.

Don't use with:
Any other medicines without consulting your doctor or pharmacist.

POSSIBLE ADVERSE REACTIONS OR SIDE EFFECTS

SYMPTOMS	WHAT TO DO
Life-threatening:	
In case of overdose, see previous column.	
Common:	
Mild skin reactions (slight stinging, mild redness, tenderness or slight swelling in treated area).	No action necessary. If they continue, call doctor.
Infrequent:	
Skin rash, burning, red skin, severe skin reaction. If too much of drug absorbed into body: hallucinations, diarrhea, nausea and vomiting, unusual bleeding, fever, muscle pain, flu-like symptoms.	Discontinue. Call doctor right away.
Rare:	
Lightening of normal skin at application site.	Continue. Call doctor when convenient.

WARNINGS & PRECAUTIONS

Don't use if:
- Warts are crumbled and bleeding.
- If warts have just been biopsied or had other surgery performed on them.
- If you are allergic to condyloma acuminatum agents.

Before you start, consult your doctor:
If you have used one of these drugs previously and have a new outbreak of warts.

Over age 60:
No special problems expected.

Pregnancy:
Consult doctor. Pregnancy risk factor not designated for podophyllum. Imiquimod is risk category B and podofilox is risk category C. See category list on page xxiii.

Breast-feeding:
It is not known if drugs pass into milk. Avoid drugs or discontinue nursing until you finish medicine. Consult doctor for advice on maintaining milk supply.

Infants & children:
Efficacy and safety have not been established.

Prolonged use:
Increased risk of adverse reactions.

Skin & sunlight:
No problems expected.

Driving, piloting or hazardous work:
No problems expected.

Discontinuing:
No problems expected. Discontinue medicine once warts are healed.

Others:
- Advise any doctor whom you consult that you are using this medicine.
- Keep medicine away from unaffected skin, eyes, nose and mouth. Wash hands before and after using.
- Don't bandage or cover the treated warts with material that is occlusive. If covering is needed, use cotton gauze or cotton underwear.
- Don't use medicine on moles or birthmarks.
- Don't use near heat or open flame.
- Do not apply more of the medicine than prescribed. It will increase risk of side effects.
- Avoid sexual contact while medicine is on the warts.
- Imiquimod may weaken contraceptive devices such as cervical caps, condoms and diaphragms and reduce their contraceptive effect.
- Recurrence of genital warts is common after treatment.

POSSIBLE INTERACTION WITH OTHER DRUGS

GENERIC NAME OR DRUG CLASS	COMBINED EFFECT
Other topical medicines used in same skin area.	Increases risk of side effects. Avoid.

POSSIBLE INTERACTION WITH OTHER SUBSTANCES

INTERACTS WITH	COMBINED EFFECT
Alcohol:	No special problems expected.
Beverages:	No special problems expected.
Cocaine:	No special problems expected.
Foods:	No special problems expected.
Marijuana:	No special problems expected.
Tobacco:	No special problems expected.

CONTRACEPTIVES, ORAL

GENERIC AND BRAND NAMES

See complete list of generic and brand names in the *Generic and Brand Name Directory*, page 877.

BASIC INFORMATION

Habit forming? No
Prescription needed? Yes
Available as generic? No
Drug class: Female sex hormone, contraceptive (oral)

 ## USES

- Prevents pregnancy.
- Regulates menstrual periods.
- May be used to treat acne vulgaris in females.

 ## DOSAGE & USAGE INFORMATION

How to take:
Tablet—Swallow with liquid or food to lessen stomach irritation.

When to take:
At same time each day according to prescribed instructions, usually for 21 days of 28-day cycle.

If you forget a dose:
Call doctor's office for advice about additional protection against pregnancy.

What drug does:
- Alters mucus at cervix entrance to prevent sperm entry.
- Alters uterus lining to resist implantation of fertilized egg.
- Creates same chemical atmosphere in blood that exists during pregnancy, suppressing pituitary hormones which stimulate ovulation.

Time lapse before drug works:
10 days or more to provide contraception.

Don't take with:
- Tobacco
- Any other medicine without consulting your doctor or pharmacist.

 ## OVERDOSE

SYMPTOMS:
Drowsiness, nausea, vomiting, vaginal bleeding.
WHAT TO DO:
Overdose unlikely to threaten life. If person takes much larger amount than prescribed, call doctor, poison control center or hospital emergency room for instructions.

 ## POSSIBLE ADVERSE REACTIONS OR SIDE EFFECTS

SYMPTOMS	WHAT TO DO
Life-threatening: Stroke, chest pain, coughing blood, sudden severe headache, severe leg pain, shortness of breath.	Seek emergency treatment immediately.
Common: Brown blotches on skin; vaginal discharge, itch; fluid retention; breakthrough bleeding; acne.	Continue. Call doctor when convenient.
Infrequent: • Headache; pain, swelling in leg (possible blood clots in leg vein); muscle, joint pain; depression; severe abdominal pain; bulging eyes; fainting; frequent urination; breast lumps.	Discontinue. Call doctor right away.
• Blue tinge to objects, lights; appetite change; nausea; bloating; vomiting; pain; changed sex drive.	Continue. Call doctor when convenient.
Rare: • Jaundice, rash, hives, itch, fever, hypercalcemia in breast cancer, intolerance of contact lenses, excess hair growth, voice change, enlarged clitoris in women.	Discontinue. Call doctor right away.
• Amenorrhea, insomnia, hair loss.	Continue. Call doctor when convenient.

 ## WARNINGS & PRECAUTIONS

Don't take if:
- You are allergic to any female hormone.
- You have had heart disease, blood clots or stroke.
- You have liver disease.
- You have cancer of breast, uterus or ovaries.
- You have unexplained vaginal bleeding.
- You smoke cigarettes.

Before you start, consult your doctor:
- If you have fibrocystic disease of breast.
- If you have migraine headaches.
- If you have fibroid tumors of uterus.
- If you have epilepsy.

- If you have asthma.
- If you have high blood pressure.
- If you will have surgery within 2 months, including dental surgery, requiring general or spinal anesthesia.
- If you have endometriosis.
- If you have diabetes.
- If you have sickle-cell anemia.
- If you are over age 35.

Over age 60:
Not used.

Pregnancy:
Discontinue at first sign of pregnancy. Risk category X (see page xxiii).

Breast-feeding:
Drug passes into milk. Avoid drug or discontinue nursing.

Infants & children:
Not recommended.

Prolonged use:
- Gallstones.
- Gradual blood pressure rise.
- Possible difficulty becoming pregnant after discontinuing.
- Talk to your doctor about the need for follow-up medical examinations or laboratory studies to check blood pressure, liver function, pap smear.

Skin & sunlight:
One or more drugs in this group may cause rash or intensify sunburn in areas exposed to sun or ultraviolet light (photosensitivity reaction). Avoid overexposure. Notify doctor if reaction occurs.

Driving, piloting or hazardous work:
No problems expected.

Discontinuing:
Don't become pregnant for 6 months after discontinuing.

Others:
- Failure to take oral contraceptives for 1 day may cancel pregnancy protection. If you forget a dose, use other contraceptive measures and call doctor for instructions on re-starting oral contraceptive.
- May interfere with the accuracy of some medical tests.
- May cause some vitamin deficiencies.

POSSIBLE INTERACTION WITH OTHER DRUGS

GENERIC NAME OR DRUG CLASS	COMBINED EFFECT
Ampicillin	Decreased contraceptive effect.
Anticoagulants*	Decreased anticoagulant effect.

Anticonvulsants, hydantoin*	Decreased contraceptive effect.
Antidepressants, tricyclic*	Increased toxicity of antidepressants.
Antidiabetics* oral	Decreased antidiabetic effect.
Antifibronolytic agents*	Increased possibility of blood clotting.
Anti-inflammatory drugs nonsteroidal (NSAIDs)*	Decreased contraceptive effect.
Antihistamines*	Decreased contraceptive effect.
Barbiturates*	Decreased contraceptive effect.
Chloramphenicol	Decreased contraceptive effect.
Clofibrate	Decreased clofibrate effect.
Dextrothyroxine	Decreased dextrothyroxine effect.
Guanethidine	Decreased guanethidine effect.
Hypoglycemics, oral*	Decreased effect of hypoglycemics.
Insulin	Possibly decreased insulin effect.
Insulin lispro	May need increased dosage of insulin.
Meperidine	Increased meperidine effect.

Continued on page 912

POSSIBLE INTERACTION WITH OTHER SUBSTANCES

INTERACTS WITH	COMBINED EFFECT
Alcohol:	No proven problems.
Beverages:	No proven problems.
Cocaine:	No proven problems.
Foods: Salt.	Increased edema (fluid retention).
Marijuana:	Increased bleeding between periods. Avoid.
Tobacco:	Possible heart attack, blood clots and stroke. If you take "the pill," *don't smoke*.

*See Glossary

CONTRACEPTIVES, VAGINAL (Spermicides)

GENERIC AND BRAND NAMES

See complete list of generic and brand names in the *Generic and Brand Name Directory,* page 878.

BASIC INFORMATION

Habit forming? No
Prescription needed? Not for most
Available as generic? Most aren't
Drug class: Contraceptive (vaginal)

 USES

- Provides a degree of protection against pregnancy.
- May help to protect against some sexually transmitted diseases, such as those caused by chlamydia, gardnerella, mycoplasma, neisseria, trichomonas, ureaplasma and possibly herpes virus, but not HIV.

 DOSAGE & USAGE INFORMATION

How to take:
- Read package insert carefully. Some cautions to remember:
- Do not douche for 6 to 8 hours after intercourse.
- Do not remove sponge, cervical cap or diaphragm for 6 to 8 hours after intercourse.
- Follow product label instructions for storage.

When to take:
Consistently with every sexual exposure.

If you forget to use:
Contact your doctor to consider using another form of pregnancy protection, such as the "morning-after" pill.

What drug does:
Forms a chemical barrier between sperm in semen and the mucous membranes in the vagina. The chemical acts to inactivate viable sperm and also kills some bacteria, viruses, yeast and fungus.

Time lapse before vaginal contraceptive works:
- Immediate for foam, gels, jellies and sponges.
- 5 to 15 minutes for film and suppositories.

Don't use with:
Not applicable.

 OVERDOSE

SYMPTOMS:
None expected.

 POSSIBLE ADVERSE REACTIONS OR SIDE EFFECTS

SYMPTOMS	WHAT TO DO
Life-threatening:	
Toxic shock syndrome (chills; fever; skin rash; muscle aches; extreme weakness; confusion; redness of vagina, inside of mouth, nose, throat or eyes). (Very rare.)	Seek emergency treatment immediately.
Common:	
None expected.	
Infrequent:	
None expected.	
Rare:	
Vaginal discharge, irritation or rash; painful urination; cloudy or bloody urine.	Discontinue. Call doctor right away.

WARNINGS & PRECAUTIONS

Don't take if:
You are allergic to any form of octoxynol, nonoxynol or benzalkonium chloride.

Before you start, consult your doctor:
If you desire complete protection against pregnancy, a combination of methods gives better protection than vaginal contraceptives alone.

Over age 60:
Adverse reactions and side effects may be more frequent and severe than in younger persons.

Pregnancy:
Risk factor not designated. See categories on page xxiii and consult doctor.

Breast-feeding:
Safety not established. Consult doctor.

Infants & children:
Not recommended.

Prolonged use:
Allergic reactions and irritation more likely.

Skin & sunlight:
No problems expected.

Driving, piloting or hazardous work:
No special problems expected.

Discontinuing:
No special problems expected.

Others:
- Failure rate when used alone is relatively high. Therefore a vaginal cream, sponge, suppository, foam, gel, jelly or other product should be used with a mechanical barrier, such as a condom, cervical cap, vaginal diaphragm or other form of pregnancy protection.
- Don't use a cervical cap, sponge or diaphragm during menstruation. Consider using a condom instead if additional protection is desired.
- Vaginal contraceptives usually also have spermicidal effects and may partially protect against sexually transmitted diseases.

POSSIBLE INTERACTION WITH OTHER DRUGS

GENERIC NAME OR DRUG CLASS	COMBINED EFFECT
Topical vaginal medications that include any of the following: sulfa drugs, soaps or disinfectants, nitrates*, permanganates, lanolin, hydrogen peroxide, iodides, cotton dressings, aluminum citrates, salicylates*	Spermicidal activity may be reduced or negated. Avoid combinations.
Vaginal douche products	May prevent spermicidal effect. Avoid until 8 hours following intercourse.

POSSIBLE INTERACTION WITH OTHER SUBSTANCES

INTERACTS WITH	COMBINED EFFECT
Alcohol:	None expected.
Beverages:	None expected.
Cocaine:	None expected.
Foods:	None expected.
Marijuana:	None expected.
Tobacco:	None expected.

*See Glossary

CROMOLYN

BRAND NAMES

Crolom	Opticrom
Fivent	PMS-Sodium
Gastrocrom	Cromoglycate
Intal	Rynacrom
Nalcrom	Sodium
Nasalcrom	Cromoglycate
Novo-Cromolyn	Vistacrom

BASIC INFORMATION

Habit forming? No
Prescription needed? Yes, for some
Available as generic? Yes, for some
**Drug class: Nasal decongestant,
  anti-inflammatory (nonsteroidal)**

 USES

- Powdered form and nebulizer solution prevent asthma attacks. Will not stop an active asthma attack.
- Eye drops treat inflammation of covering to eye and cornea.
- Nasal spray reduces nasal allergic symptoms.
- Capsules may help prevent allergic symptoms.

 DOSAGE & USAGE INFORMATION

How to take:
Inhaler
Follow instructions enclosed with inhaler. Don't swallow cartridges for inhaler. Gargle and rinse mouth after inhalations.
Eye drops
- Wash hands.
- Apply pressure to inside corner of eye with middle finger.
- Continue pressure for 1 minute after placing medicine in eye.
- Tilt head backward. Pull lower lid away from eye with index finger of the same hand.
- Drop eye drops into pouch and close eye. Don't blink.

Continued next column

 OVERDOSE

SYMPTOMS:
Increased side effects and adverse reactions listed.
WHAT TO DO:
Overdose unlikely to threaten life. If person inhales much larger amount than prescribed, call doctor, poison control center or hospital emergency room for instructions.

- Keep eyes closed for 1 to 2 minutes.
- Don't touch applicator tip to any surface (including the eye). If you accidentally touch tip, clean with warm soap and water.
- Keep container tightly closed.
- Keep cool, but don't freeze.
- Wash hands immediately after using.

Nasal solution
Follow prescription instructions.
Capsules
Open capsule and dissolve contents in 4 ounces of hot water, then add equal amount of cold water. Drink all the liquid.

When to take:
At the same times each day. If you also use a bronchodilator inhaler, use the bronchodilator before the cromolyn.

If you forget a dose:
Take as soon as you remember up to 2 hours late. If more than 2 hours, wait for next scheduled dose (don't double this dose).

What drug does:
Blocks histamine release from mast cells.

Time lapse before drug works:
- For inhaler forms: 4 weeks for prevention of asthma attacks. However, if taken 10-15 minutes after exercise or exposure to known allergens, may prevent wheezing.
- 1 to 2 weeks for nasal symptoms; only a few days for eye symptoms.

Don't take with:
Any other medicine without consulting your doctor or pharmacist.

 POSSIBLE ADVERSE REACTIONS OR SIDE EFFECTS

SYMPTOMS	WHAT TO DO
Life-threatening:	
Hives, rash, intense itching, faintness soon after a dose (anaphylaxis).	Seek emergency treatment immediately.
Common:	
Inhaler—cough, stuffy nose, dry mouth or throat; nasal—burning or stinging inside nose, increased sneezing; oral—diarrhea, headache.	Continue. Call doctor when convenient.
Infrequent:	
Inhaler—hoarseness, watery eyes; nasal— headache, bad taste, postnasal drip; oral— stomach pain, nausea, insomnia, rash.	Continue. Call doctor when convenient.

Rare:

Inhaler—rash, hives, swallowing difficulty, increased wheezing, joint pain or swelling, weakness, muscle pain, difficult or painful urination, difficulty breathing; nasal—difficulty swallowing, hives, itching, skin rash, facial swelling, wheezing, nosebleed; oral—cough, difficulty swallowing, facial swelling, wheezing, breathing difficulty.

Discontinue. Call doctor right away.

WARNINGS & PRECAUTIONS

Don't take if:
You use the dry powder form of cromolyn and if you are allergic to cromolyn, lactose, milk or milk products.

Before you start, consult your doctor:
- If you plan to become pregnant within medication period.
- If you have kidney or liver disease.

Over age 60:
Adverse reactions and side effects may be more frequent and severe than in younger persons.

Pregnancy:
No proven harm to unborn child, but avoid if possible. Consult doctor. Risk category B (see page xxiii).

Breast-feeding:
Effects unknown. Confer with your doctor.

Infants & children:
Use only under medical supervision.

Prolonged use:
Consult doctor on a regular basis while using this drug.

Skin & sunlight:
No problems expected.

Driving, piloting or hazardous work:
No problems expected.

Discontinuing:
Don't discontinue without doctor's approval if drug is used to prevent asthma symptoms. Dosages of other drugs may need to be adjusted.

Others:
- Inhaler must be cleaned and work well for drug to be effective.
- Treatment with inhalation cromolyn does not stop an acute asthma attack and may aggravate it.
- Advise any doctor or dentist whom you consult about the use of this medicine.
- Be sure you and the doctor discuss benefits and risks of this drug before starting.
- Call doctor if symptoms worsen or new symptoms develop with use of this medicine.
- Wear a medical identification that indicates the use of this medicine.
- Use medicine only as directed. Don't increase or decrease dosage without doctor's approval.

POSSIBLE INTERACTION WITH OTHER DRUGS

GENERIC NAME OR DRUG CLASS	COMBINED EFFECT
None significant.	

POSSIBLE INTERACTION WITH OTHER SUBSTANCES

INTERACTS WITH	COMBINED EFFECT
Alcohol:	None expected.
Beverages:	None expected.
Cocaine:	None expected.
Foods:	None expected.
Marijuana:	None expected.
Tobacco:	None expected, but tobacco smoke aggravates asthma and eye irritation. Avoid.

267

CYCLANDELATE

BRAND NAMES

Cyclospasmol   Cyraso-400

BASIC INFORMATION

Habit forming? No
Prescription needed?
  U.S.: Yes
  Canada: No
Available as generic? Yes
Drug class: Vasodilator

USES

May improve poor blood flow to extremities.

DOSAGE & USAGE INFORMATION

How to take:
Tablet or capsule—Swallow with liquid. If you can't swallow whole, crumble tablet or open capsule and take with liquid or food.

When to take:
At the same time each day.

If you forget a dose:
Take as soon as you remember up to 2 hours late. If more than 2 hours, wait for next scheduled dose (don't double this dose).

What drug does:
Increases blood flow by relaxing and expanding blood-vessel walls.

Time lapse before drug works:
3 weeks.

Don't take with:
Any other medicine without consulting your doctor or pharmacist.

OVERDOSE

SYMPTOMS:
Severe headache, dizziness; nausea, vomiting; flushed, hot face.
WHAT TO DO:
Overdose unlikely to threaten life. If person takes much larger amount than prescribed, call doctor, poison control center or hospital emergency room for instructions.

POSSIBLE ADVERSE REACTIONS OR SIDE EFFECTS

SYMPTOMS	WHAT TO DO
Life-threatening:	
In case of overdose, see previous column.	
Common:	
None expected.	
Infrequent:	
• Rapid heartbeat.	Discontinue. Call doctor right away.
• Dizziness; headache; weakness; flushed face; tingling in face, fingers or toes; unusual sweating.	Continue. Call doctor when convenient.
• Belching, heartburn, nausea or stomach pain.	Continue. Tell doctor at next visit.
Rare:	
None expected.	

WARNINGS & PRECAUTIONS

Don't take if:
You have had allergic reaction to cyclandelate.

Before you start, consult your doctor:
• If you have glaucoma.
• If you have had heart attack or stroke.

Over age 60:
Adverse reactions and side effects may be more frequent and severe than in younger persons.

Pregnancy:
Consult doctor. Risk category C (see page xxiii).

Breast-feeding:
No proven problems. Consult doctor.

Infants & children:
Not recommended.

Prolonged use:
No problems expected.

Skin & sunlight:
No problems expected.

Driving, piloting or hazardous work:
Avoid if you feel dizzy or weak. Otherwise, no problems expected.

Discontinuing:
Don't discontinue without doctor's advice until you complete prescribed dose, even though symptoms diminish or disappear.

Others:
Response to drug varies. If your symptoms don't improve after 3 weeks of use, consult doctor.

 ## POSSIBLE INTERACTION WITH OTHER DRUGS

GENERIC NAME OR DRUG CLASS	COMBINED EFFECT
None expected.	

 ## POSSIBLE INTERACTION WITH OTHER SUBSTANCES

INTERACTS WITH	COMBINED EFFECT
Alcohol:	None expected.
Beverages:	None expected.
Cocaine:	Decreased cyclandelate effect. Avoid.
Foods:	None expected.
Marijuana:	None expected.
Tobacco:	May decrease cyclandelate effect.

CYCLIZINE

BRAND NAMES

Marezine   Marzine

BASIC INFORMATION

Habit forming? No
Prescription needed?
  U.S.: No
  Canada: Yes
Available as generic? No
Drug class: Antiemetic, antimotion
  sickness

USES

Prevention and treatment for motion sickness.

DOSAGE & USAGE INFORMATION

How to take:
Tablet—Swallow with liquid or food to lessen
stomach irritation. If you can't swallow whole,
crumble tablet and chew or take with liquid or
food.

When to take:
30 minutes to 1 hour before traveling.

If you forget a dose:
Take as soon as you remember. Wait 4 hours
for next dose.

What drug does:
Reduces sensitivity of nerve endings in inner
ear, blocking messages to brain's vomiting
center.

Time lapse before drug works:
30 to 60 minutes.

Don't take with:
Any other medicine without consulting your
doctor or pharmacist.

OVERDOSE

SYMPTOMS:
**Drowsiness, confusion, incoordination,
stupor, coma, weak pulse, shallow breathing,
hallucinations.**
WHAT TO DO:
• **Dial 911 (emergency) or 0 (operator) for an
ambulance or medical help. Then give first
aid immediately.**
• **See emergency information on inside
covers.**

POSSIBLE ADVERSE REACTIONS OR SIDE EFFECTS

SYMPTOMS	WHAT TO DO
Life-threatening: In case of overdose, see previous column.	
Common: Drowsiness.	Continue. Tell doctor at next visit.
Infrequent: • Headache, diarrhea or constipation, nausea, fast heartbeat.	Continue. Call doctor when convenient.
• Dry mouth, nose, throat; dizziness.	Continue. Tell doctor at next visit.
Rare: • Rash or hives, jaundice.	Discontinue. Call doctor right away.
• Restlessness, excitement, insomnia, blurred vision, frequent or difficult urination, hallucinations.	Continue. Call doctor when convenient.
• Appetite loss, nausea.	Continue. Tell doctor at next visit.

WARNINGS & PRECAUTIONS

Don't take if:
• You are allergic to meclizine, buclizine or
cyclizine.
• You have taken a monoamine oxidase (MAO)
inhibitor* in the past 2 weeks.

Before you start, consult your doctor:
• If you have glaucoma.
• If you have prostate enlargement.
• If you have reacted badly to any antihistamine
• If you have asthma.

Over age 60:
Adverse reactions and side effects may be more
frequent and severe than in younger persons,
especially impaired urination from enlarged
prostate gland.

Pregnancy:
Consult doctor. Risk category B (see page xxiii).

Breast-feeding:
Drug passes into milk. Avoid drug or discontinue
nursing until you finish medicine. Consult doctor
for advice on maintaining milk supply.

Infants & children:
Avoid if under age 6.

Prolonged use:
No problems expected.

Skin & sunlight:
No problems expected.

Driving, piloting or hazardous work:
Don't fly aircraft. Don't drive until you learn how medicine affects you. Don't work around dangerous machinery. Don't climb ladders or work in high places. Danger increases if you drink alcohol or take medicine affecting alertness and reflexes, such as antihistamines, tranquilizers, sedatives, pain medicine, narcotics and mind-altering drugs.

Discontinuing:
No problems expected.

Others:
- Some products contain tartrazine dye. Avoid if allergic (especially aspirin hypersensitivity).
- May interfere with the accuracy of some medical tests.

POSSIBLE INTERACTION WITH OTHER DRUGS

GENERIC NAME OR DRUG CLASS	COMBINED EFFECT
Amphetamines*	May decrease drowsiness caused by cyclizine.
Anticholinergics*	Increased effect of both drugs.
Antidepressants, tricyclic*	Increased effect of both drugs.
Carteolol	Decreased antihistamine effect.
Clozapine	Toxic effect on the central nervous system.
Dronabinol	Increased cyclizine effect.
Ethinamate	Dangerous increased effects of ethinamate. Avoid combining.
Fluoxetine	Increased depressant effects of both drugs.
Guanfacine	May increase depressant effects of either drug.
Leucovorin	High alcohol content of leucovorin may cause adverse effects.

Methyprylon	Increased sedative effect, perhaps to dangerous level. Avoid.
Monoamine oxidase (MAO) inhibitors*	Increased cyclizine effect.
Nabilone	Greater depression of central nervous system.
Narcotics*	Increased effect of both drugs.
Pain relievers*	Increased effect of both drugs.
Sedatives*	Increased effect of both drugs.
Sertraline	Increased depressive effect of both drugs.
Sleep inducers*	Increased effect of both drugs.
Sotalol	Increased antihistamine effect.
Tranquilizers*	Increased effect of both drugs.

POSSIBLE INTERACTION WITH OTHER SUBSTANCES

INTERACTS WITH	COMBINED EFFECT
Alcohol:	Increased sedation. Avoid.
Beverages: Caffeine drinks.	May decrease drowsiness.
Cocaine:	None expected.
Foods:	None expected.
Marijuana:	Increased drowsiness, dry mouth.
Tobacco:	None expected.

CYCLOBENZAPRINE

BRAND NAMES

Cycoflex   Flexeril

BASIC INFORMATION

Habit forming? No
Prescription needed? Yes
Available as generic? Yes
Drug class: Muscle relaxant

USES

Treatment for pain and limited motion caused by spasms in voluntary muscles.

DOSAGE & USAGE INFORMATION

How to take:
Tablet—Swallow with liquid.

When to take:
At the same time each day or according to label instructions.

If you forget a dose:
Take as soon as you remember. Wait 4 hours for next dose.

What drug does:
Blocks body's pain messages to brain. May also sedate.

Time lapse before drug works:
30 to 60 minutes.

Continued next column

OVERDOSE

SYMPTOMS:
Drowsiness, confusion, difficulty concentrating, visual problems, vomiting, blood pressure drop, low body temperature, weak and rapid pulse, convulsions, coma.
WHAT TO DO:
- **Dial 911 (emergency) or 0 (operator) for an ambulance or medical help. Then give first aid immediately.**
- **If patient is unconscious and not breathing, give mouth-to-mouth breathing. If there is no heartbeat, use cardiac massage and mouth-to-mouth breathing (CPR). Don't try to make patient vomit. If you can't get help quickly, take patient to nearest emergency facility.**
- **See emergency information on inside covers.**

Don't take with:
Nonprescription drugs without consulting doctor.

POSSIBLE ADVERSE REACTIONS OR SIDE EFFECTS

SYMPTOMS	WHAT TO DO
Life-threatening:	
In case of overdose, see previous column.	
Common:	
Drowsiness, dizziness, dry mouth.	Continue. Call doctor when convenient.
Infrequent:	
• Blurred vision, fast heartbeat.	Discontinue. Call doctor right away.
• Insomnia, numbness in extremities, bad taste in mouth, fatigue, nausea, sweating.	Continue. Call doctor when convenient.
Rare:	
• Unsteadiness, confusion, depression, hallucinations, rash, itch, swelling, breathing difficulty.	Discontinue. Call doctor right away.
• Difficult urination, rash.	Continue. Call doctor when convenient.

WARNINGS & PRECAUTIONS

Don't take if:
- You are allergic to any skeletal muscle relaxant*.
- You have taken a monoamine oxidase (MAO) inhibitor* in last 2 weeks.
- You have had a heart attack within 6 weeks, or suffer from congestive heart failure.
- You have an overactive thyroid.

Before you start, consult your doctor:
- If you have a heart problem.
- If you have reacted to tricyclic anti-depressants.
- If you have glaucoma.
- If you have a prostate condition and urination difficulty.
- If you intend to pilot aircraft.

Over age 60:
Adverse reactions and side effects may be more frequent and severe than in younger persons. Avoid extremes of heat and cold.

Pregnancy:
No problems expected. Consult doctor. Risk category B (see page xxiii).

Breast-feeding:
Drug may pass into milk. Avoid drug or discontinue nursing until you finish medicine. Consult doctor for advice on maintaining milk supply.

Infants & children:
Don't use for children younger than 15.

Prolonged use:
Do not take for longer than 2 to 3 weeks.

Skin & sunlight:
No special problems expected.

Driving, piloting or hazardous work:
Don't drive or pilot aircraft until you learn how medicine affects you. Don't work around dangerous machinery. Don't climb ladders or work in high places. Danger increases if you drink alcohol or take medicine affecting alertness and reflexes.

Discontinuing:
May be unnecessary to finish medicine. Follow doctor's instructions.

Others:
No problems expected.

POSSIBLE INTERACTION WITH OTHER DRUGS

GENERIC NAME OR DRUG CLASS	COMBINED EFFECT
Anticholinergics*	Increased anticholinergic effect.
Antidepressants*	Increased sedation.
Antihistamines*	Increased antihistamine effect.
Barbiturates*	Increased sedation.
Central nervous system (CNS) depressants*	Increased sedation.
Cimetidine	Possible increased cyclobenzaprine effect.
Cisapride	Decreased cyclobenzaprine effect.
Clonidine	Decreased clonidine effect.
Dronabinol	Increased effect of dronabinol on central nervous system. Avoid combination.
Guanethidine	Decreased guanethidine effect.
Methyldopa	Decreased methyldopa effect.

Mind-altering drugs*	Increased mind-altering effect.
Monoamine oxidase (MAO) inhibitors*	High fever, convulsions, possible death.
Narcotics*	Increased sedation.
Pain relievers*	Increased pain reliever effect.
Procainamide	Possible increased conduction disturbance.
Quinidine	Possible increased conduction disturbance.
Rauwolfia alkaloids*	Decreased effect of rauwolfia alkaloids.
Sedatives*	Increased sedative effect.
Sleep inducers*	Increased sedation.
Tranquilizers*	Increased tranquilizer effect.

POSSIBLE INTERACTION WITH OTHER SUBSTANCES

INTERACTS WITH	COMBINED EFFECT
Alcohol:	Depressed brain function. Avoid.
Beverages:	None expected.
Cocaine:	Decreased cyclobenzaprine effect.
Foods:	None expected.
Marijuana:	Occasional use—Drowsiness. Frequent use—Severe mental and physical impairment.
Tobacco:	None expected.

CYCLOPENTOLATE (Ophthalmic)

BRAND NAMES

Ak-Pentolate
Cyclogyl
I-Pentolate
Minims
  Cyclopentolate

Ocu-Pentolate
Pentolair
Spectro-Pentolate

BASIC INFORMATION

Habit forming? No
Prescription needed? Yes
Available as generic? Yes
Drug class: Cycloplegic, mydriatic

 USES

- Enlarges (dilates) pupil.
- Temporarily paralyzes the normal pupil accommodation to light before eye examinations and to treat some eye conditions.

 DOSAGE & USAGE INFORMATION

How to use:
Eye drops
- Wash hands.
- Apply pressure to inside corner of eye with middle finger.
- Continue pressure for 1 minute after placing medicine in eye.
- Tilt head backward. Pull lower lid away from eye with index finger of the same hand.
- Drop eye drops into pouch and close eye. Don't blink.
- Keep eyes closed for 1 to 2 minutes.
- Don't touch applicator tip to any surface (including the eye). If you accidentally touch tip, clean with warm soap and water.
- Keep container tightly closed.
- Keep cool, but don't freeze.
- Wash hands immediately after using.

When to use:
As directed on bottle.

Continued next column

 OVERDOSE

SYMPTOMS:
None expected.
WHAT TO DO:
Not intended for internal use. If child accidentally swallows, call poison control center.

If you forget a dose:
Use as soon as you remember.

What drug does:
Blocks sphincter muscle of the iris and ciliary body.

Time lapse before drug works:
Within 30 to 60 minutes. Effects usually disappear in 24 hours.

Don't use with:
Other eye medicines such as carbachol, demecarium, echothiopate, isoflurophate, physostigmine, pilocarpine without doctor's approval.

 POSSIBLE ADVERSE REACTIONS OR SIDE EFFECTS

SYMPTOMS	WHAT TO DO
Life-threatening: None expected.	
Common: • Increased sensitivity to light. • Burning eyes.	Continue. Call doctor when convenient. Continue. Tell doctor at next visit.
Infrequent: None expected.	
Rare (extremely): Symptoms of excess medicine absorbed by the body—Clumsiness, confusion, fever, flushed face, hallucinations, rash, slurred speech, swollen stomach (children), drowsiness, fast heartbeat.	Discontinue. Call doctor right away.

CYCLOPENTOLATE (Ophthalmic)

WARNINGS & PRECAUTIONS

Don't use if:
You are allergic to cyclopentolate.

Before you start, consult your doctor:
• If medicine is for a brain-damaged child or child with Down syndrome.
• If prescribed for a child with spastic paralysis.

Over age 60:
No problems expected.

Pregnancy:
Avoid if possible. Consult doctor. Risk category C (see page xxiii).

Breast-feeding:
Safety unestablished. Avoid if possible. Consult doctor.

Infants & children:
Use only under close medical supervision.

Prolonged use:
Avoid. May increase absorption into body.

Skin & sunlight:
No special problems expected.

Driving, piloting or hazardous work:
Don't drive or pilot aircraft until you learn how medicine affects you. Don't work around dangerous machinery. Don't climb ladders or work in high places. Danger increases if you drink alcohol or take medicine affecting alertness and reflexes, such as antihistamines, tranquilizers, sedatives, pain medicine, narcotics and mind-altering drugs.

Discontinuing:
If effects last longer than 36 hours after last drops, consult doctor.

Others:
• Keep medicine cool, but don't freeze.
• Wear sunglasses to protect eyes from sunlight and bright light

POSSIBLE INTERACTION WITH OTHER DRUGS

GENERIC NAME OR DRUG CLASS	COMBINED EFFECT
Clinically significant interactions with oral or injected medicines unlikely.	

POSSIBLE INTERACTION WITH OTHER SUBSTANCES

INTERACTS WITH	COMBINED EFFECT
Alcohol:	None expected.
Beverages:	None expected.
Cocaine:	None expected.
Foods:	None expected.
Marijuana:	None expected.
Tobacco:	None expected.

CYCLOPHOSPHAMIDE

BRAND NAMES

Cytoxan   Procytox
Neosar

BASIC INFORMATION

Habit forming? No
Prescription needed? Yes
Available as generic? No
Drug class: Immunosuppressant, anti-neoplastic

 USES

* Treatment for cancer.
* Treatment for severe rheumatoid arthritis.
* Treatment for blood-vessel disease.
* Treatment for skin disease.

 DOSAGE & USAGE INFORMATION

How to take:
Tablet or liquid—Swallow with liquid. If you can't swallow whole, crumble tablet and take with liquid or food.

When to take:
Works best if taken first thing in morning. Should be taken on an empty stomach. However, may take with food to lessen stomach irritation. Don't take at bedtime.

If you forget a dose:
Take as soon as you remember up to 12 hours late. If more than 12 hours, wait for next scheduled dose (don't double this dose).

What drug does:
* Kills cancer cells.
* Suppresses spread of cancer cells.
* Suppresses immune system.

Time lapse before drug works:
7 to 10 days continual use.

Don't take with:
Any other medicine without consulting your doctor or pharmacist.

 OVERDOSE

SYMPTOMS:
Bloody urine, water retention, weight gain, severe infection.
WHAT TO DO:
Overdose unlikely to threaten life. If person takes much larger amount than prescribed, call doctor, poison control center or hospital emergency room for instructions.

 POSSIBLE ADVERSE REACTIONS OR SIDE EFFECTS

SYMPTOMS	WHAT TO DO
Life-threatening:	
Hives, rash, intense itching, faintness soon after a dose (anaphylaxis).	Seek emergency treatment immediately.
Common:	
• Sore throat, fever.	Continue, but call doctor right away.
• Dark skin, nails; nausea; appetite loss; vomiting; missed menstrual period.	Continue. Call doctor when convenient.
Infrequent:	
• Rash, hives, itch; shortness of breath; rapid heartbeat; cough; blood in urine, painful urination; pain in side; bleeding, bruising; increased sweating; hoarseness; foot or ankle swelling.	Continue, but call doctor right away.
• Confusion, agitation, headache, dizziness, flushed face, stomach pain, joint pain, fatigue, weakness, diarrhea.	Continue. Call doctor when convenient.
Rare:	
• Mouth, lip sores; black stool; unusual thirst; jaundice.	Continue, but call doctor right away.
• Blurred vision, increased urination, hair loss.	Continue. Call doctor when convenient.

 WARNINGS & PRECAUTIONS

Don't take if:
* You are allergic to any alkylating agent.
* You have an infection.
* You have bloody urine.
* You will have surgery within 2 months, including dental surgery, requiring general or spinal anesthesia.

Before you start, consult your doctor:
- If you have impaired liver or kidney function.
- If you have impaired bone marrow or blood cell production.
- If you have had chemotherapy or x-ray therapy.
- If you have taken cortisone drugs in the past year.
- If you plan to become pregnant.

Over age 60:
Adverse reactions and side effects may be more frequent and severe than in younger persons. To reduce risk of chemical bladder inflammation, drink 8 to 10 glasses of water daily.

Pregnancy:
Risk to unborn child outweighs drug benefits. Don't use. Risk category D (see page xxiii).

Breast-feeding:
Drug passes into milk. Avoid drug or discontinue nursing until you finish medicine. Consult doctor for advice on maintaining milk supply.

Infants & children:
Use only under medical supervision.

Prolonged use:
- Development of fibrous lung tissue.
- Possible jaundice.
- Swelling of feet, lower legs.
- Cancer.
- Infertility in men.
- Talk to your doctor about the need for follow-up medical examinations or laboratory studies to check complete blood counts (white blood cell count, platelet count, red blood cell count, hemoglobin, hematocrit), urine, liver function.

Skin & sunlight:
No problems expected.

Driving, piloting or hazardous work:
Avoid if you feel dizzy or have blurred vision. Otherwise, no problems expected.

Discontinuing:
Don't discontinue without consulting doctor. Dose may require gradual reduction if you have taken drug for a long time. Doses of other drugs may also require adjustment.

Others:
- Frequently causes hair loss. After treatment ends, hair should grow back.
- Avoid vaccinations.

 ## POSSIBLE INTERACTION WITH OTHER DRUGS

GENERIC NAME OR DRUG CLASS	COMBINED EFFECT
Allopurinol or other medicines to treat gout	Possible anemia; decreased anti-gout effect.
Antidiabetics, oral*	Increased antidiabetic effect.
Bone marrow depressants,* other	Increased bone marrow depressant effect.
Clozapine	Toxic effect on bone marrow.
Cyclosporine	May increase risk of infection.
Digoxin	Possible decreased digoxin absorption.
Immuno-suppressants,* other	Increased risk of infection.
Insulin	Increased insulin effect.
Levamisole	Increased risk of bone marrow depression.
Lovastatin	Increased heart and kidney damage.
Phenobarbital	Increased cyclophosphamide effect.
Probenecid	Increased blood uric acid.
Sulfinpyrazone	Increased blood uric acid.
Tiopronin	Increased risk of toxicity to bone marrow.

 ## POSSIBLE INTERACTION WITH OTHER SUBSTANCES

INTERACTS WITH	COMBINED EFFECT
Alcohol:	No problems expected.
Beverages:	No problems expected. Drink at least 2 quarts fluid every day.
Cocaine:	Increased danger of brain damage.
Foods:	None expected.
Marijuana:	Increased impair-ment of immunity.
Tobacco:	None expected.

*See Glossary

CYCLOPLEGIC, MYDRIATIC (Ophthalmic)

GENERIC AND BRAND NAMES

ATROPINE
Atropair
Atropine Care Eye
  Drops and Ointment
Atropine Sulfate
  S.O.P.
Atropisol
Atrosulf
Isopto Atropine
I-Tropine
Minims Atropine
Ocu-Tropine

HOMATROPINE
AK Homatropine
I-Homatrine
I-Homatropine
Isopto
  Homatropine
Minims
  Homatropine
Spectro-
  Homatropine
SCOPOLAMINE
Isopto Hyoscine

BASIC INFORMATION

Habit forming? No
Prescription needed? Yes
Available as generic? Yes, some
Drug class: Cycloplegic, mydriatic

 ## USES

- Dilates pupil of the eye.
- Used before some eye examinations, before and after some eye surgical procedures and, rarely, to treat some eye problems such as glaucoma.

 ## DOSAGE & USAGE INFORMATION

How to use:
Eye drops
- Wash hands.
- Apply pressure to inside corner of eye with middle finger.
- Continue pressure for 1 minute after placing medicine in eye.
- Tilt head backward. Pull lower lid away from eye with index finger of the same hand.
- Drop eye drops into pouch and close eye. Don't blink.
- Keep eyes closed for 1 to 2 minutes.

Continued next column

 ## OVERDOSE

SYMPTOMS:
None expected.
WHAT TO DO:
Not intended for internal use. If child accidentally swallows, call poison control center.

Eye ointment
- Wash hands.
- Pull lower lid down from eye to form a pouch.
- Squeeze tube to apply thin strip of ointment into pouch.
- Close eye for 1 to 2 minutes.
- Don't touch applicator tip to any surface (including the eye). If you accidentally touch tip, clean with warm soap and water.
- Keep container tightly closed.
- Keep cool, but don't freeze.
- Wash hands immediately after using.

When to use:
As directed on label.

If you forget a dose:
Use as soon as you remember.

What drug does:
Blocks normal response to sphincter muscle of the iris of the eye and the accommodative muscle of the ciliary body.

Time lapse before drug works:
Begins within 1 minute. Residual effects may last up to 14 days.

Don't use with:
Other eye medicines such as carbachol, demecarium, echothiopate, isoflurophate, physostigmine, pilocarpine.

 ## POSSIBLE ADVERSE REACTIONS OR SIDE EFFECTS

SYMPTOMS	WHAT TO DO
Life-threatening: None expected.	
Common: • Increased sensitivity to light. • Burning eyes.	Continue. Call doctor when convenient. Continue. Tell doctor at next visit.
Infrequent: None expected.	
Rare (extremely): Symptoms of excess medicine absorbed by the body—Clumsiness, confusion, fever, flushed face, hallucinations, rash, slurred speech, swollen stomach (children), unusual drowsiness, fast heartbeat.	Discontinue. Call doctor right away.

278

CYCLOPLEGIC, MYDRIATIC (Ophthalmic)

WARNINGS & PRECAUTIONS

Don't use if:
You are allergic to cyclopentolate.

Before you start, consult your doctor:
- If medicine is for a brain-damaged child or child with Down's syndrome.
- If prescribed for a child with spastic paralysis.

Over age 60:
No problems expected.

Pregnancy:
Decide with your doctor if drug benefits justify risk to unborn child. Risk category C (see page xxiii).

Breast-feeding:
Safety unestablished. Avoid if possible.

Infants & children:
Use only under close medical supervision.

Prolonged use:
Avoid. May increase absorption into body.

Skin & sunlight:
No special problems expected.

Driving, piloting or hazardous work:
Don't drive or pilot aircraft until you learn how medicine affects you. Don't work around dangerous machinery. Don't climb ladders or work in high places. Danger increases if you drink alcohol or take medicine affecting alertness and reflexes, such as antihistamines, tranquilizers, sedatives, pain medicine, narcotics and mind-altering drugs.

Discontinuing:
Effects may last up to 14 days later.

Others:
- Keep medicine cool, but don't freeze.
- Wear sunglasses to protect eyes from sunlight and bright light

POSSIBLE INTERACTION WITH OTHER DRUGS

GENERIC NAME OR DRUG CLASS	COMBINED EFFECT
Clinically significant interactions with oral or injected medicines unlikely.	

POSSIBLE INTERACTION WITH OTHER SUBSTANCES

INTERACTS WITH	COMBINED EFFECT
Alcohol:	None expected.
Beverages:	None expected.
Cocaine:	None expected.
Foods:	None expected.
Marijuana:	None expected.
Tobacco:	None expected.

CYCLOSERINE

BRAND NAMES

Seromycin

BASIC INFORMATION

Habit forming? No
Prescription needed? Yes
Available as generic? No
Drug class: Antibacterial

 USES

- Treats urinary tract infections.
- Treats tuberculosis.

 DOSAGE & USAGE INFORMATION

How to take:
Capsules—Swallow with liquid or food to lessen stomach irritation. If you can't swallow whole, open capsule and take with liquid or food.

When to take:
- Once or twice daily.
- At the same time each day after meals to prevent stomach irritation.

If you forget a dose:
Take as soon as you remember up to 2 hours late. If more than 2 hours, wait for next scheduled dose (don't double this dose).

What drug does:
Interferes with bacterial wall synthesis and keeps germs from multiplying.

Time lapse before drug works:
3 to 4 hours.

Don't take with:
Any other medicine without consulting your doctor or pharmacist.

 OVERDOSE

SYMPTOMS:
Seizures.
WHAT TO DO:
- Dial 911 (emergency) or 0 (operator) for an ambulance or medical help. Then give first aid immediately.
- See emergency information on inside covers.

 POSSIBLE ADVERSE REACTIONS OR SIDE EFFECTS

SYMPTOMS	WHAT TO DO
Life-threatening: Seizures, muscle twitching or trembling.	Seek emergency treatment immediately.
Common: Gum inflammation, pale skin, depression, confusion, dizziness, restlessness, anxiety, nightmares, severe headache, drowsiness.	Continue, but call doctor right away.
Infrequent: Visual changes; skin rash; numbness, tingling or burning in hands and feet; jaundice; eye pain.	Continue. Call doctor when convenient.
Rare: Seizures, thoughts of suicide.	Discontinue. Seek emergency treatment.

WARNINGS & PRECAUTIONS

Don't take if:
- You are a frequent user of alcohol.
- You have a convulsive disorder.

Before you start, consult your doctor:
- If you are depressed.
- If you have kidney disease.
- If you have severe anxiety.

Over age 60:
Adverse reactions and side effects may be more frequent and severe than in younger persons. You may need smaller doses for shorter periods of time.

Pregnancy:
Decide with your doctor if drug benefits justify risk to unborn child. Risk category C (see page xxiii).

Breast-feeding:
Drug passes into milk. Avoid drug or discontinue nursing until you finish medicine. Consult doctor for advice on maintaining milk supply.

Infants & children:
Use only under close medical supervision.

Prolonged use:
- May cause liver or kidney damage.
- May cause anemia.

Skin & sunlight:
No special problems expected.

Driving, piloting or hazardous work:
Don't drive or pilot aircraft until you learn how medicine affects you. Don't work around dangerous machinery. Don't climb ladders or work in high places. Danger increases if you drink alcohol or take medicine affecting alertness and reflexes.

Discontinuing:
Don't discontinue without consulting doctor. Dose may require gradual reduction if you have taken drug for a long time. Doses of other drugs may also require adjustment.

Others:
- May have to take anticonvulsants, sedatives and/or pyridoxine to prevent or minimize toxic effects on the brain.
- If you must take more than 500 mg per day, toxicity is much more likely to occur.
- Talk to your doctor about taking pyridoxine as a supplement.

POSSIBLE INTERACTION WITH OTHER DRUGS

GENERIC NAME OR DRUG CLASS	COMBINED EFFECT
Ethionamide	Increased risk of seizures.
Isoniazid	Increased risk of central nervous system effects.
Pyridoxine	Reduces effects of pyridoxine. Since pyridoxine is a vital vitamin, patients on cycloserine require pyridoxine supplements to prevent anemia or peripheral neuritis.

POSSIBLE INTERACTION WITH OTHER SUBSTANCES

INTERACTS WITH	COMBINED EFFECT
Alcohol:	Toxic. May increase risk of seizures. Avoid.
Beverages:	None expected. All beverages except those with alcohol.
Cocaine:	Toxic. Avoid.
Foods:	None expected.
Marijuana:	May increase risk of seizures.
Tobacco:	May decrease effect of cycloserine.

CYCLOSPORINE

BRAND NAMES

Neoral   Sandimmune

BASIC INFORMATION

Habit forming? No
Prescription needed? Yes
Available as generic? No
Drug class: Immunosuppressant

 ## USES

- Suppresses the immune response in patients who have transplants of the heart, lung, kidney, liver, pancreas. Cyclosporine treats rejection as well as helps prevent it.
- Treatment for severe psoriasis when regular treatment is ineffective or not appropriate.

 ## DOSAGE & USAGE INFORMATION

How to take:
- Oral solution—Take after meals with liquid to decrease stomach irritation. May mix with milk, chocolate milk or orange juice. Don't mix in styrofoam cups. Use special dropper for exact dosage.
- Capsules—Take with water or other fluid. Don't break capsule open.

When to take:
At the same time each day, according to instructions on prescription label.

If you forget a dose:
Take as soon as you remember up to 2 hours late. If more than 2 hours, wait for next scheduled dose (don't double this dose).

What drug does:
Exact mechanism is unknown, but believed to inhibit interluken II to affect T-lymphocytes.

Time lapse before drug works:
3 to 3-1/2 hours.

Don't take with:
Any other medicine without consulting your doctor or pharmacist.

 ## OVERDOSE

SYMPTOMS:
Irregular heartbeat, seizures, coma.
WHAT TO DO:
- Dial 911 (emergency) or 0 (operator) for an ambulance or medical help. Then give first aid immediately.
- See emergency information on inside covers.

 ## POSSIBLE ADVERSE REACTIONS OR SIDE EFFECTS

SYMPTOMS	WHAT TO DO
Life-threatening:	
Seizures, wheezing with shortness of breath, convulsions.	Discontinue. Seek emergency treatment.
Common:	
• Gum inflammation, blood in urine, jaundice, tremors.	Continue. Call doctor when convenient.
• Increased hair growth.	Continue. Tell doctor at next visit.
Infrequent:	
• Fever, chills, sore throat, shortness of breath.	Call doctor right away.
• Frequent urination, headache, leg cramps.	Continue. Call doctor when convenient.
Rare:	
• Confusion, irregular heartbeat, numbness of hands and feet, nervousness, face flushing, severe abdominal pain, weakness.	Call doctor right away.
• Acne, headache.	Continue. Call doctor when convenient.

 ## WARNINGS & PRECAUTIONS

Don't take if:
- You have chicken pox.
- You have shingles (herpes zoster).

Before you start, consult your doctor:
- If you have liver problems.
- If you have an infection.
- If you have kidney disease.

Over age 60:
No special problems expected.

Pregnancy:
Decide with your doctor if drug benefits justify risk to unborn child. Risk category C (see page xxiii).

Breast-feeding:
Drug passes into milk. Avoid drug or discontinue nursing until you finish medicine. Consult doctor for advice on maintaining milk supply.

Infants & children:
No problems expected.

Prolonged use:
- Can cause reduced function of kidney.
- Talk to your doctor about the need for follow-up medical examinations or laboratory studies to check blood pressure, kidney function, liver function.

Skin & sunlight:
No problems expected.

Driving, piloting or hazardous work:
Don't drive or pilot aircraft until you learn how medicine affects you. Don't work around dangerous machinery. Don't climb ladders or work in high places. Danger increases if you drink alcohol or take medicine affecting alertness and reflexes.

Discontinuing:
Don't discontinue without consulting doctor. You probably will require this medicine for the remainder of your life.

Others:
- Request regular laboratory studies to measure levels of potassium and cyclosporine in blood and to evaluate liver and kidney function.
- Check blood pressure. Cyclosporine sometimes causes hypertension.
- Don't store solution in the refrigerator.
- Avoid any immunizations except those specifically recommended by your doctor.
- Maintain good dental hygiene. Cyclosporine can cause gum problems.
- Kidney toxicity occurs commonly after 12 months of taking cyclosporine.
- Don't mix in styrofoam cups.

POSSIBLE INTERACTION WITH OTHER DRUGS

GENERIC NAME OR DRUG CLASS	COMBINED EFFECT
Androgens	Increased effect of cyclosporine.
Anticonvulsants*	Decreased effect of cyclosporine.
Cimetidine	Increased effect of cyclosporine.
Danazol	Increased effect of cyclosporine.
Diltiazem	Increased effect of cyclosporine.
Diuretics, potassium-sparing	Increased effect of cyclosporine.
Erythromycin	Increased effect of cyclosporine.
Estrogens	Increased effect of cyclosporine.

Fluconazole	Increased effect of cyclosporine. Cyclosporine dosage must be adjusted.
HMG-CoA reductase inhibitors	Increased risk of muscle and kidney problems.
Immuno-suppressants* (adrenocorticoids, azathioprine, chlorambucil, cyclophosphamide, mercaptopurine, muromonab-CD3)	May increase risk of infection.
Itraconazole	Increased cyclosporine toxicity.
Ketoconazole	Increased risk of toxicity to kidney.
Leukotriene modifiers	Increased effect of cyclosporine.
Losartan	Increased potassium levels.
Lovastatin	Increased heart and kidney damage.
Medicines that may be toxic to kidneys (gold*, NSAIDs*, sulfonamides*)	Increased risk of toxicity to kidneys.
Nimodipine	Increased cyclosporine toxicity.

Continued on page 912

POSSIBLE INTERACTION WITH OTHER SUBSTANCES

INTERACTS WITH	COMBINED EFFECT
Alcohol:	May increase possibility of toxic effects. Avoid.
Beverages: Grapefruit juice.	Increased cyclosporine effect.
Cocaine:	May increase possibility of toxic effects. Avoid.
Foods:	None expected.
Marijuana:	May increase possibility of toxic effects. Avoid.
Tobacco:	May increase possibility of toxic effects. Avoid.

*See Glossary

DANAZOL

BRAND NAMES

Cyclomen   Danocrine

BASIC INFORMATION

Habit forming? No
Prescription needed? Yes
Available as generic? No
Drug class: Gonadotropin inhibitor

 USES

Treatment of endometriosis, fibrocystic breast disease, angioneurotic edema except in pregnant women, gynecomastia, infertility, excessive menstruation, precocious puberty.

 DOSAGE & USAGE INFORMATION

How to take:
Capsule—Swallow with liquid or food to lessen stomach irritation. If you can't swallow whole, open capsule and take with liquid or food.

When to take:
At the same times each day.

If you forget a dose:
Take as soon as you remember (don't double dose).

What drug does:
Partially prevents output of pituitary follicle-stimulating hormone and lutenizing hormone reducing estrogen production.

Time lapse before drug works:
- 2 to 3 months to treat endometriosis.
- 1 to 2 months to treat other disorders.

Don't take with:
- Birth control pills.
- Any other medicine without consulting your doctor or pharmacist.

 OVERDOSE

SYMPTOMS:
None expected.
WHAT TO DO:
Overdose unlikely to threaten life. If person takes much larger amount than prescribed, call doctor, poison control center or hospital emergency room for instructions.

 POSSIBLE ADVERSE REACTIONS OR SIDE EFFECTS

SYMPTOMS	WHAT TO DO
Life-threatening: None expected.	
Common: Menstrual irregularities.	Continue. Call doctor when convenient.
Infrequent: • Unnatural hair growth in women, nosebleeds, bleeding gums, sore throat and chills.	Discontinue. Call doctor right away.
• Dizziness; deepened voice; hoarseness; flushed or red skin; muscle cramps; enlarged clitoris; decreased testicle size; vaginal burning, itching; swollen feet; decreased breast size; increased or decreased sex drive.	Continue. Call doctor when convenient.
• Headache, acne, weight gain, vision changes.	Continue. Tell doctor at next visit.
Rare: Jaundice, flushing, sweating, vaginitis, rash, nausea, vomiting, constipation, abdominal pain.	Discontinue. Call doctor right away.

DANAZOL

WARNINGS & PRECAUTIONS

Don't take if:
- You become pregnant.
- You have breast cancer.

Before you start, consult your doctor:
- If you take birth control pills.
- If you have diabetes.
- If you have heart disease.
- If you have epilepsy.
- If you have kidney disease.
- If you have liver disease.
- If you have migraine headaches.

Over age 60:
Adverse reactions and side effects may be more frequent and severe than in younger persons.

Pregnancy:
Risk to unborn child outweighs drug benefits. Don't use. Stop if you get pregnant. Risk category X (see page xxiii).

Breast-feeding:
Unknown whether medicine filters into milk. Consult doctor.

Infants & children:
Not recommended.

Prolonged use:
- Required for full effect. Don't discontinue without consulting doctor.
- Talk to your doctor about the need for follow-up medical examinations or laboratory studies to check liver function, mammogram.

Skin & sunlight:
No problems expected.

Driving, piloting or hazardous work:
No problems expected.

Discontinuing:
Don't discontinue without consulting doctor. Menstrual periods may be absent for 2 to 3 months after discontinuation.

Others:
- May alter blood sugar levels in diabetic persons.
- May interfere with the accuracy of some medical tests.

POSSIBLE INTERACTION WITH OTHER DRUGS

GENERIC NAME OR DRUG CLASS	COMBINED EFFECT
Anticoagulants, oral*	Increased anticoagulant effect.
Antidiabetic agents, oral*	Decreased antidiabetic effect.
Cyclosporine	Increased risk of kidney damage.
Insulin	Decreased insulin effect.

POSSIBLE INTERACTION WITH OTHER SUBSTANCES

INTERACTS WITH	COMBINED EFFECT
Alcohol:	Excessive nervous system depression. Avoid.
Beverages: Caffeine.	Rapid, irregular heartbeat. Avoid.
Cocaine:	May interfere with expected action of danazol. Avoid.
Foods:	No problems expected.
Marijuana:	May interfere with expected action of danazol. Avoid.
Tobacco:	Rapid, irregular heartbeat. Avoid. Increased leg cramps.

*See Glossary

DANTROLENE

BRAND NAMES

Dantrium

BASIC INFORMATION

Habit forming? No
Prescription needed? Yes
Available as generic? No
Drug class: Muscle relaxant, antispastic

 ## USES

- Relieves muscle spasticity caused by diseases such as multiple sclerosis, cerebral palsy, stroke.
- Relieves muscle spasticity caused by injury to spinal cord.
- Relieves or prevents excess body temperature brought on by some surgical procedures.

 ## DOSAGE & USAGE INFORMATION

How to take:
Capsules—Swallow with liquid.

When to take:
Once a day for muscle spasticity during first 6 days. Later, every 6 hours. For excess body temperature, follow label instructions.

If you forget a dose:
Take as soon as you remember up to 2 hours late. If more than 2 hours, wait for next scheduled dose (don't double this dose).

Continued next column

 ## OVERDOSE

SYMPTOMS:
Shortness of breath, bloody urine, chest pain, convulsions.
WHAT TO DO:
- **Dial 911 (emergency) or 0 (operator) for an ambulance or medical help. Then give first aid immediately.**
- **If patient is unconscious and not breathing, give mouth-to-mouth breathing. If there is no heartbeat, use cardiac massage and mouth-to-mouth breathing (CPR). Don't try to make patient vomit. If you can't get help quickly, take patient to nearest emergency facility.**
- **See emergency information on inside covers.**

What drug does:
Acts directly on muscles to prevent excess contractions.

Time lapse before drug works:
1 or more weeks.

Don't take with:
Any other medicine without consulting your doctor or pharmacist.

 ## POSSIBLE ADVERSE REACTIONS OR SIDE EFFECTS

SYMPTOMS	WHAT TO DO
Life-threatening:	
Seizure.	Seek emergency treatment immediately.
Common:	
Drowsiness, dizziness, weakness.	Discontinue. Call doctor right away.
Infrequent:	
• Rash, hives; black or bloody stools; chest pain; fast heartbeat; backache; blood in urine; painful, swollen feet; chills; fever; shortness of breath.	Discontinue. Call doctor right away.
• Depression, confusion, headache, slurred speech, insomnia, nervousness, diarrhea, blurred vision, difficult swallowing, appetite loss, difficult urination, decreased sexual function in males.	Continue. Call doctor when convenient.
Rare:	
• Jaundice, abdominal cramps, double vision.	Discontinue. Call doctor right away.
• Constipation.	Continue. Call doctor when convenient.

WARNINGS & PRECAUTIONS

Don't take if:
You are allergic to dantrolene or any muscle relaxant or antispastic medication.

Before you start, consult your doctor:
• If you have liver disease.
• If you have heart disease.
• If you have lung disease (especially emphysema).
• If you are over age 35.
• If you will have surgery within 2 months, including dental surgery, requiring general or spinal anesthesia.

Over age 60:
Adverse reactions and side effects may be more frequent and severe than in younger persons.

Pregnancy:
Decide with your doctor if drug benefits justify risk to unborn child. Risk category C (see page xxiii).

Breast-feeding:
Avoid nursing or discontinue until you finish drug. Consult doctor.

Infants & children:
Only under close medical supervision.

Prolonged use:
Recommended periodically during prolonged use—Blood counts, G6PD* tests, liver function studies.

Skin & sunlight:
No special problems expected.

Driving, piloting or hazardous work:
Don't drive or pilot aircraft until you learn how medicine affects you. Don't work around dangerous machinery. Don't climb ladders or work in high places. Danger increases if you drink alcohol or take medicine affecting alertness and reflexes, such as antihistamines, tranquilizers, sedatives, pain medicine, narcotics and mind-altering drugs.

Discontinuing:
Don't discontinue without consulting doctor. Dose may require gradual reduction if you have taken drug for a long time. Doses of other drugs may also require adjustment.

Others:
• No problems expected.
• Advise any doctor or dentist whom you consult that you take this medicine.

POSSIBLE INTERACTION WITH OTHER DRUGS

GENERIC NAME OR DRUG CLASS	COMBINED EFFECT
Central nervous system (CNS) depressants *	Increased sedation, low blood pressure. Avoid.
Dronabinol	Increased effect of dronabinol on central nervous system. Avoid.

POSSIBLE INTERACTION WITH OTHER SUBSTANCES

INTERACTS WITH	COMBINED EFFECT
Alcohol:	Increased sedation, low blood pressure. Avoid.
Beverages:	No problems expected.
Cocaine:	Increased spasticity. Avoid.
Foods:	No problems expected.
Marijuana:	Increased spasticity. Avoid.
Tobacco:	May interfere with absorption of medicine.

DAPSONE

BRAND NAMES

Avlosulfon   DDS

BASIC INFORMATION

Habit forming? No
Prescription needed? Yes
Available as generic? Yes
Drug class: Antibacterial (antileprosy),
  sulfone

USES

- Treatment of dermatitis herpetiformis.
- Treatment of leprosy.
- Prevention and treatment of pneumocystis carnii pneumonia.
- Other uses include granuloma annulare, pemphigoid, pyoderma gangrenosum, polychondritis, eye ulcerations, systemic lupus erythematosus.

DOSAGE & USAGE INFORMATION

How to take:
Tablet—Swallow with liquid or food to lessen stomach irritation.

When to take:
Once a day at same time.

If you forget a dose:
Take as soon as you remember up to 2 hours late. If more than 2 hours, wait for next scheduled dose (don't double this dose).

Continued next column

OVERDOSE

SYMPTOMS:
Bleeding, vomiting, seizures, cyanosis, coma.
WHAT TO DO:
- Dial 911 (emergency) or 0 (operator) for an ambulance or medical help. Then give first aid immediately.
- If patient is unconscious and not breathing, give mouth-to-mouth breathing. If there is no heartbeat, use cardiac massage and mouth-to-mouth breathing (CPR). Don't try to make patient vomit. If you can't get help quickly, take patient to nearest emergency facility.
- See emergency information on inside covers.

What drug does:
Inhibits enzymes. Kills leprosy germs.

Time lapse before drug works:
- 3 years for leprosy.
- 1 to 2 weeks for dermatitis herpetiformis.

Don't take with:
Any other medicine without consulting your doctor or pharmacist.

POSSIBLE ADVERSE REACTIONS OR SIDE EFFECTS

SYMPTOMS	WHAT TO DO
Life-threatening: In case of overdose, see previous column.	
Common:	
• Rash, abdominal pain.	Discontinue. Call doctor right away.
• Appetite loss.	Continue. Call doctor when convenient.
Infrequent: Pale.	Discontinue. Call doctor right away.
Rare:	
• Dizziness; mental changes; sore throat; fever; difficult breathing; bleeding; jaundice; numbness, tingling, pain or burning in hands or feet; swelling of feet, hands, eyelids; blurred vision; anemia; peeling skin.	Discontinue. Call doctor right away.
• Headache; itching; nausea; vomiting; blue fingernails, lips.	Continue. Call doctor when convenient.

WARNINGS & PRECAUTIONS

Don't take if:
- You have G6PD* deficiency.
- You are allergic to furosemide, thiazide diuretics, sulfonureas, carbonic anhydrase inhibitors, sulfonamides.

Before you start, consult your doctor:
- If you take any other medicine.
- If you are anemic.
- If you have liver or kidney disease.
- If you are Negro or Caucasian with Mediterranean heritage.
- If you will have surgery within 2 months, including dental surgery, requiring general or spinal anesthesia.

Over age 60:
Adverse reactions and side effects may be more frequent and severe than in younger persons.

Pregnancy:
Decide with your doctor if drug benefits justify risk to unborn child. Risk category C (see page xxiii).

Breast-feeding:
Consult doctor. Avoid drug or discontinue nursing.

Infants & children:
Under close medical supervision only.

Prolonged use:
- Request liver function studies.
- Talk to your doctor about the need for follow-up medical examinations or laboratory studies to check complete blood counts (white blood cell count, platelet count, red blood cell count, hemoglobin, hematocrit).

Skin & sunlight:
May cause rash or intensify sunburn in areas exposed to sun or ultraviolet light (photosensitivity reaction). Avoid overexposure. Notify doctor if reaction occurs.

Driving, piloting or hazardous work:
Don't drive or pilot aircraft until you learn how medicine affects you. Don't work around dangerous machinery. Don't climb ladders or work in high places. Danger increases if you drink alcohol or take medicine affecting alertness and reflexes, such as antihistamines, tranquilizers, sedatives, pain medicine, narcotics and mind-altering drugs.

Discontinuing:
Don't discontinue without consulting doctor. Dose may require gradual reduction if you have taken drug for a long time. Doses of other drugs may also require adjustment.

Others:
- Dapsone may rarely cause liver damage.
- For full effect you may need to take dapsone for many months or years.

 POSSIBLE INTERACTION WITH OTHER DRUGS

GENERIC NAME OR DRUG CLASS	COMBINED EFFECT
Aminobenzoic acid (PABA)	Decreased dapsone effect. Avoid.
Antivirals, HIV/AIDS*	Increased risk of peripheral neuropathy. Reduced absorption of both drugs.
Dideoxyinosine (ddI)	Decreased dapsone effect.
Hemolytics*	May increase adverse effects on blood cells.
Methotrexate	May increase blood toxicity.
Probenecid	Increased toxicity of dapsone.
Pyrimethamine	May increase blood toxicity.
Rifampin	Decreased effect of dapsone.
Trimethoprim	May increase blood toxicity.

 POSSIBLE INTERACTION WITH OTHER SUBSTANCES

INTERACTS WITH	COMBINED EFFECT
Alcohol:	Increased chance of toxicity to liver.
Beverages:	No problems expected.
Cocaine:	Increased chance of toxicity. Avoid.
Foods:	No problems expected.
Marijuana:	Increased chance of toxicity. Avoid.
Tobacco:	May interfere with absorption of medicine.

*See Glossary

DECONGESTANTS (Ophthalmic)

GENERIC AND BRAND NAMES

ANTAZOLINE
  Vasocon-A
NAPHAZOLINE
  Ak-Con
  Albalon
  Albalon Liquifilm
  Allerest
  Allergy Drops
  Clear Eyes
  Comfort Eye Drops
  Degest 2
  Estivin II
  I-Naphline
  Murine Plus
  Muro's Opcon
  Nafazair
  Naphcon
  Naphcon A
  Naphcon Forte
  Ocu-Zoline
  Vasoclear
  Vasoclear A
  Vasocon
  Vasocon Regular

OXYMETAZOLINE
  OcuClear
  Visine L.R.
TETRAHYDROZILINE
  Visine

BASIC INFORMATION

Habit forming? No
Prescription needed? Yes, for some
Available as generic? Yes
Drug class: Decongestant (ophthalmic)

 ## USES

Treats eye redness, itching, burning or other irritation due to dust, colds, allergies, rubbing eyes, wearing contact lenses, swimming or eye strain from close work, watching TV, reading.

 ## OVERDOSE

SYMPTOMS:
None expected.
WHAT TO DO:
Not intended for internal use. If child accidentally swallows, call poison control center.

 ## DOSAGE & USAGE INFORMATION

How to use:
Eye drops
- Wash hands.
- Apply pressure to inside corner of eye with middle finger.
- Tilt head backward. Pull lower lid away from eye with index finger of the same hand.
- Drop eye drops into pouch and close eye. Don't blink.
- Keep eyes closed for 1 to 2 minutes.
- Continue pressure for 1 minute after placing medicine in eye.
- Don't touch applicator tip to any surface (including the eye). If you accidentally touch tip, clean with warm soap and water.
- Keep container tightly closed.
- Keep cool, but don't freeze.
- Wash hands immediately after using.

When to use:
As directed. Usually every 3 or 4 hours.

If you forget a dose:
Use as soon as you remember.

What drug does:
Acts on small blood vessels to make them constrict or become smaller.

Time lapse before drug works:
2 to 10 minutes.

Don't use with:
Other eye drops without consulting your doctor.

 ## POSSIBLE ADVERSE REACTIONS OR SIDE EFFECTS

SYMPTOMS	WHAT TO DO
Life-threatening: None expected.	
Common: Increased eye irritation.	Discontinue. Call doctor right away.
Infrequent: None expected.	
Rare: Blurred vision, large pupils, weakness, drowsiness, decreased body temperature, slow heartbeat, dizziness, headache, nervousness, nausea.	Discontinue. Call doctor right away.

DECONGESTANTS (Ophthalmic)

WARNINGS & PRECAUTIONS

Don't use if:
You are allergic to any decongestant eye drops.

Before you start, consult your doctor:
- If you take antidepressants or maprolitine.
- If you have glaucoma, eye disease, infection or injury.
- If you have heart disease, high blood pressure, thyroid disease.

Over age 60:
No problems expected.

Pregnancy:
Decide with your doctor if drug benefits justify risk to unborn child. Risk category C (see page xxiii).

Breast-feeding:
No problems expected, but check with doctor.

Infants & children:
Don't use.

Prolonged use:
Don't use for more than 3 or 4 days.

Skin & sunlight:
No problems expected.

Driving, piloting or hazardous work:
No problems expected.

Discontinuing:
May not need all the medicine in container. If symptoms disappear, stop using.

Others:
- Keep cool, but don't freeze.
- Check with your doctor if eye irritation continues or becomes worse.

POSSIBLE INTERACTION WITH OTHER DRUGS

GENERIC NAME OR DRUG CLASS	COMBINED EFFECT
Clinically significant interactions with oral or injected medicines unlikely.	

POSSIBLE INTERACTION WITH OTHER SUBSTANCES

INTERACTS WITH	COMBINED EFFECT
Alcohol:	None expected.
Beverages:	None expected.
Cocaine:	None expected.
Foods:	None expected.
Marijuana:	None expected.
Tobacco:	Smoke may increase eye irritation. Avoid.

DEHYDROEPIANDROSTERONE (DHEA)

BRAND NAMES

Numerous brand names are available

BASIC INFORMATION

Habit forming? No
Prescription needed? No
Available as generic? Yes
Drug class: Adrenal steroid

 ## USES

DHEA is a steroid produced in the human body by the adrenal glands (which sit on top of each kidney). DHEA concentration peaks at about age 20 and then decreases progressively with age. Supplements are sold as an anti-aging remedy claimed by some, to improve energy, strength, and immunity. DHEA is also said to increase muscle and decrease fat. Studies to date do not provide a clear picture of the risks and benefits of DHEA.

 ## DOSAGE & USAGE INFORMATION

How to take:
For tablet or capsule—Follow instructions on the label or consult your doctor or pharmacist. Different brands supply different doses. DHEA, as a product, is marketed as a dietary supplement and is not reviewed by the U.S. Food & Drug Administration (FDA) for effectiveness and safety. The best dosage amounts are unknown. Use with caution.

When to take:
At the same times each day according to label directions.

If you forget a dose:
Follow label instructions for your particular brand of DHEA. Usually you can take a medication as soon as you remember up to 2 hours late. If more than 2 hours, wait for the next scheduled dose (don't double this dose).

Continued next column

 ## OVERDOSE

SYMPTOMS:
It is unknown what symptoms may occur.
WHAT TO DO:
If person takes much larger amount than prescribed, call doctor, poison control center or hospital emergency room for instructions.

What drug does:
- Although it is not known whether DHEA itself causes hormonal effects, the body breaks DHEA down into two hormones—estrogen and testosterone. Some people's bodies make large amounts of estrogen and testosterone from DHEA, while others make smaller amounts.
- Hormone supplements may not have the same effects on the body as naturally produced hormones have, because the body processes them differently. Higher doses of supplements may result in higher amounts of hormones in the blood than are healthy.

Time lapse before drug works:
Effectiveness will vary from person to person and will also depend on the reason for taking DHEA, such as for a chronic health problem.

Don't take with:
Any prescription or nonprescription medicine without consulting your doctor or pharmacist.

 ## POSSIBLE ADVERSE REACTIONS OR SIDE EFFECTS

SYMPTOMS	WHAT TO DO
Life-threatening: None expected.	
Common: Unknown.	
Infrequent: In women: acne, hair loss, facial hair growth (hirsutism), deepening of voice (the last two may be irreversible).	Discontinue. Call doctor when convenient.
Rare: Unknown. If symptoms occur that you are concerned about, talk to your doctor or pharmacist. Further research may uncover other side effects.	

WARNINGS & PRECAUTIONS

Don't use if:
You are allergic to DHEA.

Before you start, consult your doctor:
- If you have any chronic health problem.
- If you have a family history of cancer.
- If you are allergic to any medication, food or other substance.
- If you have or have had prostate, ovarian, breast, cervical or uterine cancer.

Over age 60:
A lower starting dosage may be recommended until a response is determined.

Pregnancy:
Decide with your doctor if any possible benefits of DHEA justify risk to unborn child. Risk category is unknown since DHEA is not regulated by the FDA (see page xxiii).

Breast-feeding:
It is unknown if DHEA passes into milk. Avoid it or discontinue nursing until you finish medicine. Consult doctor for advice on maintaining milk supply.

Infants & children:
Not recommended for children.

Prolonged use:
Effects are unknown. More research is needed to determine long-term effects of DHEA use.

Skin & sunlight:
No problems expected.

Driving, piloting or hazardous work:
No problems expected.

Discontinuing:
No problems expected, but effects after long-term use are unknown.

Others:
- Advise any doctor or dentist whom you consult that you take DHEA.
- DHEA is not researched carefully as yet for use in humans. Most research has been performed on animals. Studies are ongoing to find more definite answers about its effect on aging, muscles, and the immune system. Studies in men and women have shown an improvement in the feeling of well being. Studies in AIDS patients and those with multiple sclerosis also have shown improvement in well being, but without an outcome change.

- Researchers are concerned that DHEA supplements may cause high levels of estrogen or testosterone in some people. The body's own testosterone plays a role in prostate cancer and high levels of naturally produced estrogen are suspected of increasing breast cancer risk. The effect of DHEA is unknown.

POSSIBLE INTERACTION WITH OTHER DRUGS

GENERIC NAME OR DRUG CLASS	COMBINED EFFECT
All medications	Effects are unknown. Talk to your doctor or pharmacist.

POSSIBLE INTERACTION WITH OTHER SUBSTANCES

INTERACTS WITH	COMBINED EFFECT
Alcohol:	Unknown.
Beverages:	No special problems expected.
Cocaine:	Problems not known. Best to avoid.
Foods:	No special problems expected.
Marijuana:	Problems not known. Best to avoid.
Tobacco:	Unknown.

DESMOPRESSIN

BRAND NAMES

DDAVP   Stimate

BASIC INFORMATION

Habit forming? No
Prescription needed? Yes
Available as generic? No
Drug class: Antidiuretic, antihemorrhagic

 ## USES

- Prevents and controls symptoms associated with central diabetes insipidus.
- Treats primary nocturnal enuresis (bedwetting during sleep).

 ## DOSAGE & USAGE INFORMATION

How to take:
- Nasal spray—Fill the rhinyle (a flexible, calibrated catheter) with a measured dose of the nasal spray. Blow on the other end of the catheter to deposit the solution deep in the nasal cavity. For infants and children, an air-filled syringe may be used.
- Tablet—Swallow with liquid.

When to take:
At the same time each day, according to instructions on prescription label.

If you forget a dose:
Take as soon as you remember up to 2 hours late. If more than 2 hours, wait for next scheduled dose. Don't double this dose.

What drug does:
Increases water reabsorption in the kidney and decreases urine output.

Time lapse before drug works:
Within 1 hour. Effect may last from 6 to 24 hours.

Don't take with:
Any other medicine without consulting your doctor or pharmacist.

 ## OVERDOSE

SYMPTOMS:
Confusion, coma, seizures.
WHAT TO DO:
Overdose unlikely to threaten life. If person takes much larger amount than prescribed, call doctor, poison control center or hospital emergency room for instructions.

 ## POSSIBLE ADVERSE REACTIONS OR SIDE EFFECTS

SYMPTOMS	WHAT TO DO
Life-threatening: None expected.	
Common: None expected.	
Infrequent: Flushing or redness of skin, headache, nausea, nasal congestion.	Continue. Call doctor when convenient.
Rare: Water intoxication—confusion, drowsiness, headache, seizures, rapid weight gain, decreased urination (very rare).	Discontinue. Seek emergency treatment.

WARNINGS & PRECAUTIONS

Don't take if:
You know that you are sensitive to desmopressin.

Before you start, consult your doctor:
- If you have allergic rhinitis.
- If you have nasal congestion.
- If you have a cold or other upper respiratory infection or are dehydrated.
- If you have heart disease or high blood pressure.
- If you have had cystic fibrosis.

Over age 60:
Increased risk of water intoxication.

Pregnancy:
No proven harm to unborn child, but avoid if possible. Consult doctor. Risk category B (see page xxiii).

Breast-feeding:
Drug passes into milk. Avoid drug or discontinue nursing until you finish medicine. Consult doctor for advice on maintaining milk supply.

Infants & children:
More sensitive to effect. Use only under close medical supervision.

Prolonged use:
May require increasing dosage for same effect.

Skin & sunlight:
No special problems expected.

Driving, piloting or hazardous work:
Don't drive or pilot aircraft until you learn how medicine affects you. Don't work around dangerous machinery. Don't climb ladders or work in high places. Danger increases if you drink alcohol or take medicine affecting alertness and reflexes.

Discontinuing:
No special problems expected.

Others:
- Advise any doctor or dentist whom you consult that you take this medicine.
- Fluid intake may need to be adjusted.

POSSIBLE INTERACTION WITH OTHER DRUGS

GENERIC NAME OR DRUG CLASS	COMBINED EFFECT
Carbamazepine	May increase desmopressin effect.
Chlorpropamide	May increase desmopressin effect.
Clofibrate	May increase desmopressin effect.
Demeclocycline	May decrease desmopressin effect.
Lithium	May decrease desmopressin effect.
Norepinephrine	May decrease desmopressin effect.

POSSIBLE INTERACTION WITH OTHER SUBSTANCES

INTERACTS WITH	COMBINED EFFECT
Alcohol:	May decrease desmopressin effect.
Beverages: Caffeine drinks.	May decrease desmopressin effect.
Cocaine:	May decrease desmopressin effect.
Foods:	None expected.
Marijuana:	May decrease desmopressin effect.
Tobacco:	May decrease desmopressin effect.

DEXTROMETHORPHAN

BRAND NAMES

See complete list of brand names in the *Generic and Brand Name Directory*, page 878.

BASIC INFORMATION

Habit forming? No
Prescription needed? No
Available as generic? Yes
Drug class: Cough suppressant, antitussive

 ## USES

Suppresses cough associated with allergies or infections such as colds, bronchitis, flu and lung disorders. Used in many cough, cold and allergy combination medicines.

 ## DOSAGE & USAGE INFORMATION

How to take:
- Chewable tablet—Chew well before swallowing.
- Oral suspension, lozenges or syrups—Take as directed on label.
- Capsules—Swallow with liquid.

When to take:
As needed, no more often than every 4 hours.

If you forget a dose:
Take as soon as you remember. Wait 4 hours for next dose.

What drug does:
Reduces sensitivity of brain's cough control center, suppressing urge to cough.

Time lapse before drug works:
15 to 30 minutes.

Don't take with:
Any other medicine without consulting your doctor or pharmacist.

 ## OVERDOSE

SYMPTOMS:
Euphoria, overactivity, sense of intoxication, visual and auditory hallucinations, lack of coordination, stagger, stupor, shallow breathing.
WHAT TO DO:
- **Dial 911 (emergency) or 0 (operator) for an ambulance or medical help. Then give first aid immediately.**
- **See emergency information on inside covers.**

 ## POSSIBLE ADVERSE REACTIONS OR SIDE EFFECTS

SYMPTOMS	WHAT TO DO
Life-threatening: None expected.	
Common: None expected.	
Infrequent: Mild dizziness or drowsiness, nausea, stomach cramps.	Continue. Call doctor when convenient.
Rare: None expected.	

WARNINGS & PRECAUTIONS

Don't take if:
You are allergic to any cough syrup containing dextromethorphan.

Before you start, consult your doctor:
• If you have asthma attacks.
• If you have impaired liver function.

Over age 60:
Adverse reactions and side effects may be more frequent and severe than in younger persons. You may require smaller doses for shorter periods of time.

Pregnancy:
Dooide with your doctor if drug benefits justify risk to unborn child. Risk category C (see page xxiii).

Breast-feeding:
No proven problems. Consult doctor.

Infants & children:
Use only as label directs.

Prolonged use:
No problems expected.

Skin & sunlight:
No problems expected.

Driving, piloting or hazardous work:
Don't drive or pilot aircraft until you learn how medicine affects you. Don't work around dangerous machinery. Don't climb ladders or work in high places. Danger increases if you drink alcohol or take medicine affecting alertness and reflexes, such as antihistamines, tranquilizers, sedatives, pain medicine, narcotics and mind-altering drugs.

Discontinuing:
May be unnecessary to finish medicine. Follow doctor's instructions.

Others:
• If cough persists or if you cough blood or brown-yellow, thick mucus, call your doctor.
• Excessive use may lead to functional dependence.

POSSIBLE INTERACTION WITH OTHER DRUGS

GENERIC NAME OR DRUG CLASS	COMBINED EFFECT
Doxepin (topical)	Increased risk of toxicity of both drugs.
Monozmine oxidase (MAO) inhibitors*	Disorientation, high fever, drop in blood pressure and loss of consciousness.
Sedatives* and other central nervous system (CNS) depressants*	Increased sedative effect of both drugs.

POSSIBLE INTERACTION WITH OTHER SUBSTANCES

INTERACTS WITH	COMBINED EFFECT
Alcohol:	None expected.
Beverages:	None expected.
Cocaine:	Decreased dextromethorphan effect. Avoid.
Foods:	None expected.
Marijuana:	None expected.
Tobacco:	None expected.

DEXTROTHYROXINE

BRAND NAMES

Choloxin

BASIC INFORMATION

Habit forming? No
Prescription needed? Yes
Available as generic? No
Drug class: Antihyperlipidemic, thyroid hormone

USES

- Lowers blood cholesterol and low-density lipoproteins in patients who don't respond to low-fat diet and weight loss alone.
- Treats hypothyroidism in patients with heart disease.

DOSAGE & USAGE INFORMATION

How to take:
Tablets—Swallow with liquid. If you can't swallow whole, crumble tablet and take with liquid or food. Instructions to take on empty stomach mean 1 hour before or 2 hours after eating.

When to take:
According to your doctor's instructions.

If you forget a dose:
Take as soon as you remember up to 2 hours late. If more than 2 hours, wait for next scheduled dose (don't double this dose).

What drug does:
Increases breakdown of LDL (low-density lipoprotein).

Time lapse before drug works:
1 to 2 months.

Don't take with:
Any other medicines (including over-the-counter drugs such as cough and cold medicines, laxatives, antacids, diet pills, caffeine, nose drops or vitamins) without consulting your doctor.

OVERDOSE

SYMPTOMS:
None expected.
WHAT TO DO:
Overdose unlikely to threaten life. If person takes much larger amount than prescribed, call doctor, poison control center or hospital emergency room for instructions.

POSSIBLE ADVERSE REACTIONS OR SIDE EFFECTS

SYMPTOMS	WHAT TO DO
Life-threatening: None expected.	
Common: • Tremor, headache, irritability, insomnia.	Discontinue. Call doctor right away.
• Appetite change, diarrhea, leg cramps, menstrual irregularities, fever, heat sensitivity, unusual sweating, weight loss.	Continue. Call doctor when convenient.
Infrequent: Hives, rash, vomiting, chest pain, rapid and irregular heartbeat, shortness of breath.	Discontinue. Call doctor right away.
Rare: None expected.	

WARNINGS & PRECAUTIONS

Don't take if:
- You have had a heart attack within 6 weeks.
- You have no thyroid deficiency, but want to use this to lose weight.

Before you start, consult your doctor:
- If you have heart disease or high blood pressure.
- If you have diabetes.
- If you have Addison's disease, have had adrenal gland deficiency or use epinephrine, ephedrine or isoproterenol for asthma.

Over age 60:
More sensitive to thyroid hormone. May need smaller doses.

Pregnancy:
Consult doctor. Risk category B (see page xxiii).

Breast-feeding:
Present in milk. Considered safe if dose is correct.

Infants & children:
Use only under medical supervision.

Prolonged use:
- No problems expected, if dose is correct.
- Talk to your doctor about the need for follow-up medical examinations or laboratory studies to check serum cholesterol and triglycerides.

Skin & sunlight:
No problems expected.

Driving, piloting or hazardous work:
No problems expected.

Discontinuing:
Don't discontinue without consulting doctor.
Dose may require gradual reduction if you have
taken drug for a long time. Doses of other drugs
may also require adjustment.

Others:
- Digestive upsets, tremors, cramps,
  nervousness, insomnia or diarrhea may
  indicate need for dose adjustment.
- Advise any doctor or dentist whom you consult
  that you take this medicine.
- May affect results in some medical tests.
- Stay on a low-fat diet.

POSSIBLE INTERACTION WITH OTHER DRUGS

GENERIC NAME OR DRUG CLASS	COMBINED EFFECT
Adrenocorticoids, systemic	Requires dose adjustment to prevent adreno-corticoid deficiency.
Amphetamines*	Increased amphetamine effect.
Anticoagulants, oral*	Increased anticoagulant effect.
Antidepressants, tricyclic*	Increased anti-depressant effect. Irregular heartbeat.
Antidiabetics*	Antidiabetic may require adjustment.
Aspirin (large doses, continuous use)	Increased dextrothyroxine effect.
Barbiturates*	Decreased barbiturate effect.
Beta-adrenergic blocking agents*	Possible decreased beta blocker effect.
Cholestyramine	Decreased dextrothyroxine effect.
Colestipol	Decreased dextrothyroxine effect.

Contraceptives, oral*	Decreased dextrothyroxine effect.
Dexfenfluramine	May require dosage change as weight loss occurs.
Digitalis preparations*	Decreased digitalis effect.
Ephedrine	Increased ephedrine effect.
Epinephrine	Increased epinephrine effect.
Estrogens*	Decreased dextrothyroxine effect.
Methylphenidate	Increased methylphenidate effect.
Phenytoin	Possible decreased dextrothyroxine effect.

POSSIBLE INTERACTION WITH OTHER SUBSTANCES

INTERACTS WITH	COMBINED EFFECT
Alcohol:	None expected.
Beverages:	None expected.
Cocaine:	Excess stimulation. Avoid.
Foods: Soybeans.	Heavy consumption interferes with thyroid function.
Marijuana:	None expected.
Tobacco:	None expected.

DICYCLOMINE

BRAND NAMES

See complete list of brand names in the *Generic and Brand Name Directory*, page 880.

BASIC INFORMATION

Habit forming? No
Prescription needed? Yes
Available as generic? Yes
Drug class: Antispasmodic, anticholinergic

USES

- Reduces spasms of digestive system, bladder and urethra.
- Treats irritable bowel syndrome.

DOSAGE & USAGE INFORMATION

How to take:
Tablet, syrup or capsule—Swallow with liquid or food to lessen stomach irritation.

When to take:
30 minutes before meals (unless directed otherwise by doctor).

If you forget a dose:
Take as soon as you remember up to 2 hours late. If more than 2 hours, wait for next scheduled dose (don't double this dose).

What drug does:
Blocks nerve impulses at parasympathetic nerve endings, preventing muscle contractions and gland secretions of organs involved.

Time lapse before drug works:
15 to 30 minutes.

Don't take with:
Any other medicine without consulting your doctor or pharmacist.

OVERDOSE

SYMPTOMS:
Dilated pupils, blurred vision, rapid pulse and breathing, dizziness, fever, hallucinations, confusion, slurred speech, agitation, flushed face, convulsions, coma.
WHAT TO DO:
- **Dial 911 (emergency) or 0 (operator) for an ambulance or medical help. Then give first aid immediately.**
- **See emergency information on inside covers.**

POSSIBLE ADVERSE REACTIONS OR SIDE EFFECTS

SYMPTOMS	WHAT TO DO
Life-threatening:	
Hives, rash, intense itching, faintness soon after a dose (anaphylaxis).	Seek emergency treatment immediately.
Common:	
• Confusion, delirium, rapid heartbeat.	Discontinue. Call doctor right away.
• Nausea, vomiting.	Discontinue. Call doctor when convenient.
• Constipation, loss of taste, decreased sweating.	Continue. Tell doctor at next visit.
• Dry ears, nose, throat, mouth.	No action necessary.
Infrequent:	
• Headache, difficult urination, nasal congestion, altered taste.	Continue. Call doctor when convenient.
• Lightheadedness.	Discontinue. Call doctor right away.
Rare:	
Rash or hives, eye pain, blurred vision.	Discontinue. Call doctor right away.

WARNINGS & PRECAUTIONS

Don't take if:
- You are allergic to any anticholinergic.
- You have trouble with stomach bloating.
- You have difficulty emptying your bladder completely.
- You have narrow-angle glaucoma.
- You have severe ulcerative colitis.

Before you start, consult your doctor:
- If you have open-angle glaucoma.
- If you have angina, chronic bronchitis or asthma.
- If you have hiatal hernia, liver disease, kidney or thyroid disease, enlarged prostate, myasthenia gravis, peptic ulcer.
- If you will have surgery within 2 months, including dental surgery, requiring general or spinal anesthesia.

Over age 60:
Adverse reactions and side effects may be more frequent and severe than in younger persons.

Pregnancy:
Decide with your doctor whether drug benefits justify risk to unborn child. Risk category C (see page xxiii).

Breast-feeding:
Drug passes into milk and decreases milk flow. Avoid drug or discontinue nursing until you finish medicine. Consult doctor for advice on maintaining milk supply.

Infants & children:
Use only under medical supervision.

Prolonged use:
Chronic constipation, possible fecal impaction. Consult doctor immediately.

Skin & sunlight:
No problems expected.

Driving, piloting or hazardous work:
Use disqualifies you for piloting aircraft. Otherwise, no problems expected.

Discontinuing:
May be unnecessary to finish medicine. Follow doctor's instructions.

Others:
Advise any doctor or dentist whom you consult that you take this medicine.

POSSIBLE INTERACTION WITH OTHER DRUGS

GENERIC NAME OR DRUG CLASS	COMBINED EFFECT
Adrenocorticoids, systemic	Possible glaucoma.
Amantadine	Increased dicyclomine effect.
Antacids*	Decreased dicyclomine effect.
Anticholinergics, other*	Increased dicyclomine effect.
Antidepressants, tricyclic*	Increased dicyclomine effect. Increased sedation.
Antidiarrheals*	Decreased dicyclomine effect.
Antihistamines*	Increased dicyclomine effect.
Attapulgite	Decreased dicyclomine effect.
Buclizine	Increased dicyclomine effect.
Digitalis	Possible decreased absorption of digitalis.
Haloperidol	Increased internal eye pressure.
Ketoconazole	Decreased ketoconazole effect.
Meperidine	Increased dicyclomine effect.
Methylphenidate	Increased dicyclomine effect.
Monoamine oxidase (MAO) inhibitors*	Increased dicyclomine effect.
Nitrates*	Increased internal eye pressure.
Nizatidine	Increased nizatidine effect.
Orphenadrine	Increased dicyclomine effect.
Phenothiazines*	Increased dicyclomine effect.
Pilocarpine	Loss of pilocarpine effect in glaucoma treatment.
Potassium supplements*	Possible intestinal ulcers with oral potassium tablets.
Quinidine	Increased dicyclomine effect.
Sedatives* or central nervous system (CNS) depressants*	Increased sedative effect of both drugs.
Vitamin C	Decreased dicyclomine effect. Avoid large doses of vitamin C.

POSSIBLE INTERACTION WITH OTHER SUBSTANCES

INTERACTS WITH	COMBINED EFFECT
Alcohol:	None expected.
Beverages:	None expected.
Cocaine:	Excessively rapid heartbeat. Avoid.
Foods:	None expected.
Marijuana:	Drowsiness and dry mouth.
Tobacco:	None expected.

DIFENOXIN & ATROPINE

BRAND NAMES

Motofen

BASIC INFORMATION

Habit forming? Yes
Prescription needed? Yes
Available as generic? No
Drug class: Antidiarrheal

 ## USES

- Reduces spasms of digestive system.
- Treats severe diarrhea.

 ## DOSAGE & USAGE INFORMATION

How to take:
Tablet—Swallow with liquid or food to lessen stomach irritation.

When to take:
After each loose stool or every 3 to 4 hours. No more than 5 tablets in 12 hours.

If you forget a dose:
Take as soon as you remember. Don't double this dose.

What drug does:
- Blocks nerve impulses at parasympathetic nerve endings, preventing muscle contractions and gland secretions of organs involved.
- Acts on brain to decrease spasm of smooth muscle.

Time lapse before drug works:
40 to 60 minutes.

Continued next column

 ## OVERDOSE

SYMPTOMS:
Dilated pupils, rapid pulse and breathing, dizziness, fever, hallucinations, confusion, slurred speech, agitation, flushed face, convulsions, coma.
WHAT TO DO:
- Dial 911 (emergency) or 0 (operator) for an ambulance or medical help. Then give first aid immediately.
- See emergency information on inside covers.

Don't take with:
Any medicine that will decrease mentalalertness or reflexes, such as alcohol, other mind-altering drugs, cough/cold medicines, antihistamines, allergy medicine, sedatives, tranquilizers (sleeping pills or "downers") barbiturates, seizure medicine, narcotics, other prescription medicines for pain, muscle relaxants, anesthetics.

 ## POSSIBLE ADVERSE REACTIONS OR SIDE EFFECTS

SYMPTOMS	WHAT TO DO
Life-threatening:	
Shortness of breath, agitation, nervousness.	Discontinue. Seek emergency treatment.
Common:	
Dizziness, drowsiness.	Continue. Call doctor when convenient.
Infrequent:	
• Bloating; constipation; appetite loss; abdominal pain; blurred vision; warm, flushed skin; fast heartbeat; dry mouth.	Discontinue. Call doctor right away.
• Frequent urination, lightheadedness, dry skin, headache, insomnia.	Continue. Call doctor when convenient.
Rare:	
Weakness, confusion, fever.	Continue. Call doctor when convenient.

 ## WARNINGS & PRECAUTIONS

Don't take if:
- You are allergic to any anticholinergic.
- You have trouble with stomach bloating, difficulty emptying your bladder completely, narrow-angle glaucoma, severe ulcerative colitis.
- You are dehydrated.

Before you start, consult your doctor:
- If you have open-angle glaucoma, angina, chronic bronchitis, asthma, liver disease, hiatal hernia, enlarged prostate, myasthenia gravis, peptic ulcer.
- If you will have surgery within 2 months, including dental surgery, requiring general or spinal anesthesia.

Over age 60:
Adverse reactions and side effects may be more frequent and severe than in younger persons.

Pregnancy:
Decide with your doctor whether drug benefits justify risk to unborn child. Risk category C (see page xxiii).

Breast-feeding:
Drug passes into milk. Avoid drug or discontinue nursing until you finish medicine. Consult doctor for advice on maintaining milk supply.

Infants & children:
Use only under medical supervision.

Prolonged use:
- Chronic constipation, possible fecal impaction. Consult doctor immediately.
- Talk to your doctor about the need for follow-up medical examinations or laboratory studies to check liver function.

Skin & sunlight:
No problems expected.

Driving, piloting or hazardous work:
Use disqualifies you for piloting aircraft. Don't drive until you learn how medicine affects you. Don't work around dangerous machinery. Don't climb ladders or work in high places. Danger increases if you drink alcohol or take medicine affecting alertness and reflexes, such as antihis-tamines, tranquilizers, sedatives, pain medicine, narcotics and mind-altering drugs.

Discontinuing:
May be unnecessary to finish medicine. Follow doctor's instructions.

Others:
Atropine included at doses below therapeutic level to prevent abuse.

POSSIBLE INTERACTION WITH OTHER DRUGS

GENERIC NAME OR DRUG CLASS	COMBINED EFFECT
Addictive substances (narcotics,* others)	Increased chance of abuse.
Amantadine	Increased atropine effect.
Anticholinergics, other*	Increased atropine effect.
Antidepressants, tricyclic (TCA)*	Increased atropine effect. Increased sedation.
Antihistamines*	Increased atropine effect.
Antihypertensives*	Increased sedation.
Clozapine	Toxic effect on the central nervous system.
Cortisone drugs*	Increased internal eye pressure.
Ethinamate	Dangerous increased effects of ethinamate. Avoid combining.
Fluoxetine	Increased depressant effects of both drugs.
Guanfacine	May increase depressant effects of either drug.
Haloperidol	Increased internal eye pressure.
Leucovorin	High alcohol content of leucovorin may cause adverse effects.
Meperidine	Increased atropine effect.
Methylphenidate	Increased atropine effect.
Methyprylon	Increased sedative effect, perhaps to dangerous level. Avoid.
Monozmine oxidase (MAO) inhibitors*	Increased atropine effect.
Nabilone	Greater depression of central nervous system.
Naltrexone	Triggers withdrawal symptoms.
Narcotics*	Increased sedation. Avoid.

Continued on page 912

POSSIBLE INTERACTION WITH OTHER SUBSTANCES

INTERACTS WITH	COMBINED EFFECT
Alcohol:	Increased sedation. Avoid.
Beverages:	None expected.
Cocaine:	Excessively rapid heartbeat. Avoid.
Foods:	None expected.
Marijuana:	Drowsiness and dry mouth.
Tobacco:	May increase diarrhea. Avoid.

*See Glossary

DIGITALIS PREPARATIONS
(Digitalis Glycosides)

GENERIC AND BRAND NAMES

DIGITOXIN
  Crystodigin

DIGOXIN
  Lanoxicaps
  Lanoxin
  Novodigoxin

BASIC INFORMATION

Habit forming? No
Prescription needed? Yes
Available as generic? Yes
Drug class: Digitalis preparation

 ## USES

- Strengthens weak heart muscle contractions to prevent congestive heart failure.
- Corrects irregular heartbeat.

 ## DOSAGE & USAGE INFORMATION

How to take:
- Tablet or capsule—Swallow with liquid. If you can't swallow whole, crumble tablet or open capsule and take with liquid or food.
- Liquid—Dilute dose in beverage before swallowing.

When to take:
At the same time each day.

If you forget a dose:
Take as soon as you remember up to 12 hours late. If more than 12 hours, wait for next scheduled dose (don't double this dose).

What drug does:
- Strengthens heart muscle contraction.
- Delays nerve impulses to heart.

Time lapse before drug works:
May require regular use for a week or more.

Continued next column

 ## OVERDOSE

SYMPTOMS:
Nausea, vomiting, diarrhea, vision disturbances, halos around lights, fatigue, irregular heartbeat, confusion, hallucinations, convulsions.
WHAT TO DO:
- Dial 911 (emergency) or 0 (operator) for an ambulance or medical help. Then give first aid immediately.
- See emergency information on inside covers.

Don't take with:
Nonprescription drugs without consulting doctor.

 ## POSSIBLE ADVERSE REACTIONS OR SIDE EFFECTS

SYMPTOMS	WHAT TO DO
Life-threatening: In case of overdose, see previous column.	
Common: Appetite loss, diarrhea.	Continue. Call doctor when convenient.
Infrequent: Extreme drowsiness, lethargy, disorientation, headache, fainting.	Discontinue. Call doctor right away.
Rare: • Rash, hives, cardiac arrhythmias, hallucinations, psychosis.	Discontinue. Call doctor right away.
• Double or yellow-green vision; enlarged, sensitive male breasts; tiredness; weakness; depression; decreased sex drive.	Continue. Call doctor when convenient.

 ## WARNINGS & PRECAUTIONS

Don't take if:
- You are allergic to any digitalis preparation.
- Your heartbeat is slower than 50 beats per minute.

Before you start, consult your doctor:
- If you have taken another digitalis preparation in past 2 weeks.
- If you have taken a diuretic within 2 weeks.
- If you have liver or kidney disease.
- If you have a thyroid disorder.
- If you will have surgery within 2 months, including dental surgery, requiring general or spinal anesthesia.

Over age 60:
Adverse reactions and side effects may be more frequent and severe than in younger persons.

Pregnancy:
Decide with you doctor if drug benefits justify risk to unborn child. Risk category C (see page xxiii).

Breast-feeding:
Drug filters into milk. May harm child. Avoid.

Infants & children:
Use only under medical supervision.

Prolonged use:
Talk to your doctor about the need for follow-up medical examinations or laboratory studies to check ECG*, liver function, kidney function, serum electrolytes.

Skin & sunlight:
No problems expected.

Driving, piloting or hazardous work:
Possible vision disturbances. Otherwise, no problems expected.

Discontinuing:
Don't stop without doctor's advice.

Others:
Some digitalis products contain tartrazine dye. Avoid, especially if you are allergic to aspirin.

POSSIBLE INTERACTION WITH OTHER DRUGS

GENERIC NAME OR DRUG CLASS	COMBINED EFFECT
Adrenocorticoids, systemic	Dangerous potassium depletion. Possible digitalis toxicity.
Amiodarone	Increased digitalis effect.
Amphotericin B	Decreased potassium. Increased toxicity of amphotericin B.
Antacids*	Decreased digitalis effect.
Anticonvulsants, hydantoin*	Increased digitalis effect at first, then decreased.
Anticholinergics*	Possible increased digitalis effect.
Attapulgite	May decrease effectiveness of digitalis.
Beta-adrenergic blocking agents*	Increased digitalis effect.
Beta-agonists*	Increased risk of heartbeat irregularity.
Calcium supplements*	Decreased digitalis effects.
Carteolol	Can either increase or decrease heart rate. Improves irregular heartbeat.
Cholestyramine	Decreased digitalis effect.
Colestipol	Decreased digitalis effect.

Dextrothyroxine	Decreased digitalis effect.
Disopyramide	Possible decreased digitalis effect.
Diuretics*	Possible digitalis toxicity. Excessive potassium loss that may cause irregular heartbeat.
Ephedrine	Disturbed heart rhythm. Avoid.
Epinephrine	Disturbed heart rhythm. Avoid.
Erythromycins*	May increase digitalis absorption.
Flecainide	May increase digitalis blood level.
Fluoxetine	May cause confusion, agitation, convulsions and high blood pressure. Avoid combining.
Hydroxychloroquine	Possible increased digitalis toxicity.
Itraconazole	Possible toxic levels of digitalis.
Laxatives*	Decreased digitalis effect.
Metformin	Increased metformin effect.

Continued on page 913

POSSIBLE INTERACTION WITH OTHER SUBSTANCES

INTERACTS WITH	COMBINED EFFECT
Alcohol:	None expected.
Beverages: Caffeine drinks.	Irregular heartbeat. Avoid.
Cocaine:	Irregular heartbeat. Avoid.
Foods: Prune juice, bran cereals, foods high in fiber.	Decreased digitalis effect.
Marijuana:	Decreased digitalis effect.
Tobacco:	Irregular heartbeat. Avoid.

*See Glossary

DIMETHYL SULFOXIDE (DMSO)

BRAND NAMES

Rimso-50

BASIC INFORMATION

Habit forming? No
Prescription needed? Yes
Available as generic? Yes
Drug class: Anti-inflammatory (local)

 ## USES

When applied directly to the bladder's membrane lining, DMSO relieves symptoms of bladder inflammation.

 ## DOSAGE & USAGE INFORMATION

How to use:
Under doctor's guidance, directly instill into urinary bladder using a catheter or aseptic syringe. Allow to remain in bladder about 15 minutes, then void. *Note:* Follow doctor's instructions.

When to use:
Follow doctor's instructions.

If you forget a dose:
Take as soon as you remember up to 2 hours late. If more than 2 hours, wait for next scheduled dose (don't double this dose).

What drug does:
Reduces inflammation by unknown mechanism.

Time lapse before drug works:
Works quickly (within minutes).

Don't take with:
Any other medicines (including over-the-counter drugs such as cough and cold medicines, laxatives, antacids, diet pills, caffeine, nose drops or vitamins) without consulting your doctor.

 ## OVERDOSE

SYMPTOMS:
None expected.
WHAT TO DO:
Overdose unlikely to threaten life. If person takes much larger amount than prescribed, call doctor, poison control center or hospital emergency room for instructions.

 ## POSSIBLE ADVERSE REACTIONS OR SIDE EFFECTS

SYMPTOMS	WHAT TO DO
Life-threatening: Breathing difficulty.	Seek emergency treatment immediately.
Common: Garlic-like taste for up to 72 hours.	No action necessary.
Infrequent: Vision problems (not documented in humans, but well documented in animals).	Continue. Call doctor when convenient.
Rare: Nasal congestion, itching, hives, facial swelling.	Discontinue. Seek emergency treatment.

DIMETHYL SULFOXIDE (DMSO)

WARNINGS & PRECAUTIONS

Don't use if:
- You have a bladder malignancy.
- You are allergic to DMSO.

Before you start, consult your doctor:
If you have visual problems.

Over age 60:
No special problems expected.

Pregnancy:
Decide with you doctor if drug benefits justify risk to unborn child. Risk category C (see page xxiii).

Breast-feeding:
Effect not documented. Consult your doctor.

Infants & children:
Not recommended.

Prolonged use:
Talk to your doctor about the need for follow-up medical examinations or laboratory studies to check liver and kidney function, complete blood counts (white blood cell count, platelet count, red blood cell count, hemoglobin, hematocrit) and vision.

Skin & sunlight:
No special problems expected.

Driving, piloting or hazardous work:
No special problems expected.

Discontinuing:
No special problems expected.

Others:
Although readily available in impure forms, DMSO has not proven effective or safe for sprains, strains, arthritis, scleroderma, gout, skin infections, burns or other uses. Many studies are underway for safety and efficacy for conditions other than bladder inflammation.

POSSIBLE INTERACTION WITH OTHER DRUGS

GENERIC NAME OR DRUG CLASS	COMBINED EFFECT
Any other drug used inside the bladder	Increased effect of both medicines.

POSSIBLE INTERACTION WITH OTHER SUBSTANCES

INTERACTS WITH	COMBINED EFFECT
Alcohol:	No special problems expected.
Beverages:	No special problems expected.
Cocaine:	No special problems expected.
Foods:	No special problems expected.
Marijuana:	No special problems expected.
Tobacco:	No special problems expected.

DIPHENIDOL

BRAND NAMES

Vontrol

BASIC INFORMATION

Habit forming? No
Prescription needed? Yes
Available as generic? No
Drug class: Antiemetic, antivertigo

 ## USES

- Prevents motion sickness.
- Controls nausea and vomiting (do not use during pregnancy).

 ## DOSAGE & USAGE INFORMATION

How to take:
Tablet—Swallow with liquid or food to lessen stomach irritation. If you can't swallow whole, crumble tablet and chew or take with liquid or food.

When to take:
30 to 60 minutes before traveling.

If you forget a dose:
Take as soon as you remember. Wait 4 hours for next dose.

What drug does:
Reduces sensitivity of nerve endings in inner ear, blocking messages to brain's vomiting center.

Time lapse before drug works:
30 to 60 minutes.

Don't take with:
Any other medicine without consulting your doctor or pharmacist.

 ## OVERDOSE

SYMPTOMS:
Drowsiness, confusion, incoordination, weak pulse, shallow breathing, stupor, coma.
WHAT TO DO:
- Dial 911 (emergency) or 0 (operator) for an ambulance or medical help. Then give first aid immediately.
- See emergency information on inside covers.

 ## POSSIBLE ADVERSE REACTIONS OR SIDE EFFECTS

SYMPTOMS	WHAT TO DO
Life-threatening:	
In case of overdose, see previous column.	
Common:	
Drowsiness.	Continue. Tell doctor at next visit.
Infrequent:	
• Headache, diarrhea or constipation, heartburn.	Continue. Call doctor when convenient.
• Dry mouth, nose or throat; dizziness.	Continue. Tell doctor at next visit.
Rare:	
• Hallucinations, confusion.	Discontinue. Seek emergency treatment.
• Rash or hives, depression, jaundice.	Discontinue. Call doctor right away.
• Restlessness; excitement; insomnia; blurred vision; urgent, painful or difficult urination.	Continue. Call doctor when convenient.
• Appetite loss, nausea, weakness.	Continue. Tell doctor at next visit.

WARNINGS & PRECAUTIONS

Don't take if:
- You have severe kidney disease.
- You are allergic to diphenidol or meclizine.

Before you start, consult your doctor:
- If you have prostate enlargement.
- If you have glaucoma.
- If you have heart disease.
- If you have intestinal obstruction or ulcers in the gastrointestinal tract.
- If you have kidney disease.
- If you have low blood pressure.
- If you will have surgery within 2 months, including dental surgery, requiring general or spinal anesthesia.

Over age 60:
Adverse reactions and side effects may be more frequent and severe than in younger persons.

Pregnancy:
Decide with your doctor whether drug benefits justify risk to unborn child. Risk category C (see page xxiii).

Breast-feeding:
Drug passes into milk. Avoid drug or discontinue nursing until you finish medicine. Consult doctor for advice on maintaining milk supply.

Infants & children:
No problems expected.

Prolonged use:
No problems expected.

Skin & sunlight:
No problems expected.

Driving, piloting or hazardous work:
Don't fly aircraft. Don't drive until you learn how medicine affects you. Don't work around dangerous machinery. Don't climb ladders or work in high places. Danger increases if you drink alcohol or take medicine affecting alertness and reflexes, such as antihistamines, tranquilizers, sedatives, pain medicine, narcotics and mind-altering drugs.

Discontinuing:
No problems expected.

Others:
No problems expected.

POSSIBLE INTERACTION WITH OTHER DRUGS

GENERIC NAME OR DRUG CLASS	COMBINED EFFECT
Anticonvulsants*	Increased effect of both drugs.
Antidepressants, tricyclic*	Increased sedative effect of both drugs.
Antihistamines*	Increased sedative effect of both drugs.
Atropine	Increased chance of toxic effect of atropine and atropine-like medicines.
Narcotics*	Increased sedative effect of both drugs.
Sedatives*	Increased sedative effect of both drugs.
Tranquilizers*	Increased sedative effect of both drugs.

POSSIBLE INTERACTION WITH OTHER SUBSTANCES

INTERACTS WITH	COMBINED EFFECT
Alcohol:	Increased sedation. Avoid.
Beverages: Caffeine.	May decrease drowsiness.
Cocaine:	Increased chance of toxic effects of cocaine. Avoid.
Foods:	None expected.
Marijuana:	Increased drowsiness, dry mouth.
Tobacco:	None expected.

DIPHENOXYLATE & ATROPINE

BRAND NAMES

Diphenatol	Lomotil
Lofene	Lonox
Logen	Lo-Trol
Lomanate	Nor-Mil

BASIC INFORMATION

Habit forming? Yes
Prescription needed? Yes
Available as generic? Yes
Drug class: Antidiarrheal

USES

Relieves diarrhea and intestinal cramps.

DOSAGE & USAGE INFORMATION

How to take:
- Tablet—Swallow with liquid or food to lessen stomach irritation.
- Drops or liquid—Follow label instructions and use marked dropper.

When to take:
No more often than directed on label.

If you forget a dose:
Take as soon as you remember up to 2 hours late. If more than 2 hours, wait for next scheduled dose (don't double this dose).

What drug does:
Blocks digestive tract's nerve supply, which reduces propelling movements.

Continued next column

OVERDOSE

SYMPTOMS:
Excitement, constricted pupils, shallow breathing, coma.
WHAT TO DO:
- **Dial 911 (emergency) or 0 (operator) for an ambulance or medical help. Then give first aid immediately.**
- **If patient is unconscious and not breathing, give mouth-to-mouth breathing. If there is no heartbeat, use cardiac massage and mouth-to-mouth breathing (CPR). Don't try to make patient vomit. If you can't get help quickly, take patient to nearest emergency facility.**
- **See emergency information on inside covers.**

Time lapse before drug works:
May require 12 to 24 hours of regular doses to control diarrhea.

Don't take with:
Any other medicine without consulting your doctor or pharmacist.

POSSIBLE ADVERSE REACTIONS OR SIDE EFFECTS

SYMPTOMS	WHAT TO DO
Life-threatening: Hives, rash, intense itching, faintness soon after a dose (anaphylaxis).	Seek emergency treatment immediately.
Common: None expected.	
Infrequent: Dry mouth or skin, numbness of hands or feet, dizziness, depression, rash or itch, blurred vision, decreased urination, drowsiness, headache, swollen gums (these symptoms usually mean too much of the drug has been taken).	Discontinue. Call doctor right away.
Rare: Severe stomach pain, nausea, vomiting, constipation, bloating, loss of appetite.	Discontinue. Call doctor right away.

WARNINGS & PRECAUTIONS

Don't take if:
- You are allergic to diphenoxylate and atropine or any narcotic or anticholinergic.
- You have jaundice.
- You have infectious diarrhea or antibiotic-associated diarrhea.
- Patient is younger than 2.

Before you start, consult your doctor:
- If you have had liver problems.
- If you have ulcerative colitis.
- If you plan to become pregnant within medication period.
- If you have any medical disorder.
- If you take any medication, including nonprescription drugs.

Over age 60:
Adverse reactions and side effects may be more frequent and severe than in younger persons.

Pregnancy:
Decide with your doctor if drug benefits justify risk to unborn child. Risk category C (see page xxiii).

Breast-feeding:
Drug passes into milk. Avoid drug or discontinue nursing until you finish medicine. Consult doctor for advice on maintaining milk supply.

Infants & children:
Don't give to children under 2 years of age. Use only under doctor's supervision for children older than 2.

Prolonged use:
- May be habit forming if larger doses than recommended are taken for a long period of time.
- Talk to your doctor about the need for follow-up medical examinations or laboratory studies to check liver function.

Skin & sunlight:
No problems expected.

Driving, piloting or hazardous work:
Don't drive or pilot aircraft until you learn how medicine affects you. Don't work around dangerous machinery. Don't climb ladders or work in high places. Danger increases if you drink alcohol or take medicine affecting alertness and reflexes.

Discontinuing:
- May be unnecessary to finish medicine. Follow doctor's instructions.
- After discontinuing, consult doctor if you experience muscle cramps, nausea, vomiting, trembling, stomach cramps or unusual sweating.

Others:
If diarrhea lasts longer than 2 days, discontinue and call doctor.

 POSSIBLE INTERACTION WITH OTHER DRUGS

GENERIC NAME OR DRUG CLASS	COMBINED EFFECT
Barbiturates*	Increased effect of both drugs.
Clozapine	Toxic effect on the central nervous system.
Ethinamate	Dangerous increased effects of ethinamate. Avoid combining.
Fluoxetine	Increased depressant effects of both drugs.
Guanfacine	May increase depressant effects of either drug.
Leucovorin	High alcohol content of leucovorin may cause adverse effects.
Methyprylon	Increased sedative effect, perhaps to dangerous level. Avoid.
Monozmine oxidase (MAO) inhibitors*	May increase blood pressure excessively.
Naltrexone	Triggers withdrawal symptoms.
Narcotics*	Increased sedation. Avoid.
Sedatives*	Increased effect of both drugs.
Sertraline	Increased depressive effects of both drugs.
Tranquilizers*	Increased effect of both drugs.

 POSSIBLE INTERACTION WITH OTHER SUBSTANCES

INTERACTS WITH	COMBINED EFFECT
Alcohol:	Depressed brain function. Avoid.
Beverages:	None expected.
Cocaine:	Decreased effect of diphenoxylate and atropine.
Foods:	None expected.
Marijuana:	None expected.
Tobacco:	None expected.

*See Glossary

DIPYRIDAMOLE

BRAND NAMES

Apo-Dipyridamole   Novodipiradol
Dipimol   Persantine
Dipridacot   Pyridamole

BASIC INFORMATION

Habit forming? No
Prescription needed?
  U.S.: Yes
  Canada: No
Available as generic? Yes
Drug class: Platelet aggregation inhibitor

 ## USES

- May reduce frequency and intensity of angina attacks.
- May reduce the risk of blood clots after heart surgery.

 ## DOSAGE & USAGE INFORMATION

How to take:
Tablet—Swallow with a full glass of water. If you can't swallow whole, crumble tablet and take with liquid.

When to take:
1 hour before or 2 hours after meals.

If you forget a dose:
Take as soon as you remember up to 2 hours late. If more than 2 hours, wait for next scheduled dose (don't double this dose).

Continued next column

 ## OVERDOSE

SYMPTOMS:
Decreased blood pressure; weak, rapid pulse; cold, clammy skin; collapse.
WHAT TO DO:
- Dial 911 (emergency) or 0 (operator) for an ambulance or medical help. Then give first aid immediately.
- If patient is unconscious and not breathing, give mouth-to-mouth breathing. If there is no heartbeat, use cardiac massage and mouth-to-mouth breathing (CPR). Don't try to make patient vomit. If you can't get help quickly, take patient to nearest emergency facility.
- See emergency information on inside covers.

What drug does:
- Probably dilates blood vessels to increase oxygen to heart.
- May reduce platelet clumping, which causes blood clots.

Time lapse before drug works:
3 months of continual use.

Don't take with:
Any other medicine without consulting your doctor or pharmacist.

 ## POSSIBLE ADVERSE REACTIONS OR SIDE EFFECTS

SYMPTOMS	WHAT TO DO
Life-threatening:	
In case of overdose, see previous column.	
Common:	
Dizziness.	Continue. Call doctor when convenient.
Infrequent:	
• Fainting, headache.	Discontinue. Call doctor right away.
• Red flush, rash, nausea, vomiting, cramps, weakness.	Continue. Call doctor when convenient.
Rare:	
Chest pain.	Discontinue. Call doctor right away.

DIPYRIDAMOLE

WARNINGS & PRECAUTIONS

Don't take if:
- You are allergic to dipyridamole.
- You are recovering from a heart attack.

Before you start, consult your doctor:
- If you have low blood pressure.
- If you have liver disease.

Over age 60:
Begin treatment with small doses.

Pregnancy:
No proven harm to unborn child. Avoid if possible. Consult doctor. Risk category B (see page xxiii).

Breast-feeding:
No proven problems. Consult doctor.

Infants & children:
Not recommended.

Prolonged use:
Talk to your doctor about the need for follow-up medical examinations or laboratory studies.

Skin & sunlight:
No problems expected.

Driving, piloting or hazardous work:
Avoid if you feel dizzy. Otherwise, no problems expected.

Discontinuing:
Don't discontinue without doctor's advice until you complete prescribed dose, even though symptoms diminish or disappear.

Others:
- Drug increases your ability to be active without angina pain. Avoid excessive physical exertion that might injure heart.
- Advise any doctor or dentist whom you consult that you take this medicine.

POSSIBLE INTERACTION WITH OTHER DRUGS

GENERIC NAME OR DRUG CLASS	COMBINED EFFECT
Anticoagulants, oral*	Increased anticoagulant effect. Bleeding tendency.
Aspirin and combination drugs containing aspirin	Increased dipyridamole effect. Dose may need adjustment.

POSSIBLE INTERACTION WITH OTHER SUBSTANCES

INTERACTS WITH	COMBINED EFFECT
Alcohol:	May lower blood pressure excessively.
Beverages:	None expected.
Cocaine:	No proven problems.
Foods:	Decreased dipyridamole absorption unless taken 1 hour before eating.
Marijuana:	Daily use— Decreased dipyridamole effect.
Tobacco: Nicotine.	May decrease dipyridamole effect.

DISOPYRAMIDE

BRAND NAMES

Norpace
Norpace CR
Rythmodan
Rythmodan-LA

BASIC INFORMATION

Habit forming? No
Prescription needed? Yes
Available as generic? Yes
Drug class: Antiarrhythmic

USES

Corrects heart rhythm disorders.

DOSAGE & USAGE INFORMATION

How to take:
* Extended-release tablet or capsule—Swallow with liquid. Do not crush tablet or open capsule.
* Capsule—Swallow with liquid. If you can't swallow whole, ask your pharmacist to prepare a liquid suspension for your use.

When to take:
At the same times each day.

If you forget a dose:
Take as soon as you remember up to 2 hours late. If more than 2 hours, wait for next scheduled dose (don't double this dose).

What drug does:
Delays nerve impulses to heart to regulate heartbeat.

Continued next column

OVERDOSE

SYMPTOMS:
Blood-pressure drop, irregular heartbeat, apnea, loss of consciousness.
WHAT TO DO:
* Dial 911 (emergency) or 0 (operator) for an ambulance or medical help. Then give first aid immediately.
* If patient is unconscious and not breathing, give mouth-to-mouth breathing. If there is no heartbeat, use cardiac massage and mouth-to-mouth breathing (CPR). Don't try to make patient vomit. If you can't get help quickly, take patient to nearest emergency facility.
* See emergency information on inside covers.

Time lapse before drug works:
Begins in 30 to 60 minutes. Must use for 5 to 7 days to determine effectiveness.

Don't take with:
Any other medicine without consulting your doctor or pharmacist.

POSSIBLE ADVERSE REACTIONS OR SIDE EFFECTS

SYMPTOMS	WHAT TO DO
Life-threatening:	
Hives, rash, intense itching, faintness soon after a dose (anaphylaxis).	Seek emergency treatment immediately.
Common:	
• Hypoglycemia (cold sweats, fast heartbeat, extreme hunger, shakiness and nervousness, anxiety, cool and pale skin, drowsiness, headache).	Discontinue. Call doctor right away.
• Dry mouth, constipation, painful or difficult urination, rapid weight gain, blurred vision.	Continue. Call doctor when convenient.
Infrequent:	
• Dizziness, fainting, confusion, chest pain, nervousness, depression, slow or fast heartbeat.	Discontinue. Call doctor right away.
• Swollen feet.	Continue. Call doctor when convenient.
Rare:	
• Shortness of breath, psychosis.	Discontinue. Seek emergency treatment.
• Rash, sore throat, fever, headache, jaundice, muscle weakness.	Discontinue. Call doctor right away.
• Eye pain, diminished sex drive, numbness or tingling of hands and feet, bleeding tendency.	Continue. Call doctor when convenient.

WARNINGS & PRECAUTIONS

Don't take if:
* You are allergic to disopyramide or any antiarrhythmic.
* You have second- or third-degree heart block.
* You have heart failure.

Before you start, consult your doctor:
- If you react unfavorably to other anti-arrhythmic drugs.
- If you have had heart disease.
- If you have low blood pressure.
- If you have liver disease.
- If you have glaucoma.
- If you have enlarged prostate.
- If you have myasthenia gravis.
- If you take digitalis preparations or diuretics.

Over age 60:
- May require reduced dose.
- More likely to have difficulty urinating or be constipated.
- More likely to have blood pressure drop.

Pregnancy:
Decide with your doctor if drug benefits justify risk to unborn child. Risk category C (see page xxiii).

Breast-feeding:
Drug passes into milk. Avoid drug or discontinue nursing until you finish medicine. Consult doctor for advice on maintaining milk supply.

Infants & children:
Safety not established. Don't use.

Prolonged use:
Talk to your doctor about the need for follow-up medical examinations or laboratory studies to check liver function, kidney function, ECG*, blood pressure, serum potassium.

Skin & sunlight:
May cause rash or intensify sunburn in areas exposed to sun or ultraviolet light photosensitivity reaction). Avoid overexposure. Notify doctor if reaction occurs.

Driving, piloting or hazardous work:
Don't drive or pilot aircraft until you learn how medicine affects you. Don't work around dangerous machinery. Don't climb ladders or work in high places. Danger increases if you drink alcohol or take medicine affecting alertness and reflexes, such as antihistamines, tranquilizers, sedatives, pain medicine, narcotics, or mind-altering drugs.

Discontinuing:
Don't discontinue without doctor's advice until you complete prescribed dose, even though symptoms diminish or disappear.

Others:
If new illness, injury or surgery occurs, tell doctors of disopyramide use.

POSSIBLE INTERACTION WITH OTHER DRUGS

GENERIC NAME OR DRUG CLASS	COMBINED EFFECT
Antiarrhythmics*	May increase effect and toxicity of each drug.
Anticholinergics*	Increased anticholinergic effect.
Anticoagulants, oral*	Possible increased anticoagulant effect.
Antihypertensives*	Increased anti-hypertensive effect.
Cisapride	Decreased disopyramide effect.
Encainide	Increased effect of toxicity on the heart muscle.
Flecainide	Possible irregular heartbeat.
Nicardipine	May cause dangerously slow, fast or irregular heartbeat.
Nimodipine	May cause dangerous irregular, slow or fast heartbeat.
Phenobarbital	Increased metabolism, decreased disopyramide effect.
Phenytoin	Increased metabolism, decreased disopyramide effect.
Propafenone	Increased effect of both drugs and increased risk of toxicity.
Rifampin	Increased metabolism, decreased disopyramide effect.
Tocainide	Increased likelihood of adverse reactions with either drug.

POSSIBLE INTERACTION WITH OTHER SUBSTANCES

INTERACTS WITH	COMBINED EFFECT
Alcohol:	Decreased blood pressure and blood sugar. Use caution.
Beverages:	None expected.
Cocaine:	Irregular heartbeat.
Foods:	None expected.
Marijuana:	Unpredictable. May decrease disopyramide effect.
Tobacco:	May decrease disopyramide effect.

*See Glossary

DISULFIRAM

BRAND NAMES

Antabuse

BASIC INFORMATION

Habit forming? No
Prescription needed? Yes
Available as generic? Yes
Drug class: None

USES

Treatment for alcoholism. Will not cure alcoholism, but is a powerful deterrent to drinking.

DOSAGE & USAGE INFORMATION

How to take:
Tablet—Swallow with liquid.

When to take:
Morning or bedtime. Avoid if you have used *any* alcohol, tonics, cough syrups, fermented vinegar, after-shave lotion or backrub solutions within 12 hours.

If you forget a dose:
Take as soon as you remember up to 12 hours late. If more than 12 hours, wait for next scheduled dose (don't double this dose).

What drug does:
In combination with alcohol, produces a metabolic change that causes severe, temporary toxicity.

Time lapse before drug works:
3 to 12 hours.

Continued next column

OVERDOSE

SYMPTOMS:
Memory loss, behavior disturbances, lethargy, confusion and headaches; nausea, vomiting, stomach pain and diarrhea; weakness and unsteady walk; temporary paralysis.
WHAT TO DO:
- **Dial 911 (emergency) or 0 (operator) for an ambulance or medical help. Then give first aid immediately.**
- **See emergency information at end of book.**

Don't take with:
- Nonprescription drugs that contain *any* alcohol.
- Any other central nervous system (CNS) depressant drugs*.

POSSIBLE ADVERSE REACTIONS OR SIDE EFFECTS

SYMPTOMS	WHAT TO DO
Life-threatening:	
In case of overdose, see previous column.	
Common:	
Drowsiness.	Continue. Tell doctor at next visit.
Infrequent:	
• Eye pain, vision changes, abdominal discomfort, throbbing headache, numbness in hands and feet.	Continue. Call doctor when convenient.
• Mood change, decreased sexual ability in men, tiredness.	Continue. Tell doctor at next visit.
• Bad taste in mouth (metal or garlic).	No action necessary.
Rare:	
Rash, jaundice.	Discontinue. Call doctor right away.

WARNINGS & PRECAUTIONS

Don't take if:
- You are allergic to disulfiram (alcohol-disulfiram combination is not an allergic reaction).
- You have used alcohol in any form or amount within 12 hours.
- You have taken paraldehyde within 1 week.
- You have heart disease.

Before you start, consult your doctor:
- If you have allergies.
- If you plan to become pregnant within medication period.
- If no one has explained to you how disulfiram reacts with alcohol.
- If you think you cannot avoid drinking.
- If you have diabetes, epilepsy, liver or kidney disease.
- If you take other drugs.

Over age 60:
Adverse reactions and side effects may be more frequent and severe than in younger persons.

Pregnancy:
Decide with your doctor if drug benefits justify risk to unborn child. Risk category C (see page xxiii).

Breast-feeding:
Studies inconclusive. Consult your doctor.

Infants & children:
Not recommended.

Prolonged use:
Periodic blood cell counts and liver function tests recommended if you take this drug a long time.

Skin & sunlight:
No problems expected.

Driving, piloting or hazardous work:
Avoid if you feel drowsy or have vision side effects. Otherwise, no restrictions.

Discontinuing:
Don't discontinue without consulting doctor. Dose may require gradual reduction if you have taken drug for a long time. Doses of other drugs may also require adjustment. Avoid alcohol at least 14 days following last dose.

Others:
- Check all liquids that you take or rub on for presence of alcohol.
- Advise any doctor or dentist whom you consult that you take this medicine.

POSSIBLE INTERACTION WITH OTHER DRUGS

GENERIC NAME OR DRUG CLASS	COMBINED EFFECT
Anticoagulants*	Possible unexplained bleeding.
Anticonvulsants*	Excessive sedation.
Barbiturates*	Excessive sedation.
Central nervous system (CNS) depressants*	Increased depressive effect.
Clozapine	Toxic effect on the central nervous system.
Guanfacine	May increase depressant effects of either drug.
Isoniazid	Unsteady walk and disturbed behavior.
Leucovorin	High alcohol content of leucovorin may cause disulfiram reaction*.
Methyprylon	Increased sedative effect, perhaps to dangerous level. Avoid.
Metronidazole	Disulfiram reaction*.
Nabilone	Greater depression of central nervous system.
Sedatives*	Excessive sedation.
Theophylline	Increased theophylline effect; possibly toxic levels.

POSSIBLE INTERACTION WITH OTHER SUBSTANCES

INTERACTS WITH	COMBINED EFFECT
Alcohol: *Any* form or amount.	Possible life-threatening toxicity. See disulfiram reaction*.
Beverages: Punch or fruit drink that may contain alcohol.	Disulfiram reaction*.
Cocaine:	Increased disulfiram effect.
Foods: Sauces, fermented vinegar, marinades, desserts or other foods prepared with *any* alcohol.	Disulfiram reaction*.
Marijuana:	None expected.
Tobacco:	None expected.

DIURETICS, LOOP

GENERIC AND BRAND NAMES

BUMETADINE
  Bumex
ETHACRYNIC ACID
  Edecrin
FUROSEMIDE
  Apo-Furosemide
  Furoside
  Lasix
  Lasix Special
  Myrosemide
  Novosemide
  Uritol

TORSEMIDE
  Demadex

BASIC INFORMATION

Habit forming? No
Prescription needed? Yes
Available as generic? Yes
Drug class: Diuretic (loop), antihypertensive

USES

- Lowers high blood pressure.
- Decreases fluid retention.

DOSAGE & USAGE INFORMATION

How to take:
Tablet or liquid—Swallow with liquid. If you can't swallow whole, crumble tablet and take with liquid or food.

When to take:
- 1 dose a day—Take after breakfast.
- More than 1 dose a day—Take last dose no later than 6 p.m. unless otherwise directed.

If you forget a dose:
- 1 dose a day—Take as soon as you remember up to 12 hours late. If more than 12 hours, wait for next scheduled dose (don't double this dose).

Continued next column

OVERDOSE

SYMPTOMS:
Weakness, lethargy, dizziness, confusion, nausea, vomiting, leg muscle cramps, thirst, stupor, deep sleep, weak and rapid pulse, cardiac arrest.
WHAT TO DO:
- **Dial 911 (emergency) or 0 (operator) for an ambulance or medical help. Then give first aid immediately.**
- **See emergency information on inside covers.**

- More than 1 dose a day—Take as soon as you remember up to 2 hours late. If more than 2 hours, wait for next scheduled dose (don't double this dose).

What drug does:
Increases elimination of sodium, potassium and water from body. Decreased body fluid reduces blood pressure.

Time lapse before drug works:
1 hour to increase water loss. Requires 2 to 3 weeks to lower blood pressure.

Don't take with:
- Nonprescription drugs with aspirin.
- Any other medicine without consulting your doctor.

POSSIBLE ADVERSE REACTIONS OR SIDE EFFECTS

SYMPTOMS	WHAT TO DO
Life-threatening: In case of overdose, see previous column.	
Common: Dizziness.	Continue. Call doctor when convenient.
Infrequent: Mood change, fatigue, appetite loss, diarrhea, irregular heartbeat, muscle cramps, low blood pressure, abdominal pain, weakness.	Discontinue. Call doctor right away.
Rare: Rash or hives, yellow vision, ringing in ears, hearing loss, sore throat, fever, dry mouth, thirst, side or stomach pain, nausea, vomiting, unusual bleeding or bruising, joint pain, jaundice, numbness or tingling in hands or feet.	Discontinue. Call doctor right away.

WARNINGS & PRECAUTIONS

Don't take if:
You are allergic to loop diuretics.

Before you start, consult your doctor:
- If you are taking any other prescription or nonprescription medicine.
- If you are allergic to any sulfa drug.
- If you have liver or kidney disease.
- If you have gout, diabetes or impaired hearing.
- If you will have surgery within 2 months, including dental surgery, requiring general or spinal anesthesia.

Over age 60:
Adverse reactions and side effects may be more frequent and severe than in younger persons.

Pregnancy:
Risk factors vary for drugs in this group. See category list on page xxiii and consult doctor.

Breast-feeding:
Drug filters into milk. May harm child. Avoid.

Infants & children:
Use only under medical supervision.

Prolonged use:
- Impaired balance of water and salt, with low potassium level in blood and body tissues.
- Possible diabetes.

Skin & sunlight:
One or more drugs in this group may cause rash or intensify sunburn in areas exposed to sun or ultraviolet light (photosensitivity reaction). Avoid overexposure. Notify doctor if reaction occurs.

Driving, piloting or hazardous work:
Avoid if you feel dizzy; otherwise no problems expected.

Discontinuing:
Don't discontinue without doctor's advice until you complete prescribed dose, even though symptoms diminish or disappear.

Others:
Frequent laboratory studies to monitor potassium level in blood recommended. Eat foods rich in potassium or take potassium supplements. Consult doctor.

POSSIBLE INTERACTION WITH OTHER DRUGS

GENERIC NAME OR DRUG CLASS	COMBINED EFFECT
Adrenocorticoids, systemic	Potassium depletion.
Allopurinol	Decreased allopurinol effect.
Amiodarone	Increased risk of heartbeat irregularity due to low potassium.
Angiotensin-converting enzyme (ACE) inhibitors*	Possible excessive potassium in blood.
Anticoagulants*	Abnormal clotting.
Antidepressants, tricyclic*	Excessive blood pressure drop.
Antidiabetics, oral*	Decreased anti-diabetic effect.

Antihypertensives*	Increased anti-hypertensive effect. Dosages may require adjustment.
Anti-inflammatory drugs, nonsteroidal (NSAIDs)*	Decreased diuretic effect.
Antivirals, HIV/AIDS*	Increased risk of pancreatitis with furosemide.
Barbiturates*	Low blood pressure.
Beta-adrenergic blocking agents*	Increased anti-hypertensive effect. Dosages may require adjustment.
Corticosteroids*	Decreased potassium.
Digitalis preparations*	Excessive potassium loss could lead to serious heart rhythm disorders.
Diuretics, other*	Increased diuretic effect.
Hypokalemia-causing medicines*	Increased risk of excessive potassium loss.
Insulin	Decreased insulin effect.
Lithium	Increased lithium toxicity.
Metformin	Increased metformin effect with furosemide.
Narcotics*	Dangerous low blood pressure. Avoid.

Continued on page 913

POSSIBLE INTERACTION WITH OTHER SUBSTANCES

INTERACTS WITH	COMBINED EFFECT
Alcohol:	Blood pressure drop. Avoid.
Beverages:	None expected.
Cocaine:	Dangerous blood pressure drop. Avoid.
Foods:	None expected.
Marijuana:	Increased thirst and urinary frequency, fainting.
Tobacco:	Decreased furosemide effect.

*See Glossary

DIURETICS, POTASSIUM-SPARING

GENERIC AND BRAND NAMES

AMILORIDE
  Midamor

TRIAMTERENE
  Dyrenium

SPIRONOLACTONE
  Aldactone
  Novospiroton

BASIC INFORMATION

Habit forming? No
Prescription needed? Yes
Available as generic? Yes
Drug class: Diuretic, antihypertensive, antihypokalemic

 USES

- Treatment for high blood pressure (hypertension) and congestive heart failure. Decreases fluid retention and prevents potassium loss.
- Treatment for hypokalemia (low potassium), polycystic ovary syndrome and hirsutism in women.

 DOSAGE & USAGE INFORMATION

How to take:
Capsule or tablet—Swallow with liquid. If you can't swallow whole, open capsule or crush tablet and take with liquid or food. May take with meal to lessen stomach irritation.

When to take:
At the same times each day. May interfere with sleep if taken after 6 p.m.

Continued next column

 OVERDOSE

SYMPTOMS:
Rapid, irregular heartbeat; confusion; shortness of breath; nervousness; extreme weakness; stupor; coma.
WHAT TO DO:
- **Dial 911 (emergency) or 0 (operator) for an ambulance or medical help. Then give first aid immediately.**
- **If patient is unconscious and not breathing, give mouth-to-mouth breathing. If there is no heartbeat, use cardiac massage and mouth-to-mouth breathing (CPR). Don't try to make patient vomit. If you can't get help quickly, take patient to nearest emergency facility.**
- **See emergency information on inside covers.**

If you forget a dose:
Take as soon as you remember. If it is almost time for the next dose, wait for next scheduled dose (don't double this dose).

What drug does:
- Blocks exchange of certain chemicals in the kidneys so sodium and water are excreted. Conserves potassium.
- In polycystic ovary syndrome and hirsutism, blocks androgen hormones.

Time lapse before drug works:
2 to 4 hours.

Don't take with:
Any other medicine without consulting your doctor or pharmacist.

 POSSIBLE ADVERSE REACTIONS OR SIDE EFFECTS

SYMPTOMS	WHAT TO DO
Life-threatening:	
In case of overdose, see previous column.	
Common:	
Headache, nausea, appetite loss, vomiting, mild diarrhea.	Continue. Call doctor when convenient.
Infrequent:	
Dizziness, headache, muscle cramps, dry mouth, decreased sexual drive, muscle cramps, constipation.	Continue. Call doctor when convenient.
Rare:	
Shortness of breath, skin rash or itch (with amiloride); cough or hoarseness, painful urination, back or side pain (with triamterene and spironolactone); potassium changes (confusion, dry mouth, breathing difficulty, irregular heartbeat, unusual tiredness or weakness, mood or mental changes, muscle cramps, tingling in body); red, burning, inflamed feeling of tongue (with triamterene).	Discontinue. Call doctor right away.

 WARNINGS & PRECAUTIONS

Don't take if:
- You are allergic to potassium-sparing diuretics.
- Your serum potassium level is high.

Before you start, consult your doctor:
- If you have diabetes.
- If you have heart disease, kidney or liver disease or gout.

Over age 60:
Adverse reactions and side effects may be more frequent and severe than in younger persons. More likely to exceed safe potassium blood levels.

Pregnancy:
Avoid if possible. Consult doctor. Risk category B (see page xxiii).

Breast-feeding:
Drug may pass into milk. Avoid drug or discontinue nursing until you finish medicine. Consult doctor for advice on maintaining milk supply.

Infants & children:
No special problems expected.

Prolonged use:
Talk to your doctor about the need for follow-up medical examinations or laboratory studies to check blood pressure, kidney function, ECG* and serum electrolytes.

Skin & sunlight:
One or more of these drugs may cause increased sensitivity to sunlight (photosensitivity reaction). Avoid overexposure. If reaction occurs, notify doctor.

Driving, piloting or hazardous work:
Don't drive or pilot aircraft until you learn how medicine affects you. Don't work around dangerous machinery. Don't climb ladders or work in high places. Danger increases if you drink alcohol or take medicine affecting alertness and reflexes.

Discontinuing:
Don't discontinue without doctor's advice until you complete prescribed dose, even though symptoms diminish or disappear.

Others:
- Periodic physical checkups and potassium-level tests recommended.
- Advise any doctor or dentist whom you consult that you take this medicine.
- If you experience an illness with severe vomiting and diarrhea, consult doctor.
- A special diet may be recommended in addition to this medicine. Follow doctor's advice.

POSSIBLE INTERACTION WITH OTHER DRUGS

GENERIC NAME OR DRUG CLASS	COMBINED EFFECT
Amantadine	Increased effect of amantadine (with triamterene).
Angiotensin-converting enzyme (ACE) inhibitors*	Possible excessive potassium in blood.
Anticoagulants*, oral	Decreased anticoagulant effect.
Antigout drugs*	Decreased antigout effect.
Antihypertensives*	Increased effect of both drugs.
Anti-inflammatory drugs, nonsteroidal (NSAIDs)*	Increased potassium levels.
Cyclosporine	Increased potassium levels.
Digoxin	Increased digoxin effect (with spironolactone).
Diuretics*, other	Increased effect of both drugs.
Folic acid	Decreased effect of folic acid.
Lithium	Possible lithium toxicity.
Metformin	Increased metformin effect.
Potassium supplements*	Increased potassium levels.

POSSIBLE INTERACTION WITH OTHER SUBSTANCES

INTERACTS WITH	COMBINED EFFECT
Alcohol:	Increased blood pressure drop. Avoid.
Beverages: Low-salt milk.	Possible excess potassium levels. Low-salt milk has extra potassium.
Cocaine:	Blood pressure rise. Avoid.
Foods: Salt substitutes.	Possible excess potassium levels.
Marijuana:	None expected.
Tobacco:	None expected.

DIURETICS, POTASSIUM-SPARING & HYDROCHLOROTHIAZIDE

GENERIC AND BRAND NAMES

AMILODINE &
HYDROCHLORO-
THIAZIDE
Moduret
Moduretic
SPIRONOLACTONE
& HYDROCHLORO-
THIAZIDE
Aldactazide
Spirozide

TRIAMTERENE &
HYDROCHLORO-
THIAZIDE
Apo-Triazide
Diazide
Maxzide
Novo-Triamzide

BASIC INFORMATION

Habit forming? No
Prescription needed? Yes
Available as generic? Yes
Drug class: Diuretic, antihypertensive, antihypokalemic

USES

- Treats, but does not cure, high blood pressure (hypertension) and congestive heart failure. Decreases fluid retention and prevents potassium loss.
- Treatment for hypokalemia (low potassium).

DOSAGE & USAGE INFORMATION

How to take:
Capsule or tablet—Swallow with liquid. Take with meals or milk if stomach irritation occurs.

When to take:
At the same time or times each day. May interfere with sleep if taken after 6 p.m.

Continued next column

OVERDOSE

SYMPTOMS: Rapid, irregular heartbeat; confusion; shortness of breath; nervousness; extreme weakness.
WHAT TO DO:
- **Dial 911 (emergency) or 0 (operator) for ambulance or medical help. Give first aid immediately.**
- **If patient is unconscious and not breathing, give mouth-to-mouth breathing. If no heartbeat, use cardiac massage and mouth-to-mouth breathing (CPR). Don't make patient vomit. If you can't get help quickly, take patient to nearest emergency facility.**
- **See emergency information on inside covers.**

If you forget a dose:
Take as soon as you remember. If it is almost time for the next dose, wait for next scheduled dose (don't double this dose).

What drug does:
This is a combination of 2 diuretics that blocks exchange of certain chemicals in the kidneys so sodium and water are excreted. Conserves potassium.

Time lapse before drug works:
Starts in 2 to 4 hours; several days for full effect.

Don't take with:
Any other medicine without consulting your doctor or pharmacist. This includes any nonprescription medicines for colds, coughs, hay fever, sinus problems, appetite control or asthma.

POSSIBLE ADVERSE REACTIONS OR SIDE EFFECTS

SYMPTOMS	WHAT TO DO
Life-threatening: In case of overdose, see previous column.	
Common: Nausea or mild vomiting, appetite loss, stomach cramps, mild diarrhea, constipation (with amiloride).	Continue. Call doctor when convenient.
Infrequent: Dizziness, muscle cramps, headache, skin sensitive to sun, dry mouth, decreased interest in sex. With spironolactone—tender breasts, deepening of voice, menstrual changes, and increased hair growth in females; breast enlargement in males; increased sweating in both sexes.	Continue. Call doctor when convenient.
Rare: Black, tarry or bloody stools; blood in urine; pain or difficulty in urinating; fever or chills; pain in back, side or joints; spots, rash or hives on skin; severe stomach pain; unusual bleeding or bruising, yellow skin or eyes; potassium changes (confusion, dry mouth, breathing difficulty, irregular heartbeat,	Discontinue. Call doctor right away.

unusual tiredness or weakness, mood or mental changes, muscle cramps, tingling in body); red, burning, inflamed feeling of tongue (with triamterene).

WARNINGS & PRECAUTIONS

Don't take if:
- You are allergic to potassium-sparing or thiazide diuretics* or sulfa drugs*.
- Your serum potassium level is high.

Before you start, consult your doctor:
- If you have diabetes or lupus erythematosus.
- If you have menstrual problems (in females) or enlarged breast (in males).
- If you have heart or blood vessel disease, kidney or liver disease, pancreatitis or gout.

Over age 60:
Adverse reactions and side effects may be more frequent and severe than in younger persons. More likely to exceed safe potassium blood levels.

Pregnancy:
Does not control pregnancy symptoms of swollen hands and feet. Avoid if possible. Consult doctor. Risk category B (see page xxiii).

Breast-feeding:
Drug passes into milk. Avoid drug or discontinue nursing until you finish medicine. Consult doctor for advice on maintaining milk supply.

Infants & children:
Unknown effect. Use only with doctor's approval.

Prolonged use:
Talk to your doctor about the need for follow-up medical examinations or laboratory studies to check blood pressure, kidney function, ECG* and serum electrolytes.

Skin & sunlight:
One or more of these drugs may cause increased sensitivity to sunlight (photosensitivity reaction). Avoid overexposure. If reaction occurs, notify doctor.

Driving, piloting or hazardous work:
Don't drive or pilot aircraft until you learn how medicine affects you. Don't work around dangerous machinery. Don't climb ladders or work in high places. Danger increases if you drink alcohol or take medicine affecting alertness and reflexes, such as antihistamines, tranquilizers, sedatives, pain medicine, narcotics and mind-altering drugs.

Discontinuing:
Don't discontinue without doctor's approval, even though symptoms diminish or disappear.

Others:
- Your doctor may prescribe a special diet.
- Advise any doctor or dentist whom you consult that you take this medicine.
- If you experience an illness with severe vomiting or diarrhea, consult doctor.

POSSIBLE INTERACTION WITH OTHER DRUGS

GENERIC NAME OR DRUG CLASS	COMBINED EFFECT
Amantadine	Increased effect of amantadine (with triamterene).
Angiotensin-converting enzyme (ACE) inhibitors*	Possible excessive potassium in blood.
Anticoagulants*, oral	Decreased anticoagulant effect.
Antigout drugs*	Decreased antigout effect.
Antihypertensives*	Increased effect of both drugs.
Anti-inflammatory drugs, nonsteroidal (NSAIDs)*	Increased potassium levels.
Cholestyramine	Decreased diuretic effect. Take 1 hour before diuretic.

Continued on page 913

POSSIBLE INTERACTION WITH OTHER SUBSTANCES

INTERACTS WITH	COMBINED EFFECT
Alcohol:	Increased blood pressure drop. Avoid.
Beverages: Low-salt milk.	Possible excess potassium levels. Low-salt milk has extra potassium.
Cocaine:	Blood pressure rise. Avoid.
Foods: Salt substitutes.	Possible excess potassium levels.
Marijuana:	None expected.
Tobacco:	None expected.

GENERIC AND BRAND NAMES

See complete list of generic and brand names in the *Generic and Brand Name Directory*, page 880.

BASIC INFORMATION

Habit forming? No
Prescription needed? Yes
Available as generic? Yes, for some.
Drug class: Antihypertensive, diuretic (thiazide)

USES

- Controls, but doesn't cure, high blood pressure.
- Reduces fluid retention (edema) caused by conditions such as heart disorders and liver disease.

DOSAGE & USAGE INFORMATION

How to take:
Tablet, capsule or liquid—Swallow with liquid. If you can't swallow whole, crumble tablet or open capsule and take with liquid or food. Don't exceed dose.

When to take:
At the same time each day.

If you forget a dose:
Take as soon as you remember up to 2 hours late. If more than 2 hours, wait for next scheduled dose (don't double this dose).

What drug does:
- Forces sodium and water excretion, reducing body fluid.
- Relaxes muscle cells of small arteries.
- Reduced body fluid and relaxed arteries lower blood pressure.

Continued next column

OVERDOSE

SYMPTOMS:
Cramps, weakness, drowsiness, weak pulse, coma.
WHAT TO DO:
- **Dial 911 (emergency) or 0 (operator) for an ambulance or medical help. Then give first aid immediately.**
- **See emergency information on inside covers.**

Time lapse before drug works:
4 to 6 hours. May require several weeks to lower blood pressure.

Don't take with:
Nonprescription drugs without consulting doctor.

POSSIBLE ADVERSE REACTIONS OR SIDE EFFECTS

SYMPTOMS	WHAT TO DO
Life-threatening:	
In case of overdose, see previous column.	
Common:	
Muscle cramps.	Discontinue. Call doctor right away.
Infrequent:	
• Blurred vision, severe abdominal pain, nausea, vomiting, irregular heartbeat, weak pulse.	Discontinue. Call doctor right away.
• Dizziness, mood changes, headaches, weakness, tiredness, weight changes, decreased sex drive, diarrhea.	Continue. Call doctor when convenient.
• Dry mouth, thirst.	Continue. Tell doctor at next visit.
Rare:	
• Rash or hives.	Discontinue. Seek emergency treatment.
• Jaundice, joint pain, black stools.	Discontinue. Call doctor right away.
• Sore throat, fever.	Continue. Tell doctor at next visit.

WARNINGS & PRECAUTIONS

Don't take if:
You are allergic to any thiazide diuretic drug.

Before you start, consult your doctor:
- If you are allergic to any sulfa drug or tartrazine dye.
- If you have gout, systemic lupus erythematosis.
- If you have liver, pancreas, diabetes or kidney disorder.

Over age 60:
Adverse reactions and side effects may be more frequent and severe than in younger persons, especially dizziness and excessive potassium loss.

Pregnancy:
Risk factors vary for drugs in this group. See category list on page xxiii and consult doctor.

Breast-feeding:
Drug passes into milk. Avoid drug or discontinue nursing.

Infants & children:
No problems expected.

Prolonged use:
- You may need medicine to treat high blood pressure for the rest of your life.
- Talk to your doctor about the need for follow-up medical examinations or laboratory studies to check blood sugar, kidney function, blood pressure, serum electrolytes.

Skin & sunlight:
One or more drugs in this group may cause rash or intensify sunburn in areas exposed to sun or ultraviolet light (photosensitivity reaction). Avoid overexposure. Notify doctor if reaction occurs.

Driving, piloting or hazardous work:
Don't drive or pilot aircraft until you learn how medicine affects you. Don't work around dangerous machinery. Don't climb ladders or work in high places. Danger increases if you drink alcohol or take medicine affecting alertness and reflexes, such as antihistamines, tranquilizers, sedatives, pain medicine, narcotics and mind-altering drugs.

Discontinuing:
Don't discontinue without medical advice.

Others:
- Hot weather and fever may cause dehydration and drop in blood pressure. Dose may require temporary adjustment. Weigh daily and report any unexpected weight decreases to your doctor.
- May cause rise in uric acid, leading to gout.
- May cause blood-sugar rise in diabetics.
- May affect results in some medical tests.
- Advise any doctor or dentist whom you consult that you take this medicine.

POSSIBLE INTERACTION WITH OTHER DRUGS

GENERIC NAME OR DRUG CLASS	COMBINED EFFECT
Adrenocorticoids, systemic	Potassium depletion.
Allopurinol	Decreased allopurinol effect.
Amiodarone	Increased risk of heartbeat irregularity due to low potassium.
Amphotericin B	Increased potassium.
Angiotensin-converting enzyme (ACE) inhibitors*	Decreased blood pressure.

Antidepressants, tricyclic*	Dangerous drop in blood pressure. Avoid combination unless under medical supervision.
Antidiabetic agents, oral*	Increased blood sugar.
Antihypertensives*	Increased hypertensive effect.
Antivirals, HIV/AIDS*	Increased risk of pancreatitis.
Barbiturates*	Increased anti-hypertensive effect.
Beta-adrenergic blocking agents*	Increased anti-hypertensive effect. Dosages of both drugs may require adjustments.
Calcium supplements*	Increased calcium in blood.
Carteolol	Increased anti-hypertensive effect.
Cholestyramine	Decreased anti-hypertensive effect.
Colestipol	Decreased anti-hypertensive effect.
Digitalis preparations*	Excessive potassium loss that causes dangerous heart rhythms.
Diuretics, thiazide*, other	Increased effect of other thiazide diuretics.

Continued on page 914

POSSIBLE INTERACTION WITH OTHER SUBSTANCES

INTERACTS WITH	COMBINED EFFECT
Alcohol:	Dangerous blood pressure drop.
Beverages:	None expected.
Cocaine	Increased risk of heart block and high blood pressure.
Foods: Licorice.	Excessive potassium loss that causes dangerous heart rhythms.
Marijuana:	May increase blood pressure.
Tobacco:	None expected.

*See Glossary

DIVALPROEX

BRAND NAMES

Depakote   Epival
Depakote Sprinkle

BASIC INFORMATION

Habit forming? No
Prescription needed? Yes
Available as generic? No
Drug class: Anticonvulsant

USES

- Controls petit mal (absence) seizures in treatment of epilepsy.
- Treats the manic episodes associated with bipolar disorder.
- Treats migraine headaches.

DOSAGE & USAGE INFORMATION

How to take:
Delayed-release capsule or delayed-release tablet—Swallow with liquid or food to lessen stomach irritation. Do not crumble capsule or crush tablet.

When to take:
One to three times a day as directed by your doctor.

If you forget a dose:
Take as soon as you remember. Don't ever double dose.

What drug does:
Increases concentration of gamma aminobutyric acid, which inhibits nerve transmission in parts of brain.

Continued next column

OVERDOSE

SYMPTOMS:
Coma.
WHAT TO DO:
- Dial 911 (emergency) or 0 (operator) for an ambulance or medical help. Then give first aid immediately.
- If patient is unconscious and not breathing, give mouth-to-mouth breathing. If there is no heartbeat, use cardiac massage and mouth-to-mouth breathing (CPR). Don't try to make patient vomit. If you can't get help quickly, take patient to nearest emergency facility.
- See emergency information on inside covers.

Time lapse before drug works:
1 to 4 hours.

Don't take with:
Any other medicine without consulting your doctor or pharmacist.

POSSIBLE ADVERSE REACTIONS OR SIDE EFFECTS

SYMPTOMS	WHAT TO DO
Life-threatening: In case of overdose, see previous column.	
Common: Loss of appetite, indigestion, nausea, vomiting, stomach cramps, diarrhea, tremor, unusual weight gain or loss, menstrual changes.	Continue. Call doctor when convenient.
Infrequent: Clumsiness or unsteadiness, constipation, skin rash, dizziness, drowsiness, unusual excitement or irritability.	Continue. Call doctor when convenient.
Rare: Mood or behavior changes; continued nausea, vomiting and appetite loss; increase in number of seizures; swelling of face, feet or legs; yellow skin or eyes; tiredness or weakness; back-and-forth eye movements (nystagmus); seeing double or seeing spots; severe stomach cramps; unusual bleeding or bruising.	Continue, but call doctor right away.

WARNINGS & PRECAUTIONS

Don't take if:
You are allergic to divalproex or valproic acid.

Before you start, consult your doctor:
- If you have blood, kidney or liver disease.
- If you will have surgery within 2 months, including dental surgery, requiring general or spinal anesthesia.

Over age 60:
Adverse reactions and side effects may be more frequent and severe than in younger persons.

Pregnancy:
Risk to unborn child outweighs drug benefits. Don't use. Risk category D (see page xxiii).

Breast-feeding:
Unknown effect. Consult doctor.

Infants & children:
Under close medical supervision only.

Prolonged use:
Request periodic blood tests, liver and kidney function tests.

Skin & sunlight:
No problems expected.

Driving, piloting or hazardous work:
Don't drive or pilot aircraft until you learn how medicine affects you. Don't work around dangerous machinery. Don't climb ladders or work in high places. Danger increases if you drink alcohol or take medicine affecting alertness and reflexes, such as antihistamines, tranquilizers, sedatives, pain medicine, narcotics and mind-altering drugs.

Discontinuing:
Don't discontinue without consulting doctor. Dose may require gradual reduction if you have taken drug for a long time. Doses of other drugs may also require adjustment.

Others:
- Advise any doctor or dentist whom you consult that you take this medicine.
- Be sure you and the doctor discuss benefits and risks of this drug before starting.
- Wear a medical identification that indicates the use of this medicine.
- Use as directed. Don't increase or decrease dosage without doctor's approval.

POSSIBLE INTERACTION WITH OTHER DRUGS

GENERIC NAME OR DRUG CLASS	COMBINED EFFECT
Anticoagulants*	Increases chance of bleeding.
Aspirin	Increases chance of bleeding.
Central nervous system (CNS) depressants*	Increases sedative effect.
Clonazepam	May cause or prolong seizure.
Dipyridamole	Increases chance of bleeding.
Monoamine oxidase (MAO) inhibitors*	Increases sedative effect.
Nabilone	Greater depression of central nervous system.
Phenobarbital	Increases chance of toxicity.
Phenytoin	Unpredictable. May require increased or decreased dosage.
Primidone	Increases chance of toxicity.
Sertraline	Increased depressive effect of both drugs.
Sulfinpyrazone	Increases chance of bleeding.

POSSIBLE INTERACTION WITH OTHER SUBSTANCES

INTERACTS WITH	COMBINED EFFECT
Alcohol:	Deep sedation. Avoid.
Beverages:	No problems expected.
Cocaine:	Increased brain sensitivity. Avoid.
Foods:	No problems expected.
Marijuana:	Increased brain sensitivity. Avoid.
Tobacco:	Increased brain sensitivity. Avoid.

*See Glossary

DONEPEZIL

BRAND NAMES

Aricept

BASIC INFORMATION

Habit forming? No
Prescription needed? Yes
Available as generic? No
Drug class: Cholinesterase inhibitor

 USES

Treatment for symptoms of mild to moderate
Alzheimer's disease. May improve memory,
reasoning and other cognitive functions slightly
in some patients or slow the progress of
Alzheimer's disease. It will not reverse the
disease.

 DOSAGE & USAGE INFORMATION

How to take:
Tablet—Swallow with liquid. It may be taken with
or without food. If you are unable to swallow
whole, crumble tablet and take with liquid or
food.

When to take:
Once a day at bedtime.

If you forget a dose:
Skip the missed dose and wait for next
scheduled dose (don't double this dose).

Continued next column

 OVERDOSE

SYMPTOMS:
**Severe nausea and vomiting, excessive
saliva, sweating, blood pressure decrease,
slow heartbeat, collapse, convulsions,
muscle weakness (including respiratory
muscles, which could lead to death).**
WHAT TO DO:
• **Dial 911 (emergency) or 0 (operator) for an
ambulance or medical help. Then give first
aid immediately.**
• **If patient is unconscious and not breathing,
use cardiac massage and mouth-to-mouth
breathing (CPR). Don't try to make patient
vomit. If you can't get help quickly, take
patient to nearest emergency facility.**
• **See emergency information on inside
covers.**

What drug does:
Slows breakdown of a brain chemical (acetylcholine) that gradually disappears from the
brains of people with Alzheimer's disease.

Time lapse before drug works:
May take several weeks before beneficial results
are observed. Dosage may be increased after 4
to 6 weeks if needed.

Don't take with:
Any other medication without consulting your
doctor or pharmacist. All possible drug
interactions have not been studied.

 POSSIBLE ADVERSE REACTIONS OR SIDE EFFECTS

SYMPTOMS	WHAT TO DO
Life-threatening: In case of overdose, see previous column.	
Common: Nausea, vomiting, diarrhea, insomnia, muscle cramps.	Continue. Call doctor when convenient.
Infrequent: Headache, weight loss, appetite decrease, depression, faintness, dizziness, drowsiness, joint pain, unusual tiredness, unusual bruising or bleeding, frequent urination.	Continue. Call doctor when convenient.
Rare: Problems with speech, unsteadiness, bloating, irregular heartbeat, changes in stool color, increased sweating, vision changes or eye irritation, increased libido, changes in blood pressure, incontinence, mood changes, mental changes, itching or other skin irritations, flushing or hot flashes, abdominal or chest pain, breathing difficulty.	Continue, but call doctor right away.

WARNINGS & PRECAUTIONS

Don't take if:
You are allergic to donepezil, tacrine or acridine derivatives*.

Before you start, consult your doctor:
- If you have heart disease.
- If you have a history of ulcer disease or are at risk of developing ulcers.
- If you have a history of liver disease or urinary tract disorder.
- If you have glaucoma.
- If you have epilepsy or seizure disorder.
- If you have a history of asthma or chronic obstructive pulmonary disease.

Over age 60:
No problems expected.

Pregnancy:
Unknown effect. Drug is usually not prescribed for women of childbearing age. Risk category C (see page xxiii).

Breast-feeding:
Unknown effect. Drug is not recommended for women of childbearing age.

Infants & children:
Not used in this age group.

Prolonged use:
- Drug may lose its effectiveness. Schedule regular visits with the doctor to determine if drug continues its effectiveness
- Talk to your doctor about the need for follow-up medical examinations or laboratory studies to check blood chemistries and liver function.

Skin & sunlight:
No problems expected.

Driving, piloting or hazardous work:
Don't drive or pilot aircraft until you learn how medicine affects you. Don't work around dangerous machinery. Don't climb ladders or work in high places. Danger increases if you drink alcohol or take other medicines affecting alertness and reflexes such as antihistamines, tranquilizers, sedatives, pain medicine, narcotics and mind-altering drugs.

Discontinuing:
Do not discontinue drug unless advised by doctor. Abrupt decreases in dosage may cause a cognitive decline.

Others:
- Advise any doctor or dentist whom you consult that you take this medicine.
- May affect the results in some medical tests.
- Do not increase dosage without doctor's approval.

 ## POSSIBLE INTERACTION WITH OTHER DRUGS

GENERIC NAME OR DRUG CLASS	COMBINED EFFECT
Anticholinergics*	Decreased anticholinergic effect.
Anti-inflammatories, nonsteroidal (NSAIDs)	May increase gastric acid secretions.
Enzyme inducers*	May decrease effect of donepezil.
Ketoconazole	May interact, but effect is unknown.
Quinidine	May interact, but effect is unknown.

 ## POSSIBLE INTERACTION WITH OTHER SUBSTANCES

INTERACTS WITH	COMBINED EFFECT
Alcohol:	None expected.
Beverages:	None expected.
Cocaine:	None expected.
Foods:	None expected.
Marijuana:	None expected.
Tobacco:	None expected.

*See Glossary

DORZOLAMIDE

BRAND NAMES

Cosopt   Trusopt

BASIC INFORMATION

Habit forming? No
Prescription needed? Yes
Available as generic? No
Drug class: Antiglaucoma (ophthalmic)

 USES

- Treatment for open-angle glaucoma (increased pressure in the eye).
- Treatment for ocular hypertension.

 DOSAGE & USAGE INFORMATION

How to use:
Eye drops
- Wash hands.
- Tilt head back.
- Press finger gently on the skin right under the lower eyelid; pull the eyelid away from the eye to make a space or small pocket.
- Drop the medicine into this pocket, then let go of the skin and gently close the eyes; don't blink.
- Keep the eyes closed and apply pressure to the inner corner of the eye with your finger for 1 to 2 minutes.
- Wash hands again after using the drops.
- To keep the solution germ-free, do not allow the applicator tip to touch the skin or eye.

When to use:
Normally used 3 times a day (about 8 hours apart). Always use as directed by your doctor.

If you forget a dose:
Use as soon as you remember. If it is almost time for the next dose, wait for next dose (don't double this dose).

Continued next column

 OVERDOSE

SYMPTOMS:
None expected.
WHAT TO DO:
Overdose unlikely to threaten life. If person use much larger amount than prescribed or if a child accidentally swallows, call doctor, poison control center or hospital emergency room for instructions.

What drug does:
This medicine is a topically applied carbonic anhydrase inhibitor that helps decrease production of aqueous humor (the fluid in the eye) and lowers the pressure inside the eye.

Time lapse before drug works:
30 to 60 minutes.

Don't take with:
Any other medicine (oral or topical) without consulting your doctor or pharmacist.

 POSSIBLE ADVERSE REACTIONS OR SIDE EFFECTS

SYMPTOMS	WHAT TO DO
Life-threatening: None expected.	
Common:	
• Allergic reaction (redness, itching or swelling of eye or eyelid); feeling of something in the eye; continued or severe sensitivity to light.	Discontinue. Call doctor right away.
• Bitter taste; burning, stinging or discomfort when medicine is used; increased sensitivity to light.	Continue. Call doctor when convenient.
Infrequent: Blurred vision, dryness or mild tearing of eyes, tiredness or weakness, headache.	Continue. Call doctor when convenient.
Rare: Blood in urine; ongoing nausea or vomiting; pain in back, side or abdomen; eye pain; severe or continued tearing; skin rash.	Discontinue. Call doctor right away.

WARNINGS & PRECAUTIONS

Don't use if:
You are allergic to dorzolamide or any sulfonamide* medications.

Before you start, consult your doctor:
• If you have kidney or liver disease.
• If you wear soft contact lenses. The amount of time you use the soft contact lenses may need to be reduced.
• If you are allergic to any medication, food, or other substances.

Over age 60:
No special problems expected.

Pregnancy:
Decide with your doctor whether drug benefits justify risk to unborn child. Risk category C (see page xxiii).

Breast-feeding:
Unknown effect. Avoid drug or discontinue nursing until you finish medicine. Consult doctor for advice on maintaining milk supply.

Infants & children:
Safety and dosage have not been established. Use only under medical supervision.

Prolonged use:
Schedule regular appointments with your doctor for eye examinations to be sure the medication is controlling the glaucoma.

Skin & sunlight:
No special problems expected.

Driving, piloting or hazardous work:
Don't drive a motor vehicle or pilot aircraft until you learn how medicine affects you. Don't work around dangerous machinery. Don't climb ladders or work in high places.

Discontinuing:
Don't discontinue without consulting your doctor.

Others:
• Don't let the medicine's applicator touch the eye or surrounding skin. If it does, it can become contaminated by common bacteria known to cause eye infections that can cause serious damage to the eye.
• If you develop an eye infection or experience an injury to the eye, consult your doctor about the continued use of that particular container of your medicine. It may have become contaminated.
• Advise any doctor or dentist whom you consult that you use this medicine.
• Wear sunglasses when outside in sunlight.

POSSIBLE INTERACTION WITH OTHER DRUGS

GENERIC NAME OR DRUG CLASS	COMBINED EFFECT
Amphetamines	Increased risk of side effects.
Mecamylamine	Increased risk of side effects.
Other topical eye medicines	One medicine may "wash out" the other. Use the two at least 10 minutes apart.
Quinidine	Increased risk of side effects.

POSSIBLE INTERACTION WITH OTHER SUBSTANCES

INTERACTS WITH	COMBINED EFFECT
Alcohol:	No special problems expected.
Beverages:	No special problems expected.
Cocaine:	No special problems expected.
Foods:	No special problems expected.
Marijuana:	No special problems expected.
Tobacco:	No special problems expected.

DOXEPIN (Topical)

BRAND NAMES

Zonalon

BASIC INFORMATION

Habit forming? No
Prescription needed? Yes
Available as generic? No
Drug class: Antipruritic (topical)

 ## USES

Treats itching of the skin caused by certain types of eczema (an inflammation of the skin).

 ## DOSAGE & USAGE INFORMATION

How to use:
Cream—Apply a thin layer to the affected area of skin and gently rub it in. Do not cover the treated area with a bandage or other dressing.

When to use:
4 times a day. Allow 3 to 4 hours between applications. Not to be used longer than 8 days.

If you forget a dose:
Use as soon as you remember. If it is almost time for the next dose, wait for the next scheduled dose (don't double this dose).

Continued next column

 ## OVERDOSE

SYMPTOMS:
An overdose of topical medicine is unlikely to occur, but if too much is applied, it can be absorbed into the system.
- **Mild effects include blurred vision, drowsiness, very dry mouth, decreased awareness or responsiveness.**
- **More severe effects include irregular or fast heartbeat, enlarged pupils, jerking movements, dizziness, fainting, abdominal pain or swelling, weak or feeble pulse, high fever or low temperature, vomiting, incurable constipation, seizures, breathing difficulty, unconsciousness.**

WHAT TO DO:
- **Dial 911 (emergency) or 0 (operator) for an ambulance or medical help. Then give first aid immediately.**
- **See emergency information on inside covers.**

What drug does:
The exact mechanism is unknown. It appears to block histamine* reactions, which can cause the itching. The drug also has a sedating effect on some people, which can help to relieve the itching symptoms. Variable and sometimes significant amounts of the drug are absorbed through the skin.

Time lapse before drug works:
May take up to 8 days for maximum benefit.

Don't take with:
Any other oral or topical medication without consulting your doctor or pharmacist. This includes nonprescription drugs such as cold or allergy remedies that may contain alcohol or antihistamines. They increase the risk of drowsiness.

 ## POSSIBLE ADVERSE REACTIONS OR SIDE EFFECTS

SYMPTOMS	WHAT TO DO
Life-threatening:	
In case of overdose, see previous column.	
Common:	
• Swelling of the skin where drug is applied; worsening of the itching; burning, tingling or crawling feeling in the skin.	Discontinue. Call doctor right away.
• Stinging of skin where drug is applied, dryness or tightness of skin, taste changes, dizziness, drowsiness, dry mouth or lips, thirst, emotional changes, fatigue, headache.	Continue. Call doctor when convenient.
Infrequent:	
Scaling or cracking of the skin, nausea, anxiety, irritation.	Continue. Call doctor when convenient.
Rare:	
Fever.	Discontinue. Call doctor right away.

Note: Though the drug is applied topically, it is absorbed into the bloodstream and can cause systemic reactions. Adverse reactions are more likely in patients who use the drug on more than 10% of their body surface.

WARNINGS & PRECAUTIONS

Don't use if:
You are allergic to doxepin.

Before you start, consult your doctor:
- If you have narrow-angle glaucoma.
- If you are allergic to any other medications.
- If you have a problem with urinary retention.

Over age 60:
No special problems expected.

Pregnancy:
Consult doctor. Risk category B (page xxiii).

Breast-feeding:
Drug passes into milk. Avoid drug or discontinue nursing until you finish medicine. Consult doctor for advice on maintaining milk supply.

Infants & children:
Safety in children has not been established. Use only under close medical supervision.

Prolonged use:
Don't use for more than 8 days unless directed by doctor. Longer use can increase the risk of side effects or adverse reactions.

Skin & sunlight:
No special problems expected.

Driving, piloting or hazardous work:
Don't drive or pilot aircraft until you learn how medicine affects you. Don't work around dangerous machinery. Don't climb ladders or work in high places. Danger increases if you drink alcohol or take medicine affecting alertness and reflexes.

Discontinuing:
To be sure of maximum benefit, don't discontinue this medicine before the treatment has been completed unless advised to do so by your doctor.

Others:
- Use medicine only on affected area. It is not to be used in the mouth, the eyes or the vagina.
- Advise any doctor or dentist whom you consult that you are using this medicine.
- If your skin condition doesn't improve within 8 days, consult doctor.
- Use medicine only as directed. Do not increase or reduce dosage without doctor's approval.

POSSIBLE INTERACTION WITH OTHER DRUGS

GENERIC NAME OR DRUG CLASS	COMBINED EFFECT
Antidepressants*	Increased risk of toxicity of both drugs.
Carbamazepine	Increased risk of toxicity of both drugs.
Central nervous system (CNS) depressants*	Increased sedation. May need dosage adjustment.
Cimetidine	Increased risk of doxepin toxicity.
Dextromethorphan	Increased risk of toxicity of both drugs.
Flecainide	Increased risk of toxicity of both drugs.
Monoamine oxidase (MAO) inhibitors*	Potentially life-threatening. Allow 14 days between use of the 2 drugs.
Phenothiazines*	Increased risk of toxicity of both drugs.
Propafenone	Increased risk of toxicity of both drugs.
Quinidine	Increased risk of toxicity of both drugs.

POSSIBLE INTERACTION WITH OTHER SUBSTANCES

INTERACTS WITH	COMBINED EFFECT
Alcohol:	Increased sedative effect. Avoid.
Beverages:	No special problems expected.
Cocaine:	Problems not known. Best to avoid.
Foods:	No special problems expected.
Marijuana:	Problems not known. Best to avoid.
Tobacco:	No special problems expected.

*See Glossary

DRONABINOL (THC, Marijuana)

BRAND NAMES

Marinol

BASIC INFORMATION

Habit forming? Yes
Prescription needed? Yes
Available as generic? No
Drug class: Antiemetic

 ## USES

- Prevents nausea and vomiting that may accompany taking anticancer medication (cancer chemotherapy). Should not be used unless other antinausea medicines fail.
- Appetite stimulant. Used to treat appetite loss in AIDS patients.

 ## DOSAGE & USAGE INFORMATION

How to take:
Capsule—Swallow with liquid.

When to take:
Under supervision, a total of no more than 4 to 6 doses per day, every 2 to 4 hours after cancer chemotherapy for prescribed number of days.

If you forget a dose:
Take as soon as you remember up to 2 hours late. If more than 2 hours, wait for next scheduled dose (don't double this dose).

What drug does:
Affects nausea and vomiting center in brain to make it less irritable following cancer chemotherapy. Exact mechanism is unknown.

Time lapse before drug works:
2 to 4 hours.

Don't take with:
Nonprescription drugs without consulting doctor.

 ## OVERDOSE

SYMPTOMS:
Pounding, rapid heart rate; high or low blood pressure; confusion; hallucinations; drastic mood changes; nervousness or anxiety.
WHAT TO DO:
Overdose unlikely to threaten life. If person takes much larger amount than prescribed, call doctor, poison control center or hospital emergency room for instructions.

 ## POSSIBLE ADVERSE REACTIONS OR SIDE EFFECTS

SYMPTOMS	WHAT TO DO
Life-threatening:	
In case of overdose, see previous column.	
Common:	
• Rapid, pounding heartbeat.	Discontinue. Call doctor right away.
• Dizziness, irritability, drowsiness, euphoria, decreased coordination.	Continue. Call doctor when convenient.
• Red eyes, dry mouth.	No action necessary.
Infrequent:	
• Depression, anxiety, nervousness, headache, hallucinations, dramatic mood changes.	Discontinue. Call doctor right away.
• Blurred or changed vision.	Continue. Call doctor when convenient.
Rare:	
• Rapid heartbeat, fainting, frequent or difficult urination, convulsions, shortness of breath.	Discontinue. Call doctor right away.
• Paranoia, nausea, loss of appetite, dizziness when standing after sitting or lying down, diarrhea.	Continue. Call doctor when convenient.

 ## WARNINGS & PRECAUTIONS

Don't take if:
- Your nausea and vomiting is caused by anything other than cancer chemotherapy.
- You are sensitive or allergic to any form of marijuana or sesame oil.
- Your cycle of chemotherapy is longer than 7 consecutive days. Harmful side effects may occur.

Before you start, consult your doctor:
- If you have heart disease or high blood pressure.
- If you are an alcoholic or drug addict.
- If you are pregnant or intend to become pregnant.
- If you are nursing an infant.
- If you have schizophrenia or a manic-depressive disorder.

Over age 60:
Adverse reactions and side effects may be more frequent and severe than in younger persons.

Pregnancy:
Decide with your doctor if drug benefits justify risk to unborn child. Risk category C (see page xxiii).

Breast-feeding:
Drug passes into milk. Avoid drug or discontinue nursing until you finish medicine. Consult doctor about maintaining milk supply.

Infants & children:
Not recommended.

Prolonged use:
- Avoid. Habit forming.
- Talk to your doctor about the need for follow-up medical examinations or laboratory studies to check heart function.

Skin & sunlight:
No problems expected.

Driving, piloting or hazardous work:
Don't drive or pilot aircraft until you learn how medicine affects you. Don't work around dangerous machinery. Don't climb ladders or work in high places. Danger increases if you drink alcohol or take medicine affecting alertness and reflexes, such as antihistamines, tranquilizers, sedatives, pain medicine, narcotics and mind-altering drugs.

Discontinuing:
Withdrawal effects such as irritability, insomnia, restlessness, sweating, diarrhea, hiccups, loss of appetite and hot flashes may follow abrupt withdrawal within 12 hours. Should they occur, these symptoms will probably subside within 96 hours.

Others:
Store in refrigerator.

POSSIBLE INTERACTION WITH OTHER DRUGS

GENERIC NAME OR DRUG CLASS	COMBINED EFFECT
Anesthetics*	Oversedation.
Anticonvulsants*	Oversedation.
Antidepressants, tricyclic*	Oversedation.
Antihistamines*	Oversedation.
Barbiturates*	Oversedation.
Clozapine	Toxic effect on the central nervous system.
Ethinamate	Dangerous increased effects of ethinamate. Avoid combining.
Fluoxetine	Increased depressant effects of both drugs.
Guanfacine	May increase depressant effects of either drug.
Leucovorin	High alcohol content of leucovorin may cause adverse effects.
Methyprylon	Increased sedative effect, perhaps to dangerous level. Avoid.
Molindone	Increased effects of both drugs. Avoid.
Muscle relaxants*	Oversedation.
Nabilone	Greater depression of central nervous system.
Narcotics*	Oversedation.
Sedatives*	Oversedation.
Sertraline	Increased depressive effects of both drugs.
Tranquilizers*	Oversedation.

POSSIBLE INTERACTION WITH OTHER SUBSTANCES

INTERACTS WITH	COMBINED EFFECT
Alcohol:	Oversedation.
Beverages:	No problems expected.
Cocaine:	No problems expected.
Foods:	No problems expected.
Marijuana:	Oversedation.
Tobacco:	No problems expected.

EPHEDRINE

BRAND NAMES

See complete list of brand names in the *Generic and Brand Name Directory*, page 880.

BASIC INFORMATION

Habit forming? No
Prescription needed?
  Low Strength: No
  High Strength: Yes
Available as generic? Yes, for some.
Drug class: Sympathomimetic

 ## USES

- Relieves bronchial asthma.
- Decreases congestion of breathing passages.
- Suppresses allergic reactions.

 ## DOSAGE & USAGE INFORMATION

How to take:
- Tablet or capsule—Swallow with liquid. You may chew or crush tablet.
- Extended-release tablets or capsules—Swallow each dose whole.
- Syrup—Take as directed on bottle.
- Drops—Dilute dose in beverage.

When to take:
As needed, no more often than every 4 hours. To prevent insomnia, take last dose at least 2 hours before bedtime.

If you forget a dose:
Take up to 2 hours late. If more than 2 hours, wait for next dose (don't double this dose).

What drug does:
- Prevents cells from releasing allergy-causing chemicals (histamines).
- Relaxes muscles of bronchial tubes.
- Decreases blood vessel size and blood flow, thus causing decongestion.

Continued next column

 ## OVERDOSE

SYMPTOMS:
Severe anxiety, confusion, delirium, muscle tremors, rapid and irregular pulse.
WHAT TO DO:
- **Dial 911 (emergency) or 0 (operator) for an ambulance or medical help. Then give first aid immediately.**
- **See emergency information on inside covers.**

Time lapse before drug works:
30 to 60 minutes.

Don't take with:
- Nonprescription drugs with ephedrine, pseudoephedrine or epinephrine.
- Nonprescription drugs for cough, cold, allergy or asthma without consulting doctor.

 ## POSSIBLE ADVERSE REACTIONS OR SIDE EFFECTS

SYMPTOMS	WHAT TO DO
Life-threatening:	
In case of overdose, see previous column.	
Common:	
• Nervousness, headache, paleness, rapid heartbeat.	Continue. Call doctor when convenient.
• Insomnia.	Continue. Tell doctor at next visit.
Infrequent:	
• Irregular heartbeat.	Discontinue. Call doctor right away.
• Dizziness, appetite loss, nausea, vomiting, painful or difficult urination.	Continue. Call doctor when convenient.
Rare:	
None expected.	

 ## WARNINGS & PRECAUTIONS

Don't take if:
You are allergic to ephedrine or any sympathomimetic* drug.

Before you start, consult your doctor:
- If you have high blood pressure.
- If you have diabetes.
- If you have overactive thyroid gland.
- If you have difficulty urinating.
- If you have taken any MAO inhibitor in past 2 weeks.
- If you have taken digitalis preparations in the last 7 days.
- If you will have surgery within 2 months, including dental surgery, requiring general or spinal anesthesia.

Over age 60:
More likely to develop high blood pressure, heart-rhythm disturbances, angina and to feel drug's stimulant effects.

Pregnancy:
Decide with your doctor if drug benefits justify risk to unborn child. Risk category C (see page xxiii).

Breast-feeding:
Drug passes into milk. Avoid drug or discontinue nursing until you finish medicine. Consult doctor for advice on maintaining milk supply.

Infants & children:
No problems expected.

Prolonged use:
- Excessive doses—Rare toxic psychosis.
- Men with enlarged prostate gland may have more urination difficulty.

Skin & sunlight:
No problems expected.

Driving, piloting or hazardous work:
Avoid if you feel dizzy. Otherwise, no problems expected.

Discontinuing:
May be unnecessary to finish medicine. Follow doctor's instructions.

Others:
No problems expected.

POSSIBLE INTERACTION WITH OTHER DRUGS

GENERIC NAME OR DRUG CLASS	COMBINED EFFECT
Adrenocorticoids, systemic	Decreased adrenocorticoid effect.
Antidepressants, tricyclic*	Increased effect of ephedrine. Excessive stimulation of heart and blood pressure.
Antihypertensives*	Decreased antihypertensive effect.
Beta-adrenergic blocking agents*	Decreased effects of both drugs.
Dextrothyroxine	Increased ephedrine effect.
Digitalis preparations*	Serious heart rhythm disturbances.
Epinephrine	Increased epinephrine effect.
Ergot preparations*	Serious blood pressure rise.
Furazolidine	Sudden, severe increase in blood pressure.
Guanadrel	Decreased effect of both drugs.
Guanethidine	Decreased effect of both drugs.
Methyldopa	Possible increased blood pressure.
Monoamine oxidase (MAO) inhibitors*	Increased ephedrine effect. Dangerous blood pressure rise.
Nitrates*	Possible decreased effects of both drugs.
Phenothiazines*	Possible increased ephedrine toxicity. Possible decreased ephedrine effect.
Pseudoephedrine	Increased pseudoephedrine effect.
Rauwolfia	Decreased rauwolfia effect.
Sympathomimetics*	Increased ephedrine effect.
Terazosin	Decreases effectiveness of terazosin.
Theophylline	Increased gastrointestinal intolerance.

POSSIBLE INTERACTION WITH OTHER SUBSTANCES

INTERACTS WITH	COMBINED EFFECT
Alcohol:	None expected.
Beverages: Caffeine drinks.	Nervousness or insomnia.
Cocaine:	High risk of heartbeat irregularities and high blood pressure.
Foods:	None expected.
Marijuana:	Rapid heartbeat, possible heart rhythm disturbance.
Tobacco:	None expected.

ERGOLOID MESYLATES

BRAND NAMES

Gerimal   Hydergine LC
Hydergine   Niloric

BASIC INFORMATION

Habit forming? No
Prescription needed? Yes
Available as generic? Yes
Drug class: Ergot preparation

USES

Treatment for reduced alertness, poor memory, confusion, depression or lack of motivation in the elderly.

DOSAGE & USAGE INFORMATION

How to take:
- Tablet or capsule—Swallow with liquid. If you can't swallow whole, crumble tablet or open capsule and take with liquid or food.
- Liquid—Take as directed on label.
- Sublingual tablets—Dissolve tablet under tongue.

When to take:
At the same times each day.

If you forget a dose:
Take as soon as you remember up to 2 hours late. If more than 2 hours, wait for next scheduled dose (don't double this dose).

What drug does:
Stimulates brain-cell metabolism to increase use of oxygen and nutrients.

Time lapse before drug works:
Gradual improvements over 3 to 4 months.

Continued next column

OVERDOSE

SYMPTOMS:
Headache, flushed face, nasal congestion, nausea, vomiting, blood pressure drop, blurred vision, weakness, collapse, coma.
WHAT TO DO:
- **Dial 911 (emergency) or 0 (operator) for an ambulance or medical help. Then give first aid immediately.**
- **See emergency information on inside covers.**

Don't take with:
- Nonprescription drugs containing alcohol without consulting doctor.
- Any other medication without consulting your doctor or pharmacist.

POSSIBLE ADVERSE REACTIONS OR SIDE EFFECTS

SYMPTOMS	WHAT TO DO
Life-threatening: In case of overdose, see previous column.	
Common: Runny nose, skin flushing, headache.	Continue. Tell doctor at next visit.
Infrequent: • Slow heartbeat, tingling fingers.	Discontinue. Call doctor right away.
• Blurred vision.	Continue. Call doctor when convenient.
Rare: • Fainting.	Discontinue. Seek emergency treatment.
• Rash, nausea, vomiting, stomach cramps, dizziness when getting up, drowsiness, soreness under tongue, appetite loss.	Continue. Call doctor when convenient.

ERGOLOID MESYLATES

WARNINGS & PRECAUTIONS

Don't use if:
- If you are allergic to any ergot preparation.
- Your heartbeat is less than 60 beats per minute.
- Your systolic blood pressure is consistently below 100.

Before you start, consult your doctor:
- If you have had low blood pressure.
- If you have liver disease.
- If you have severe mental illness.

Over age 60:
Primarily used in persons older than 60. Results unpredictable, but many patients show improved brain function.

Pregnancy:
Decide with your doctor if drug benefits justify risk to unborn child. Risk category C (see page xxiii).

Breast-feeding:
Risk to nursing child outweighs drug benefits. Don't use.

Infants & children:
Not recommended.

Prolonged use:
Talk to your doctor about the need for follow-up medical examinations or laboratory studies.

Skin & sunlight:
No problems expected.

Driving, piloting or hazardous work:
Avoid if you feel dizzy, faint or have blurred vision. Otherwise, no problems expected.

Discontinuing:
No problems expected.

Others:
May lessen your body's ability to adjust to cold temperatures.

POSSIBLE INTERACTION WITH OTHER DRUGS

GENERIC NAME OR DRUG CLASS	COMBINED EFFECT
Ergot preparations, other	May cause decreased circulation to arms, legs, feet and hands. Avoid.
Sympathomimetics*	May cause decreased circulation to arms, legs, feet and hands. Avoid.

POSSIBLE INTERACTION WITH OTHER SUBSTANCES

INTERACTS WITH	COMBINED EFFECT
Alcohol:	Use caution. May drop blood pressure excessively.
Beverages:	None expected.
Cocaine:	Overstimulation. Avoid.
Foods:	None expected.
Marijuana:	Decreased effect of ergot alkaloids.
Tobacco:	Decreased ergoloid effect. Don't smoke.

ERGONOVINE

BRAND NAMES

Ergometrine   Ergotrate Maleate
Ergotrate

BASIC INFORMATION

Habit forming? No
Prescription needed? Yes
Available as generic? Yes
Drug class: Ergot preparation (uterine stimulant)

 USES

Retards excessive post-delivery bleeding.

 DOSAGE & USAGE INFORMATION

How to take:
Tablet—Swallow with liquid or food to lessen stomach irritation.

When to take:
At the same times each day.

If you forget a dose:
Don't take missed dose and don't double next one. Wait for next scheduled dose.

What drug does:
Causes smooth muscle cells of uterine wall to contract and surround bleeding blood vessels of relaxed uterus.

Time lapse before drug works:
Tablets—20 to 30 minutes.

Don't take with:
Any other medicine without consulting your doctor or pharmacist.

 OVERDOSE

SYMPTOMS:
Vomiting, diarrhea, weak pulse, low blood pressure, difficult breathing, angina, convulsions.
WHAT TO DO:
* **Dial 911 (emergency) or 0 (operator) for an ambulance or medical help. Then give first aid immediately.**
* **If patient is unconscious and not breathing, give mouth-to-mouth breathing. If there is no heartbeat, use cardiac massage and mouth-to-mouth breathing (CPR). Don't try to make patient vomit. If you can't get help quickly, take patient to nearest emergency facility.**
* **See emergency information on inside covers.**

 POSSIBLE ADVERSE REACTIONS OR SIDE EFFECTS

SYMPTOMS	WHAT TO DO
Life-threatening:	
In case of overdose, see previous column.	
Common:	
Nausea, vomiting, severe lower abdominal menstrual-like cramps.	Discontinue. Call doctor right away.
Infrequent:	
• Confusion, ringing in ears, diarrhea, muscle cramps.	Discontinue. Call doctor right away.
• Unusual sweating.	Continue. Call doctor when convenient.
Rare:	
Sudden, severe headache; shortness of breath; chest pain; numb, cold hands and feet.	Discontinue. Seek emergency treatment.

ERGONOVINE

WARNINGS & PRECAUTIONS

Don't take if:
You are allergic to any ergot preparation.

Before you start, consult your doctor:
- If you have coronary artery or blood vessel disease.
- If you have liver or kidney disease.
- If you have high blood pressure.
- If you have postpartum infection.

Over age 60:
Not recommended.

Pregnancy:
Risk to unborn child outweighs drug benefits. Don't use. Risk category X (see page xxIII).

Breast-feeding:
Drug passes into milk. Avoid drug or discontinue nursing until you finish medicine. Consult doctor for advice on maintaining milk supply.

Infants & children:
Not recommended.

Prolonged use:
Talk to your doctor about the need for follow-up medical examinations or laboratory studies to check blood pressure, ECG*.

Skin & sunlight:
No problems expected.

Driving, piloting or hazardous work:
No problems expected.

Discontinuing:
May be unnecessary to finish medicine. Follow doctor's instructions.

Others:
Drug should be used for short time only following childbirth or miscarriage.

POSSIBLE INTERACTION WITH OTHER DRUGS

GENERIC NAME OR DRUG CLASS	COMBINED EFFECT
Beta-adrenergic blocking agents*	Possible vasospasm (peripheral and cardiac).
Ergot preparations, other	May cause decreased circulation to arms, legs, feet and hands. Avoid.
Sympathomimetics*	May cause decreased circulation to arms, legs, feet and hands. Avoid.

POSSIBLE INTERACTION WITH OTHER SUBSTANCES

INTERACTS WITH	COMBINED EFFECT
Alcohol:	None expected.
Beverages:	None expected.
Cocaine:	None expected.
Foods:	None expected.
Marijuana:	None expected.
Tobacco:	Decreased ergonovine effect. Don't smoke.

*See Glossary

ERGOTAMINE

BRAND NAMES

Cafergot	Ergostat
Cafergot-PB	Gotamine
Cafertine	Gynergen
Cafetrate	Medihaler
Ercaf	Ergotamine
Ergo-caff	Migergot
Ergomar	Wigraine

BASIC INFORMATION

Habit forming? No
Prescription needed? Yes
Available as generic? No
Drug class: Vasoconstrictor, ergot preparation

USES

Relieves pain of migraines and other headaches caused by dilated blood vessels. Will not prevent headaches.

DOSAGE & USAGE INFORMATION

How to take:
- Tablet—Swallow with liquid. If you can't swallow whole, crumble tablet and take with liquid or food.
- Sublingual tablet—Don't swallow whole. Let dissolve under tongue. Don't eat or drink while tablet is dissolving.
- Suppositories—Remove wrapper and moisten suppository with water. Gently insert larger end into rectum. Push well into rectum with finger.
- Aerosol inhaler—Use only as directed on prescription label.
- Lie down in quiet, dark room after taking.

Continued next column

OVERDOSE

SYMPTOMS:
Tingling, cold extremities and muscle pain. Progresses to nausea, vomiting, diarrhea, cold skin, rapid and weak pulse, severe numbness of extremities, confusion, convulsions, coma.
WHAT TO DO:
- **Dial 911 (emergency) or 0 (operator) for an ambulance or medical help. Then give first aid immediately.**
- **See emergency information on inside covers.**

When to take:
At first sign of vascular or migraine headache.

If you forget a dose:
Take as soon as you remember. Wait 4 hours for next dose.

What drug does:
Constricts blood vessels in the head.

Time lapse before drug works:
30 to 60 minutes.

Don't take with:
Any other medicine without consulting your doctor or pharmacist.

POSSIBLE ADVERSE REACTIONS OR SIDE EFFECTS

SYMPTOMS	WHAT TO DO
Life-threatening: In case of overdose, see previous column.	
Common: • Dizziness, nausea, diarrhea, vomiting, increased frequency or severity of headaches.	Continue. Call doctor when convenient.
• Feet and ankle swelling.	Discontinue. Call doctor right away.
Infrequent: Itchy or swollen skin; cold, pale hands or feet; pain or weakness in arms, legs, back.	Discontinue. Call doctor right away.
Rare: Anxiety or confusion; red or purple blisters, especially on hands, feet; change in vision; extreme thirst; stomach pain or bloating; unusually fast or slow heartbeat; chest pain; numbness or tingling in face, fingers, toes.	Discontinue. Call doctor right away.

WARNINGS & PRECAUTIONS

Don't take if:
You are allergic to any ergot preparation.

Before you start, consult your doctor:
- If you plan to become pregnant within medication period.
- If you have an infection.
- If you have angina, heart problems, high blood pressure, hardening of the arteries or vein problems.
- If you have kidney or liver disease.
- If you are allergic to other spray inhalants.

Over age 60:
Adverse reactions and side effects may be more frequent and severe than in younger persons.

Pregnancy:
Risk to unborn child outweighs drug benefits. Don't use. Risk category X (see page xxiii).

Breast-feeding:
Drug filters into milk. May harm child. Avoid.

Infants & children:
Studies inconclusive on harm to children. Consult your doctor.

Prolonged use:
Cold skin, muscle pain, gangrene of hands and feet. This medicine not intended for uninterrupted use.

Skin & sunlight:
No problems expected.

Driving, piloting or hazardous work:
Don't drive or pilot aircraft until you learn how medicine affects you. Don't work around dangerous machinery. Don't climb ladders or work in high places. Danger increases if you drink alcohol or take medicine affecting alertness and reflexes, such as antihistamines, tranquilizers, sedatives, pain medicine, narcotics and mind-altering drugs.

Discontinuing:
May be unnecessary to finish medicine. Follow doctor's instructions.

Others:
- Impaired blood circulation can lead to gangrene in intestines or extremities. Never exceed recommended dose.
- May affect results in some medical tests.

POSSIBLE INTERACTION WITH OTHER DRUGS

GENERIC NAME OR DRUG CLASS	COMBINED EFFECT
Amphetamines*	Dangerous blood pressure rise.
Beta-adrenergic blocking agents*	Narrowed arteries in heart if ergotamine is taken in high doses.
Ephedrine	Dangerous blood pressure rise.
Epinephrine	Dangerous blood pressure rise.
Ergot preparations, other	May cause decreased circulation to arms, legs, feet and hands. Avoid.
Erythromycin	Decreased ergotamine effect.
Nitroglycerin	Decreased nitroglycerin effect.
Pseudoephedrine	Dangerous blood pressure rise.
Sumatriptan	Increased vasoconstriction. Delay 24 hours between drugs.
Sympathomimetics*	May cause decreased circulation to arms, legs, feet and hands. Avoid.
Troleandomycin	Decreased ergotamine effect.

POSSIBLE INTERACTION WITH OTHER SUBSTANCES

INTERACTS WITH	COMBINED EFFECT
Alcohol:	Dilates blood vessels. Makes headache worse.
Beverages: Caffeine drinks.	May help relieve headache.
Cocaine:	Decreased ergotamine effect.
Foods: Any to which you are allergic.	May make headache worse. Avoid.
Marijuana:	Occasional use—Cool extremities. Regular use—Persistent chill.
Tobacco:	Decreased effect of ergotamine. Makes headache worse.

ERGOTAMINE, BELLADONNA & PHENOBARBITAL

BRAND NAMES

Bellergal   Bellergal Spacetabs
Bellergal-S

BASIC INFORMATION

Habit forming? Yes
Prescription needed? Yes
Available as generic? No
Drug class: Analgesic, antispasmodic, vasoconstrictor

USES

- Reduces anxiety or nervous tension (low dose).
- Prevents vascular headaches.

DOSAGE & USAGE INFORMATION

How to take:
- Tablet or extended-release tablet—Swallow with liquid, or let dissolve under tongue.
- Lie down in quiet, dark room after taking.

When to take:
At first sign of vascular or migraine headache.

If you forget a dose:
Take as soon as you remember. Wait 4 hours for next dose.

What drug does:
- Constricts blood vessels in the head.
- Blocks nerve impulses at parasympathetic nerve endings, preventing muscle contractions and gland secretions of organs involved.

Continued next column

OVERDOSE

SYMPTOMS:
Tingling, cold extremities; muscle pain; nausea; vomiting; diarrhea; cold skin; rapid and weak pulse; severe numbness of extremities; confusion; dilated pupils; rapid pulse and breathing; dizziness; fever; hallucinations; slurred speech; agitation; flushed face; convulsions; coma.
WHAT TO DO:
- Dial 911 (emergency) or 0 (operator) for an ambulance or medical help. Then give first aid immediately.
- See emergency information on inside covers.

Time lapse before drug works:
15 to 30 minutes.

Don't take with:
Nonprescription drugs without consulting doctor.

POSSIBLE ADVERSE REACTIONS OR SIDE EFFECTS

SYMPTOMS	WHAT TO DO
Life-threatening:	
In case of overdose, see previous column.	
Common:	
• Flushed skin, fever, drowsiness, bloating, depression, frequent urination.	Discontinue. Call doctor right away.
• Constipation, dizziness, drowsiness, "hangover" effect, increased frequency or severity of headaches.	Continue. Call doctor when convenient.
Infrequent:	
• Swollen feet and ankles, numbness or tingling in hands or feet, cold hands and feet, rash.	Discontinue. Call doctor right away.
• Nasal congestion, altered taste.	Continue. Call doctor when convenient.
Rare:	
Jaundice, weak legs, swallowing difficulty, dry mouth, increased sensitivity to sunlight, nausea, vomiting, decreased sweating.	Discontinue. Call doctor right away.

WARNINGS & PRECAUTIONS

Don't take if:
- You are allergic to any barbiturate, tartrazine dye, anticholinergic or ergot preparation.
- You have porphyria, trouble with stomach bloating, difficulty emptying your bladder completely, narrow-angle glaucoma, severe ulcerative colitis, enlarged prostate.

Before you start, consult your doctor:
- If you have epilepsy; kidney, thyroid or liver damage; anemia; chronic pain; open-angle glaucoma; angina; fast heartbeat; heart problems; high blood pressure; hardening of the arteries; vein problems; chronic bronchitis; asthma; hiatal hernia; enlarged prostate; myasthenia gravis; peptic ulcer; an infection.
- If you plan to become pregnant within medication period.

344

ERGOTAMINE, BELLADONNA & PHENOBARBITAL

- If you will have surgery within 2 months, including dental surgery, requiring general or spinal anesthesia.

Over age 60:
Adverse reactions and side effects may be more frequent and severe than in younger persons.

Pregnancy:
Risk to unborn child outweighs drug benefits. Don't use. Risk category X (see page xxiii).

Breast-feeding:
Drug passes into milk. Avoid drug or discontinue nursing until you finish medicine. Consult doctor for advice on maintaining milk supply.

Infants & children:
Not recommended.

Prolonged use:
- May cause addiction, anemia, chronic intoxication.
- May lower body temperature, making exposure to cold temperatures hazardous.
- Chronic constipation, possible fecal impaction.
- Cold skin, muscle pain, gangrene of hands and feet. This medicine not intended for uninterrupted use.

Skin & sunlight:
One or more drugs in this group may cause rash or intensify sunburn in areas exposed to sun or ultraviolet light (photosensitivity reaction). Avoid overexposure. Notify doctor if reaction occurs.

Driving, piloting or hazardous work:
Don't drive or pilot aircraft until you learn how medicine affects you. Don't work around dangerous machinery. Don't climb ladders or work in high places. Danger increases if you drink alcohol or take medicine affecting alertness and reflexes, such as antihistamines, tranquilizers, sedatives, pain medicine, narcotics and mind-altering drugs.

Discontinuing:
May be unnecessary to finish medicine. Follow doctor's instructions. If you develop withdrawal symptoms of hallucinations, agitation or sleeplessness after discontinuing, call doctor right away.

Others:
- Impaired blood circulation can lead to gangrene in intestines or extremities. Never exceed recommended dose.
- May affect results in some medical tests.

POSSIBLE INTERACTION WITH OTHER DRUGS

GENERIC NAME OR DRUG CLASS	COMBINED EFFECT
Amantadine	Increased belladonna effect.

Amphetamines*	Dangerous blood pressure rise.
Anticholinergics, other*	Increased belladonna effect.
Anticoagulants, oral*	Decreased anticoagulant effect.
Anticonvulsants*	Changed seizure patterns.
Antidepressants, tricyclic*	Decreased antidepressant effect. Possible dangerous oversedation.
Antidiabetics, oral*	Increased phenobarbital effect.
Antihistamines*	Dangerous sedation. Avoid.
Aspirin	Decreased aspirin effect.
Beta-adrenergic blocking agents*	Narrowed arteries in heart if taken in large doses.
Contraceptives, oral*	Decreased contraceptive effect.
Cortisone drugs*	Decreased cortisone effect. Increased internal eye pressure.
Digitoxin	Decreased digitoxin effect.
Doxycycline	Decreased doxycycline effect.
Dronabinol	Increased effect of drugs.

Continued on page 914

POSSIBLE INTERACTION WITH OTHER SUBSTANCES

INTERACTS WITH	COMBINED EFFECT
Alcohol:	Possible fatal oversedation. Avoid.
Beverages:	None expected.
Cocaine:	Excessively rapid heartbeat. Avoid.
Foods:	None expected.
Marijuana:	Drowsiness and dry mouth, excessive sedation. Avoid.
Tobacco:	None expected.

*See Glossary

345

ERYTHROMYCINS

GENERIC AND BRAND NAMES

See complete list of generic and brand names in the *Generic and Brand Name Directory*, page 880.

BASIC INFORMATION

Habit forming? No
Prescription needed? Yes
Available as generic? Yes
Drug class: Antibacterial

USES

Treatment of infections responsive to erythromycin.

DOSAGE & USAGE INFORMATION

How to take:
- Tablet or capsule—Swallow with liquid. You may chew or crush.
- Extended-release tablets or capsules—Swallow each dose whole.
- Oral suspension—Shake well before using. Use dropper supplied with prescription or use a specially marked measuring spoon to measure dose.

When to take:
At the same times each day, 1 hour before or 2 hours after eating. May be taken with food if stomach upset occurs.

If you forget a dose:
- If you take 3 or more doses daily—Take as soon as you remember. Return to regular schedule.
- If you take 2 doses daily—Take as soon as you remember. Wait 5 to 6 hours for next dose. Return to regular schedule.

What drug does:
Prevents growth and reproduction of susceptible bacteria.

Continued next column

OVERDOSE

SYMPTOMS:
Nausea, vomiting, abdominal discomfort, diarrhea.
WHAT TO DO:
Overdose unlikely to threaten life. If person takes much larger amount than prescribed, call doctor, poison control center or hospital emergency room for instructions.

Time lapse before drug works:
2 to 5 days.

Don't take with:
Any other medicine without consulting your doctor or pharmacist.

POSSIBLE ADVERSE REACTIONS OR SIDE EFFECTS

SYMPTOMS	WHAT TO DO
Life-threatening: None expected.	
Common: Mild nausea.	Continue. Call doctor when convenient.
Infrequent: • Mild diarrhea, stomach cramps or vomiting; sore mouth or tongue; skin dryness, irritation or stinging (with use of skin solution).	Continue. Call doctor when convenient.
• Fever with severe nausea and vomiting, severe stomach pain, unusual tiredness or weakness, yellow eyes or skin; allergic skin reaction (skin rash, redness or itch).	Discontinue. Call doctor right away.
Rare: Irregular or slow heartbeat, any hearing loss, fainting.	Discontinue. Call doctor right away.

WARNINGS & PRECAUTIONS

Don't take if:
- You are allergic to any erythromycin.
- You have had liver disease or impaired liver function.

Before you start, consult your doctor:
If you have taken erythromycin estolate in the past.

Over age 60:
Adverse reactions and side effects may be more frequent and severe than in younger persons, especially skin reactions around genitals and anus.

Pregnancy:
Decide with your doctor if drug benefits justify risk to unborn child. Risk category C (see page xxiii).

Breast-feeding:
Drug passes into milk. Avoid drug or discontinue nursing until you finish medicine. Consult doctor for advice on maintaining milk supply.

Infants & children:
Use only under medical supervision.

Prolonged use:
- You may become more susceptible to infections caused by germs not responsive to erythromycin.
- Talk to your doctor about the need for follow-up medical examinations or laboratory studies to check liver function.

Skin & sunlight:
No problems expected.

Driving, piloting or hazardous work:
No problems expected.

Discontinuing:
You must take full dose at least 10 consecutive days for streptococcal or staphylococcal infections.

Others:
Advise any doctor or dentist whom you consult that you take this medicine.

POSSIBLE INTERACTION WITH OTHER DRUGS

GENERIC NAME OR DRUG CLASS	COMBINED EFFECT
Aminophylline	Increased effect of aminophylline in blood.
Antihistamines, nonsedating	Serious heart rhythm problems with astemizole or terfenadine. Avoid.
Astemizole	Increased risk of heart toxicity.
Caffeine	Increased effect of caffeine.
Carbamazepine	Increased risk of carbamazepine toxicity.
Cefixime	Decreased antibiotic effect of cefixime.
Cyclosporins	May increase cyclosporin toxicity.
Hepatotoxics*	Increased risk of liver toxicity.
HMG-CoA reductase inhibitors	Increased risk of muscle and kidney problems.
Ketoconazole	Possible heartbeat irregularity
Leukotriene modifiers	Decreased effect of zafirlukast.
Lincomycins*	Decreased lincomycin effect.
Oxtriphylline	Increased level of oxtriphylline in blood.
Penicillins*	Decreased penicillin effect.
Sibutramine	Increased sibutramine effect.
Theophylline	Increased level of theophylline in blood.
Warfarin	Increased risk of bleeding.
Zafirlukast	Decreased effect of zafirlukast.

POSSIBLE INTERACTION WITH OTHER SUBSTANCES

INTERACTS WITH	COMBINED EFFECT
Alcohol:	Possible liver damage.
Beverages:	None expected.
Cocaine:	None expected.
Foods: Wines, syrup, acidic fruits or juices (if taken with).	Decreased antibiotic effect.
Marijuana:	None expected.
Tobacco:	None expected.

*See Glossary

ESTRAMUSTINE

BRAND NAMES

Emcyt

BASIC INFORMATION

Habit forming? No
Prescription needed? Yes
Available as generic? No
Drug class: Antineoplastic

USES

Treats prostate cancer.

DOSAGE & USAGE INFORMATION

How to take:
Capsule—Swallow with liquid. If you can't swallow whole, open capsule and take with liquid or food. Instructions to take on empty stomach mean 1 hour before or 2 hours after eating.

When to take:
According to doctor's instructions. Try to take 1 hour before or 2 hours after eating or drinking any milk products.

If you forget a dose:
Skip dose. Never double dose.

What drug does:
Suppresses growth of cancer cells.

Time lapse before drug works:
Within 20 hours.

Don't take with:
Any other medicines (including over-the-counter drugs such as cough and cold medicines, laxatives, antacids, diet pills, caffeine, nose drops or vitamins) without consulting your doctor.

OVERDOSE

SYMPTOMS:
None expected.
WHAT TO DO:
Overdose unlikely to threaten life. If person takes much larger amount than prescribed, call doctor, poison control center or hospital emergency room for instructions.

POSSIBLE ADVERSE REACTIONS OR SIDE EFFECTS

SYMPTOMS	WHAT TO DO
Life-threatening: Sudden headaches, chest pain, shortness of breath, leg pain, vision changes, slurred speech.	Seek emergency treatment immediately.
Common: • Skin rash, itching.	Discontinue. Call doctor right away.
• Increased sun sensitivity.	Decrease sun exposure. Call doctor when convenient.
• Diarrhea, dizziness, nausea, vomiting, headache, swelling in hands or feet.	Continue. Call doctor when convenient.
Infrequent: • Joint or muscle pain, difficulty swallowing, sore throat and fever, peeling skin, jaundice.	Discontinue. Call doctor right away.
• Mouth or tongue irritation, breast tenderness or enlargement, decreased interest in sex.	Continue. Call doctor when convenient.
Rare: Bloody urine, hearing loss, back pain, abdominal pain.	Discontinue. Call doctor right away.

348

ESTRAMUSTINE

WARNINGS & PRECAUTIONS

Don't take if:
You have active thrombophlebitis.

Before you start, consult your doctor:
- If you have jaundice.
- If you have history of thrombophlebitis.
- If you have peptic ulcer.
- If you have mental depression.
- If you have migraine headaches.
- If you have or recently had chicken pox.
- If you have shingles (herpes zoster).
- If you have had a recent heart attack.

Over age 60:
Adverse reactions and side effects may be more frequent and severe than in younger persons. You may need smaller doses for shorter periods of time.

Pregnancy:
Used in men only.

Breast-feeding:
Used in men only.

Infants & children:
Not used.

Prolonged use:
Talk to your doctor about the need for follow-up medical examinations or laboratory studies to check complete blood counts (white blood cell count, platelet count, red blood cell count, hemoglobin, hematocrit), blood pressure, liver function, serum acid, serum calcium and alkaline phosphatase.

Skin & sunlight:
No problems expected.

Driving, piloting or hazardous work:
No special problems expected.

Discontinuing:
No special problems expected.

Others:
- Advise any doctor or dentist whom you consult that you take this medicine.
- May affect results in some medical tests.
- May decrease sperm count in males.

POSSIBLE INTERACTION WITH OTHER DRUGS

GENERIC NAME OR DRUG CLASS	COMBINED EFFECT
Calcium supplements*	Decreased absorption of estramustine.
Hepatotoxic medications*	Increased risk of liver toxicity.

POSSIBLE INTERACTION WITH OTHER SUBSTANCES

INTERACTS WITH	COMBINED EFFECT
Alcohol:	Increased "hangover effect" and other gastrointestinal symptoms.
Beverages: Milk and milk products.	Decreased absorption of estramustine.
Cocaine:	No special problems expected.
Foods: Foods high in calcium.	Decreased absorption of estramustine.
Marijuana:	No special problems expected.
Tobacco:	Increased risk of heart attack and blood clots.

*See Glossary

349

ESTROGENS

GENERIC AND BRAND NAMES

See complete list of generic and brand names in *Generic and Brand Name Directory*, page 880.

BASIC INFORMATION

Habit forming? No
Prescription needed? Yes
Available as generic? Yes
Drug class: Female sex hormone (estrogen)

USES

- Treatment for estrogen deficiency.
- Treatment for symptoms of menopause and menstrual cycle irregularity.
- Treatment for estrogen-deficiency osteoporosis (bone softening from calcium loss).
- Treatment for vulvar squamous hyperplasia.
- Treatment for atrophic vaginitis.
- Treatment for prostate cancer.
- Reduces the risk of heart attack.

DOSAGE & USAGE INFORMATION

How to take:
- Tablet or capsule—Take with or after food to reduce nausea. Swallow with liquid. If you can't swallow whole, crumble tablet or open capsule and take with liquid or food.
- Vaginal cream or suppositories—Use as directed on label.
- By injection under medical supervision.
- Transdermal patches—Follow package instructions.
- Vaginal insert—Follow package instructions.

When to take:
- Oral estrogen—Take at the same time each day.
- Creams, suppositories, injections or patches—Follow label instructions.

Continued next column

OVERDOSE

SYMPTOMS:
Nausea, vomiting, fluid retention, breast enlargement and discomfort, abnormal vaginal bleeding.
WHAT TO DO:
Overdose unlikely to threaten life. If person takes much larger amount than prescribed, call doctor, poison control center or hospital emergency room for instructions.

If you forget a dose:
Take as soon as you remember up to 12 hours late. If more than 12 hours, wait for next scheduled dose (don't double this dose).

What drug does:
- Restores normal estrogen level in tissues.
- Combined with progestins for contraception.

Time lapse before drug works:
10 to 20 days.

Don't take with:
Any other medicine without consulting your doctor or pharmacist.

POSSIBLE ADVERSE REACTIONS OR SIDE EFFECTS

SYMPTOMS	WHAT TO DO
Life-threatening:	
Profuse bleeding.	Seek emergency treatment.
Common:	
• Stomach cramps.	Discontinue. Call doctor right away.
• Appetite loss.	Continue. Call doctor when convenient.
• Nausea; diarrhea; swollen feet and ankles; tender, swollen breasts; acne; intolerance of contact lenses; change in menstruation.	Continue. Tell doctor at next visit.
Infrequent:	
• Rash, stomach or side pain, joint or muscle pain, bloody skin blisters, breast lumps.	Discontinue. Call doctor right away.
• Depression, dizziness, migraine headache, irritability, vomiting.	Continue. Call doctor when convenient.
• Brown blotches, hair loss, vaginal discharge or bleeding, changes in sex drive.	Continue. Tell doctor at next visit.
Rare:	
• Jaundice, hypercalcemia in breast cancer.	Discontinue. Call doctor right away.
• Involuntary movements.	

WARNINGS & PRECAUTIONS

Don't take if:
- You are allergic to any estrogen-containing drugs.
- You have impaired liver function.
- You have had blood clots, stroke or heart attack.
- You have unexplained vaginal bleeding.

Before you start, consult your doctor:
- If you have had cancer of the breast or reproductive organs, fibrocystic breast disease, fibroid tumors of the uterus or endometriosis.
- If you have had migraine headaches, epilepsy or porphyria.
- If you have diabetes, high blood pressure, asthma, congestive heart failure, kidney disease or gallstones.
- If you plan to become pregnant within 3 months.

Over age 60:
Controversial. You and your doctor must decide if risks of drug outweigh benefits.

Pregnancy:
Risk to unborn child outweighs benefits of drug. Don't use. Risk category X (see page xxiii).

Breast-feeding:
Drug filters into milk. May harm child. Avoid.

Infants & children:
Not recommended.

Prolonged use:
- Increased growth of fibroid tumors of uterus. Possible association with cancer of uterus.
- Talk to your doctor about the need for follow-up medical examinations or laboratory studies to check pap smear, liver function, mammogram.

Skin & sunlight:
One or more drugs in this group may cause rash or intensify sunburn in areas exposed to sun or ultraviolet light (photosensitivity reaction). Avoid overexposure. Notify doctor if reaction occurs.

Driving, piloting or hazardous work:
No problems expected.

Discontinuing:
You may need to discontinue estrogens periodically. Consult your doctor.

Others:
- In rare instances, may cause blood clot in lung, brain or leg. Symptoms are sudden severe headache, coordination loss, vision change, chest pain, breathing difficulty, slurred speech, pain in legs or groin. Seek emergency treatment immediately.
- Carefully read the paper called "Information for the Patient" that was given to you with your prescription. If you lose it, ask your pharmacist for a copy.

POSSIBLE INTERACTION WITH OTHER DRUGS

GENERIC NAME OR DRUG CLASS	COMBINED EFFECT
Adrenocorticoids, systemic	Increased adreno-corticoid effect.
Alpha adrenergic receptor blockers	Decreased effect of alpha adrenergic blocker.
Anticoagulants, oral*	Decreased anti-coagulant effect.
Anticonvulsants, hydantoin*	Decreased estrogen effect.
Antidepressants, tricyclic*	Increased toxicity of antidepressants.
Antidiabetics, oral*	Unpredictable increase or decrease in blood sugar.
Antifibrinolytic agents*	Increased possibility of blood clotting.
Antivirals, HIV/AIDS*	Increased risk of pancreatitis.
Carbamazepine	Decreased estrogen effect.
Clofibrate	Decreased clofibrate effect.
Dextrothyroxine	Decreased dextrothyroxine effect.
Guanfacine	May decrease antihypertensive effects of guanfacine.
Insulin	Possible decreased insulin effect. May require dosage adjustment.

Continued on page 915

POSSIBLE INTERACTION WITH OTHER SUBSTANCES

INTERACTS WITH	COMBINED EFFECT
Alcohol:	None expected.
Beverages: Grapefruit juice.	Possible increased estrogen effect.
Cocaine:	No proven problems.
Foods:	None expected.
Marijuana:	Possible menstrual irregularities and bleeding between periods.
Tobacco:	Increased risk of blood clots leading to stroke or heart attack.

ETHCHLORVYNOL

BRAND NAMES

Placidyl

BASIC INFORMATION

Habit forming? Yes
Prescription needed? Yes
Available as generic? No
Drug class: Sleep inducer (hypnotic)

USES

Treatment of insomnia for short periods.
Prolonged use is not recommended.

DOSAGE & USAGE INFORMATION

How to take:
Capsules—Take with food or milk to lessen side effects.

When to take:
At or near bedtime.

If you forget a dose:
Bedtime dose—If you forget your once-a-day bedtime dose, don't take it more than 3 hours late.

What drug does:
Affects brain centers that control waking and sleeping.

Time lapse before drug works:
30 to 60 minutes.

Don't take with:
Any other medicine without consulting your doctor or pharmacist.

OVERDOSE

SYMPTOMS:
Excitement, delirium, incoordination, shortness of breath, slow heartbeat, excessive drowsiness, deep coma.
WHAT TO DO:
- Dial 911 (emergency) or 0 (operator) for an ambulance or medical help. Then give first aid immediately.
- If patient is unconscious and not breathing, give mouth-to-mouth breathing. If there is no heartbeat, use cardiac massage and mouth-to-mouth breathing (CPR). Don't try to make patient vomit. If you can't get help quickly, take patient to nearest emergency facility.
- See emergency information on inside covers.

POSSIBLE ADVERSE REACTIONS OR SIDE EFFECTS

SYMPTOMS	WHAT TO DO
Life-threatening: In case of overdose, see previous column.	
Common:	
• Indigestion, nausea, vomiting, stomach pain.	Discontinue. Call doctor right away.
• Blurred vision, dizziness.	Continue. Call doctor when convenient.
• Unpleasant taste in mouth, fatigue, weakness.	Continue. Tell doctor at next visit.
Infrequent: Jitters, clumsiness, unsteadiness, drowsiness, confusion, rash, hives, unusual bleeding or bruising, facial numbness.	Discontinue. Call doctor right away.
Rare: Slow heartbeat, difficult breathing, fainting, jaundice, slurred speech, trembling, uncontrolled eye movements.	Discontinue. Call doctor right away.

WARNINGS & PRECAUTIONS

Don't take if:
- You are allergic to any hypnotic.
- You have porphyria.
- Patient is younger than 12.

Before you start, consult your doctor:
- If you plan to become pregnant within medication period.
- If you have kidney or liver disease.

Over age 60:
Adverse reactions and side effects, especially a "hangover" effect, may be more frequent and severe than in younger persons.

Pregnancy:
Decide with your doctor if drug benefits justify risk to unborn child. Risk category C (see page xxiii).

Breast-feeding:
No problems expected, but observe child and ask doctor for guidance.

Infants & children:
Not recommended.

Prolonged use:
Impaired vision.

Skin & sunlight:
No problems expected.

Driving, piloting or hazardous work:
Don't drive or pilot aircraft until you learn how medicine affects you. Don't work around dangerous machinery. Don't climb ladders or work in high places. Danger increases if you drink alcohol or take medicine affecting alertness and reflexes.

Discontinuing:
- Don't discontinue without consulting doctor. Dose may require gradual reduction if you have taken drug for a long time. Doses of other drugs may also require adjustment.
- Many side effects may occur when you stop taking this drug, including irritability, muscle twitching, hallucinations or seizures. Consult your doctor.

Others:
No problems expected.

POSSIBLE INTERACTION WITH OTHER DRUGS

GENERIC NAME OR DRUG CLASS	COMBINED EFFECT
Anticoagulants, oral*	Decreased anticoagulant effect.
Antidepressants, tricyclic* (especially amitriptyline)	Delirium and deep sedation.
Antihistamines*	Increased antihistamine effect.
Clozapine	Toxic effect on the central nervous system.
Ethinamate	Dangerous increased effects of ethinamate. Avoid combining.
Fluoxetine	Increased depressant effects of both drugs.
Guanfacine	May increase depressant effects of either drug.
Leucovorin	High alcohol content of leucovorin may cause adverse effects.

Methyprylon	Increased sedative effect, perhaps to dangerous level. Avoid.
Molindone	Increased sedative effect.
Monoamine oxidase (MAO) inhibitors*	Increased sedation.
Nabilone	Greater depression of central nervous system.
Narcotics*	Increased narcotic effect.
Pain relievers*	Increased effect of pain reliever.
Sedatives*	Increased sedative effect.
Sertraline	Increased depressive effects of both drugs.
Tranquilizers*	Increased tranquilizer effect.

POSSIBLE INTERACTION WITH OTHER SUBSTANCES

INTERACTS WITH	COMBINED EFFECT
Alcohol:	Excessive depressant and sedative effect. Avoid.
Beverages:	None expected.
Cocaine:	Decreased ethchlorvynol effect.
Foods:	None expected.
Marijuana:	Occasional use— Drowsiness, unsteadiness, depressed function. Frequent use— Severe drowsiness, impaired physical and mental function.
Tobacco:	None expected.

ETHIONAMIDE

BRAND NAMES

Trecator-SC

BASIC INFORMATION

Habit forming? No
Prescription needed? Yes
Available as generic? No
Drug class: Antimycobacterial
 (antituberculosis)

 ## USES

Treats tuberculosis. Used in combination with other antituberculosis drugs such as isoniazid, streptomycin, rifampin, ethambutol.

 ## DOSAGE & USAGE INFORMATION

How to take:
Tablets—Swallow with liquid or food to lessen stomach irritation. If you can't swallow whole, crumble tablet and take with liquid or food.

When to take:
Usually every 8 to 12 hours, with or after meals.

If you forget a dose:
Take as soon as you remember up to 2 hours late. If more than 2 hours, wait for next scheduled dose. Don't double this dose.

What drug does:
Kills germs that cause tuberculosis.

Time lapse before drug works:
Within 3 hours.

Don't take with:
Any other medicine without consulting your doctor or pharmacist.

 ## OVERDOSE

SYMPTOMS:
None expected.
WHAT TO DO:
Overdose unlikely to threaten life. If person takes much larger amount than prescribed, call doctor, poison control center or hospital emergency room for instructions.

 ## POSSIBLE ADVERSE REACTIONS OR SIDE EFFECTS

SYMPTOMS	WHAT TO DO
Life-threatening:	
None expected.	
Common:	
• Vomiting.	Discontinue. Call doctor right away.
• Dizziness, sore mouth, nausea, metallic taste.	Continue. Call doctor when convenient.
Infrequent:	
Jaundice (yellow eyes and skin); numbness, tingling, pain in hands or feet; depression; confusion.	Discontinue. Call doctor right away.
Rare:	
• Hunger, shakiness, rapid heartbeat; blurred vision; vision changes; skin rash.	Discontinue. Call doctor right away.
• Gradual swelling in the neck (thyroid gland).	Continue. Call doctor when convenient.
• Enlargement of breasts (male).	No action necessary.

ETHIONAMIDE

WARNINGS & PRECAUTIONS

Don't take if:
You know you are hypersensitive to ethionamide.

Before you start, consult your doctor:
• If you have diabetes mellitus.
• If you have liver disease.

Over age 60:
No information available.

Pregnancy:
Decide with your doctor if drug benefits justify risk to unborn child. Risk category C (see page xxiii).

Breast-feeding:
Effect not documented. Consult your family doctor or pediatrician.

Infants & children:
Effect not documented. Consult your family doctor or pediatrician.

Prolonged use:
No special problems expected.

Skin & sunlight:
No special problems expected.

Driving, piloting or hazardous work:
Don't drive or pilot aircraft until you learn how medicine affects you. Don't work around dangerous machinery. Don't climb ladders or work in high places. Danger increases if you drink alcohol or take medicine affecting alertness and reflexes.

Discontinuing:
Don't discontinue without consulting doctor.

Others:
• Advise any doctor or dentist whom you consult that you take this medicine.
• Request occasional laboratory studies for liver function.
• Request occasional eye examinations.
• Treatment may take months or years.
• You should take pyridoxine (vitamin B-6) supplements while taking ethionamide.

POSSIBLE INTERACTION WITH OTHER DRUGS

GENERIC NAME OR DRUG CLASS	COMBINED EFFECT
Antivirals, HIV/AIDS*	Increased risk of peripheral neuropathy.
Cycloserine	Increased risk of seizures.
Pyridoxine	Increased excretion by kidney. (Should take pyridoxine supplements while on ethionamide to prevent development of neuritis in feet and hands).

POSSIBLE INTERACTION WITH OTHER SUBSTANCES

INTERACTS WITH	COMBINED EFFECT
Alcohol:	Increased incidence of liver diseases.
Beverages: Any alcoholic beverage.	Increased incidence of liver diseases.
Cocaine:	None expected.
Foods:	None expected.
Marijuana:	No interaction expected, but may slow body's recovery.
Tobacco:	No interaction expected, but may slow body's recovery.

ETIDRONATE

BRAND NAMES

Didronel   EHDP

BASIC INFORMATION

Habit forming? No
Prescription needed? Yes
Available as generic? No
Drug class: Antihypercalcemic

USES

- Treats Paget's disease of the bone.
- Aids healing following hip replacement or spinal cord injury.

DOSAGE & USAGE INFORMATION

How to take:
Tablet—Swallow with water. Do not take with milk.

When to take:
According to doctor's instructions. Take 1 hour before or 2 hours after eating.

If you forget a dose:
Take as soon as you remember up to 6 hours late. If more than 6 hours, wait for next dose (don't double this dose).

What drug does:
Unknown. Appears to retard bone loss and stimulates bone formation.

Time lapse before drug works:
- Paget's disease—1 month.
- Other uses—1 day to several months.

Don't take with:
Any other medicine without consulting your doctor or pharmacist.

OVERDOSE

SYMPTOMS:
None expected.
WHAT TO DO:
Overdose unlikely to threaten life. If person takes much larger amount than prescribed, call doctor, poison control center or hospital emergency room for instructions.

POSSIBLE ADVERSE REACTIONS OR SIDE EFFECTS

SYMPTOMS	WHAT TO DO
Life-threatening: None expected.	
Common: Tenderness or pain in bones, diarrhea, nausea.	Continue. Call doctor when convenient.
Infrequent: None expected.	
Rare: Rash; hives; swelling of hands, feet, lips, throat.	Discontinue. Call doctor right away.

WARNINGS & PRECAUTIONS

Don't take if:
You are allergic to etidronate or alendronate.

Before you start, consult your doctor:
If you have kidney disease, heart failure, bone fractures or colitis.

Over age 60:
No special problems expected.

Pregnancy:
Consult doctor. Risk category B (see page xxiii).

Breast-feeding:
Safety not established. Consult doctor.

Infants & children:
Use only under supervision of a medical professional.

Prolonged use:
No special problems expected.

Skin & sunlight:
No special problems expected.

Driving, piloting or hazardous work:
No special problems expected.

Discontinuing:
Don't discontinue without doctor's advice, even though symptoms diminish or disappear.

Others:
* Medicine may be prescribed for 2 weeks, stopped for 2 to 3 months, then started again.
* Have regular check-ups with your doctor even if you currently are not undergoing treatment.

POSSIBLE INTERACTION WITH OTHER DRUGS

GENERIC NAME OR DRUG CLASS	COMBINED EFFECT
Antacids*	Decreased effect of etidronate.
Mineral supplements*	Decreased effect of etidronate.

POSSIBLE INTERACTION WITH OTHER SUBSTANCES

INTERACTS WITH	COMBINED EFFECT
Alcohol:	None expected.
Beverages: Milk.	Decreased effect of etidronate.
Cocaine:	None expected.
Foods: Dairy products or foods containing high levels of calcium.	Decreased effect of etidronate.
Marijuana:	None expected.
Tobacco:	None expected.

*See Glossary

ETOPOSIDE

BRAND NAMES

VePesid   VP-16

BASIC INFORMATION

Habit forming? No
Prescription needed? Yes
Available as generic? No
Drug class: Antineoplastic

 USES

- Treats testicle, lung and bladder cancer.
- Treats Hodgkin's disease and some other forms of cancer.

 DOSAGE & USAGE INFORMATION

How to take:
- Capsules—Swallow with liquid. If you can't swallow whole, open capsule and take with liquid or food. Instructions to take on empty stomach mean 1 hour before or 2 hours after eating.
- Injection—Given under doctor's supervision.

When to take:
According to your doctor's instructions.

If you forget a dose:
Skip this dose. Never double dose. Resume regular schedule.

What drug does:
Inhibits DNA in cancer cells.

Time lapse before drug works:
Unpredictable.

Don't take with:
Any other medicines (including over-the-counter drugs such as cough and cold medicines, laxatives, antacids, diet pills, caffeine, nose drops or vitamins) without consulting your doctor.

 OVERDOSE

SYMPTOMS:
Rapid pulse, shortness of breath, wheezing, fainting, coma.
WHAT TO DO:
- Dial 911 (emergency) or 0 (operator) for an ambulance or medical help. Then give first aid immediately.
- See emergency information on inside covers.

 POSSIBLE ADVERSE REACTIONS OR SIDE EFFECTS

SYMPTOMS	WHAT TO DO
Life-threatening:	
In case of overdose, see previous column.	
Common:	
• Appetite loss, nausea, vomiting.	Continue. Call doctor when convenient.
• Loss of hair	No action necessary.
Infrequent:	
Symptoms of low white blood cell count and low platelet count: black, tarry stools; bloody urine; cough; chills or fever; low back pain; bruising.	Discontinue. Call doctor right away.
Rare:	
Mouth sores.	Continue. Call doctor when convenient.

WARNINGS & PRECAUTIONS

Don't take if:
* You have chicken pox.
* You have shingles (herpes zoster).

Before you start, consult your doctor:
If you have liver or kidney disease.

Over age 60:
No special problems expected.

Pregnancy:
Risk to unborn child outweighs drug benefits. Don't use. Risk category D (see page xxiii).

Breast-feeding:
Drug passes into milk. Avoid drug or discontinue nursing until you finish medicine. Consult doctor for advice on maintaining milk supply.

Infants & children:
Effect not documented. Consult your doctor.

Prolonged use:
* Talk to your doctor about the need for follow-up medical examinations or laboratory studies to check complete blood counts (white blood cell count, platelet count, red blood cell count, hemoglobin, hematocrit).
* Check mouth frequently for ulcers.

Skin & sunlight:
No problems expected.

Driving, piloting or hazardous work:
Avoid if you feel confused, drowsy or dizzy.

Discontinuing:
May still experience symptoms of bone marrow depression, such as: blood in stools, fever or chills, blood spots under the skin, back pain, hoarseness, bloody urine. If any of these occur, call your doctor right away.

Others:
* Advise any doctor or dentist whom you consult that you take this medicine.
* May affect results in some medical tests.
* Etoposide may be used in combinations with other antineoplastic treatment plans. The incidence and severity of side effects may be different when used in combinations such as doxorubicin, procarbazine and etoposide (APE); etoposide, cyclophosphamide, doxorubicin and vincristine (CAVE, ECHO, CAPO, EVAC or VOCA); cyclophosphamide, doxorubicin and etoposide (CAE or ACE); cisplatin, bleomycin, doxorubicin and etoposide; cisplatin, bleomycin and etoposide; cisplatin and etoposide. For further information regarding these combinations, consult your doctor.

POSSIBLE INTERACTION WITH OTHER DRUGS

GENERIC NAME OR DRUG CLASS	COMBINED EFFECT
Angiotensin-converting enzyme (ACE) inhibitors*	May increase bone marrow depression or make kidney damage more likely.
Antineoplastic (cancer-treating) drugs*	May increase bone marrow depression or make kidney damage more likely.
Clozapine	Toxic effect on bone marrow.
Tiopronin	Increased risk of toxicity to bone marrow.
Vaccines, live or killed virus	Increased likelihood of toxicity or reduced effectiveness of vaccine. Wait 3 months to 1 year after etoposide treatment before getting vaccine.

POSSIBLE INTERACTION WITH OTHER SUBSTANCES

INTERACTS WITH	COMBINED EFFECT
Alcohol:	Increased likelihood of adverse reactions. Avoid.
Beverages:	No special problems expected.
Cocaine:	Increased likelihood of adverse reactions. Avoid.
Foods:	No special problems expected.
Marijuana:	Increased likelihood of adverse reactions. Avoid.
Tobacco:	No special problems expected.

*See Glossary

FELBAMATE

BRAND AND GENERIC NAMES

FBM   Felbatol

BASIC INFORMATION

Habit forming? No
Prescription needed? Yes
Available as generic? No
Drug class: Anticonvulsant

USES

- Treatment for partial epileptic seizures.
- Treatment for Lennox-Gastaut syndrome (a severe form of epilepsy in children).

DOSAGE & USAGE INFORMATION

How to take:
- Tablet—Swallow with liquid. May be taken with food to lessen stomach upset unless the doctor has directed taking on an empty stomach.
- Oral suspension—Shake bottle well before measuring. Use specially marked measuring device to measure each dose accurately. Don't measure with a regular household teaspoon.

When to take:
At the same times each day. Your doctor will determine the best schedule. Dosages will gradually be increased over the first 3 weeks.

If you forget a dose:
Take as soon as you remember up to 2 hours late. If more than 2 hours, wait for next scheduled dose (don't double this dose).

What drug does:
- Decreases the frequency of partial seizures that start in a localized part of the brain, including those that progress into more generalized grand mal seizures.
- Decreases seizure activity and improves quality of life in children with Lennox-Gastaut syndrome.

Continued next column

OVERDOSE

SYMPTOMS:
Gastric distress, increased heart rate.
WHAT TO DO:
Overdose unlikely to threaten life. If person takes much larger amount than prescribed, call doctor, poison control center or hospital emergency room for instructions.

Time lapse before drug works:
May take several weeks for maximum effectiveness.

Don't take with:
Any other prescription or nonprescription drug without consulting your doctor.

POSSIBLE ADVERSE REACTIONS OR SIDE EFFECTS

SYMPTOMS	WHAT TO DO
Life-threatening: None expected.	
Common:	
• Fever, red or purple spots on skin, walking in unusual manner.	Continue, but call doctor right away.
• Abdominal pain, taste changes, constipation, sleeping difficulty, dizziness, headache, nausea or vomiting, indigestion, appetite loss.	Continue. Call doctor when convenient.
Infrequent:	
• Mood or mental changes, clumsiness, skin rash, tremor.	Continue, but call doctor right away.
• Vision changes, diarrhea, drowsiness, coughing or sneezing, ear pain or fullness, runny nose, weight loss.	Continue. Call doctor when convenient.
Rare:	
Black or tarry stools, bloody or dark-colored urine, unusual bruising or bleeding, breathing difficulty, wheezing, pain or tightness in chest, sore throat, mouth or lip sores, swollen face, swollen or painful glands or lymph nodes, yellow skin or eyes, chills, general tired feeling, continuing headache or abdominal pain, hives, itching, muscle cramps, stuffy nose, skin reaction to sunlight.	Continue, but call doctor right away.

WARNINGS & PRECAUTIONS

Don't take if:
You are allergic to felbamate.

Before you start, consult your doctor:
- If you have a sensitivity to other carbamate drugs*, other medications or other substances.
- If you have any blood disorder.
- If you have a history of bone marrow depression.
- If you have or have had any liver disease.

Over age 60:
Adverse reactions and side effects may be more frequent and severe than in younger persons.

Pregnancy:
Decide with your doctor if drug benefits justify risks to unborn child. Risk category B (see page xxiii).

Breast-feeding:
Drug passes into milk. Unknown effect. Consult your doctor.

Infants & children:
Give only under close medical supervision.

Prolonged use:
Talk to your doctor about the need for follow-up medical examinations or laboratory studies to check complete blood counts (white blood cell count, platelet count, red blood cell count, hemoglobin, hematocrit), iron concentrations and liver function studies.

Skin & sunlight:
No problems expected.

Driving, piloting or hazardous work:
Don't drive or pilot aircraft until you learn how medicine affects you. Don't work around dangerous machinery. Don't climb ladders or work in high places. Danger increases if you drink alcohol or take other medicines affecting alertness and reflexes such as antihistamines, tranquilizers, sedatives, pain medicine, narcotics and mind-altering drugs.

Discontinuing:
Don't discontinue without doctor's approval due to risk of increased seizure activity.

Others:
- Felbamate may cause serious side effects including blood problems and liver problems (rarely fatal). Decide with your doctor if drug benefits justify risks.
- Advise any doctor or dentist whom you consult that you take this medicine.
- Felbamate may be used alone or combined with other antiepileptic drugs. The dosages of other antiepileptic drugs you currently use will be reduced to minimize side effects and adverse reactions due to interactions.
- Wear medical identification that indicates the use of this medicine.

POSSIBLE INTERACTION WITH OTHER DRUGS

GENERIC NAME OR DRUG CLASS	COMBINED EFFECT
Carbamazepine	Increased side effects and adverse reactions.
Phenytoin	Increased side effects and adverse reactions.
Valproic acid	Increased side effects and adverse reactions.

POSSIBLE INTERACTION WITH OTHER SUBSTANCES

INTERACTS WITH	COMBINED EFFECT
Alcohol:	None expected.
Beverages:	None expected.
Cocaine:	None expected.
Foods:	None expected.
Marijuana:	None expected.
Tobacco:	None expected.

*See Glossary

FIBRATES

GENERIC AND BRAND NAMES

CLOFIBRATE
Abitrate
Atromid-S
Claripex
Novofibrate

FENOFIBRATE
Lipidil
Tricor

BASIC INFORMATION

Habit forming? No
Prescription needed? Yes
Available as generic? Yes
Drug class: Antihyperlipidemic

 ## USES

Reduces fatty substances in the blood (triglycerides).

 ## DOSAGE & USAGE INFORMATION

How to take:
Capsule—Swallow with liquid or food to lessen stomach irritation.

When to take:
At the same times each day.

If you forget a dose:
Take as soon as you remember up to 2 hours late. If more than 2 hours, wait for next scheduled dose (don't double this dose).

What drug does:
Inhibits formation of fatty substances.

Time lapse before drug works:
3 months or more.

Don't take with:
Any other medicine without consulting your doctor or pharmacist.

 ## OVERDOSE

SYMPTOMS:
Diarrhea, headache, muscle pain.
WHAT TO DO:
Overdose unlikely to threaten life. If person takes much larger amount than prescribed, call doctor, poison control center or hospital emergency room for instructions.

 ## POSSIBLE ADVERSE REACTIONS OR SIDE EFFECTS

SYMPTOMS	WHAT TO DO
Life-threatening: None expected.	
Common: None expected.	
Infrequent:	
• Chest pain, shortness of breath, irregular heartbeat.	Discontinue. Seek emergency treatment.
• Nausea, flu-like illness, vomiting.	Discontinue. Call doctor right away.
• Diarrhea, abdominal pain, belching, constipation, muscle aches and pains.	Continue. Call doctor when convenient.
Rare:	
• Cardiac arrhythmias, angina.	Discontinue. Seek emergency treatment.
• Rash, itch; mouth or lip sores; sore throat; swollen feet, legs; blood in urine; painful urination; fever; chills; anemia.	Discontinue. Call doctor right away.
• Dizziness, weakness, drowsiness, muscle cramps, headache, diminished sex drive, hair loss, dry mouth, bloating or stomach pain, chronic indigestion, loss of appetite, nausea, unusual bleeding or bruising, unusual tiredness, vomiting, yellow eyes or skin.	Continue. Call doctor when convenient.

WARNINGS & PRECAUTIONS

Don't take if:
- You are allergic to any fibrates.
- You have had serious liver disease.

Before you start, consult your doctor:
- If you have had liver or kidney disease.
- If you have had peptic ulcer disease.
- If you have had gallbladder disease or gallstones.
- If you have diabetes.

Over age 60:
Adverse reactions and side effects may be more frequent and severe than in younger persons. May develop flu-like symptoms.

Pregnancy:
Decide with your doctor if drug benefits justify risk to unborn child. Risk category C (see page xxiii).

Breast-feeding:
May harm child. Avoid. Consult doctor.

Infants & children:
Not recommended.

Prolonged use:
- May cause gallbladder infection.
- Possible cause of stomach cancer.
- Talk to your doctor about the need for follow-up medical examinations or laboratory studies to check complete blood counts (white blood cell count, platelet count, red blood cell count, hemoglobin, hematocrit) and serum low-density lipoprotein.

Skin & sunlight:
May cause rash or intensify sunburn in areas exposed to sun or ultraviolet light (photosensitivity reaction). Avoid overexposure. Notify doctor if reaction occurs.

Driving, piloting or hazardous work:
Avoid if you feel drowsy or dizzy. Otherwise, no problems expected.

Discontinuing:
Don't discontinue without doctor's advice until you complete prescribed dose, even though symptoms diminish or disappear.

Others:
- Periodic blood cell counts and liver-function studies recommended if you take clofibrate for a long time.
- Some studies question effectiveness. Many studies warn of toxicity.

POSSIBLE INTERACTION WITH OTHER DRUGS

GENERIC NAME OR DRUG CLASS	COMBINED EFFECT
Anticoagulants, oral*	Increased anticoagulant effect. Dose reduction of anticoagulant necessary.
Antidiabetics, oral*	Increased antidiabetic effect.
Contraceptives, oral*	Decreased fibrate effect.
Cyclosporine	May cause kidney problems, or worsen them.
Desmopressin	May decrease desmopressin effect.
Dexfenfluramine	May require dosage change as weight loss occurs.
Estrogens*	Decreased fibrate effect.
Furosemide	Possible toxicity of both drugs.
HMG-CoA reductase inhibitors	May cause muscle or kidney problems or make them worse.
Insulin	Increased insulin effect
Insulin lispro	May need decreased dosage of insulin.
Probenecid	Increased effect and toxicity of fibrate.
Thyroid hormones*	Increased fibrate effect.
Ursodiol	Decreased effect of ursodiol.

POSSIBLE INTERACTION WITH OTHER SUBSTANCES

INTERACTS WITH	COMBINED EFFECT
Alcohol:	None expected.
Beverages:	None expected.
Cocaine:	None expected.
Foods: Fatty foods.	Decreased fibrate effect.
Marijuana:	None expected.

FINASTERIDE

BRAND NAMES

Propecia   Proscar

BASIC INFORMATION

Habit forming? No
Prescription needed? Yes
Available as generic? No
Drug class: Dihydrotestosterone inhibitor

 ## USES

- Treats noncancerous enlargement of the prostate gland in men (benign prostatic hypertrophy or BPH).
- Theoretically, may prevent the development of prostate cancer.
- Treatment of male pattern hair loss in men only.

 ## DOSAGE & USAGE INFORMATION

How to take:
Tablets—Swallow with liquid. If you can't swallow whole, crumble tablet and take with liquid or food.

When to take:
Once a day or as directed, with or without meals.

If you forget a dose:
Take as soon as you remember up to 2 hours late. If more than 2 hours, wait for next scheduled dose (don't double this dose).

What drug does:
Inhibits the enzyme needed for the conversion of testosterone to dihydrotestosterone. Dihydrotestosterone is required for the development of benign prostatic hypertrophy.

Time lapse before drug works:
- May require up to 6 months for full therapeutic effect for BPH.
- For treatment of hair loss, may not see any benefit for 3 months or more.

Don't take with:
Any other medicine without consulting your doctor or pharmacist, especially nonprescription decongestants.

 ## OVERDOSE

SYMPTOMS:
None expected.
WHAT TO DO:
Overdose unlikely to threaten life.

 ## POSSIBLE ADVERSE REACTIONS OR SIDE EFFECTS

SYMPTOMS	WHAT TO DO
Life-threatening: None expected.	
Common: None expected.	
Infrequent: Decreased volume of ejaculation, back or stomach pain, headache.	Continue. Call doctor when convenient.
Rare: Impotence, decreased libido, breast enlargement and tenderness, allergic reaction (skin rash, swelling of lips).	Continue. Call doctor when convenient.

WARNINGS & PRECAUTIONS

Don't take if:
- You are allergic to finasteride.
- You are a female or a child.

Before you start, consult your doctor:
- If you have not had a blood test to check for prostate cancer.
- If your sexual partner is pregnant or may become pregnant.
- If you have a liver disorder.
- If you have reduced urinary flow.
- If you have large residual urinary volume.

Over age 60:
No special problems expected.

Pregnancy:
- Not recommended for women.
- Pregnant women should not handle the crushed tablets.
- Ask your doctor if you should avoid exposure to mate's semen if he takes finasteride.
- Risk category X (see page xxiii).

Breast-feeding:
Not recommended for women.

Infants & children:
Not recommended.

Prolonged use:
Talk to your doctor about the need for follow-up medical examinations or laboratory studies to check the effectiveness of the treatment.

Skin & sunlight:
No special problems expected.

Driving, piloting or hazardous work:
No special problems expected.

Discontinuing:
Don't discontinue without medical advice.

Others:
- Advise any doctor or dentist whom you consult that you take this medicine.
- May affect results of some medical tests.
- For those who respond well, the drug must be continued indefinitely.

POSSIBLE INTERACTION WITH OTHER DRUGS

GENERIC NAME OR DRUG CLASS	COMBINED EFFECT
None expected.	

POSSIBLE INTERACTION WITH OTHER SUBSTANCES

INTERACTS WITH	COMBINED EFFECT
Alcohol:	No proven problems.
Beverages:	No proven problems.
Cocaine:	No proven problems.
Foods:	No proven problems.
Marijuana:	No proven problems.
Tobacco:	No proven problems.

*See Glossary

FLAVOXATE

BRAND NAMES

Urispas

BASIC INFORMATION

Habit forming? No
Prescription needed? Yes
Available as generic? No
Drug class: Antispasmodic (urinary tract)

 USES

Relieves urinary pain, urgency, nighttime urination, unusual frequency of urination associated with urinary system disorders.

 DOSAGE & USAGE INFORMATION

How to take:
Tablet—Swallow with liquid or food to lessen stomach irritation.

When to take:
30 minutes before meals (unless directed otherwise by doctor).

If you forget a dose:
Take as soon as you remember up to 2 hours late. If more than 2 hours, wait for next scheduled dose (don't double this dose).

What drug does:
Blocks nerve impulses at smooth muscle nerve endings, preventing muscle contractions and gland secretions of organs involved.

Time lapse before drug works:
15 to 30 minutes.

Don't take with:
Any other medicine without consulting your doctor or pharmacist.

 OVERDOSE

SYMPTOMS:
Dilated pupils, rapid pulse and breathing, dizziness, fever, hallucinations, confusion, slurred speech, agitation, flushed face, convulsions, coma.
WHAT TO DO:
* **Dial 911 (emergency) or 0 (operator) for an ambulance or medical help. Then give first aid immediately.**
* **See emergency information on inside covers.**

 POSSIBLE ADVERSE REACTIONS OR SIDE EFFECTS

SYMPTOMS	WHAT TO DO
Life-threatening:	
In case of overdose, see previous column.	
Common:	
• Confusion, delirium, rapid heartbeat.	Discontinue. Call doctor right away.
• Nausea, vomiting, less perspiration, drowsiness.	Continue. Call doctor when convenient.
• Constipation.	Continue. Tell doctor at next visit.
• Dry ears, nose, throat.	No action necessary.
Infrequent:	
• Unusual excitement, irritability, restlessness, clumsiness, hallucinations.	Discontinue. Call doctor right away.
• Headache, increased sensitivity to light, painful or difficult urination.	Continue. Call doctor when convenient.
Rare:	
• Shortness of breath.	Discontinue. Seek emergency treatment.
• Rash or hives; eye pain; blurred vision; sore throat, fever, mouth sores; abdominal pain.	Discontinue. Call doctor right away.
• Dizziness.	Continue. Call doctor when convenient.

WARNINGS & PRECAUTIONS

Don't take if:
- You are allergic to any anticholinergic.
- You have trouble with stomach bloating.
- You have difficulty emptying your bladder completely.
- You have narrow-angle glaucoma.
- You have severe ulcerative colitis.

Before you start, consult your doctor:
- If you have open-angle glaucoma.
- If you have angina.
- If you have chronic bronchitis or asthma.
- If you have liver disease.
- If you have hiatal hernia.
- If you have enlarged prostate.
- If you have myasthenia gravis.
- If you have peptic ulcer.
- If you will have surgery within 2 months, including dental surgery, requiring general or spinal anesthesia.

Over age 60:
Adverse reactions and side effects, particularly mental confusion, may be more frequent and severe than in younger persons.

Pregnancy:
Consult doctor. Risk category B (see page xxiii).

Breast-feeding:
Drug passes into milk. Avoid drug or discontinue nursing until you finish medicine. Consult doctor for advice on maintaining milk supply.

Infants & children:
Use only under medical supervision.

Prolonged use:
Chronic constipation, possible fecal impaction. Consult doctor immediately.

Skin & sunlight:
No problems expected.

Driving, piloting or hazardous work:
Use disqualifies you for piloting aircraft. Don't drive until you learn how medicine affects you. Don't work around dangerous machinery. Don't climb ladders or work in high places. Danger increases if you drink alcohol or take medicine affecting alertness and reflexes, such as antihistamines, tranquilizers, sedatives, pain medicine, narcotics and mind-altering drugs.

Discontinuing:
May be unnecessary to finish medicine. Follow doctor's instructions.

Others:
No problems expected.

 ## POSSIBLE INTERACTION WITH OTHER DRUGS

GENERIC NAME OR DRUG CLASS	COMBINED EFFECT
Antimuscarinics*	Increased effect of flavoxate.
Central nervous system (CNS) depressants, other*	Increased effect of both drugs.
Clozapine	Toxic effect on the central nervous system.
Ethinamate	Dangerous increased effects of ethinamate. Avoid combining.
Fluoxetine	Increased depressant effects of both drugs.
Guanfacine	May increase depressant effects of either drug.
Leucovorin	High alcohol content of leucovorin may cause adverse effects.
Methyprylon	Increased sedative effect, perhaps to dangerous level. Avoid.
Nabilone	Greater depression of central nervous system.
Nizatidine	Increased nizatidine effect.
Sertraline	Increased depressive effects of both drugs.

 ## POSSIBLE INTERACTION WITH OTHER SUBSTANCES

INTERACTS WITH	COMBINED EFFECT
Alcohol:	None expected.
Beverages:	None expected.
Cocaine:	Excessively rapid heartbeat. Avoid.
Foods:	None expected.
Marijuana:	Drowsiness, dry mouth.
Tobacco:	None expected.

*See Glossary

FLECAINIDE ACETATE

BRAND NAMES

Tambocor

BASIC INFORMATION

Habit forming? No
Prescription needed? Yes
Available as generic? No
Drug class: Antiarrhythmic

USES

Stabilizes irregular heartbeat.

DOSAGE & USAGE INFORMATION

How to take:
Tablet—Swallow with liquid. If you can't swallow whole, crumble tablet and take with liquid or food.

When to take:
At the same time each day, according to instructions on prescription label. Take tablets approximately 12 hours apart.

If you forget a dose:
Take as soon as you remember up to 4 hours late. If more than 4 hours, wait for next scheduled dose (don't double this dose).

What drug does:
Decreases conduction of abnormal electrical activity in the heart muscle or its regulating systems.

Continued next column

OVERDOSE

SYMPTOMS:
Low blood pressure or unconsciousness, irregular or rapid heartbeat, sleepiness, tremor, sweating.
WHAT TO DO:
- **Dial 911 (emergency) or 0 (operator) for an ambulance or medical help. Then give first aid immediately.**
- **If patient is unconscious and not breathing, give mouth-to-mouth breathing. If there is no heartbeat, use cardiac massage and mouth-to-mouth breathing (CPR). Don't try to make patient vomit. If you can't get help quickly, take patient to nearest emergency facility.**
- **See emergency information on inside covers.**

Time lapse before drug works:
1 to 6 hours. May need doses daily for 2 to 3 days for maximum effect.

Don't take with:
Any other medicine without consulting your doctor or pharmacist.

POSSIBLE ADVERSE REACTIONS OR SIDE EFFECTS

SYMPTOMS	WHAT TO DO
Life-threatening: In case of overdose, see previous column.	
Common: Blurred vision, dizziness.	Continue. Call doctor when convenient.
Infrequent:	
• Chest pain, irregular heartbeat.	Discontinue. Seek emergency treatment.
• Shakiness, rash, nausea, vomiting.	Continue, but call doctor right away.
• Anxiety; depression; weakness; headache; appetite loss; weakness in muscles, bones, joints; swollen feet, ankles or legs; loss of taste; numbness or tingling in hands or feet, abdominal pain.	Continue. Call doctor when convenient.
• Constipation.	Continue. Tell doctor at next visit.
Rare:	
• Shortness of breath.	Discontinue. Seek emergency treatment.
• Sore throat, jaundice, fever.	Continue, but call doctor right away.

WARNINGS & PRECAUTIONS

Don't take if:
You are allergic to flecainide or a local anesthetic such as novocaine, xylocaine or other drug whose generic name ends with "caine."

Before you start, consult your doctor:
- If you have kidney disease.
- If you have liver disease.
- If you have had a heart attack in past 3 weeks.
- If you have a pacemaker.

Over age 60:
Adverse reactions and side effects may be more frequent and severe than in younger persons.

Pregnancy:
Decide with your doctor whether drug benefits justify risk to unborn child. Risk category C (see page xxiii).

Breast-feeding:
Drug passes into milk. Avoid drug or discontinue nursing until you finish medicine. Consult doctor for advice on maintaining milk supply.

Infants & children:
Not recommended. Safety and dosage have not been established.

Prolonged use:
Talk to your doctor about the need for follow-up medical examinations or laboratory studies to check complete blood counts (white blood cell count, platelet count, red blood cell count, hemoglobin, hematocrit), ECG*.

Skin & sunlight:
No problems expected.

Driving, piloting or hazardous work:
Don't drive or pilot aircraft until you learn how medicine affects you. Don't work around dangerous machinery. Don't climb ladders or work in high places. Danger increases if you drink alcohol or take medicine affecting alertness and reflexes, such as antihistamines, tranquilizers, sedatives, pain medicine, narcotics and mind-altering drugs.

Discontinuing:
Don't discontinue without consulting doctor. Dose may require gradual reduction if you have taken drug for a long time. Doses of other drugs may also require adjustment.

Others:
Wear identification bracelet or carry an identification card with inscription of medicine you take.

POSSIBLE INTERACTION WITH OTHER DRUGS

GENERIC NAME OR DRUG CLASS	COMBINED EFFECT
Antacids* (high dose)	Possible increased flecainide acetate effect.
Antiarrhythmics, other*	Possible irregular heartbeat.
Beta-adrenergic blocking agents*	Possible decreased efficiency of heart muscle contraction, leading to congestive heart failure.
Bone marrow depressants*	Possible decreased production of blood cells in bone marrow.
Carbonic anhydrase inhibitors*	Possible increased flecainide acetate effect.
Cimetidine	Increased effect of flecainide.
Digitalis preparations*	Possible increased digitalis effect. Possible irregular heartbeat.
Disopyramide	Possible decreased efficiency of heart muscle contraction, leading to congestive heart failure.
Doxepin (topical)	Increased risk of toxicity of both drugs.
Nicardipine	Possible increased effect and toxicity of each drug.
Paroxetine	Increased effect of both drugs.
Propafenone	Increased effect of both drugs and increased risk of toxicity.
Sodium bicarbonate	Possible increased flecainide acetate effect.
Verapamil	Possible decreased efficiency of heart muscle contraction, leading to congestive heart failure.

POSSIBLE INTERACTION WITH OTHER SUBSTANCES

INTERACTS WITH	COMBINED EFFECT
Alcohol:	May further depress normal heart function.
Beverages: Caffeine-containing beverages.	Possible decreased flecainide effect.
Cocaine:	Possible decreased flecainide effect.
Foods:	None expected.
Marijuana:	Possible decreased flecainide effect.
Tobacco:	Possible decreased flecainide effect.

FLUCONAZOLE

BRAND NAMES

Diflucan

BASIC INFORMATION

Habit forming? No
Prescription needed? Yes
Available as generic? No
Drug class: Antifungal

USES

- Treats meningitis.
- Treats candidiasis (thrush) whether in the mouth, esophagus or vagina or widely disseminated throughout the body.

DOSAGE & USAGE INFORMATION

How to take:
Tablets—Swallow with liquid. If you can't swallow whole, crumble tablet and take with liquid or food. Instructions to take on empty stomach mean 1 hour before or 2 hours after eating.

When to take:
Once a day, probably for 10 to 12 weeks, depending on the disease being treated and your kidney function status.

If you forget a dose:
Take as soon as you remember up to 2 hours late. If more than 2 hours, wait for next scheduled dose (don't double this dose).

What drug does:
Changes the cell membranes of susceptible fungus germs.

Time lapse before drug works:
1 to 2 hours. Several weeks of treatment are necessary for full benefit.

Don't take with:
Other antifungal drugs in the azole family (ketoconazole, miconazole or itraconazole).

OVERDOSE

SYMPTOMS:
Overdose not expected to threaten life, but if accidental or purposeful overdose occurs, follow the directions below.
WHAT TO DO:
- **Dial 911 (emergency) or 0 (operator) for an ambulance or medical help. Then give first aid immediately.**
- **See emergency information on inside covers.**

POSSIBLE ADVERSE REACTIONS OR SIDE EFFECTS

SYMPTOMS	WHAT TO DO
Life-threatening: In case of overdose, see previous column.	
Common: None expected.	
Infrequent: Diarrhea, nausea, vomiting.	Continue. Call doctor when convenient.
Rare: Skin rash, blistering, peeling skin, dark urine, yellow skin or eyes, abdominal pain, unusual bleeding or bruising.	Discontinue. Call doctor right away.

WARNINGS & PRECAUTIONS

Don't take if:
You are allergic to similar drugs, such as ketoconazole, miconazole or itraconazole.

Before you start, consult your doctor:
• If you have kidney disease.
• If you have liver disease.

Over age 60:
No studies available, but dosage may need adjustment if there is any age-related kidney impairment

Pregnancy:
Decide with your doctor if drug benefits justify risk to unborn child. Risk category C (see page xxiii).

Breast-feeding:
Safety not established. Consult doctor.

Infants & children:
Safety not established. Consult doctor.

Prolonged use:
No special problems expected.

Skin & sunlight:
No special problems expected.

Driving, piloting or hazardous work:
No special problems expected

Discontinuing:
Don't discontinue without consulting doctor. Dose may require gradual reduction if you have taken drug for a long time. Doses of other drugs may also require adjustment.

Others:
• Advise any doctor or dentist whom you consult that you take this medicine.
• May affect results of some medical tests.
• Does not alter male hormone activity. (A similar drug, ketoconazole, does alter male hormone activity.)

POSSIBLE INTERACTION WITH OTHER DRUGS

GENERIC NAME OR DRUG CLASS	COMBINED EFFECT
Antidiabetics, oral*	Greater than expected drop in blood sugar. If any antidiabetic agent is taken with fluconazole, blood sugars must be monitored carefully.
Antihistamines, nonsedating	May cause serious heart rhythm problems with astemizole or terfenadine. Avoid.
Cyclosporine	Increased cyclosporine effect.
Phenytoin	Increased phenytoin effect.
Rifampin	Decreased fluconazole effect.
Warfarin	Increased warfarin effect.

POSSIBLE INTERACTION WITH OTHER SUBSTANCES

INTERACTS WITH	COMBINED EFFECT
Alcohol:	None expected.
Beverages:	None expected.
Cocaine:	None expected.
Foods:	None expected.
Marijuana:	None expected.
Tobacco:	None expected.

FLUOROQUINOLONES

GENERIC AND BRAND NAMES

CIPROFLOXACIN
  Cipro
ENOXACIN
  Penetrex
GREPAFLOXACIN
  Raxar
LEVOFLOXACIN
  Levaquin
LOMEFLOXACIN
  Maxaquin

NORFLOXACIN
  Noroxin
OFLOXACIN
  Floxin
SPARFLOXACIN
  Zagam
TROVAFLOXACIN
  Trovan

BASIC INFORMATION

Habit forming? No
Prescription needed? Yes
Available as generic? No
Drug class: Antibacterial

USES

Treats a wide range of bacteria that may cause diarrhea, pneumonia, skin and soft tissue infections, urinary tract infections, bone infections.

DOSAGE & USAGE INFORMATION

How to take:
- Tablets—Take with full glass of water. Take enoxacin and ofloxacin on empty stomach. Ciprofloxacin, levofloxacin, lomefloxacin and norfloxacin may be taken with or without meals.
- Oral suspension—Take as directed on label.

When to take:
As directed by your doctor.

Continued next column

OVERDOSE

SYMPTOMS:
Confusion and hallucinations, headache, abdominal pain, convulsions.
WHAT TO DO:
- **Dial 911 (emergency) or 0 (operator) for an ambulance or medical help. Then give first aid immediately.**
- **If patient is unconscious and not breathing, give mouth-to-mouth breathing. If there is no heartbeat, use cardiac massage and mouth-to-mouth breathing (CPR). Don't try to make patient vomit. If you can't get help quickly, take patient to nearest emergency facility.**
- **See emergency information on inside covers.**

If you forget a dose:
Take as soon as you remember up to 2 hours late. If more than 2 hours, wait for next scheduled dose (don't double this dose).

What drug does:
Destroys bacteria in the body, probably by promoting DNA breakage in germs.

Time lapse before drug works:
1 to 2 weeks for most infections, but some infections may take 6 weeks or more for cure.

Don't take with:
Any other medicine without consulting your doctor or pharmacist.

POSSIBLE ADVERSE REACTIONS OR SIDE EFFECTS

SYMPTOMS	WHAT TO DO
Life-threatening: Hives, rash, intense itching, faintness soon after a dose (anaphylaxis).	Seek emergency treatment immediately.
Common: Skin reaction when exposed to sunlight (blisters, burning, sunburn, itching).	Discontinue. Call doctor right away.
Infrequent: Dizziness, light-headedness, headache, nervousness, drowsiness or insomnia, stomach pain, diarrhea, nausea or vomiting, changes in taste, vaginal itching.	Continue. Call doctor when convenient.
Rare: Agitation, confusion, hallucinations, tremors, skin rash or redness, shortness of breath, neck or face swelling, bloody or cloudy urine, swelling of feet or legs, tendon problems (inflammation, pain, rupture), seizures.	Discontinue. Call doctor right away.

WARNINGS & PRECAUTIONS

Don't take if:
You are allergic to fluoroquinolones or quinolone derivatives.

Before you start, consult your doctor:
- If you have any disorder of the central nervous system such as epilepsy or stroke.
- If you have liver or kidney disease.

Over age 60:
Adverse reactions and side effects may be more frequent and severe than in younger persons. You may need smaller doses for shorter periods of time.

Pregnancy:
Decide with your doctor if drug benefits justify risk to unborn child. Risk category C (see page xxiii).

Breast-feeding:
Drug passes into milk. Avoid drug or discontinue nursing until you finish medicine. Consult doctor for advice on maintaining milk supply.

Infants & children:
Not recommended. Can impair bone growth and development.

Prolonged use:
Usually not prescribed for long-term use.

Skin & sunlight:
One or more drugs in this group may cause rash or intensify sunburn in areas exposed to sun or ultraviolet light (photosensitivity reaction). Avoid overexposure. Notify doctor if reaction occurs.

Driving, piloting or hazardous work:
Don't drive or pilot aircraft until you learn how medicine affects you. Don't work around dangerous machinery. Don't climb ladders or work in high places. Danger increases if you drink alcohol or take medicine affecting alertness and reflexes, such as antihistamines, tranquilizers, sedatives, pain medicine, narcotics and mind-altering drugs.

Discontinuing:
Don't discontinue without consulting doctor or completing prescribed dosage. Call doctor if symptoms occur after you stop drug (stomach cramps, diarrhea that is watery or bloody).

Others:
- May affect accuracy of laboratory test values for SGOT*, serum bilirubin, serum creatinine and LDH*.
- If tendon problems develop, rest and refrain from exercise.
- Drink plenty of fluids while taking drug.
- Advise any doctor or dentist whom you consult that you take this medicine.

POSSIBLE INTERACTION WITH OTHER DRUGS

GENERIC NAME OR DRUG CLASS	COMBINED EFFECT
Aminophylline	Increased risk of aminophylline toxicity.
Antacids*	Decreased fluoro-quinolone effect.

Antidiabetic agents*	Adverse diabetic reactions with levofloxacin.
Antivirals, HIV/AIDS*	Decreased antibiotic effect.
Caffeine	With enoxacin or norfloxacin— Increased risk of central nervous system side effects.
Carbonic anhydrase inhibitors*	May cause kidney dysfunction.
Cyclosporine	Risk of kidney toxicity.
Didanosine	Decreased fluoro-quinolone effect.
Ferrous sulfate	Decreased fluoro-quinolone effect.
Oxtriphylline	Increased risk of oxtriphylline toxicity.
Probenecid	May cause kidney dysfunction.
QT interval prolongation causing drugs*	May cause heart rhythm problems with sparfloxacin.
Sucralfate	Decreased fluoro-quinolone effect.

Continued on page 915

POSSIBLE INTERACTION WITH OTHER SUBSTANCES

INTERACTS WITH	COMBINED EFFECT
Alcohol:	Increased possibility of central nervous system side effects.
Beverages: Caffeine drinks.	Increased effect of caffeine.
Cocaine:	Increased possibility of central nervous system side effects.
Foods: Dairy foods.	Decreased effect of fluoroquinolone.
Marijuana:	Increased possibility of central nervous system side effects.
Tobacco:	Increased possibility of central nervous system side effects.

*See Glossary

FLUOROURACIL (Topical)

BRAND NAMES

5-FU   Fluoroplex
Efudex

BASIC INFORMATION

Habit forming? No
Prescription needed? Yes
Available as generic? No
Drug class: Antineoplastic (topical)

USES

- Treats precancerous actinic keratoses on skin.
- Treats superficial basal cell carcinomas (skin cancers that don't spread to distant organs and, therefore, do not threaten life).

DOSAGE & USAGE INFORMATION

How to use:
- Apply with cotton-tipped applicator.
- Cream, lotion, ointment—Bathe and dry area before use. Apply small amount and rub gently.
- Wash hands (if fingertips are used to apply) after applying medicine to other parts of body.

When to use:
Once or twice a day or as directed by doctor.

If you forget a dose:
Apply as soon as you remember. Resume basic schedule.

What drug does:
Selectively destroys actively proliferating cells.

Time lapse before drug works:
2 to 3 days.

Don't use with:
Other topical medications unless prescribed by your doctor.

OVERDOSE

SYMPTOMS:
None expected.
WHAT TO DO:
Not for internal use. If child accidentally swallows, call poison control center.

POSSIBLE ADVERSE REACTIONS OR SIDE EFFECTS

SYMPTOMS	WHAT TO DO
Life-threatening None expected.	
Common • Skin redness or swelling.	Discontinue. Call doctor right away.
• After 1 or 2 weeks of use—Skin itching or oozing; rash, tenderness, soreness.	Continue. Call doctor when convenient.
Infrequent Skin darkening or scaling.	Continue. Call doctor when convenient.
Rare Watery eyes.	Discontinue. Call doctor right away.

FLUOROURACIL (Topical)

 WARNINGS & PRECAUTIONS

Don't use if:
You are allergic to fluorouracil.

Before you start, consult your doctor:
- If you have cloasma or acne rosacea.
- If you have any other skin problems.

Over age 60:
No problems expected.

Pregnancy:
Consult doctor. Risk category X (see page xxiii).

Breast-feeding:
Avoid drug or discontinue nursing until you finish medicine. Consult doctor for advice on maintaining milk supply.

Infants & children:
No problems expected, but check with doctor.

Prolonged use:
No problems expected, but check with doctor.

Skin & sunlight:
May cause rash or intensify sunburn in areas exposed to sun or ultraviolet light (photosensitivity reaction). Avoid overexposure. Notify doctor if reaction occurs.

Driving, piloting or hazardous work:
No problems expected, but check with doctor.

Discontinuing:
Pink, smooth area remains after treatment (usually fades in 1 to 2 months).

Others:
- Skin lesions may need biopsy before treatment.
- Keep medicine out of eyes or mouth.
- Heat and moisture in bathroom medicine cabinet can cause breakdown of medicine. Store someplace else.

 POSSIBLE INTERACTION WITH OTHER DRUGS

GENERIC NAME OR DRUG CLASS	COMBINED EFFECT
None significant.	

 POSSIBLE INTERACTION WITH OTHER SUBSTANCES

INTERACTS WITH	COMBINED EFFECT
Alcohol:	None expected.
Beverages:	None expected.
Cocaine:	None expected.
Foods:	None expected.
Marijuana:	None expected.
Tobacco:	None expected.

FLUOXETINE

BRAND NAMES

Prozac

BASIC INFORMATION

Habit forming? No
Prescription needed? Yes
Available as generic? No
Drug class: Antidepressant (selective serotonin reuptake inhibitor)

USES

- Treats mental depression, particularly in people who do not tolerate tricyclic antidepressants.
- Treats obsessive-compulsive disorder.
- Treats bulimia.

DOSAGE & USAGE INFORMATION

How to take:
- Capsules—Swallow with liquid or food to lessen stomach irritation. If you can't swallow whole, open capsule and take with liquid or food.
- Oral solution—Follow instructions on prescription.

When to take:
In the morning at the same time each day.

If you forget a dose:
Take as soon as you remember up to 2 hours late. If more than 2 hours, wait for next scheduled dose (don't double this dose).

What drug does:
Affects serotonin, one of the chemicals in the brain called neurotransmitters, that plays a role in emotions and psychological disturbances.

Time lapse before drug works:
1 to 3 weeks.

Continued next column

OVERDOSE

SYMPTOMS:
Seizures, agitation, violent vomiting.
WHAT TO DO:
- **Dial 911 (emergency) or 0 (operator) for an ambulance or medical help. Then give first aid immediately.**
- **See emergency information at end of book.**

Don't take with:
- Any monoamine oxidase (MAO) inhibitor* or within 14 days of stopping one. To do so may result in a serious or fatal reaction.
- Any other medicine without consulting your doctor or pharmacist.

POSSIBLE ADVERSE REACTIONS OR SIDE EFFECTS

SYMPTOMS	WHAT TO DO
Life-threatening: Rash, itchy skin, breathing difficulty (allergic reaction), chest pain.	Seek emergency treatment immediately.
Common: Diarrhea, nervousness, drowsiness, headache, increased sweating, insomnia, anxiety.	Continue. Call doctor when convenient.
Infrequent: • Chills, fever, joint or muscle pain, enlarged lymph glands, unusual excitability, blurred vision, chest pain.	Discontinue. Call doctor right away.
• Nightmares, taste changes, vision changes, decreased sex drive, dry mouth, skin flushing, urinating frequently, painful menstruation, stuffy nose, tremors.	Continue. Call doctor when convenient.
Rare: • Seizures. (convulsions).	Discontinue. Seek emergency treatment.
• Fast heartbeat; abdominal pain; signs of low blood sugar (anxiety, nervousness, chills, increased sweating, difficulty concentrating).	Discontinue. Call doctor right away.
• Nausea, vomiting, constipation, cough, increased appetite.	Continue. Call doctor when convenient.

WARNINGS & PRECAUTIONS

Don't take if:
You are allergic to fluoxetine.

Before you start, consult your doctor:
- If you have a history of seizure disorders.
- If you have severe liver or kidney disease.

Over age 60:
Adverse reactions and side effects may be more frequent and severe than in younger persons. You may need smaller doses for shorter periods of time.

Pregnancy:
Don't take unless essential. Consult doctor. Risk category B (see page xxiii).

Breast-feeding:
Unknown effects. Consult doctor.

Infants & children:
Not recommended.

Prolonged use:
No problems expected, but stay under a doctor's care as long as you take this medicine.

Skin & sunlight:
No problems expected.

Driving, piloting or hazardous work:
Don't drive or pilot aircraft until you learn how medicine affects you. Don't work around dangerous machinery. Don't climb ladders or work in high places. Danger increases if you drink alcohol or take medicine affecting alertness and reflexes.

Discontinuing:
Don't discontinue without consulting doctor. Dose may require gradual reduction if you have taken drug for a long time. Doses of other drugs may also require adjustment.

Others:
- Advise any doctor or dentist whom you consult about the use of this medicine.
- For dry mouth, suck on sugarless hard candy or chew sugarless gum. If dry mouth persists, see your dentist.

POSSIBLE INTERACTION WITH OTHER DRUGS

GENERIC NAME OR DRUG CLASS	COMBINED EFFECT
Anticoagulants, oral*	Increased risk of bleeding.
Anticonvulsants*	Increased risk of anticonvulsant toxicity.
Antidepressants, tricyclic*	Increased levels of tricyclic antidepressant; possible toxicity.
Bupropion	Increased risk of seizures.
Central nervous system (CNS) depressants*	Increased depressant effects of both drugs.
Clozapine	Increased risk of adverse clozapine reactions.
Dexfenfluramine	May cause serotonin syndrome*. Avoid.
Lithium	Risk of increased lithium effect.
Monoamine oxidase (MAO) inhibitors*	May cause confusion, agitation, convulsions, high blood pressure. Possibly life-threatening. Allow 4-5 weeks between use of these drugs.
Selegiline	Increased risk of adverse effects. May lead to convulsions and hypertensive crisis. Let 14 days elapse between taking the 2 drugs.

POSSIBLE INTERACTION WITH OTHER SUBSTANCES

INTERACTS WITH	COMBINED EFFECT
Alcohol:	Possible toxicity of both drugs. Avoid.
Beverages:	Decreases effect of fluoxetine.
Cocaine:	Decreases effect of fluoxetine.
Foods:	None expected.
Marijuana:	Decreases effect of fluoxetine.
Tobacco:	Decreases effect of fluoxetine.

*See Glossary

FLUTAMIDE

BRAND NAMES

Euflex   Eulexin

BASIC INFORMATION

Habit forming? No
Prescription needed? Yes
Available as generic? No
Drug class: Antineoplastic

 USES

Treats prostate cancer when used with leuteinizing hormone-releasing hormone (LHRH).

 DOSAGE & USAGE INFORMATION

How to take:
Tablet or capsule—Swallow with liquid.

When to take:
According to doctor's instructions.

If you forget a dose:
Take as soon as you remember up to 2 hours late. If more than 2 hours, wait for next scheduled dose (don't double this dose).

What drug does:
Interferes with utilization of androgen (testosterone) by body cells.

Time lapse before drug works:
2 hours.

Don't take with:
Any other medicines (including over-the-counter drugs such as cough and cold medicines, laxatives, antacids, diet pills, caffeine, nose drops or vitamins) without consulting your doctor.

 OVERDOSE

SYMPTOMS:
None expected.
WHAT TO DO:
Overdose unlikely to threaten life. If person takes much larger amount than prescribed, call doctor, poison control center or hospital emergency room for instructions.

 POSSIBLE ADVERSE REACTIONS OR SIDE EFFECTS

SYMPTOMS	WHAT TO DO
Life-threatening: None expected.	
Common: Decreased sex drive, diarrhea, appetite loss, sweating and hot flashes, nausea, vomiting.	Continue. Call doctor when convenient.
Infrequent: Hands and feet tingling or numb, swollen breasts, swollen feet and legs.	Continue. Call doctor when convenient.
Rare: Jaundice (yellow eyes and skin).	Continue. Call doctor right away.

WARNINGS & PRECAUTIONS

Don't take if:
You can't tolerate flutamide.

Before you start, consult your doctor:
If you have liver disease.

Over age 60:
Adverse reactions and side effects may be more frequent and severe than in younger persons. You may need smaller doses for shorter periods of time.

Pregnancy:
Not intended for use in women. Risk category D (see page xxiii).

Breast-feeding:
Not intended for use in women.

Infants & children:
Not intended for use in infants and children.

Prolonged use:
Talk to your doctor about the need for follow-up medical examinations or laboratory studies to check liver function.

Skin & sunlight:
May cause rash or intensify sunburn in areas exposed to sun or ultraviolet light (photosensitivity reaction). Avoid overexposure. Notify doctor if reaction occurs.

Driving, piloting or hazardous work:
No problems expected.

Discontinuing:
No special problems expected. Don't discontinue drug without doctor's approval.

Others:
- Advise any doctor or dentist whom you consult that you take this medicine.
- May affect results in some medical tests.
- May decrease sperm count.

 POSSIBLE INTERACTION WITH OTHER DRUGS

GENERIC NAME OR DRUG CLASS	COMBINED EFFECT
None significant.	

 POSSIBLE INTERACTION WITH OTHER SUBSTANCES

INTERACTS WITH	COMBINED EFFECT
Alcohol:	Jaundice more likely.
Beverages:	No special problems expected.
Cocaine:	No special problems expected.
Foods:	No special problems expected.
Marijuana:	No special problems expected.
Tobacco:	No special problems expected.

FLUVOXAMINE

BRAND NAMES

Luvox

BASIC INFORMATION

Habit forming? No
Prescription needed? Yes
Available as generic? No
Drug class: Antiobsessional agent

 USES

- Used to relieve the symptoms of obsessive-compulsive disorder (OCD), including recurrent disturbing thoughts (obsessions) and/or repetitive, ritualized behaviors (compulsions).
- Treatment for other disorders as determined by your doctor.

 DOSAGE & USAGE INFORMATION

How to take:
Tablet–Swallow with liquid. May be taken with or without food.

When to take:
1 dose a day–Take at bedtime. 2 doses a day–Take one at bedtime and one in the morning. Dosages may be increased gradually every 4-7 days to achieve maximum benefits.

If you forget a dose:
- 1 dose a day–Skip the missed dose and wait for the next scheduled dose (don't double this dose).
- 2 doses a day–Take as soon as you remember if it is almost time for the next dose, then skip the missed dose and wait for your next scheduled dose (don't double this dose).

What drug does:
Affects serotonin, one of the chemicals in the brain called neurotransmitters, that plays a role in emotions and psychological disturbances.

Continued next column

 OVERDOSE

SYMPTOMS:
Diarrhea, dizziness, drowsiness, vomiting, slow or irregular heartbeat, seizures, breathing difficulty, coma.
WHAT TO DO:
- **Dial 911 (emergency) or 0 (operator) for an ambulance or medical help. Then give first aid immediately.**
- **See emergency information at end of book.**

Time lapse before drug works:
May take several weeks for full effectiveness.

Don't take with:
- Any other medication without consulting your doctor or pharmacist.
- Any monoamine oxidase (MAO) inhibitor* or within 14 days of stopping one. May result in a serious or fatal reaction.

 POSSIBLE ADVERSE REACTIONS OR SIDE EFFECTS

SYMPTOMS	WHAT TO DO
Life-threatening:	
In case of overdose, see previous column.	
Common:	
• Diarrhea, dizziness, nervousness, unusual tiredness or weakness, twitching or jerking movements, impotence, loss of sexual desire.	Discontinue. Call doctor right away.
• Constipation, dry mouth, drowsiness, headache, nausea, runny nose, trouble sleeping, loss of appetite, heartburn, flushing, increased sweating, weight loss, frequent urination, taste changes.	Continue. Call doctor when convenient.
• Yawning.	No action necessary.
Infrequent:	
• Mood or behavior changes, agitation, blurred vision, fast or pounding heartbeat, urination problems, skin rash or hives, uncontrolled excitable behavior, breathing problems, vomiting, shakiness, trouble swallowing, anxiety, forgetfulness.	Discontinue. Call doctor right away.
• Chills, swelling of hands or feet, gas, weight gain.	Continue. Call doctor when convenient.

Rare:
Unusual bleeding or bruising, chest pain, cold hands or feet, restlessness, clumsiness or unsteadiness, unusual feeling of well-being, hallucinations, eye problems, sensitivity to light, black or tarry stools, bloody vomit, swollen glands, menstrual changes.

Discontinue. Call doctor right away.

WARNINGS & PRECAUTIONS

Don't take if:
You are allergic to fluvoxamine.

Before you start, consult your doctor:
- If you have a seizure disorder, heart disease, kidney or liver disease.
- If you have or have had a history of drug dependence or drug abuse.
- If you have a history of mood disorders or thoughts of suicide.
- If you are allergic to any other medication, food or other substance.

Over age 60:
Adverse reactions and side effects may be more frequent and severe than in younger persons. Lower dosages may to be prescribed.

Pregnancy:
Decide with your doctor if drug benefits justify risks to unborn child. Risk category C (see page xxiii).

Breast-feeding:
Drug passes into milk. Avoid drug or discontinue nursing until you finish medicine. Consult doctor for advice on maintaining milk supply.

Infants & children:
Not recommended for children under age 8.

Prolonged use:
No special problems expected. Schedule regular doctor visits to determine if drug is continuing to be effective in controlling symptoms of OCD.

Skin & sunlight:
May cause rash or intensify sunburn in areas exposed to sun or ultraviolet light (photosensitivity). Avoid overexposure and use sunscreen. Consult doctor if reaction occurs.

Driving, piloting or hazardous work:
Don't drive or pilot aircraft until you learn how medicine affects you. Don't work around dangerous machinery. Don't climb ladders or work in high places. Danger increases if you drink alcohol or take other medicines affecting alertness and reflexes such as antihistamines, tranquilizers, sedatives, pain medicine, narcotics and mind-altering drugs.

Discontinuing:
Since obsessive-compulsive disorder is a chronic condition, you may have a recurrence of symptoms if drug is discontinued.

Others:
Advise any doctor or dentist whom you consult that you take this medicine.

POSSIBLE INTERACTION WITH OTHER DRUGS

GENERIC NAME OR DRUG CLASS	COMBINED EFFECT
Anticoagulants, oral*	Increased risk of bleeding.
Antidepressants, tricyclic*	Increased antidepressant effect.
Antihistamines, nonsedating	May cause serious heart rhythm problems with astemizole or terfenadine. Avoid.
Astemizole	Serious heart problems. Avoid.
Benzodiazepines*	Increased benzodiazepine effect.
Beta-adrenergic blocking agents*	Increased beta blocker effect.
Carbamazepine	Possible toxicity of carbamazepine.
Clozapine	Increased risk of adverse reactions.
Dexfenfluramine	May cause serotonin syndrome*. Avoid.
Lithium	Increased risk of seizures.
Methadone	Increased methadone effect.

Continued on page 915

POSSIBLE INTERACTION WITH OTHER SUBSTANCES

INTERACTS WITH	COMBINED EFFECT
Alcohol:	Unknown. Avoid.
Beverages:	None expected.
Cocaine:	Unknown. Avoid.
Foods:	None expected.
Marijuana:	Increased sedation. Avoid.
Tobacco:	Decreased fluvoxamine effect.

FOLIC ACID (Vitamin B-9)

BRAND NAMES

Apo-Folic   Novo-Folacid
Folvite
Numerous other multiple vitamin-mineral supplements. Check labels.

BASIC INFORMATION

Habit forming? No
Prescription needed?
  High strength: Yes
  Vitamin mixtures: No
Available as generic? Yes
Drug class: Vitamin supplement

 USES

- Dietary supplement to promote normal growth, development and good health.
- Dietary supplement during pregnancy to prevent spinal defects.
- Treatment for anemias due to folic acid deficiency occurring from alcoholism, liver disease, hemolytic anemia, sprue, infants on artificial formula, pregnancy, breast feeding and use of oral contraceptives.
- Some studies have found that folic acid supplementation alone or in combination with other vitamins taken before conception and during early pregnancy may reduce the incidence of neural tube defects in infants.

 DOSAGE & USAGE INFORMATION

How to take:
Tablet—Swallow with liquid or food to lessen stomach irritation. If you can't swallow whole, crumble tablet and take with liquid or food.

When to take:
At the same time each day.

If you forget a dose:
Take when you remember. Don't double next dose. Resume regular schedule.

What drug does:
Essential to normal red blood cell formation.

Continued next column

 OVERDOSE

SYMPTOMS:
None expected.
WHAT TO DO:
Overdose unlikely to threaten life.

Time lapse before drug works:
Not determined.

Don't take with:
Any other medicine without consulting your doctor or pharmacist.

 POSSIBLE ADVERSE REACTIONS OR SIDE EFFECTS

SYMPTOMS	WHAT TO DO
Life-threatening: None expected.	
Common: Large dose may produce yellow urine.	Continue. Tell doctor at next visit.
Infrequent: None expected.	
Rare: Rash, itching, bronchospasm.	Discontinue. Call doctor right away.

WARNINGS & PRECAUTIONS

Don't take if:
You are allergic to any B vitamin.

Before you start, consult your doctor:
- If you have liver disease.
- If you have pernicious anemia. (Folic acid corrects anemia, but nerve damage of pernicious anemia continues.)

Over age 60:
No problems expected.

Pregnancy:
No problems expected. Consult doctor. Risk category A (see page xxiii)

Breast-feeding:
No problems expected. Consult doctor.

Infants & children:
No problems expected.

Prolonged use:
No problems expected.

Skin & sunlight:
No problems expected.

Driving, piloting or hazardous work:
No problems expected.

Discontinuing:
Don't discontinue without doctor's advice until you complete prescribed dose, even though symptoms diminish or disappear.

Others:
- Folic acid removed by kidney dialysis. Dialysis patients should increase intake to 300% of RDA or take as directed.
- A balanced diet should provide all the folic acid a healthy person needs and make supplements unnecessary. Best sources are green, leafy vegetables; fruits; liver and kidney.

POSSIBLE INTERACTION WITH OTHER DRUGS

GENERIC NAME OR DRUG CLASS	COMBINED EFFECT
Analgesics*	Decreased effect of folic acid.
Anticonvulsants, hydantoin*	Decreased effect of folic acid. Possible increased seizure frequency.
Chloramphenicol	Possible decreased folic acid effect.
Contraceptives, oral*	Decreased effect of folic acid.
Cortisone drugs*	Decreased effect of folic acid.
Methotrexate	Decreased effect of folic acid.
Para-aminosalicylic acid (PAS)	Decreased effect of folic acid.
Pyrimethamine	Decreased effect of folic acid.
Sulfasalazine	Decreased dietary absorption of folic acid.
Triamterene	Decreased effect of folic acid.
Trimethoprim	Decreased effect of folic acid.
Zinc supplements	Increased need for zinc.

POSSIBLE INTERACTION WITH OTHER SUBSTANCES

INTERACTS WITH	COMBINED EFFECT
Alcohol:	None expected.
Beverages:	None expected.
Cocaine:	None expected.
Foods:	None expected.
Marijuana:	None expected.
Tobacco:	None expected.

FURAZOLIDONE

BRAND NAMES

Furoxone   Furoxone Liquid

BASIC INFORMATION

Habit forming? No
Prescription needed? Yes
Available as generic? No
**Drug class: Antiprotozoal, antibacterial
(antibiotic)**

 ## USES

- As an adjunct in treating most germs that
  infect the gastrointestinal tract such as
  cholera, salmonellosis, E. coli, proteus
  infections, and other bacterial causes of
  diarrhea.
- Treats giardiasis.

 ## DOSAGE & USAGE INFORMATION

How to take:
- Liquid—Use a measuring spoon to ensure
  correct dose.
- Tablet—Swallow with liquid or food to lessen
  stomach irritation. If you can't swallow whole,
  crumble tablet and take with liquid or food.

When to take:
At the same time each day, according to
instructions on prescription label.

If you forget a dose:
Take as soon as you remember up to 2 hours
late. If more than 2 hours, wait for next
scheduled dose. Don't double this dose.

What drug does:
Kills microscopic germs.

Time lapse before drug works:
Immediate.

Don't take with:
Any other medicine without consulting your
doctor or pharmacist.

 ## OVERDOSE

SYMPTOMS:
None expected.
WHAT TO DO:
**Overdose unlikely to threaten life. If person
takes much larger amount than prescribed,
call doctor, poison control center or hospital
emergency room for instructions.**

 ## POSSIBLE ADVERSE REACTIONS OR SIDE EFFECTS

SYMPTOMS	WHAT TO DO
Life-threatening:	
None expected except when taken with forbidden foods (see Possible Interaction with Other Substances).	
Common:	
• Nausea, vomiting.	Continue. Call doctor when convenient.
• Dark yellow or brown urine.	No action necessary.
Infrequent:	
• Abdominal pain.	Discontinue. Call doctor right away.
• Headache.	Continue. Call doctor when convenient.
Rare:	
Sore throat, fever, skin rash, itching, joint pain.	Discontinue. Call doctor right away.

WARNINGS & PRECAUTIONS

Don't take if:
- You have G6PD* deficiency.
- You have hypersensitivity to furazolidone, nitrofurantoin (Furadantin), or nitrofurazone (Furacin).

Before you start, consult your doctor:
If you are taking any other prescription or nonprescription medicine.

Over age 60:
No special problems expected.

Pregnancy:
Decide with your doctor if drug benefits justify risk to unborn child. Risk category C (see page xxiii).

Breast-feeding:
Drug may pass into milk. Avoid drug or discontinue nursing until you finish medicine. Consult doctor for advice on maintaining milk supply.

Infants & children:
Don't use for infants without specific instructions from your doctor.

Prolonged use:
No special problems expected.

Skin & sunlight:
No special problems expected.

Driving, piloting or hazardous work:
No special problems expected.

Discontinuing:
Food restrictions outlined in Possible Interaction with Other Substances must be continued for at least 2 weeks after furazolidone is discontinued.

Others:
- Should not be taken with foods or drinks high in tyramine (see Possible Interaction with Other Substances).
- Advise any doctor or dentist whom you consult that you take this medicine.

POSSIBLE INTERACTION WITH OTHER DRUGS

GENERIC NAME OR DRUG CLASS	COMBINED EFFECT
Antidepressants, tricyclic*	Sudden, severe increase in blood pressure.
Monoamine oxidase (MAO) inhibitors*	Sudden, severe increase in blood pressure.
Sumatriptan	Adverse effects unknown. Avoid.
Sympathomimetics*	Sudden, severe increase in blood pressure.

POSSIBLE INTERACTION WITH OTHER SUBSTANCES

INTERACTS WITH	COMBINED EFFECT
Alcohol:	Flushed face, shortness of breath, fever, tightness in chest. Avoid.
Beverages: Any alcoholic beverage.	Flushed face, shortness of breath, fever, tightness in chest. Avoid.
Cocaine:	High blood pressure. Avoid.
Foods: Aged cheese; dark beer; red wine (especially Chianti); sherry; liqueurs; caviar; yeast or protein extracts; fava beans; smoked or pickled meat, poultry, fish; pepperoni, salami, summer sausage; over-ripe fruit.	Sudden, severe high blood pressure that may be life-threatening. Avoid.
Marijuana:	High blood pressure. Avoid.
Tobacco:	No special problems expected.

GABAPENTIN

BRAND NAMES

Neurontin

BASIC INFORMATION

Habit forming? No
Prescription needed? Yes
Available as generic? No
Drug class: Anticonvulsant, antiepileptic

 ## USES

Treatment for partial (focal) epileptic seizures. Used in combination with other antiepileptic drugs.

 ## DOSAGE & USAGE INFORMATION

How to take:
Capsule—Swallow with liquid. May be taken with or without food.

When to take:
Your doctor will determine the best schedule. Dosages will be increased rapidly over the first 3 days of use. Further increases may be necessary to achieve maximum benefits.

If you forget a dose:
Take as soon as you remember. If it is almost time for the next dose, skip the missed dose and wait for your next scheduled dose (don't double this dose).

What drug does:
The exact mechanism is unknown. The anticonvulsant action may result from an altered transport of brain amino acids. Amino acids play an important part in chemical reactions within the cells.

Time lapse before drug works:
May take several weeks for effectiveness.

Don't take with:
Any other prescription or nonprescription drug without consulting your doctor.

 ## OVERDOSE

SYMPTOMS:
Double vision, slurred speech, drowsiness, tiredness, diarrhea.
WHAT TO DO:
Overdose unlikely to threaten life. If person takes much larger amount than prescribed, call doctor, poison control center or hospital emergency room for instructions.

 ## POSSIBLE ADVERSE REACTIONS OR SIDE EFFECTS

SYMPTOMS	WHAT TO DO
Life-threatening: None expected.	
Common: Sleepiness, dizziness, fatigue, clumsiness, lack of coordination.	Continue. Call doctor when convenient.
Infrequent: Rapid eye movement (nystagmus), double or blurred vision.	Continue. Call doctor when convenient.
Rare: Rash; nervousness; depression; twitching or swelling in hands, feet or legs; runny nose; dry or sore throat; nausea; vomiting, coughing; dry mouth; constipation; impotence; increased appetite, weight gain; muscle or back ache; forgetfulness; indigestion.	Continue. Call doctor when convenient.

WARNINGS & PRECAUTIONS

Don't take if:
You are allergic to gabapentin.

Before you start, consult your doctor:
If you have kidney disease.

Over age 60:
No special problems expected.

Pregnancy:
Decide with your doctor if drug benefits justify risks to unborn child. Risk category C (see page xxiii).

Breast-feeding:
It is unknown if drug passes into milk. Consult your doctor.

Infants & children:
Not recommended for children under age 12.

Prolonged use:
No special problems expected. Follow-up laboratory blood studies may be recommended by your doctor.

Skin & sunlight:
No problems expected.

Driving, piloting or hazardous work:
Don't drive or pilot aircraft until you learn how medicine affects you. Don't work around dangerous machinery. Don't climb ladders or work in high places. Danger increases if you drink alcohol or take other medicines affecting alertness and reflexes such as antihistamines, tranquilizers, sedatives, pain medicine, narcotics and mind-altering drugs.

Discontinuing:
Don't discontinue without doctor's approval due to risk of increased seizure activity.

Others:
- Advise any doctor or dentist whom you consult that you take this medicine.
- Side effects of gabapentin are usually mild to moderate. Because it is normally used with other anticonvulsant drugs, additional side effects may also occur. If they do, discuss them with your doctor.

POSSIBLE INTERACTION WITH OTHER DRUGS

GENERIC NAME OR DRUG CLASS	COMBINED EFFECT
Antacids*	Allow at least 2 hours between the 2 drugs.

POSSIBLE INTERACTION WITH OTHER SUBSTANCES

INTERACTS WITH	COMBINED EFFECT
Alcohol:	None expected.
Beverages:	None expected.
Cocaine:	None expected.
Foods:	None expected.
Marijuana:	None expected.
Tobacco:	None expected.

GEMFIBROZIL

BRAND NAMES

Lopid

BASIC INFORMATION

Habit forming? No
Prescription needed? Yes
Available as generic? Yes
Drug class: Antihyperlipidemic

USES

Reduces fatty substances in the blood
(triglycerides).

DOSAGE & USAGE INFORMATION

How to take:
Tablet or capsule—Swallow with liquid or food to
lessen stomach irritation.

When to take:
At the same times each day.

If you forget a dose:
Take as soon as you remember up to 2 hours
late. If more than 2 hours, wait for next
scheduled dose (don't double this dose).

What drug does:
Inhibits formation of fatty substances.

Time lapse before drug works:
3 months or more.

Don't take with:
Any other medicine without consulting your
doctor or pharmacist.

OVERDOSE

SYMPTOMS:
Diarrhea, headache, muscle pain.
WHAT TO DO:
**Overdose unlikely to threaten life. If person
takes much larger amount than prescribed,
call doctor, poison control center or hospital
emergency room for instructions.**

POSSIBLE ADVERSE REACTIONS OR SIDE EFFECTS

SYMPTOMS	WHAT TO DO
Life-threatening: None expected.	
Common: Indigestion.	Continue. Call doctor when convenient.
Infrequent: Chest pain, shortness of breath, irregular heartbeat, nausea, vomiting, diarrhea, stomach pain.	Discontinue. Call doctor right away.
Rare: • Rash, itch; sores in mouth, on lips; sore throat; swollen feet, legs; blood in urine; painful urination; fever; chills.	Discontinue. Call doctor right away.
• Dizziness, headache, drowsiness, muscle cramps, dry skin, backache, unusual tiredness, decreased sex drive.	Continue. Call doctor when convenient.

WARNINGS & PRECAUTIONS

Don't take if:
You are allergic to any antihyperlipidemic.

Before you start, consult your doctor:
- If you have had liver or kidney disease.
- If you have had peptic-ulcer disease.
- If you have diabetes.

Over age 60:
Adverse reactions and side effects may be more frequent and severe than in younger persons.

Pregnancy:
Decide with your doctor if drug benefits justify risks to unborn child. Risk category C (see page xxiii).

Breast-feeding:
May harm child. Avoid. Consult doctor.

Infants & children:
Not recommended.

Prolonged use:
Periodic blood cell counts and liver function studies recommended if you take gemfibrozil for a long time.

Skin & sunlight:
No problems expected.

Driving, piloting or hazardous work:
Avoid if you feel drowsy or dizzy. Otherwise, no problems expected.

Discontinuing:
Don't discontinue without doctor's advice until you complete prescribed dose.

Others:
- Some studies question effectiveness. Many studies warn against toxicity.
- May affect results in some medical tests.

POSSIBLE INTERACTION WITH OTHER DRUGS

GENERIC NAME OR DRUG CLASS	COMBINED EFFECT
Anticoagulants, oral*	Increased anti-coagulant effect. Dose reduction of anticoagulant necessary.
Antidiabetics, oral*	Increased antidiabetic effect.
Contraceptives, oral*	Decreased gemfibrozil effect.
Dexfenfluramine	May require dosage change as weight loss occurs.
Estrogens*	Decreased gemfibrozil effect.
Furosemide	Possible toxicity of both drugs.
HMG-CoA reductase inhibitors	Increased risk of muscle inflammation and kidney failure.
Insulin	Increased insulin effect.
Lovastatin	Increased risk of kidney problems.
Thyroid hormones*	Increased gemfibrozil effect.

POSSIBLE INTERACTION WITH OTHER SUBSTANCES

INTERACTS WITH	COMBINED EFFECT
Alcohol:	None expected.
Beverages:	None expected.
Cocaine:	Decreased effect of gemfibrozil. Avoid.
Foods: Fatty foods.	Decreased gemfibrozil effect.
Marijuana:	None expected.
Tobacco:	Decreased gemfibrozil absorption. Avoid.

GLUCAGON

BRAND NAMES

Glucagon for Injection

BASIC INFORMATION

Habit forming? No
Prescription needed? Yes
Available as generic? Yes
Drug class: Antihypoglycemic, diagnostic aid

 USES

- Treats low blood sugar (hypoglycemia) in diabetics.
- Used as antidote for overdose of beta-adrenergic blockers, quinidine and tricyclic antidepressants.

 DOSAGE & USAGE INFORMATION

How to take:
Injection—As directed by your doctor.

When to take:
When there are signs of low blood sugar (anxiety; chills; cool, pale skin; hunger; nausea; tremors; sweating; weakness; stomach pain; confusion; drowsiness; fast heartbeat; continuing headache; unsteady walk; unusual tiredness or weakness; vision changes; unconsciousness) in diabetics who don't respond to eating some form of sugar.

If you forget a dose:
Single dose only.

What drug does:
Forces liver to make more sugar and release it into the bloodstream.

Continued next column

 OVERDOSE

SYMPTOMS:
Nausea, vomiting, severe weakness, irregular heartbeat, hoarseness, cramps.
WHAT TO DO:
- Dial 911 (emergency) or 0 (operator) for an ambulance or medical help. Then give first aid immediately.
- See emergency information on inside covers.

Time lapse before drug works:
- For hypoglycemic condition—5 to 20 minutes.
- For muscle relaxant—1 to 10 minutes.

Don't take with:
Any other medicines (including over-the-counter drugs such as cough and cold medicines, laxatives, antacids, diet pills, caffeine, nose drops or vitamins) without consulting your doctor.

 POSSIBLE ADVERSE REACTIONS OR SIDE EFFECTS

SYMPTOMS	WHAT TO DO
Life-threatening:	
Unconsciousness.	Seek emergency treatment immediately.
Common:	
Nausea.	Continue. Call doctor when convenient.
Infrequent:	
Lightheadedness, breathing difficulty, skin rash.	Discontinue. Call doctor right away.
Rare:	
None expected.	

WARNINGS & PRECAUTIONS

Don't take if:
You can't tolerate glucagon.

Before you start, consult your doctor:
* If you are allergic to beef or pork.
* If you have phoochromocytoma.*

Over age 60:
No special problems expected.

Pregnancy:
No proven harm to unborn child, but avoid if possible. Consult doctor. Risk category B (see page xxiii).

Breast feeding:
No special problems expected. Consult doctor.

Infants & children:
No special problems expected.

Prolonged use:
To be used intermittently and not for prolonged periods.

Skin & sunlight:
No problems expected.

Driving, piloting or hazardous work:
Don't drive or pilot aircraft until you learn how medicine affects you. Don't work around dangerous machinery. Don't climb ladders or work in high places. Danger increases if you drink alcohol or take medicine affecting alertness and reflexes.

Discontinuing:
No special problems expected.

Others:
* May affect results in some medical tests.
* Explain to other family members how to inject glucagon.
* Before injecting, try to eat some form of sugar, such as glucose tablets, corn syrup, honey, orange juice, hard candy or sugar cubes.
* Store unmixed glucagon at room temperature. Store mixed glucagon in refrigerator, but don't freeze. Mixed solution is only good for 48 hours.
* Check expiration date regularly and replace drug before it expires.

POSSIBLE INTERACTION WITH OTHER DRUGS

GENERIC NAME OR DRUG CLASS	COMBINED EFFECT
Anticoagulants*	Increased anticoagulant effect.

POSSIBLE INTERACTION WITH OTHER SUBSTANCES

INTERACTS WITH	COMBINED EFFECT
Alcohol:	Decreased glucagon effect.
Beverages:	No special problems expected.
Cocaine:	Increased adverse reactions.
Foods: Sugar, fruit juice, candy.	Enhances glucagon effect.
Marijuana:	Increased adverse reactions.
Tobacco:	No special problems expected.

GLYCOPYRROLATE

BRAND NAMES

Robinul   Robinul Forte

BASIC INFORMATION

Habit forming? No
Prescription needed? Yes
Available as generic? Yes
Drug class: Antispasmodic, anticholinergic

 ## USES

- Reduces spasms of digestive system.
- Reduces production of saliva during dental procedures.
- Treats peptic ulcer by reducing gastric acid secretion.

 ## DOSAGE & USAGE INFORMATION

How to take:
Tablet—Swallow with liquid. If you can't swallow whole, crumble tablet and take with small amount of liquid or food.

When to take:
30 minutes before meals (unless directed otherwise by doctor).

If you forget a dose:
Wait for next scheduled dose (don't double this dose).

What drug does:
Blocks nerve impulses at parasympathetic nerve endings, preventing smooth (involuntary) muscle contractions and gland secretions of organs involved.

Time lapse before drug works:
15 to 30 minutes.

Don't take with:
Any other medicine without consulting your doctor or pharmacist.

 ## OVERDOSE

SYMPTOMS:
Dry mouth, blurred vision, low blood pressure, decreased breathing rate, rapid heartbeat, flushed skin, drowsiness.
WHAT TO DO:
- Dial 911 (emergency) or 0 (operator) for an ambulance or medical help. Then give first aid immediately.
- See emergency information on inside covers.

 ## POSSIBLE ADVERSE REACTIONS OR SIDE EFFECTS

SYMPTOMS	WHAT TO DO
Life-threatening: Hives, rash, intense itching, faintness soon after a dose (anaphylaxis).	Seek emergency treatment immediately.
Common: Dry mouth, loss of taste, constipation, difficult urination.	Continue. Call doctor when convenient.
Infrequent: • Confusion; dizziness; drowsiness; eye pain; headache; rash; sleep disturbance such as nightmares, frequent waking; nausea; vomiting; rapid heart-beat; lightheadedness.	Discontinue. Call doctor right away.
• Insomnia, blurred vision, diminished sex drive, decreased sweating, nasal congestion, altered taste.	Continue. Call doctor when convenient.
Rare: Rash, hives.	Discontinue. Call doctor right away.

 ## WARNINGS & PRECAUTIONS

Don't take if:
- You are allergic to any anticholinergic.
- You have trouble with stomach bloating.
- You have difficulty emptying your bladder completely.
- You have narrow-angle glaucoma.
- You have severe ulcerative colitis.

Before you start, consult your doctor:
- If you have open-angle glaucoma.
- If you have angina, chronic bronchitis or asthma, liver disease, hiatal hernia, enlarged prostate, myasthenia gravis, peptic ulcer, kidney or thyroid disease.
- If you will have surgery within 2 months, including dental surgery, requiring general or spinal anesthesia.

Over age 60:
Adverse reactions and side effects may be more frequent and severe than in younger persons.

Pregnancy:
Consult doctor. Risk category B (see page xxiii).

Breast-feeding:
Drug passes into milk and decreases milk flow. Avoid drug or discontinue nursing until you finish medicine. Consult doctor for advice on maintaining milk supply.

Infants & children:
Use only under medical supervision.

Prolonged use:
Chronic constipation, possible fecal impaction. Consult doctor immediately.

Skin & sunlight:
No problems expected.

Driving, piloting or hazardous work:
Use disqualifies you for piloting aircraft. Otherwise, no problems expected.

Discontinuing:
May be unnecessary to finish medicine. Follow doctor's instructions.

Others:
- Heatstroke more likely if you become overheated during exertion.
- Advise any doctor or dentist whom you consult that you take this medicine.

POSSIBLE INTERACTION WITH OTHER DRUGS

GENERIC NAME OR DRUG CLASS	COMBINED EFFECT
Adrenocorticoids, systemic	Possible glaucoma.
Antacids*	Decreased glycopyrrolate absorption effect.
Amantadine	Increased glycopyrrolate effect.
Anticholinergics, other*	Increased glycopyrrolate effect.
Antidepressants, tricyclic*	Increased glycopyrrolate effect.
Antidiarrheals*	Decreased glycopyrrolate absorption effect.
Attapulgite	Decreased effect of anticholinergic.
Buclizine	Increased glycopyrrolate effect.
Digitalis	Possible decreased absorption of digitalis.
Haloperidol	Increased internal eye pressure.

Ketoconazole	Decreased ketoconazole effect.
Meperidine	Increased glycopyrrolate effect.
Methylphenidate	Increased anticholinergic effect.
Molindone	Increased nizatidine effect.
Monoamine oxidase (MAO) inhibitors*	Increased glycopyrrolate effect.
Orphenadrine	Increased glycopyrrolate effect
Phenothiazines	Increased glycopyrrolate effect.
Pilocarpine	Increased glycopyrrolate effect. Loss of pilocarpine effect in glaucoma treatment.
Potassium chloride tabs	Increased side effects of potassium tablets.
Quinidine	Increased glycopyrrolate effect.
Retocunazole	Decreased absorption of both.
Sedatives* or central nervous system (CNS) depressants*	Increased sedative effect of both drugs.
Vitamin C	Increased glycopyrrolate effect. Avoid large vitamin C doses.

POSSIBLE INTERACTION WITH OTHER SUBSTANCES

INTERACTS WITH	COMBINED EFFECT
Alcohol:	None expected.
Beverages:	None expected.
Cocaine:	Excessively rapid heartbeat.
Foods:	None exected.
Marijuana:	Drowsiness and dry mouth.
Tobacco:	None expected.

*See Glossary

GOLD COMPOUNDS

GENERIC AND BRAND NAMES

AURANOFIN
Ridaura-Oral

GOLD SODIUM
THIOMOLATE
Myocrisin

BASIC INFORMATION

Habit forming? No
Prescription needed? Yes
Available as generic? No
Drug class: Gold compounds

 ## USES

Treatment for rheumatoid arthritis and juvenile arthritis.

 ## DOSAGE & USAGE INFORMATION

How to take:
- Capsules—Swallow with full glass of fluid. Follow prescription directions. Taking too much can cause serious adverse reactions.
- Injections—Under medical supervision.

When to take:
Once or twice daily, morning and night.

If you forget a dose:
Take as soon as you remember up to 6 hours late, then go back to usual schedule.

What drug does:
Modifies disease activity of rheumatoid arthritis by mechanisms not yet understood.

Time lapse before drug works:
3 to 6 months.

Don't take with:
Any other medicine without consulting your doctor or pharmacist.

 ## OVERDOSE

SYMPTOMS:
Confusion, delirium, numbness and tingling in feet and hands.
WHAT TO DO:
- **Induce vomiting with syrup of ipecac if available.**
- **Dial 911 (emergency) or 0 (operator) for an ambulance or medical help. Then give first aid immediately.**
- **See emergency information on inside covers.**

 ## POSSIBLE ADVERSE REACTIONS OR SIDE EFFECTS

SYMPTOMS	WHAT TO DO
Life-threatening:	
Hives, rash, intense itching, faintness soon after a dose (anaphylaxis).	Seek emergency treatment immediately.
Common:	
• Itch; hives; sores or white spots in mouth, throat; appetite loss; diarrhea; vomiting; skin rashes; fever.	Discontinue. Call doctor right away.
• Indigestion, constipation.	Continue. Call doctor when convenient.
Infrequent:	
• Excessive fatigue; sore tongue, mouth or gums; metallic or odd taste; unusual bleeding or bruising; blood in urine; vaginal discharge; flushing; fainting; dizziness; sweating after injection.	Discontinue. Call doctor right away.
• Hair loss; pain in muscles, bones and joints (with injections).	Continue. Call doctor when convenient.
Rare:	
• Blood in stool, difficult breathing, coughing, seizures.	Discontinue. Seek emergency treatment.
• Abdominal pain, jaundice, numbness or tingling in hands or feet, muscle weakness.	Discontinue. Call doctor right away.
• "Pink eye."	Continue. Call doctor when convenient.

WARNINGS & PRECAUTIONS

Don't take if:
- You have history of allergy to gold or other metals.
- You have any blood disorder.
- You have kidney disease.

Before you start, consult your doctor:
- If you are pregnant or may become pregnant.
- If you have lupus erythematosus.
- If you have Sjögren's syndrome.
- If you have chronic skin disease.
- If you are debilitated.
- If you have blood dyscrasias.

Over age 60:
Adverse reactions and side effects may be more frequent and severe than in younger persons.

Pregnancy:
Decide with your doctor if drug benefits justify risks to unborn child. Risk category C (see page xxiii).

Breast-feeding:
Drug may filter into milk, causing side effects in infants. Avoid. Consult doctor.

Infants & children:
Not recommended. Safety and dosage have not been established.

Prolonged use:
Request periodic laboratory studies of blood counts, urine and liver function. These should be done before use and at least once a month during treatment.

Skin & sunlight:
- One or more drugs in this group may cause rash or intensify sunburn in areas exposed to sun or ultraviolet light (photosensitivity reaction). Avoid overexposure. Notify doctor if reaction occurs.
- Blue-gray pigmentation in skin exposed to sunlight.

Driving, piloting or hazardous work:
Avoid if you have serious adverse reactions or side effects. Otherwise, no problems expected.

Discontinuing:
Don't discontinue without doctor's advice until you complete prescribed dose.

Others:
- Side effects and adverse reactions may appear during treatment or for many months after discontinuing.
- Gold has been shown to cause kidney tumors and kidney cancer in animals given excessive doses.
- May interfere with the accuracy of some medical tests.

POSSIBLE INTERACTION WITH OTHER DRUGS

GENERIC NAME OR DRUG CLASS	COMBINED EFFECT
Bone marrow depressants*	Increased risk of toxicity of both drugs.
Hepatotoxics*	Increased risk of toxicity of both drugs.
Nephrotoxics*	Increased risk of toxicity of both drugs.
Penicillamine	Increased likelihood of kidney damage.
Phenytoin	Increased phenytoin blood levels. Phenytoin dosage may require adjustment.

POSSIBLE INTERACTION WITH OTHER SUBSTANCES

INTERACTS WITH	COMBINED EFFECT
Alcohol:	None expected.
Beverages:	None expected.
Cocaine:	None expected.
Foods:	None expected.
Marijuana:	None expected.
Tobacco:	None expected.

*See Glossary

GRISEOFULVIN

BRAND NAMES

Fulvicin P/G
Fulvicin U/F
Grifulvin V
Grisactin

Grisactin Ultra
Grisovin-FP
Gris-PEG

BASIC INFORMATION

Habit forming? No
Prescription needed? Yes
Available as generic? Yes
Drug class: Antifungal

USES

Treatment for fungal infections susceptible to griseofulvin.

DOSAGE & USAGE INFORMATION

How to take:
- Tablet or capsule—Swallow with liquid or food to lessen stomach irritation. If you can't swallow whole, crumble tablet or open capsule and take with liquid or food.
- Liquid—Follow label instructions.

When to take:
With or immediately after meals.

If you forget a dose:
Take as soon as you remember up to 2 hours late. If more than 2 hours, wait for next scheduled dose (don't double this dose).

What drug does:
Prevents fungi from growing and reproducing.

Time lapse before drug works:
2 to 10 days for skin infections. 2 to 4 weeks for infections of fingernails or toenails. Complete cure of either may require several months.

Don't take with:
Any other medicine without consulting your doctor or pharmacist.

OVERDOSE

SYMPTOMS:
Nausea, vomiting, diarrhea. In sensitive individuals, severe diarrhea may occur without overdosing.
WHAT TO DO:
Overdose unlikely to threaten life. If person takes much larger amount than prescribed, call doctor, poison control center or hospital emergency room for instructions.

POSSIBLE ADVERSE REACTIONS OR SIDE EFFECTS

SYMPTOMS	WHAT TO DO
Life-threatening:	
In case of overdose, see previous column.	
Common:	
Headache.	Continue. Tell doctor at next visit.
Infrequent:	
• Confusion; rash, hives, itch; mouth or tongue irritation; soreness; nausea; vomiting; diarrhea; stomach pain.	Discontinue. Call doctor right away.
• Insomnia, tiredness.	Continue. Call doctor when convenient.
Rare:	
Sore throat, fever, numbness or tingling in hands or feet, cloudy urine, sensitivity to sunlight, yellow skin or eyes, sensitivity of skin to sunlight (these symptoms are more likely to occur with high doses taken for long periods).	Discontinue. Call doctor right away.

WARNINGS & PRECAUTIONS

Don't take if:
- You are allergic to any antifungal medicine.
- You are allergic to penicillin.
- You have liver disease.
- You have porphyria.
- The infection is minor and will respond to less potent drugs.

Before you start, consult your doctor:
- If you plan to become pregnant within medication period.
- If you have liver disease.
- If you have lupus.

Over age 60:
Adverse reactions and side effects may be more frequent and severe than in younger persons.

Pregnancy:
Risk to unborn child outweighs drug benefits. Don't use. Risk category X (see page xxiii).

Breast-feeding:
No problems expected, but consult your doctor.

Infants & children:
Not recommended for children younger than 2.

Prolonged use:
- You may become susceptible to infections caused by germs not responsive to griseofulvin.
- Talk to your doctor about the need for follow-up medical examinations or laboratory studies to check complete blood counts (white blood cell count, platelet count, red blood cell count, hemoglobin, hematocrit), liver function, kidney function.

Skin & sunlight:
May cause rash or intensify sunburn in areas exposed to sun or ultraviolet light (photosensitivity reaction). Avoid overexposure. Notify doctor if reaction occurs.

Driving, piloting or hazardous work:
- Don't drive if you feel dizzy or have vision problems.
- Don't pilot aircraft.

Discontinuing:
Don't discontinue without doctor's advice until you complete prescribed dose, even though symptoms diminish or disappear.

Others:
- Periodic laboratory blood studies and liver and kidney function tests recommended.
- Advise any doctor or dentist whom you consult that you take this medicine.

 ## POSSIBLE INTERACTION WITH OTHER DRUGS

GENERIC NAME OR DRUG CLASS	COMBINED EFFECT
Anticoagulants, oral*	Decreased anti-anticoagulant effect.
Barbiturates*	Decreased griseofulvin effect.
Contraceptives, oral*	Decreased contraceptive effect.
Photosensitizing medications*	Increased sun hazard.

 ## POSSIBLE INTERACTION WITH OTHER SUBSTANCES

INTERACTS WITH	COMBINED EFFECT
Alcohol:	Increased intoxication. Possible disulfiram reaction.*
Beverages:	None expected.
Cocaine:	None expected.
Foods:	None expected, but foods high in fat will improve drug absorption.
Marijuana:	None expected.
Tobacco:	None expected.

GUAIFENESIN

BRAND NAMES

See complete list of brand names in the *Generic and Brand Name Directory*, page 880.

BASIC INFORMATION

Habit forming? No
Prescription needed? No
Available as generic? Yes
Drug class: Expectorant

USES

Loosens mucus in respiratory passages from allergies and infections (hay fever, cough, cold).

DOSAGE & USAGE INFORMATION

How to take:
- Tablet or capsule—Swallow with liquid. If you can't swallow whole, crumble tablet or open capsule and take with liquid or food.
- Extended-release tablet or extended-release capsule—Swallow with liquid.
- Syrup, oral solution or lozenge—Take as directed on label. Follow with 8 oz. water.

When to take:
As needed, no more often than every 4 hours.

If you forget a dose:
Take as soon as you remember. Wait 4 hours for next dose.

What drug does:
Increases production of watery fluids to thin mucus so it can be coughed out or absorbed.

Time lapse before drug works:
15 to 30 minutes. Regular use for 5 to 7 days necessary for maximum benefit.

Don't take with:
Any other medicine without consulting your doctor or pharmacist.

OVERDOSE

SYMPTOMS:
Drowsiness, mild weakness, nausea, vomiting.
WHAT TO DO:
Overdose unlikely to threaten life. If person takes much larger amount than prescribed, call doctor, poison control center or hospital emergency room for instructions.

POSSIBLE ADVERSE REACTIONS OR SIDE EFFECTS

SYMPTOMS	WHAT TO DO
Life-threatening: None expected.	
Common: None expected.	
Infrequent: Drowsiness, rash, stomach pain, diarrhea, nausea.	Continue. Call doctor when convenient.
Rare: None expected.	

WARNINGS & PRECAUTIONS

Don't take if:
You are allergic to any cough or cold preparation containing guaifenesin.

Before you start, consult your doctor:
If you are allergic to any medicine, food or other substance.

Over age 60:
Adverse reactions and side effects may be more frequent and severe than in younger persons. For drug to work, you must drink 8 to 10 glasses of fluid per day.

Pregnancy:
Decide with your doctor if drug benefits justify risks to unborn child. Risk category C (see page xxiii).

Breast-feeding:
No proven problems. Consult your doctor.

Infants & children:
No problems expected.

Prolonged use:
No problems expected.

Skin & sunlight:
No problems expected.

Driving, piloting or hazardous work:
Avoid if you feel drowsy. Otherwise, no problems expected.

Discontinuing:
May be unnecessary to finish medicine. Discontinue when symptoms disappear. If symptoms persist more than 1 week, consult doctor.

Others:
Some guaifenesin syrup products contain alcohol. Read labels for alcohol content if you want to avoid these products.

POSSIBLE INTERACTION WITH OTHER DRUGS

GENERIC NAME OR DRUG CLASS	COMBINED EFFECT
Anticoagulants*	Possible risk of bleeding.

POSSIBLE INTERACTION WITH OTHER SUBSTANCES

INTERACTS WITH	COMBINED EFFECT
Alcohol:	No proven problems.
Beverages:	You must drink 8 to 10 glasses of fluid per day for drug to work.
Cocaine:	No proven problems.
Foods:	None expected.
Marijuana:	No proven problems.
Tobacco:	No proven problems.

GUANABENZ

BRAND NAMES

Wytensin

BASIC INFORMATION

Habit forming? No
Prescription needed? Yes
Available as generic? No
Drug class: Antihypertensive

 ## USES

Controls, but doesn't cure, high blood pressure.

 ## DOSAGE & USAGE INFORMATION

How to take:
Tablet—Swallow with liquid or food to lessen stomach irritation. If you can't swallow whole, crumble tablet and take with liquid or food.

When to take:
At the same times each day.

If you forget a dose:
Take as soon as you remember up to 2 hours late. If more than 2 hours, wait for next scheduled dose (don't double this dose).

What drug does:
• Relaxes muscle cells of small arteries.
• Slows heartbeat.

Time lapse before drug works:
1 hour.

Don't take with:
Any other medicine without consulting your doctor or pharmacist.

 ## OVERDOSE

SYMPTOMS:
Severe dizziness, slow heartbeat, unusual tiredness or weakness, pinpoint pupils, fainting, coma.
WHAT TO DO:
• **Dial 911 (emergency) or 0 (operator) for an ambulance or medical help. Then give first aid immediately.**
• **If patient is unconscious and not breathing, give mouth-to-mouth breathing. If there is no heartbeat, use cardiac massage and mouth-to-mouth breathing (CPR). Don't try to make patient vomit. If you can't get help quickly, take patient to nearest emergency facility.**
• **See emergency information on inside covers.**

 ## POSSIBLE ADVERSE REACTIONS OR SIDE EFFECTS

SYMPTOMS	WHAT TO DO
Life-threatening:	
In case of overdose, see previous column.	
Common:	
• Dry mouth, drowsiness.	Continue. Call doctor when convenient.
• Insomnia, weakness.	Continue. Tell doctor at next visit.
Infrequent:	
• Irregular heartbeat, shakiness in hands.	Discontinue. Call doctor right away.
• Dizziness, appetite loss, nausea, vomiting, painful or difficult urination, headache.	Continue. Call doctor when convenient.
Rare:	
Decreased sex drive.	Continue. Call doctor when convenient.

 ## WARNINGS & PRECAUTIONS

Don't take if:
You are allergic to any sympathomimetic drug.

Before you start, consult your doctor:
• If you have blood disease.
• If you have heart disease.
• If you have liver disease.
• If you have diabetes or overactive thyroid.
• If you will have surgery within 2 months, including dental surgery, requiring general or spinal anesthesia.

Over age 60:
Adverse reactions and side effects may be more frequent and severe than in younger persons. Hot weather may cause need to reduce dosage.

Pregnancy:
Decide with your doctor if drug benefits justify risks to unborn child. Risk category C (see page xxiii).

Breast-feeding:
Unknown effect. Consult doctor.

Infants & children:
Not recommended.

Prolonged use:
Side effects tend to diminish. Request uric acid and kidney function studies periodically.

Skin & sunlight:
No problems expected.

Driving, piloting or hazardous work:
Avoid if you feel dizzy; otherwise, no problems expected.

Discontinuing:
Don't discontinue without consulting doctor. Dose may require gradual reduction if you have taken drug for a long time. Doses of other drugs may also require adjustment. Abruptly discontinuing may cause anxiety, chest pain, salivation, headache, abdominal cramps, fast heartbeat, increased sweating, tremors, insomnia.

Others:
- Stay away from high-sodium foods. Lose weight if you are overweight.
- May interfere with the accuracy of some medical tests.

POSSIBLE INTERACTION WITH OTHER DRUGS

GENERIC NAME OR DRUG CLASS	COMBINED EFFECT
Angiotensin-converting enzyme (ACE) inhibitors*	Possible excessive potassium in blood.
Antihypertensives, other*	Decreases blood pressure more than either alone. May be beneficial, but requires dosage adjustment.
Beta-adrenergic blocking agents*	Blood pressure control more difficult.
Central nervous system (CNS) depressants* (sedatives,* sleeping pills,* tranquilizers,* antidepressants,* narcotics*)	Increased brain depression. Avoid.
Clozapine	Toxic effect on the central nervous system.
Diuretics*	Decreases blood pressure more than either alone. May be beneficial, but requires dosage adjustment.
Ethinamate	Dangerous increased effects of ethinamate. Avoid combining.
Fluoxetine	Increased depressant effects of both drugs.
Guanfacine	May increase depressant effects of either drug.
Leucovorin	High alcohol content of leucovorin may cause adverse effects.
Methyprylon	Increased sedative effect, perhaps to dangerous level. Avoid.
Nabilone	Greater depression of central nervous system.
Nicardipine	Blood pressure drop. Dosages may require adjustment.
Nimodipine	Dangerous blood pressure drop.
Sertraline	Increased depressive effects of both drugs.

POSSIBLE INTERACTION WITH OTHER SUBSTANCES

INTERACTS WITH	COMBINED EFFECT
Alcohol:	Oversedation. Avoid.
Beverages: Caffeine.	Overstimulation. Avoid.
Cocaine:	Overstimulation. Avoid.
Foods: Salt.	Decrease salt intake to increase beneficial effects of guanabenz.
Marijuana:	Overstimulation. Avoid.
Tobacco:	Decreased guanabenz effect.

*See Glossary

GUANADREL

BRAND NAMES

Hylorel

BASIC INFORMATION

Habit forming? No
Prescription needed? Yes
Available as generic? No
Drug class: Antihypertensive

 USES

Controls, but doesn't cure, high blood pressure.

 DOSAGE & USAGE INFORMATION

How to take:
Tablet—Swallow with liquid or food to lessen stomach irritation. If you can't swallow whole, crumble tablet and take with liquid or food.

When to take:
At the same time each day.

If you forget a dose:
Take as soon as you remember up to 2 hours late. If more than 2 hours, wait for next scheduled dose (don't double this dose).

What drug does:
Relaxes muscle cells of small arteries.

Time lapse before drug works:
4 to 6 hours. May need to take for lifetime.

Don't take with:
Any other medicine without consulting your doctor or pharmacist.

 OVERDOSE

SYMPTOMS:
Severe blood pressure drop; fainting; blurred vision; slow, weak pulse; cold, sweaty skin; loss of consciousness.
WHAT TO DO:
* **Dial 911 (emergency) or 0 (operator) for an ambulance or medical help. Then give first aid immediately.**
* **See emergency information on inside covers.**

 POSSIBLE ADVERSE REACTIONS OR SIDE EFFECTS

SYMPTOMS	WHAT TO DO
Life-threatening:	
In case of overdose, see previous column.	
Common:	
• Diarrhea, more bowel movements, fatigue, weakness.	Continue. Call doctor when convenient.
• Dizziness, lower sex drive, feet and ankle swelling, drowsiness.	Continue. Tell doctor at next visit.
• Stuffy nose, dry mouth.	No action necessary.
Infrequent:	
• Rash, blurred vision, drooping eyelids, chest pain or shortness of breath, muscle pain or tremor.	Discontinue. Call doctor right away.
• Nausea or vomiting, headache.	Continue. Call doctor when convenient.
• Impotence, nighttime urination.	Continue. Tell doctor at next visit.
Rare:	
Decreased white blood cells causing sore throat, fever.	Discontinue. Call doctor right away.

 WARNINGS & PRECAUTIONS

Don't take if:
* You are allergic to guanadrel.
* You have taken MAO inhibitors* within 2 weeks.

Before you start, consult your doctor:
* If you have stroke or heart disease.
* If you have asthma.
* If you have had kidney disease.
* If you have peptic ulcer or chronic acid indigestion.
* If you will have surgery within 2 months, including dental surgery, requiring general or spinal anesthesia.

Over age 60:
Adverse reactions and side effects may be more frequent and severe than in younger persons. Start with small doses and monitor blood pressure frequently.

Pregnancy:
No proven harm to unborn child. Avoid if possible. Consult doctor. Risk category B (see page xxiii).

Breast-feeding:
No proven harm to nursing infant. Avoid if possible. Consult doctor.

Infants & children:
Not recommended.

Prolonged use:
- Due to drug's cumulative effect, dose will require adjustment to prevent wide fluctuations in blood pressure.
- Talk to your doctor about the need for follow-up medical examinations or laboratory studies.

Skin & sunlight:
No problems expected.

Driving, piloting or hazardous work:
Don't drive or pilot aircraft until you learn how medicine affects you. Don't work around dangerous machinery. Don't climb ladders or work in high places. Danger increases if you drink alcohol or take medicine affecting alertness and reflexes, such as antihistamines, tranquilizers, sedatives, pain medicine, narcotics and mind-altering drugs.

Discontinuing:
Don't discontinue without consulting doctor. Dose may require gradual reduction if you have taken drug for a long time. Doses of other drugs may also require adjustment.

Others:
- Hot weather further lowers blood pressure, particularly in patients over 60.
- Advise any doctor or dentist whom you consult that you take this medicine.

POSSIBLE INTERACTION WITH OTHER DRUGS

GENERIC NAME OR DRUG CLASS	COMBINED EFFECT
Angiotensin-converting enzyme (ACE) inhibitors*	Possible excessive potassium in blood.
Antidepressants, tricyclic*	Decreased effect of guanadrel.
Antihypertensives, other*	Increased effect of guanadrel.
Beta-adrenergic blocking agents*	Increased likelihood of dizziness and fainting.
Carteolol	Increased anti-hypertensive effect.
Contraceptives, oral*	Increased side effects of oral contraceptives.
Central nervous system (CNS) depressants* (anticonvulsants,* antihistamines,* muscle relaxants,* narcotics,* sedatives,* tranquilizers*)	Decreased effect of guanadrel.

	COMBINED EFFECT
Diuretics*	Increased likelihood of dizziness and fainting.
Haloperidol	Decreased effect of guanadrel.
Insulin	Increased insulin effect.
Loxapine	Decreased effect of guanadrel.
Monoamine oxidase (MAO) inhibitors*	Severe high blood pressure. Avoid.
Nicardipine	Blood pressure drop. Dosages may require adjustment.
Nimodipine	Dangerous blood pressure drop.
Phenothiazines*	Decreased effect of guanadrel.
Rauwolfia alkaloids*	Increased likelihood of dizziness and fainting.
Sotalol	Increased anti-hypertensive effect.
Sympathomimetics*	Decreased effect of guanadrel.
Terazosin	Decreases effectiveness of terazosin.
Thioxanthenes*	Decreased effect of guanadrel.
Trimeprazine	Decreased effect of guanadrel.

POSSIBLE INTERACTION WITH OTHER SUBSTANCES

INTERACTS WITH	COMBINED EFFECT
Alcohol:	Decreased effect of guanadrel. Avoid.
Beverages: Caffeine.	Decreased effect of guanadrel.
Cocaine:	Increased risk of heart block and high blood pressure.
Foods:	No problems expected.
Marijuana:	Higher blood pressure. Avoid.
Tobacco:	Higher blood pressure. Avoid.

GUANETHIDINE

BRAND NAMES

Apo-Guanethidine   Ismelin

BASIC INFORMATION

Habit forming? No
Prescription needed? Yes
Available as generic? Yes
Drug class: Antihypertensive

 ## USES

Reduces high blood pressure.

 ## DOSAGE & USAGE INFORMATION

How to take:
Tablet—Swallow with liquid. If you can't swallow tablet whole, crumble and take with liquid or food.

When to take:
At the same time each day.

If you forget a dose:
Take as soon as you remember up to 2 hours late. If more than 2 hours, wait for next scheduled dose (don't double this dose).

What drug does:
Displaces norepinephrine—hormone necessary to maintain small blood vessel tone. Blood vessels relax and high blood pressure drops.

Time lapse before drug works:
Regular use for several weeks may be necessary to determine effectiveness.

Don't take with:
- Nonprescription drugs containing alcohol without consulting doctor.
- Any other medicine without consulting your doctor or pharmacist.

 ## OVERDOSE

SYMPTOMS:
Severe blood pressure drop; fainting; blurred vision; slow, weak pulse; cold, sweaty skin; loss of consciousness.
WHAT TO DO:
- Dial 911 (emergency) or 0 (operator) for an ambulance or medical help. Then give first aid immediately.
- See emergency information on inside covers.

 ## POSSIBLE ADVERSE REACTIONS OR SIDE EFFECTS

SYMPTOMS	WHAT TO DO
Life-threatening:	
In case of overdose, see previous column.	
Common:	
• Unusually slow heartbeat.	Discontinue. Call doctor right away.
• Diarrhea; more bowel movements; swollen feet, legs; fatigue, weakness.	Continue. Call doctor when convenient.
• Dizziness, lower sex drive.	Continue. Tell doctor at next visit.
• Stuffy nose, dry mouth.	No action necessary.
Infrequent:	
• Rash, blurred vision, drooping eyelids, chest pain or shortness of breath, muscle pain or tremor.	Discontinue. Call doctor right away.
• Nausea or vomiting, headache.	Continue. Call doctor when convenient.
• Impotence, nighttime urination, hair loss.	Continue. Tell doctor at next visit.
Rare:	
Decreased white blood cells causing sore throat, fever.	Discontinue. Call doctor right away.

 ## WARNINGS & PRECAUTIONS

Don't take if:
- You are allergic to guanethidine.
- You have taken MAO inhibitors within 2 weeks.

Before you start, consult your doctor:
- If you have had stroke or heart disease.
- If you have asthma.
- If you have had kidney disease.
- If you have peptic ulcer or chronic acid indigestion.
- If you will have surgery within 2 months, including dental surgery, requiring general or spinal anesthesia.

Over age 60:
Adverse reactions and side effects may be more frequent and severe than in younger persons. Start with small doses and monitor blood pressure frequently.

Pregnancy:
Decide with your doctor if drug benefits justify risk to unborn child. Risk category C (see page xxiii).

Breast-feeding:
Unknown effect. Consult doctor.

Infants & children:
Not recommended.

Prolonged use:
- Due to drug's cumulative effect, dose will require adjustment to prevent wide fluctuations in blood pressure.
- Talk to your doctor about the need for follow-up medical examinations or laboratory studies.

Skin & sunlight:
No problems expected.

Driving, piloting or hazardous work:
Don't drive or pilot aircraft until you learn how medicine affects you. Don't work around dangerous machinery. Don't climb ladders or work in high places. Danger increases if you drink alcohol or take medicine affecting alertness and reflexes, such as antihistamines, tranquilizers, sedatives, pain medicine, narcotics and mind-altering drugs.

Discontinuing:
Don't discontinue without consulting doctor. Dose may require gradual reduction if you have taken drug for a long time. Doses of other drugs may also require adjustment.

Others:
Hot weather further lowers blood pressure.

 POSSIBLE INTERACTION WITH OTHER DRUGS

GENERIC NAME OR DRUG CLASS	COMBINED EFFECT
Amphetamines*	Decreased guanethidine effect.
Angiotensin-converting enzyme (ACE) inhibitors*	Possible excessive potassium in blood.
Antidepressants, tricyclic*	Decreased guanethidine effect.
Antidiabetics, oral*	Increased guanethidine effect.
Antihistamines*	Decreased guanethidine effect.
Carteolol	Increased anti-hypertensive effect.
Contraceptives, oral*	Decreased guanethidine effect. Increased side effects of oral contraceptives.
Digitalis preparations*	Slower heartbeat.
Diuretics, thiazide*	Increased guanethidine effect.

Haloperidol	Decreased guanethidine effect.
Indapamide	Possible increased effects of both drugs. When monitored carefully, combination may be beneficial in controlling hypertension.
Insulin	Increased insulin effect.
Loxapine	Decreased effect of guanethidine.
Minoxidil	Dosage adjustments may be necessary to keep blood pressure at proper level.
Monoamine oxidase (MAO) inhibitors*	Increased blood pressure.
Nicardipine	Blood pressure drop. Dosages may require adjustment.
Nimodipine	Dangerous blood pressure drop.
Phenothiazines*	Decreased guanethidine effect.

Continued on page 916

 POSSIBLE INTERACTION WITH OTHER SUBSTANCES

INTERACTS WITH	COMBINED EFFECT
Alcohol:	Use caution. Decreases blood pressure.
Beverages: Carbonated drinks.	Use sparingly. Sodium content increases blood pressure.
Cocaine:	Increased risk of heart block and high blood pressure.
Foods: Spicy or acid foods.	Avoid if subject to indigestion or peptic ulcer.
Marijuana:	Excessively low blood pressure. Avoid.
Tobacco:	Possible blood pressure rise. Avoid.

*See Glossary

GUANETHIDINE & HYDROCHLOROTHIAZIDE

BRAND NAMES

Esimil   Ismelin-Esidrix

BASIC INFORMATION

Habit forming? No
Prescription needed? Yes
Available as generic? No
Drug class: Antihypertensive, diuretic

USES

- Controls, but doesn't cure, high blood pressure.
- Reduces fluid retention (edema).

DOSAGE & USAGE INFORMATION

How to take:
Tablet—Swallow with liquid. If you can't swallow whole, crumble tablet and take with liquid or food.

When to take:
At the same time each day.

If you forget a dose:
Take as soon as you remember up to 2 hours late. If more than 2 hours, wait for next scheduled dose (don't double this dose).

What drug does:
- Forces sodium and water secretion, reducing body fluid.
- Displaces norepinephrine—hormone necessary to maintain small blood vessel tone. Blood vessels relax and high blood pressure drops.

Time lapse before drug works:
Regular use for several weeks may be necessary to determine effectiveness.

Continued next column

OVERDOSE

SYMPTOMS:
Cramps, weakness, drowsiness, blurred vision, weak pulse, severe blood pressure drop, fainting, cold and sweaty skin, loss of consciousness, coma.
WHAT TO DO:
- **Dial 911 (emergency) or 0 (operator) for an ambulance or medical help. Then give first aid immediately.**
- **See emergency information on inside covers.**

Don't take with:
- Nonprescription drugs containing alcohol without consulting doctor.
- Any other medicine without consulting your doctor or pharmacist.

POSSIBLE ADVERSE REACTIONS OR SIDE EFFECTS

SYMPTOMS	WHAT TO DO
Life-threatening:	
Chest pain, shortness of breath, irregular heartbeat.	Discontinue. Seek emergency treatment.
Common:	
• Slow heartbeat, swollen feet and ankles, fatigue, weakness.	Discontinue. Call doctor right away.
• Dizziness, stuffy nose, dry mouth, diarrhea, diminished sex drive.	Continue. Call doctor when convenient.
Infrequent:	
• Mood change, rash or hives, blurred vision, drooping eyelids, muscle pain or tremors.	Discontinue. Call doctor right away.
• Increased nighttime urination, abdominal pain, vomiting, nausea, headache, weakness.	Continue. Call doctor when convenient.
• Impotence, nighttime urination, hair loss.	Continue. Tell doctor at next visit.
Rare:	
• Decreased white blood cells causing sore throat, fever; jaundice.	Discontinue. Call doctor right away.
• Weight gain or loss.	Continue. Call doctor when convenient.

WARNINGS & PRECAUTIONS

Don't take if:
- You are allergic to any thiazide diuretic drug or guanethidine.
- You have taken MAO inhibitors within 2 weeks.

Before you start, consult your doctor:
- If you are allergic to any sulfa drug.
- If you have gout, asthma, liver, pancreas or kidney disorder, peptic ulcer or chronic acid indigestion.
- If you have had stroke or heart disease.
- If you will have surgery within 2 months, including dental surgery, requiring general or spinal anesthesia.

GUANETHIDINE & HYDROCHLOROTHIAZIDE

Over age 60:
Adverse reactions and side effects may be more frequent and severe than in younger persons, especially dizziness and excessive potassium loss.

Pregnancy:
Decide with your doctor if drug benefits justify risk to unborn child. Risk category C (see page xxiii).

Breast-feeding:
Drug passes into milk. Avoid drug or discontinue nursing until you finish medicine. Consult doctor for advice on maintaining milk supply.

Infants & children:
Not recommended.

Prolonged use:
- Due to drug's cumulative effect, dose will require adjustment to prevent wide fluctuations in blood pressure.
- Talk to your doctor about the need for follow-up medical examinations or laboratory studies.

Skin & sunlight:
One or more drugs in this group may cause rash or intensify sunburn in areas exposed to sun or ultraviolet light (photosensitivity reaction). Avoid overexposure. Notify doctor if reaction occurs.

Driving, piloting or hazardous work:
Don't drive or pilot aircraft until you learn how medicine affects you. Don't work around dangerous machinery. Don't climb ladders or work in high places. Danger increases if you drink alcohol or take medicine affecting alertness and reflexes, such as antihistamines, tranquilizers, sedatives, pain medicine, narcotics and mind-altering drugs.

Discontinuing:
Don't discontinue without consulting doctor. Dose may require gradual reduction if you have taken drug for a long time. Doses of other drugs may also require adjustment.

Others:
- Hot weather and fever may cause dehydration and drop in blood pressure. Dose may require temporary adjustment. Weigh daily and report any unexpected weight decreases to your doctor.
- May cause rise in uric acid, leading to gout.
- May cause blood sugar rise in diabetics.

 ## POSSIBLE INTERACTION WITH OTHER DRUGS

GENERIC NAME OR DRUG CLASS	COMBINED EFFECT
Allopurinol	Decreased allopurinol effect.
Amphetamines*	Decreased guanethidine effect.

Antidepressants, tricyclic*	Dangerous drop in blood pressure. Avoid combination unless under medical supervision.
Antihistamines*	Decreased guanethidine effect.
Barbiturates*	Increased hydrochlorothiazide effect.
Beta-adrenergic blocking agents*	Increased anti-hypertensive effect. Dosages of both drugs may require adjustments.
Carteolol	Increased anti-hypertensive effect.
Cholestyramine	Decreased hydrochlorothiazide effect.
Contraceptives, oral*	Decreased guanethidine effect.

Continued on page 916

 ## POSSIBLE INTERACTION WITH OTHER SUBSTANCES

INTERACTS WITH	COMBINED EFFECT
Alcohol:	Use caution Decreases blood pressure.
Beverages: Carbonated drinks.	Use sparingly. Sodium content increases blood pressure.
Cocaine:	Raises blood pressure. Avoid.
Foods: Spicy or acid foods.	Avoid if subject to indigestion or peptic ulcer.
Licorice.	Excessive potassium loss that causes dangerous heart rhythms.
Marijuana:	Effect on blood pressure unpredictable.
Tobacco:	Possible blood pressure rise. Avoid.

*See Glossary

GUANFACINE

BRAND NAMES

Tenex

BASIC INFORMATION

Habit forming? No
Prescription needed? Yes
Available as generic? No
Drug class: Antihypertensive

 ## USES

Treats high blood pressure, usually in combination with a diuretic drug.

 ## DOSAGE & USAGE INFORMATION

How to take:
Tablets—Swallow with liquid or food to lessen stomach irritation. If you can't swallow whole, crumble tablet and take with liquid or food.

When to take:
Usually at bedtime to minimize daytime drowsiness.

If you forget a dose:
Take as soon as you remember up to 2 hours late. If more than 2 hours, wait for next scheduled dose (don't double this dose).

What drug does:
- Decreases stimulating effects of the sympathetic nervous system on the heart, kidneys and arteries throughout the body.
- Decreases both systolic and diastolic blood pressure.

Time lapse before drug works:
Within 1 week.

Don't take with:
Any other medicine without consulting your doctor or pharmacist.

 ## OVERDOSE

SYMPTOMS:
Difficulty breathing, loss of consciousness, dizziness, very slow heartbeat.
WHAT TO DO:
- Dial 911 (emergency) or 0 (operator) for an ambulance or medical help. Then give first aid immediately.
- See emergency information on inside covers.

 ## POSSIBLE ADVERSE REACTIONS OR SIDE EFFECTS

SYMPTOMS	WHAT TO DO
Life-threatening: Shortness of breath.	Seek emergency treatment immediately.
Common:	
• Decreased sexual function, drowsiness, constipation.	Continue. Call doctor when convenient.
• Increased dental problems because of dry mouth and less salivation.	Consult your dentist about a prevention program.
Infrequent:	
• Confusion, dizziness or fainting, slow heartbeat.	Continue, but call doctor right away.
• Mental depression, eye irritation, insomnia, tiredness or weakness, headache, nausea and/or vomiting.	Continue. Call doctor when convenient.
Rare: May occur if medicine is abruptly discontinued— Anxiety, chest pain, heartbeat irregularities, excess salivation, sleep problems, nervousness, sweating.	Seek emergency treatment.

 ## WARNINGS & PRECAUTIONS

Don't take if:
You have had a recent heart attack.

Before you start, consult your doctor:
- If you have heart disease or liver disease.
- If you have coronary insufficiency.
- If you have mental depression.

Over age 60:
None significant.

Pregnancy:
No proven harm to unborn child, but avoid if possible. Consult doctor. Risk category B (see page xxiii).

Breast-feeding:
Effect not documented. Consult your doctor.

Infants & children:
Effect not documented. Consult your pediatrician.

Prolonged use:
Talk to your doctor about the need for follow-up medical examinations or laboratory studies to check blood pressure.

Skin & sunlight:
No problems expected.

Driving, piloting or hazardous work:
Don't drive or pilot aircraft until you learn how medicine affects you. Don't work around dangerous machinery. Don't climb ladders or work in high places. Danger increases if you drink alcohol or take medicine affecting alertness and reflexes.

Discontinuing:
- Don't discontinue without consulting doctor. Dose may require gradual reduction if you have taken drug for a long time. Doses of other drugs may also require adjustment.
- May occur if medicine is discontinued abruptly: anxiety, chest pain, heartbeat irregularities, excess salivation, sleep problems, nervousness, sweating.

Others:
- This medication works better if you attempt to reduce your weight to normal, exercise regularly, restrict salt in your diet and reduce stress wherever possible. Continue taking medicine even when you feel good.
- Adverse reactions are usually dose-related and diminish when dosage is reduced.

POSSIBLE INTERACTION WITH OTHER DRUGS

GENERIC NAME OR DRUG CLASS	COMBINED EFFECT
Antihypertensives, other*	May increase effects of guanfacine and other medicines.
Anti-inflammatory drugs, nonsteroidal (NSAIDs)*	May decrease anti-hypertensive effects of guanfacine.
Carteolol	Increased anti-hypertensive effect.
Central nervous system (CNS) depressants*	Increases depressant effect of both drugs.
Clozapine	Toxic effect on the central nervous system.
Estrogens*	May decrease anti-hypertensive effects of guanfacine.
Ethinamate	Dangerous increased effects of ethinamate. Avoid combining.
Fluoxetine	Increased depressant effects of both drugs.

Leucovorin	High alcohol content of leucovorin may cause adverse effects.
Lisinopril	Increased anti-hypertensive effect. Dosage of each may require adjustment.
Methyprylon	Increased sedative effect, perhaps to dangerous level. Avoid.
Nabilone	Greater depression of central nervous system.
Nicardipine	Blood pressure drop. Dosages may require adjustment.
Nimodipine	Dangerous blood pressure drop.
Propafenone	Increased effect of both drugs and increased risk of toxicity.
Sertraline	Increased depressive effects of both drugs.
Sotalol	Increased anti-hypertensive effect.

Continued on page 916

POSSIBLE INTERACTION WITH OTHER SUBSTANCES

INTERACTS WITH	COMBINED EFFECT
Alcohol:	Excess use may lead to dangerous drop in blood pressure.
Beverages: Any containing caffeine, such as coffee, tea or cocoa.	May decrease anti-hypertensive effect of guanfacine.
Cocaine:	Increased risk of heart block and high blood pressure.
Foods:	None expected.
Marijuana:	May decrease anti-hypertensive effect of guanfacine.
Tobacco:	May decrease anti-hypertensive effect of guanfacine

*See Glossary

HALOPERIDOL

BRAND NAMES

Apo-Haloperidol
Haldol
Haldol Decanoate
Haldol LA

Halperon
Novo-Peridol
Peridol
PMS Haloperidol

BASIC INFORMATION

Habit forming? No
Prescription needed? Yes
Available as generic? Yes
Drug class: Antipsychotic

 ## USES

- Reduces severe anxiety, agitation and psychotic behavior.
- Treatment for Tourette's syndrome
- Treatment for infantile autism.
- Treatment for Huntington's chorea.

 ## DOSAGE & USAGE INFORMATION

How to take:
- Tablet—Swallow with liquid. If you can't swallow whole, crumble tablet and take with liquid or food.
- Drops—Dilute dose in beverage before swallowing.

When to take:
At the same times each day.

Continued next column

 ## OVERDOSE

SYMPTOMS:
Weak, rapid pulse; shallow, slow breathing; tremor or muscle weakness; very low blood pressure; convulsions; deep sleep ending in coma.
WHAT TO DO:
- Dial 911 (emergency) or 0 (operator) for an ambulance or medical help. Then give first aid immediately.
- If patient is unconscious and not breathing, give mouth-to-mouth breathing. If there is no heartbeat, use cardiac massage and mouth-to-mouth breathing (CPR). Don't try to make patient vomit. If you can't get help quickly, take patient to nearest emergency facility.
- See emergency information at end of book.

If you forget a dose:
Take as soon as you remember up to 2 hours late. If more than 2 hours, wait for next scheduled dose (don't double this dose).

What drug does:
Corrects an imbalance in nerve impulses from brain; blocks effect of dopamine*.

Time lapse before drug works:
Up to 4 weeks.

Don't take with:
- Nonprescription drugs without consulting doctor.
- Any other medicine without consulting your doctor or pharmacist.

 ## POSSIBLE ADVERSE REACTIONS OR SIDE EFFECTS

SYMPTOMS	WHAT TO DO
Life-threatening: High fever, rapid pulse, profuse sweating, muscle rigidity, confusion and irritability, seizures.	Discontinue. Seek emergency treatment.
Common: • Jerky or involuntary movements, especially of the face, lips, jaw, tongue; slow-frequency tremor of head or limbs, especially while moving; muscle rigidity, lack of facial expression and slow inflexible movements.	Discontinue. Call doctor right away.
• Pacing or restlessness; intermittent spasms of muscles of face, eyes, tongue, jaw, neck, body or limbs.	Continue. Call doctor when convenient.
Infrequent: Dry mouth, blurred vision, constipation, difficulty urinating; sedation, low blood pressure, dizziness.	Continue. Call doctor when convenient.
Rare: Other symptoms not listed above.	Continue. Call doctor when convenient.

WARNINGS & PRECAUTIONS

Don't take if:
- You have ever been allergic to haloperidol.
- You are depressed.
- You have Parkinson's disease.
- Patient is younger than 3 years old.

Before you start, consult your doctor:
- If you take sedatives, sleeping pills, tranquilizers, antidepressants, antihistamines, narcotics or mind-altering drugs.
- If you have a history of mental depression.
- If you have had kidney or liver problems.
- If you have diabetes, epilepsy, glaucoma, high blood pressure or heart disease, prostate trouble, overactive thyroid or asthma.
- If you drink alcoholic beverages frequently.

Over age 60:
Adverse reactions and side effects may be more frequent and severe than in younger persons.

Pregnancy:
Decide with your doctor if drug benefits justify risk to unborn child. Risk category C (see page xxiii).

Breast-feeding:
Drug passes into milk. Avoid drug or discontinue nursing until you finish medicine. Consult doctor about maintaining milk supply.

Infants & children:
Not recommended. Side effects may be more common.

Prolonged use:
- May develop tardive dyskinesia (involuntary movements of jaws, lips and tongue).
- Talk to your doctor about the need for follow-up medical examinations or laboratory studies to check blood pressure, liver function.

Skin & sunlight:
- May cause rash or intensify sunburn in areas exposed to sun or ultraviolet light (photosensitivity). Avoid overexposure and use sunscreen. Consult doctor if reaction occurs.
- Avoid getting overheated. The drug affects body temperature and sweating.

Driving, piloting or hazardous work:
Don't drive or pilot aircraft until you learn how medicine affects you. Don't work around dangerous machinery. Don't climb ladders or work in high places. Danger increases if you drink alcohol or take medicine affecting alertness and reflexes.

Discontinuing:
Don't discontinue without consulting doctor. Dose may require gradual reduction if you have taken drug for a long time. Doses of other drugs may also require adjustment.

Others:
- For dry mouth, suck on sugarless hard candy or chew sugarless gum. If dry mouth persists, consult your dentist
- Advise any doctor or dentist whom you consult that you take this medicine.

POSSIBLE INTERACTION WITH OTHER DRUGS

GENERIC NAME OR DRUG CLASS	COMBINED EFFECT
Anticholinergics*	Increased anticholinergic effect. May cause elevated pressure within the eye.
Anticonvulsants*	Changed seizure pattern.
Antidepressants*	Excessive sedation.
Antihistamines*	Excessive sedation.
Antihypertensives*	May cause severe blood pressure drop.
Barbiturates*	Excessive sedation.
Buproplon	Increased risk of seizures.
Central nervous system (CNS) depressants*	Increased CNS depression; increased blood pressure drop.
Clozapine	Toxic effect on the nervous system.

Continued on page 916

POSSIBLE INTERACTION WITH OTHER SUBSTANCES

INTERACTS WITH	COMBINED EFFECT
Alcohol:	Excessive sedation and depressed brain function. Avoid.
Beverages:	None expected.
Cocaine:	Decreased effect of haloperidol. Avoid.
Foods:	None expected.
Marijuana:	Occasional use—Increased sedation. Frequent use—Possible toxic psychosis.
Tobacco:	None expected.

*See Glossary

HISTAMINE H₂ RECEPTOR ANTAGONISTS

GENERIC AND BRAND NAMES

CIMETIDINE
  Apo-Cimetidine
  Novocimetine
  Peptol
  Tagamet
  Tagamet HB
FAMOTIDINE
  Mylanta-AR
  Pepcid
  Pepcid AC
  Ulcidine

NIZATIDINE
  Axid
RANITIDINE
  Apo-Ranitidine
  Zantac
  Zantac 75
  Zantac-C
  Zantac Efferdose
  Zantac Geldose

BASIC INFORMATION

Habit forming? No
Prescription needed? Yes, for some
Available as generic? No
Drug class: Histamine H₂ antagonist

USES

- Treatment for duodenal and gastric ulcers and other conditions in which stomach produces excess hydrochloric acid.
- Treatment for and prevention of heartburn.
- Maintenance of healing of erosive esophagitis.

DOSAGE & USAGE INFORMATION

How to take:
- Chewable tablet (Pepcid AC)—Chew thoroughly and swallow with water.
- Tablet, capsule or liquid—Swallow with liquid.
- Oral suspension or effervescent tablets for oral solution—Follow instructions on label.

When to take:
- 1 dose per day—Take at bedtime.
- 2 or more doses per day—Take at the same times each day.

Continued next column

OVERDOSE

SYMPTOMS:
Confusion, slurred speech, breathing difficulty, rapid heartbeat, delirium.
WHAT TO DO:
Overdose unlikely to threaten life. If person takes much larger amount than prescribed, call doctor, poison control center or hospital emergency room for instructions.

If you forget a dose:
Take as soon as you remember up to 2 hours late. If more than 2 hours, wait for next scheduled dose (don't double this dose).

What drug does:
Blocks histamine release so stomach secretes less acid.

Time lapse before drug works:
- Begins in 30 minutes. May require several days to relieve pain.
- Lower dosages in nonprescription medicines may take 45 minutes ro relieve heartburn.

Don't take with:
Any other medicine without consulting your doctor or pharmacist.

POSSIBLE ADVERSE REACTIONS OR SIDE EFFECTS

SYMPTOMS	WHAT TO DO
Life-threatening:	
In case of overdose, see previous column.	
Common:	
None expected.	
Infrequent:	
• Dizziness or headache, diarrhea.	Continue. Call doctor when convenient.
• Diminished sex drive, unusual milk flow in females, hair loss.	Continue. Tell doctor at next visit.
Rare:	
• Confusion; rash, hives; sore throat, fever; slow, fast or irregular heartbeat; unusual bleeding or bruising; muscle cramps or pain; fatigue; weakness.	Discontinue. Call doctor right away.
• Constipation.	Continue. Call doctor when convenient.

WARNINGS & PRECAUTIONS

Don't take if:
You are allergic to any histamine H₂ antagonist.

Before you start, consult your doctor:
- If you plan to become pregnant while on medication.
- If you take aspirin. Aspirin may irritate stomach.

Over age 60:
Adverse reactions and side effects may be more frequent and severe than in younger persons.

Pregnancy:
Risk factors vary for drugs in this group. See category list on page xxiii and consult doctor.

HISTAMINE H₂ RECEPTOR ANTAGONISTS

Breast-feeding:
Drug passes into milk. Avoid drug or discontinue nursing until you finish medicine. Consult doctor about maintaining milk supply.

Infants & children:
Not recommended.

Prolonged use:
- Possible liver damage.
- Talk to your doctor about the need for follow-up medical examinations or laboratory studies to check blood levels of vitamin B-12.

Skin & sunlight:
No problems expected.

Driving, piloting or hazardous work:
Don't drive or pilot aircraft until you learn how medicine affects you. Don't work around dangerous machinery. Don't climb ladders or work in high places. Danger increases if you drink alcohol or take medicine affecting alertness and reflexes, such as antihistamines, tranquilizers, sedatives, pain medicine, narcotics and mind-altering drugs.

Discontinuing:
Don't discontinue without consulting a doctor. Dose may require gradual reduction if you have taken drug for a long time. Doses of other drugs may also require adjustment.

Others:
- Patients on kidney dialysis—Take at end of dialysis treatment.
- May interfere with the accuracy of some medical tests.

POSSIBLE INTERACTION WITH OTHER DRUGS

GENERIC NAME OR DRUG CLASS	COMBINED EFFECT
Alprazolam	Increased effect and toxicity of alprazolam.
Antacids*	Decreased absorption of histamine H₂ receptor antagonist.
Anticoagulants, oral*	Increased anticoagulant effect.
Anticholinergics*	Increased histamine H₂ receptor antagonist effect.
Antivirals, HIV/AIDS*	Increased antiviral effect with cimetidine.
Azelastine	Increased azelastine effect.
Bupropion	Increased bupropion effect.

Carbamazepine	Increased effect and toxicity of carbamazepine.
Carmustine (BCNU)	Severe impairment of red blood cell production; some interference with white blood cell formation.
Chlordiazepoxide	Increased effect and toxicity of chlordiazepoxide.
Cisapride	Decreased histamine H₂ receptor effect.
Citalopram	Increased effect of citalopram.
Diazepam	Increased effect and toxicity of diazepam.

Continued on page 917

POSSIBLE INTERACTION WITH OTHER SUBSTANCES

INTERACTS WITH	COMBINED EFFECT
Alcohol:	No interactions expected, but alcohol may slow body's recovery. Avoid.
Beverages: Milk.	Enhanced effectiveness. Small amounts useful for taking medication.
Caffeine drinks.	May increase acid secretion and delay healing.
Cocaine:	Decreased effect of histamine H₂ receptor antagonist.
Foods:	Enhanced effectiveness. Protein-rich foods should be eaten in moderation to minimize secretion of stomach acid.
Marijuana:	Increased chance of low sperm count. Marijuana may slow body's recovery. Avoid.
Tobacco:	Reversed effect of histamine H₂ receptor antagonist. Tobacco may slow body's recovery. Avoid.

HMG-CoA REDUCTASE INHIBITORS

GENERIC AND BRAND NAMES

ATORVASTATIN
  Lipitor
CERIVASTATIN
  Baycol
FLUVASTATIN
  Lescol
LOVASTATIN
  Mevacor
  Mevinolin

PRAVASTATIN
  Eptastatin
  Pravachol
SIMVASTATIN
  Epistatin
  Synvinolin
  Zocor

BASIC INFORMATION

Habit forming? No
Prescription needed? Yes
Available as generic? No
Drug class: Antihyperlipidemic

USES

- Lowers blood cholesterol levels caused by low-density lipoproteins (LDL) in persons who haven't improved by exercising, dieting or using other measures.
- Used in combination with a low-fat diet to slow the progression of atherosclerosis in patients with coronary heart disease and high cholesterol levels.
- Lowers triglyceride levels.

DOSAGE & USAGE INFORMATION

How to take:
Tablet or capsule—Swallow with liquid. If you can't swallow whole, crumble tablet and take with liquid or food.

When to take:
According to directions on prescription.

If you forget a dose:
Take as soon as you remember up to 2 hours late. If more than 2 hours, wait for next scheduled dose (don't double this dose).

Continued next column

OVERDOSE

SYMPTOMS:
None expected.
WHAT TO DO:
Overdose not expected to threaten life. If person takes much larger amount than prescribed, call doctor, poison control center or hospital emergency room for instructions.

What drug does:
Inhibits an enzyme in the liver.

Time lapse before drug works:
2 to 4 weeks.

Don't take with:
- A high-fat diet.
- Any other medicine without consulting your doctor or pharmacist.

POSSIBLE ADVERSE REACTIONS OR SIDE EFFECTS

SYMPTOMS	WHAT TO DO
Life-threatening: None expected.	
Common: None expected.	
Infrequent:	
• Aching muscles, fever, blurred vision.	Discontinue. Call doctor right away.
• Constipation, nausea, tiredness, weakness, dizziness, skin rash, headache, diarrhea, heartburn.	Continue. Call doctor when convenient.
Rare:	
• Muscle or stomach pain, unusual tiredness or weakness.	Discontinue. Call doctor right away.
• Impotence, insomnia.	Continue. Call doctor when convenient.

WARNINGS & PRECAUTIONS

Don't take if:
You are allergic to any HMG-CoA reductase inhibitor.

Before you start, consult your doctor:
- If you take immunosuppressive drugs, particularly following an organ transplant.
- If you have low blood pressure.
- If you have hormone abnormalities.
- If you have an active infection.
- If you have active liver disease.
- If you have a seizure disorder.
- If you have a history of alcohol abuse.
- If you have had recent surgery.

Over age 60:
Likely to be more sensitive to drug.

Pregnancy:
Consult doctor. Risk category X (see page xxiii).

Breast-feeding:
Discontinue nursing until you finish medicine. Consult doctor for advice on maintaining milk supply.

Infants & children:
Not recommended for children.

Prolonged use:
Talk to your doctor about the need for follow-up medical examinations or laboratory studies to check liver function, serum cholesterol, eyes.

Skin & sunlight:
No problems expected.

Driving, piloting or hazardous work:
No special problems expected.

Discontinuing:
Don't discontinue without consulting doctor. Dose may require gradual reduction if you have taken drug for a long time. Doses of other drugs may also require adjustment.

Others:
- Request liver function tests and eye examinations before beginning this medicine and repeat every 2 to 6 months.
- Advise any doctor or dentist whom you consult that you take this medicine.
- Use an effective form of birth control while taking this drug. Notify your doctor immediately if you become pregnant.

POSSIBLE INTERACTION WITH OTHER DRUGS

GENERIC NAME OR DRUG CLASS	COMBINED EFFECT
Antifungals, azole*	Increased effect of HMG-CoA reductase inhibitor.
Cholestyramine	Decreased effect of HMG-CoA reductase inhibitor if taken at same time.
Colestipol	Decreased effect of HMG-CoA reductase inhibitor if taken at same time.
Cyclosporine	Increased risk of muscle and kidney problems.
Digoxin	Increased digoxin effect.
Diltiazem	Increased effect of HMG-CoA inhibitor.
Erythromycins*	Increased risk of muscle and kidney problems.
Gemfibrozil	Increased risk of muscle and kidney problems and muscle inflammation.
Immunosuppressants*	Increased risk of muscle or kidney problems.
Niacin	Increased risk of muscle and kidney problems.

POSSIBLE INTERACTION WITH OTHER SUBSTANCES

INTERACTS WITH	COMBINED EFFECT
Alcohol:	Best to avoid alcohol while taking this drug.
Beverages:	None expected.
Cocaine:	None expected.
Foods:	None expected.
Marijuana:	None expected.
Tobacco:	None expected.

*See Glossary

HYDRALAZINE

BRAND NAMES

Apresoline   Novo-Hylazin

BASIC INFORMATION

Habit forming? No
Prescription needed? Yes
Available as generic? Yes
Drug class: Antihypertensive

USES

Treatment for high blood pressure and congestive heart failure.

DOSAGE & USAGE INFORMATION

How to take:
Tablet—Swallow with liquid. If you can't swallow whole, crumble tablet and take with liquid or food.

When to take:
At the same time each day. Should be taken with food.

If you forget a dose:
Take as soon as you remember up to 2 hours late. If more than 2 hours, wait for next scheduled dose (don't double this dose).

What drug does:
Relaxes and expands blood vessel walls, lowering blood pressure.

Time lapse before drug works:
Regular use for several weeks may be necessary to determine drug's effectiveness.

Continued next column

OVERDOSE

SYMPTOMS:
Rapid and weak heartbeat, fainting, extreme weakness, cold and sweaty skin, flushing.
WHAT TO DO:
- **Dial 911 (emergency) or 0 (operator) for an ambulance or medical help. Then give first aid immediately.**
- **If patient is unconscious and not breathing, give mouth-to-mouth breathing. If there is no heartbeat, use cardiac massage and mouth-to-mouth breathing (CPR). Don't try to make patient vomit. If you can't get help quickly, take patient to nearest emergency facility.**
- **See emergency information on inside covers.**

Don't take with:
- Nonprescription drugs containing alcohol without consulting doctor.
- Any other medicine without consulting your doctor or pharmacist.

POSSIBLE ADVERSE REACTIONS OR SIDE EFFECTS

SYMPTOMS	WHAT TO DO
Life-threatening:	
In case of overdose, see previous column.	
Common:	
• Nausea or vomiting, rapid or irregular heartbeat.	Discontinue. Call doctor right away.
• Headache, diarrhea, appetite loss, painful or difficult urination.	Continue. Tell doctor at next visit.
Infrequent:	
• Hives or rash, flushed face, sore throat, fever, chest pain, swelling of lymph glands, skin blisters, swelling in feet or legs, joint pain.	Discontinue. Call doctor right away.
• Confusion, dizziness, anxiety, depression, joint pain, general discomfort or weakness, fever, muscle pain, chest pain.	Continue. Call doctor when convenient.
• Watery eyes and irritation, constipation.	Continue. Tell doctor at next visit.
Rare:	
• Weakness and faintness when arising from bed or chair, jaundice.	Discontinue. Call doctor right away.
• Numbness or tingling in hands or feet, nasal congestion, impotence.	Continue. Call doctor when convenient.

WARNINGS & PRECAUTIONS

Don't take if:
- You are allergic to hydralazine or tartrazine dye.
- You have history of coronary artery disease or rheumatic heart disease.

Before you start, consult your doctor:
- If you feel pain in chest, neck or arms on physical exertion.
- If you have had lupus.
- If you have had a stroke.

- If you have had kidney disease or impaired kidney function.
- If you will have surgery within 2 months, including dental surgery, requiring general or spinal anesthesia.

Over age 60:
Adverse reactions and side effects may be more frequent and severe than in younger persons.

Pregnancy:
Decide with your doctor if drug benefits justify risk to unborn child. Risk category C (see page xxiii).

Breast-feeding:
Drug filters into milk. May harm child. Avoid.

Infants & children:
Not recommended.

Prolonged use:
- May cause lupus (arthritis-like illness).
- Possible psychosis.
- May cause numbness, tingling in hands or feet.
- Talk to your doctor about the need for follow-up medical examinations or laboratory studies to check blood pressure, complete blood counts (white blood cell count, platelet count, red blood cell count, hemoglobin, hematocrit), ANA titers*.

Skin & sunlight:
No problems expected.

Driving, piloting or hazardous work:
Don't drive or pilot aircraft until you learn how medicine affects you. Don't work around dangerous machinery. Don't climb ladders or work in high places. Danger increases if you drink alcohol or take medicine affecting alertness and reflexes, such as antihistamines, tranquilizers, sedatives, pain medicine, narcotics and mind-altering drugs.

Discontinuing:
Don't discontinue without doctor's advice until you complete prescribed dose, even though symptoms diminish or disappear.

Others:
- Vitamin B-6 diet supplement may be advisable. Consult doctor.
- Some products contain tartrazine dye. Avoid, especially if you are allergic to aspirin.
- May interfere with the accuracy of some medical tests.

POSSIBLE INTERACTION WITH OTHER DRUGS

GENERIC NAME OR DRUG CLASS	COMBINED EFFECT
Amphetamines*	Decreased hydralazine effect.

Antihypertensives, other*	Increased anti-hypertensive effect.
Anti-inflammatory drugs, nonsteroidal (NSAIDs)*	Decreased effect of hydralazine.
Antivirals, HIV/AIDS*	Increased risk of peripheral neuropathy.
Carteolol	Increased anti-hypertensive effect.
Diazoxide & other anti-hypertensive drugs	Increased anti-hypertensive effect.
Diuretics, oral*	Increased effects of both drugs. When monitored carefully, combination may be beneficial in controlling hypertension.
Guanfacine	Increased effects of both drugs.
Lisinopril	Increased anti-hypertensive effect. Dosage of each may require adjustment.
Monoamine oxidase (MAO) inhibitors*	Increased hydralazine effect.
Nicardipine	Blood pressure drop. Dosages may require adjustment.
Nimodipine	Dangerous blood pressure drop.

Continued on page 918

POSSIBLE INTERACTION WITH OTHER SUBSTANCES

INTERACTS WITH	COMBINED EFFECT
Alcohol:	May lower blood pressure excessively. Use extreme caution.
Beverages:	None expected.
Cocaine:	Increased risk of heart block and high blood pressure.
Foods:	Increased hydralazine absorption.
Marijuana:	Weakness on standing.
Tobacco:	Possible angina attacks.

HYDRALAZINE & HYDROCHLOROTHIAZIDE

BRAND NAMES

Apresazide
Apresoline-
  Esidrix

Aprozide
Hydra-zide

BASIC INFORMATION

Habit forming? No
Prescription needed? Yes
Available as generic? Yes
Drug class: Antihypertensive, diuretic

USES

- Controls, but doesn't cure, high blood pressure.
- Reduces fluid retention (edema).

DOSAGE & USAGE INFORMATION

How to take:
Tablet or capsule—Swallow with liquid. If you can't swallow whole, crumble tablet or open capsule and take with liquid or food.

When to take:
At the same time each day.

If you forget a dose:
Take as soon as you remember up to 2 hours late. If more than 2 hours, wait for next scheduled dose (don't double this dose).

Continued next column

OVERDOSE

SYMPTOMS:
Cramps, drowsiness, weak pulse, rapid and weak heartbeat, fainting, extreme weakness, cold and sweaty skin, coma.
WHAT TO DO:
- **Dial 911 (emergency) or 0 (operator) for an ambulance or medical help. Then give first aid immediately.**
- **If patient is unconscious and not breathing, give mouth-to-mouth breathing. If there is no heartbeat, use cardiac massage and mouth-to-mouth breathing (CPR). Don't try to make patient vomit. If you can't get help quickly, take patient to nearest emergency facility.**
- **See emergency information on inside covers.**

What drug does:
- Forces sodium and water excretion, reducing body fluid.
- Relaxes and expands blood vessel walls, lowering blood pressure.
- Reduced body fluid and relaxed arteries lower blood pressure.

Time lapse before drug works:
Regular use for several weeks may be necessary to determine drug's effectiveness.

Don't take with:
- Nonprescription drugs containing alcohol without consulting doctor.
- Any other medicine without consulting your doctor or pharmacist.

POSSIBLE ADVERSE REACTIONS OR SIDE EFFECTS

SYMPTOMS	WHAT TO DO
Life-threatening:	
Chest pain, irregular and fast heartbeat, weak pulse.	Discontinue. Seek emergency treatment.
Common:	
• Nausea, vomiting.	Discontinue. Call doctor right away.
• Headache, diarrhea, appetite loss, frequent urination, dry mouth, thirst.	Continue. Call doctor when convenient.
Infrequent:	
• Rash; black, bloody or tarry stool; red or flushed face; sore throat, fever, mouth sores; constipation; lymph glands swelling; blurred vision; skin blisters; swelling in feet or legs.	Discontinue. Call doctor right away.
• Dizziness; confusion; watery eyes; weight gain or loss; joint, muscle or chest pain; depression; anxiety; fever.	Continue. Call doctor when convenient.
Rare:	
• Weakness and faintness when arising from bed or chair, jaundice.	Discontinue. Call doctor right away.
• Numbness or tingling in hands or feet, nasal congestion, impotence.	Continue. Call doctor when convenient.

HYDRALAZINE & HYDROCHLOROTHIAZIDE

 WARNINGS & PRECAUTIONS

Don't take if:
- You are allergic to hydralazine, any thiazide diuretic drug or tartrazine dye.
- You have history of coronary artery disease or rheumatic heart disease.

Before you start, consult your doctor:
- If you feel pain in chest, neck or arms on physical exertion.
- If you are allergic to any sulfa drug.
- If you have had lupus or a stroke.
- If you have gout, liver, pancreas or kidney disorder.
- If you will have surgery within 2 months, including dental surgery, requiring general or spinal anesthesia.

Over age 60:
Adverse reactions and side effects may be more frequent and severe than in younger persons, especially dizziness and excessive potassium loss.

Pregnancy:
Decide with your doctor if drug benefits justify risk to unborn child. Risk category C (see page xxiii).

Breast-feeding:
Drug passes into milk. Avoid drug or discontinue nursing until you finish medicine. Consult doctor for advice on maintaining milk supply.

Infants & children:
Not recommended.

Prolonged use:
- May cause lupus (arthritis-like illness).
- Possible psychosis.
- May cause numbness, tingling in hands or feet.
- Talk to your doctor about the need for follow-up medical examinations or laboratory studies to check blood pressure, complete blood counts (white blood cell count, platelet count, red blood cell count, hemoglobin, hematocrit), ANA titers*.

Skin & sunlight:
One or more drugs in this group may cause rash or intensify sunburn in areas exposed to sun or ultraviolet light (photosensitivity reaction). Avoid overexposure. Notify doctor if reaction occurs.

Driving, piloting or hazardous work:
Don't drive or pilot aircraft until you learn how medicine affects you. Don't work around dangerous machinery. Don't climb ladders or work in high places. Danger increases if you drink alcohol or take medicine affecting alertness and reflexes, such as antihistamines, tranquilizers, sedatives, pain medicine, narcotics and mind-altering drugs.

Discontinuing:
Don't discontinue without consulting doctor's advice until you complete prescribed dose, even though symptoms diminish or disappear.

Others:
- Vitamin B-6 diet supplement may be advisable. Consult doctor.
- Hot weather and fever may cause dehydration and drop in blood pressure. Dose may require temporary adjustment. Weigh daily and report any unexpected weight decreases to your doctor.
- May cause rise in uric acid, leading to gout.
- May cause blood sugar rise in diabetics.

 POSSIBLE INTERACTION WITH OTHER DRUGS

GENERIC NAME OR DRUG CLASS	COMBINED EFFECT
Acebutolol	Decreased anti-hypertensive effect of acebutolol.
Allopurinol	Decreased allopurinol effect.
Amphetamines*	Decreased hydralazine effect.
Antidepressants, tricyclic*	Dangerous drop in blood pressure. Avoid combination unless under medical supervision.

Continued on page 918

 POSSIBLE INTERACTION WITH OTHER SUBSTANCES

INTERACTS WITH	COMBINED EFFECT
Alcohol:	May lower blood pressure excessively. Use extreme caution.
Beverages:	None expected.
Cocaine:	Dangerous blood pressure rise. Avoid.
Foods: Licorice.	Excessive potassium loss that causes dangerous heart rhythms.
Marijuana:	Weakness on standing. May increase blood pressure.
Tobacco:	Possible angina attacks.

HYDROCORTISONE (Rectal)

BRAND NAMES

Anucort	Cortiment-40
Anusol-H.C.	Dermolate
Cort-Dome High	Hemril-HC
Potency	Proctocort
Corticaine	Rectocort
Cortiment-10	

BASIC INFORMATION

Habit forming? No
Prescription needed? Yes
Available as generic? Yes, for some
**Drug class: Anti-inflammatory, steroidal
(rectal); anesthetic (rectal)**

USES

In or around the rectum to relieve swelling,
itching and pain for hemorrhoids (piles) and
other rectal conditions. Frequently used after
hemorrhoid surgery.

DOSAGE & USAGE INFORMATION

How to use:
* Follow instructions in package.
* Rectal cream or ointment—Apply to surface of
rectum with fingers. Insert applicator into
rectum no farther than halfway and apply
inside. Wash applicator with warm soapy
water or discard.
* Suppository—Remove wrapper and moisten
with water. Lie on side. Push blunt end of
suppository into rectum with finger. If
suppository is too soft, run cold water over it or
put in refrigerator for 15 to 45 minutes before
using.
* Aerosol foam—Read patient instructions.
Don't insert into rectum. Use the special
applicator and wash carefully after using.

When to use:
Follow instructions in package or when needed.

Continued next column

OVERDOSE

SYMPTOMS:
None expected.
WHAT TO DO:
**Not intended for internal use. If child
accidentally swallows, call poison control
center.**

If you forget a dose:
Use as soon as you remember.

What drug does:
* Reduces inflammation.
* Relieves pain and itching.

Time lapse before drug works:
5 to 15 minutes.

Don't use with:
Other rectal medicines without consulting your
doctor.

POSSIBLE ADVERSE REACTIONS OR SIDE EFFECTS

SYMPTOMS	WHAT TO DO
Life-threatening None expected.	
Common None expected.	
Infrequent	
• Nervousness, trembling, hives, rash, itch, inflammation or tenderness not present before application, slow heartbeat.	Discontinue. Call doctor right away.
• Dizziness, blurred vision, swollen feet.	Continue. Call doctor when convenient.
Rare	
• Blood in urine.	Discontinue. Call doctor right away.
• Increased or painful urination.	Continue. Call doctor when convenient.

WARNINGS & PRECAUTIONS

Don't use if:
You are allergic to any topical anesthetic.

Before you start, consult your doctor:
- If you have skin infection at site of treatment.
- If you have had severe or extensive skin disorders such as eczema or psoriasis.
- If you have bleeding hemorrhoids.

Over age 60:
Adverse reactions and side effects may be more frequent and severe than in younger persons.

Pregnancy:
Decide with your doctor if drug benefits justify risk to unborn child. Risk category C (see page xxiii).

Breast-feeding:
No problems expected. Consult doctor.

Infants & children:
Don't use without careful medical supervision. Too much may be absorbed into the blood stream and affect growth.

Prolonged use:
Possible excess absorption. Don't use longer than 3 days for any one problem.

Skin & sunlight:
No problems expected.

Driving, piloting or hazardous work:
No problems expected.

Discontinuing:
May be unnecessary to finish medicine. Follow doctor's instructions.

Others:
- Report any rectal bleeding to your doctor.
- Keep cool, but don't freeze.

POSSIBLE INTERACTION WITH OTHER DRUGS

GENERIC NAME OR DRUG CLASS	COMBINED EFFECT
Sulfa drugs*	Decreased anti-infective effect of sulfa drugs.

POSSIBLE INTERACTION WITH OTHER SUBSTANCES

INTERACTS WITH	COMBINED EFFECT
Alcohol:	None expected.
Beverages:	None expected.
Cocaine:	Possible nervous system toxicity. Avoid.
Foods:	None expected.
Marijuana:	None expected.
Tobacco:	None expected.

*See Glossary

HYDROXYCHLOROQUINE

BRAND NAMES

Plaquenil

BASIC INFORMATION

Habit forming? No
Prescription needed? Yes
Available as generic? No
Drug class: Antiprotozoal, antirheumatic

 USES

- Treatment for protozoal infections, such as malaria and amebiasis.
- Treatment for some forms of arthritis and lupus.

 DOSAGE & USAGE INFORMATION

How to take:
Tablet—Swallow with food or milk to lessen stomach irritation.

When to take:
- Depends on condition. Is adjusted during treatment.
- Malaria prevention—Begin taking medicine 2 weeks before entering areas where malaria is present and until 8 weeks after return.

If you forget a dose:
- 1 or more doses a day—Take as soon as you remember up to 2 hours late. If more than 2 hours, wait for next scheduled dose (don't double this dose).
- 1 dose weekly—Take as soon as possible, then return to regular dosing schedule.

What drug does:
- Inhibits parasite multiplication.
- Decreases inflammatory response in diseased joint.

Time lapse before drug works:
1 to 2 hours.

Continued next column

 OVERDOSE

SYMPTOMS:
Severe breathing difficulty, drowsiness, faintness, headache, seizures.
WHAT TO DO:
- **Dial 911 (emergency) or 0 (operator) for an ambulance or medical help. Then give first aid immediately.**
- **See emergency information on inside covers.**

Don't take with:
Any other medicine without consulting your doctor or pharmacist.

 POSSIBLE ADVERSE REACTIONS OR SIDE EFFECTS

SYMPTOMS	WHAT TO DO
Life-threatening:	
In case of overdose, see previous column.	
Common:	
Headache, appetite loss, abdominal pain.	Continue. Tell doctor at next visit.
Infrequent:	
• Blurred vision, changes in vision.	Discontinue. Call doctor right away.
• Rash or itch, diarrhea, nausea, vomiting, hair loss, blue-black skin or mouth, dizziness, nervousness.	Continue. Call doctor when convenient.
Rare:	
• Mood or mental changes, seizures, sore throat, fever, unusual bleeding or bruising, muscle weakness, convulsions.	Discontinue. Call doctor right away.
• Ringing or buzzing in ears, hearing loss.	Continue. Call doctor when convenient.

WARNINGS & PRECAUTIONS

Don't take if:
You are allergic to chloroquine or hydroxychloroquine.

Before you start, consult your doctor:
- If you plan to become pregnant within the medication period.
- If you have blood disease.
- If you have eye or vision problems.
- If you have a G6PD* deficiency.
- If you have liver disease.
- If you have nerve or brain disease (including seizure disorders).
- If you have porphyria.
- If you have psoriasis.
- If you have stomach or intestinal disease.
- If you drink more than 3 oz. of alcohol daily.

Over age 60:
Adverse reactions and side effects may be more frequent and severe than in younger persons.

Pregnancy:
Decide with your doctor if drug benefits justify risk to unborn child. Risk category C (see page xxiii).

Breast-feeding:
Drug passes into milk. Avoid drug or discontinue nursing. Consult doctor for advice on maintaining milk supply.

Infants & children:
Not recommended. Dangerous.

Prolonged use:
- Permanent damage to the retina (back part of the eye) or nerve deafness.
- Talk to your doctor about the need for follow-up medical examinations or laboratory studies to check complete blood counts (white blood cell count, platelet count, red blood cell count, hemoglobin, hematocrit), eyes.

Skin & sunlight:
No special problems expected.

Driving, piloting or hazardous work:
Don't drive or pilot aircraft until you learn how medicine affects you. Don't work around dangerous machinery. Don't climb ladders or work in high places. Danger increases if you drink alcohol or take medicine affecting alertness and reflexes.

Discontinuing:
Don't discontinue without doctor's advice until you complete prescribed dose, even though symptoms diminish or disappear.

Others:
- Periodic physical and blood examinations recommended.
- If you are in a malaria area for a long time, you may need to change to another preventive drug every 2 years.

POSSIBLE INTERACTION WITH OTHER DRUGS

GENERIC NAME OR DRUG CLASS	COMBINED EFFECT
Estrogens*	Possible liver toxicity.
Gold compounds*	Risk of severe rash and itch.
Kaolin	Decreased absorption of hydroxychloroquine.
Magnesium trisilicate	Decreased absorption of hydroxychloroquine.
Penicillamine	Possible blood or kidney toxicity.

POSSIBLE INTERACTION WITH OTHER SUBSTANCES

INTERACTS WITH	COMBINED EFFECT
Alcohol:	Possible liver toxicity. Avoid.
Beverages:	None expected.
Cocaine:	None expected.
Foods:	None expected.
Marijuana:	None expected.
Tobacco:	None expected.

*See Glossary

HYDROXYUREA

BRAND NAMES

Droxia   Hydrea

BASIC INFORMATION

Habit forming? No
Prescription needed? Yes
Available as generic? Yes
Drug class: Antineoplastic

USES

- Treats head, neck, ovarian and cervical cancer.
- Treats leukemia, melanoma and polycythemia vera.
- Treats sickle cell disease.

DOSAGE & USAGE INFORMATION

How to take:
Capsules—Swallow with liquid. If you can't swallow whole, open capsule and take with liquid or food. Instructions to take on empty stomach mean 1 hour before or 2 hours after eating.

When to take:
According to doctor's instructions.

If you forget a dose:
Skip this dose. Never double dose. Resume regular schedule.

What drug does:
Probably interferes with synthesis of DNA.

Time lapse before drug works:
2 hours.

Don't take with:
Any other medicines (including over-the-counter drugs such as cough and cold medicines, laxatives, antacids, diet pills, caffeine, nose drops or vitamins) without consulting your doctor.

OVERDOSE

SYMPTOMS:
Black, tarry stools; fainting; seizures.
WHAT TO DO:
- **Dial 911 (emergency) or 0 (operator) for an ambulance or medical help. Then give first aid immediately.**
- **See emergency information on inside covers.**

POSSIBLE ADVERSE REACTIONS OR SIDE EFFECTS

SYMPTOMS	WHAT TO DO
Life-threatening:	
In case of overdose, see previous column.	
Common:	
• Skin rash, fever, chills, cough, back pain.	Discontinue. Call doctor right away.
• Diarrhea, drowsiness, nausea, vomiting.	Continue. Call doctor when convenient.
Infrequent:	
Mouth sores, bruising, constipation, red skin.	Discontinue. Call doctor right away.
Rare:	
Confusion, hallucinations, headache, swollen feet.	Continue. Call doctor when convenient.

WARNINGS & PRECAUTIONS

Don't take if:
- You have chicken pox.
- You have shingles (herpes zoster).

Before you start, consult your doctor:
- If you have anemia.
- If you have gout.
- If you have an infection.
- If you have kidney disease.

Over age 60:
Adverse reactions and side effects may be more frequent and severe than in younger persons. You may need smaller doses for shorter periods of time.

Pregnancy:
Decide with your doctor if drug benefits justify risk to unborn child. Risk category C (see page xxiii).

Breast-feeding:
Drug passes into milk. Avoid drug or discontinue nursing until you finish medicine. Consult doctor for advice on maintaining milk supply.

Infants & children:
Effect not documented. Consult your pediatrician.

Prolonged use:
Talk to your doctor about the need for follow-up medical examinations or laboratory studies to check kidney function, complete blood counts (white blood cell count, platelet count, red blood cell count, hemoglobin, hematocrit) and serum uric acid.

Skin & sunlight:
No problems expected.

Driving, piloting or hazardous work:
Avoid if you feel confused, drowsy or dizzy.

Discontinuing:
May still experience symptoms of bone marrow depression, such as: blood in stools, fever or chills, blood spots under the skin, back pain, hoarseness, bloody urine. If any of these occur, call your doctor right away.

Others:
- Advise any doctor or dentist whom you consult that you take this medicine.
- May affect results in some medical tests.

 ## POSSIBLE INTERACTION WITH OTHER DRUGS

GENERIC NAME OR DRUG CLASS	COMBINED EFFECT
Bone marrow depressants, other*	Dangerous suppression of bone marrow activity
Clozapine	Toxic effect on bone marrow.
Levamisole	Increased risk of bone marrow depression.
Probenecid	May require increased dosage to treat gout.
Sulfinpyrazone	May require increased dosage to treat gout.
Tiopronin	Increased risk of toxicity to bone marrow.
Vaccines, live or killed virus	Increased risk of side effects.

 ## POSSIBLE INTERACTION WITH OTHER SUBSTANCES

INTERACTS WITH	COMBINED EFFECT
Alcohol:	No special problems expected.
Beverages:	No special problems expected.
Cocaine:	Increased confusion. Avoid.
Foods:	No special problems expected.
Marijuana:	Increased confusion. Avoid.
Tobacco:	No special problems expected.

HYDROXYZINE

BRAND NAMES

Anxanil
Apo-Hydroxyzine
Atarax

Multipax
Novo-Hydroxyzin
Vistaril

BASIC INFORMATION

Habit forming? No
Prescription needed? Yes
Available as generic? Yes
Drug class: Tranquilizer, antihistamine

USES

- Treatment for anxiety, tension and agitation.
- Relieves itching from allergic reactions.

DOSAGE & USAGE INFORMATION

How to take:
- Tablet, syrup or capsule—Swallow with liquid. If you can't swallow whole, crumble tablet or open capsule and take with liquid or food.
- Liquid—If desired, dilute dose in beverage before swallowing.

When to take:
At the same times each day.

If you forget a dose:
Take as soon as you remember up to 2 hours late. If more than 2 hours, wait for next scheduled dose (don't double this dose).

What drug does:
Blocks action of histamine after an allergic response triggers histamine release. Histamines cause itching, sneezing, runny nose and eyes and other symptoms.

Time lapse before drug works:
15 to 30 minutes.

Don't take with:
Any other medicine without consulting your doctor or pharmacist.

OVERDOSE

SYMPTOMS:
Drowsiness, unsteadiness, agitation, purposeless movements, tremor, convulsions.
WHAT TO DO:
- **Dial 911 (emergency) or 0 (operator) for an ambulance or medical help. Then give first aid immediately.**
- **See emergency information at end of book.**

POSSIBLE ADVERSE REACTIONS OR SIDE EFFECTS

SYMPTOMS	WHAT TO DO
Life-threatening: In case of overdose, see previous column.	
Common: Drowsiness; dizziness; dryness of mouth, nose or throat; nausea.	Continue. Call doctor when convenient.
Infrequent: • Change in vision, clumsiness, rash.	Discontinue. Call doctor right away.
• Less tolerance for contact lenses, painful or difficult urination.	Continue. Call doctor when convenient.
• Appetite loss. at next visit.	Continue. Tell doctor
Rare: Nightmares, agitation, irritability, sore throat, fever, rapid heartbeat, unusual bleeding or bruising, fatigue, weakness, confusion, fainting, seizures.	Discontinue. Call doctor right away.

WARNINGS & PRECAUTIONS

Don't take if:
You are allergic to any antihistamine.

Before you start, consult your doctor:
- If you have asthma or kidney disease.
- If you will have surgery within 2 months, including dental surgery, requiring general or spinal anesthesia.

Over age 60:
- Adverse reactions and side effects may be more frequent and severe than in younger persons.
- Drug likely to increase urination difficulty caused by enlarged prostate gland.

Pregnancy:
Decide with your doctor if drug benefits justify risk to unborn child. Risk category C (see page xxiii).

Breast-feeding:
Drug passes into milk. Avoid drug or discontinue nursing until you finish medicine. Consult doctor for advice on maintaining milk supply.

Infants & children:
Use only under medical supervision.

Prolonged use:
Tolerance* develops and reduces effectiveness.

Skin & sunlight:
No problems expected.

Driving, piloting or hazardous work:
Don't drive or pilot aircraft until you learn how medicine affects you. Don't work around dangerous machinery. Don't climb ladders or work in high places. Danger increases if you drink alcohol or take medicine affecting alertness and reflexes, such as antihistamines, tranquilizers, sedatives, pain medicine, narcotics and mind-altering drugs.

Discontinuing:
Don't discontinue without consulting doctor. Dose may require gradual reduction if you have taken drug for a long time. Doses of other drugs may also require adjustment.

Others:
Advise any doctor or dentist whom you consult that you take this medicine.

POSSIBLE INTERACTION WITH OTHER DRUGS

GENERIC NAME OR DRUG CLASS	COMBINED EFFECT
Antidepressants, tricyclic*	Increased effects of both drugs.
Antihistamines*	Increased hydroxyzine effect.
Attapulgite	Decreased hydroxyzine effect.
Carteolol	Decreased antihistamine effect.
Central nervous system (CNS) depressants*	Greater depression of central nervous system.
Clozapine	Toxic effect on the central nervous system.
Fluoxetine	Increased depressant effects of both drugs.
Guanfacine	May increase depressant effects of either drug.
Leucovorin	High alcohol content of leucovorin may cause adverse effects.
Narcotics*	Increased effects of both drugs.
Pain relievers*	Increased effects of both drugs.
Sertraline	Increased depressive effects of both drugs.
Sotalol	Increased antihistamine effect.

POSSIBLE INTERACTION WITH OTHER SUBSTANCES

INTERACTS WITH	COMBINED EFFECT
Alcohol:	Increased sedation and intoxication. Use with caution.
Beverages: Caffeine drinks.	Decreased tranquilizer effect of hydroxyzine.
Cocaine:	Decreased hydroxyzine effect. Avoid.
Foods:	None expected.
Marijuana:	None expected.
Tobacco:	None expected.

HYOSCYAMINE

BRAND NAMES

Anaspaz
Anaspaz PB
Atrohist Plus
Barbidonna
Barbidonna 2
Belladenal
Bellafoline
Cystospaz
Cystospaz-M
Gastrosed
Kinesed

Levbid
Levsin
Levsin S/L
Levsinex
Levsinex Timecaps
Neoquess
Phenahist TR
Phenchlor SHA
Ru-Tuss
Stahist

BASIC INFORMATION

Habit forming? No
Prescription needed?
  Low strength: No
  High strength: Yes
Available as generic? No
Drug class: Antispasmodic, anticholinergic

 ## USES

Reduces spasms of digestive system, bladder
and urethra.

 ## DOSAGE & USAGE INFORMATION

How to take:
- Tablet or liquid—Swallow with liquid or food to
  lessen stomach irritation. You may chew or
  crush tablets.
- Extended-release capsules or tablets—
  Swallow each dose whole.
- Drops—Dilute dose in beverage before
  swallowing.

When to take:
30 minutes before meals (unless directed
otherwise by doctor).

Continued next column

 ## OVERDOSE

SYMPTOMS:
**Dilated pupils, rapid pulse and breathing,
dizziness, fever, hallucinations, confusion,
slurred speech, agitation, flushed face,
convulsions, coma.**
WHAT TO DO:
- **Dial 911 (emergency) or 0 (operator) for an
  ambulance or medical help. Then give first
  aid immediately.**
- **See emergency information on inside
  covers.**

If you forget a dose:
Take as soon as you remember up to 2 hours
late. If more than 2 hours, wait for next
scheduled dose (don't double this dose).

What drug does:
Blocks nerve impulses at parasympathetic nerve
endings, preventing muscle contractions and
gland secretions of organs involved.

Time lapse before drug works:
15 to 30 minutes.

Don't take with:
- Antacids* or antidiarrheals*.
- Any other medicine without consulting your
  doctor or pharmacist.

 ## POSSIBLE ADVERSE REACTIONS OR SIDE EFFECTS

SYMPTOMS	WHAT TO DO
Life-threatening:	
In case of overdose, see previous column.	
Common:	
Confusion, delirium, rapid heartbeat.	Discontinue. Call doctor right away.
Nausea, vomiting, decreased sweating.	Continue. Call doctor when convenient.
Constipation.	Continue. Tell doctor at next visit.
Dryness in ears, nose, throat, mouth.	No action necessary.
Infrequent:	
Headache, painful or difficult urination, nasal congestion, altered taste.	Continue. Call doctor when convenient.
Lightheadedness.	Discontinue. Call doctor right away.
Rare:	
Rash or hives, eye pain, blurred vision.	Discontinue. Call doctor right away.

 ## WARNINGS & PRECAUTIONS

Don't take if:
- You are allergic to any anticholinergic.
- You have trouble with stomach bloating.
- You have difficulty emptying your bladder
  completely.
- You have narrow-angle glaucoma.
- You have severe ulcerative colitis.

Before you start, consult your doctor:
- If you have open-angle glaucoma.
- If you have angina.
- If you have chronic bronchitis or asthma.
- If you have hiatal hernia.
- If you have liver, kidney or thyroid disease.
- If you have enlarged prostate.
- If you have myasthenia gravis.
- If you have peptic ulcer.
- If you will have surgery within 2 months, including dental surgery, requiring general or spinal anesthesia.

Over age 60:
Adverse reactions and side effects may be more frequent and severe than in younger persons.

Pregnancy:
Decide with your doctor if drug benefits justify risk to unborn child. Risk category C (see page xxiii).

Breast-feeding:
Drug passes into milk and decreases milk flow. Avoid drug or discontinue nursing until you finish medicine. Consult doctor for advice on maintaining milk supply.

Infants & children:
Use only under medical supervision.

Prolonged use:
Chronic constipation, possible fecal impaction. Consult doctor immediately.

Skin & sunlight:
No problems expected.

Driving, piloting or hazardous work:
Use disqualifies you for piloting aircraft. Otherwise, no problems expected.

Discontinuing:
May be unnecessary to finish medicine. Follow doctor's instructions.

Others:
Advise any doctor or dentist whom you consult that you take this medicine.

POSSIBLE INTERACTION WITH OTHER DRUGS

GENERIC NAME OR DRUG CLASS	COMBINED EFFECT
Amantadine	Increased hyoscyamine effect.
Anticholinergics, other*	Increased hyoscyamine effect.
Antidepressants, tricyclic*	Increased hyoscyamine effect.
Antihistamines*	Increased hyoscyamine effect.
Cortisone drugs*	Increased internal eye pressure.
Haloperidol	Increased internal eye pressure.
Ketoconazole	Decreased ketoconazole effect.
Meperidine	Increased hyoscyamine effect.
Methylphenidate	Increased hyoscyamine effect.
Molindone	Increased anticholinergic effect
Monoamine oxidase (MAO) inhibitors*	Increased hyoscyamine effect..
Nizatidine	Increased nizatidine effect.
Orphenadrine	Increased hyoscyamine effect.
Phenothiazines*	Increased hyoscyamine effect.
Pilocarpine	Loss of pilocarpine effect in glaucoma treatment.
Sedatives* or central nervous system (CNS) depressants*	Increased sedative effect of both drugs.
Vitamin C	Decreased hyoscyamine effect. Avoid large doses of vitamin C.

POSSIBLE INTERACTION WITH OTHER SUBSTANCES

INTERACTS WITH	COMBINED EFFECT
Alcohol:	None expected.
Beverages:	None expected.
Cocaine:	Excessively rapid heartbeat. Avoid.
Foods:	None expected.
Marijuana:	Drowsiness and dry mouth.
Tobacco:	None expected.

*See Glossary

IMMUNOSUPPRESSIVE AGENTS

GENERIC AND BRAND NAMES

MYCOPHENOLATE   **TACROLIMUS**
  CellCept   Prograf

BASIC INFORMATION

Habit forming? No
Prescription needed? Yes
Available as generic? No
Drug class: Immunosuppressant

 ## USES

Helps to suppress the immune system and prevent rejection in patients who have undergone organ transplants.

 ## DOSAGE & USAGE INFORMATION

How to take:
- Oral suspension—Take as directed on label.
- Tablet or capsule—Swallow with liquid. Do not open capsule or crush tablet. Tacrolimus may be taken with or without food. Take mycophenolate on an empty stomach (1 hour before or 2 hours after a meal).

When to take:
At the same times each day, according to instructions on prescription label.

If you forget a dose:
Take as soon as you remember. If it is almost time for the next dose, wait for next scheduled dose (don't double this dose). Consult doctor if you are unsure about dosing schedule.

What drug does:
Tacrolimus and myclophenolate are 2 different types of immunsuppressive drugs. They suppress immune reactions (to transplanted organs) in certain cells by inhibiting their growth.

Time lapse before drug works:
3 to 3-1/2 hours. May take several weeks to evaluate effectiveness against organ rejection.

Continued next column

 ## OVERDOSE

SYMPTOMS:
Increased severity of adverse reactions, coma, delirium.
WHAT TO DO:
- **Dial 911 (emergency) or 0 (operator) for an ambulance or medical help. Then give first aid immediately.**
- **See emergency information on inside covers.**

Don't take with:
Any other medicine without consulting your doctor or pharmacist.

 ## POSSIBLE ADVERSE REACTIONS OR SIDE EFFECTS

SYMPTOMS	WHAT TO DO
Life-threatening:	
In case of overdose, see previous column.	
Common:	
• Infections (fever, chills, hoarseness, cough, trouble urinating, back or side pain); headache; tingling or numbness of hands or feet; chest pain; blood in urine; trouble sleeping; trembling of hands; shortness of breath.	Continue, but call doctor right away.
• Mild back pain, constipation or diarrhea, stomach pain, heartburn.	Continue. Call doctor when convenient.
Infrequent:	
• Bloody vomit; anxiety; nervousness; white patches on mouth, tongue or throat; weakness; seizures.	Continue, but call doctor right away.
• Hair loss or excess hair growth, nausea, mild vomiting, skin rash or itch, muscle or joint pain, dizziness.	Continue. Call doctor when convenient.
Rare:	
• Bloody, black or tarry stools; small red spots on skin; unusual bleeding or bruising; irregular heartbeat.	Continue, but call doctor right away.
• Mood or mental changes, any other side effects not listed.	Continue. Call doctor when convenient

 ## WARNINGS & PRECAUTIONS

Don't take if:
You are allergic to mycophenolate or tacrolimus.

Before you start, consult your doctor:
- If you have liver or kidney disease.
- If you have a digestive system disease.
- If you have an infection.
- If you have chickenpox (or have recently been exposed) or herpes zoster (shingles).

Over age 60:
No special problems expected.

Pregnancy:
Decide with your doctor if drug benefits justify risk to unborn child. Risk category C (see page xxiii).

Breast-feeding:
Tacrolimus passes into milk; mycophenolate may pass into milk. Avoid drugs or discontinue nursing until you finish medicine. Consult doctor for advice on maintaining milk supply.

Infants & children:
Safety and effectiveness of mycophenolate are not established. Tacrolimus has been used successfully in liver transplants in pediatric patients.

Prolonged use:
- Can cause reduced function of kidneys.
- Can increase risk of developing lymphoma (cancer of lymph glands).
- Talk to your doctor about the need for follow-up medical examinations or laboratory studies to check blood concentration of drug, kidney function, liver function, potassium levels, drug's effectiveness and adverse reactions.

Skin & sunlight:
No special problems expected.

Driving, piloting or hazardous work:
Don't drive or pilot aircraft until you learn how medicine affects you. Don't work around dangerous machinery. Don't climb ladders or work in high places. Danger increases if you drink alcohol or take medicine affecting alertness and reflexes.

Discontinuing:
Don't discontinue without consulting doctor. You probably will require this medicine for the remainder of your life.

Others:
- Advise any doctor or dentist whom you consult that you take this drug. May interfere with results of some medical tests.
- Wear medical identification stating that you have had a transplant and take this drug.
- Check blood pressure routinely at home. Drug may sometimes cause hypertension.
- Avoid any immunizations except those specifically recommended by your doctor.
- Maintain good dental hygiene. Immunosuppression can cause gum problems.

POSSIBLE INTERACTION WITH OTHER DRUGS

GENERIC NAME OR DRUG CLASS	COMBINED EFFECT
Acyclovir	Increased effect of mycophenolate.
Antacids*	Decreased effect of mycophenolate.
Cholestyramine	Decreased effect of mycophenolate.
Diuretics, potassium-sparing*	Increased risk of potassium toxicity.
Enzyme inducers*	Decreased effect of tacrolimus.
Enzyme inhibitors*	Increased effect of tacrolimus.
Gancyclovir	Increased effect of mycophenolate.
Immunosuppressants*, other	Increased immuno-suppressive effect.
Nephrotoxic medications*	Increased risk of kidney problems.
Potassium supplements	Increased risk of potassium toxicity.
Probenecid	Increased effect of mycophenolate.
Troglitazone	Decreased effect of tacrolimus.
Vaccinations	Avoid unless doctor approves.

POSSIBLE INTERACTION WITH OTHER SUBSTANCES

INTERACTS WITH	COMBINED EFFECT
Alcohol:	May increase possibility of toxic effects. Avoid.
Beverages: Grapefruit juice.	Increased effect and toxicity of drug. Avoid.
Cocaine:	May increase possibility of toxic effects. Avoid.
Foods:	No special problems expected.
Marijuana:	May increase possibility of toxic effects. Avoid.
Tobacco:	No special problems expected.

*See Glossary

INDAPAMIDE

BRAND NAMES

Lozide   Lozol

BASIC INFORMATION

Habit forming? No
Prescription needed? Yes
Available as generic? Yes
Drug class: Antihypertensive, diuretic

 ## USES

- Controls, but doesn't cure, high blood pressure.
- Reduces fluid retention (edema) caused by conditions such as heart disorders.

 ## DOSAGE & USAGE INFORMATION

How to take:
Tablet—Swallow with liquid or food to lessen stomach irritation.

When to take:
At the same times each day, usually at bedtime.

If you forget a dose:
Bedtime dose—If you forget your once-a-day bedtime dose, don't take it more than 3 hours late. Never double dose.

What drug does:
Forces kidney to excrete more sodium and causes excess salt and fluid to be excreted.

Time lapse before drug works:
2 hours for effect to begin. May require 1 to 4 weeks for full effects.

Continued next column.

 ## OVERDOSE

SYMPTOMS:
Nausea, vomiting, diarrhea, very dry mouth, thirst, weakness, excessive fatigue, very rapid heart rate, weak pulse.
WHAT TO DO:
- **Dial 911 (emergency) or 0 (operator) for an ambulance or medical help. Then give first aid immediately.**
- **If patient is unconscious and not breathing, give mouth-to-mouth breathing. If there is no heartbeat, use cardiac massage and mouth-to-mouth breathing (CPR). Don't try to make patient vomit. If you can't get help quickly, take patient to nearest emergency facility.**
- **See emergency information on inside covers.**

Don't take with:
Any other medicine without consulting your doctor or pharmacist.

 ## POSSIBLE ADVERSE REACTIONS OR SIDE EFFECTS

SYMPTOMS	WHAT TO DO
Life-threatening:	
In case of overdose, see previous column.	
Common:	
• Excessive tiredness or weakness, muscle cramps.	Discontinue. Call doctor right away.
• Frequent urination.	Continue. Tell doctor at next visit.
Infrequent:	
Insomnia, mood change, dizziness on changing position, headache, excessive thirst, diarrhea, appetite loss, nausea, dry mouth, decreased sex drive.	Continue. Call doctor when convenient.
Rare:	
• Weak pulse.	Discontinue. Seek emergency treatment.
• Itching, rash, hives, irregular heartbeat.	Discontinue. Call doctor right away.

 ## WARNINGS & PRECAUTIONS

Don't take if:
- You are allergic to indapamide or to any sulfa drug or thiazide diuretic.*
- You have severe kidney disease.

Before you start, consult your doctor:
- If you have severe kidney disease.
- If you have diabetes.
- If you have gout.
- If you have liver disease.
- If you will have surgery within 2 months, including dental surgery, requiring general or spinal anesthesia.
- If you have lupus erythematosus.
- If you are pregnant or plan to become pregnant.

Over age 60:
Adverse reactions and side effects may be more frequent and severe than in younger persons.

Pregnancy:
Consult doctor. Risk category B (see page xxiii).

Breast-feeding:
Unknown effect on child. Consult doctor.

Infants & children:
Use only under close medical supervision.

Prolonged use:
Request laboratory studies for blood sugar, BUN*, uric acid and serum electrolytes (potassium and sodium).

Skin & sunlight:
May cause rash or intensify sunburn in areas exposed to sun or ultraviolet light (photosensitivity reaction). Avoid overexposure. Notify doctor if reaction occurs.

Driving, piloting or hazardous work:
Don't drive or pilot aircraft until you learn how medicine affects you. Don't work around dangerous machinery. Don't climb ladders or work in high places. Danger increases if you drink alcohol or take medicine affecting alertness and reflexes, such as antihistamines, tranquilizers, sedatives, pain medicine, narcotics and mind-altering drugs.

Discontinuing:
Don't discontinue without consulting doctor. Dose may require gradual reduction if you have taken drug for a long time. Doses of other drugs may also require adjustment.

Others:
No problems expected.

 ## POSSIBLE INTERACTION WITH OTHER DRUGS

GENERIC NAME OR DRUG CLASS	COMBINED EFFECT
Adrenocorticoids, systemic	Possible excessive potassium loss.
Allopurinol	Decreased allopurinol effect.
Amiodarone	Increased risk of heartbeat irregularity due to low potassium.
Amphotericin B	Increased potassium.
Angiotensin-converting enzyme (ACE) inhibitors*	Decreased blood pressure. Possible excessive potassium in blood.
Antidepressants, tricyclic*	Dangerous drop in blood pressure.
Antidiabetic agents, oral*	Increased blood sugar.
Antihypertensives, other*	Increased anti-hypertensive effect.
Barbiturates*	Increased indapamide effect.
Beta-adrenergic blocking agents*	Increased effect of indapamide.

Calcium supplements*	Increased calcium in blood.
Carteolol	Increased anti-hypertensive effect.
Cholestyramine	Decreased indapamide effect.
Colestipol	Decreased indapamide effect.
Digitalis preparations*	Excessive potassium loss that may cause dangerous heart rhythms.
Diuretics, thiazide*	Increased effect of thiazide diuretics.
Indomethacin	Decreased indapamide effect.
Lithium	High risk of lithium toxicity.
Monoamine oxidase (MAO) inhibitors*	Increased indapamide effect.
Nicardipine	Dangerous blood pressure drop. Dosages may require adjustment.
Nimodipine	Dangerous blood pressure drop.

Continued on page 918

 ## POSSIBLE INTERACTION WITH OTHER SUBSTANCES

INTERACTS WITH	COMBINED EFFECT
Alcohol:	Dangerous blood pressure drop. Avoid.
Beverages:	No problems expected.
Cocaine:	Increased risk of heart block and high blood pressure.
Foods: Licorice.	Excessive potassium loss that may cause dangerous heart rhythms.
Marijuana:	Reduced effectiveness of indapamide. Avoid.
Tobacco:	Reduced effectiveness of indapamide. Avoid.

INSULIN

BRAND NAMES

See complete list of brand names in the *Generic and Brand Name Directory*, page 882.

BASIC INFORMATION

Habit forming? No
Prescription needed? No
Available as generic? Yes
Drug class: Antidiabetic

USES

Controls diabetes, a complex metabolic disorder, in which the body does not manufacture insulin.

DOSAGE & USAGE INFORMATION

How to take:
Must be taken by injection under the skin. Use disposable, sterile needles. Rotate injection sites.

When to take:
At the same time each day.

If you forget a dose:
Take as soon as you remember. Wait at least 4 hours for next dose. Resume regular schedule.

What drug does:
Facilitates passage of blood sugar through cell membranes so sugar is usable.

Time lapse before drug works:
30 minutes to 8 hours, depending on type of insulin used.

Continued next column

OVERDOSE

SYMPTOMS:
Low blood sugar (hypoglycemia)—Anxiety; chills, cold sweats, pale skin; drowsiness; excess hunger; headache; nausea; nervousness; fast heartbeat; shakiness; unusual tiredness or weakness.
WHAT TO DO:
- **Eat some type of sugar immediately, such as orange juice, honey, sugar cubes, crackers, sandwich.**
- **If patient loses consciousness, give glucagon if you have it and know how to use it.**
- **Otherwise, dial 911 (emergency) or 0 (operator) for an ambulance or medical help. Then give first aid immediately.**
- **See emergency information on inside covers.**

Don't take with:
Any other medicine without consulting your doctor or pharmacist.

POSSIBLE ADVERSE REACTIONS OR SIDE EFFECTS

SYMPTOMS	WHAT TO DO
Life-threatening: Hives, rash, intense itching, faintness soon after a dose (anaphylaxis).	Seek emergency treatment immediately.
Common: None expected.	
Infrequent:	
• Symptoms of low blood sugar— nervousness, hunger (excessive), cold sweats, rapid pulse, anxiety, cold skin, chills, confusion, concentration loss, drowsiness, headache, nausea, weakness, shakiness, vision changes.	Seek treatment (eat some form of quick-acting sugar— glucose tablets, sugar, fruit juice, corn syrup, honey).
• Symptoms of high blood sugar— increased urination, unusual thirst, dry mouth, drowsiness, flushed or dry skin, fruit-like breath odor, appetite loss, stomach pain or vomiting, tiredness, trouble breathing, increased blood sugar level.	Seek emergency treatment immediately.
• Swelling, redness, itch or warmth at injection site.	Continue. Call doctor when convenient.
Rare: None expected.	

WARNINGS & PRECAUTIONS

Don't take if:
- Your diagnosis and dose schedule is not established.
- You don't know how to deal with overdose emergencies.

Before you start, consult your doctor:
- If you are allergic to insulin.
- If you take MAO inhibitors.
- If you have liver or kidney disease or low thyroid function.

Over age 60:
Guard against hypoglycemia. Repeated episodes can cause permanent confusion and abnormal behavior.

Pregnancy:
Adhere rigidly to diabetes treatment program. Risk category B (see page xxiii).

Breast-feeding:
No problems expected. Consult doctor.

Infants & children:
Use only under medical supervision.

Prolonged use:
Talk to your doctor about the need for follow-up medical examinations or laboratory studies to check blood sugar, serum potassium, urine.

Skin & sunlight:
No problems expected.

Driving, piloting or hazardous work:
No problems expected after dose is established.

Discontinuing:
Don't discontinue without doctor's advice until you complete prescribed dose, even though symptoms diminish or disappear.

Others:
- Diet and exercise affect how much insulin you need. Work with your doctor to determine accurate dose.
- Notify your doctor if you skip a dose, overeat, have fever or infection.
- Notify doctor if you develop symptoms of high blood sugar: drowsiness, dry skin, orange fruit-like odor to breath, increased urination, appetite loss, unusual thirst.
- Never freeze insulin.
- May interfere with the accuracy of some medical tests.

POSSIBLE INTERACTION WITH OTHER DRUGS

GENERIC NAME OR DRUG CLASS	COMBINED EFFECT
Adrenocorticoids, systemic	Decreased insulin effect.
Anticonvulsants, hydantoin*	Decreased insulin effect.
Antidiabetics, oral*	Increased antibiabetic effect.
Beta-adrenergic blocking agents*	Possible increased difficulty in regulating blood sugar levels.
Bismuth subsalicylate	Increased insulin effect. May require dosage adjustment.
Carteolol	Hypoglycemic effects may be prolonged.
Contraceptives, oral*	Decreased insulin effect.
Dexfenfluramine	May require dosage change as weight loss occurs.
Diuretics, thiazide*	Decreased insulin effect.
Furosemide	Decreased insulin effect.
Monoamine oxidase (MAO) inhibitors*	Increased insulin effect.
Nicotine	Increased insulin effect.
Oxyphenbutazone	Increased insulin effect.
Phenylbutazone	Increased insulin effect.
Salicylates*	Increased insulin effect.
Smoking deterrents	May require insulin dosage adjustment.
Sulfa drugs*	Increased insulin effect.
Tetracyclines*	Increased insulin effect.
Thyroid hormones*	Decreased insulin effect.

POSSIBLE INTERACTION WITH OTHER SUBSTANCES

INTERACTS WITH	COMBINED EFFECT
Alcohol:	Increased insulin effect. May cause hypoglycemia and brain damage.
Beverages:	None expected.
Cocaine:	May cause brain damage.
Foods:	None expected.
Marijuana:	Possible increase in blood sugar.
Tobacco:	Decreased insulin absorption.

*See Glossary

INSULIN LISPRO

BRAND NAMES

Humalog

BASIC INFORMATION

Habit forming? No
Prescription needed? Yes
Available as generic? No
Drug class: Antidiabetic

 ## USES

Controls diabetes, a complex metabolic disorder in which the body does not manufacture insulin.

 ## DOSAGE & USAGE INFORMATION

How to take:
Must be taken by injection under the skin. Use disposable, sterile needles. Rotate injection sites. Always follow instruction provided with the product.

When to take:
At the same times each day. If taken at meal-time, use it within a 15 minute period prior to the meal. May need to be taken in combination with a long-acting insulin to prevent hyperglycemia.

If you forget a dose:
Take as soon as you remember. Wait at least 4 hours for next dose. Resume regular schedule.

Continued next column

 ## OVERDOSE

SYMPTOMS:
Low blood sugar (hypoglycemia)—Anxiety; chills, cold sweats, pale skin; drowsiness; excessive hunger; headache; nausea; nervousness; fast heartbeat; shakiness; unusual tiredness or weakness.
WHAT TO DO:
- **Eat some type of sugar immediately, such as fruit juice, nondiet sodas, candy (such as 5 Lifesavers), one cup of milk, glucose tablets.**
- **If patient loses consciousness, give glucagon if you have it and know how to use it.**
- **Otherwise, dial 911 (emergency) or 0 (operator) for an ambulance or medical help. Then give first aid immediately.**
- **See emergency information on inside covers.**

What drug does:
Facilitates passage of blood sugar through cell membranes so sugar is usable. The drug helps keep your blood sugar levels from going too high after you eat.

Time lapse before drug works:
30 minutes to 1 hour, which is faster than regular insulin; the duration of action is 3 to 4 hours.

Don't take with:
Any other medicine without consulting your doctor or pharmacist.

 ## POSSIBLE ADVERSE REACTIONS OR SIDE EFFECTS

SYMPTOMS	WHAT TO DO
Life-threatening: Hives, rash, intense itching, faintness, swelling, breathing difficulty soon after a dose (anaphylaxis).	Seek emergency treatment immediately.
Common: None expected.	
Infrequent: • Symptoms of low blood sugar— nervousness, hunger (excessive), cold sweats, rapid pulse, anxiety, cold skin, chills, confusion, concentration loss, drowsiness, headache, nausea, weakness, shakiness, vision changes.	Seek treatment (eat some form of quick-acting sugar— glucose tablets, sugar, fruit juice, corn syrup, honey).
• Symptoms of high blood sugar— increased urination, unusual thirst, dry mouth, drowsiness, flushed or dry skin, fruit-like breath odor, appetite loss, stomach pain or vomiting, tiredness, trouble breathing, increased blood sugar level.	Seek emergency treatment immediately.
• Swelling, redness, itch or warmth at injection site; other skin changes at injection site (e.g., thinning or thickened skin).	Continue. Call doctor when convenient.

Rare:

Dry mouth, excessive thirst, weak or fast pulse, heartbeat irregularities, mental or mood changes, nausea or vomiting, unusual tiredness or weakness, muscle cramps (may be symptoms of hypokalemla).

Continue, but call doctor right away.

WARNINGS & PRECAUTIONS

Don't take if:
- Your diagnosis and dose schedule are not established.
- You don't know how to deal with overdose emergencies.

Before you start, consult your doctor:
- If you are allergic to insulin or have allergies to any medicines or other substances.
- If you take MAO inhibitors*.
- If you have liver or kidney disease or low thyroid function.

Over age 60:
Insulin requirements may change. The family should notify the doctor if abnormal behavior or confusion occurs in an older person.

Pregnancy:
Adhere rigidly to diabetes treatment program. Risk category B (see page xxiii).

Breast-feeding:
No problems expected. Consult doctor.

Infants & children:
Use only under medical supervision.

Prolonged use:
Talk to your doctor about the need for follow-up medical examinations or laboratory studies to check blood sugar, serum potassium, urine.

Skin & sunlight:
No problems expected.

Driving, piloting or hazardous work:
No problems expected after dose is established. Need to be cautious if signs of hypoglycemia occur.

Discontinuing:
Don't discontinue without doctor's advice, even though symptoms diminish or disappear.

Others:
- Diet and exercise affect how much insulin you need. Work with your doctor to determine accurate dose. Monitor your glucose levels as directed.
- Notify your doctor if you have a fever, infection, diarrhea, or experience vomiting.
- Advise any doctor or dentist whom you consult that you take this medicine.
- Never freeze insulin.
- Wear medical identification that indicates you have diabetes and take insulin.
- You and your family should educate yourselves about diabetes.
- May interfere with the accuracy of some medical tests.

POSSIBLE INTERACTION WITH OTHER DRUGS

GENERIC NAME OR DRUG CLASS	COMBINED EFFECT
Antidiabetics, oral*	Increased antidiabetic effect.
Hyperglycemia-causing agents*	May need increased dosage of insulin.
Hypoglycemia-causing agents*	May need decreased dosage of insulin.
Insulin	May need dosage adjustment.
Sympatholytics*	Increased insulin effect.
Smoking deterrents	May require insulin dosage adjustment.

POSSIBLE INTERACTION WITH OTHER SUBSTANCES

INTERACTS WITH	COMBINED EFFECT
Alcohol:	Increased insulin effect. May cause hypoglycemia and brain damage.
Beverages:	None expected.
Cocaine:	May cause brain damage.
Foods:	None expected. Follow your diabetic diet instructions.
Marijuana:	Possible increase in blood sugar.
Tobacco:	Decreased insulin absorption.

IODOQUINOL

BRAND NAMES

Diiodohydroxyquin   Yodoquinol
Diodoquin   Yodoxin
Diquinol

BASIC INFORMATION

Habit forming? No
Prescription needed? Yes
Available as generic? Yes
Drug class: Antiprotozoal, antiparasitic

 USES

Treatment for intestinal amebiasis and balantidiasis.

 DOSAGE & USAGE INFORMATION

How to take:
Tablets—Mix with applesauce or chocolate syrup if unable to swallow tablets.

When to take:
Three times daily after meals for 20 days. Treatment may be repeated after 2 to 3 weeks.

If you forget a dose:
Take as soon as you remember up to 2 hours late. If more than 2 hours, wait for next scheduled dose (don't double this dose).

What drug does:
Kills amoeba (microscopic parasites) in intestinal tract.

Time lapse before drug works:
May require full course of treatment (20 days) to cure.

Don't take with:
Any other medication without consulting your doctor or pharmacist.

 OVERDOSE

SYMPTOMS:
- Prolonged dosing at high level may produce blurred vision, muscle pain, eye pain, numbness and tingling in hands or feet.
- Single overdosage unlikely to threaten life.

WHAT TO DO:
If person takes much larger amount than prescribed, call doctor, poison control center or hospital emergency room for instructions.

 POSSIBLE ADVERSE REACTIONS OR SIDE EFFECTS

SYMPTOMS	WHAT TO DO
Life-threatening:	
In case of overdose, see previous column.	
Common:	
Diarrhea, nausea, vomiting, abdominal pain.	Continue. Call doctor when convenient.
Infrequent:	
• Clumsiness, rash, hives, itching, blurred vision, muscle pain, numbness or tingling in hands or feet, chills, fever, weakness.	Discontinue. Call doctor right away.
• Swelling of neck. (thyroid gland)	Continue. Call doctor when convenient.
Rare:	
Dizziness, headache, rectal itching.	Continue. Call doctor when convenient.

WARNINGS & PRECAUTIONS

Don't take if:
You have kidney or liver disease.

Before you start, consult your doctor:
If you have optic atrophy or thyroid disease.

Over age 60:
Adverse reactions and side effects may be more frequent and severe than in younger persons.

Pregnancy:
Decide with your doctor if drug benefits justify risk to unborn child. Risk category C (see page xxiii).

Breast-feeding:
No proven problems, but avoid if possible. Discontinue nursing until you finish medicine. Consult doctor for advice on maintaining milk supply.

Infants & children:
Not recommended. Safety and dosage has not been established.

Prolonged use:
Not recommended.

Skin & sunlight:
No problems expected.

Driving, piloting or hazardous work:
No problems expected.

Discontinuing:
Don't discontinue without consulting doctor.

Others:
- Thyroid tests may be inaccurate for as long as 6 months after discontinuing iodoquinol treatment.
- May interfere with the accuracy of some medical tests.

POSSIBLE INTERACTION WITH OTHER DRUGS

GENERIC NAME OR DRUG CLASS	COMBINED EFFECT
None expected.	

POSSIBLE INTERACTION WITH OTHER SUBSTANCES

INTERACTS WITH	COMBINED EFFECT
Alcohol:	None expected.
Beverages:	None expected.
Cocaine:	None expected.
Foods:	Taking with food may decrease gastrointestinal side effects.
Marijuana:	None expected.
Tobacco:	None expected.

IPECAC

BRAND NAMES

Ipecac Syrup   Quelidrine Cough

BASIC INFORMATION

Habit forming? No
Prescription needed? No
Available as generic? Yes
Drug class: Emetic

 ## USES

- Used in emergencies to induce vomiting after medication overdose and in some instances of poisoning.
- Don't use if suspected substance to be vomited is strychnine or a corrosive such as lye, kerosene, gasoline, bleach, strong acid or cleaning fluid.

How to take:
- Call doctor, poison control center or emergency room before giving ipecac to any one.
- Don't give to an unconscious or semiconscious person.
- Syrup, undiluted—Carefully follow instructions on the bottle.
- Drink water immediately after taking ipecac.
- Place person in a head-down position to prevent aspiration of vomitus.

When to take:
- Upon discovery of accidental or intentional poisoning or overdose.
- May repeat in 30 minutes if vomiting doesn't occur with first ipecac dose.
- Don't give more than 2 doses.

If you forget a dose:
One-time use only.

Continued next column

 ## OVERDOSE

SYMPTOMS:
Watery diarrhea, breathing difficulty, stiff muscles.
WHAT TO DO:
- **Dial 911 (emergency) or 0 (operator) for an ambulance or medical help. Then give first aid immediately.**
- **See emergency information on inside covers.**

What drug does:
Irritates stomach lining and stimulates the vomiting center in the brain.

Time lapse before drug works:
20 minutes.

Don't take with:
Any other medicines (including over-the-counter drugs such as cough and cold medicines, laxatives, antacids, diet pills, caffeine, nose drops or vitamins) without consulting your doctor.

 ## POSSIBLE ADVERSE REACTIONS OR SIDE EFFECTS

SYMPTOMS	WHAT TO DO
Life-threatening: Heartbeat irregularity.	Seek emergency treatment immediately.
Common: None expected.	
Infrequent: None expected.	
Rare: None expected.	

WARNINGS & PRECAUTIONS

Don't take if:
You are drunk from any source.

Before you start, consult your doctor:
If you have heart disease (ipecac can be poisonous to a damaged heart).

Over age 60:
No special problems expected.

Pregnancy:
No studies done. Unknown effect. Consult doctor. Risk category C (see page xxiii).

Breast-feeding:
Consult your doctor.

Infants & children:
Give only after consulting doctor or poison control center.

Prolonged use:
Not intended for long-term use.

Skin & sunlight:
No problems expected.

Driving, piloting or hazardous work:
Don't drive or pilot aircraft until you learn how medicine affects you. Don't work around dangerous machinery. Don't climb ladders or work in high places. Danger increases if you drink alcohol or take medicine affecting alertness and reflexes.

Discontinuing:
No special problems expected.

Others:
- If you are instructed to also use activated charcoal, don't use until after ipecac has induced vomiting.
- Don't give more than 2 doses to anyone.
- Don't use ipecac as a means of inducing vomiting to lose weight. It can be toxic to the heart and cause death as a result of chronic use.

POSSIBLE INTERACTION WITH OTHER DRUGS

GENERIC NAME OR DRUG CLASS	COMBINED EFFECT
Antiemetics*	Decreased ipecac effect. Possible ipecac toxicity.
Charcoal, activated	Improves treatment. If taken for the same overdose, charcoal should follow vomiting induced by ipecac.
Other medicines or herbs to cause vomiting	Decreased ipecac effect.

POSSIBLE INTERACTION WITH OTHER SUBSTANCES

INTERACTS WITH	COMBINED EFFECT
Alcohol:	Avoid. Vomiting while drunk can be dangerous.
Beverages: Carbonated.	Stomach distention. Avoid.
Milk.	Decreased ipecac effect.
Cocaine:	Avoid.
Foods:	No problems expected.
Marijuana:	Avoid. Aspiration of vomitus could be fatal.
Tobacco:	No problems expected.

*See Glossary

IPRATROPIUM

BRAND NAMES

Apo-Ipravent
Atrovent
Combivent
Kendral-Ipratropium

BASIC INFORMATION

Habit forming? No
Prescription needed? Yes
Available as generic? No
Drug class: Bronchodilator, anticholinergic

 ## USES

- Treats asthma, bronchitis and emphysema.
- Should not be used alone for acute asthma attacks. May be used with inhalation forms of albuterol or fenoterol.
- May be used to treat rhinorrhea (runny nose).

 ## DOSAGE & USAGE INFORMATION

How to use:
- By inhalation. Follow printed instructions on package.
- Avoid contact with eyes.
- Allow 1 minute between inhalations.

When to take:
Follow your doctor's instructions.

If you forget a dose:
Take as soon as you remember up to 2 hours late. If more than 2 hours, wait for next scheduled dose (don't double this dose).

What drug does:
Dilates bronchial tubes or nasal passages by direct effect on them.

Time lapse before drug works:
None. Effect begins right away.

Don't take with:
Any other medicines (including over-the-counter drugs such as cough and cold medicines, laxatives, antacids, diet pills, caffeine, nose drops or vitamins) without consulting your doctor.

 ## OVERDOSE

SYMPTOMS:
None likely.
WHAT TO DO:
Overdose unlikely to threaten life. If person takes much larger amount than prescribed, call doctor, poison control center or hospital emergency room for instructions.

 ## POSSIBLE ADVERSE REACTIONS OR SIDE EFFECTS

SYMPTOMS	WHAT TO DO
Life-threatening: Pounding heartbeat.	Discontinue. Call doctor right away.
Common: Cough, headache, dizziness, nervousness, nausea.	Continue. Call doctor when convenient.
Infrequent: Blurred vision, difficult urination, stuffy nose, insomnia, tremors, weakness.	Continue. Call doctor when convenient.
Rare: Skin rash, ulcers on lips or in mouth, hives.	Discontinue. Call doctor right away.

WARNINGS & PRECAUTIONS

Don't take if:
You are sensitive to belladonna or atropine.

Before you start, consult your doctor:
- If you have prostate trouble.
- If you have glaucoma.
- If you have severe dental problems.

Over age 60:
Adverse reactions and side effects may be more frequent and severe than in younger persons. You may need smaller doses for shorter periods of time.

Pregnancy:
Consult doctor. Risk category B (see page xxiii).

Breast-feeding:
No special problems expected. Consult doctor.

Infants & children:
Effect not documented. Consult your pediatrician.

Prolonged use:
Decreases saliva flow and may increase cavities, gum disease, thrush and discomfort.

Skin & sunlight:
No problems expected.

Driving, piloting or hazardous work:
Avoid if you feel confused, drowsy or dizzy.

Discontinuing:
No special problems expected.

Others:
- Advise any doctor or dentist whom you consult that you take this medicine.
- Allow 5-minute intervals between ipratropium inhalations and inhalations of cromolyn, cortisone or other inhalant medicines.
- Check with doctor if this medicine doesn't bring relief within 30 minutes.

POSSIBLE INTERACTION WITH OTHER DRUGS

GENERIC NAME OR DRUG CLASS	COMBINED EFFECT
Anticholinergics*	Increased anticholinergic effect.
Cromolyn (inhalation form)	Wait 5 minutes before using cromolyn.

POSSIBLE INTERACTION WITH OTHER SUBSTANCES

INTERACTS WITH	COMBINED EFFECT
Alcohol:	No special problems expected.
Beverages:	No special problems expected.
Cocaine:	Excess central nervous system stimulation. Avoid.
Foods:	No special problems expected.
Marijuana:	Decreased ipratropium effect.
Tobacco:	Decreased ipratropium effect.

IRON SUPPLEMENTS

GENERIC AND BRAND NAMES

See complete list of generic and brand names in the *Generic and Brand Name Directory*, page 882.

BASIC INFORMATION

Habit forming? No
Prescription needed?
  With folic acid: Yes
  Without folic acid: No
Available as generic? Yes
Drug class: Mineral supplement (iron)

USES

Treatment for dietary iron deficiency or iron-deficiency anemia from other causes.

DOSAGE & USAGE INFORMATION

How to take:
- Tablet, capsule or syrup—Swallow with liquid or food to lessen stomach irritation. If you can't swallow whole, crumble tablet or open capsule and take with liquid or food. Place medicine far back on tongue to avoid staining teeth.
- Extended-release capsule—Swallow whole with liquid. Do not crush.
- Chewable tablets—Chew well before swallowing.
- Liquid—Dilute dose in beverage before swallowing and drink through a straw.

When to take:
1 hour before or 2 hours after eating.

If you forget a dose:
Take up to 2 hours late. If more than 2 hours, wait for next dose (don't double this dose).

Continued next column

OVERDOSE

SYMPTOMS:
- **Moderate overdose—Stomach pain, vomiting, diarrhea, black stools, lethargy.**
- **Serious overdose—Weakness and collapse; pallor, weak and rapid heartbeat; shallow breathing; convulsions and coma.**

WHAT TO DO:
- **Dial 911 (emergency) or 0 (operator) for an ambulance or medical help. Then give first aid immediately.**
- **See emergency information on inside covers.**

What drug does:
Stimulates bone marrow's production of hemoglobin (red blood cell pigment that carries oxygen to body cells).

Time lapse before drug works:
3 to 7 days. May require 3 weeks for maximum benefit.

Don't take with:
- Multiple vitamin and mineral supplements.
- Any other medicine without consulting your doctor or pharmacist.

POSSIBLE ADVERSE REACTIONS OR SIDE EFFECTS

SYMPTOMS	WHAT TO DO
Life-threatening: In case of overdose, see last column.	
Common:	
• Stomach pain that is continuing.	Discontinue. Call doctor right away.
• Dark green or black stool, teeth stained with liquid iron, constipation, diarrhea, mild nausea or vomiting.	Continue. Call doctor when convenient.
Infrequent: None expected.	
Rare:	
• Throat pain on swallowing, chest pain, cramps, blood in stool or black stool that has sticky constistency.	Discontinue. Call doctor right away.
• Darkened urine, heartburn.	Continue. Call doctor when convenient.

WARNINGS & PRECAUTIONS

Don't take if:
- You are allergic to any iron supplement or tartrazine dye.
- You take iron injections.
- You have acute hepatitis, hemosiderosis or hemochromatosis (conditions involving excess iron in body).
- You have hemolytic anemia.

Before you start, consult your doctor:
- If you plan to become pregnant while on medication.
- If you have had stomach surgery.
- If you have had peptic ulcer, enteritis or colitis.

Over age 60:
May cause hemochromatosis (iron storage disease) with bronze skin, liver damage, diabetes, heart problems and impotence.

Pregnancy:
Take only if your doctor advises. Risk category C (see page xxiii).

Breast-feeding:
No problems expected. Take only if your doctor confirms you have a dietary deficiency or an iron-deficiency anemia.

Infants & children:
Use only under medical supervision. Overdose common and dangerous. Keep out of children's reach.

Prolonged use:
- May cause hemochromatosis (iron storage disease) with bronze skin, liver damage, diabetes, heart problems and impotence.
- Talk to your doctor about the need for follow-up medical examinations or laboratory studies to check complete blood counts (white blood cell count, platelet count, red blood cell count, hemoglobin, hematocrit), serum iron, total iron-binding capacity.

Skin & sunlight:
No problems expected.

Driving, piloting or hazardous work:
No problems expected.

Discontinuing:
May be unnecessary to finish medicine. Follow doctor's instructions.

Others:
- Liquid form stains teeth. Mix with water or juice to lessen the effect. Brush with baking soda or hydrogen peroxide to help remove stain.
- Some products contain tartrazine dye. Avoid, especially if you are allergic to aspirin.
- May interfere with the accuracy of some medical tests.
- If using extended-release form or coated tablet and your stools don't turn black, consult doctor. The tablet may not be breaking down, and an underdose may result.

POSSIBLE INTERACTION WITH OTHER DRUGS

GENERIC NAME OR DRUG CLASS	COMBINED EFFECT
Acetohydroxamic acid	Decreased effects of both drugs.
Allopurinol	Possible excess iron storage in liver.
Antacids*	Poor iron absorption.
Chloramphenicol	Decreased effect of iron. Interferes with formation of red blood cells and hemoglobin.
Cholestyramine	Decreased iron effect.
Etidronate	Decreased etidronate effect. Take at least 2 hours after iron supplement.
H₂ antagonists*	Decreased iron effect.
Iron supplements, other*	Possible excess iron storage in liver.
Tetracyclines*	Decreased tetracycline effect. Take iron 3 hours before or 2 hours after taking tetracycline.
Vitamin E	Decreased iron and vitamin E effect.
Zinc supplements	Increased need for zinc.

POSSIBLE INTERACTION WITH OTHER SUBSTANCES

INTERACTS WITH	COMBINED EFFECT
Alcohol:	Increased iron absorption. May cause organ damage. Avoid or use in moderation.
Beverages: Milk, tea.	Decreased iron effect.
Cocaine:	None expected.
Foods: Dairy foods, eggs, whole-grain bread and cereal.	Decreased iron effect.
Marijuana:	None expected.
Tobacco:	None expected.

ISOMETHEPTENE, DICHLORALPHENAZONE & ACETAMINOPHEN

BRAND NAMES

Amidrine	Migquin
I.D.A.	Migrapap
Iso-Acetazone	Migratine
Isocom	Migrazone
Midchlor	Migrend
Midquin	Migrex
Midrin	Mitride

BASIC INFORMATION

Habit forming? No
Prescription needed? Yes
Available as generic? No
Drug class: Analgesic, sedative, vascular headache suppressant

USES

Treatment of vascular (throbbing or migraine type) and tension headaches.

DOSAGE & USAGE INFORMATION

How to take:
Capsules—Take with fluid. Usual dose—2 capsules at start, then 1 every hour until fully relieved. Don't exceed 5 capsules in 12 hours.

When to take:
At first sign of headache.

If you forget a dose:
Use as soon as you remember.

What drug does:
Causes blood vessels in head to constrict or become narrower. Acetaminophen relieves pain by effects on hypothalamus—the part of the brain that helps regulate body heat and receives body's pain messages.

Time lapse before drug works:
30-60 minutes.

Continued next column

OVERDOSE

SYMPTOMS:
Stomach upsets, irritability, sweating, severe diarrhea, convulsions, coma.
WHAT TO DO:
- Dial 911 (emergency) or 0 (operator) for an ambulance or medical help. Then give first aid immediately.
- See emergency information on inside covers.

Don't take with:
Any medicine that will decrease mental alertness or reflexes, such as alcohol, other mind-altering drugs, cough/cold medicines, antihistamines, allergy medicine, sedatives, tranquilizers (sleeping pills or "downers") barbiturates, seizure medicine, narcotics, other prescription medicine for pain, muscle relaxants, anesthetics.

POSSIBLE ADVERSE REACTIONS OR SIDE EFFECTS

SYMPTOMS	WHAT TO DO
Life-threatening: In case of overdose, see previous column.	
Common: Dizziness, drowsiness.	Continue. Call doctor when convenient.
Infrequent: Diarrhea, vomiting, nausea, abdominal cramps, upper abdominal pain.	Discontinue. Call doctor right away.
Rare: Rash; itchy skin; sore throat, fever, mouth sores; unusual bleeding or bruising; weakness; jaundice.	Discontinue. Call doctor right away.

WARNINGS & PRECAUTIONS

Don't take if:
- You are allergic to acetaminophen or any other component of this combination medicine.
- Your symptoms don't improve after 2 days use. Call your doctor.

Before you start, consult your doctor:
If you have kidney disease, liver damage, glaucoma, heart or blood vessel disorder, hypertension, alcoholism (active).

Over age 60:
Don't exceed recommended dose. You can't eliminate drug as efficiently as younger persons.

Pregnancy:
Decide with your doctor if drug benefits justify risk to unborn child. Risk category C (see page xxiii).

Breast-feeding:
No proven harm to nursing infant. Consult doctor.

Infants & children:
Give under careful medical supervision only.

ISOMETHEPTENE, DICHLORALPHENAZONE & ACETAMINOPHEN

Prolonged use:
- May affect blood system and cause anemia. Limit use to 5 days for children 12 and under, and 10 days for adults.
- Talk to your doctor about the need for follow-up medical examinations or laboratory studies to check complete blood counts (white blood cell count, platelet count, red blood cell count, hemoglobin, hematocrit), liver function.

Skin & sunlight:
No problems expected.

Driving, piloting or hazardous work:
Avoid if you feel drowsy. Otherwise, no restrictions.

Discontinuing:
Discontinue in 2 days if symptoms don't improve.

Others:
No problems expected.

 POSSIBLE INTERACTION WITH OTHER DRUGS

GENERIC NAME OR DRUG CLASS	COMBINED EFFECT
Anticoagulants, oral*	May increase anticoagulant effect. If combined frequently, prothrombin time should be monitored.
Anti-inflammatory drugs, nonsteroidal (NSAIDs)*	Long-term combined effect (3 years or longer) increases chance of damage to kidney, including malignancy.
Aspirin or other salicylates*	Long-term combined effect (3 years or longer) increases chance of damage to kidney, including malignancy.
Beta-adrenergic blocking agents*	Narrowed arteries in heart if taken in large doses.
Central nervous system (CNS) depressants*	Increased sedative effect.
Monoamine oxidase (MAO) inhibitors*	Sudden increase in blood pressure.

Phenacetin	Long-term combined effect (3 years or longer) increases chance of damage to kidney, including malignancy.
Phenobarbital	Quicker elimination and decreased effect of acetaminophen.
Tetracyclines* (effervescent granules or tablets)	May slow tetracycline absorption. Space doses 2 hours apart.
Zidovudine (AZT)	Increased toxic effect of zidovudine.

 POSSIBLE INTERACTION WITH OTHER SUBSTANCES

INTERACTS WITH	COMBINED EFFECT
Alcohol:	Drowsiness. Toxicity to liver. Avoid.
Beverages:	None expected.
Cocaine:	None expected. However, cocaine may slow body's recovery. Avoid.
Foods:	None expected.
Marijuana:	Increased pain relief. However, marijuana may slow body's recovery. Avoid.
Tobacco:	May decrease medicine's effectiveness. Avoid.

ISONIAZID

BRAND NAMES

INH
Isotamine
Laniazid
Nydrazid

PMS Isoniazid
Rifamate
Tubizid

BASIC INFORMATION

Habit forming? No
Prescription needed? Yes
Available as generic? Yes
Drug class: Antitubercular

 ## USES

Kills tuberculosis germs.

 ## DOSAGE & USAGE INFORMATION

How to take:
* Tablet—Swallow with liquid to lessen stomach irritation.
* Syrup—Follow label directions.

When to take:
At the same time each day.

If you forget a dose:
Take as soon as you remember up to 12 hours late. If more than 12 hours, wait for next scheduled dose (don't double this dose).

What drug does:
Interferes with TB germ metabolism. Eventually destroys the germ.

Continued next column

 ## OVERDOSE

SYMPTOMS:
Difficult breathing, convulsions, coma.
WHAT TO DO:
* **Dial 911 (emergency) or 0 (operator) for an ambulance or medical help. Then give first aid immediately.**
* **If patient is unconscious and not breathing, give mouth-to-mouth breathing. If there is no heartbeat, use cardiac massage and mouth-to-mouth breathing (CPR). Don't try to make patient vomit. If you can't get help quickly, take patient to nearest emergency facility.**
* **See emergency information on inside covers.**

Time lapse before drug works:
3 to 6 months. You may need to take drug as long as 2 years.

Don't take with:
Any other medication without consulting your doctor or pharmacist.

 ## POSSIBLE ADVERSE REACTIONS OR SIDE EFFECTS

SYMPTOMS	WHAT TO DO
Life-threatening:	
In case of overdose, see previous column.	
Common:	
• Muscle pain and pain in joints, tingling or numbness in extremities, jaundice.	Discontinue. Call doctor right away.
• Confusion, unsteady walk.	Continue. Call doctor when convenient.
Infrequent:	
• Swollen glands, nausea, indigestion, diarrhea, vomiting.	Discontinue. Call doctor right away.
• Dizziness, appetite loss.	Continue. Call doctor when convenient.
Rare:	
• Rash, fever, impaired vision, anemia with fatigue, weakness, fever, sore throat, unusual bleeding or bruising.	Discontinue. Call doctor right away.
• Breast enlargement or discomfort.	Continue. Tell doctor at next visit.

 ## WARNINGS & PRECAUTIONS

Don't take if:
You are allergic to isoniazid.

Before you start, consult your doctor:
* If you plan to become pregnant within medication period.
* If you are allergic to athionamide, pyrazinamide or nicotinic acid.
* If you drink alcohol.
* If you have liver or kidney disease.
* If you have epilepsy, diabetes or lupus.

Over age 60:
Adverse reactions and side effects, especially jaundice, may be more frequent and severe than in younger persons. Kidneys may be less efficient.

Pregnancy:
Decide with your doctor if drug benefits justify risk to unborn child. Risk category C (see page xxiii).

ISONIAZID

Breast-feeding:
Drug passes into milk. Avoid drug or discontinue nursing until you finish medicine. Consult doctor for advice on maintaining milk supply.

Infants & children:
Use only under medical supervision.

Prolonged use:
- Numbness and tingling of hands and feet.
- Talk to your doctor about the need for follow-up medical examinations or laboratory studies to check liver function, eyes.

Skin & sunlight:
No problems expected.

Driving, piloting or hazardous work:
Avoid if you feel dizzy. Otherwise, no problems expected.

Discontinuing:
Don't discontinue without doctor's advice until you complete prescribed dose, even though symptoms diminish or disappear.

Others:
- Diabetic patients may have false blood sugar tests.
- Periodic liver function tests and laboratory blood studies recommended.
- Prescription for vitamin B-6 (pyridoxine) recommended to prevent nerve damage.

 POSSIBLE INTERACTION WITH OTHER DRUGS

GENERIC NAME OR DRUG CLASS	COMBINED EFFECT
Acetaminophen	Increased risk of liver damage.
Adrenocorticoids, systemic	Decreased isoniazid effect.
Alfentanil	Prolonged duration of alfentanil effect (undesirable).
Antacids* (aluminum-containing)	Decreased absorption of isoniazid.
Anticholinergics*	May increase pressure within eyeball.
Anticoagulants, oral*	Increased anticoagulant effect.
Antidiabetics*	Increased anti-diabetic effect.
Antihypertensives*	Increased anti-hypertensive effect.
Antivirals, HIV/AIDS*	Increased risk of peripheral neuropathy.

Carbamazepine	Increased risk of liver damage.
Cycloserine	Increased risk of central nervous system effects.
Disulfiram	Increased effect of disulfiram.
Laxatives*	Decreased absorption and effect of isoniazid.
Hepatotoxics*	Increased risk of liver damage.
Ketoconazole	Increased risk of liver damage
Narcotics*	Increased narcotic effect.
Phenytoin	Increased phenytoin effect.
Pyridoxine (Vitamin B-6)	Decreased chance of nerve damage in extremities.
Rifampin	Increased isoniazid toxicity to liver.
Sedatives*	Increased sedative effect.
Stimulants*	Increased stimulant effect.

 POSSIBLE INTERACTION WITH OTHER SUBSTANCES

INTERACTS WITH	COMBINED EFFECT
Alcohol:	Increased incidence of liver disease and seizures.
Beverages:	None expected.
Cocaine:	None expected.
Foods: Swiss or Cheshire cheese, fish.	Red or itching skin, fast heartbeat. Seek emergency treatment.
Marijuana:	No interactions expected, but marijuana may slow body's recovery.
Tobacco:	No interactions expected, but tobacco may slow body's recovery.

*See Glossary

ISOPROTERENOL & PHENYLEPHRINE

BRAND NAMES

Duo-Medihaler

BASIC INFORMATION

Habit forming? No
Prescription needed? Yes
Available as generic? No
Drug class: Sympathomimetic, bronchodilator

USES

- Temporary relief of congestion of nose, sinuses and throat caused by allergies, colds or sinusitis.
- Treatment for breathing difficulty from acute asthma, bronchitis and emphysema.

DOSAGE & USAGE INFORMATION

How to take:
Aerosol inhaler—Don't inhale more than twice per dose. Follow package instructions.

When to take:
As needed, no more often than every 4 hours.

If you forget a dose:
Take as soon as you remember. Wait 4 hours for next dose. Don't double this dose.

What drug does:
- Dilates constricted bronchial tubes, improving air flow.
- Stimulates heart muscle and dilates blood vessels.

Time lapse before drug works:
2 to 4 minutes.

Continued next column

OVERDOSE

SYMPTOMS:
Headache, blood pressure rise, slow and forceful pulse, nervousness, rapid or irregular heartbeat, fainting, sweating, tremor, vomiting, chest pain, convulsions, coma.
WHAT TO DO:
- Dial 911 (emergency) or 0 (operator) for an ambulance or medical help. Then give first aid immediately.
- See emergency information on inside covers.

Don't take with:
Nonprescription drugs for asthma, cough, cold, allergy, appetite suppressants, sleeping pills or drugs containing caffeine without consulting doctor.

POSSIBLE ADVERSE REACTIONS OR SIDE EFFECTS

SYMPTOMS	WHAT TO DO
Life-threatening:	
In case of overdose, see previous column.	
Common:	
• Insomnia, nervousness, restlessness.	Continue. Call doctor when convenient.
• Pink or red saliva or sputum.	No action necessary.
Infrequent:	
• Increased sweating.	Continue. Call doctor when convenient.
• Dizziness, headache, shakiness, weakness, red or flushed face, vomiting, nausea, pale skin.	Continue. Call doctor when convenient.
Rare:	
Tingling hands or feet, chest pain, irregular heartbeat.	Discontinue. Call doctor right away.

WARNINGS & PRECAUTIONS

Don't take if:
- You are allergic to any sympathomimetic*, including some diet pills.
- You have serious heart-rhythm disorder.
- You have taken a monoamine oxidase (MAO) inhibitor* in past 2 weeks.

Before you start, consult your doctor:
- If you have high blood pressure, heart disease, or take a digitalis preparation.
- If you have diabetes or overactive thyroid.
- If you use epinephrine.
- If your heartbeat is faster than 100 beats per minute.

Over age 60:
You may be more sensitive to drug's stimulant effects. Use with caution if you have hardening of the arteries.

Pregnancy:
Decide with your doctor if drug benefits justify risk to unborn child. Risk category C (see page xxiii).

Breast-feeding:
Effect unknown. Consult doctor.

Infants & children:
Use only under close supervision.

Prolonged use:
- May cause functional dependence.
- Salivary glands may swell.

Skin & sunlight:
No problems expected.

Driving, piloting or hazardous work:
Use caution if you feel dizzy or nervous.

Discontinuing:
Discontinue if drug fails to provide relief after 2 or 3 days. Consult doctor.

Others:
No problems expected.

POSSIBLE INTERACTION WITH OTHER DRUGS

GENERIC NAME OR DRUG CLASS	COMBINED EFFECT
Acebutolol	Decreased effect of both drugs.
Amphetamines*	Increased nervousness.
Antiasthmatics*	Nervous stimulation.
Antidepressants*	Increased effect of both drugs.
Antihypertensives*	Increased anti-hypertensive effect.
Beta-adrenergic blocking agents*	Decreased effect of both drugs.
Digitalis	Increased risk of serious heart disturbances.
Ephedrine	Increased ephedrine effect.
Epinephrine	Increased chance of serious heart disturbances.
Ergoloid mesylates	Blood vessel restriction.
Ergonovine	Increased vasocon-striction.
Ergotamine	Blood vessel restriction.
Furazolidine	Sudden, severe increase in blood pressure.
Maprotiline	Increase risk of serious heart disturbances.
Methyldopa	Decreased methyldopa effect.
Monoamine oxidase (MAO) inhibitors*	Dangerous blood pressure rise.
Nicotine	Decreased effect of isoproterenol and phenylephrine.
Nitrates*	Possible decreased effect of both drugs.
Oxprenolol	Decreased effect of both drugs.
Sedatives*	Decreased sedative effect.
Sympathomimetics, other*	Increased effect of both drugs, especially harmful side effects.
Terazosin	Decreases effectiveness of terazosin.
Theophylline	Possible increased effect and toxicity of both drugs.
Tranquilizers*	Decreased tranquilizer effect.

POSSIBLE INTERACTION WITH OTHER SUBSTANCES

INTERACTS WITH	COMBINED EFFECT
Alcohol:	Decreased isoproterenol effect.
Beverages: Caffeine drinks.	Overstimulation. Avoid.
Cocaine:	High risk of heartbeat irregularities and high blood pressure. Overstimulation of brain. Avoid.
Foods:	None expected.
Marijuana:	Increased antiasthmatic effect of isoproterenol.
Tobacco:	None expected.

ISOTRETINOIN

BRAND NAMES

Accutane   Accutane Roche

BASIC INFORMATION

Habit forming? No
Prescription needed? Yes
Available as generic? No
Drug classification: Antiacne (systemic)

USES

- Decreases cystic acne formation in severe cases.
- Treats certain other skin disorders involving an overabundance of outer skin layer.

DOSAGE & USAGE INFORMATION

How to take:
Capsule—Swallow with liquid or food to lessen stomach irritation. If you can't swallow whole, open capsule and take with liquid or food.

When to take:
Twice a day. Follow prescription directions.

If you forget a dose:
Take as soon as you remember up to 2 hours late. If more than 2 hours, wait for next scheduled dose and double dose.

What drug does:
Reduces sebaceous gland activity and size.

Time lapse before drug works:
May require 15 to 20 weeks to experience full benefit.

Don't take with:
- Vitamin A or supplements containing Vitamin A.
- Any other medication without consulting your doctor or pharmacist.

OVERDOSE

SYMPTOMS:
None reported.
WHAT TO DO:
Overdose unlikely to threaten life. If person takes much larger amount than prescribed, call doctor, poison control center or hospital emergency room for instructions.

POSSIBLE ADVERSE REACTIONS OR SIDE EFFECTS

SYMPTOMS	WHAT TO DO
Life-threatening: None expected.	
Common:	
• Burning, red, itching eyes; lip scaling; burning pain; nosebleeds.	Discontinue. Call doctor right away.
• Itchy skin.	Continue. Call doctor when convenient.
• Dry mouth.	Continue. Tell doctor at next visit. (Suck ice or chew gum.)
Infrequent:	
• Rash, infection, nausea, vomiting.	Discontinue. Call doctor right away.
• Pain in muscles, bones, joints; hair thinning; tiredness.	Continue. Call doctor when convenient.
Rare:	
• Severe stomach pain, bleeding gums, blurred vision, severe diarrhea, continuing headache, vomiting, eye pain, rectal bleeding, yellow skin or eyes.	Discontinue. Call doctor right away.
• Mild headache, increased sensitivity to light, stomach upset, peeling of skin on palms or soles of feet, tiredness.	Continue. Call doctor when convenient.

WARNINGS & PRECAUTIONS

Don't take if:
- You are allergic to isotretinoin, etretinate, tretinoin or vitamin A derivatives.
- You are pregnant or plan pregnancy.
- *You are even able to bear children. Read, understand and follow the patient information enclosure with your prescription.*

Before you start, consult your doctor:
- If you have diabetes.
- If you or any member of family have high triglyceride levels in blood.

Over age 60:
Adverse reactions and side effects may be more frequent and severe than in younger persons.

Pregnancy:
Causes birth defects in fetus. Don't use. Risk category X (see page xxiii).

Breast-feeding:
Effect unknown. Not recommended. Consult doctor.

Infants & children:
Not recommended.

Prolonged use:
- Possible damage to cornea.
- Talk to your doctor about the need for follow-up medical examinations or laboratory studies to check complete blood counts (white blood cell count, platelet count, red blood cell count, hemoglobin, hematocrit), liver function, blood lipids, blood sugar.

Skin & sunlight:
May cause rash or intensify sunburn in areas exposed to sun or ultraviolet light (photosensitivity reaction). Avoid overexposure. Notify doctor if reaction occurs.

Driving, piloting or hazardous work:
Use caution if there is a decrease in your night vision or you are unable to see well. Consult doctor.

Discontinuing:
Single course of treatment is usually all that's needed. If second course required, wait 8 weeks after completing first course.

Others:
- Use only for severe cases of cystic acne that have not responded to less hazardous forms of acne treatment.
- May interfere with the accuracy of some medical tests.
- Don't donate blood for at least 30 days after discontinuing medicine.
- Acne may worsen at the start of treatment.

- Contact lens wearers may experience discomfort during treatment with this drug.
- **If you are planning pregnancy or at risk of pregnancy, don't take this drug.**

POSSIBLE INTERACTION WITH OTHER DRUGS

GENERIC NAME OR DRUG CLASS	COMBINED EFFECT
Antiacne topical preparations* (other), cosmetics (medicated), skin preparations with alcohol, soaps or cleansers (abrasive)	Severe skin irritation.
Etretinate	Increased chance of toxicity of each drug.
Tetracyclines*	Increased risk of developing pseudo-tumor cerebri.*
Topical drugs or cosmetics	May interact with isotretinoin.
Tretinoin	Increased chance of toxicity.
Vitamin A	Additive toxic effect of each. Avoid.

POSSIBLE INTERACTION WITH OTHER SUBSTANCES

INTERACTS WITH	COMBINED EFFECT
Alcohol:	Significant increase in triglycerides in blood. Avoid.
Beverages:	No problems expected.
Cocaine:	Increased chance of toxicity of isotretinoin. Avoid.
Foods:	No problems expected.
Marijuana:	Increased chance of toxicity of isotretinoin. Avoid.
Tobacco:	May decrease absorption of medicine. Avoid tobacco while in treatment.

ISOXSUPRINE

BRAND NAMES

Vasodilan   Vasoprine

BASIC INFORMATION

Habit forming? No
Prescription needed? Yes
Available as generic? Yes
Drug class: Vasodilator

USES

- May improve poor blood circulation.
- Management of premature labor.
- Treatment for painful menstruation.

DOSAGE & USAGE INFORMATION

How to take:
Tablet—Swallow with liquid or food to lessen stomach irritation. If you can't swallow whole, crumble tablet and take with liquid or food.

When to take:
At the same times each day.

If you forget a dose:
Take as soon as you remember up to 2 hours late. If more than 2 hours, wait for next scheduled dose (don't double this dose).

What drug does:
Expands blood vessels, increasing flow and permitting distribution of oxygen and nutrients.

Time lapse before drug works:
1 hour.

Continued next column

OVERDOSE

SYMPTOMS:
Headache, dizziness, flush, vomiting, weakness, sweating, fainting, shortness of breath, coma.
WHAT TO DO:
- Dial 911 (emergency) or 0 (operator) for an ambulance or medical help. Then give first aid immediately.
- If patient is unconscious and not breathing, give mouth-to-mouth breathing. If there is no heartbeat, use cardiac massage and mouth-to-mouth breathing (CPR). Don't try to make patient vomit. If you can't get help quickly, take patient to nearest emergency facility.
- See emergency information on inside covers.

Don't take with:
Any other medication without consulting your doctor or pharmacist.

POSSIBLE ADVERSE REACTIONS OR SIDE EFFECTS

SYMPTOMS	WHAT TO DO
Life-threatening: In case of overdose, see previous column.	
Common: None expected.	
Infrequent: Nausea, vomiting.	Continue. Call doctor when convenient.
Rare: Rapid or irregular heartbeat, rash, chest pain, shortness of breath.	Discontinue. Call doctor right away.

WARNINGS & PRECAUTIONS

Don't take if:
- You are allergic to any vasodilator.
- You have any bleeding disease.

Before you start, consult your doctor:
- If you have high blood pressure, hardening of the arteries or heart disease.
- If you plan to become pregnant within medication period.
- If you have glaucoma.

Over age 60:
Adverse reactions and side effects may be more frequent and severe than in younger persons.

Pregnancy:
Decide with your doctor whether drug benefits justify risk to unborn child. Risk category C (see page xxiii).

Breast-feeding:
No problems expected, but consult doctor.

Infants & children:
Not recommended.

Prolonged use:
Talk to your doctor about the need for follow-up medical examinations or laboratory studies.

Skin & sunlight:
No problems expected.

Driving, piloting or hazardous work:
Avoid if you feel dizzy or faint. Otherwise, no problems expected.

Discontinuing:
Don't discontinue without doctor's advice until you complete prescribed dose, even though symptoms diminish or disappear.

Others:
- Be cautious when arising from lying or sitting position, when climbing stairs, or if dizziness occurs.
- May interfere with the accuracy of some medical tests.

POSSIBLE INTERACTION WITH OTHER DRUGS

GENERIC NAME OR DRUG CLASS	COMBINED EFFECT
None significant.	

POSSIBLE INTERACTION WITH OTHER SUBSTANCES

INTERACTS WITH	COMBINED EFFECT
Alcohol:	None expected.
Beverages: Milk	Decreased stomach irritation.
Cocaine:	Decreased blood circulation to extremities. Avoid.
Foods:	None expected.
Marijuana:	Rapid heartbeat.
Tobacco:	Decreased isoxsuprine effect; nicotine constricts blood vessels.

ITRACONAZOLE

BRAND NAMES

Sporanox

BASIC INFORMATION

Habit forming? No
Prescription needed? Yes
Available as generic? No
Drug class: Antifungal

 USES

Treatment for fungal infections including blastomycosis, histoplasmosis, onychomycosis (infection of the nail plate), candidiasis and others.

 DOSAGE & USAGE INFORMATION

How to take:
Capsule—Swallow with liquid. Take at mealtime.

When to take:
At the same time each day.

If you forget a dose:
- For once-a-day dosage, take as soon as you remember up to 12 hours late. If more than 12 hours, wait for next scheduled dose (don't double this dose).
- For twice-a-day dosage, take as soon as you remember up to 2 hours late. If more than 2 hours, wait for next scheduled dose (don't double this dose).

What drug does:
Prevents fungi from growing and reproducing.

Time lapse before drug works:
May require several weeks or months, possibly years for some fungal infections.

Don't take with:
- Histamine H_2 receptor antagonists, antacids or didanosine. Take them at least 2 hours after any dose of itraconazole.
- Any other prescription or nonprescription drug without consulting your doctor.

 OVERDOSE

SYMPTOMS:
None reported.
WHAT TO DO:
Overdose unlikely to threaten life. If person takes much larger amount than prescribed, call doctor, poison control center or hospital emergency room for instructions.

 POSSIBLE ADVERSE REACTIONS OR SIDE EFFECTS

SYMPTOMS	WHAT TO DO
Life-threatening: None expected.	
Common: None expected.	
Infrequent:	
• Skin rash.	Discontinue. Call doctor right away.
• Abdominal pain, constipation or diarrhea, nausea, vomiting, appetite loss, headache.	Continue. Call doctor when convenient.
Rare: Yellow skin or eyes, pale stools, dark or amber urine, unusual tiredness or weakness.	Discontinue. Call doctor right away.

WARNINGS & PRECAUTIONS

Don't take if:
You are allergic to itraconazole, ketoconazole, fluconazole or miconazole.

Before you start, consult your doctor:
- If you have liver disease.
- If you have reduced stomach acidity (achlorhydria or hypochlorhydria).

Over age 60:
Adverse reactions and side effects may be more frequent and severe than in younger persons.

Pregnancy:
Decide with your doctor if drug benefits justify risk to unborn child. Risk category C (see page xxiii).

Breast-feeding:
Drug passes into milk. Avoid drug or discontinue nursing until you finish medicine. Consult doctor for advice on maintaining milk supply.

Infants & children:
Give only under close medical supervision.

Prolonged use:
Request periodic liver function studies.

Skin & sunlight:
No problems expected.

Driving, piloting or hazardous work:
No problems expected.

Discontinuing:
May be unnecessary to finish medicine. Follow doctor's instructions.

Others:
- Advise any doctor or dentist whom you consult that you take this medicine.
- May affect the results in some medical tests.

POSSIBLE INTERACTION WITH OTHER DRUGS

GENERIC NAME OR DRUG CLASS	COMBINED EFFECT
Antacids*	Decreased itraconazole absorption.
Anticoagulants*, oral	Increased anticoagulant effect.
Antidiabetics*, oral	Increased risk of hypoglycemia.
Antihistamines, nonsedating	Serious heart rhythm problems with astemizole or terfenadine. Avoid.
Antivirals, HIV/AIDS*	Decreased itraconazole absorption.
Astemizole	Possible cardiac toxicity and death. Avoid combining.
Carbamazepine	Decreased itraconazole effect.
Cisapride	Heartbeat irregularities. Avoid.
Cyclosporine	Possible toxic levels of cyclosporine.
Digoxin	Possible toxic levels of digoxin.
Histamine H$_2$ receptor antagonists	Decreased itraconazole absorption.
Isoniazid	Decreased anticoagulant effect.
Rifampin	Decreased itraconazole effect.
Phenytoin	Decreased itraconazole effect.
Warfarin	Increased warfarin effect.

POSSIBLE INTERACTION WITH OTHER SUBSTANCES

INTERACTS WITH	COMBINED EFFECT
Alcohol:	None expected.
Beverages:	None expected.
Cocaine:	None expected.
Foods:	None expected.
Marijuana:	None expected.
Tobacco:	None expected.

KANAMYCIN

BRAND NAMES

Kantrex

BASIC INFORMATION

Habit forming? No
Prescription needed? Yes
Available as generic? No
Drug class: Bowel preparation

 ## USES

- To cleanse bowel of bacteria prior to intestinal surgery.
- Treats hepatic coma.

 ## DOSAGE & USAGE INFORMATION

How to take:
Capsules—Swallow with liquid. If you can't swallow whole, open capsule and take with liquid or food. Instructions to take on empty stomach mean 1 hour before or 2 hours after eating.

When to take:
At the same time each day, according to instructions on prescription label.

If you forget a dose:
Take as soon as you remember up to 2 hours late. If more than 2 hours, wait for next scheduled dose (don't double this dose).

What drug does:
Kills susceptible bacteria in the intestines.

Time lapse before drug works:
15 to 30 minutes.

Don't take with:
Any other medication without consulting your doctor or pharmacist.

 ## OVERDOSE

SYMPTOMS:
Clumsiness, dizziness, seizures, coma.
WHAT TO DO:
- **Dial 911 (emergency) or 0 (operator) for an ambulance or medical help. Then give first aid immediately.**
- **See emergency information on inside covers.**

 ## POSSIBLE ADVERSE REACTIONS OR SIDE EFFECTS

SYMPTOMS	WHAT TO DO
Life-threatening: In case of overdose, see previous column.	
Common: Mouth irritation or soreness, nausea.	Continue. Call doctor when convenient.
Infrequent: Vomiting.	Discontinue. Call doctor right away.
Rare: Decreased urine, hearing loss, ringing in ears, clumsiness, unsteadiness, skin rash.	Discontinue. Call doctor right away.

WARNINGS & PRECAUTIONS

Don't take if:
- You are allergic to kanamycin.
- You can't tolerate any aminoglycoside.

Before you start, consult your doctor:
- If you have hearing difficulty.
- If you have intestinal obstruction.
- If you have severe kidney disease.
- If you have ulcerative colitis.

Over age 60:
Adverse reactions and side effects may be more frequent and severe than in younger persons. You may need smaller doses for shorter periods of time.

Pregnancy:
Consult doctor. Risk category D (see page xxiii).

Breast-feeding:
No special problems expected. Consult doctor.

Infants & children:
Not recommended for prolonged use.

Prolonged use:
Not recommended for prolonged use.

Skin & sunlight:
No problems expected.

Driving, piloting or hazardous work:
Avoid if you feel confused, drowsy or dizzy.

Discontinuing:
Not recommended for prolonged use.

Others:
No problems expected.

 ## POSSIBLE INTERACTION WITH OTHER DRUGS

GENERIC NAME OR DRUG CLASS	COMBINED EFFECT
None significant.	

 ## POSSIBLE INTERACTION WITH OTHER SUBSTANCES

INTERACTS WITH	COMBINED EFFECT
Alcohol:	No special problems expected.
Beverages:	No special problems expected.
Cocaine:	No special problems expected.
Foods:	No special problems expected.
Marijuana:	No special problems expected.
Tobacco:	No special problems expected.

*See Glossary

KAOLIN & PECTIN

BRAND NAMES

Donnagel-MB   K-C
Kao-Con   K-P
Kaotin   K-Pek
Kapectolin   Parapectolin
Kapectolin with
  Paregoric

BASIC INFORMATION

Habit forming? No
Prescription needed? No
Available as generic? Yes
Drug class: Antidiarrheal

USES

Treats mild to moderate diarrhea. Used in
conjunction with fluids, appropriate diet and rest.
Treats symptoms only. Does not cure any
disorder that causes diarrhea.

DOSAGE & USAGE INFORMATION

How to take:
Liquid—Swallow prescribed dosage (without
diluting) after each loose bowel movement.

When to take:
After each loose bowel movement.

If you forget a dose:
Take when you remember.

What drug does:
Makes loose stools less watery, but may not
prevent loss of fluids.

Time lapse before drug works:
15 to 30 minutes.

Don't take with:
Any other medication without consulting your
doctor or pharmacist.

OVERDOSE

SYMPTOMS:
Fecal impaction.
WHAT TO DO:
Overdose unlikely to threaten life. If person
takes much larger amount than prescribed,
call doctor, poison control center or hospital
emergency room for instructions.

POSSIBLE ADVERSE REACTIONS OR SIDE EFFECTS

SYMPTOMS	WHAT TO DO
Life-threatening: None expected.	
Common: None expected.	
Infrequent: None expected.	
Rare: Constipation (mild).	Continue. Call doctor when convenient.

WARNINGS & PRECAUTIONS

Don't take if:
You are allergic to kaolin or pectin.

Before you start, consult your doctor:
- If patient is child or infant.
- If you have any chronic medical problem with heart disease, peptic ulcer, asthma or others.
- If you have fever over 101F.

Over age 60:
Fluid loss caused by diarrhea, especially if taking other medicines, may lead to serious disability. Consult doctor.

Pregnancy:
Consult doctor. Risk category C (see page xxiii).

Breast-feeding:
No problems expected.

Infants & children:
Fluid loss caused by diarrhea in infants and children can cause serious dehydration. Consult doctor before giving any medicine for diarrhea.

Prolonged use:
Not recommended.

Skin & sunlight:
No problems expected.

Driving, piloting or hazardous work:
No problems expected.

Discontinuing:
May be unnecessary to finish medicine. Follow doctor's Instructions.

Others:
Consult doctor about fluids, diet and rest.

POSSIBLE INTERACTION WITH OTHER DRUGS

GENERIC NAME OR DRUG CLASS	COMBINED EFFECT
Digoxin	Decreases absorption of digoxin. Separate doses by at least 2 hours.
Lincomycins*	Decreases absorption of lincomycin. Separate doses by at least 2 hours.
All other oral medicines	May decrease absorption of other medicines. Separate doses by at least 2 hours.

POSSIBLE INTERACTION WITH OTHER SUBSTANCES

INTERACTS WITH	COMBINED EFFECT
Alcohol:	Increased diarrhea. Prevents action of kaolin and pectin.
Beverages:	No problems expected.
Cocaine:	Aggravates underlying disease. Avoid.
Foods:	No problems expected.
Marijuana:	Aggravates underlying disease. Avoid.
Tobacco:	Aggravates underlying disease. Avoid.

*See Glossary

KAOLIN, PECTIN, BELLADONNA & OPIUM

BRAND NAMES

Amogel PG	Kapectolin PG
Donnagel-PG	Quiagel PG
Donnapectolin-PG	

BASIC INFORMATION

Habit forming? Yes
Prescription needed? Yes
Available as generic? No
Drug class: Narcotic, antidiarrheal, antispasmodic

 USES

Treats mild to moderate diarrhea. Used in conjunction with fluids, appropriate diet and rest. Treats symptoms only. Does not cure any disorder that causes diarrhea.

 DOSAGE & USAGE INFORMATION

How to take:
Liquid—Swallow prescribed dosage (without diluting) after each loose bowel movement.

When to take:
As needed for diarrhea, no more often than every 4 hours.

If you forget a dose:
Take when you remember.

Continued next column

 OVERDOSE

SYMPTOMS:
Fecal impaction, rapid pulse, dizziness, fever, hallucinations, confusion, slurred speech, agitation, flushed face, convulsions, deep sleep, slow breathing, slow pulse, warm skin, constricted pupils, coma.
WHAT TO DO:
- **Dial 911 (emergency) or 0 (operator) for an ambulance or medical help. Then give first aid immediately.**
- **If patient is unconscious and not breathing, give mouth-to-mouth breathing. If there is no heartbeat, use cardiac massage and mouth-to-mouth breathing (CPR). Don't try to make patient vomit. If you can't get help quickly, take patient to nearest emergency facility.**
- **See emergency information on inside covers.**

What drug does:
- Blocks nerve impulses at parasympathetic nerve endings, preventing muscle contractions and gland secretions of organs involved.
- Makes loose stools less watery, but may not prevent loss of fluids.
- Anesthetizes surface membranes of intestines and blocks nerve impulses.

Time lapse before drug works:
15 to 30 minutes.

Don't take with:
Any other medication without consulting your doctor or pharmacist.

 POSSIBLE ADVERSE REACTIONS OR SIDE EFFECTS

SYMPTOMS	WHAT TO DO
Life-threatening:	
Unusually rapid heartbeat (over 100), difficult breathing, slow heartbeat (under 50/minute).	Discontinue. Seek emergency treatment.
Common (with large dosage):	
Weakness, increased sweating, red or flushed face, lightheadedness, headache, dry mouth, dry skin, drowsiness, dizziness, frequent urination, decreased sweating, constipation, confusion, tiredness.	Continue. Call doctor when convenient.
Infrequent:	
• Reduced taste sense, nervousness, eyes, sensitive to sunlight, blurred vision.	Discontinue. Call doctor right away.
• Diminished sex drive, memory loss.	Continue. Call doctor when convenient.
Rare:	
Bloating, abdominal cramps and vomiting, eye pain, hallucinations, shortness of breath, rash, itchy skin, slow heartbeat.	Discontinue. Call doctor right away.

 WARNINGS & PRECAUTIONS

Don't take if:
- You are allergic to any anticholinergic, narcotic, kaolin or pectin.
- You have trouble with stomach bloating, difficulty emptying your bladder completely, narrow-angle glaucoma, severe ulcerative colitis.

KAOLIN, PECTIN, BELLADONNA & OPIUM

Before you start, consult your doctor:
- If you have open-angle glaucoma, angina, chronic bronchitis or asthma, hiatal hernia, liver disease, enlarged prostate, myasthenia gravis, peptic ulcer, impaired liver or kidney function, fever over 101F, any chronic medical problem with heart disease, peptic ulcer, asthma or others.
- If patient is child or infant.
- If you will have surgery within 2 months, including dental surgery, requiring general or spinal anesthesia.

Over age 60:
- Adverse reactions and side effects may be more frequent and severe than in younger persons.
- More likely to be drowsy, dizzy, unsteady or constipated.
- Fluid loss caused by diarrhea, especially if taking other medicines, may lead to serious disability. Consult doctor.

Pregnancy:
Decide with your doctor if drug benefits justify risk to unborn child. Risk category C (see page xxiii).

Breast-feeding:
Drug passes into milk. Avoid drug or discontinue nursing until you finish medicine. Consult doctor for advice on maintaining milk supply.

Infants & children:
Fluid loss caused by diarrhea in infants and children can cause serious dehydration. Consult doctor before giving any medicine for diarrhea.

Prolonged use:
- Causes psychological and physical dependence. Not recommended.
- Talk to your doctor about the need for follow-up medical examinations or laboratory studies to check liver function, kidney function.

Skin & sunlight:
No special problems expected.

Driving, piloting or hazardous work:
Don't drive or pilot aircraft until you learn how medicine affects you. Don't work around dangerous machinery. Don't climb ladders or work in high places. Danger increases if you drink alcohol or take medicine affecting alertness and reflexes, such as antihistamines, tranquilizers, sedatives, pain medicine, narcotics and mind-altering drugs.

Discontinuing:
May be unnecessary to finish medicine. Follow doctor's instructions.

Others:
- Great potential for abuse.
- Consult doctor about fluids, diet and rest.

POSSIBLE INTERACTION WITH OTHER DRUGS

GENERIC NAME OR DRUG CLASS	COMBINED EFFECT
Amantadine	Increased belladonna effect.
Analgesics*	Increased analgesic effect.
Antidepressants*	Increased sedative effect.
Antihistamines*	Increased sedative effect.
Carteolol	Increased narcotic effect. Dangerous sedation.
Central nervous system (CNS) depressants*	Increased depressant effect of both.
Cortisone drugs*	Increased internal eye pressure.
Digoxin	Decreases absorption of digoxin. Separate doses by at least 2 hours.
Haloperidol	Increased internal eye pressure.

Continued on page 918

POSSIBLE INTERACTION WITH OTHER SUBSTANCES

INTERACTS WITH	COMBINED EFFECT
Alcohol:	Increases alcohol's intoxicating effect, increased diarrhea, prevents action of kaolin and pectin. Avoid.
Beverages:	No problems expected.
Cocaine:	Aggravates underlying disease. Avoid.
Foods:	No problems expected.
Marijuana:	Impairs physical and mental performance, aggravates underlying disease. Avoid.
Tobacco:	Aggravates underlying disease. Avoid.

*See Glossary

KERATOLYTICS

GENERIC AND BRAND NAMES

See complete list of generic and brand names in the *Generic and Brand Name Directory*, page 882.

BASIC INFORMATION

Habit forming? No
Prescription needed? Yes, on some.
Available as generic? Yes
Drug class: Keratolytic, antiacne (topical), antiseborrheic

 ## USES

Treatment for acne, psoriasis, ichthyosis, keratosis, folliculitis, flat warts, eczema, urticaria, calluses, corns, seborrheic dermatitis, dandruff.

 ## DOSAGE & USAGE INFORMATION

How to use:
Cream, gel, lotion, ointment, pads, plaster, shampoo, soap, topical solution, suspension—Always follow instructions on the label or use as directed by your doctor.

When to use:
At the same time each day or as needed.

If you forget an application:
Use as soon as you remember.

What drug does:
Keratolytics are drugs that soften, loosen and remove keratin (the tough outer layer of the skin).

Time lapse before drug works:
2 to 3 weeks. May require 6 weeks for maximum improvement.

Don't use with:
- Benzoyl peroxide. Apply 12 hours apart.
- Any other medicine without consulting your doctor or pharmacist.

 ## OVERDOSE

SYMPTOMS:
None expected.
WHAT TO DO:
If person swallows drug, call doctor, poison control center or hospital emergency room for instructions.

 ## POSSIBLE ADVERSE REACTIONS OR SIDE EFFECTS

SYMPTOMS	WHAT TO DO
Life-threatening: None expected.	
Common: • Pigment change in treated area, warmth or stinging, peeling.	Continue. Tell doctor at next visit.
• Sensitivity to wind or cold.	No action necessary.
Infrequent: Blistering, crusting, severe burning, swelling, skin irritation that begins after treatment.	Discontinue. Call doctor right away.
Rare: Symptoms of systemic toxicity (diarrhea, nausea, dizziness, headache, breathing difficulty, tiredness, weakness).	Discontinue. Call doctor right away.

WARNINGS & PRECAUTIONS

Don't take if:
- You are allergic to resorcinol or salicyclic acid.
- You are sunburned or windburned or have an open skin wound, skin irritation or infection.

Before you start, consult your doctor:
- If you have eczema.
- If you have diabetes mellitus.
- If you have peripheral vascular disease (blood vessel disease).

Over age 60:
No problems expected.

Pregnancy:
Risk factors vary for drugs in this group. See category list on page xxiii and consult doctor.

Breast-feeding:
No problems expected. Consult doctor.

Infants & children:
Not recommended. Increased risk of toxicity.

Prolonged use:
No problems expected.

Skin & sunlight:
No special problems expected.

Driving, piloting or hazardous work:
No problems expected.

Discontinuing:
Follow your doctor's instructions or the directions on the label.

Others:
- Acne may get worse before improvement starts in 2 or 3 weeks. Don't wash face more than 2 or 3 times daily.
- Keep medicine away from mouth or eyes. If it accidentally gets into the eyes, flush immediately with clear water.
- Keep medicine away from heat or flame.

POSSIBLE INTERACTION WITH OTHER DRUGS

GENERIC NAME OR DRUG CLASS	COMBINED EFFECT
Anti-acne topical preparations (other)	Severe skin irritation.
Cosmetics (medicated)	Severe skin irritation.
Skin preparations with alcohol	Severe skin irritation.
Soaps or cleansers (abrasive)	Severe skin irritation.

POSSIBLE INTERACTION WITH OTHER SUBSTANCES

INTERACTS WITH	COMBINED EFFECT
Alcohol:	None expected.
Beverages:	None expected.
Cocaine:	None expected.
Foods:	None expected.
Marijuana:	None expected.
Tobacco:	None expected.

KETOCONAZOLE

BRAND NAMES

Nizoral

BASIC INFORMATION

Habit forming? No
Prescription needed? Yes
Available as generic? No
Drug class: Antifungal

 ## USES

Treatment of fungus infections susceptible to ketoconazole.

 ## DOSAGE & USAGE INFORMATION

How to take:
Tablet or oral suspension—Swallow with liquid or food to lessen stomach irritation. If you can't swallow whole, crumble tablet and take with liquid or food.

When to take:
At same time once a day.

If you forget a dose:
Take as soon as you remember up to 2 hours late. If more than 2 hours, wait for next scheduled dose (don't double this dose).

What drug does:
Prevents fungi from growing and reproducing.

Time lapse before drug works:
8 to 10 months or longer.

Don't take with:
Any other medication without consulting your doctor or pharmacist.

 ## POSSIBLE ADVERSE REACTIONS OR SIDE EFFECTS

SYMPTOMS	WHAT TO DO

Life-threatening:
None expected.

Continued next column

 ## OVERDOSE

SYMPTOMS:
Nausea, vomiting, diarrhea.
WHAT TO DO:
Overdose unlikely to threaten life. If person takes much larger amount than prescribed, call doctor, poison control center or hospital emergency room for instructions.

Common:
None expected.

Infrequent:

Nausea or vomiting, diarrhea.	Continue. Call doctor when convenient.

Rare:

• Pale stools, abdominal pain, dark or amber urine, jaundice, rash or itchy skin.	Discontinue. Call doctor right away.
• Diminished sex drive in males, swollen breasts in males, tiredness, weakness, appetite loss, increased sensitivity to light, drowsiness, dizziness, headache, insomnia.	Continue. Call doctor when convenient.

 ## WARNINGS & PRECAUTIONS

Don't take if:
You are allergic to ketoconazole, fluconazole, itraconazole or miconazole.

Before you start, consult your doctor:
• If you have absence of stomach acid (achlorhydria).
• If you have liver disease.

Over age 60:
Adverse reactions and side effects may be more frequent and severe than in younger persons.

Pregnancy:
Decide with your doctor if drug benefits justify risk to unborn child. Risk category C (see page xxiii).

Breast-feeding:
Drug passes into milk. Avoid drug or discontinue nursing until you finish medicine. Consult doctor for advice on maintaining milk supply.

Infants & children:
Only under close medical supervision.

Prolonged use:
Request liver-function studies.

Skin & sunlight:
No special problems expected.

Driving, piloting or hazardous work:
Don't drive or pilot aircraft until you learn how medicine affects you. Don't work around dangerous machinery. Don't climb ladders or work in high places. Danger increases if you drink alcohol or take medicine affecting alertness and reflexes, such as antihistamines, tranquilizers, sedatives, pain medicine, narcotics and mind-altering drugs.

Discontinuing:
May be unnecessary to finish medicine. Follow doctor's instructions.

Others:
May interfere with some medical tests.

POSSIBLE INTERACTION WITH OTHER DRUGS

GENERIC NAME OR DRUG CLASS	COMBINED EFFECT
Adrenocorticoids, systemic	Decreased ketoconazole effect.
Antacids*	Decreased absorption of ketoconazole.
Anticoagulants, oral*	Increased anticoagulant effect.
Anticholinergics*	Decreased absorption of ketoconazole.
Antihistamines, nonsedating	Serious heart ryhthm problems with astemizole or terfenadine. Avoid.
Antivirals, HIV/AIDS*	Reduced absorption of both drugs. Increased risk of pancreatitis.
Astemizole	Heart problems. Never combine.
Atropine	Decreased absorption of ketoconazole.
Belladonna	Decreased absorption of ketoconazole.
Cimetidine	Decreased absorption of ketoconazole.
Cisapride	Heartbeat irregularities. Avoid.
Clidinium	Decreased absorption of ketoconazole.
Cyclosporine	Increased risk of toxicity to kidney.
Famotidine	Reduced absorption of ketoconazole. Take famatodine at least 2 hours after any dose of ketoconazole.
Glycopyrrolate	Decreased absorption of ketoconazole.
Hepatotoxic medications*	Increased risk of toxicity to kidney.
Histamine H$_2$ receptor antagonists	Decreased absorption of ketoconazole.

Hyoscyamine	Decreased absorption of ketoconazole.
Hypoglycemics, oral*	Increased effect of oral hypoglycemics.
Isoniazid	Decreased effect of ketoconazole.
Methscopolamine	Decreased absorption of ketoconazole.
Methylprednisolone	Increased effect of methylprednisolone.
Nizatidine	Decreased absorption of ketoconazole.
Omeprazole	Decreased absorption of ketoconazole.
Phenytoin	May alter effect of both drugs.
Propantheline	Decreased absorption of ketoconazole.
Ranitidine	Decreased absorption of ketoconazole.
Rifampin	Decreased effect of ketoconazole.
Scopolamine	Decreased absorption of ketoconazole.
Sibutramine	Increased effect of sibutramine.
Sodium bicarbonate	Decreased absorption of ketoconazole.

POSSIBLE INTERACTION WITH OTHER SUBSTANCES

INTERACTS WITH	COMBINED EFFECT
Alcohol:	Increased chance of liver damage and disulfiram reaction.*
Beverages:	No problems expected.
Cocaine:	Decreased ketoconazole effect. Avoid.
Foods:	No problems expected.
Marijuana:	Decreased ketoconazole effect. Avoid.
Tobacco:	Decreased ketoconazole effect. Avoid.

*See Glossary

LAMOTRIGINE

BRAND NAMES

Lamictal

BASIC INFORMATION

Habit forming? No
Prescription needed? Yes
Available as generic? No
Drug class: Anticonvulsant, antiepileptic

 USES

Treatment for partial (focal) epileptic seizures. May be used in combination with other antiepileptic drugs.

 DOSAGE & USAGE INFORMATION

How to take:
Tablets—Swallow with liquid. May be taken with or without food.

When to take:
Your doctor will determine the best schedule. Dosages may be increased gradually over the first few weeks of use to achieve maximum benefits.

If you forget a dose:
Take as soon as you remember. If it is almost time for the next dose, then skip the missed dose and wait for your next scheduled dose (don't double this dose).

What drug does:
The exact mechanism is unknown. The anticonvulsant action may result from a decrease in the release of stimulatory neurotransmitters (substances that stimulate nerve cells).

Time lapse before drug works:
May take several weeks for effectiveness.

Don't take with:
Any other prescription or nonprescription drug without consulting your doctor.

 OVERDOSE

SYMPTOMS:
Severe drowsiness, severe headache, severe dizziness, coma.
WHAT TO DO:
- **Dial 911 (emergency) or 0 (operator) for an ambulance or medical help. Then give first aid immediately.**
- **See emergency information on inside covers.**

 POSSIBLE ADVERSE REACTIONS OR SIDE EFFECTS

SYMPTOMS	WHAT TO DO
Life-threatening:	
In case of overdose, see previous column.	
Common:	
• Skin rash, double vision or blurred vision, clumsiness.	Continue, but call doctor right away.
• Dizziness, nausea or vomiting, headache, drowsiness.	Continue. Call doctor when convenient.
Infrequent:	
Anxiety, depression, confusion, irritability, other mood or mental changes, increase in seizure activity, back-and-forth eye movements (nystagmus).	Continue, but call doctor right away.
Rare:	
• Swelling (hands, face, mouth, feet); breathing difficulty; tiredness or weakness; fever; chills; sore throat; unusual bruising or bleeding; skin peeling, blistering or loosening; muscle cramps or pain; sores on mouth or lips; small red or purple dots on skin.	Continue, but call doctor right away.
• Slurred speech, indigestion, runny nose, trembling, trouble sleeping, weakness.	Continue. Call doctor when convenient.

WARNINGS & PRECAUTIONS

Don't take if:
You are allergic to lamotrigine.

Before you start, consult your doctor:
- If you have kidney or liver disease.
- If you have any heart disorder.
- If you are allergic to any medication, food, or other substance.

Over age 60:
No special problems expected.

Pregnancy:
Decide with your doctor if drug benefits justify risks to unborn child. Risk category C (see page xxiii).

Breast-feeding:
Drug passes into milk. Avoid drug or discontinue nursing until you finish medicine. Consult doctor for advice on maintaining milk supply.

Infants & children:
Safety not established for children under age 16. Use only under close medical supervision.

Prolonged use:
Schedule regular visits to your doctor to determine if drug is continuing to be effective in controlling seizures. Follow-up laboratory blood studies may be recommended by your doctor.

Skin & sunlight:
No special problems expected.

Driving, piloting or hazardous work:
Don't drive or pilot aircraft until you learn how medicine affects you. Don't work around dangerous machinery. Don't climb ladders or work in high places. Danger increases if you drink alcohol or take other medicines affecting alertness and reflexes, such as antihistamines, tranquilizers, sedatives, pain medicine, narcotics and mind-altering drugs.

Discontinuing:
Don't discontinue without doctor's approval due to risk of increased seizure activity. Dosage may need to be gradually reduced.

Others:
- Advise any doctor or dentist whom you consult that you take this medicine.
- Use as directed. Don't increase or decrease dosage without doctor's approval.
- Wear medical identification stating that you have a seizure disorder and take this medication.
- A skin rash may indicate a serious, and potentially life-threatening, medical problem. If a skin rash develops, it is usually during the first 4 to 6 weeks after treatment with the drug is started. Call your doctor promptly if you develop any skin rash.

POSSIBLE INTERACTION WITH OTHER DRUGS

GENERIC NAME OR DRUG CLASS	COMBINED EFFECT
Carbamazepine	Decreased effect of lamotrigine. Increase in risk of side effects.
Central nervous system (CNS) depressants*	Increased sedation.
Folate antagonists*, other	Folic acid deficiency.
Phenobarbital	Decreased effect of lamotrigine.
Phenytoin	Decreased effect of lamotrigine.
Primidone	Decreased effect of lamotrigine.
Valproic acid	Increased effect of lamotrigine. May increase risk of skin rash.

POSSIBLE INTERACTION WITH OTHER SUBSTANCES

INTERACTS WITH	COMBINED EFFECT
Alcohol:	Increased sedation. Avoid.
Beverages:	No special problems expected.
Cocaine:	Problems not known. Best to avoid.
Foods:	No special problems expected.
Marijuana:	Problems not known. Best to avoid.
Tobacco:	No special problems expected.

*See Glossary

LAXATIVES, BULK-FORMING

GENERIC AND BRAND NAMES

See complete list of generic and brand names in the *Generic and Brand Name Directory*, page 883.

BASIC INFORMATION

Habit forming? No
Prescription needed? No
Available as generic? Yes
Drug class: Laxative, bulk-forming

USES

For short-term relief of simple constipation (bowel movements that are abnormally difficult or infrequent). Normal frequency of bowel movements may vary from 2 to 3 times a day to 2 to 3 times a week. Laxatives treat the symptoms of constipation, not the cause.

DOSAGE & USAGE INFORMATION

How to take:
Powder, oral solution, tablets, capsules, granules, chewable tablets, caramels, effervescent powder, wafers—Follow package instructions. Swallow with full glass of water or fruit juice. Drink 6 to 8 glasses of water each day in addition to one taken with each dose. Mix all powders thoroughly to avoid any risk of unmixed powder causing intestinal blockage.

When to take:
As directed on the label or according to doctor's instructions.

If you forget a dose:
Take as soon as you remember.

What drug does:
Adds dietary fiber that is not digested. Once in the intestine, it helps to increase fecal bulk, lubricate and soften the intestinal contents and facilitate the passage of stools.

Continued next column

OVERDOSE

SYMPTOMS:
Weakness, increased sweating, confusion, irregular heartbeat, muscle cramps.
WHAT TO DO:
Overdose unlikely to threaten life. If person takes much larger amount than prescribed, call doctor, poison control center or hospital emergency room for instructions.

Time lapse before drug works:
May work in 12 to 24 hours. Sometimes does not work for 2 to 3 days.

Don't take with:
- Any other medicine without consulting your doctor or pharmacist.
- Don't take within 2 hours of taking another medicine. Laxative interferes with absorption of medicine.

POSSIBLE ADVERSE REACTIONS OR SIDE EFFECTS

SYMPTOMS	WHAT TO DO
Life-threatening: None expected.	
Common: None expected.	
Infrequent: Mild stomach cramps, throat irritation with liquid form.	Continue. Call doctor when convenient.
Rare: Allergic skin rash or itching, trouble breathing, swallowing difficulty.	Discontinue. Call doctor right away.

WARNINGS & PRECAUTIONS

Don't take if:
- You have symptoms of appendicitis (abdominal pain, cramping, soreness, bloating, nausea and vomiting). Consult doctor.
- You have dysphagia (swallowing difficulty).
- You are allergic to bulk-forming laxatives.
- You have missed a bowel movement for just 1 or 2 days.

Before you start, consult your doctor:
- If you are allergic to any medicine, food, or other substance or have a family history of allergies.
- If you have diabetes or heart or kidney disease.
- If you have hypertension (high blood pressure) and the laxative contains sodium.
- If you have an intestinal obstruction or undiagnosed rectal bleeding.
- If you are taking other laxatives.

Over age 60:
No special problems expected.

Pregnancy:
Most bulk-forming laxatives contain sodium or sugars, which may cause fluid retention. Risk factors vary or may not be designated for these laxatives. Read categories on page xxiii and consult doctor.

Breast-Feeding:
No special problems expected. Consult doctor.

Infants & children:
- Don't give to children under age 6 without doctor's approval. Young children are not able to describe their symptoms accurately, and a proper diagnosis needs to be made before starting any treatment.
- Don't give to a child who refuses to have a bowel movement (toileting refusal). May force a painful bowel movement and cause the child to hold back even more. Consult doctor.
- For children over age 6, follow package instructions or doctor's directions for correct dosage amount.

Prolonged use:
Don't take for more than 1 week unless under doctor's supervision. Bulk-form laxatives are sometimes used for long-term therapy.

Skin & sunlight:
No special problems expected.

Driving, piloting or hazardous work:
No special problems expected.

Discontinuing:
May be unnecessary to finish medicine. Follow doctor's instructions or instructions on label.

Others:
- Don't give to "flush out" the system or as a "tonic."
- Use as directed. Don't increase or decrease dosage without doctor's approval.
- Excessive use of laxatives in a teenager may indicate an eating disorder such as anorexia nervosa or bulimia nervosa. Consult doctor.
- If there is a sudden change in bowel habits or bowel function that lasts longer than 2 weeks, consult doctor.

POSSIBLE INTERACTION WITH OTHER DRUGS

GENERIC NAME OR DRUG CLASS	COMBINED EFFECT
Antacids*	Irritation of stomach or small intestine.
Anticoagulants*	Decreased anticoagulant effect. Take 2 hours apart.
Digitalis preparations*	Decreased digitalis effect. Take 2 hours apart.
Diuretics, potassium-sparing*	Decreased potassium effect.
Potassium supplements*	Decreased potassium effect.
Salicylates*	Decreased salicylate effect. Take 2 hours apart.
Tetracyclines*	Decreased tetracycline effect. Take 2 hours apart.

POSSIBLE INTERACTION WITH OTHER SUBSTANCES

INTERACTS WITH	COMBINED EFFECT
Alcohol:	No special problems expected.
Beverages:	No special problems expected.
Cocaine:	No special problems expected.
Foods:	No special problems expected.
Marijuana:	No special problems expected.
Tobacco:	No special problems expected.

LAXATIVES, OSMOTIC

GENERIC AND BRAND NAMES

See complete list of generic and brand names in the *Generic and Brand Name Directory*, page 884.

BASIC INFORMATION

Habit forming? No
Prescription needed? No
Available as generic? Yes
Drug class: Laxative, hyperosmotic

 ## USES

For short-term relief of simple constipation (bowel movements that are abnormally difficult or infrequent). Normal frequency of bowel movements may vary from 2 to 3 times a day to 2 to 3 times a week. Laxatives treat the symptoms of constipation, not the cause.

 ## DOSAGE & USAGE INFORMATION

How to take:
- Oral solution, tablets, crystals, effervescent powder, milk of magnesia—Follow package instructions. Swallow with full glass of water or fruit juice. A second glass of liquid is often recommended for best effect. Drink 6 to 8 glasses of water each day, in addition to one taken with each dose.
- Enema or suppositories—Read and follow package instructions.

When to take:
Since drug produces stool within 30 minutes to 3 hours following a dose, take it at a time that will not interfere with sleep or other scheduled activities. Don't take late in the day on an empty stomach.

If you forget a dose:
Take as soon as you remember.

Continued next column

 ## OVERDOSE

SYMPTOMS:
Weakness, increased sweating, confusion, irregular heartbeat, muscle cramps.
WHAT TO DO:
Overdose unlikely to threaten life. If person takes much larger amount than prescribed, call doctor, poison control center or hospital emergency room for instructions.

What drug does:
Draws water into the bowel from surrounding tissue to help loosen and soften the stool and increases bowel action.

Time lapse before drug works:
- Oral forms—30 minutes to 3 hours. May take longer if taken with a meal.
- Rectal forms—2 to 15 minutes.

Don't take with:
- Any other medicine without consulting your doctor or pharmacist.
- Don't take within 2 hours of taking another medicine. Laxative interferes with absorption of medicine.

 ## POSSIBLE ADVERSE REACTIONS OR SIDE EFFECTS

SYMPTOMS	WHAT TO DO
Life-threatening: None expected.	
Common: None expected.	
Infrequent:	
• Belching, cramps, nausea, diarrhea, increased thirst.	Continue. Call doctor when convenient.
• Rectal bleeding, burning, itching or pain (with rectal forms).	Discontinue. Call doctor right away.
Rare:	
When used too often or dose is too high—Confusion, irregular heartbeat, muscle cramps, unusual tiredness or weakness, dehydration.	Discontinue. Call doctor right away.

 ## WARNINGS & PRECAUTIONS

Don't take if:
- You are having symptoms of appendicitis (abdominal pain, cramping, soreness, bloating, nausea and vomiting). Consult doctor.
- You are allergic to osmotic laxatives.
- You have missed a bowel movement for just 1 or 2 days.

Before you start, consult your doctor:
- If you are allergic to any medicine, food or other substance or have a family history of allergies.
- If you have hypertension (high blood pressure) and the laxative contains sodium.
- If you have an intestinal obstruction, undiagnosed rectal bleeding or a colostomy or ileostomy.

- If you have diabetes or heart or kidney disease.
- If you are taking other laxatives.

Over age 60:
- Rectal solutions could cause excess fluid in the body. Consult doctor before using.
- No special problems expected with laxatives taken by mouth.

Pregnancy:
Risk factors vary or may not be designated for these laxatives. Read categories on page xxiii and consult doctor.

Breast-feeding:
No special problems expected. Consult doctor.

Infants & children:
- Don't give to children under age 6 without doctor's approval. Young children are not able to describe their symptoms accurately, and a proper diagnosis needs to be made before starting any treatment.
- Don't give to a child who refuses to have a bowel movement (toileting refusal). May force a painful bowel movement and cause the child to hold back even more. Consult doctor.
- For children over age 6, follow package instructions or doctor's directions for correct dosage amount.

Prolonged use:
Don't take for more than 1 week unless under doctor's supervision. May cause laxative dependence in which normal bowel function depends on the laxative to produce a bowel movement.

Skin & sunlight:
No special problems expected.

Driving, piloting or hazardous work:
No special problems expected.

Discontinuing:
May be unnecessary to finish medicine. Follow doctor's instructions or instructions on label.

Others:
- Don't give to "flush out" the system or as a "tonic."
- Use as directed. Don't increase or decrease dosage without doctor's approval.
- Excessive use of laxatives in a teenager may indicate an eating disorder such as anorexia nervosa or bulimia nervosa. Consult doctor.
- If there is a sudden change in bowel habits or bowel function that lasts longer than 2 weeks, consult doctor.

POSSIBLE INTERACTION WITH OTHER DRUGS

GENERIC NAME OR DRUG CLASS	COMBINED EFFECT
Antacids*	Irritation of stomach or small intestine.
Anticoagulants*	Decreased anticoagulant effect with aluminum- or magnesium-containing laxatives. Avoid.
Ciprofloxacin	Decreased ciprofloxacin effect with magnesium-containing laxatives. Avoid.
Digitalis preparations*	Decreased digitalis effect with aluminum- or magnesium-containing laxatives. Avoid.
Diuretics, potassium-sparing*	Decreased potassium effect.
Etidronate	Decreased etidronate effect if taken with magnesium-containing laxatives. Take 2 hours apart.
Phenothiazines*	Decreased phenothiazine effect with aluminum- or magnesium-containing laxatives. Avoid.
Potassium supplements*	Decreased potassium effect.
Sodium polystyrene	Fluid imbalance in body with magnesium- containing laxatives. Avoid.
Tetracyclines*	Decreased tetracycline effect. Take 2 hours apart.

POSSIBLE INTERACTION WITH OTHER SUBSTANCES

INTERACTS WITH	COMBINED EFFECT
Alcohol:	No special problems.
Beverages:	No special problems.
Cocaine:	No special problems.
Foods:	No special problems.
Marijuana:	No special problems.
Tobacco:	No special problems.

LAXATIVES, SOFTENER/LUBRICANT

GENERIC AND BRAND NAMES

See complete list of generic and brand names in the *Generic and Brand Name Directory*, page 884.

BASIC INFORMATION

Habit forming? No
Prescription needed? No
Available as generic? Yes
Drug class: Laxative (stool softener-emollient), lubricant

 ## USES

For short-term relief of simple constipation (bowel movements that are abnormally difficult or infrequent). Normal frequency of bowel movements may vary from 2 to 3 times a day to 2 to 3 times a week. Laxatives treat the symptoms of constipation, not the cause.

 ## DOSAGE & USAGE INFORMATION

How to take:
- Tablets, capsules, syrup, chewable tablets, oral solution—Follow package instructions. Swallow with full glass of water, fruit juice or milk. Drink 6 to 8 glasses of water each day in addition to one taken with each dose.
- Enema or suppositories—Read and follow package instructions.

When to take:
Produces stool within 30 minutes to 3 hours following a dose. Take drug at a time that will not interfere with sleep or scheduled activities. Don't take late in the day on an empty stomach.

If you forget a dose:
Take as soon as you remember.

Continued next column

 ## OVERDOSE

SYMPTOMS:
Weakness, increased sweating, confusion, irregular heartbeat, muscle cramps.
WHAT TO DO:
Overdose unlikely to threaten life. If person takes much larger amount than prescribed, call doctor, poison control center or hospital emergency room for instructions.

What drug does:
Softener laxatives help liquids mix into the stool to help prevent hard stool masses. Lubricant laxatives coat the stool surface with a thin film that helps ease the passage of the stool through the intestines.

Time lapse before drug works:
- When taken by mouth, usually works within 1 to 2 days after first dose, but may take 3 to 5 days for full effectiveness.
- Rectal dosage forms work in 2 to 15 minutes.

Don't take with:
- Any other medicine without consulting your doctor or pharmacist.
- Other stool softener laxatives or mineral oil.
- Don't take within 2 hours of taking another medicine. Laxative interferes with absorption of medicine.

 ## POSSIBLE ADVERSE REACTIONS OR SIDE EFFECTS

SYMPTOMS	WHAT TO DO
Life-threatening: None expected.	
Common: None expected.	
Infrequent: • Mild stomach cramps, throat irritation with liquid forms, diarrhea.	Continue. Call doctor when convenient.
• Rectal bleeding, burning, itching or pain (with rectal forms).	Discontinue. Call doctor right away.
Rare: Skin rash.	Discontinue. Call doctor right away.

 ## WARNINGS & PRECAUTIONS

Don't take if:
- You have symptoms of appendicitis (abdominal pain, cramping, soreness, bloating, nausea and vomiting). Consult doctor.
- You are allergic to a softener-emollient or lubricant laxative.
- You have missed a bowel movement for just 1 or 2 days.

Before you start, consult your doctor:
- If you are allergic to any medicine, food or other substance or have a family history of allergies.
- If you have hypertension (high blood pressure) and the laxative contains sodium.
- If you have an intestinal obstruction, undiagnosed rectal bleeding or a colostomy or ileostomy.
- If you are taking other laxatives.
- If you have diabetes or heart or kidney disease.
- If you are taking other laxatives.
- You have dysphagia (swallowing difficulty) and want to take mineral oil.

Over age 60:
Oral mineral oil is not recommended for bedridden elderly patients; otherwise, no special problems expected.

Pregnancy:
Risk factors vary or may not be designated for these laxatives. Read categories on page xxiii and consult doctor.

Breast-feeding:
No special problems expected. Consult doctor.

Infants & children:
- Don't give to children under age 6 without doctor's approval. Young children are not able to describe their symptoms accurately, and a proper diagnosis needs to be made before starting any treatment.
- Don't give to a child who refuses to have a bowel movement (toileting refusal). May force a painful bowel movement and cause the child to hold back even more. Consult doctor.
- For children over age 6, follow package instructions or doctor's directions for correct dosage amount.

Prolonged use:
Don't take for more than 1 week unless under doctor's supervision.

Skin & sunlight:
No special problems expected.

Driving, piloting or hazardous work:
No special problems expected.

Discontinuing:
May be unnecessary to finish medicine. Follow doctor's instructions or instructions on label.

Others:
- Don't give to "flush out" the system or as a "tonic."
- Use as directed. Don't increase or decrease dosage without doctor's approval.
- Excessive use of laxatives in a teenager may indicate an eating disorder such as anorexia nervosa or bulimia nervosa. Consult doctor.
- If there is a sudden change in bowel habits or bowel function that lasts longer than 2 weeks, consult doctor.

 POSSIBLE INTERACTION WITH OTHER DRUGS

GENERIC NAME OR DRUG CLASS	COMBINED EFFECT
Antacids*	Irritation of stomach or small intestine.
Anticoagulants*	Decreased anti-coagulant effect with mineral oil.
Contraceptives, oral*	Decreased contraceptive effect with mineral oil.
Danthron	Increased danthron effect.
Digitalis preparations*	Decreased digitalis effect with mineral oil.
Diuretics, potassium-sparing*	Decreased potassium effect.
Phenophthalein	Increased phenophthalein effect.
Potassium supplements*	Decreased potassium effect.
Vitamins A, D, E, K	Decreased vitamin effect with mineral oil.

 POSSIBLE INTERACTION WITH OTHER SUBSTANCES

INTERACTS WITH	COMBINED EFFECT
Alcohol:	No special problems expected.
Beverages:	No special problems expected.
Cocaine:	No special problems expected.
Foods:	No special problems expected.
Marijuana:	No special problems expected.
Tobacco:	No special problems expected.

LAXATIVES, STIMULANT

GENERIC AND BRAND NAMES

See complete list of generic and brand names in the *Generic and Brand Name Directory*, page 884.

BASIC INFORMATION

Habit forming? Potentially
Prescription needed? No
Available as generic? Yes
Drug class: Laxative (stimulant)

USES

For short-term relief of simple constipation (bowel movements that are abnormally difficult or infrequent). Normal frequency of bowel movements may vary from 2 to 3 times a day to 2 to 3 times a week. Laxatives treat the symptoms of constipation, not the cause.

DOSAGE & USAGE INFORMATION

How to take:
- Tablets, chewable tablets, syrup, chewing gum, oral solution, granules, fluidextract, emulsion, wafers—Follow package instructions. Swallow with full glass of water, fruit juice or milk. Give child 6 to 8 glasses of fluid each day in addition to the one taken with each dose to keep stool soft. Give on an empty stomach. Results may be delayed if given with food.
- Enema—Lubricate rectal area with petroleum jelly before inserting enema applicator. Insert carefully to avoid damage to rectal wall. To mix powder for rectal solution, follow instructions on package.
- Suppository—Remove wrapper and moisten suppository with water. Gently insert tapered end into rectum. Push well into rectum with finger. Retain in rectum 20 to 30 minutes.

Continued next column

OVERDOSE

SYMPTOMS:
Weakness, increased sweating, confusion, irregular heartbeat, muscle cramps.
WHAT TO DO:
Overdose unlikely to threaten life. If person takes much larger amount than prescribed, call doctor, poison control center or hospital emergency room for instructions.

When to take:
Usually at bedtime on an empty stomach, unless directed otherwise. Castor oil is usually taken late in the day, as it works within 2 to 6 hours.

If you forget a dose:
Take as soon as you remember.

What drug does:
Acts on smooth muscles of intestinal wall to cause vigorous bowel movement.

Time lapse before drug works:
Oral form within 6 to 10 hours (castor oil 2 to 6 hours). Rectal form within15 minutes to 1 hour.

Don't take with:
- Any other medicine without consulting your doctor or pharmacist.
- Don't take within 2 hours of another medicine. Laxative interferes with absorption of medicine.

POSSIBLE ADVERSE REACTIONS OR SIDE EFFECTS

SYMPTOMS	WHAT TO DO
Life-threatening: None expected.	
Common: None expected.	
Infrequent:	
• Belching, cramps, nausea, diarrhea, throat irritation.	Continue. Call doctor when convenient.
• Rectal bleeding, burning, itching or pain (with rectal forms).	Discontinue. Call doctor right away.
Rare: Confusion, irregular heartbeat, muscle cramps, unusual tiredness or weakness; pink to red color of urine and stools (with phenolphthalein); pink, red or violet to brown urine color (with cascara, danthron or senna); yellow to brown color of urine (with cascara, phenolphthalein or senna); skin rash (allergy).	Discontinue. Call doctor right away.

WARNINGS & PRECAUTIONS

Don't take if:
- You have symptoms of appendicitis (abdominal pain, cramping, soreness, bloating, nausea and vomiting). Consult doctor.
- You are allergic to a stimulant laxative.
- You have missed a bowel movement for just 1 or 2 days.

Before you start, consult your doctor:
- If you are a allergic to any medicine, food or other substance or have a family history of allergies.
- If you have hypertension (high blood pressure) and the laxative contains sodium.
- If you have an intestinal obstruction or undiagnosed rectal bleeding.
- If you have diabetes or heart or kidney disease.
- If you are taking other laxatives.

Over age 60:
Excessive use of stimulant laxatives may cause excess loss of body fluid, resulting in weakness and lack of coordination.

Pregnancy:
Risk factors vary or may not be designated for these laxatives. Read categories on page xxiii and consult doctor.

Breast-feeding:
Some of the stimulant laxatives may pass into breast milk. Consult doctor.

Infants & children:
- Don't give to children under age 6 without doctor's approval. Young children are not able to describe their symptoms accurately, and a proper diagnosis needs to be made before starting any treatment.
- Don't give to a child who refuses to have a bowel movement (toileting refusal). May force a painful bowel movement and cause the child to hold back even more. Consult doctor.
- For children over age 6, follow package instructions or doctor's directions for correct dosage amount.

Prolonged use:
Don't take for more than 1 week unless under doctor's supervision.

Skin & sunlight:
No special problems expected.

Driving, piloting or hazardous work:
No special problems expected.

Discontinuing:
May be unnecessary to finish medicine. Follow doctor's instructions or instructions on label.

Others:
- Don't give to "flush out" the system or as a "tonic."
- Use as directed. Don't increase or decrease dosage without doctor's approval.
- Excessive use of laxatives in a teenager may indicate an eating disorder such as anorexia nervosa or bulimia nervosa. Consult doctor.
- If there is a sudden change in bowel habits or bowel function that lasts longer than 2 weeks, consult doctor.

POSSIBLE INTERACTION WITH OTHER DRUGS

GENERIC NAME OR DRUG CLASS	COMBINED EFFECT
Antacids*	Irritation of stomach or small intestine.
Diuretics, potassium-sparing*	Decreased potassium effect.
Histamine H$_2$ receptor antagonists*	Stomach irritation with bisacodyl. Take 1 hour apart.
Potassium supplements*	Decreased potassium effect.

POSSIBLE INTERACTION WITH OTHER SUBSTANCES

INTERACTS WITH	COMBINED EFFECT
Alcohol:	No special problems expected.
Beverages: Milk.	Stomach irritation with bisacodyl. Take 1 hour apart.
Cocaine:	No special problems expected.
Foods:	No special problems expected.
Marijuana:	No special problems expected.
Tobacco:	No special problems expected.

LEUCOVORIN

BRAND NAMES

Citrocovorin Calcium	Folinic Acid
Citrovorum Factor	Wellcovorin

BASIC INFORMATION

Habit forming? No
Prescription needed? Yes
Available as generic? Yes
Drug class: Antianemic

 USES

- Antidote to folic acid antagonists.
- Treats anemia.

 DOSAGE & USAGE INFORMATION

How to take:
Tablets—Swallow with liquid or food to lessen stomach irritation. If you can't swallow whole, crumble tablet and take with liquid or food.

When to take:
At the same time each day, according to instructions on prescription label.

If you forget a dose:
Take as soon as you remember up to 2 hours late. If more than 2 hours, wait for next scheduled dose (don't double this dose).

What drug does:
Favors development of DNA, RNA and protein synthesis.

Time lapse before drug works:
20 to 30 minutes.

Don't take with:
Any other medicine without consulting your doctor or pharmacist.

 OVERDOSE

SYMPTOMS:
Unlikely to threaten life. If overdose is suspected, follow instructions below.
WHAT TO DO:
- Dial 911 (emergency) or 0 (operator) for an ambulance or medical help. Then give first aid immediately.
- See emergency information on inside covers.

 POSSIBLE ADVERSE REACTIONS OR SIDE EFFECTS

SYMPTOMS	WHAT TO DO
Life-threatening:	
Wheezing.	Seek emergency treatment immediately.
Common:	
None expected.	
Infrequent:	
None expected.	
Rare:	
Skin rash, hives.	Discontinue. Call doctor right away.

WARNINGS & PRECAUTIONS

Don't take if:
• You have pernicious anemia.
• You have vitamin B-12 deficiency.

Before you start, consult your doctor:
• If you have acid urine, acites, dehydration.
• If you have kidney function impairment.

Over age 60:
Adverse reactions and side effects may be more frequent and severe than in younger persons. You may need smaller doses for shorter periods of time.

Pregnancy:
Recommended for the treatment of megalo-blastic anemia caused by pregnancy. Decide with your doctor if drug benefits justify risk to unborn child. Risk category C (see page xxiii).

Breast-feeding:
No problems expected. Consult doctor.

Infants & children:
May increase frequency of seizures. Avoid if possible.

Prolonged use:
No problems expected.

Skin & sunlight:
No problems expected.

Driving, piloting or hazardous work:
Don't drive or pilot aircraft until you learn how medicine affects you. Don't work around dangerous machinery. Don't climb ladders or work in high places. Danger increases if you drink alcohol or take medicine affecting alertness and reflexes.

Discontinuing:
Don't discontinue without consulting doctor. Dose may require gradual reduction if you have taken drug for a long time. Doses of other drugs may also require adjustment.

Others:
No problems expected.

POSSIBLE INTERACTION WITH OTHER DRUGS

GENERIC NAME OR DRUG CLASS	COMBINED EFFECT
Anticonvulsants, barbiturate and hydantoin*	Large doses of leucovorin may counteract the effects of these medicines.
Central nervous system (CNS) depressants*	High alcohol content of leucovorin may cause adverse effects.
Fluorouracil	Increased levels of fluorouracil.
Primidone	Large doses of leucovorin may counteract the effects of both drugs.

POSSIBLE INTERACTION WITH OTHER SUBSTANCES

INTERACTS WITH	COMBINED EFFECT
Alcohol:	Increased adverse reactions of both.
Beverages:	None expected.
Cocaine:	Increased adverse reactions of both drugs.
Foods:	None expected.
Marijuana:	Increased adverse reactions of both drugs.
Tobacco:	Increased adverse reactions of both.

LEUKOTRIENE MODIFIERS

GENERIC AND BRAND NAMES

MONTELUKAST
  Singulair
ZAFIRLUKAST
  Accolate

ZILEUTON
  Zyflo

BASIC INFORMATION

Habit forming? No
Prescription needed? Yes
Available as generic? No
Drug class: Antiasthmatic

 USES

Treatment of mild to moderate asthma. Not used to treat an active asthma attack. May be used with other asthma medications as directed by your doctor. Montelukast is used for prophylaxis (preventive) and chronic treatment of asthma.

 DOSAGE & USAGE INFORMATION

How to take:
* Chewable tablets—(Montelukast) cherry flavor, recommended for children 6 to 15 years old.
* Tablets—Swallow with water, with or without food, except for zafirlukast which must be taken on an empty stomach 1 hour before or 2 hours after a meal.

When to take:
* Montelukast—At the same times each day.
* Zafirlukast—Twice a day at the same times.
* Zileuton—Four times a day at the same times.

If you forget a dose:
Take as soon as you remember, up to 2 hours late. If more than 2 hours, wait for next scheduled dose. Do not double doses.

What drug does:
Inhibits inflammatory cells associated with asthma. Inhibits reflex reactions to irritants, exercise and cold.

Continued next column

 OVERDOSE

SYMPTOMS:
It is unknown what symptoms may occur.
WHAT TO DO:
If person uses much larger amount than prescribed, call doctor, poison control center or hospital emergency room for instructions.

Time lapse before drug works:
30 minutes to 4 hours.

Don't take with:
Any other prescription or nonprescription drug without consulting your doctor or pharmacist.

 POSSIBLE ADVERSE REACTIONS OR SIDE EFFECTS

SYMPTOMS	WHAT TO DO
Life-threatening: None expected.	
Common: Headache, stomach upset, nausea.	Continue. Call doctor when convenient.
Infrequent: Weak feeling, pain in abdomen, headache, unusual tiredness, cough, dental pain, dizziness, heartburn, fever, nasal congestion, skin rash.	Continue. Call doctor when convenient.
Rare: Liver problems (yellow eyes or skin, fatigue, symptoms of flu, nausea, itching, pain in upper right abdominal area).	Discontinue. Call doctor right away.

WARNINGS & PRECAUTIONS

Don't take if:
You are allergic to this medication.

Before you start, consult your doctor:
- If you have any other medical problem.
- If you have a liver or kidney disease.
- If you have a history of alcoholism.

Over age 60:
In some cases older patients taking zafirlukast experienced more infections; otherwise, no problems expected.

Pregnancy:
Decide with your doctor whether drug benefits justify risk to unborn child. Montelukast and zafirlukast—risk category B; zileuton—risk category C (see page xxiii).

Breast-feeding:
- Montelukast and zileuton—It is unknown if drug passes into milk. Avoid drug or discontinue nursing until you finish medicine. Consult doctor for advice on maintaining milk supply.
- Zafirlukast—Drug passes into milk. Avoid drug or discontinue nursing until you finish medicine.

Infants & children:
- Montelukast is approved for children 6 years and older.
- Zafirlukast is approved for children over 12 years.
- Zileuton should only be given under close supervision, especially to children under 12 years old.

Prolonged use:
Schedule regular visits with your doctor to determine if the drug continues its effectiveness in controlling asthma symptoms.

Skin & sunlight:
No problems expected.

Driving, piloting or hazardous work:
No problems expected.

Discontinuing:
Don't discontinue without consulting doctor.

Others:
- In a few rare instances, patients taking zafirlukast while having their oral steroid dosage reduced developed Churg-Strauss syndrome (a rare and sometimes fatal condition). It is not known if the problem is caused by zafirlukast. Symptoms of Churg-Strauss syndrome are similar to those caused by flu. Before starting zafirlukast and reducing oral steroids, discuss the benefits and risk factors with your doctor.
- Advise any doctor or dentist you consult that you take this medicine.

- Talk to your doctor if your asthma attacks are not being controlled by the usual dosage of your fast-acting bronchodilator.
- This drug may affect results in some medical tests.
- This drug should be taken every day, even if you are not having asthma symptoms.

POSSIBLE INTERACTION WITH OTHER DRUGS

GENERIC NAME OR DRUG CLASS	COMBINED EFFECT
Astemizole	Effect unknown. Consult doctor.
Beta adrenergic blocking agents	Increased beta blocker effect.
Calcium channel blockers	Increased effect of calcium channel blocker.
Carbamazepine	Increased effect of carbamazepine.
Cisapride	Increased effect of cisapride.
Cyclosporine	Increased effect of cyclosporine.
Erythromycin	Decreased effect of zafirlukast.
Phenobarbital	Decreased effect of montelukast.
Phenytoin	Increased effect of phenytoin.
Tolbutamide	Increased effect of tolbutamide.
Warfarin	Increased effect of warfarin.

POSSIBLE INTERACTION WITH OTHER SUBSTANCES

INTERACTS WITH	COMBINED EFFECT
Alcohol:	None expected.
Beverages:	None expected.
Cocaine:	Effects unknown. Avoid.
Foods:	None expected.
Marijuana:	Effects unknown. Avoid.
Tobacco:	None expected.

*See Glossary

LEVAMISOLE

BRAND NAMES

Ergamisol

BASIC INFORMATION

Habit forming? No
Prescription needed? Yes
Available as generic? No
Drug class: Anticancer treatment adjunct

USES

- Treats colorectal cancer when used in combination with fluorouracil.
- Treats malignant melanoma after surgical removal when there is no evidence of spread to organs other than the skin.

DOSAGE & USAGE INFORMATION

How to take:
Tablet—Swallow with liquid or food to lessen stomach irritation. If you can't swallow whole, crumble tablet and take with liquid or food.

When to take:
At the same time each day, according to instructions on prescription label.

If you forget a dose:
Don't take until you notify your doctor.

What drug does:
Acts to help restore the immune system. May activate T-cell lymphocytes and other white cells. Also elevates mood.

Time lapse before drug works:
1-1/2 to 2 hours.

Don't take with:
Any other medicine without consulting your doctor or pharmacist.

OVERDOSE

SYMPTOMS:
None expected.
WHAT TO DO:
Overdose unlikely to threaten life. If person takes much larger amount than prescribed, call doctor, poison control center or hospital emergency room for instructions.

POSSIBLE ADVERSE REACTIONS OR SIDE EFFECTS

SYMPTOMS	WHAT TO DO
Life-threatening: Fever, muscle aches, headache, cough, hoarseness, sore throat, painful or difficult urination, low back or side pain.	Seek emergency treatment.
Common: • Diarrhea, metallic taste, nausea, joint or muscle pain, skin rash, insomnia, mental depression, nightmares, sleepiness or tiredness, increased dental problems.	Continue. Call doctor when convenient.
• Hair loss.	No action necessary.
Infrequent: Mouth, tongue and lip sores.	Call doctor right away.
Rare: Unsteady gait while walking; blurred vision; confusion; tremors; tingling or numbness in hands, feet or face; seizures; smacking and puckering of lips; uncontrolled tongue movements.	Call doctor right away.

WARNINGS & PRECAUTIONS

Don't take if:
You are allergic to levamisole.

Before you start, consult your doctor:
- If you take other drugs for cancer.
- If you have an active infection.
- If you have a seizure disorder.
- If you have allergies to other medications.

Over age 60:
No special problems expected.

Pregnancy:
Adequate studies not yet done. Consult your doctor. Risk category C (see page xxiii).

Breast-feeding:
Effect unknown. Consult doctor.

Infants & children:
Effect not documented. Consult your doctor.

Prolonged use:
No special problems expected.

Skin & sunlight:
No special problems expected.

Driving, piloting or hazardous work:
No special problems expected.

Discontinuing:
Don't discontinue without consulting doctor. Dose may require gradual reduction if you have taken drug for a long time. Doses of other drugs may also require adjustment.

Others:
- Advise any doctor or dentist whom you consult that you take this medicine.
- Defer dental treatments until your blood count is normal. Pay particular attention to dental hygiene. You may be subject to additional risk of oral infection, delayed healing and bleeding.
- Avoid aspirin. May increase risk of internal bleeding.
- Avoid constipation. May increase risk of internal bleeding.

POSSIBLE INTERACTION WITH OTHER DRUGS

GENERIC NAME OR DRUG CLASS	COMBINED EFFECT
Anticoagulants*	Increased risk of bleeding.
Aspirin	Increased risk of bleeding.
Bone marrow depressants*	Increased risk of bone marrow depression.

POSSIBLE INTERACTION WITH OTHER SUBSTANCES

INTERACTS WITH	COMBINED EFFECT
Alcohol:	Increased risk of gastritis and internal bleeding.
Beverages:	None expected.
Cocaine:	Increased risk of mental disturbances. Avoid.
Foods:	None expected.
Marijuana:	None expected.
Tobacco:	None expected.

LEVOCARNITINE

BRAND NAMES

Carnitor   VitaCarn
L-Carnitine

BASIC INFORMATION

Habit forming? No
Prescription needed? Yes
Available as generic? Yes
Drug class: Nutritional supplement

 ## USES

Treats carnitine deficiency, a genetic impairment preventing normal utilization from diet.

 ## DOSAGE & USAGE INFORMATION

How to take:
- Oral solution—Take after meals with liquid to decrease stomach irritation.
- Tablets—Swallow with liquid or food to lessen stomach irritation. If you can't swallow whole, crumble tablet and take with liquid or food.
- Injection—Given by medical professional.

When to take:
Immediately following or during meals to reduce stomach irritation.

If you forget a dose:
Take as soon as you remember up to 2 hours late. If more than 2 hours, wait for next scheduled dose (don't double this dose).

What drug does:
Facilitates normal use of fat to produce energy. Dietary source is meat and milk.

Time lapse before drug works:
Immediate action.

Don't take with:
Any other medicine without consulting your doctor or pharmacist.

 ## OVERDOSE

SYMPTOMS:
Severe muscle weakness.
WHAT TO DO:
- Dial 911 (emergency) or 0 (operator) for an ambulance or medical help. Then give first aid immediately.
- See emergency information on inside covers.

 ## POSSIBLE ADVERSE REACTIONS OR SIDE EFFECTS

SYMPTOMS	WHAT TO DO
Life-threatening: None expected.	
Common: Changed body odor.	Continue. Call doctor when convenient.
Infrequent: Diarrhea, abdominal pain, nausea, vomiting.	Continue, but call doctor right away.
Rare: None expected.	

WARNINGS & PRECAUTIONS

Don't take if:
No contraindications.

Before you start, consult your doctor:
No documented reasons not to take.

Over age 60:
No problems expected.

Pregnancy:
No proven harm to unborn child, but avoid if possible. Consult doctor. Risk category B (see page xxiii).

Breast-feeding:
No problems expected. Consult doctor.

Infants & children:
No problems expected. Deficiency can cause impaired growth and development.

Prolonged use:
Talk to your doctor about the need for follow-up medical examinations or laboratory studies to check triglycerides.

Skin & sunlight:
No problems expected.

Driving, piloting or hazardous work:
No problems expected.

Discontinuing:
Don't discontinue without consulting doctor. Dose may require gradual reduction if you have taken drug for a long time. Doses of other drugs may also require adjustment.

Others:
Health food store "vitamin B-T" contains dextro- and levo-carnitine which completely negates the effectiveness of levocarnitine (L-carnitine). Only the L-carnitine form is effective in levocarnitine deficiency.

POSSIBLE INTERACTION WITH OTHER DRUGS

GENERIC NAME OR DRUG CLASS	COMBINED EFFECT
Valproic acid	Decreased levocarnitine effect. Patients taking valproic acid may need to take the supplement levocarnitine.

POSSIBLE INTERACTION WITH OTHER SUBSTANCES

INTERACTS WITH	COMBINED EFFECT
Alcohol:	None expected.
Beverages:	None expected.
Cocaine:	None expected.
Foods:	None expected.
Marijuana:	None expected.
Tobacco:	None expected.

LEVODOPA

BRAND NAMES

Dopar   Larodopa

BASIC INFORMATION

Habit forming? No
Prescription needed? Yes
Available as generic? Yes
Drug class: Antiparkinsonism

USES

Controls Parkinson's disease symptoms such as rigidity, tremor and unsteady gait.

DOSAGE & USAGE INFORMATION

How to take:
Tablet or capsule—Swallow with liquid or food to lessen stomach irritation. If you can't swallow whole, crumble tablet or open capsule and take with liquid or food.

When to take:
At the same times each day.

If you forget a dose:
Take as soon as you remember up to 2 hours late. If more than 2 hours, wait for next scheduled dose (don't double this dose).

What drug does:
Restores chemical balance necessary for normal nerve impulses.

Continued next column

OVERDOSE

SYMPTOMS:
Muscle twitch, spastic eyelid closure, nausea, vomiting, diarrhea, irregular and rapid pulse, weakness, fainting, confusion, agitation, hallucination, coma.
WHAT TO DO:
- **Dial 911 (emergency) or 0 (operator) for an ambulance or medical help. Then give first aid immediately.**
- **If patient is unconscious and not breathing, give mouth-to-mouth breathing. If there is no heartbeat, use cardiac massage and mouth-to-mouth breathing (CPR). Don't try to make patient vomit. If you can't get help quickly, take patient to nearest emergency facility.**
- **See emergency information on inside covers.**

Time lapse before drug works:
2 to 3 weeks to improve; 6 weeks or longer for maximum benefit.

Don't take with:
Any other medication without consulting your doctor or pharmacist.

POSSIBLE ADVERSE REACTIONS OR SIDE EFFECTS

SYMPTOMS	WHAT TO DO
Life-threatening:	
In case of overdose, see previous column.	
Common:	
• Mood change, diarrhea, depression, anxiety.	Continue. Call doctor when convenient.
• Dry mouth, body odor.	No action necessary.
• Uncontrollable body movements.	Discontinue. Call doctor right away.
Infrequent:	
• Fainting, severe dizziness, headache, insomnia, nightmares, itchy skin, rash, nausea, vomiting, irregular heartbeat, eyelid spasm.	Discontinue. Call doctor right away.
• Flushed face, muscle twitching, discolored or dark urine, difficult urination, blurred vision, appetite loss.	Continue. Call doctor when convenient.
• Constipation, tiredness.	Continue. Tell doctor at next visit.
Rare:	
• High blood pressure.	Discontinue. Call doctor right away.
• Upper abdominal pain, anemia, increased sex drive.	Continue. Call doctor when convenient.

WARNINGS & PRECAUTIONS

Don't take if:
- You are allergic to levodopa or carbidopa.
- You have taken a monoamine oxidase (MAO) inhibitor* in past 2 weeks.
- You have glaucoma (narrow-angle type).

Before you start, consult your doctor:
- If you have diabetes or epilepsy.
- If you have had high blood pressure, heart or lung disease.
- If you have had liver or kidney disease.
- If you have a peptic ulcer.
- If you have malignant melanoma.

- If you will have surgery within 2 months, including dental surgery, requiring general or spinal anesthesia.

Over age 60:
Adverse reactions and side effects may be more frequent and severe than in younger persons.

Pregnancy:
Decide with your doctor if drug benefits justify risk to unborn child. Risk category C (see page xxiii).

Breast-feeding:
Drug filters into milk. May harm child. Avoid.

Infants & children:
Not recommended.

Prolonged use:
- May lead to uncontrolled movements of head, face, mouth, tongue, arms or legs.
- Talk to your doctor about the need for follow-up medical examinations or laboratory studies to check complete blood counts (white blood cell count, platelet count, red blood cell count, hemoglobin, hematocrit), kidney function, liver function.

Skin & sunlight:
No problems expected.

Driving, piloting or hazardous work:
Don't drive or pilot aircraft until you learn how medicine affects you. Don't work around dangerous machinery. Don't climb ladders or work in high places. Danger increases if you drink alcohol or take medicine affecting alertness and reflexes, such as antihistamines, tranquilizers, sedatives, pain medicine, narcotics and mind-altering drugs.

Discontinuing:
Don't discontinue without doctor's advice until you complete prescribed dose, even though symptoms diminish or disappear.

Others:
Expect to start with small dose and increase gradually to lessen frequency and severity of adverse reactions.

POSSIBLE INTERACTION WITH OTHER DRUGS

GENERIC NAME OR DRUG CLASS	COMBINED EFFECT
Albuterol	Increased risk of heartbeat irregularity.
Antidepressants, tricyclic (TCA)*	Decreased blood pressure. Weakness and faintness when arising from bed or chair.
Anticonvulsants hydantoin*	Decreased levodopa effect.
Antihypertensives*	Decreased blood pressure and levodopa effect.
Antiparkinsonism drugs, other*	Increased levodopa effect.
Bupropion	Increased levodopa effect.
Guanfacine	Increased effects of both drugs.
Haloperidol	Decreased levodopa effect.
MAO inhibitors*	Dangerous rise in blood pressure.
Methyldopa	Decreased levodopa effect.
Molindone	Decreased levodopa effect.
Olanzapine	May decrease levodopa effect.
Papaverine	Decreased levodopa effect.
Phenothiazines*	Decreased levodopa effect.
Phenytoin	Decreased levodopa effect.
Pyridoxine (Vitamin B-6)	Decreased levodopa effect.
Rauwolfia alkaloids*	Decreased levodopa effect.
Selegiline	May require reduced dosage of levodopa.

POSSIBLE INTERACTION WITH OTHER SUBSTANCES

INTERACTS WITH	COMBINED EFFECT
Alcohol:	None expected.
Beverages:	None expected.
Cocaine:	Increased risk of heartbeat irregularity.
Foods: High-protein diet.	Decreased levodopa effect.
Marijuana:	Increased fatigue, lethargy, fainting.
Tobacco:	None expected.

LEVONORGESTREL

BRAND NAMES

Norplant

BASIC INFORMATION

Habit forming? No
Prescription needed? Yes
Available as generic? No
Drug class: Female sex hormone (progestin)

 USES

Highly effective long-term reversible contraceptive method.

 DOSAGE & USAGE INFORMATION

How to take:
Administered by means of implants consisting of six flexible closed capsules (about the size of matchsticks) that are inserted beneath the skin on the inside of the upper arm. Implantation is done by a health-care professional within seven days of the start of the last menstrual period. The drug slowly diffuses into the bloodstream, delivering a nearly constant level of levonorgestrel to the body for up to 5 years.

When to take:
Implanted when long-term (up to 5 years) contraception is desired.

If you forget a dose:
Not a concern.

What drug does:
Inhibits ovulation so that eggs are not produced regularly. Causes the mucus of the cervix to thicken, preventing the sperm from reaching the egg if one is produced.

Time lapse before drug works:
24 hours

Don't take with:
Any other medicine without consulting your doctor or pharmacist.

 OVERDOSE

SYMPTOMS:
None expected.

 POSSIBLE ADVERSE REACTIONS OR SIDE EFFECTS

SYMPTOMS	WHAT TO DO
Life-threatening: None expected.	
Common: Increased, decreased, irregular or prolonged menstruation; spotting between periods.	Call doctor when convenient.
Infrequent: Headache, acne.	Call doctor when convenient.
Rare: • Severe bleeding, infection with pus at implant site, vaginal infection.	Call doctor right away.
• Swelling, numbness, discoloration or tenderness at implant site; breast discharge or tenderness; weight gain or loss; excess hair growth; hair loss from scalp; nausea; dizziness; muscle or abdominal pain; appetite changes; nervousness; depression.	Call doctor when convenient.

WARNINGS & PRECAUTIONS

Don't take if:
- You are allergic to any progestin hormone.
- You are or suspect you might be pregnant.
- You have liver disease or liver tumors.
- You have unexplained vaginal bleeding.
- You have breast cancer.
- You have now, or have a history of, blood clots in the legs, lungs or eyes.

Before you start, consult your doctor:
- If you have a condition that could be aggravated by fluid retention.
- If you have a history of depression or emotional disorders.

Over age 60:
Not recommended.

Pregnancy:
If pregnancy occurs, the capsules should be removed. Risk category X (see page xxiii).

Breast-feeding:
Drug passes into milk. Consult your doctor about the advisability of breast-feeding.

Infants & children:
Not recommended.

Prolonged use:
- No problems expected.
- Capsules should be removed at end of five years. New capsules may be implanted if continuing contraception is desired.

Skin & sunlight:
No problems expected.

Driving, piloting or hazardous work:
No problems expected.

Discontinuing:
- Must be removed by a health-care professional.
- May be removed at your request at any time for any reason.
- Removal should be considered if you will be immobile for a long time due to illness or surgery.

Others:
- Review patient information booklet before you have Norplant implanted. You will be given a form to sign indicating you have received information on the risks and benefits of the implants.
- May affect results of some medical tests.
- Does not protect against sexually transmitted diseases. For additional protection, couples may also use condoms and/or spermicidal agents.
- Fertility returns shortly after implants are removed, usually within two weeks.
- Have blood pressure checked by your doctor 3 months after implant.

 POSSIBLE INTERACTION WITH OTHER DRUGS

GENERIC NAME OR DRUG CLASS	COMBINED EFFECT
Phenytoin	Decreased contraceptive effect.
Carbamazepine	Decreased contraceptive effect.
Barbiturates*	Decreased contraceptive effect.
Phenylbutazone	Decreased contraceptive effect.
Isoniazid	Decreased contraceptive effect.
Rifampin	Decreased contraceptive effect.

 POSSIBLE INTERACTION WITH OTHER SUBSTANCES

INTERACTS WITH	COMBINED EFFECT
Alcohol:	None expected.
Beverages:	None expected.
Cocaine:	None expected.
Foods:	None expected.
Marijuana:	None expected.
Tobacco:	None expected, but consult doctor.

LINCOMYCIN

BRAND NAMES

Lincocin

BASIC INFORMATION

Habit forming? No
Prescription needed? Yes
Available as generic? Yes
Drug class: Antibacterial

 ## USES

Treatment of bacterial infections that are susceptible to lincomycin.

 ## DOSAGE & USAGE INFORMATION

How to take:
Capsule—Swallow with liquid 1 hour before or 2 hours after eating. Drink 8 ounces of water with each dose.

When to take:
At the same times each day.

If you forget a dose:
Take as soon as you remember up to 2 hours late. If more than 2 hours, wait for next scheduled dose (don't double this dose).

What drug does:
Destroys susceptible bacteria. Does not kill viruses.

Time lapse before drug works:
3 to 5 days.

Don't take with:
Any other medication without consulting your doctor or pharmacist.

 ## OVERDOSE

SYMPTOMS:
Severe nausea, vomiting, diarrhea.
WHAT TO DO:
Overdose unlikely to threaten life. If person takes much larger amount than prescribed, call doctor, poison control center or hospital emergency room for instructions.

 ## POSSIBLE ADVERSE REACTIONS OR SIDE EFFECTS

SYMPTOMS	WHAT TO DO
Life-threatening:	
Hives, wheezing, faintness, itching, coma.	Seek emergency treatment.
Common:	
Bloating	Discontinue. Call doctor right away.
Infrequent:	
• Unusual thirst; vomiting; stomach cramps; severe and watery diarrhea with blood or mucus; painful, swollen joints; jaundice; fever; tiredness; weakness; weight loss.	Discontinue. Call doctor right away.
• Itch around groin, rectum or armpits; white patches in mouth; vaginal discharge, itching.	Continue. Call doctor when convenient.
Rare:	
Skin rash.	Discontinue. Call doctor right away.

WARNINGS & PRECAUTIONS

Don't take if:
- You are allergic to lincomycins.
- You have had ulcerative colitis.
- Prescribed for infant under 1 month old.

Before you start, consult your doctor:
- If you have had yeast infections of mouth, skin or vagina.
- If you will have surgery within 2 months, including dental surgery, requiring general or spinal anesthesia.
- If you have kidney or liver disease.
- If you have allergies of any kind.

Over age 60:
Adverse reactions and side effects may be more frequent and severe than in younger persons.

Pregnancy:
Decide with your doctor if drug benefits justify risk to unborn child. Risk category C (see page xxiii).

Breast-feeding:
Drug passes into milk. Avoid drug or discontinue nursing until you finish medicine. Consult doctor for advice on maintaining milk supply.

Infants & children:
Don't give to infants younger than 1 month. Use for children only under medical supervision.

Prolonged use:
- Severe colitis with diarrhea and bleeding.
- You may become more susceptible to infections caused by germs not responsive to lincomycin.
- Talk to your doctor about the need for follow-up medical examinations or laboratory studies to check proctosigmoidoscopy.

Skin & sunlight:
No problems expected.

Driving, piloting or hazardous work:
No problems expected.

Discontinuing:
Don't discontinue without doctor's advice until you complete prescribed dose, even though symptoms diminish or disappear.

Others:
May interfere with the accuracy of some medical tests.

POSSIBLE INTERACTION WITH OTHER DRUGS

GENERIC NAME OR DRUG CLASS	COMBINED EFFECT
Antidiarrheal preparations*	Decreased lincomycin effect.
Attapulgite	May decrease effectiveness of lincomycin.
Chloramphenicol	Decreased lincomycin effect.
Erythromycins*	Decreased lincomycin effect.
Narcotics*	Increased risk of respiratory problems.

POSSIBLE INTERACTION WITH OTHER SUBSTANCES

INTERACTS WITH	COMBINED EFFECT
Alcohol:	None expected.
Beverages:	None expected.
Cocaine:	None expected.
Foods:	None expected.
Marijuana:	None expected.
Tobacco:	None expected.

LITHIUM

BRAND NAMES

Carbolith	Lithane
Cibalith-S	Lithizine
Duralith	Lithobid
Eskalith	Lithonate
Eskalith CR	Lithotabs

BASIC INFORMATION

Habit forming? No
Prescription needed? Yes
Available as generic? Yes
Drug class: Mood stabilizer

 ## USES

- Normalizes mood and behavior in bipolar (manic-depressive) disorder.
- Treats alcohol toxicity and addiction.
- Treats schizoid personality disorders.

 ## DOSAGE & USAGE INFORMATION

How to take:
- Tablet or capsule—Swallow with liquid or food to lessen stomach irritation. If you can't swallow whole, crumble tablet or open capsule and take with liquid or food. Drink 2 or 3 quarts liquid per day, especially in hot weather.
- Extended-release tablets—Swallow each dose whole. Do not crush.
- Syrup—Take at mealtime. Follow with 8 oz. water.

When to take:
At the same times each day, preferably at mealtime.

If you forget a dose:
Take as soon as you remember up to 2 hours late. If more than 2 hours, wait for next scheduled dose (don't double this dose).

Continued next column

 ## OVERDOSE

SYMPTOMS:
Moderate overdose increases some side effects and may cause diarrhea, nausea. Large overdose may cause vomiting, muscle weakness, convulsions, stupor and coma.
WHAT TO DO:
- **Dial 911 (emergency) or 0 (operator) for an ambulance or medical help. Then give first aid immediately.**
- **See emergency information at end of book.**

What drug does:
May correct chemical imbalance in brain's transmission of nerve impulses that influence mood and behavior.

Time lapse before drug works:
1 to 3 weeks. May require 3 months before depressive phase of illness improves.

Don't take with:
Any other medication without consulting your doctor or pharmacist.

 ## POSSIBLE ADVERSE REACTIONS OR SIDE EFFECTS

SYMPTOMS	WHAT TO DO
Life-threatening:	
In case of overdose, see previous column.	
Common:	
• Dizziness, diarrhea, nausea, vomiting, shakiness, tremor.	Continue. Call doctor when convenient.
• Dry mouth, thirst, decreased sexual ability, increased urination, anorexia.	Continue. Tell doctor at next visit.
Infrequent:	
• Rash, stomach pain, fainting, heartbeat irregularities, shortness of breath, ear noises.	Discontinue. Call doctor right away.
• Swollen hands, feet; slurred speech; thyroid impairment (coldness; dry, puffy skin; muscle aches; headache; weight gain; fatigue; menstrual irregularities, acnelike eruptions.	Continue. Call doctor when convenient.
• Drowsiness, confusion, weakness.	Continue. Tell doctor at next visit.
Rare:	
• Blurred vision, eye pain.	Discontinue. Call doctor right away.
• Jerking of arms and legs, worsening of psoriasis, hair loss.	Continue. Call doctor when convenient.

 ## WARNINGS & PRECAUTIONS

Don't take if:
- You are allergic to lithium or tartrazine dye.
- You have kidney or heart disease.
- Patient is younger than 12.

Before you start, consult your doctor:
- About all medications you take.
- If you plan to become pregnant within medication period.

LOMUSTINE

BRAND NAMES

CCNU   CeeNU

BASIC INFORMATION

Habit forming? No
Prescription needed? Yes
Available as generic? No
Drug class: Antineoplastic

 USES

- Treats brain cancer and Hodgkin's lymphoma.
- Sometimes used to treat breast, lung, skin and gastrointestinal cancer.

 DOSAGE & USAGE INFORMATION

How to take:
Capsules—Swallow with liquid. If you can't swallow whole, open capsule and take with liquid or food. Instructions to take on empty stomach mean 1 hour before or 2 hours after eating. Note: There may be two or more different types of capsules in the container. This is not an error.

When to take:
According to doctor's instructions. Usual course of treatment requires single dosage repeated every 6 weeks.

If you forget a dose:
Take as soon as you remember. Don't ever double doses.

What drug does:
Interferes with growth of cancer cells.

Time lapse before drug works:
None. Works immediately.

Don't take with:
Any other medicines (including over-the-counter drugs such as cough and cold medicines, laxatives, antacids, diet pills, caffeine, nose drops or vitamins) without consulting your doctor

 OVERDOSE

SYMPTOMS:
Decreased urine (kidney failure); high fever, chills (infection); bloody or black stools (bleeding).
WHAT TO DO:
- **Dial 911 (emergency) or 0 (operator) for an ambulance or medical help. Then give first aid immediately.**
- **See emergency information on inside covers.**

 POSSIBLE ADVERSE REACTIONS OR SIDE EFFECTS

SYMPTOMS	WHAT TO DO
Life-threatening:	
In case of overdose, see previous column.	
Common:	
• Fever, chills, difficult urination, unusual bleeding.	Continue. Call doctor when convenient.
• Appetite loss, nausea, hair loss.	No action necessary.
Infrequent:	
• Anemia, confusion, slurred speech, mouth sores, skin rash.	Continue. Call doctor when convenient.
• Darkened skin.	No action necessary.
Rare:	
• Jaundice (yellow skin and eyes), cough.	Continue. Call doctor when convenient.
• Shortness of breath.	Discontinue. Call doctor right away.

WARNINGS & PRECAUTIONS

Don't take if:
- You have chicken pox.
- You have shingles (herpes zoster).

Before you start, consult your doctor:
- If you have an infection.
- If you have kidney disease.
- If you have had previous cancer chemotherapy or radiation treatment.

Over age 60:
Adverse reactions and side effects may be more frequent and severe than in younger persons. You may need smaller doses for shorter periods of time.

Pregnancy:
Risk to unborn child outweighs drug benefits. Don't use. Risk category D (see page xxiii).

Breast-feeding:
Drug passes into milk. Avoid drug or discontinue nursing until you finish medicine. Consult doctor for advice on maintaining milk supply.

Infants & children:
Effect not documented. Consult your doctor.

Prolonged use:
Talk to your doctor about the need for follow-up medical examinations or laboratory studies to check kidney function, liver function and complete blood counts (white blood cell count, platelet count, red blood cell count, hemoglobin, hematocrit).

Skin & sunlight:
No problems expected.

Driving, piloting or hazardous work:
Don't drive or pilot aircraft until you learn how medicine affects you. Don't work around dangerous machinery. Don't climb ladders or work in high places. Danger increases if you drink alcohol or take medicine affecting alertness and reflexes.

Discontinuing:
Call doctor if any of these occur after discontinuing: black or tarry stools, bloody urine, hoarseness, bleeding or bruising, fever or chills.

Others:
- Advise any doctor or dentist whom you consult that you take this medicine.
- May affect results in some medical tests.
- Most adverse reactions and side effects are unavoidable.
- Avoid immunizations, if possible.
- Avoid persons with infections.
- Check with doctor about brushing or flossing teeth.
- Avoid contact sports.

POSSIBLE INTERACTION WITH OTHER DRUGS

GENERIC NAME OR DRUG CLASS	COMBINED EFFECT
Antineoplastic drugs, other*	Increased chance of drug toxicity.
Blood dyscrasia-causing medicines*	Adverse effect on bone marrow, causing decreased white cells and platelets.
Bone marrow depressants*, other	Increased risk of bone marrow depression.
Clozapine	Toxic effect on bone marrow.
Levamisole	Increased risk of bone marrow depression.
Tiopronin	Increased risk of toxicity to bone marrow.
Vaccines, live or killed virus	Increased chance of toxicity or reduced effectiveness of vaccine. Wait 3 to 12 months after lomustine treatment before getting vaccination.

POSSIBLE INTERACTION WITH OTHER SUBSTANCES

INTERACTS WITH	COMBINED EFFECT
Alcohol:	Increased chance of liver damage.
Beverages:	No special problems expected.
Cocaine:	Increased chance of central nervous system toxicity.
Foods:	No special problems expected.
Marijuana:	No special problems expected.
Tobacco:	No special problems expected.

*See Glossary

LOPERAMIDE

BRAND NAMES

Apo-Loperamide
  Caplets
Imodium
Imodium A-D
Imodium Advanced

Kaopectate II
  Caplets
Pepto Diarrhea
  Control

BASIC INFORMATION

Habit forming? No, unless taken in high
  doses for long periods.
Prescription needed? Yes, for some
Available as generic? Yes
Drug class: Antidiarrheal

USES

- Treats mild to moderate diarrhea. Used in
  conjunction with fluids, appropriate diet and
  rest. Treats symptoms only. Does not cure any
  disorder that causes diarrhea.
- Treats chronic diarrhea associated with
  inflammatory bowel disease.

DOSAGE & USAGE INFORMATION

How to take:
- Tablet or capsule—Swallow with food to
  lessen stomach irritation.
- Liquid—Follow label instructions and use
  marked dropper.

When to take:
No more often than directed on label.

If you forget a dose:
Take as soon as you remember up to 2 hours
late. If more than 2 hours, wait for next
scheduled dose (don't double this dose).

What drug does:
Blocks digestive tract's nerve supply, which
reduces irritability and contractions in intestinal
tract.

Continued next column

OVERDOSE

SYMPTOMS:
Constipation, lethargy, drowsiness or
unconsciousness.
WHAT TO DO:
Overdose unlikely to threaten life. If person
takes much larger amount than prescribed,
call doctor, poison control center or hospital
emergency room for instructions.

Time lapse before drug works:
1 to 2 hours.

Don't take with:
Any other medication without consulting your
doctor or pharmacist.

POSSIBLE ADVERSE REACTIONS OR SIDE EFFECTS

SYMPTOMS	WHAT TO DO
Life-threatening: None expected.	
Common: None expected.	
Infrequent: None expected.	
Rare:	
• Drowsiness, dizziness, dry mouth.	Continue. Call doctor when convenient.
• Nausea, vomiting, bloating, constipation, appetite loss, rash, abdominal pain.	Discontinue. Call doctor right away.

WARNINGS &
PRECAUTIONS

Don't take if:
- You have severe colitis.
- You have colitis resulting from antibiotic treatment or infection.
- You are allergic to loperamide.

Before you start, consult your doctor:
- If you are dehydrated from fluid loss caused by diarrhea.
- If you have liver disease.

Over age 60:
Adverse reactions and side effects may be more frequent and severe than in younger persons.

Pregnancy:
No proven harm. Avoid if possible. Consult doctor. Risk category B (see page xxiii).

Breast-feeding:
No proven problems, but avoid if possible or discontinue nursing until you finish medicine. Consult doctor for advice on maintaining milk supply.

Infants & children:
Don't give to infants or toddlers. Use only under doctor's supervision for children older than 2.

Prolonged use:
Habit forming at high dose.

Skin & sunlight:
No problems expected.

Driving, piloting or hazardous work:
Don't drive or pilot aircraft until you learn how medicine affects you. Don't work around dangerous machinery. Don't climb ladders or work in high places. Danger increases if you drink alcohol or take medicine affecting alertness and reflexes.

Discontinuing:
- May be unnecessary to finish medicine. Follow doctor's instructions.
- After discontinuing, consult doctor if you experience muscle cramps, nausea, vomiting, trembling, stomach cramps or unusual sweating.

Others:
If acute diarrhea lasts longer than 48 hours, discontinue and call doctor. In chronic diarrhea, loperamide is unlikely to be effective if diarrhea doesn't improve in 10 days.

 POSSIBLE INTERACTION
WITH OTHER DRUGS

GENERIC NAME OR DRUG CLASS	COMBINED EFFECT
Antibiotics*	Increased risk of diarrhea.
Narcotic analgesics	Increased risk of severe constipation.

 POSSIBLE INTERACTION
WITH OTHER SUBSTANCES

INTERACTS WITH	COMBINED EFFECT
Alcohol:	Depressed brain function. Avoid.
Beverages:	None expected.
Cocaine:	Decreased loperamide effect.
Foods:	None expected.
Marijuana:	None expected.
Tobacco:	None expected.

LORACARBEF

BRAND NAMES

Lorabid

BASIC INFORMATION

Habit forming? No
Prescription needed? Yes
Available as generic? No
Drug class: Antibacterial

 ## USES

Treatment for bacterial infections of the upper respiratory tract, lower respiratory tract, urinary tract, skin and skin structure.

 ## DOSAGE & USAGE INFORMATION

How to take:
- Capsule—Swallow with liquid. If you can't swallow whole, open capsule and take with liquid. Instructions to take on an empty stomach mean 1 hour before or 2 hours after eating.
- Oral suspension—Follow label instructions for mixing the powder with water. Instructions to take on an empty stomach mean 1 hour before or 2 hours after eating.

When to take:
At the same times each day.

If you forget a dose:
Take as soon as you remember up to 2 hours late. If more than 2 hours, wait for next scheduled dose (don't double this dose).

What drug does:
Kills bacteria susceptible to loracarbef.

Time lapse before drug works:
May require several days to affect infection.

Don't take with:
Any other prescription or nonprescription drug without consulting your doctor.

 ## OVERDOSE

SYMPTOMS:
Nausea, vomiting, diarrhea or abdominal cramps.
WHAT TO DO:
Overdose unlikely to threaten life. If person takes much larger amount than prescribed, call doctor, poison control center or hospital emergency room for instructions.

 ## POSSIBLE ADVERSE REACTIONS OR SIDE EFFECTS

SYMPTOMS	WHAT TO DO
Life-threatening: Hives, rash, intense itching, faintness soon after a dose (anaphylaxis); difficulty in breathing.	Seek emergency treatment immediately.
Common: Abdominal pain, diarrhea, nausea and vomiting, loss of appetite	Continue. Call doctor when convenient.
Infrequent: Itching, skin rash.	Discontinue. Call doctor right away.
Rare: Dizziness, drowsiness, insomnia, nervousness, vaginal itching and discharge.	Continue. Call doctor when convenient.

WARNINGS & PRECAUTIONS

Don't take if:
You are allergic to loracarbef, penicillins* or cephalosporins*.

Before you start, consult your doctor:
• If you have kidney disease.
• If you have a history of colitis.

Over age 60:
Adverse reactions and side effects may be more frequent and severe than in younger persons. You may need smaller doses for shorter periods of time.

Pregnancy:
Consult doctor. Risk category B (see page xxiii)

Breast-feeding:
Effect not documented. Consult your doctor.

Infants & children:
Not recommended for patients under 6 months of age.

Prolonged use:
• Kills beneficial bacteria that protect body against other germs. Unchecked germs may cause secondary infections
• Talk to your doctor about the need for follow-up medical examinations or laboratory studies.

Skin & sunlight:
No problems expected.

Driving, piloting or hazardous work:
Avoid if you feel dizzy or drowsy. Otherwise, no problems expected.

Discontinuing:
Don't discontinue without doctor's advice until you complete prescribed dose, even though symptoms diminish or disappear.

Others:
• Advise any doctor or dentist whom you consult that you take this medicine.
• May affect the results in some medical tests.

POSSIBLE INTERACTION WITH OTHER DRUGS

GENERIC NAME OR DRUG CLASS	COMBINED EFFECT
Probenecid	Increased loracarbef effect.

POSSIBLE INTERACTION WITH OTHER SUBSTANCES

INTERACTS WITH	COMBINED EFFECT
Alcohol:	None expected.
Beverages:	None expected.
Cocaine:	None expected.
Foods:	None expected.
Marijuana:	None expected.
Tobacco:	None expected.

LOXAPINE

BRAND NAMES

Loxapac   Loxitane C
Loxitane

BASIC INFORMATION

Habit forming? No
Prescription needed? Yes
Available as generic? Yes
Drug class: Tranquilizer, antidepressant

 ## USES

- Treats serious mental illness.
- Treats anxiety and depression.

 ## DOSAGE & USAGE INFORMATION

How to take:
- Oral solution—Take after meals with liquid to decrease stomach irritation.
- Tablets—Swallow with liquid or food to lessen stomach irritation. If you can't swallow whole, crumble tablet and take with liquid or food.
- Capsules—Swallow with liquid or food to lessen stomach irritation. If you can't swallow whole, open capsule and take with liquid or food.

When to take:
At the same times each day, according to instructions on prescription label.

If you forget a dose:
Take as soon as you remember up to 2 hours late. If more than 2 hours, wait for next scheduled dose (don't double this dose).

What drug does:
Probably blocks the effects of dopamine* in the brain.

Time lapse before drug works:
1/2 to 3 hours.

Don't take with:
Any other medicine without consulting your doctor or pharmacist.

 ## OVERDOSE

SYMPTOMS:
Dizziness, drowsiness, severe shortness of breath, muscle spasms, coma.
WHAT TO DO:
- **Dial 911 (emergency) or 0 (operator) for an ambulance or medical help. Then give first aid immediately.**
- **See emergency information at end of book.**

 ## POSSIBLE ADVERSE REACTIONS OR SIDE EFFECTS

SYMPTOMS	WHAT TO DO
Life-threatening:	
Severe shortness of breath, skin rash, heartbeat irregularities, profuse sweating, fever, convulsions (rare).	Seek emergency treatment immediately.
Common:	
• Increased dental problems because of dry mouth and less salivation.	Consult your dentist about a prevention program.
• Swallowing difficulty, expressionless face, stiff arms and legs, dizziness.	Discontinue. Call doctor right away.
Infrequent:	
• Chewing movements with lip smacking, loss of balance, shuffling walk, tremor of fingers and hands, uncontrolled tongue movements.	Discontinue. Call doctor right away.
• Constipation, difficult urination, blurred vision, confusion, loss of sex drive, headache, insomnia, menstrual irregularities, weight gain, light sensitivity, nausea.	Continue. Call doctor when convenient.
Rare:	
Rapid heartbeat, fever, sore throat, jaundice, unusual bleeding.	Discontinue. Call doctor right away.

 ## WARNINGS & PRECAUTIONS

Don't take if:
- You are an alcoholic.
- You have liver disease.

Before you start, consult your doctor:
- If you have a seizure disorder.
- If you have an enlarged prostate, glaucoma, Parkinson's disease, heart disease.

Over age 60:
Adverse reactions and side effects may be more frequent and severe than in younger persons. You may need smaller doses for shorter periods of time.

Pregnancy:
Decide with your doctor if drug benefits justify risk to unborn child. Risk category C (see page xxiii).

Breast-feeding:
Drug may pass into milk. Avoid drug or discontinue nursing until you finish medicine. Consult doctor for advice on maintaining milk supply.

Infants & children:
Not recommended.

Prolonged use:
Talk to your doctor about the need for follow-up medical examinations or laboratory studies to check complete blood counts (white blood cell count, platelet count, red blood cell count, hemoglobin, hematocrit), liver function, eyes.

Skin & sunlight:
May cause rash or intensify sunburn in areas exposed to sun or ultraviolet light (photosensitivity reaction). Avoid overexposure and use sunscreen. Notify doctor if reaction occurs.

Driving, piloting or hazardous work:
Don't drive or pilot aircraft until you learn how medicine affects you. Don't work around dangerous machinery. Don't climb ladders or work in high places. Danger increases if you drink alcohol or take medicine affecting alertness and reflexes.

Discontinuing:
- Don't discontinue without consulting doctor. Dose may require gradual reduction if you have taken drug for a long time. Doses of other drugs may also require adjustment.
- These symptoms may occur after medicine has been discontinued: dizziness; nausea; abdominal pain; uncontrolled movements of mouth, tongue and jaw.

Others:
Use careful oral hygiene.

POSSIBLE INTERACTION WITH OTHER DRUGS

GENERIC NAME OR DRUG CLASS	COMBINED EFFECT
Anticonvulsants*	Decreased effect of anticonvulsant.
Antidepressants, tricyclic*	May increase toxic effects of both drugs.
Bupropion	Increased risk of seizures.
Central nervous system (CNS) depressants*	Increased sedative effects of both drugs.
Clozapine	Toxic effect on the central nervous system.
Epinephrine	Rapid heart rate and severe drop in blood pressure.

Extrapyramidal reaction*-causing drugs	Increased risk of side effects.
Fluoxetine	Increased depressant effects of both drugs.
Guanadrel	Decreased effect of guanadrel.
Guanethidine	Decreased effect of guanethidine.
Guanfacine	Increased effects of both drugs.
Haloperidol	May increase toxic effects of both drugs.
Leucovorin	High alcohol content of leucovorin may cause adverse effects.
Methyldopa	May increase toxic effects of both drugs.
Metoclopramide	May increase toxic effects of both drugs.
Molindone	May increase toxic effects of both drugs.
Pemoline	Increased central nervous stimulation.
Pergolide	Decreased pergolide effect.
Phenothiazines*	May increase toxic effects of both drugs.
Pimozide	May increase toxic effects of both drugs.

Continued on page 919

POSSIBLE INTERACTION WITH OTHER SUBSTANCES

INTERACTS WITH	COMBINED EFFECT
Alcohol:	May decrease effect of loxapine. Avoid.
Beverages:	None expected.
Cocaine:	May increase toxicity of both drugs. Avoid.
Foods:	None expected.
Marijuana:	May increase toxicity of both drugs. Avoid.
Tobacco:	May increase toxicity.

*See Glossary

MACROLIDE ANTIBIOTICS

GENERIC AND BRAND NAMES

AZITHROMYCIN
  Zithromax
CLARITHROMYCIN
  Biaxin

DIRITHROMYCIN
  Dynabac

BASIC INFORMATION

Habit forming? No
Prescription needed? Yes
Available as generic? No
Drug class: Antibiotic (macrolide),
  antibiotic (erythromycin)

USES

Treatment for mild to moderate bacterial infections responsive to macrolide antibiotics. These include bronchitis, tonsillitis, some pneumonias, ear infections, skin infections (e.g., acne), sinusitis, streptococcal sore throat, urethritis and others. Note: Erythromycin is also a macrolide antibiotic. See individual chart for information.

DOSAGE & USAGE INFORMATION

How to take:
- Enteric-coated tablet or delayed release tablet—Swallow with liquid. Do not crush or chew tablet.
- Tablet or capsule—Swallow with liquid. If you can't swallow whole, crumble tablet or open capsule and take with food or water.
- Oral suspension—Swallow with liquid.

When to take:
At the same time each day. Take azithromycin on an empty stomach, 1 hour before or 2 hours after a meal. Clarithromycin may be taken with or without food. Take dirithromycin with food or within 1 hour after eating.

Continued next column

OVERDOSE

SYMPTOMS:
Possibly diarrhea, nausea, vomiting, abdominal pain.
WHAT TO DO:
Overdose unlikely to threaten life. If person takes much larger amount than prescribed, call doctor, poison control center or hospital emergency room for instructions.

If you forget a dose:
Take as soon as you remember. If it is almost time for the next dose, wait for that dose (don't double this dose) and resume regular schedule.

What drug does:
Prevents growth and reproduction of susceptible bacteria.

Time lapse before drug works:
Usually 2 to 5 days. Some infections may require 10 days or longer of therapy to resolve.

Don't take with:
Any other prescription or nonprescription drug without consulting your doctor or pharmacist.

POSSIBLE ADVERSE REACTIONS OR SIDE EFFECTS

SYMPTOMS	WHAT TO DO
Life-threatening:	
Rare allergic reaction—Breathing difficulty; swelling of hands, feet, face, mouth, neck; skin rash; temporary deafness.	Discontinue. Seek emergency treatment.
Common:	
None expected.	
Infrequent:	
Nausea, vomiting, abdominal discomfort, diarrhea.	Continue. Call doctor when convenient.
Rare:	
• Headache, dizziness.	Continue. Call doctor when convenient.
• Allergic reaction (skin rash, itching).	Discontinue. Call right away.

WARNINGS & PRECAUTIONS

Don't take if:
You are allergic to macrolide antibiotics.

Before you start, consult your doctor:
- If you have impaired liver or kidney function.
- If you are allergic to any medication, food or other substance.

Over age 60:
No special problems expected.

Pregnancy:
Risk factors vary for drugs in this group. See page xxiii and consult doctor.

Breast-feeding:
One or more of these drugs may pass into milk. Avoid drug or discontinue nursing until you finish medicine. Consult doctor for advice on maintaining milk supply.

Infants & children:
Give only under close medical supervision to those under age 12. Young children may not complain or recognize adverse effects of drug. Observe child closely for any reactions

Prolonged use:
Not recommended. Medicine is discontinued once the infection is cured.

Skin & sunlight:
No special problems expected.

Driving, piloting or hazardous work:
Avoid if you experience dizziness. Otherwise, no problems expected.

Discontinuing:
Don't discontinue without doctor's advice until you complete prescribed dose, even though symptoms diminish or disappear.

Others:
- Advise any doctor or dentist whom you consult that you take this medicine.
- May affect the results of some medical tests.

POSSIBLE INTERACTION WITH OTHER DRUGS

GENERIC NAME OR DRUG CLASS	COMBINED EFFECT
Antacids*, aluminum- or magnesium-containing	Take one hour apart.
Astemizole	May increase risk of heart rhythm problems.
Benzodiazepines	Increased effect of benzodiazepine.
Bromocriptine	Increased effect of bromocriptine.
Carbamazepine	Increased effect of carbamazepine.
Cyclosporine	Increased effect of cyclosporine.
Digoxin	Increased effect of digoxin.
Disopyramide	Unknown effect. Use with caution.
Histamine H₂ receptor antagonists*	Increased effect of antibiotic.
Lovastatin	Unknown effect. Use with caution.
Rifabutin	Decreased effect of antibiotic.
Rifampin	Decreased effect of antibiotic.
Tacrolimus	Increased effect of tacrolimus.
Theophylline	Increased effect of theophylline.
Triazolam	Increased risk of toxicity.
Warfarin	Increased risk of bleeding.
Zidovudine	Decreased effect of zidovudine.

POSSIBLE INTERACTION WITH OTHER SUBSTANCES

INTERACTS WITH	COMBINED EFFECT
Alcohol:	No proven problems.
Beverages:	No proven problems.
Cocaine:	No proven problems.
Foods:	No proven problems.
Marijuana:	No proven problems.
Tobacco:	No proven problems.

MAPROTILINE

BRAND NAMES

Ludiomil

BASIC INFORMATION

Habit forming? No
Prescription needed? Yes
Available as generic? Yes
Drug class: Antidepressant

 USES

Treatment for depression or anxiety associated with depression.

 DOSAGE & USAGE INFORMATION

How to take:
Tablet—Swallow with liquid.

When to take:
At the same time each day, usually bedtime.

If you forget a dose:
Bedtime dose—If you forget your once-a-day bedtime dose, don't take it more than 3 hours late. If more than 3 hours, wait for next scheduled dose. Don't double this dose.

What drug does:
Probably affects part of brain that controls messages between nerve cells.

Time lapse before drug works:
Begins in 1 to 2 weeks. May require 4 to 6 weeks for maximum benefit.

Continued next column

 OVERDOSE

SYMPTOMS:
Respiratory failure, fever, cardiac arrhythmia, muscle stiffness, drowsiness, hallucinations, convulsions, coma.
WHAT TO DO:
- **Dial 911 (emergency) or 0 (operator) for an ambulance or medical help. Then give first aid immediately.**
- **If patient is unconscious and not breathing, give mouth-to-mouth breathing. If there is no heartbeat, use cardiac massage and mouth-to-mouth breathing (CPR). Don't try to make patient vomit. If you can't get help quickly, take patient to nearest emergency facility.**
- **See emergency information at end of book.**

Don't take with:
Nonprescription drugs without consulting your doctor or pharmacist.

 POSSIBLE ADVERSE REACTIONS OR SIDE EFFECTS

SYMPTOMS	WHAT TO DO
Life-threatening: Seizures.	Seek emergency treatment immediately.
Common:	
• Tremor.	Discontinue. Call doctor right away.
• Headache, dry mouth or unpleasant taste, constipation or diarrhea, nausea, indigestion, fatigue, weakness, drowsiness, nervousness, anxiety, excessive sweating.	Continue. Call doctor when convenient.
• Insomnia, craving sweets.	Continue. Tell doctor at next visit.
Infrequent:	
• Hallucinations, shakiness, dizziness, fainting, blurred vision, eye pain, vomiting, irregular heartbeat or slow pulse, inflamed tongue, abdominal pain, jaundice, hair loss, rash, chills, joint pain, palpitations, hiccups, vision changes.	Discontinue. Call doctor right away.
• Painful or difficult urination; fatigue; decreased sex drive; abnormal dreams; nasal congestion; back pain; muscle aches; frequent urination; painful, absent or irregular menstruation.	Continue. Call doctor when convenient.
Rare: Itchy skin; sore throat; jaundice; fever; involuntary movements of jaw, lips and tongue; nightmares; confusion; swollen breasts in men.	Discontinue. Call doctor right away.

WARNINGS & PRECAUTIONS

Don't take if:
- You are allergic to tricyclic antidepressants.
- You drink alcohol.
- You have had a heart attack within 6 weeks.
- You have glaucoma.
- You have taken a monoamine oxidase (MAO) inhibitor* within 2 weeks.

Before you start, consult your doctor:
- If you will have surgery within 2 months, including dental surgery, requiring general or spinal anesthesia.
- If you have an enlarged prostate, heart disease or high blood pressure, stomach or intestinal problems, overactive thyroid, asthma, liver disease, schizophrenia, urinary retention, respiratory disorders, seizure disorders, diabetes, kidney disease.

Over age 60:
More likely to develop urination difficulty and side effects such as hallucinations, shakiness, dizziness, fainting, headache or insomnia.

Pregnancy:
Consult doctor. Risk category B (see page xxiii).

Breast-feeding:
Drug passes into milk. Avoid drug or discontinue nursing until you finish medicine. Consult doctor for advice on maintaining milk supply.

Infants & children:
Don't give to children younger than 12.

Prolonged use:
Request blood cell counts, liver function studies; monitor blood pressure closely.

Skin & sunlight:
May cause rash or intensify sunburn in areas exposed to sun or ultraviolet light (photosensitivity reaction). Avoid overexposure and use sunscreen. Notify doctor if reaction occurs.

Driving, piloting or hazardous work:
Don't drive or pilot aircraft until you learn how medicine affects you. Don't work around dangerous machinery. Don't climb ladders or work in high places. Danger increases if you drink alcohol or take medicine affecting alertness and reflexes.

Discontinuing:
Don't discontinue without consulting doctor. Dose may require gradual reduction if you have taken drug for a long time. Doses of other drugs may also require adjustment.

Others:
- Advise any doctor or dentist whom you consult that you take this drug.
- For dry mouth, suck sugarless hard candy or chew sugarless gum. If dry mouth persists, consult your dentist.

POSSIBLE INTERACTION WITH OTHER DRUGS

GENERIC NAME OR DRUG CLASS	COMBINED EFFECT
Anticholinergics*	Increased sedation.
Antihistamines*	Increased antihistamine effect.
Barbiturates*	Decreased anti-depressant effect.
Benzodiazepines*	Increased sedation.
Bupropion	Increased risk of seizures.
Central nervous system (CNS) depressants*	Increased sedation.
Cimetidine	Possible increased antidepressant effect and toxicity.
Clonidine	Decreased clonidine effect.
Clozapine	Toxic effect on the central nervous system.
Disulfiram	Delirium.
Diuretics, thiazide*	Increased maprotiline effect.
Ethchlorvynol	Delirium.
Fluoxetine	Increased depressant effects of both drugs.

Continued on page 919

POSSIBLE INTERACTION WITH OTHER SUBSTANCES

INTERACTS WITH	COMBINED EFFECT
Alcohol: Beverages or medicines with alcohol.	Excessive intoxication. Avoid.
Beverages:	None expected.
Cocaine:	Excessive intoxication. Avoid.
Foods:	None expected.
Marijuana:	Excessive drowsiness. Avoid.
Tobacco:	May decrease absorption of maprotiline. Avoid.

MASOPROCOL

BRAND NAMES

Actinex

BASIC INFORMATION

Habit forming? No
Prescription needed? Yes
Available as generic? No
Drug class: Antineoplastic (topical)

 ## USES

Treats actinic keratoses (scaly, flat or slightly raised skin lesions).

 ## DOSAGE & USAGE INFORMATION

How to take:
Cream—Wash and dry the skin where lesions are located. Massage cream into affected area. Wash hands immediately after use.

When to take:
Use at the same times each day.

If you forget a dose:
Apply as soon as you remember, then resume regular schedule.

What drug does:
Selectively destroys actively proliferating cells.

Time lapse before drug works:
1 to 2 months.

Don't take with:
Other topical prescription or nonprescription drugs without consulting your doctor.

 ## OVERDOSE

SYMPTOMS:
None reported.
WHAT TO DO:
Not for internal use. If child accidently swallows, call poison control center.

 ## POSSIBLE ADVERSE REACTIONS OR SIDE EFFECTS

SYMPTOMS	WHAT TO DO
Life-threatening: None expected.	
Common:	
• Redness and swelling of otherwise normal skin.	Discontinue. Call doctor right away.
• Skin reactions including itching, redness, dryness, flaking where medicine applied.	Continue. Call doctor when convenient.
• Temporary burning sensation right after application.	No action necessary.
Infrequent:	
• Allergic reaction to sulfites—bluish skin, severe dizziness, faintness, wheezing, breathing difficulty.	Discontinue. Seek emergency help.
• Swelling, soreness, persistent burning in treated area.	Continue. Call doctor when convenient.
Rare:	
Bleeding, oozing, blistering skin.	Discontinue. Call doctor right away.

WARNINGS & PRECAUTIONS

Don't take if:
You are allergic to masoprocol.

Before you start, consult your doctor:
If you have a sulfite sensitivity.

Over age 60:
No problems expected.

Pregnancy:
Consult doctor. Risk category B (see page xxiii).

Breast-feeding:
Effect not documented. Consult your doctor.

Infants & children:
Not used in this age group.

Prolonged use:
Effects of long-term use unknown. Visit doctor on a regular basis to determine effectiveness of treatment.

Skin & sunlight:
Drug does not cause sensitivity to sunlight. However, keratoses are related to sun exposure, so avoid sunlight when possible.

Driving, piloting or hazardous work:
No problems expected.

Discontinuing:
No problems expected.

Others:
- If you accidently get masoprocol in your eye, promptly wash the eye with water.
- The cream may stain your clothing.
- Get doctor's approval before using cosmetics or make-up on the skin area you are treating.
- Leave the treated skin areas exposed. Don't cover them with a bandage or a dressing.

POSSIBLE INTERACTION WITH OTHER DRUGS

GENERIC NAME OR DRUG CLASS	COMBINED EFFECT
None significant.	

POSSIBLE INTERACTION WITH OTHER SUBSTANCES

INTERACTS WITH	COMBINED EFFECT
Alcohol:	None expected.
Beverages:	None expected.
Cocaine:	None expected.
Foods:	None expected.
Marijuana:	None expected.
Tobacco:	None expected.

MECAMYLAMINE

BRAND NAMES

Inversine

BASIC INFORMATION

Habit forming? No
Prescription needed? Yes
Available as generic? No
Drug class: Antihypertensive

 USES

Helps control, but doesn't cure, high blood pressure.

 DOSAGE & USAGE INFORMATION

How to take:
Tablets—Swallow with liquid. If you can't swallow whole, crumble tablet and take with liquid or food. Instructions to take on empty stomach mean 1 hour before or 2 hours after eating.

When to take:
* At the same time each day, according to instructions on prescription label.
* Usually twice a day, every 8 or 12 hours apart. Follow label directions.

If you forget a dose:
Take as soon as you remember up to 2 hours late. If more than 2 hours, wait for next scheduled dose (don't double this dose).

What drug does:
Blocks transmission of electrical impulse where two nerve cells connect. Causes constricted blood vessels to relax.

Time lapse before drug works:
30 minutes to 2 hours.

Don't take with:
Any other medicines (including over-the-counter drugs such as cough and cold medicines, laxatives, antacids, diet pills, caffeine, nose drops or vitamins) without consulting your doctor.

 OVERDOSE

SYMPTOMS:
Confusion, excitement, seizures, coma.
WHAT TO DO:
* Dial 911 (emergency) or 0 (operator) for an ambulance or medical help. Then give first aid immediately.
* See emergency information on inside covers.

 POSSIBLE ADVERSE REACTIONS OR SIDE EFFECTS

SYMPTOMS	WHAT TO DO
Life-threatening:	
In case of overdose, see previous column.	
Common:	
Dizziness upon arising from chair or bed, blurred vision, decreased sex drive, dry mouth, enlarged pupils, constipation.	Continue. Call doctor when convenient.
Infrequent:	
• Confusion, depression, tremors, shortness of breath.	Discontinue. Call doctor right away.
• Difficult urination, tiredness.	Continue. Tell doctor at next visit.
Rare:	
Appetite loss, nausea and vomiting.	Continue. Tell doctor at next visit.

WARNINGS & PRECAUTIONS

Don't take if:
You are allergic to mecamylamine.

Before you start, consult your doctor:
- If you have heart disease.
- If you had a recent heart attack.
- If you have glaucoma or gout.
- If you have kidney disease.

Over age 60:
Adverse reactions and side effects may be more frequent and severe than in younger persons. You may need smaller doses for shorter periods of time.

Pregnancy:
Decide with your doctor if drug benefits justify risk to unborn child. Risk category C (see page xxiii).

Breast-feeding:
Effect unknown. Consult doctor.

Infants & children:
Effect not documented. Consult your pediatrician.

Prolonged use:
Talk to your doctor about the need for follow-up medical examinations or laboratory studies to check blood pressure, kidney function and heart function.

Skin & sunlight:
No problems expected.

Driving, piloting or hazardous work:
Avoid if you feel confused, drowsy or dizzy.

Discontinuing:
Don't discontinue without consulting doctor. Dose may require gradual reduction if you have taken drug for a long time. Doses of other drugs may also require adjustment.

Others:
- Advise any doctor or dentist whom you consult that you take this medicine.
- May affect results in some medical tests.
- Get up slowly from chair or bed.
- Dosage may need to be adjusted for hot weather or heavy exercise.

POSSIBLE INTERACTION WITH OTHER DRUGS

GENERIC NAME OR DRUG CLASS	COMBINED EFFECT
Ambenonium	Swallowing difficulty.
Antacids*	Prolonged effect of mecamylamine.
Antibiotics*	Decreased antibiotic effect.
Alkalizers, urine*	Prolonged effect of mecamylamine.
Neostigmine	Swallowing difficulty.
Nimodipine	Dangerous blood pressure drop.
Pyridostigmine	Swallowing difficulty.
Sodium bicarbonate	Increased mecamylamine effect.
Sulfa drugs*	Decreased antibiotic effect.

POSSIBLE INTERACTION WITH OTHER SUBSTANCES

INTERACTS WITH	COMBINED EFFECT
Alcohol:	Increased likelihood of fainting.
Beverages:	No special problems expected.
Cocaine:	Increased central nervous system stimulation. Avoid.
Foods: Food with high salt or sodium.	Decreased effectiveness of mecamylamine.
Marijuana:	Increased central nervous system stimulation. Avoid.
Tobacco:	No special problems expected.

MECHLORETHAMINE (Topical)

BRAND NAMES

Mustargen

BASIC INFORMATION

Habit forming? No
Prescription needed? Yes
Available as generic? No
Drug class: Antineoplastic (topical)

 ## USES

- Treats mycosis fungoides.
- Treats other malignancies (by injection).

 ## DOSAGE & USAGE INFORMATION

How to use:
- Solution—Mix according to doctor's instructions. Don't inhale vapors or powder.
- Shower and rinse before treatment.
- Use rubber gloves to apply over entire body.
- Avoid contact with eyes, nose and mouth.
- Ointment—Use according to doctor's instructions.

When to use:
Usually once a day.

If you forget a dose:
Notify your doctor.

What drug does:
Destroys cells that produce mycosis fungoides.

Time lapse before drug works:
None. Works immediately.

Don't use with:
Any other medicines (including over-the-counter drugs such as cough and cold medicines, laxatives, antacids, diet pills, caffeine, nose drops or vitamins) without consulting your doctor.

 ## OVERDOSE

SYMPTOMS:
None expected for topical solutions.
WHAT TO DO:
Not intended for internal use. If child accidentally swallows, call poison control center.

 ## POSSIBLE ADVERSE REACTIONS OR SIDE EFFECTS

SYMPTOMS	WHAT TO DO
Life-threatening: Immediate hives, shortness of breath.	Seek emergency treatment immediately.
Common: Darkening, dry skin.	Continue. Tell doctor at next visit.
Infrequent: Allergic reaction with rash, itching, hives.	Seek emergency treatment immediately.
Rare: None expected.	

WARNINGS & PRECAUTIONS

Don't use if:
You are allergic to mechlorethamine.

Before you start, consult your doctor:
- If you have chicken pox.
- If you have shingles (herpes zoster).
- If you have skin infection.

Over age 60:
No special problems expected.

Pregnancy:
Risk to unborn child outweighs drug benefits. Don't use. Risk category D (see page xxiii).

Breast-feeding:
Drug may be absorbed and pass into milk. Avoid drug or discontinue nursing until you finish medicine. Consult doctor for advice on maintaining milk supply.

Infants & children:
Effect unknown. Consult doctor.

Prolonged use:
- Allergic or hypersensitive reactions more likely.
- Talk to your doctor about the need for follow-up medical examinations or laboratory studies to check liver function, complete blood counts (white blood cell count, platelet count, red blood cell count, hemoglobin, hematocrit) and hearing tests.

Skin & sunlight:
No problems expected.

Driving, piloting or hazardous work:
Don't drive or pilot aircraft until you learn how medicine affects you. Don't work around dangerous machinery. Don't climb ladders or work in high places. Danger increases if you drink alcohol or take medicine affecting alertness and reflexes.

Discontinuing:
No special problems expected.

Others:
- Advise any doctor or dentist whom you consult that you take this medicine.
- May affect results in some medical tests.
- Don't use if solution is discolored.

POSSIBLE INTERACTION WITH OTHER DRUGS

GENERIC NAME OR DRUG CLASS	COMBINED EFFECT
None significant.	

POSSIBLE INTERACTION WITH OTHER SUBSTANCES

INTERACTS WITH	COMBINED EFFECT
Alcohol:	None expected.
Beverages:	None expected.
Cocaine:	None expected.
Foods:	None expected.
Marijuana:	None expected.
Tobacco:	None expected.

MECLIZINE

BRAND NAMES

Antivert	Dramamine II
Antivert/25	D-Vert 15
Antivert/50	D-Vert 30
Bonamine	Meni-D
Bonine	Ru-Vert-M

BASIC INFORMATION

Habit forming? No
Prescription needed?
U.S.: No, for some
Canada: Yes
Available as generic? Yes
Drug class: Antihistamine, antiemetic, anti-motion sickness

 ## USES

- Prevents motion sickness.
- Treatment for vertigo.

 ## DOSAGE & USAGE INFORMATION

How to take:
- Tablet or capsule—Swallow with liquid or food to lessen stomach irritation. If you can't swallow whole, crumble tablet or open capsule and take with liquid or food.
- Chewable tablet—May be chewed, swallowed whole or mixed with food.

When to take:
30 minutes to 1 hour before traveling or as directed by doctor.

If you forget a dose:
Take as soon as you remember. Wait 4 hours for next dose.

What drug does:
Reduces sensitivity of nerve endings in inner ear, blocking messages to brain's vomiting center.

Continued next column

 ## OVERDOSE

SYMPTOMS:
Drowsiness, confusion, incoordination, stupor, coma, weak pulse, shallow breathing, hallucinations.
WHAT TO DO:
- **Dial 911 (emergency) or 0 (operator) for an ambulance or medical help. Then give first aid immediately.**
- **See emergency information on inside covers.**

Time lapse before drug works:
30 to 60 minutes.

Don't take with:
Any other medicine without consulting your doctor or pharmacist.

 ## POSSIBLE ADVERSE REACTIONS OR SIDE EFFECTS

SYMPTOMS	WHAT TO DO
Life-threatening:	
In case of overdose, see previous column.	
Common:	
Drowsiness.	Continue. Tell doctor at next visit.
Infrequent:	
• Headache, diarrhea or constipation, fast heartbeat.	Continue. Call doctor when convenient.
• Dry mouth, nose, throat.	Continue. Tell doctor at next visit.
Rare:	
• Rash, hives.	Discontinue. Call doctor right away.
• Restlessness, excitement, insomnia, blurred vision, frequent and difficult urination, hallucinations.	Continue. Call doctor when convenient.
• Appetite loss, nausea.	Continue. Tell doctor at next visit.

 ## WARNINGS & PRECAUTIONS

Don't take if:
- You are allergic to meclizine, buclizine or cyclizine.
- You have taken a monoamine oxidase (MAO) inhibitor* in the past 2 weeks.

Before you start, consult your doctor:
- If you have glaucoma.
- If you have prostate enlargement.
- If you have reacted badly to any antihistamine.

Over age 60:
Adverse reactions and side effects may be more frequent and severe than in younger persons, especially impaired urination from enlarged prostate gland.

Pregnancy:
Consult doctor. Risk category B (see page xxiii).

Breast-feeding:
Drug passes into milk. Avoid drug or discontinue nursing until you finish medicine. Consult doctor for advice on maintaining milk supply.

MECLIZINE

Infants & children:
Safety not established. Avoid if under age 12.

Prolonged use:
No problems expected.

Skin & sunlight:
No problems expected.

Driving, piloting or hazardous work:
Don't fly aircraft. Don't drive until you learn how medicine affects you. Don't work around dangerous machinery. Don't climb ladders or work in high places. Danger increases if you drink alcohol or take medicine affecting alertness and reflexes, such as antihistamines, tranquilizers, sedatives, pain medicine, narcotics and mind-altering drugs.

Discontinuing:
No problems expected.

Others:
Some products contain tartrazine dye. Avoid, especially if you are allergic to aspirin.

 POSSIBLE INTERACTION WITH OTHER DRUGS

GENERIC NAME OR DRUG CLASS	COMBINED EFFECT
Amphetamines*	May decrease drowsiness caused by meclizine.
Anticholinergics*	Increased effect of both drugs.
Antidepressants, tricyclic*	Increased effect of both drugs.
Carteolol	Decreased antihistamine effect.
Cisapride	Decreased meclizine effect.
Clozapine	Toxic effect on the central nervous system.
Dronabinol	Increases meclizine effect.
Ethinamate	Dangerous increased effects of ethinamate. Avoid combining.
Fluoxetine	Increased depressant effects of both drugs.
Guanfacine	May increase depressant effects of either drug.
Leucovorin	High alcohol content of leucovorin may cause adverse effects.
Methyprylon	Increased sedative effect, perhaps to dangerous level. Avoid.
Monoamine oxidase (MAO) inhibitors*	Increased meclizine effect.
Nabilone	Greater depression of central nervous system.
Narcotics*	Increased effect of both drugs.
Pain relievers*	Increased effect of both drugs.
Sedatives*	Increased effect of both drugs.
Sertraline	Increased depressive effects of both drugs.
Sleep inducers*	Increased effect of both drugs.
Sotalol	Increased antihistamine effect.
Tranquilizers*	Increased effect of both drugs.

 POSSIBLE INTERACTION WITH OTHER SUBSTANCES

INTERACTS WITH	COMBINED EFFECT
Alcohol:	Increased sedation. Avoid.
Beverages: Caffeine drinks.	May decrease drowsiness.
Cocaine:	None expected.
Foods:	None expected.
Marijuana:	Increased drowsiness, dry mouth.
Tobacco:	None expected.

*See Glossary

513

MELATONIN

BRAND NAMES

Numerous brand names are available

BASIC INFORMATION

Habit forming? No
Prescription needed? No
Available as generic? Yes
Drug class: Hormone

 ## USES

- Melatonin is a hormone produced in the human body by the pineal gland and secreted at night. In most people, the melatonin levels are highest during the normal hours of sleep. The levels increase rapidly in the late evening, peaking after midnight and decreasing toward morning.
- Jet lag: Some research studies have shown that taking melatonin before a flight and continuing for a few days after arrival at the destination helped control jet lag symptoms of fatigue and sleep disturbances. Appears to work best after plane trips that crossed more than six time zones. Timing of doses very important for effectiveness.
- Insomnia and restless leg syndrome: Some research studies have shown that taking melatonin about 2 hours before bedtime decreased the time needed to fall asleep and improved quality of sleep (less wakefulness).
- Other claims that it can slow aging, fight disease, and enhance one's sex life have been less studied and more difficult to prove.

 ## DOSAGE & USAGE INFORMATION

How to take:
For tablet or capsule—Follow instructions on the label or consult your doctor or pharmacist. Different brands supply different doses. Melatonin, as a product, is marketed as a dietary supplement and is not reviewed by the U.S. Food & Drug Administration (FDA) for effectiveness and safety. The melatonin products being sold are made

Continued next column

 ## OVERDOSE

SYMPTOMS:
It is unknown what symptoms may occur.
WHAT TO DO:
If person takes much larger amount than prescribed, call doctor, poison control center or hospital emergency room for instructions.

from animal pineal glands or synthesized. The best dosage amounts are unknown. Use with caution.

When to take:
At the same time each day according to label directions. It is recommended that melatonin be taken at night before bedtime.

If you forget a dose:
Follow label instructions for your particular brand of melatonin. Usually you can take a medication as soon as you remember up to 2 hours late. If more than 2 hours, wait for the next scheduled dose (don't double this dose).

What drug does:
- Glands in the body make chemicals called hormones and release them into the bloodstream. Hormones taken as supplements also end up in the bloodstream. In either case, the blood then carries hormones to different parts of the body. There, hormones influence the way organs and tissues work.
- Hormone supplements may not have the same effects on the body as naturally produced hormones have, because the body processes them differently. Higher doses of supplements may result in higher amounts of hormones in the blood than are healthy.

Time lapse before drug works:
Effectiveness will vary from person to person and will also depend on the reason for taking melatonin.

Don't take with:
Any prescription or nonprescription medicine without consulting your doctor or pharmacist.

 ## POSSIBLE ADVERSE REACTIONS OR SIDE EFFECTS

SYMPTOMS	WHAT TO DO
Life-threatening: None expected.	
Common: Unknown.	
Infrequent: Drowsiness, confusion, headache or grogginess may occur the following morning.	Reduce dosage or discontinue taking.
Rare: Unknown. If symptoms occur that you are concerned about, talk to your doctor or pharmacist. Further research may uncover other side effects.	

WARNINGS & PRECAUTIONS

Don't use if:
You are allergic to melatonin.

Before you start, consult your doctor:
- If you have any chronic health problem.
- If you have high blood pressure (hypertension) or cardiovascular disease. Some studies in animals suggest that melatonin may constrict blood vessels (a condition that could be dangerous for people with these conditions).
- If you are allergic to any medication, food or other substance.

Over age 60:
A lower starting dosage is often recommended until a response is determined.

Pregnancy:
Melatonin is not recommended for pregnant women. Decide with your doctor if drug benefits justify risk to unborn child. Risk category is unknown since melatonin is not regulated by the FDA (see page xxiii).

Breast-feeding:
It is unknown if drug passes into milk. Avoid drug or discontinue nursing until you finish medicine. Consult doctor for advice on maintaining milk supply.

Infants & children:
Not recommended for children.

Prolonged use:
Effects are unknown. More research is needed to determine long-term effects of melatonin use.

Skin & sunlight:
No problems expected.

Driving, piloting or hazardous work:
Since it causes drowsiness, don't drive or pilot aircraft until you learn how medicine affects you. Don't work around dangerous machinery. Don't climb ladders or work in high places. Danger increases if you drink alcohol or take medicine affecting alertness and reflexes.

Discontinuing:
No problems expected.

Others:
- Advise any doctor or dentist whom you consult that you take melatonin.
- Melatonin is not researched carefully as yet, but there does not appear to be any particular problems. Some studies are promising as to its effect on health.
- Before starting melatonin, talk to your doctor about your sleep problems or try other things that can help sleep, such as avoidance of caffeine, chocolate, and especially, alcohol in any amount.

POSSIBLE INTERACTION WITH OTHER DRUGS

GENERIC NAME OR DRUG CLASS	COMBINED EFFECT
All medications	Effects are unknown. Talk to your doctor or pharmacist.

POSSIBLE INTERACTION WITH OTHER SUBSTANCES

INTERACTS WITH	COMBINED EFFECT
Alcohol:	Disrupts the night-time melatonin effect. Avoid.
Beverages:	No special problems expected.
Cocaine:	Problems not known. Best to avoid.
Foods:	No special problems expected.
Marijuana:	Problems not known. Best to avoid.
Tobacco:	Smoking can disrupt your normal melatonin cycle. Avoid.

MELPHALAN

BRAND NAMES

Alkeran
L-PAM

Phenylalanine
Mustard

BASIC INFORMATION

Habit forming? No
Prescription needed? Yes
Available as generic? No
Drug class: Antineoplastic

 ## USES

- Treatment for some kinds of cancer.
- Suppresses immune response after organ transplantation and in immune disorders.

 ## DOSAGE & USAGE INFORMATION

How to take:
Tablet—Swallow with liquid after light meal. Don't drink fluids with meals. Drink extra fluids between meals. Avoid sweet or fatty foods.

When to take:
At the same time each day.

If you forget a dose:
Take as soon as you remember. Don't ever double dose.

What drug does:
Inhibits abnormal cell reproduction. May suppress immune system.

Continued next column

 ## OVERDOSE

SYMPTOMS:
Bleeding, chills, fever, collapse, stupor, seizure.
WHAT TO DO:
- **Dial 911 (emergency) or 0 (operator) for an ambulance or medical help. Then give first aid immediately.**
- **If patient is unconscious and not breathing, give mouth-to-mouth breathing. If there is no heartbeat, use cardiac massage and mouth-to-mouth breathing (CPR). Don't try to make patient vomit. If you can't get help quickly, take patient to nearest emergency facility.**
- **See emergency information on inside covers.**

Time lapse before drug works:
Up to 6 weeks for full effect.

Don't take with:
Any other medicine without consulting your doctor or pharmacist.

 ## POSSIBLE ADVERSE REACTIONS OR SIDE EFFECTS

SYMPTOMS	WHAT TO DO
Life-threatening:	
In case of overdose, see previous column.	
Common:	
• Unusual bleeding or bruising, mouth sores with sore throat, chills and fever, black stools, sores in mouth and lips, back pain.	Continue, but call doctor right away.
• Hair loss, joint pain, menstrual. irregularities.	Continue. Call doctor when convenient.
• Nausea, vomiting, diarrhea (unavoidable), tiredness, weakness.	Continue. Tell doctor at next visit.
Infrequent:	
• Skin rash.	Continue, but call doctor right away.
• Mental confusion, shortness of breath.	Continue. Call doctor when convenient.
• Cough.	Continue. Tell doctor at next visit.
Rare:	
Jaundice, swelling in feet or legs.	Continue, but call doctor right away.

WARNINGS & PRECAUTIONS

Don't take if:
- You have had hypersensitivity to alkylating antineoplastic drugs.
- Your physician has not explained serious nature of your medical problem and risks of taking this medicine.

Before you start, consult your doctor:
- If you have gout.
- If you have had kidney stones.
- If you have active infection.
- If you have impaired kidney or liver function.
- If you have taken other antineoplastic drugs or had radiation treatment in last 3 weeks.
- If you have herpes zoster or chicken pox (or been exposed).

Over age 60:
Adverse reactions and side effects may be more frequent and severe than in younger persons.

Pregnancy:
Consult doctor. Risk category D (see page xxiii).

Breast-feeding:
Safety not established. Consult doctor.

Infants & children:
Use only under special medical supervision at center experienced in anticancer drugs.

Prolonged use:
- Adverse reactions more likely the longer drug is required.
- Talk to your doctor about the need for follow-up medical examinations or laboratory studies to check complete blood counts (white blood cell count, platelet count, red blood cell count, hemoglobin, hematocrit), kidney function.

Skin & sunlight:
No problems expected.

Driving, piloting or hazardous work:
No problems expected.

Discontinuing:
Don't discontinue without doctor's advice until you complete prescribed dose, even though symptoms diminish or disappear. Some side effects may follow discontinuing. Report to doctor blurred vision, convulsions, confusion, persistent headache, fever or chills, blood in urine, unusual bleeding.

Others:
- May cause sterility.
- May increase chance of developing leukemia.

POSSIBLE INTERACTION WITH OTHER DRUGS

GENERIC NAME OR DRUG CLASS	COMBINED EFFECT
Antigout drugs*	Decreased antigout effect.
Antineoplastic drugs, other*	Increased effect of all drugs (may be beneficial).
Bone marrow depressants*	Increased risk of bone marrow toxicity.
Chloramphenicol	Increased likelihood of toxic effects of both drugs.
Clozapine	Toxic effect on bone marrow.
Lovastatin	Increased heart and kidney damage.
Probenecid	Increased likelihood of bone marrow toxicity.
Sulfinpyrazone	Increased likelihood of bone marrow toxicity.
Tiopronin	Increased risk of toxicity to bone marrow.
Vaccines, live or killed	Increased likelihood of toxicity or reduced effectiveness of vaccine.

POSSIBLE INTERACTION WITH OTHER SUBSTANCES

INTERACTS WITH	COMBINED EFFECT
Alcohol:	May increase chance of intestinal bleeding.
Beverages:	No problems expected.
Cocaine:	Increases chance of toxicity.
Foods:	Reduces irritation in stomach.
Marijuana:	No problems expected.
Tobacco:	Increases lung toxicity.

MEPROBAMATE

BRAND NAMES

See complete list of brand names in the *Generic and Brand Name Directory*, page 885.

BASIC INFORMATION

Habit forming? Yes
Prescription needed? Yes
Available as generic? Yes
Drug class: Tranquilizer, antianxiety agent

 ## USES

Reduces mild anxiety, tension and insomnia.

 ## DOSAGE & USAGE INFORMATION

How to take:
- Tablet—Swallow with liquid.
- Extended-release capsules—Swallow each dose whole.

When to take:
At the same times each day.

If you forget a dose:
Take as soon as you remember up to 2 hours late. If more than 2 hours, wait for next scheduled dose (don't double this dose).

What drug does:
Sedates brain centers that control behavior and emotions.

Time lapse before drug works:
1 to 2 hours.

Don't take with:
- Nonprescription drugs containing alcohol or caffeine without consulting doctor.
- Any other medicine without consulting your doctor or pharmacist.

 ## OVERDOSE

SYMPTOMS:
Dizziness, slurred speech, stagger, confusion, depressed breathing and heart function, stupor, coma.
WHAT TO DO:
- **Dial 911 (emergency) or 0 (operator) for an ambulance or medical help. Then give first aid immediately.**
- **See emergency information at end of book.**

 ## POSSIBLE ADVERSE REACTIONS OR SIDE EFFECTS

SYMPTOMS	WHAT TO DO
Life-threatening: Hives, rash, intense itching, faintness soon after a dose, wheezing (anaphylaxis).	Seek emergency treatment immediately.
Common: Dizziness, confusion, agitation, drowsiness, unsteadiness, fatigue, weakness.	Continue. Tell doctor at next visit.
Infrequent: • Rash, hives, itchy skin; change in vision; diarrhea, nausea or vomiting.	Discontinue. Call doctor right away.
• False sense of well-being, headache, slurred speech, blurred vision.	Continue. Call doctor when convenient.
Rare: Sore throat; fever; rapid, pounding, unusually slow or irregular heartbeat; difficult breathing; unusual bleeding or bruising.	Discontinue. Call doctor right away.

MEPROBAMATE

 ## WARNINGS & PRECAUTIONS

Don't take if:
- You are allergic to meprobamate, tybamate, carbromal or carisoprodol.
- You have had porphyria.
- Patient is younger than 6.

Before you start, consult your doctor:
- If you have epilepsy.
- If you have impaired liver or kidney function.
- If you have tartrazine dye allergy.
- If you suffer from drug abuse or alcoholism, active or in remission.
- If you have porphyria.

Over age 60:
Adverse reactions and side effects may be more frequent and severe than in younger persons.

Pregnancy:
Risk to unborn child outweighs drug benefits. Don't use. Risk category D (see page xxiii).

Breast-feeding:
Drug filters into milk. May cause sedation in child. Avoid.

Infants & children:
Not recommended.

Prolonged use:
- Habit forming.
- May impair blood cell production.

Skin & sunlight:
No problems expected.

Driving, piloting or hazardous work:
Don't drive or pilot aircraft until you learn how medicine affects you. Don't work around dangerous machinery. Don't climb ladders or work in high places. Danger increases if you drink alcohol or take medicine affecting alertness and reflexes, such as antihistamines, tranquilizers, sedatives, pain medicine, narcotics and mind-altering drugs.

Discontinuing:
Don't discontinue without consulting doctor. Dose may require gradual reduction if you have taken drug for a long time. Doses of other drugs may also require adjustment. Report to your doctor any unusual symptom that begins in the first week you discontinue this medicine. These symptoms may include convulsions, confusion, nightmares, insomnia.

Others:
- Advise any doctor or dentist whom you consult that you take this drug.
- For dry mouth, suck sugarless hard candy or sugarless gum. If dry mouth persists, consult your dentist.

 ## POSSIBLE INTERACTION WITH OTHER DRUGS

GENERIC NAME OR DRUG CLASS	COMBINED EFFECT
Addictive drugs*	Increased risk of addictive effect.
Antidepressants, tricyclic*	Increased antidepressant effect.
Antihistamines*	Possible excessive sedation.
Central nervous system (CNS) depressants*	Increased depressive effects of both drugs.
Monoamine oxidase (MAO) inhibitors*	Increased meprobamate effect.
Narcotics*	Increased narcotic effect.
Sertraline	Increased depressive effects of both drugs.

 ## POSSIBLE INTERACTION WITH OTHER SUBSTANCES

INTERACTS WITH	COMBINED EFFECT
Alcohol:	Dangerous increased effect of meprobamate.
Beverages: Caffeine drinks.	Decreased calming effect of meprobamate.
Cocaine:	Decreased meprobamate effect.
Foods:	None expected.
Marijuana:	Increased sedative effect of meprobamate.
Tobacco:	None expected.

MEPROBAMATE & ASPIRIN

BRAND NAMES

Epromate-M
Equagesic
Equazine-M
Heptogesic
Mepro Analgesic
Meprogese

Meprogesic
Meprogesic Q
Micrainin
Q-gesic
Tranquigesic

BASIC INFORMATION

Habit forming? Yes
Prescription needed? Yes
Available as generic? Yes
Drug class: Anti-inflammatory (nonsteroidal), analgesic, tranquilizer

 ## USES

- Reduces mild anxiety, tension and insomnia.
- Reduces pain, fever, inflammation.
- Relieves swelling, stiffness, joint pain.
- Antiplatelet effect.

 ## DOSAGE & USAGE INFORMATION

How to take:
- Tablet—Swallow with liquid.
- Effervescent tablets—Dissolve in water.

When to take:
Pain, fever, inflammation—As needed, no more often than every 4 hours.

If you forget a dose:
Take as soon as you remember up to 2 hours late. If more than 2 hours, wait for next scheduled dose (don't double this dose).

What drug does:
- Sedates brain centers which control behavior and emotions.

Continued next column

 ## OVERDOSE

SYMPTOMS:
Dizziness; slurred speech; stagger; depressed heart function; ringing in ears; nausea; vomiting; fever; deep, rapid breathing; hallucinations; convulsions; stupor; coma.
WHAT TO DO:
- **Dial 911 (emergency) or 0 (operator) for an ambulance or medical help. Then give first aid immediately.**
- **See emergency information on inside covers.**

- Affects hypothalamus, the part of the brain which regulates temperature by dilating small blood vessels in skin.
- Prevents clumping of platelets (small blood cells) so blood vessels remain open.
- Decreases prostaglandin effect.
- Suppresses body's pain messages.

Time lapse before drug works:
1 to 2 hours.

Don't take with:
- Tetracyclines.
- Nonprescription drugs containing alcohol or caffeine without consulting doctor.
- Any other medicine without consulting your doctor or pharmacist.

 ## POSSIBLE ADVERSE REACTIONS OR SIDE EFFECTS

SYMPTOMS	WHAT TO DO
Life-threatening:	
Hives, rash, intense itching, faintness soon after a dose (anaphylaxis); difficulty breathing.	Seek emergency treatment immediately
Common:	
• Nausea, vomiting.	Discontinue. Call doctor right away.
• Dizziness, confusion, agitation, drowsiness, unsteadiness, fatigue, weakness, ears ringing, heartburn, indigestion, abdominal pain.	Continue. Call doctor when convenient.
Infrequent:	
Blurred vision, headache.	Continue. Call doctor when convenient.
Rare:	
• Black, bloody or tarry stool; vomiting blood or black material; blood in urine.	Discontinue. Seek emergency treatment.
• Rash, hives, itchy skin, change in vision, fever, jaundice, mental confusion.	Discontinue. Call doctor right away.

 ## WARNINGS & PRECAUTIONS

Don't take if:
- You are allergic to meprobamate, tybamate, carbromal or carisoprodol.
- You are sensitive to aspirin.
- You have had porphyria.
- You have a peptic ulcer of stomach or duo-denum or a bleeding disorder.
- Patient is younger than 6.

Before you start, consult your doctor:
- If you have epilepsy, impaired liver or kidney function, asthma or nasal polyps.
- If you are allergic to tartrazine.
- If you have had gout, stomach or duodenal ulcers.

Over age 60:
Adverse reactions and side effects may be more frequent and severe than in younger persons. More likely to cause hidden bleeding in stomach or intestines. Watch for dark stools.

Pregnancy:
Risk to unborn child outweighs drug benefits. Don't use.

Breast-feeding:
Drug passes into milk. Avoid drug or discontinue nursing until you finish medicine. Consult doctor for advice on maintaining milk supply.

Infants & children:
Not recommended.

Prolonged use:
- Habit forming.
- May impair blood cell production.
- Kidney damage. Periodic kidney function test recommended.

Skin & sunlight:
No special problems expected.

Driving, piloting or hazardous work:
Don't drive or pilot aircraft until you learn how medicine affects you. Don't work around dangerous machinery. Don't climb ladders or work in high places. Danger increases if you drink alcohol or take medicine affecting alertness and reflexes, such as antihistamines, tranquilizers, sedatives, pain medicine, narcotics and mind-altering drugs.

Discontinuing:
Don't discontinue without consulting doctor. Dose may require gradual reduction if you have taken drug for a long time. Doses of other drugs may also require adjustment.

Others:
- Aspirin can complicate surgery; illness; pregnancy, labor and delivery.
- Urine tests for blood sugar may be inaccurate.

POSSIBLE INTERACTION WITH OTHER DRUGS

GENERIC NAME OR DRUG CLASS	COMBINED EFFECT
Acebutolol	Decreased anti-hypertensive effect of acebutolol.
Addictive drugs*	Increased risk of addictive effect.
Adrenocorticoids, systemic	Increased risk of ulcers. Increased adrenocorticoid effect.
Allopurinol	Decreased allopurinol effect.
Angiotensin-converting enzyme (ACE) inhibitors*	Decreased effect of ACE inhibitors.
Antacids*	Decreased aspirin effect.
Anticoagulants*	Increased anticoagulant effect. Abnormal bleeding.
Anticonvulsants*	Change in seizure pattern.
Antidepressants, tricyclic*	Increased anti-depressant effect.
Antidiabetics*, oral	Low blood sugar.
Anti-inflammatory drugs, nonsteroidal (NSAIDs)*	Risk of stomach bleeding and ulcers.
Aspirin, other	Likely aspirin toxicity.
Bumetanide	Possible aspirin toxicity.
Dronabinol	Increased effect of both drugs.

Continued on page 920

POSSIBLE INTERACTION WITH OTHER SUBSTANCES

INTERACTS WITH	COMBINED EFFECT
Alcohol:	Possible stomach irritation and bleeding. Dangerous increased effect of meprobamate. Avoid.
Beverages: Caffeine drinks.	Decreased calming effect of meprobamate.
Cocaine:	Decreased meprobamate effect.
Foods:	None expected.
Marijuana:	Possible increased pain relief, but marijuana may slow body's recovery. Avoid.
Tobacco:	None expected.

*See Glossary

MERCAPTOPURINE

BRAND NAMES

6-MP   Purinethol

BASIC INFORMATION

Habit forming? No
Prescription needed? Yes
Available as generic? No
Drug class: Antineoplastic,
   immunosuppressant

 ## USES

- Treatment for some kinds of cancer.
- Treatment for regional enteritis and ulcerative colitis and other immune disorders.

 ## DOSAGE & USAGE INFORMATION

How to take:
Tablet—Swallow with liquid.

When to take:
At the same time each day.

If you forget a dose:
Skip the missed dose. Don't double the next dose.

What drug does:
Inhibits abnormal cell reproduction.

Time lapse before drug works:
May require 6 weeks for maximum effect.

Don't take with:
Any other medicine without consulting your doctor or pharmacist.

 ## OVERDOSE

SYMPTOMS:
Headache, stupor, seizures.
WHAT TO DO:
- Dial 911 (emergency) or 0 (operator) for an ambulance or medical help. Then give first aid immediately.
- If patient is unconscious and not breathing, give mouth-to-mouth breathing. If there is no heartbeat, use cardiac massage and mouth-to-mouth breathing (CPR). Don't try to make patient vomit. If you can't get help quickly, take patient to nearest emergency facility.
- See emergency information on inside covers.

 ## POSSIBLE ADVERSE REACTIONS OR SIDE EFFECTS

SYMPTOMS	WHAT TO DO
Life-threatening:	
In case of overdose, see previous column.	
Common:	
• Black stools or bloody vomit.	Discontinue. Seek emergency treatment.
• Mouth sores, sore throat, unusual bleeding or bruising.	Discontinue. Call doctor right away.
• Abdominal pain, nausea, vomiting, weakness, tiredness.	Continue. Call doctor when convenient.
Infrequent:	
• Seizures.	Discontinue. Seek emergency treatment.
• Diarrhea, headache, confusion, blurred vision, shortness of breath, joint pain, blood in urine, jaundice, back pain, appetite loss, feet and leg swelling.	Discontinue. Call doctor right away.
• Cough.	Continue. Call doctor when convenient.
• Acne, boils, hair loss, itchy skin.	Continue. Tell doctor at next visit.
Rare:	
Fever and chills.	Discontinue. Call doctor right away.

 ## WARNINGS & PRECAUTIONS

Don't take if:
You are allergic to any antineoplastic.

Before you start, consult your doctor:
- If you are alcoholic.
- If you have blood, liver or kidney disease.
- If you have colitis or peptic ulcer.
- If you have gout.
- If you have an infection.
- If you plan to become pregnant within 3 months.

Over age 60:
Adverse reactions and side effects may be more frequent and severe than in younger persons.

Pregnancy:
Risk to unborn child outweighs drug benefits. Don't use. Risk category D (see page xxiii).

Breast-feeding:
Avoid drug or discontinue nursing.

Infants & children:
Use only under special medical supervision.

Prolonged use:
- Adverse reactions more likely the longer drug is required.
- Talk to your doctor about the need for follow-up medical examinations or laboratory studies to check complete blood counts (white blood cell count, platelet count, red blood cell count, hemoglobin, hematocrit), liver function, kidney function, uric acid.

Skin & sunlight:
No problems expected.

Driving, piloting or hazardous work:
Avoid if you feel dizzy, drowsy or confused. Otherwise, no problems expected.

Discontinuing:
Don't discontinue without doctor's advice until you complete prescribed dose, even though symptoms diminish or disappear. Some side effects may follow discontinuing. Report to doctor blurred vision, convulsions, confusion, persistent headache, chills or fever, bloody urine or stools, back pain, jaundice.

Others:
- Drink more water than usual to cause frequent urination.
- Don't give this medicine to anyone else for any purpose. It is a strong drug that requires close medical supervision.
- Report for frequent medical follow-up and laboratory studies.

POSSIBLE INTERACTION WITH OTHER DRUGS

GENERIC NAME OR DRUG CLASS	COMBINED EFFECT
Acetaminophen	Increased likelihood of liver toxicity.
Allopurinol	Increased toxic effect of mercaptopurine.
Anticoagulants,* oral	May increase or decrease anticoagulant effect.
Antineoplastic drugs*, other	Increased effect of both (may be desirable) or increased toxicity of each.
Chloramphenicol	Increased toxicity of each.

Clozapine	Toxic effect on bone marrow.
Cyclosporine	May increase risk of infection.
Hepatotoxic drugs*	Increased risk of liver toxicity.
Immunosuppresants*, other	Increased risk of infections and neoplasms*.
Isoniazid	Increased risk of liver damage.
Levamisole	Increased risk of bone marrow depression.
Lovastatin	Increased heart and kidney damage.
Probenecid	Increased toxic effect of mercaptopurine.
Sulfinpyrazone	Increased toxic effect of mercaptopurine.
Tiopronin	Increased risk of toxicity to bone marrow.
Vaccines, live or killed	Increased risk of toxicity or reduced effectiveness of vaccine.

POSSIBLE INTERACTION WITH OTHER SUBSTANCES

INTERACTS WITH	COMBINED EFFECT
Alcohol:	May increase chance of intestinal bleeding.
Beverages:	No problems expected.
Cocaine:	Increased chance of toxicity.
Foods:	Reduced irritation in stomach.
Marijuana:	No problems expected.
Tobacco:	Increased lung toxicity.

MESALAMINE

BRAND NAMES

5-ASA	Pentasa
Asacol	Rowasa
Mesalazine	Salofalk

BASIC INFORMATION

Habit forming? No
Prescription needed? Yes
Available as generic? No
Drug class: Anti-inflammatory (nonsteroidal)

 USES

- Treats ulcerative colitis.
- Reduces inflammatory conditions of the lower colon and rectum.

 DOSAGE & USAGE INFORMATION

How to use:
- Rectal—Use as an enema. Insert the tip of the pre-packaged medicine container into the rectum. Squeeze container to empty contents. Retain in rectum all night or as long as possible.
- Delayed-release tablet or extended-release capsule—Swallow with liquid. Do not crush or chew tablet.

When to use:
- Rectal—Each night, preferably after a bowel movement. Continue for 3 to 6 weeks according to your doctor's instructions.
- Tablet—3 to 4 times a day or as directed by doctor.

If you forget a dose:
Take as soon as you remember up to 2 hours late. If more than 2 hours, wait for next scheduled dose (don't double this dose).

What drug does:
Decreases production of arachidonic acid forms which are increased in patients with chronic inflammatory bowel disease.

Time lapse before drug works:
3 to 21 days.

Continued next column

 OVERDOSE

SYMPTOMS:
None expected.
WHAT TO DO:
No action needed.

Don't take with:
- Oral sulfasalazine concurrently. To do so may increase chances of kidney damage.
- Any other medicine without consulting your doctor or pharmacist.

 POSSIBLE ADVERSE REACTIONS OR SIDE EFFECTS

SYMPTOMS	WHAT TO DO
Life-threatening: None expected.	
Common: None expected.	
Infrequent: None expected.	
Rare:	
• Abdominal pain, bloody diarrhea, fever, skin rash, anal irritation.	Discontinue. Call doctor right away.
• Gaseousness, nausea, headache, hair loss.	Continue. Call doctor when convenient.

WARNINGS & PRECAUTIONS

Don't take if:
You are allergic to salicylates* or any medication containing sulfasalazine (such as Azulfidine) or mesalamine.

Before you start, consult your doctor:
If you have had chronic kidney disease.

Over age 60:
More sensitive to drug. Aggravates symptoms of enlarged prostate. Causes impaired thinking, hallucinations, nightmares. Consult doctor about any of these.

Pregnancy:
Consult doctor. Risk category B (see page xxiii).

Breast-feeding:
Effect unknown. Consult your doctor.

Infants & children:
Use for children only under doctor's supervision.

Prolonged use:
Talk to your doctor about the need for follow-up medical examinations or laboratory studies to check urine.

Skin & sunlight:
No problems expected.

Driving, piloting or hazardous work:
Don't drive or pilot aircraft until you learn how medicine affects you. Don't work around dangerous machinery. Don't climb ladders or work in high places. Danger increases if you drink alcohol or take medicine affecting alertness and reflexes.

Discontinuing:
Don't discontinue without consulting doctor. Dose may require gradual reduction if you have taken drug for a long time. Doses of other drugs may also require adjustment.

Others:
- Internal eye pressure should be measured regularly.
- Avoid becoming overheated.

POSSIBLE INTERACTION WITH OTHER DRUGS

GENERIC NAME OR DRUG CLASS	COMBINED EFFECT
None reported.	

POSSIBLE INTERACTION WITH OTHER SUBSTANCES

INTERACTS WITH	COMBINED EFFECT
Alcohol:	None expected.
Beverages:	None expected.
Cocaine:	None expected.
Foods:	None expected.
Marijuana:	None expected.
Tobacco:	None expected.

METFORMIN

BRAND NAMES

Glucophage

BASIC INFORMATION

Habit forming? No
Prescription needed? Yes
Available as generic? No
Drug class: Antihyperglycemic, antidiabetic

 ## USES

Treatment for hyperglycemia (excess sugar in the blood) that cannot be controlled by diet alone in patients with type II non-insulin-dependent diabetes mellitus (NIDDM).

 ## DOSAGE & USAGE INFORMATION

How to take:
Tablet—Swallow with liquid.

When to take:
Usually 2 to 3 times a day as directed by doctor. Take with meals to lessen stomach irritation. Dosage may be increased on a weekly basis until maximum benefits are achieved.

Continued next column

 ## OVERDOSE

SYMPTOMS:
- Symptoms of lactic acidosis (acid in the blood)—chills, diarrhea, fatigue, muscle pain, sleepiness, slow heartbeat, breathing difficulty, unusual weakness.
- Symptoms of hypoglycemia (low blood sugar)—stomach pain, anxious feeling, cold sweats, chills, confusion, convulsions, cool pale skin, excessive hunger, nausea or vomiting, rapid heartbeat, nervousness, shakiness, unsteady walk, unusual weakness or tiredness, vision changes, unconsciousness.

WHAT TO DO:
- For symptoms of lactic acidosis, call doctor immediately.
- For mild low blood sugar symptoms, drink or eat something containing sugar right away.
- For more severe symptoms, dial 911 (emergency) or 0 (operator) for an ambulance or medical help. Then give first aid immediately.
- See emergency information on inside covers.

If you forget a dose:
Take as soon as you remember. If it is almost time for the next dose, then skip the missed dose and wait for your next scheduled dose (don't double this dose).

What drug does:
Helps to lower blood sugar when it is too high. Treats the symptoms of diabetes, but does not cure it.

Time lapse before drug works:
May take several weeks for full effectiveness.

Don't take with:
Any other prescription or nonprescription drug without consulting your doctor or pharmacist.

 ## POSSIBLE ADVERSE REACTIONS OR SIDE EFFECTS

SYMPTOMS	WHAT TO DO
Life-threatening: In case of overdose or low blood sugar, see previous column.	
Common:	
• Stomach pain, diarrhea, vomiting.	Continue, but call doctor right away.
• Decreased appetite, changes in taste, gas, headache, weight loss, feeling of fullness or stomach discomfort, nausea.	Continue. Call doctor when convenient.
Infrequent: None expected.	
Rare: Lactic acidosis or severe low blood sugar (see symptoms under Overdose).	Discontinue. Call doctor right away or seek emergency help.

 ## WARNINGS & PRECAUTIONS

Don't take if:
You are allergic to metformin.

Before you start, consult your doctor:
- If you have any kidney or liver disease or any heart or blood vessel disorder.
- If you have any chronic health problem.
- If you have an infection, illness or any condition that can cause low blood sugar.
- If you have a history of acid in the blood (metabolic acidosis or ketoacidosis).
- If you are allergic to any medication, food or other substance.

Over age 60:
No special problems expected. A lower starting dosage may be recommended by your doctor.

Pregnancy:
Decide with your doctor if drug benefits justify risks to unborn child. Risk category B (see page xxiii).

Breast-feeding:
Drug passes into milk. Avoid drug or discontinue nursing until you finish medicine. Consult doctor for advice on maintaining milk supply.

Infants & children:
Safety and efficacy have not been established. Use only under close medical supervision.

Prolonged use:
- Schedule regular doctor visits to determine if the drug is continuing to be effective in controlling the diabetes and to check for any problems in kidney function.
- You will most likely require an antidiabetic medicine for the rest of your life.
- You will need to test your blood glucose levels several times a day, or for some, once to several times a week.

Skin & sunlight:
No special problems expected.

Driving, piloting or hazardous work:
No special problems expected.

Discontinuing:
Don't discontinue without consulting your doctor, even if you feel well. You can have diabetes without feeling any symptoms. Untreated diabetes can cause serious problems.

Others:
- Advise any doctor or dentist whom you consult that you take this medicine. Drug may interfere with the accuracy of some medical tests.
- Follow any special diet your doctor may prescribe. It can help control diabetes.
- Consult doctor if you become ill with vomiting or diarrhea.
- Use caution when exercising. Ask your doctor about an appropriate exercise program.
- Wear medical identification stating that you have diabetes and take this medication.
- Learn to recognize the symptoms of low blood sugar. You and your family need to know what to do if these symptoms occur.
- Have a glucagon kit and syringe in the event severe low blood sugar occurs. Carry a quick-acting sugar to treat symptoms of mild low blood sugar.
- High blood sugar (hyperglycemia) may occur with diabetes. Ask your doctor about symptoms to watch for and treatment steps to take.
- This drug may be discontinued temporarily prior to x-ray studies or some surgeries.
- Educate yourself about diabetes.

POSSIBLE INTERACTION WITH OTHER DRUGS

GENERIC NAME OR DRUG CLASS	COMBINED EFFECT
Amiloride	Increased metformin effect.
Calcium channel blockers*	Increased metformin effect.
Cimetidine	Increased metformin effect.
Dexfenfluramine	May require dosage change as weight loss occurs.
Digoxin	Increased metformin effect.
Furosemide	Increased metformin effect.
Hyperglycemia-causing medications*	Increased risk of hyperglycemia.
Hypoglycemia-causing medications*	Increased risk of hypoglycemia.
Morphine	Increased metformin effect.
Procainamide	Increased metformin effect.
Quinidine	Increased metformin effect.
Quinine	Increased metformin effect.
Ranitidine	Increased metformin effect.
Triamterene	Increased metformin effect.

Continued on page 920

POSSIBLE INTERACTION WITH OTHER SUBSTANCES

INTERACTS WITH	COMBINED EFFECT
Alcohol:	Increased effect of metformin. Avoid excessive amounts.
Beverages:	No special problems.
Cocaine:	No special problems.
Foods:	No special problems.
Marijuana:	No special problems.
Tobacco:	No special problems.

*See Glossary

METHENAMINE

BRAND NAMES

Hip-Rex   Mandelamine
Hiprex   Urex

BASIC INFORMATION

Habit forming? No
Prescription needed? Yes
Available as generic? Yes
Drug class: Anti-infective (urinary)

USES

Suppresses chronic urinary tract infections.

DOSAGE & USAGE INFORMATION

How to take:
- Tablet—Swallow with liquid or food to lessen stomach irritation. If you can't swallow whole, crumble tablet and take with liquid or food. If enteric-coated tablet, swallow whole.
- Liquid form—Use a measuring spoon to ensure correct dose.
- Granules—Dissolve dose in 4 oz. of water. Drink all the liquid.

When to take:
At the same times each day.

If you forget a dose:
Take as soon as you remember up to 8 hours late. If more than 8 hours, wait for next scheduled dose (don't double this dose).

What drug does:
A chemical reaction in the urine changes methenamine into formaldehyde, which destroys certain bacteria.

Continued next column

OVERDOSE

SYMPTOMS:
Bloody urine, weakness, deep breathing, stupor, coma.
WHAT TO DO:
- Dial 911 (emergency) or 0 (operator) for an ambulance or medical help. Then give first aid immediately.
- See emergency information on inside covers.

Time lapse before drug works:
Continual use for 3 to 6 months.

Don't take with:
Any other medicine without consulting your doctor or pharmacist.

POSSIBLE ADVERSE REACTIONS OR SIDE EFFECTS

SYMPTOMS	WHAT TO DO
Life-threatening:	
In case of overdose, see previous column.	
Common:	
• Rash.	Discontinue. Call doctor right away.
• Nausea, difficult urination.	Continue. Call doctor when convenient.
Infrequent:	
• Blood in urine.	Discontinue. Call doctor right away.
• Burning on urination, lower back pain.	Continue. Call doctor when convenient.
Rare:	
None expected.	

WARNINGS & PRECAUTIONS

Don't take if:
- You are allergic to methenamine.
- You have a severe impairment of kidney or liver function.
- Your urine cannot or should not be acidified (check with your doctor).

Before you start, consult your doctor:
- If you have had kidney or liver disease.
- If you plan to become pregnant within medication period.
- If you have had gout.

Over age 60:
Don't exceed recommended dose.

Pregnancy:
Decide with your doctor if drug benefits justify risk to unborn child. Risk category C (see page xxiii).

Breast-feeding:
Drug passes into milk in small amounts. Consult doctor.

Infants & children:
Use only under medical supervision.

Prolonged use:
No problems expected.

Skin & sunlight:
No problems expected.

Driving, piloting or hazardous work:
No problems expected.

Discontinuing:
Don't discontinue without doctor's advice until you complete prescribed dose, even though symptoms diminish or disappear.

Others:
Requires an acid urine to be effective. Eat more protein foods, cranberries, cranberry juice with vitamin C, plums, prunes.

POSSIBLE INTERACTION WITH OTHER DRUGS

GENERIC NAME OR DRUG CLASS	COMBINED EFFECT
Antacids*	Decreased methenamine effect.
Carbonic anhydrase inhibitors*	Decreased methenamine effect.
Citrates*	Decreases effects of methenamine.
Diuretics, thiazide*	Decreased urine acidity.
Sodium bicarbonate	Decreased methenamine effect.
Sulfadoxine and pyrimethamine	Increased risk of kidney toxicity.
Sulfa drugs*	Possible kidney damage.

POSSIBLE INTERACTION WITH OTHER SUBSTANCES

INTERACTS WITH	COMBINED EFFECT
Alcohol:	Possible brain depression. Avoid or use with caution.
Beverages: Milk and other dairy products.	Decreased methenamine effect.
Cocaine:	None expected.
Foods: Citrus, cranberries, plums, prunes.	Increased methenamine effect.
Marijuana:	Drowsiness, muscle weakness or blood pressure drop.
Tobacco:	None expected.

METHOTREXATE

BRAND NAMES

Amethopterin	Mexate
Folex	Mexate AQ
Folex PFS	Rheumatrex

BASIC INFORMATION

Habit forming? No
Prescription needed? Yes
Available as generic? Yes
Drug class: Antimetabolite, antipsoriatic

 ## USES

- Treatment for some kinds of cancer.
- Treatment for psoriasis in patients with severe problems.
- Treatment for severe rheumatoid arthritis.

 ## DOSAGE & USAGE INFORMATION

How to take:
Tablet—Swallow with liquid.

When to take:
At the same time each day.

If you forget a dose:
Skip the missed dose. Don't double the next dose.

What drug does:
Inhibits abnormal cell reproduction.

Time lapse before drug works:
May require 6 weeks for maximum effect.

Don't take with:
Any other medicine without consulting your doctor or pharmacist.

 ## OVERDOSE

SYMPTOMS:
Headache, stupor, seizures.
WHAT TO DO:
- **Dial 911 (emergency) or 0 (operator) for an ambulance or medical help. Then give first aid immediately.**
- **If patient is unconscious and not breathing, give mouth-to-mouth breathing. If there is no heartbeat, use cardiac massage and mouth-to-mouth breathing (CPR). Don't try to make patient vomit. If you can't get help quickly, take patient to nearest emergency facility.**
- **See emergency information on inside covers.**

 ## POSSIBLE ADVERSE REACTIONS OR SIDE EFFECTS

SYMPTOMS	WHAT TO DO
Life-threatening: Hives, rash, intense itching, faintness soon after a dose (anaphylaxis).	Seek emergency treatment immediately.
Common:	
• Black stools or bloody vomit.	Discontinue. Seek emergency treatment.
• Sore throat, fever, mouth sores; chills; unusual bleeding or bruising.	Discontinue. Call doctor right away.
• Abdominal pain, nausea, vomiting.	Continue. Call doctor when convenient.
Infrequent:	
• Seizures.	Discontinue. Seek emergency treatment.
• Dizziness when standing after sitting or lying, drowsiness, headache, confusion, blurred vision, shortness of breath, joint pain, blood in urine, jaundice, diarrhea, red skin, back pain.	Discontinue. Call doctor right away.
• Cough, rash, sexual difficulties in males.	Continue. Call doctor when convenient.
• Acne, boils, hair loss, itchy skin.	Continue. Tell doctor at next visit.
Rare:	
• Convulsions.	Seek emergency treatment.
• Painful urination.	Discontinue. Seek emergency treatment.

 ## WARNINGS & PRECAUTIONS

Don't take if:
You are allergic to any antimetabolite.

Before you start, consult your doctor:
- If you are alcoholic.
- If you have blood, liver or kidney disease.
- If you have colitis or peptic ulcer.
- If you have gout.
- If you have an infection.
- If you plan to become pregnant within 3 months.

Over age 60:
Adverse reactions and side effects may be more frequent and severe than in younger persons.

Pregnancy:
- Psoriasis—Risk to unborn child outweighs drug benefits. Don't use.
- Cancer—Consult doctor.
- Risk category X (see page xxiii).

Breast-feeding:
Drug passes into milk. Avoid drug or discontinue nursing.

Infants & children:
Use only under special medical supervision.

Prolonged use:
- Adverse reactions more likely the longer drug is required.
- Talk to your doctor about the need for follow-up medical examinations or laboratory studies to check liver function, kidney function, complete blood counts (white blood cell count, platelet count, red blood cell count, hemoglobin, hematocrit).

Skin & sunlight:
May cause rash or intensify sunburn in areas exposed to sun or ultraviolet light (photosensitivity reaction). Avoid overexposure. Notify doctor if reaction occurs.

Driving, piloting or hazardous work:
Avoid if you feel dizzy, drowsy or confused. Otherwise, no problems expected.

Discontinuing:
Don't discontinue without doctor's advice until you complete prescribed dose, even though symptoms diminish or disappear. Some side effects may follow discontinuing. Report to doctor blurred vision, convulsions, confusion, persistent headache.

Others:
- Drink more water than usual to cause frequent urination.
- Don't give this medicine to anyone else for any purpose. It is a strong drug that requires close medical supervision.
- Report for frequent medical follow-up and laboratory studies.

POSSIBLE INTERACTION WITH OTHER DRUGS

GENERIC NAME OR DRUG CLASS	COMBINED EFFECT
Anticoagulants,* oral	Increased anti-coagulant effect.
Anticonvulsants,* hydantoin	Possible methotrexate toxicity.
Antigout drugs*	Decreased antigout effect. Toxic levels of methotrexate.
Anti-inflammatory drugs, nonsteroidal (NSAIDs)*	Possible increased methotrexate toxicity.
Asparaginase	Decreased methotrexate effect.
Bone marrow depressants*, other	Increased risk of bone marrow depression.
Clozapine	Toxic effect on bone marrow.
Diclofenac	May increase toxicity.
Etretinate	Increased chance of toxicity to liver.
Fluorouracil	Decreased methotrexate effect.
Folic acid	Possible decreased methotrexate effect.
Isoniazid	Increased risk of liver damage.
Leukovorin calcium	Decreased methotrexate toxicity.
Levamisole	Increased risk of bone marrow depression.
Oxyphenbutazone	Possible methotrexate toxicity.
Penicillins*	Increased risk of methotrexate toxicity.
Phenylbutazone	Possible methotrexate toxicity.

Continued on page 921

POSSIBLE INTERACTION WITH OTHER SUBSTANCES

INTERACTS WITH	COMBINED EFFECT
Alcohol:	Likely liver damage. Avoid.
Beverages:	Extra fluid intake decreases chance of methotrexate toxicity.
Cocaine:	Increased chance of methotrexate adverse reactions. Avoid.
Foods:	None expected.
Marijuana:	None expected.
Tobacco:	None expected.

METHYLDOPA

BRAND NAMES

Aldomet
Apo-Methyldopa
Dopamet

Novomedopa
Nu-Medopa

BASIC INFORMATION

Habit forming? No
Prescription needed? Yes
Available as generic? Yes
Drug class: Antihypertensive

USES

Reduces high blood pressure.

DOSAGE & USAGE INFORMATION

How to take:
Liquid or tablet—Swallow with liquid. If you can't swallow whole, crumble tablet and take with liquid or food.

When to take:
At the same times each day.

If you forget a dose:
Take as soon as you remember up to 2 hours late. If more than 2 hours, wait for next scheduled dose (don't double this dose).

What drug does:
Relaxes walls of small arteries to decrease blood pressure.

Time lapse before drug works:
Continual use for 2 to 4 weeks may be necessary to determine effectiveness.

Continued next column

OVERDOSE

SYMPTOMS:
Drowsiness; exhaustion; stupor; confusion; slow, weak pulse.
WHAT TO DO:
- **Dial 911 (emergency) or 0 (operator) for an ambulance or medical help. Then give first aid immediately.**
- **If patient is unconscious and not breathing, give mouth-to-mouth breathing. If there is no heartbeat, use cardiac massage and mouth-to-mouth breathing (CPR). Don't try to make patient vomit. If you can't get help quickly, take patient to nearest emergency facility.**
- **See emergency information on inside covers.**

Don't take with:
Any other medicine without consulting your doctor or pharmacist.

POSSIBLE ADVERSE REACTIONS OR SIDE EFFECTS

SYMPTOMS	WHAT TO DO
Life-threatening: In case of overdose, see previous column.	
Common: Depression, sedation, nightmares, headache, drowsiness, weakness, stuffy nose, dry mouth, fluid retention, swollen feet or legs.	Continue. Call doctor when convenient.
Infrequent: • Fast heartbeat, fainting.	Discontinue. Call doctor right away.
• Insomnia, nausea, vomiting, diarrhea, constipation, foot and hand numbness and tingling.	Continue. Call doctor when convenient.
• Swollen breasts, diminished sex drive.	Continue. Tell doctor at next visit.
Rare: Rash, jaundice, dark urine, chills, breathing difficulty, unexplained fever, sore or "black" tongue, severe abdominal pain, decreased mental activity and memory impairment, facial paralysis, slow heartbeat, chest pain, swollen abdomen.	Discontinue. Call doctor right away.

WARNINGS & PRECAUTIONS

Don't take if:
You will have surgery within 2 months, including dental surgery, requiring general or spinal anesthesia.

Before you start, consult your doctor:
If you have liver disease.

Over age 60:
- Increased susceptibility to dizziness, unsteadiness, fainting, falling.
- Drug can produce or intensify Parkinson's disease.

Pregnancy:
No proven problems. Consult doctor. Risk category B (see page xxiii).

Breast-feeding:
No proven problems. Consult doctor.

Infants & children:
Not used.

Prolonged use:
- May cause anemia.
- Severe edema (fluid retention).
- Talk to your doctor about the need for follow-up medical examinations or laboratory studies to check complete blood counts (white blood cell count, platelet count, red blood cell count, hemoglobin, hematocrit), blood pressure, liver function.

Skin & sunlight:
May cause rash or intensify sunburn in areas exposed to sun or ultraviolet light (photosensitivity reaction). Avoid overexposure. Notify doctor if reaction occurs.

Driving, piloting or hazardous work:
Don't drive or pilot aircraft until you learn how medicine affects you. Don't work around dangerous machinery. Don't climb ladders or work in high places. Danger increases if you drink alcohol or take medicine affecting alertness and reflexes, such as antihistamines, tranquilizers, sedatives, pain medicine, narcotics and mind-altering drugs.

Discontinuing:
Don't discontinue without consulting doctor. Dose may require gradual reduction if you have taken drug for a long time. Doses of other drugs may also require adjustment.

Others:
Avoid heavy exercise, exertion, sweating.

 POSSIBLE INTERACTION WITH OTHER DRUGS

GENERIC NAME OR DRUG CLASS	COMBINED EFFECT
Amphetamines*	Decreased methyldopa effect.
Angiotensin-converting enzyme (ACE) inhibitors*	Possible excessive potassium in blood.
Anticoagulants*, oral	Increased anticoagulant effect.
Antidepressants, tricyclic*	Dangerous blood pressure rise. Decreased methyldopa effect.
Antihypertensives*	Increased antihypertensive effect.
Antivirals, HIV/AIDS*	Increased risk of pancreatitis.
Carteolol	Increased antihypertensive effect.

Clozapine	Toxic effect on the central nervous system.
Dapsone	Increased risk of adverse effect on blood cells.
Digitalis preparations*	Excessively slow heartbeat.
Diuretics, thiazide*	Increased methyldopa effect.
Ethinamate	Dangerous increased effects of ethinamate. Avoid combining.
Fluoxetine	Increased depressant effects of both drugs.
Guanfacine	May increase depressant effects of either drug.
Haloperidol	Increased sedation. Possibly dementia.
Isoniazid	Increased risk of liver damage.
Leucovorin	High alcohol content of leucovorin may cause adverse effects.
Levodopa	Increased effect of both drugs.
Loxapine	May increase toxic effects of both drugs.

Continued on page 921

 POSSIBLE INTERACTION WITH OTHER SUBSTANCES

INTERACTS WITH	COMBINED EFFECT
Alcohol:	Increased sedation. Excessive blood pressure drop. Avoid.
Beverages:	None expected.
Cocaine:	Increased risk of heart block and high blood pressure.
Foods:	None expected.
Marijuana:	Possible fainting.
Tobacco:	Possible increased blood pressure.

*See Glossary

METHYLDOPA & THIAZIDE DIURETICS

GENERIC AND BRAND NAMES

**METHYLDOPA &
CHLOROTHIAZIDE**
Aldoclor

**METHYLDOPA &
HYDROCHLORO-
THIAZIDE**
Aldoril
Novodoparil
PMS Dopazide

BASIC INFORMATION

Habit forming? No
Prescription needed? Yes
Available as generic? Yes
**Drug class: Antihypertensive, diuretic
(thiazide)**

USES

- Controls, but doesn't cure, high blood pressure.
- Reduces fluid retention (edema).

DOSAGE & USAGE INFORMATION

How to take:
Tablet—Swallow with liquid. If you can't swallow whole, crumble tablet and take with liquid or food.

When to take:
At the same times each day.

If you forget a dose:
Take as soon as you remember up to 2 hours late. If more than 2 hours, wait for next scheduled dose (don't double this dose).

Continued next column

OVERDOSE

SYMPTOMS:
Drowsiness; exhaustion; cramps; weakness; stupor; confusion; slow, weak pulse; coma.
WHAT TO DO:
- **Dial 911 (emergency) or 0 (operator) for an ambulance or medical help. Then give first aid immediately.**
- **If patient is unconscious and not breathing, give mouth-to-mouth breathing. If there is no heartbeat, use cardiac massage and mouth-to-mouth breathing (CPR). Don't try to make patient vomit. If you can't get help quickly, take patient to nearest emergency facility.**
- **See emergency information on inside covers.**

What drug does:
- Relaxes walls of small arteries to decrease blood pressure.
- Forces sodium and water excretion, reducing body fluid.
- Reduced body fluid and relaxed arteries lower blood pressure.

Time lapse before drug works:
Continual use for 2 to 4 weeks may be necessary to determine effectiveness.

Don't take with:
- Nonprescription drugs without consulting doctor.
- Any other medicine without consulting your doctor or pharmacist.

POSSIBLE ADVERSE REACTIONS OR SIDE EFFECTS

SYMPTOMS	WHAT TO DO
Life-threatening: Irregular heartbeat, weak pulse.	Discontinue. Seek emergency treatment.
Common: Depression, nightmares, drowsiness, weakness, stuffy nose, dry mouth, swollen feet and ankles, dizziness, sedation, increased thirst, muscle cramps.	Continue. Call doctor when convenient.
Infrequent: • Fast heartbeat, change in vision, abdominal pain, nervousness.	Discontinue. Call doctor right away.
• Insomnia, nausea, vomiting, diarrhea, headache, constipation.	Continue. Call doctor when convenient.
Rare: Rash, jaundice, dark urine, chills, breathing difficulty, hives, sore throat, fever, mouth sores, sore or "black" tongue, severe abdominal pain, decreased mental activity, memory impairment, facial paralysis, slow heartbeat, chest pain.	Discontinue. Call doctor right away.

METHYLDOPA & THIAZIDE DIURETICS

WARNINGS & PRECAUTIONS

Don't take if:
- You are allergic to any thiazide diuretic drug.
- You will have surgery within 2 months, including dental surgery, requiring general or spinal anesthesia.

Before you start, consult your doctor:
- If you are allergic to any sulfa drug.
- If you have gout, liver, pancreas or kidney disorder.

Over age 60:
- Increased susceptibility to dizziness, unsteadiness, fainting, falling.
- Drug can produce or intensify Parkinson's disease.

Pregnancy:
Decide with your doctor if drug benefits justify risk to unborn child. Risk category C (see page xxiii).

Breast-feeding:
Drug passes into milk. Avoid drug or discontinue nursing until you finish medicine. Consult doctor for advice on maintaining milk supply.

Infants & children:
Not recommended.

Prolonged use:
- May cause anemia.
- Severe edema (fluid retention).
- Talk to your doctor about the need for follow-up medical examinations or laboratory studies to check complete blood counts (white blood cell count, platelet count, red blood cell count, hemoglobin, hematocrit), blood pressure, liver function.

Skin & sunlight:
One or more drugs in this group may cause rash or intensify sunburn in areas exposed to sun or ultraviolet light (photosensitivity reaction). Avoid overexposure. Notify doctor if reaction occurs.

Driving, piloting or hazardous work:
Don't drive or pilot aircraft until you learn how medicine affects you. Don't work around dangerous machinery. Don't climb ladders or work in high places. Danger increases if you drink alcohol or take medicine affecting alertness and reflexes, such as antihistamines, tranquilizers, sedatives, pain medicine, narcotics and mind-altering drugs.

Discontinuing:
Don't discontinue without consulting doctor. Dose may require gradual reduction if you have taken drug for a long time. Doses of other drugs may also require adjustment.

Others:
- Hot weather and fever may cause dehydration and drop in blood pressure. Dose may require temporary adjustment. Weigh daily and report any unexpected weight decreases to your doctor.

- May cause rise in uric acid, leading to gout.
- May cause blood sugar rise in diabetics.
- Avoid heavy exercise, exertion, sweating.

POSSIBLE INTERACTION WITH OTHER DRUGS

GENERIC NAME OR DRUG CLASS	COMBINED EFFECT
Acebutolol	Increased antihypertensive effect. Dosages of both drugs may require adjustments.
Allopurinol	Decreased allopurinol effect.
Amphetamines*	Decreased methyldopa effect.
Angiotensin-converting enzyme (ACE) inhibitors*	Possible excessive potassium in blood.
Anticoagulants*, oral	Increased anticoagulant effect.
Antidepressants, tricyclic*	Dangerous changes in blood pressure. Avoid combination unless under medical supervision.

Continued on page 921

POSSIBLE INTERACTION WITH OTHER SUBSTANCES

INTERACTS WITH	COMBINED EFFECT
Alcohol:	Increased sedation. Excessive blood pressure drop. Avoid.
Beverages:	None expected.
Cocaine:	Increased risk of heart block and high blood pressure.
Foods: Licorice.	Excessive potassium loss that causes dangerous heart rhythms.
Marijuana:	May increase blood pressure.
Tobacco:	Possible increased blood pressure.

*See Glossary

METHYLERGONOVINE

BRAND NAMES

Methergine

Methylergometrine

BASIC INFORMATION

Habit forming? No
Prescription needed? Yes
Available as generic? No
Drug class: Ergot preparation (uterine stimulant)

USES

Retards excessive post-delivery bleeding.

DOSAGE & USAGE INFORMATION

How to take:
Tablet—Swallow with liquid or food to lessen stomach irritation.

When to take:
At the same times each day.

If you forget a dose:
Don't take missed dose and don't double next one. Wait for next scheduled dose.

What drug does:
Causes smooth muscle cells of uterine wall to contract and surround bleeding blood vessels of relaxed uterus.

Time lapse before drug works:
Tablets—20 to 30 minutes.

Don't take with:
Any other medicine without consulting your doctor or pharmacist.

OVERDOSE

SYMPTOMS:
Vomiting, diarrhea, weak pulse, low blood pressure, dyspnea, angina, convulsions.
WHAT TO DO:
- Dial 911 (emergency) or 0 (operator) for an ambulance or medical help. Then give first aid immediately.
- If patient is unconscious and not breathing, give mouth-to-mouth breathing. If there is no heartbeat, use cardiac massage and mouth-to-mouth breathing (CPR). Don't try to make patient vomit. If you can't get help quickly, take patient to nearest emergency facility.
- See emergency information on inside covers.

POSSIBLE ADVERSE REACTIONS OR SIDE EFFECTS

SYMPTOMS	WHAT TO DO
Life-threatening: In case of overdose, see previous column.	
Common: Nausea, vomiting, severe lower abdominal menstrual-like cramps.	Discontinue. Call doctor right away.
Infrequent: • Confusion, ringing in ears, diarrhea, muscle cramps.	Discontinue. Call doctor right away.
• Unusual sweating.	Continue. Call doctor when convenient.
Rare: Sudden, severe headache; shortness of breath; chest pain; numb, cold hands and feet.	Discontinue. Seek emergency treatment.

WARNINGS & PRECAUTIONS

Don't take if:
You are allergic to any ergot preparation.

Before you start, consult your doctor:
- If you have coronary artery or blood vessel disease.
- If you have liver or kidney disease.
- If you have high blood pressure.
- If you have postpartum infection.

Over age 60:
Not recommended.

Pregnancy:
Consult doctor. Risk category C (see page xxiii).

Breast-feeding:
Drug passes into milk. Avoid drug or discontinue nursing until you finish medicine. Consult doctor for advice on maintaining milk supply.

Infants & children:
Not recommended.

Prolonged use:
Talk to your doctor about the need for follow-up medical examinations or laboratory studies to check blood pressure, ECG*.

Skin & sunlight:
No problems expected.

Driving, piloting or hazardous work:
No problems expected.

Discontinuing:
May be unnecessary to finish medicine. Follow doctor's instructions.

Others:
Drug should be used for short time only following childbirth or miscarriage.

POSSIBLE INTERACTION WITH OTHER DRUGS

GENERIC NAME OR DRUG CLASS	COMBINED EFFECT
Antianginals*	Possible vasospasm (peripheral and cardiac)
Ergot preparations*, other	Increased methyl-ergonovine effect.

POSSIBLE INTERACTION WITH OTHER SUBSTANCES

INTERACTS WITH	COMBINED EFFECT
Alcohol:	None expected.
Beverages:	None expected.
Cocaine:	None expected.
Foods:	None expected.
Marijuana:	None expected.
Tobacco:	Decreased methylergonovine effect. Don't smoke.

METHYLPHENIDATE

BRAND NAMES

PMS Methylphenidate   Ritalin SR
Ritalin

BASIC INFORMATION

Habit forming? Yes
Prescription needed? Yes
Available as generic? Yes
Drug class: Central nervous system
stimulant, sympathomimetic

 ## USES

- Decreases overactivity and lengthens atten-tion span in children with attention-deficit hyperactivity disorder (ADHD). It is used as part of the total management plan that includes educational, social and psychological treatment.
- Treatment of depression in adults.
- Treatment for narcolepsy (uncontrollable attacks of sleepiness) and other disorders.

 ## DOSAGE & USAGE INFORMATION

How to take:
- Tablet—Swallow with liquid or food to lessen stomach irritation. If you can't swallow whole, crumble tablet and take with liquid or small amount of food.
- Extended-release tablet—Swallow whole with liquid.

Continued next column

 ## OVERDOSE

SYMPTOMS:
Rapid heartbeat, fever, confusion, vomiting, agitation, hallucinations, convulsions, coma.
WHAT TO DO:
- **Dial 911 (emergency) or 0 (operator) for an ambulance or medical help. Then give first aid immediately.**
- **If patient is unconscious and not breathing, give mouth-to-mouth breathing. If there is no heartbeat, use cardiac massage and mouth-to-mouth breathing (CPR). Don't try to make patient vomit. If you can't get help quickly, take patient to nearest emergency facility.**
- **See emergency information at end of book.**

When to take:
- At the same times each day, preferably on an empty stomach.
- Take extended-release tablet in the morning. Regular tablet often taken at breakfast and lunch. Don't take late in evening.

If you forget a dose:
Take as soon as you remember up to 2 hours late. If more than 2 hours, wait for next scheduled dose (don't double this dose).

What drug does:
Stimulates brain to improve alertness, concentration and attention span. Calms the hyperactive child.

Time lapse before drug works:
- 1 month or more for maximum effect on child.
- 30 minutes to stimulate adults.

Don't take with:
Any other medicine without consulting your doctor or pharmacist.

 ## POSSIBLE ADVERSE REACTIONS OR SIDE EFFECTS

SYMPTOMS	WHAT TO DO
Life-threatening: In case of overdose, see previous column.	
Common: Nervousness, trouble sleeping, dizziness, nausea, appetite loss, headache, drowsiness, stomach pain, weight loss.	Continue. Call doctor when convenient.
Infrequent: Rash or hives; chest pain; fast, irregular heartbeat; unusual bruising; joint pain; psychosis; uncontrollable movements; unexplained fever.	Discontinue. Call doctor right away.
Rare: Blurred vision, other vision change, sore throat, unusual tiredness, convulsions.	Discontinue. Call doctor right away.

WARNINGS & PRECAUTIONS

Don't take if:
• You are allergic to methylphenidate.
• You have glaucoma.

Before you start, consult your doctor:
• If you have epilepsy.
• It you have high blood pressure.
• If you take MAO inhibitors*.
• If you have emotional or psychotic problems.
• If you have a history of drug abuse.

Over age 60:
Adverse reactions and side effects may be more frequent and severe than in younger persons.

Pregnancy:
Decide with your doctor if drug benefits justify risk to unborn child. Risk category C (see page xxiii).

Breast-feeding:
No proven problems. Consult doctor.

Infants & children:
Use only under medical supervision for children 6 or older. Don't give to child younger than 6.

Prolonged use:
• Rare possibility of physical growth retardation in children.
• Talk to your doctor about the need for follow-up medical examinations or laboratory studies to check blood pressure, complete blood counts (white blood cell count, platelet count, red blood cell count, hemoglobin, hematocrit), growth charts.

Skin & sunlight:
No problems expected.

Driving, piloting or hazardous work:
No problems expected.

Discontinuing:
Don't discontinue abruptly. Don't discontinue without doctor's advice until you complete prescribed dose, even though symptoms diminish or disappear. Report to your doctor any new symptoms of depression, unusual behavior, unusual weakness or tiredness.

Others:
• Dose must be carefully adjusted by doctor.
• Advise any doctor or dentist whom you consult about the use of this medicine.

POSSIBLE INTERACTION WITH OTHER DRUGS

GENERIC NAME OR DRUG CLASS	COMBINED EFFECT
Anticholinergics*	Increased anticholinergic effect.
Anticoagulants*, oral	Increased anticoagulant effect.
Anticonvulsants*	Increased anticonvulsant effect.
Antidepressants, tricyclic*	Increased antidepressant effect. Decreased methylphenidate effect.
Antihypertensives*	Decreased antihypertensive effect.
Central nervous system (CNS) stimulants*	Overstimulation.
Cisapride	Decreased methylphenidate effect.
Dextrothyroxine	Increased methylphenidate effect.
Guanadrel	Decreased guanadrel effect.
Guanethidine	Decreased guanethidine effect.
Minoxidil	Decreased minoxidil effect.
Monoamine oxidase (MAO) inhibitors*	Dangerous rise in blood pressure.
Nitrates*	Possible decreased effects of both drugs.
Pimozide	May mask the cause of tics.

POSSIBLE INTERACTION WITH OTHER SUBSTANCES

INTERACTS WITH	COMBINED EFFECT
Alcohol:	None expected.
Beverages: Caffeine drinks.	May raise blood pressure.
Cocaine:	High risk of heartbeat irregularities and high blood pressure.
Foods: Foods containing tyramine*.	May raise blood pressure.
Marijuana:	None expected.
Tobacco:	None expected.

METHYSERGIDE

BRAND NAMES

Sansert

BASIC INFORMATION

Habit forming? Yes
Prescription needed? Yes
Available as generic? No
Drug class: Vasoconstrictor

 USES

Prevents migraine and other recurring vascular headaches. Not for acute attack.

 DOSAGE & USAGE INFORMATION

How to take:
Tablet—Swallow with liquid or with food to lessen stomach irritation. If you can't swallow whole, crumble tablet and take with liquid or food.

When to take:
At the same times each day.

If you forget a dose:
Don't take missed dose. Wait for next scheduled dose (don't double this dose).

What drug does:
Blocks the action of serotonin, a chemical that constricts blood vessels.

Time lapse before drug works:
About 3 weeks.

Don't take with:
Any other medicine without consulting your doctor or pharmacist.

 OVERDOSE

SYMPTOMS:
Nausea, vomiting, abdominal pain, severe diarrhea, lack of coordination, extreme thirst.
WHAT TO DO:
Overdose unlikely to threaten life. If person takes much larger amount than prescribed, call doctor, poison control center or hospital emergency room for instructions.

 POSSIBLE ADVERSE REACTIONS OR SIDE EFFECTS

SYMPTOMS	WHAT TO DO
Life-threatening:	
In case of overdose, see previous column.	
Common:	
• Itchy skin.	Discontinue. Call doctor right away.
• Nausea, vomiting, diarrhea, numbness or tingling of extremities, leg weakness, abdominal pain.	Continue. Call doctor when convenient.
• Drowsiness, constipation.	Continue. Tell doctor at next visit.
Infrequent:	
• Anxiety, agitation, hallucinations, unusually fast or slow heartbeat, dizziness.	Discontinue. Call doctor right away.
• Change in vision, nightmares, insomnia.	Continue. Call doctor when convenient.
Rare:	
• Extreme thirst, chest pain, shortness of breath, fever, pale or swollen extremities, leg cramps, lower back pain, side or groin pain, appetite loss, joint and muscle pain, rash, facial flush, painful or difficult urination.	Discontinue. Call doctor right away.
• Weight change, hair loss.	Continue. Tell doctor at next visit.

 WARNINGS & PRECAUTIONS

Don't take if:
• You are allergic to any antiserotonin*.
• You plan to become pregnant within medication period.
• You have an infection.
• You have a heart or blood vessel disease.
• You have a chronic lung disease.
• You have a collagen (connective tissue) disorder.
• You have impaired liver or kidney function.

Before you start, consult your doctor:
- If you have been allergic to any ergot preparation.
- If you have had a peptic ulcer.

Over age 60:
Adverse reactions and side effects may be more frequent and severe than in younger persons.

Pregnancy:
Consult doctor. Risk category X (see page xxiii).

Breast-feeding:
Drug probably passes into milk. Avoid drug or discontinue nursing until you finish medicine. Consult doctor for advice on maintaining milk supply.

Infants & children:
Not recommended.

Prolonged use:
- May cause fibrosis, a condition in which scar tissue is deposited on heart valves, in lung tissue, blood vessels and internal organs. After 6 months, decrease dose over 2 to 3 weeks. Then discontinue for at least 2 months for re-evaluation.
- Talk to your doctor about the need for follow-up medical examinations or laboratory studies to check retroperitoneal imaging*.

Skin & sunlight:
No problems expected.

Driving, piloting or hazardous work:
Avoid if you feel drowsy or dizzy. Otherwise, no problems expected.

Discontinuing:
- Don't discontinue without consulting doctor. Dose may require gradual reduction if you have taken drug for a long time. Doses of other drugs may also require adjustment.
- Probably should discontinue drug if you don't improve after 3 weeks use.

Others:
- Periodic laboratory tests for liver function and blood counts recommended.
- Potential for abuse.
- Some products contain tartrazine dye. Avoid, especially if you are allergic to aspirin.

POSSIBLE INTERACTION WITH OTHER DRUGS

GENERIC NAME OR DRUG CLASS	COMBINED EFFECT
Ergot preparations*	Unpredictable increased or decreased effect of either drug.
Narcotics*	Decreased narcotic effect.

POSSIBLE INTERACTION WITH OTHER SUBSTANCES

INTERACTS WITH	COMBINED EFFECT
Alcohol:	None expected. However, alcohol may trigger a migraine headache.
Beverages: Caffeine drinks.	Decreased methysergide effect.
Cocaine:	May make headache worse.
Foods:	None expected. Avoid foods to which you are allergic.
Marijuana:	No proven problems.
Tobacco:	Blood vessel constriction. Makes headache worse.

METOCLOPRAMIDE

BRAND NAMES

Apo-Metoclop	Octamide
Clopra	Octamide PFS
Emex	Reclomide
Maxeran	Reglan

BASIC INFORMATION

Habit forming? No
Prescription needed? Yes
Available as generic? Yes
Drug class: Antiemetic, dopaminergic blocker

USES

- Relieves nausea and vomiting caused by chemotherapy and drug-related postoperative factors.
- Relieves symptoms of esophagitis and stomach swelling in people with diabetes.

DOSAGE & USAGE INFORMATION

How to take:
Tablet or syrup—Swallow with liquid or food to lessen stomach irritation.

When to take:
30 minutes before symptoms expected, up to 4 times a day.

If you forget a dose:
Take as soon as you remember up to 2 hours late. If more than 2 hours, wait for next scheduled dose (don't double this dose).

Continued next column

OVERDOSE

SYMPTOMS:
Severe drowsiness, muscle spasms, mental confusion, trembling, seizure, coma.
WHAT TO DO:
- Dial 911 (emergency) or 0 (operator) for an ambulance or medical help. Then give first aid immediately.
- If patient is unconscious and not breathing, give mouth-to-mouth breathing. If there is no heartbeat, use cardiac massage and mouth-to-mouth breathing (CPR). Don't try to make patient vomit. If you can't get help quickly, take patient to nearest emergency facility.
- See emergency information on inside covers.

What drug does:
- Prevents smooth muscle in stomach from relaxing.
- Affects vomiting center in brain.

Time lapse before drug works:
30 to 60 minutes.

Don't take with:
Any other medicine without consulting your doctor or pharmacist.

POSSIBLE ADVERSE REACTIONS OR SIDE EFFECTS

SYMPTOMS	WHAT TO DO
Life-threatening: In case of overdose, see previous column.	
Common: Drowsiness, restlessness.	Continue. Call doctor when convenient.
Frequent Rash.	Continue. Call doctor when convenient.
Infrequent: • Wheezing, shortness of breath.	Discontinue. Call doctor right away.
• Dizziness; headache; insomnia; tender, swollen breasts; increased milk flow, menstrual changes; decreased sex drive.	Continue. Call doctor when convenient.
Rare: • Abnormal, involuntary movements of jaw, lips and tongue; depression; Parkinson's syndrome*.	Discontinue. Call doctor right away.
• Constipation, nausea, diarrhea, dry mouth.	Continue. Call doctor when convenient.

WARNINGS & PRECAUTIONS

Don't take if:
You are allergic to procaine, procainamide or metoclopramide.

Before you start, consult your doctor:
- If you have Parkinson's disease.
- If you have liver or kidney disease.
- If you have epilepsy.
- If you have bleeding from gastrointestinal tract or intestinal obstruction.
- If you will have surgery within 2 months, including dental surgery, requiring general or spinal anesthesia.

Over age 60:
Adverse reactions and side effects may be more frequent and severe than in younger persons.

Pregnancy:
No proven harm to unborn child. Avoid if possible. Consult doctor. Risk category B (see page xxiii).

Breast-feeding:
Unknown effect. Consult doctor.

Infants & children:
Adverse reactions more likely to occur than in adults.

Prolonged use:
Adverse reactions including muscle spasms and trembling hands more likely to occur.

Skin & sunlight:
No problems expected.

Driving, piloting or hazardous work:
Don't drive or pilot aircraft until you learn how medicine affects you. Don't work around dangerous machinery. Don't climb ladders or work in high places. Danger increases if you drink alcohol or take medicine affecting alertness and reflexes, such as antihistamines, tranquilizers, sedatives, pain medicine, narcotics and mind-altering drugs.

Discontinuing:
May be unnecessary to finish medicine. Follow doctor's instructions.

Others:
No problems expected.

POSSIBLE INTERACTION WITH OTHER DRUGS

GENERIC NAME OR DRUG CLASS	COMBINED EFFECT
Acetaminophen	Increased absorption of acetaminophen.
Anticholinergics*	Decreased metoclopramide effect.
Aspirin	Increased absorption of aspirin.
Bromocriptine	Decreased bromocriptine effect.
Butyophenone	Increased chance of muscle spasm and trembling.
Central nervous system (CNS) depressants*	Excess sedation.
Clozapine	Toxic effect on the central nervous system.
Digitalis preparations*	Decreased absorption of digitalis.

Ethinamate	Dangerous increased effects of ethinamate. Avoid combining.
Fluoxetine	Increased depressant effects of both drugs.
Guanfacine	May increase depressant effects of either drug.
Insulin	Unpredictable changes in blood glucose. Dosages may require adjustment.
Leucovorin	High alcohol content of leucovorin may cause adverse effects.
Levodopa	Increased absorption of levodopa.
Lithium	Increased absorption of lithium.
Loxapine	May increase toxic effects of both drugs.
Methyprylon	Increased sedative effect, perhaps to dangerous level. Avoid.
Nabilone	Greater depression of central nervous system.

Continued on page 922

POSSIBLE INTERACTION WITH OTHER SUBSTANCES

INTERACTS WITH	COMBINED EFFECT
Alcohol:	Excess sedation. Avoid.
Beverages: Coffee.	Decreased metoclopramide effect.
Cocaine:	Decreased metoclopramide effect.
Foods:	No problems expected.
Marijuana:	Decreased metoclopramide effect.
Tobacco:	Decreased metoclopramide effect.

*See Glossary

METRONIDAZOLE

BRAND NAMES

Apo-Metronidazole
Flagyl
Helidac
Metizol
Metric 21
Metro Cream
Metro I.V.
Metrogel

Metrogel-Vaginal
Neo-Metric
Novonidazol
PMS Metronidazole
Protostat
Satric
Trikacide

BASIC INFORMATION

Habit forming? No
Prescription needed? Yes
Available as generic? Yes
Drug class: Antiprotozoal, antibacterial (antibiotic)

 ## USES

- Treatment for infections susceptible to metronidazole, such as trichomoniasis and amebiasis.
- Treatment for bacterial infections.
- Topical—Treats acne rosacea (adult acne).
- Vaginal—Treats vaginal infections.
- Treatment (combined with other drugs) for duodenal ulcer associated with *Helicobacter pylori* infection.

 ## DOSAGE & USAGE INFORMATION

How to take:
- Cream—Apply to affected area 3 times daily.
- Tablet—Swallow with liquid or food to lessen stomach irritation. If you can't swallow whole, crumble tablet and take with liquid or food.
- Topical gel—Apply thin layer to involved area.

When to take:
- At the same times each day.
- Gel—Apply twice a day.

Continued next column

 ## OVERDOSE

SYMPTOMS:
Weakness, nausea, vomiting, diarrhea, confusion, seizures.
WHAT TO DO:
Overdose unlikely to threaten life. If person takes much larger amount than prescribed, call doctor, poison control center or hospital emergency room for instructions.

If you forget a dose:
Take as soon as you remember up to 2 hours late. If more than 2 hours, wait for next scheduled dose (don't double this dose).

What drug does:
Kills organisms causing the infection.

Time lapse before drug works:
Begins in 1 hour. May require regular use for 10 days to cure infection.

Don't take with:
- Nonprescription medicines containing alcohol.
- Any other medicine without consulting your doctor or pharmacist.

 ## POSSIBLE ADVERSE REACTIONS OR SIDE EFFECTS

SYMPTOMS	WHAT TO DO
Life-threatening:	
In case of overdose, see previous column.	
Common:	
Appetite loss, nausea, stomach pain, diarrhea, vomiting.	Continue. Call doctor when convenient.
Infrequent:	
• Dizziness, headache.	Continue. Call doctor when convenient.
• Numbness, tingling, weakness or pain in hands or feet.	Discontinue. Call doctor right away.
• Dark urine (will go away when drug is discontinued).	No action necessary.
Rare:	
• Metallic taste, unpleasant taste, dry mouth, vaginal irritation.	Continue. Call doctor when convenient.
• Unsteadiness or clumsiness; mood or mental changes; skin rash, hives, redness or itch; sore throat and fever; seizures; severe stomach or back pain.	Discontinue. Call doctor right away.

WARNINGS & PRECAUTIONS

Don't take if:
- You are allergic to metronidazole.
- You have had a blood cell or bone marrow disorder.

Before you start, consult your doctor:
- If you plan to become pregnant within medication period.
- If you have a brain or nervous system disorder.
- If you have liver or heart disease.
- If you drink alcohol.

Over age 60:
Adverse reactions and side effects may be more frequent and severe than in younger persons.

Pregnancy:
Consult doctor. Risk category B (see page xxiii).

Breast-feeding:
Drug passes into milk. Avoid drug or discontinue nursing until you finish medicine. Consult doctor for advice on maintaining milk supply.

Infants & children:
Use in children for amoeba infection only under close medical supervision.

Prolonged use:
Talk to your doctor about the need for follow-up medical examinations or laboratory studies to check for giardiasis in stools.

Skin & sunlight:
No problems expected.

Driving, piloting or hazardous work:
Avoid if you feel dizzy or unsteady. Otherwise, no problems expected.

Discontinuing:
Don't discontinue without doctor's advice until you complete prescribed dose, even though symptoms diminish or disappear.

Others:
Avoid alcohol 12 hours before and *at least* 24 hours after treatment period with metronidazole.

POSSIBLE INTERACTION WITH OTHER DRUGS

GENERIC NAME OR DRUG CLASS	COMBINED EFFECT
Anticoagulants*, oral	Increased anticoagulant effect. Possible bleeding or bruising.
Antihistamines, nonsedating	Serious heart rhythm problems with astemizole and terfenadine. Avoid.
Antivirals, HIV/AIDS*	Increased risk of peripheral neuropathy.
Cimetidine	Prolongs increased serum levels.
Disulfiram	Disulfiram reaction*. Avoid.
Nizatidine	Increased effect and toxicity of metoprolol.
Oxytetracycline	Decreased metronidazole effect.
Phenobarbital	Decreased metronidazole effect.
Phenytoin	Decreased metronidazole effect.

POSSIBLE INTERACTION WITH OTHER SUBSTANCES

INTERACTS WITH	COMBINED EFFECT
Alcohol:	Possible disulfiram reaction*. Avoid alcohol in *any* form or amount.
Beverages:	None expected.
Cocaine:	Decreased metronidazole effect. Avoid.
Foods:	None expected.
Marijuana:	None expected.
Tobacco:	None expected.

METYRAPONE

BRAND NAMES

Metopirone

BASIC INFORMATION

Habit forming? No
Prescription needed? Yes
Available as generic? No
Drug class: Antiadrenal

 ## USES

- To diagnose the function of the pituitary gland.
- Treats Cushing's disease, a disorder characterized by higher than normal concentrations of cortisol (one of the hormones secreted by the adrenal glands) in the blood.

 ## DOSAGE & USAGE INFORMATION

How to take:
- For medical testing purposes—Take the prescribed number of tablets with milk or food on the day before the scheduled test. On the day of the test, blood and urine studies will show the amount of hormones in your blood. Results of the test will help establish your diagnosis.
- For treatment of Cushing's syndrome— Swallow tablet with liquid. If you can't swallow whole, crumble tablet and take with liquid or food.

When to take:
- For medical testing—Take the prescribed number of tablets on the day before the scheduled test.
- For treatment of Cushing's disease—Take total daily amount in divided doses. Follow prescription directions carefully.

Continued next column

 ## OVERDOSE

SYMPTOMS:
Nausea (severe), vomiting, diarrhea, abdominal pain, sudden weakness, irregular heartbeat.
WHAT TO DO:
- **Dial 911 (emergency) or 0 (operator) for an ambulance or medical help. Then give first aid immediately.**
- **See emergency information on inside covers.**

If you forget a dose:
Take as soon as you remember up to 2 hours late. If more than 2 hours, wait for next scheduled dose (don't double this dose).

What drug does:
Prevents one of the chemical reactions in the production of cortisol by the adrenal glands.

Time lapse before drug works:
Approximately 1 hour.

Don't take with:
Cortisone*-like medicines for 48 hours prior to testing.

 ## POSSIBLE ADVERSE REACTIONS OR SIDE EFFECTS

SYMPTOMS	WHAT TO DO?
Life-threatening:	
In case of overdose, see previous column.	
Common:	
Dizziness, headache, nausea.	Continue. Call doctor when convenient.
Infrequent:	
Drowsiness.	Continue. Call doctor when convenient.
Rare:	
Hair loss or excess growth, decreased appetite, confusion, acne (may begin or may worsen if already present).	Continue. Call doctor when convenient.

WARNINGS & PRECAUTIONS

Don't take if:
• You have adrenal insufficiency (Addison's disease).
• You have decreased pituitary function.

Before you start, consult your doctor:
• If you are allergic to metyrapone.
• If you have porphyria.

Over age 60:
No special problems expected.

Pregnancy:
Safety not established. Take only under careful supervision of medical professional. Risk category C (see page xxiii).

Breast-feeding:
Drug may pass into milk, although controlled studies in humans have not been performed. Since the possibility exists, avoid nursing until you finish the medicine.

Infants & children:
No special problems expected.

Prolonged use:
No special problems expected.

Skin & sunlight:
No special problems expected.

Driving, piloting or hazardous work:
Don't drive or pilot aircraft until you learn how medicine affects you. Don't work around dangerous machinery. Don't climb ladders or work in high places. Danger increases if you drink alcohol or take medicine affecting alertness and reflexes.

Discontinuing:
No special problems expected.

Others:
Advise any doctor or dentist whom you consult that you take this medicine.

POSSIBLE INTERACTION WITH OTHER DRUGS

GENERIC NAME OR DRUG CLASS	COMBINED EFFECT
Antidiabetics, oral*	Increased risk of adverse reactions.
Contraceptives, oral*	Possible inaccurate test results.
Estrogens*	Possible inaccurate test results.
Insulin	Increased risk of adverse reactions.
Phenytoin	Possible inaccurate test results.

POSSIBLE INTERACTION WITH OTHER SUBSTANCES

INTERACTS WITH	COMBINED EFFECT
Alcohol:	None expected.
Beverages:	None expected.
Cocaine:	None expected.
Foods:	Increased appetite and absorption of nutrients, causing difficulty with weight control.
Marijuana:	None expected.
Tobacco:	None expected.

METYROSINE

BRAND NAMES

Demser

BASIC INFORMATION

Habit forming? No
Prescription needed? Yes
Available as generic? No
Drug class: Antihypertensive

USES

- Treatment of pheochromocytoma* (adrenal gland tumor) that causes high blood pressure.
- Preoperative medication for removal of the tumor.

DOSAGE & USAGE INFORMATION

How to take:
Capsules—Swallow with liquid. If you can't swallow whole, open capsule and take with liquid or food. Instructions to take on empty stomach mean 1 hour before or 2 hours after eating.

When to take:
- Usually 4 times a day, approximately 6 hours apart.
- If used before surgery, take for at least 5 to 7 days.

If you forget a dose:
Take as soon as you remember up to 2 hours late. If more than 2 hours, wait for next scheduled dose (don't double this dose).

What drug does:
Reduces blood pressure in patients with pheochromocytoma* by reducing synthesis of catecholamines*.

Time lapse before drug works:
2 to 3 days.

Continued next column

OVERDOSE

SYMPTOMS:
Confusion, sudden shortness of breath, hallucinations, seizures, coma.
WHAT TO DO:
- **Dial 911 (emergency) or 0 (operator) for an ambulance or medical help. Then give first aid immediately.**
- **See emergency information on inside covers.**

Don't take with:
Any other medicines (including over-the-counter drugs such as cough and cold medicines, laxatives, antacids, diet pills, caffeine, nose drops or vitamins) without consulting your doctor.

POSSIBLE ADVERSE REACTIONS OR SIDE EFFECTS

SYMPTOMS	WHAT TO DO
Life-threatening:	
In case of overdose, see previous column.	
Common:	
• Severe diarrhea, tremors, drooling, speech difficulties.	Continue. Call doctor when convenient.
• Drowsiness.	Continue. Tell doctor at next visit.
Infrequent:	
Skin rash, sexual difficulties in males.	Continue. Call doctor when convenient.
Rare:	
• Shortness of breath, itching, bloody urine, muscle spasms, swollen feet.	Discontinue. Call doctor right away.
• Depression.	Continue. Call doctor when convenient.

WARNINGS & PRECAUTIONS

Don't take if:
You are allergic to metyrosine.

Before you start, consult your doctor:
- If you have liver disease.
- If you have mental depression.
- If you have Parkinson's disease.
- If you have kidney disease.

Over age 60:
Adverse reactions and side effects may be more frequent and severe than in younger persons. You may need smaller doses for shorter periods of time.

Pregnancy:
Decide with your doctor if drug benefits justify risk to unborn child. Risk category C (see page xxiii).

Breast-feeding:
Not recommended. Consult doctor.

Infants & children:
No proven problems.

Prolonged use:
Talk to your doctor about the need for follow-up medical examinations or laboratory studies to check blood pressure, heart function, ECG*, kidney function and urinary catecholamine measurements.

Skin & sunlight:
No problems expected.

Driving, piloting or hazardous work:
Don't drive or pilot aircraft until you learn how medicine affects you. Don't work around dangerous machinery. Don't climb ladders or work in high places. Danger increases if you drink alcohol or take medicine affecting alertness and reflexes.

Discontinuing:
May experience increased energy and insomnia for a short period (2 to 7 days).

Others:
- Advise any doctor or dentist whom you consult that you take this medicine.
- May affect results in some medical tests.

POSSIBLE INTERACTION WITH OTHER DRUGS

GENERIC NAME OR DRUG CLASS	COMBINED EFFECT
Antidepressants, tricyclic*	Increased sedative effect of each.
Central nervous system (CNS) depressants*	Increased sedative effect.
Clozapine	Toxic effect on the central nervous system.
Phenothiazines*	Increased likelihood of toxic symptoms of each.
Sertraline	Increased depressive effects of both drugs.
Trimeprazine	Increased likelihood of toxic symptoms of each.

POSSIBLE INTERACTION WITH OTHER SUBSTANCES

INTERACTS WITH	COMBINED EFFECT
Alcohol:	May cause Parkinson's*-like disorder. Don't mix.
Beverages:	No special problems expected.
Cocaine:	No special problems expected.
Foods:	No special problems expected.
Marijuana:	No special problems expected.
Tobacco:	No special problems expected.

MEXILETINE

BRAND NAMES

Mexitil

BASIC INFORMATION

Habit forming? No
Prescription needed? Yes
Available as generic? Yes
Drug class: Antiarrhythmic

 ## USES

Stabilizes irregular heartbeat.

 ## DOSAGE & USAGE INFORMATION

How to take:
Capsules—Swallow whole with food, milk or antacid to lessen stomach irritation.

When to take:
At the same times each day as directed by your doctor.

If you forget a dose:
Take as soon as you remember up to 4 hours late. If more than 4 hours, wait for next scheduled dose (don't double this dose).

What drug does:
Blocks the fast sodium channel in heart tissue.

Time lapse before drug works:
30 minutes to 2 hours.

Don't take with:
Any other medicine without consulting your doctor or pharmacist.

 ## OVERDOSE

SYMPTOMS:
Nausea, vomiting, seizures, convulsions, cardiac arrest.
WHAT TO DO:
* **Dial 911 (emergency) or 0 (operator) for an ambulance or medical help. Then give first aid immediately.**
* **See emergency information on inside covers.**

 ## POSSIBLE ADVERSE REACTIONS OR SIDE EFFECTS

SYMPTOMS	WHAT TO DO
Life-threatening: Chest pain, shortness of breath, irregular or fast heartbeat.	Discontinue. Seek emergency treatment.
Common: Dizziness, anxiety, shakiness, unsteadiness when walking, heartburn, nausea, vomiting.	Discontinue. Call doctor right away.
Infrequent: • Sore throat, fever, mouth sores; blurred vision; confusion; constipation; diarrhea; headache; numbness or tingling in hands or feet; ringing in ears; unexplained bleeding or bruising; rash; slurred speech; insomnia; weakness; difficult swallowing.	Discontinue. Call doctor right away.
• Loss of taste.	Continue. Call doctor when convenient.
Rare: • Seizures.	Discontinue. Seek emergency treatment.
• Hallucinations, psychosis, memory loss, difficult breathing, swollen feet and ankles, hiccups, jaundice.	Discontinue. Call doctor right away.
• Hair loss, impotence.	Continue. Call doctor when convenient.

WARNINGS & PRECAUTIONS

Don't take if:
If you are allergic to mexiletine, lidocaine or tocainide.

Before you start, consult your doctor:
- If you have had liver or kidney disease or impaired kidney function.
- If you have had lupus.
- If you have a history of seizures.
- If you will have surgery within 2 months, including dental surgery, requiring general or spinal anesthesia.
- If you have heart disease or low blood pressure.

Over age 60:
Adverse reactions and side effects may be more frequent and severe than in younger persons. Ask doctor about smaller doses.

Pregnancy:
Decide with your doctor if drug benefits justify risk to unborn child. Risk category C (see page xxiii).

Breast-feeding:
Drug passes into milk. Avoid drug or discontinue nursing until you finish medicine. Consult doctor for advice on maintaining milk supply.

Infants & children:
Use only under close medical supervision.

Prolonged use:
- May cause lupus*-like illness.
- Talk to your doctor about the need for follow-up medical examinations or laboratory studies to check ECG*, liver function.

Skin & sunlight:
No problems expected.

Driving, piloting or hazardous work:
Use caution if you feel dizzy or weak. Otherwise, no problems expected.

Discontinuing:
Don't discontinue without consulting doctor. Dose may require gradual reduction if you have taken drug for a long time. Doses of other drugs may also require adjustment.

Others:
No problems expected.

POSSIBLE INTERACTION WITH OTHER DRUGS

GENERIC NAME OR DRUG CLASS	COMBINED EFFECT
Cimetidine	Increased mexiletine effect and toxicity.
Encainide	Increased effect of toxicity on the heart muscle.
Nicardipine	Possible increased effect and toxicity of each drug.
Phenobarbital	Decreased mexiletine effect.
Phenytoin	Decreased mexiletine effect.
Propafenone	Increased effect of both drugs and increased risk of toxicity.
Rifampin	Decreased mexiletine effect.
Urinary acidifiers* (ammonium chloride, ascorbic acid, potassium or sodium phosphate)	May decrease effectiveness of medicine.
Urinary alkalizers* (acetazolamide, antacids with calcium or magnesium, citric acid, dichlorphenamide, methazolamide, potassium citrate, sodium bicarbonate, sodium citrate)	May slow elimination of mexiletine and cause need to adjust dosage.

POSSIBLE INTERACTION WITH OTHER SUBSTANCES

INTERACTS WITH	COMBINED EFFECT
Alcohol:	Causes irregular effectiveness of mexiletine. Avoid.
Beverages: Caffeine drinks, iced drinks.	Irregular heartbeat.
Cocaine:	Decreased mexiletine effect.
Foods:	None expected.
Marijuana:	Irregular heartbeat. Avoid.
Tobacco:	Dangerous combination. May lead to liver problems and reduce excretion of mexiletine.

MIGLITOL

BRAND NAMES

Glyset

BASIC INFORMATION

Habit forming? No
Prescription needed? Yes
Available as generic? No
Drug class: Antidiabetic

 USES

Treatment for hyperglycemia (excess sugar in the blood) that cannot be controlled by diet alone in patients with type II non-insulin-dependent diabetes mellitus (NIDDM). May be used alone or in combination with other antidiabetic drugs.

 DOSAGE & USAGE INFORMATION

How to take:
Tablet—Swallow with liquid. Take at the very beginning of a meal.

When to take:
Usually 3 times a day or as directed by doctor. Dosage may be increased at 4- to 8-week intervals until maximum benefits are achieved.

Continued next column

 OVERDOSE

SYMPTOMS:
- Will not produce hypoglycemia. May cause flatulence, diarrhea, abdominal pain. Unlikely to produce serious side effects.
- Symptoms of hypoglycemia—stomach pain, anxious feeling, cold sweats, chills, confusion, convulsions, cool pale skin, excessive hunger, nausea or vomiting, rapid heartbeat, nervousness, shakiness, unsteady walk, unusual weakness or tiredness, vision changes, unconsciousness.

WHAT TO DO:
- For mild low blood sugar symptoms, drink or eat something containing dextrose or glucose (fruits, honey, starches) right away.
- For more severe symptoms, dial 911 (emergency) or 0 (operator) for an ambulance or medical help. Then give first aid immediately.
- See emergency information on inside covers.

If you forget a dose:
And your meal is finished, then skip the missed dose and wait for your next meal and next scheduled dose (don't double this dose).

What drug does:
Impedes the digestion and absorption of carbohydrates and their subsequent conversion into glucose. This improves control of blood glucose and may reduce the complications of diabetes. However, miglitol does not cure diabetes.

Time lapse before drug works:
May take several weeks for full effectiveness.

Don't take with:
Any other prescription or nonprescription drug without consulting your doctor or pharmacist. All possible drug interactions have not been studied.

 POSSIBLE ADVERSE REACTIONS OR SIDE EFFECTS

SYMPTOMS	WHAT TO DO
Life-threatening:	
In case of overdose or low blood sugar, see previous column.	
Common:	
Diarrhea, stomach cramps, gas, bloating feeling.	Continue. Call doctor when convenient.
Infrequent:	
Skin rash.	Continue. Call doctor when convenient.
Rare:	
Severe low blood sugar (see symptoms under Overdose). help.	Discontinue. Call doctor right away or seek emergency

WARNINGS & PRECAUTIONS

Don't take if:
You are allergic to miglitol.

Before you start, consult your doctor:
- If you have any kidney or liver disease or any heart or blood vessel disorder.
- If you have any chronic health problem.
- If you have an infection, illness or any condition that can cause low blood sugar.
- If you have a history of acid in the blood (metabolic acidosis or ketoacidosis).
- If you have inflammatory bowel disease or any other intestinal disorder.
- If you are allergic to any medication, food or other substance.

Over age 60:
No special problems expected.

Pregnancy:
Decide with your doctor if drug benefits justify risks to unborn child. Risk category B (see page xxiii).

Breast-feeding:
Drug passes into milk. It is not recommended for use in nursing mothers.

Infants & children:
Safety and efficacy have not been established. Use only under close medical supervision.

Prolonged use:
- Schedule regular doctor visits to determine if the drug is continuing to be effective in controlling the diabetes and to check for any problems in kidney function.
- You will most likely require an antidiabetic medicine for the rest of your life.
- You will need to test your blood glucose levels several times a day, or for some, once to several times a week.

Skin & sunlight:
No special problems expected.

Driving, piloting or hazardous work:
No special problems expected.

Discontinuing:
Don't discontinue without consulting your doctor even if you feel well. You can have diabetes without feeling any symptoms. Untreated diabetes can cause serious problems.

Others:
- Advise any doctor or dentist whom you consult that you take this medicine.
- It may interfere with the accuracy of some medical tests.
- Follow any special diet your doctor may prescribe. It can help control diabetes.
- Consult doctor if you become ill with vomiting or diarrhea while taking this drug.

- Use caution when exercising. Ask your doctor about an appropriate exercise program.
- Wear medical identification stating that you have diabetes and take this medication.
- Learn to recognize the symptoms of low blood sugar. You and your family need to know what to do if these symptoms occur.
- Have a glucagon kit and syringe in the event severe low blood sugar occurs.
- High blood sugar (hyperglycemia) may occur with diabetes. Ask your doctor about symptoms to watch for and treatment steps to take.
- Educate yourself about diabetes.

POSSIBLE INTERACTION WITH OTHER DRUGS

GENERIC NAME OR DRUG CLASS	COMBINED EFFECT
Amylase (Pancreatic enzyme)	Decreased miglitol effect.
Antidiabetic agents, sulfonylurea	May cause hypoglycemia.
Charcoal, activated	Decreased miglitol effect.
Pancreatin (Pancreatic enzyme)	Decreased miglitol effect.
Propranolol	**Decreased effect of** propranolol.
Ranitidine	Decreased effect of ranitidine.

POSSIBLE INTERACTION WITH OTHER SUBSTANCES

INTERACTS WITH	COMBINED EFFECT
Alcohol:	May increase effect of miglitol. Avoid excessive amounts.
Beverages:	No special problems.
Cocaine:	No special problems. Best to avoid.
Foods:	No special problems.
Marijuana:	No special problems. Best to avoid.
Tobacco:	People with diabetes should not smoke.

MINOXIDIL

BRAND NAMES

Loniten

BASIC INFORMATION

Habit forming? No
Prescription needed? Yes
Available as generic? Yes
Drug class: Antihypertensive

USES

- Treatment for high blood pressure in conjunction with other drugs, such as beta-adrenergic blockers and diuretics.
- Treatment for congestive heart failure.
- Can stimulate hair growth.

DOSAGE & USAGE INFORMATION

How to take:
Tablet—Swallow with liquid. If you can't swallow whole, crumble tablet and take with liquid or food.

When to take:
At the same time each day, according to instructions on prescription label.

If you forget a dose:
Take as soon as you remember up to 2 hours late. If more than 2 hours, wait for next scheduled dose (don't double this dose).

What drug does:
Relaxes small blood vessels (arterioles) so blood can pass through more easily.

Time lapse before drug works:
2 to 3 hours for effect to begin; 3 to 7 days of continuous use may be necessary for maximum blood pressure response.

Don't take with:
Any other medicine without consulting your doctor or pharmacist.

OVERDOSE

SYMPTOMS:
Low blood pressure, fainting, chest pain, shortness of breath, coma.
WHAT TO DO:
- **Dial 911 (emergency) or 0 (operator) for an ambulance or medical help. Then give first aid immediately.**
- **See emergency information on inside covers.**

POSSIBLE ADVERSE REACTIONS OR SIDE EFFECTS

SYMPTOMS	WHAT TO DO
Life-threatening:	
In case of overdose, see previous column.	
Common:	
• Excessive hair growth, flushed skin or redness.	Continue. Call doctor when convenient.
• Bloating.	Discontinue. Call doctor right away.
Infrequent:	
• Chest pain, irregular or slow heartbeat, shortness of breath, swollen feet or legs, rapid weight gain.	Discontinue. Call doctor right away.
• Numbness of hands, feet or face; headache; tender breasts; darkening of skin.	Continue. Call doctor when convenient.
Rare:	
Rash.	Discontinue. Call doctor right away.

WARNINGS & PRECAUTIONS

Don't take if:
You are allergic to minoxidil.

Before you start, consult your doctor:
* If you have had recent stroke or heart attack or angina pectoris in past 3 weeks.
* If you have impaired kidney function.
* If you have pheochromocytoma*

Over age 60:
Adverse reactions and side effects may be more frequent and severe than in younger persons.

Pregnancy:
Decide with your doctor if drug benefits justify risk to unborn child. Risk category C (see page xxiii).

Breast-feeding:
Human studies not available. Avoid if possible. Consult doctor.

Infants & children:
Not recommended. Safety and dosage have not been established.

Prolonged use:
Request periodic blood examinations that include potassium levels.

Skin & sunlight:
May cause rash or intensify sunburn in areas exposed to sun or ultraviolet light (photosensitivity reaction). Avoid overexposure. Notify doctor if reaction occurs.

Driving, piloting or hazardous work:
Avoid if you become dizzy or faint. Otherwise, no problems expected.

Discontinuing:
Don't discontinue without consulting doctor. Dose may require gradual reduction if you have taken drug for a long time. Doses of other drugs may also require adjustment.

Others:
* Check pulse regularly. If it exceeds 20 or more beats per minute over your normal rate, consult doctor immediately.
* Check blood pressure frequently.

POSSIBLE INTERACTION WITH OTHER DRUGS

GENERIC NAME OR DRUG CLASS	COMBINED EFFECT
Anesthesia	Drastic blood pressure drop.
Antihypertensives*, other	Dosage adjustments may be necessary to keep blood pressure at desired level.
Carteolol	Increased anti-hypertensive effect.
Diuretics*	Dosage adjustments may be necessary to keep blood pressure at desired level.
Estrogens*	May increase blood pressure.
Guanadrel	Weakness and faintness when arising from bed or chair.
Guanethidine	Weakness and faintness when arising from bed or chair.
Lisinopril	Increased anti-hypertensive effect. Dosage of each may require adjustment.
Nicardipine	Blood pressure drop. Dosages may require adjustment.
Nimodipine	Dangerous blood pressure drop.
Nitrates*	Drastic blood pressure drop.
Sotalol	Increased anti-hypertensive effect.
Sympathomimetics*	Possible decreased minoxidil effect.
Terazosin	Decreased effectiveness of terazosin.

POSSIBLE INTERACTION WITH OTHER SUBSTANCES

INTERACTS WITH	COMBINED EFFECT
Alcohol:	Possible excessive blood pressure drop.
Beverages:	None expected.
Cocaine:	Increased risk of heart block and high blood pressure.
Foods: Salt substitutes.	Possible excessive potassium levels in blood.
Marijuana:	Increased dizziness.
Tobacco:	May decrease minoxidil effect. Avoid.

*See Glossary

MINOXIDIL (Topical)

BRAND NAMES

Dermal   Rogaine for Men
Rogaine   Rogaine for Women
Rogaine Extra
  Strength for Men

BASIC INFORMATION

Habit forming? No
Prescription needed? No
Available as generic? No
Drug class: Hair growth stimulant

 ## USES

Treats hair loss on scalp from male and female pattern baldness (alopecia androgenetica).

 ## DOSAGE & USAGE INFORMATION

How to use:
Topical solution
- Apply only to dry hair and scalp. With the provided applicator, apply the amount prescribed to the scalp area being treated. Begin in center of the treated area.
- Wash hands immediately after use.
- Don't use a blow dryer.
- If you are using at bedtime, wait 30 minutes after applying before retiring.

When to use:
Twice a day or as directed.

If you forget a dose:
Use as soon as you remember. No need to ever double the dose.

What drug does:
Stimulates hair growth by possibly dilating small blood capillaries, thereby providing more blood to hair follicles.

Time lapse before drug works:
Varies with individuals.

Don't use with:
Any other medicine without consulting your doctor or pharmacist

 ## OVERDOSE

SYMPTOMS:
None expected.
WHAT TO DO:
Not for internal use. If child accidentally swallows, call poison control center.

 ## POSSIBLE ADVERSE REACTIONS OR SIDE EFFECTS

SYMPTOMS	WHAT TO DO
Life-threatening: Fast, irregular heartbeat (rare; represents too much absorbed into body).	Discontinue. Seek emergency treatment.
Common: None expected.	
Infrequent: Itching scalp; flaking, reddened skin.	Continue. Call doctor when convenient.
Rare: Burning scalp, skin rash, swollen face, headache, dizziness or fainting, hands and feet numb or tingling, rapid weight gain.	Discontinue. Call doctor right away.

WARNINGS & PRECAUTIONS

Don't use if:
You are allergic to minoxidil.

Before you start, consult your doctor:
- If you are allergic to anything.
- If you have heart disease or high blood pressure.
- If you have skin irritation or abrasion or severe sunburn (systemic absorption may be increased).

Over age 60:
No problems expected.

Pregnancy:
Decide with your doctor if drug benefits justify risk to unborn child. Risk category C (see page xxiii).

Breast-feeding:
Don't use.

Infants & children:
Don't use.

Prolonged use:
No problems expected.

Skin & sunlight:
No problems expected.

Driving, piloting or hazardous work:
No problems expected.

Discontinuing:
No problems expected.

Others:
- Keep away from eyes, nose and mouth. Flush with plain water if accident occurs.
- New hair will drop out when you stop using minoxidil.
- Keep solution cool, but don't freeze.

POSSIBLE INTERACTION WITH OTHER DRUGS

GENERIC NAME OR DRUG CLASS	COMBINED EFFECT
Adrenocorticoids*, topical	May cause undesirable absorption of minoxidil.
Minoxidil, oral	Increased risk of toxicity.
Petrolatum, topical	May cause undesirable absorption of minoxidil.
Retinoids*, topical	May cause undesirable absorption of minoxidil.

POSSIBLE INTERACTION WITH OTHER SUBSTANCES

INTERACTS WITH	COMBINED EFFECT
Alcohol:	None expected.
Beverages:	None expected.
Cocaine:	None expected.
Foods:	None expected.
Marijuana:	None expected.
Tobacco:	None expected.

MIRTAZAPINE

BRAND NAMES

Remeron

BASIC INFORMATION

Habit forming? Not expected
Prescription needed? Yes
Available as generic? No
Drug class: Antidepressant

 ## USES

Treats symptoms of mental depression.

 ## DOSAGE & USAGE INFORMATION

How to take:
Tablet—Swallow with liquid. May be taken with or without food.

When to take:
At the same time each day, usually in the evening before bedtime.

If you forget a dose:
Take as soon as you remember up to 12 hours late. If more than 12 hours, wait for the next scheduled dose (don't double this dose).

What drug does:
The exact mechanism is unknown. It appears to block certain chemicals in the brain, which in turn helps production of other brain chemicals that play a role in helping to relieve symptoms of depression.

Time lapse before drug works:
Will take up to several weeks to show improvement of the depression symptoms.

Don't take with:
Any other prescription or nonprescription drug without consulting your doctor or pharmacist.

 ## OVERDOSE

SYMPTOMS:
Drowsiness, disorientation, memory impairment, rapid heartbeat.
WHAT TO DO:
- **Dial 911 (emergency) or 0 (operator) for an ambulance or medical help. Then give first aid immediately.**
- **See emergency information on inside covers.**

 ## POSSIBLE ADVERSE REACTIONS OR SIDE EFFECTS

SYMPTOMS	WHAT TO DO
Life-threatening: None expected.	
Common:	
• Sleepiness, increased appetite, weight gain, dizziness, dry mouth, constipation, tiredness, increased thirst.	Continue. Call doctor when convenient.
• Abdominal pain, vomiting, joint pain, increased cough, rash, itching, agitation, anxiety, twitching, apathy.	Discontinue. Call doctor right away.
Infrequent:	
• Forgetfulness, lightheadedness.	Continue. Call doctor when convenient.
• Slow heartbeat, migraine, dehydration, weight loss, unusual weakness, pain in any part of the body, changes in menstrual periods, changes in vision or hearing, mouth sores, mood or mental changes, breathing difficulty, lack of coordination.	Discontinue. Call doctor right away.
Rare:	
• Muscle aches, strange dreams, headache.	Continue. Call doctor when convenient.
• Swelling of hands, feet or legs; infection (fever, chills, aches or pains, sore throat); swollen or discolored tongue; changes in urinary function; hives.	Discontinue. Call doctor right away.

WARNINGS & PRECAUTIONS

Don't take if:
You are allergic to mirtazapine.

Before you start, consult your doctor:
- If you have seizure disorder, heart disease, blood circulation problem or had a stroke.
- If you are dehydrated.
- If you have a history of drug dependence or drug abuse.
- If you have kidney or liver disease.
- If you have a history of mood disorders, such as mania, or thoughts of suicide.
- If you are allergic to any other medication, food or other substances.

Over age 60:
A lower starting dosage is usually recommended until a response is determined.

Pregnancy:
Decide with your doctor if drug benefits justify risk to unborn child. Risk category C (see page xxiii).

Breast-feeding:
It is unknown if drug passes into milk. Avoid drug or discontinue nursing until you finish medicine. Consult doctor for advice on maintaining milk supply.

Infants & children:
Safety in children under age 18 has not been established.

Prolonged use:
Consult with your doctor on a regular basis while taking this drug to check your progress, to discuss any increase or changes in side effects and the need for continued treatment.

Skin & sunlight:
May cause a rash or intensify sunburn in areas exposed to sun or ultraviolet light (photosensitivity reaction). Avoid excessive sun exposure. Consult doctor if reaction occurs.

Driving, piloting or hazardous work:
Don't drive or pilot aircraft until you learn how medicine affects you. Don't work around dangerous machinery. Don't climb ladders or work in high places. Danger increases if you drink alcohol or take medicine affecting alertness and reflexes.

Discontinuing:
Consult doctor before discontinuing this drug.

Others:
- Get up slowly from a sitting or lying position to avoid dizziness, faintness or lightheadedness.
- Advise any doctor or dentist whom you consult that you take this medicine.
- Do not increase or reduce dosage without doctor's approval.

POSSIBLE INTERACTION WITH OTHER DRUGS

GENERIC NAME OR DRUG CLASS	COMBINED EFFECT
Benzodiazepines	Increased sedative effect. Avoid.
Monoamine oxidase, (MAO) inhibitors	Potentially life-threatening. Allow 14 days between use of 2 drugs.
Other medications	Complete studies have not been done to evaluate interactions with other drugs, but the potential exists for a variety of possible interactions. Consult doctor.

POSSIBLE INTERACTION WITH OTHER SUBSTANCES

INTERACTS WITH	COMBINED EFFECT
Alcohol:	Increased sedative affect. Avoid.
Beverages:	None expected.
Cocaine:	Unknown effect. Best to avoid.
Foods:	None expected.
Marijuana:	Unknown effect. Best to avoid.
Tobacco:	None expected.

MISOPROSTOL

BRAND NAMES

Arthrotec   Cytotec

BASIC INFORMATION

Habit forming? No
Prescription needed? Yes
Available as generic? No
Drug class: Antiulcer agent

USES

Prevents development of stomach ulcers in persons taking nonsteroidal anti-inflammatory drugs (NSAIDs), including aspirin.

DOSAGE & USAGE INFORMATION

How to take:
Tablets—Swallow with liquid. If you can't swallow whole, crumble tablet and take with liquid or food. Instructions to take on empty stomach mean 1 hour before or 2 hours after eating.

When to take:
Usually 4 times a day while awake, with or after meals and at bedtime.

If you forget a dose:
Take as soon as you remember up to 2 hours late. If more than 2 hours, wait for next scheduled dose (don't double this dose).

What drug does:
- Improves defense against peptic ulcers by strengthening natural defenses of the stomach lining.
- Decreases stomach acid production.

Time lapse before drug works:
10 to 15 minutes.

Don't take with:
Any other medicines (including over-the-counter drugs such as cough and cold medicines, laxatives, antacids, diet pills, caffeine, nose drops or vitamins) without consulting your doctor or pharmacist.

OVERDOSE

SYMPTOMS:
None expected.
WHAT TO DO:
Overdose unlikely to threaten life. If person takes much larger amount than prescribed, call doctor, poison control center or hospital emergency room for instructions.

POSSIBLE ADVERSE REACTIONS OR SIDE EFFECTS

SYMPTOMS	WHAT TO DO
Life-threatening: None expected.	
Common: Abdominal pain, diarrhea.	Discontinue. Call doctor right away.
Infrequent:	
• Nausea or vomiting.	Continue. Call doctor when convenient.
• Constipation, headache.	Continue. Tell doctor at next visit.
Rare:	
• Gaseousness.	Continue. Tell doctor at next visit.
• Vaginal bleeding	Discontinue. Call doctor right away.

WARNINGS & PRECAUTIONS

Don't take if:
- You are allergic to any prostaglandin*.
- You are pregnant or of child-bearing age.

Before you start, consult your doctor:
- If you have epilepsy.
- If you have heart disease.
- If you have blood vessel disease of any kind.

Over age 60:
No special problems expected.

Pregnancy:
- Risk to unborn child outweighs drug benefits. Don't use.
- May also lead to serious complications in pregnant women, including excessive bleeding and future infertility.
- Risk category X (see page xxiii).

Breast-feeding:
Drug passes into milk. Avoid drug or discontinue nursing until you finish medicine. Consult doctor for advice on maintaining milk supply.

Infants & children:
Not recommended for children under 18.

Prolonged use:
Talk to your doctor about the need for follow-up medical examinations or laboratory studies to check gastric analysis.

Skin & sunlight:
No problems expected.

Driving, piloting or hazardous work:
Avoid if you feel confused, drowsy or dizzy.

Discontinuing:
No special problems expected.

Others:
Advise any doctor or dentist whom you consult that you take this medicine.

POSSIBLE INTERACTION WITH OTHER DRUGS

GENERIC NAME OR DRUG CLASS	COMBINED EFFECT
Antacids*, magnesium-containing	Severe diarrhea.

POSSIBLE INTERACTION WITH OTHER SUBSTANCES

INTERACTS WITH	COMBINED EFFECT
Alcohol:	Decreases misoprostol effect. Avoid.
Beverages: Caffeine-containing.	Decreases misoprostol effect. Avoid.
Cocaine:	Decreases misoprostol effect. Avoid.
Foods:	No special problems expected.
Marijuana:	Decreases misoprostol effect. Avoid.
Tobacco:	Decreases misoprostol effect. Avoid.

*See Glossary

MITOTANE

BRAND NAMES

Lysodren   o,p´-DDD

BASIC INFORMATION

Habit forming? No
Prescription needed? Yes
Available as generic? No
Drug class: Antineoplastic, antiadrenal

 USES

- Treatment for some kinds of cancer.
- Treatment of Cushing's disease.

 DOSAGE & USAGE INFORMATION

How to take:
Tablet—Take with liquid after light meal. Don't drink fluid with meals. Drink extra fluids between meals. Avoid sweet and fatty foods.

When to take:
At the same time each day.

If you forget a dose:
Take as soon as you remember. Don't ever double dose.

What drug does:
Suppresses adrenal cortex to prevent manufacture of excess cortisone.

Time lapse before drug works:
2 to 3 weeks for full effect.

Don't take with:
Any other medicine without consulting your doctor or pharmacist.

 OVERDOSE

SYMPTOMS:
Headache, vomiting blood, stupor, seizure.
WHAT TO DO:
- **Dial 911 (emergency) or 0 (operator) for an ambulance or medical help. Then give first aid immediately.**
- **If patient is unconscious and not breathing, give mouth-to-mouth breathing. If there is no heartbeat, use cardiac massage and mouth-to-mouth breathing (CPR). Don't try to make patient vomit. If you can't get help quickly, take patient to nearest emergency facility.**
- **See emergency information on inside covers.**

 ## POSSIBLE ADVERSE REACTIONS OR SIDE EFFECTS

SYMPTOMS	WHAT TO DO
Life-threatening:	
In case of overdose, see previous column.	
Common:	
• Darkened skin, appetite loss, nausea, vomiting.	Continue. Call doctor when convenient.
• Mental depression, drowsiness.	Continue. Tell doctor at next visit.
Infrequent:	
• Fever, chills, sore throat.	Discontinue. Seek emergency treatment.
• Unusual bleeding or bruising, difficult breathing.	Discontinue. Call doctor right away.
• Rash, hair loss, blurred vision, seeing double, cough, tiredness, weakness, dizziness when standing after sitting or lying down.	Continue. Call doctor when convenient.
Rare:	
Blood in urine.	Continue. Call doctor when convenient.

WARNINGS & PRECAUTIONS

Don't take if:
You are allergic to mitotane corticosteroids* or any antineoplastic drug.

Before you start, consult your doctor:
- If you have liver disease.
- If you have infection.

Over age 60:
Adverse reactions and side effects may be more frequent and severe than in younger persons.

Pregnancy:
Decide with your doctor whether drug benefits justify risk to unborn child. Risk category C (see page xxiii).

Breast-feeding:
Unknown if drug passes into milk. Consult doctor.

Infants & children:
Use only under care of medical supervisors who are experienced in administering anticancer drugs.

Prolonged use:
Adverse reactions more likely the longer drug is required.

Skin & sunlight:
No problems expected.

Driving, piloting or hazardous work:
No problems expected.

Discontinuing:
- Don't discontinue without consulting doctor. Dose may require gradual reduction if you have taken drug for a long time. Doses of other drugs may also require adjustment.
- Some side effects may follow discontinuing. Report any new symptoms.

Others:
No problems expected.

POSSIBLE INTERACTION WITH OTHER DRUGS

GENERIC NAME OR DRUG CLASS	COMBINED EFFECT
Adrenocorticoids, systemic	Decreased adreno-corticoid effect.
Antidepressants*	Increased central nervous system depression.
Antihistamines*	Increased central nervous system depression.
Central nervous system (CNS) depressants*	Increased sedation.
Phenytoin	Possible increased metabolism.
Spironolactone	Decreased mitotane effect.
Warfarin	Decreased warfarin effect.

POSSIBLE INTERACTION WITH OTHER SUBSTANCES

INTERACTS WITH	COMBINED EFFECT
Alcohol:	Increased depression. Avoid.
Beverages:	No problems expected.
Cocaine:	Increased toxicity. Avoid.
Foods:	Reduced irritation in stomach.
Marijuana:	No problems expected.
Tobacco:	Increased possibility of lung toxicity.

MOLINDONE

BRAND NAMES

Moban   Moban Concentrate

BASIC INFORMATION

Habit forming? No
Prescription needed? Yes
Available as generic? No
Drug class: Antipsychotic

USES

Treats severe emotional, mental or nervous problems.

DOSAGE & USAGE INFORMATION

How to take:
Tablet or solution—Swallow with liquid or food to lessen stomach irritation. If you can't swallow tablet whole, crumble and take with food or liquid.

When to take:
Follow instructions on prescription label. Doses should be evenly spaced. For example, 4 times a day means every 6 hours.

If you forget a dose:
Take as soon as you remember up to 2 hours late. If more than 2 hours, wait for next scheduled dose (don't double this dose).

What drug does:
Corrects an imbalance in nerve impulses from the brain.

Time lapse before drug works:
Some benefit seen within a week; 4 to 6 weeks for full benefit.

Don't take with:
- Antacid or medicine for diarrhea.
- Nonprescription drugs for cough, cold or allergy.

OVERDOSE

SYMPTOMS:
Stupor, convulsions, coma.
WHAT TO DO:
- **Dial 911 (emergency) or 0 (operator) for an ambulance or medical help. Then give first aid immediately.**
- **See emergency information at end of book.**

POSSIBLE ADVERSE REACTIONS OR SIDE EFFECTS

SYMPTOMS	WHAT TO DO
Life-threatening:	
High fever, rapid pulse, profuse sweating, muscle rigidity, confusion and irritability, seizures.	Discontinue. Seek emergency treatment.
Common:	
Sedation, low blood pressure and dizziness.	Continue. Call doctor when convenient.
Infrequent:	
• Jerky or involuntary movements, especially of the face, lips, jaw, tongue; slow-frequency tremor of head or limbs, especially while moving; muscle rigidity, lack of facial expression and slow, inflexible movements	Discontinue. Call doctor right away.
• Pacing or restlessness; intermittent spasms of muscles of face, eyes, tongue, jaw, neck, body or limbs; dry mouth, blurred vision, constipation, difficulty urinating.	Continue. Call doctor when convenient.
Rare:	
Other symptoms not listed above.	Continue. Call doctor when convenient.

WARNINGS & PRECAUTIONS

Don't take if:
- You are allergic to any phenothiazine.
- You have a blood or bone marrow disease.

Before you start, consult your doctor:
- If you will have surgery within 2 months, including dental surgery, requiring general or spinal anesthesia.
- If you have asthma, emphysema or other lung disorder, glaucoma, prostate trouble, seizure disorders.
- If you take nonprescription ulcer medicine, asthma medicine or amphetamines.

Over age 60:
Adverse reactions and side effects may be more frequent and severe than in younger persons. More likely to develop involuntary movement of jaws, lips, tongue; chewing. Report this to your doctor immediately. Early treatment can help.

Pregnancy:
Decide with your doctor if drug benefits justify risk to unborn child. Risk category C (see page xxiii).

Breast-feeding:
Safety not established. Consult doctor.

Infants & children:
Don't give to children younger than 2.

Prolonged use:
- May lead to tardive dyskinesia (involuntary movement of jaws, lips, tongue; chewing).
- Talk to your doctor about the need for follow-up medical examinations or laboratory studies to check kidney function, eyes.

Skin & sunlight:
Avoid getting overheated. The drug affects body temperature and sweating.

Driving, piloting or hazardous work:
Don't drive or pilot aircraft until you learn how medicine affects you. Don't work around dangerous machinery. Don't climb ladders or work in high places. Danger increases if you drink alcohol or take medicine affecting alertness and reflexes.

Discontinuing:
- Nervous and mental disorders—Don't discontinue without doctor's advice until you complete prescribed dose, even though symptoms diminish or disappear.
- Notify your doctor if any of the following occurs—Uncontrollable movements of tongue, arms and legs; lip smacking.

Others:
Advise any doctor or dentist whom you consult that you take this medicine.

 POSSIBLE INTERACTION WITH OTHER DRUGS

GENERIC NAME OR DRUG CLASS	COMBINED EFFECT
Anticholinergics*	Increased anticholinergic effect.
Antidepressants, tricyclic*	Increased molindone effect.
Antihistamines*	Increased antihistamine effect.
Appetite suppressants*	Decreased appetite suppressant effect.
Beta-adrenergic blocking agents*	Increased tranquilizer effect.
Bupropion	Increased risk of seizures.
Central nervous system (CNS) depressants*	Increased depressive effects of both drugs.
Clozapine	Toxic effect on the central nervous system.
Extrapyramidal reaction-causing medications*	Increased frequency and severity of extrapyramidal effects.
Fluoxetine	Increased depressant effects of both drugs.
Guanethidine	Decreased guanethidine effect.
Guanfacine	May increase depressant effects of either drug.
Leucovorin	High alcohol content of leucovorin may cause adverse effects.
Levodopa	Decreased levodopa effect.
Loxapine	May increase toxic effects of both drugs.
Mind-altering drugs*	Increased effect of mind-altering drugs.

Continued on page 922

 POSSIBLE INTERACTION WITH OTHER SUBSTANCES

INTERACTS WITH	COMBINED EFFECT
Alcohol:	Dangerous oversedation.
Beverages:	None expected.
Cocaine:	Decreased molindone effect. Avoid.
Foods:	None expected.
Marijuana:	Drowsiness. May increase antinausea effect.
Tobacco:	None expected.

MONOAMINE OXIDASE (MAO) INHIBITORS

GENERIC AND BRAND Names

PHENELZINE
Nardil

TRANYLCYPROMINE
Parnate

BASIC INFORMATION

Habit forming? No
Prescription needed? Yes
Available as generic? No
Drug class: MAO (monoamine oxidase)
inhibitor, antidepressant

USES

- Treatment for depression and panic disorder.
- Prevention of vascular or tension headaches.

DOSAGE & USAGE INFORMATION

How to take:
Tablet—Swallow with liquid. If you can't swallow whole, crumble tablet and take with liquid or food.

When to take:
At the same times each day.

If you forget a dose:
Take as soon as you remember up to 2 hours late. If more than 2 hours, wait for next scheduled dose (don't double this dose).

What drug does:
Inhibits nerve transmissions in brain that may cause depression.

Time lapse before drug works:
4 to 6 weeks for maximum effect.

Continued next column

OVERDOSE

SYMPTOMS:
Restlessness, agitation, excitement, fever, confusion, dizziness, heartbeat irregularities, hallucinations, sweating, breathing difficulties, insomnia, irritability, convulsions, coma.
WHAT TO DO:
- **Dial 911 (emergency) or 0 (operator) for an ambulance or medical help. Then give first aid immediately.**
- **See emergency information at end of book.**

Don't take with:
- Nonprescription diet pills; nose drops; medicine for asthma, cough, cold or allergy; medicine containing caffeine or alcohol.
- Foods containing tyramine*. Life-threatening elevation of blood pressure may result.
- Any other medicine without consulting your doctor or pharmacist.

POSSIBLE ADVERSE REACTIONS OR SIDE EFFECTS

SYMPTOMS	WHAT TO DO
Life-threatening: In case of overdose, see previous column. Also see above regarding dangers associated with tyramine.	
Common:	
Fatigue, weakness.	Continue. Call doctor when convenient.
Dizziness when changing position, restlessness, tremors, dry mouth, constipation, difficult urination, blurred vision, "sweet tooth."	Continue. Tell doctor at next visit.
Infrequent:	
Fainting, enlarged pupils, severe headache, chest pain, rapid or pounding heartbeat.	Discontinue. Seek emergency treatment.
Hallucinations, insomnia, nightmares, diarrhea, swollen feet or legs, joint pain.	Continue. Call doctor when convenient.
Diminished sex drive.	Continue. Tell doctor at next visit.
Rare: Rash, nausea, vomiting, stiff neck, jaundice, fever, increased sweating, dark urine, slurred speech, staggering gait.	Discontinue. Call doctor right away.

WARNINGS & PRECAUTIONS

Don't take if:
- You are allergic to any MAO inhibitor.
- You have heart disease, congestive heart failure, heart rhythm irregularities or high blood pressure.
- You have liver or kidney disease.

Before you start, consult your doctor:
- If you are alcoholic.
- If you have had a stroke.

- If you have diabetes, epilepsy, asthma, over-active thyroid, schizophrenia, Parkinson's disease, adrenal gland tumor.
- If you will have surgery within 2 months, including dental surgery, requiring general or spinal anesthesia.

Over age 60:
Not recommended. Adverse effects more likely.

Pregnancy:
Decide with your doctor if drug benefits justify risk to unborn child. Risk category C (see page xxiii).

Breast-feeding:
Safety not established. Consult doctor.

Infants & children:
Not recommended. Consult doctor.

Prolonged use:
- May be toxic to liver.
- Talk to your doctor about the need for follow-up medical examinations or laboratory studies to check blood pressure, liver function.

Skin & sunlight:
No special problems expected.

Driving, piloting or hazardous work:
Don't drive or pilot aircraft until you learn how medicine affects you. Don't work around dangerous machinery. Don't climb ladders or work in high places. Danger increases if you drink alcohol or take medicine affecting alertness and reflexes.

Discontinuing:
- Don't discontinue without doctor's advice until you complete prescribed dose, even though symptoms diminish or disappear.
- Follow precautions regarding foods, drinks and other medicines for 2 weeks after discontinuing.
- Adverse symptoms caused by this medicine may occur even after discontinuation. If you develop any of the symptoms listed under Overdose, notify your doctor immediately.

Others:
- May affect blood sugar levels in patients with diabetes.
- Advise any doctor or dentist whom you consult about the use of this medicine.
- Fever may indicate that MAO inhibitor dose requires adjustment.

 POSSIBLE INTERACTION WITH OTHER DRUGS

GENERIC NAME OR DRUG CLASS	COMBINED EFFECT
Amphetamines*	Blood pressure rise to life-threatening level.

Anticholinergics*	Increased anticholinergic effect.
Anticonvulsants*	Changed seizure pattern.
Antidepressants, tricyclic*	Blood pressure rise to life-threatening level. Possible fever, convulsions, delirium.
Antidiabetic agents, oral* and insulin	Excessively low blood sugar.
Antihypertensives*	Excessively low blood pressure.
Beta-adrenergic blocking agents*	Possible blood pressure rise if MAO inhibitor is discontinued after simultaneous use with acebutolol.
Bupropion	Increased risk of side effects.
Buspirone	Very high blood pressure.
Caffeine	Irregular heartbeat or high blood pressure.
Carbamazepine	Fever, seizures. Avoid.

Continued on page 922

 POSSIBLE INTERACTION WITH OTHER SUBSTANCES

INTERACTS WITH	COMBINED EFFECT
Alcohol:	Increased sedation to dangerous level.
Beverages: Caffeine drinks.	Irregular heartbeat or high blood pressure.
Drinks containing tyramine*.	Blood pressure rise to life-threatening level.
Cocaine:	Overstimulation. Possibly fatal.
Foods: Foods containing tyramine*.	Blood pressure rise to life-threatening level.
Marijuana:	Overstimulation. Avoid.
Tobacco:	No proven problems.

*See Glossary

MORICIZINE

BRAND NAMES

Ethmozine

BASIC INFORMATION

Habit forming? No
Prescription needed? Yes
Available as generic? No
Drug class: Antiarrhythmic

 ## USES

Treats severe heartbeat irregularities, primarily life-threatening ventricular tachycardia.

 ## DOSAGE & USAGE INFORMATION

How to take:
Tablets—As directed, by mouth with water.

When to take:
When directed. The first dose of this medicine is usually given in an emergency room or in the hospital under continuous monitoring.

If you forget a dose:
Take as soon as you remember up to 4 hours late. If more than 4 hours, wait for next scheduled dose (don't double this dose).

What drug does:
Affects the electrical conduction system inside the heart.

Time lapse before drug works:
Promptly, but may require up to 2 hours for full effect.

Don't take with:
Any other medicine without consulting your doctor or pharmacist.

 ## OVERDOSE

SYMPTOMS:
Fainting, chest pain, vomiting, lethargy, coma.
WHAT TO DO:
- Dial 911 (emergency) or 0 (operator) for an ambulance or medical help. Then give first aid immediately.
- See emergency information on inside covers.

 ## POSSIBLE ADVERSE REACTIONS OR SIDE EFFECTS

SYMPTOMS	WHAT TO DO
Life-threatening: In case of overdose, see previous column.	
Common: Dizziness.	Continue. Call doctor when convenient.
Infrequent: Chest pain; blurred vision; diarrhea; dry mouth; headache; numbness and tingling in arms, legs; nausea; abdominal pain.	Discontinue. Call doctor right away.
Rare: Sudden high fever.	Discontinue. Call doctor right away.

WARNINGS & PRECAUTIONS

Don't take if:
- You have pre-existing heart block.
- You have right bundle branch block.
- You are allergic to moricizine.

Before you start, consult your doctor:
- If you take any other prescription or nonprescription medicine.
- If you have liver or kidney disease.
- If you have any heart problems.

Over age 60:
No age-related adverse effects expected.

Pregnancy:
Consult doctor. Risk category B (see page xxlii).

Breast-feeding:
Drug may pass into milk. Consult doctor.

Infants & children:
No special problems expected.

Prolonged use:
No special problems expected.

Skin & sunlight:
No special problems expected.

Driving, piloting or hazardous work:
Don't drive or pilot aircraft until you learn how medicine affects you. Don't work around dangerous machinery. Don't climb ladders or work in high places. Danger increases if you drink alcohol or take medicine affecting alertness and reflexes.

Discontinuing:
No special problems expected.

Others:
The first dose of this medication is usually given while the patient is being closely monitored in an intensive care setting with cardiac monitoring or in an emergency room.

POSSIBLE INTERACTION WITH OTHER DRUGS

GENERIC NAME OR DRUG CLASS	COMBINED EFFECT
Antiarrhythmics*, other	Possible increased effects of both drugs.
Cimetidine	Increased concentration of cimetidine in the blood.
Theophylline	Decreased effect of theophylline.

POSSIBLE INTERACTION WITH OTHER SUBSTANCES

INTERACTS WITH	COMBINED EFFECT
Alcohol:	Avoid.
Beverages:	None expected.
Cocaine:	Increased irregular heartbeat. Avoid.
Foods:	None expected.
Marijuana:	Possible increased irregular heartbeat. Avoid.
Tobacco:	Possible increased irregular heartbeat. Avoid.

GENERIC AND BRAND NAMES

CARISOPRODOL	**METAXALONE**
Rela	Skalaxin
Sodol	**METHOCARBAMOL**
Soma	Carbacot
Soma Compound	Delaxin
with Codeine	Marbaxin
Sopridol	Robamol
Soridol	Robaxin
CHLORPHENESIN	Robaxisal
Maolate	Robomol
CHLORZOXAZONE	Skelex
Paraflex	
Parafon Forte	

BASIC INFORMATION

Habit forming? Possibly
Prescription needed? Yes
Available as generic? Yes, for some.
Drug class: Muscle relaxant

USES

Adjunctive treatment to rest, analgesics and physical therapy for muscle spasms.

DOSAGE & USAGE INFORMATION

How to take:
- Tablets—Swallow with liquid. If you can't swallow whole, crumble tablet and take with liquid or food. Instructions to take on empty stomach mean 1 hour before or 2 hours after eating.
- Extended-release tablets—Swallow whole with liquid. Don't crumble tablet.

When to take:
As needed, no more often than every 4 hours.

Continued next column

OVERDOSE

SYMPTOMS:
Nausea, vomiting, diarrhea, convulsions, headache. May progress to severe weakness, difficult breathing, sensation of paralysis, coma.
WHAT TO DO:
- **Dial 911 (emergency) or 0 (operator) for an ambulance or medical help. Then give first aid immediately.**
- **See emergency information on inside covers.**

If you forget a dose:
Take as soon as you remember. Wait 4 hours for next dose (don't double this dose).

What drug does:
Blocks body's pain messages to brain. Also causes sedation.

Time lapse before drug works:
30 to 60 minutes.

Don't take with:
Any other medicine without consulting your doctor or pharmacist.

POSSIBLE ADVERSE REACTIONS OR SIDE EFFECTS

SYMPTOMS	WHAT TO DO
Life-threatening:	
Hives, rash, intense itching, faintness soon after a dose (anaphylaxis); extreme weakness, transient paralysis, temporary vision loss.	Seek emergency treatment immediately.
Common:	
• Drowsiness, dizziness.	Continue. Call doctor when convenient.
• Orange or red-purple urine.	No action necessary.
Infrequent:	
• Agitation, constipation or diarrhea, nausea, cramps, vomiting, wheezing, shortness of breath, headache, depression, muscle weakness, trembling, insomnia, uncontrolled eye movements, fainting.	Discontinue. Call doctor right away.
• Blurred vision.	Continue. Call Doctor when convenient.
Rare:	
• Black, tarry or bloody stool; convulsions.	Discontinue. Seek emergency treatment.
• Rash, hives, or itch; sore throat; fever; jaundice; tiredness; weakness; hiccups.	Discontinue. Call doctor right away.

WARNINGS & PRECAUTIONS

Don't take if:
- You are allergic to any skeletal muscle relaxant.
- You have porphyria.

Before you start, consult your doctor:
- If you have had liver or kidney disease.
- If you plan pregnancy within medication period.
- If you are allergic to tartrazine dye.
- If you suffer from depression.

Over age 60:
Adverse reactions and side effects may be more frequent and severe than in younger persons.

Pregnancy:
Safety not proven. Avoid if possible. Consult doctor. Risk category C (see page xxiii).

Breast-feeding:
Drug may pass into milk. Avoid drug or discontinue nursing until you finish medicine. Consult doctor for advice on maintaining milk supply.

Infants & children:
Not recommended.

Prolonged use:
- Talk to your doctor about the need for follow-up medical examinations or laboratory studies to check liver function, kidney function, complete blood counts (white blood cell count, platelet count, red blood cell count, hemoglobin, hematocrit).
- Safety beyond 8 weeks of treatment not established.

Skin & sunlight:
No problems expected.

Driving, piloting or hazardous work:
Don't drive or pilot aircraft until you learn how medicine affects you. Don't work around dangerous machinery. Don't climb ladders or work in high places. Danger increases if you drink alcohol or take medicine affecting alertness and reflexes, such as antihistamines, tranquilizers, sedatives, pain medicine, narcotics and mind-altering drugs.

Discontinuing:
Don't discontinue without doctor's advice until you complete prescribed dose, even though symptoms diminish or disappear.

Others:
- May affect results in some medical tests.
- Advise any doctor or dentist whom you consult that you take this medicine.

POSSIBLE INTERACTION WITH OTHER DRUGS

GENERIC NAME OR DRUG CLASS	COMBINED EFFECT
Antidepressants*	Increased sedation.
Antihistamines*	Increased sedation.
Clozapine	Toxic effect on the central nervous system.
Central nervous system (CNS) depressants*	Increased depressive effects of both drugs.
Dronabinol	Increased effect of dronabinol on central nervous system. Avoid combination.
Mind-altering drugs*	Increased sedation.
Muscle relaxants*, others	Increased sedation.
Narcotics*	Increased sedation.
Sedatives*	Increased sedation.
Sertraline	Increased depressive effects of both drugs.
Sleep inducers*	Increased sedation.
Tranquilizers*	Increased sedation.

POSSIBLE INTERACTION WITH OTHER SUBSTANCES

INTERACTS WITH	COMBINED EFFECT
Alcohol:	Increased sedation.
Beverages:	None expected.
Cocaine:	Lack of coordination, increased sedation.
Foods:	None expected.
Marijuana:	Lack of coordination, drowsiness, fainting.
Tobacco:	None expected.

NABILONE

BRAND NAMES

Cesamet

BASIC INFORMATION

Habit forming? No
Prescription needed? Yes
Available as generic? No
Drug class: Antiemetic

USES

- Treats nausea and vomiting.
- Prevents nausea and vomiting in patients receiving cancer chemotherapy.

DOSAGE & USAGE INFORMATION

How to take:
Capsule—Swallow with liquid. If you can't swallow whole, open capsule and take with liquid or food.

When to take:
At the same times each day, according to instructions on prescription label.

If you forget a dose:
Take as soon as you remember up to 2 hours late. If more than 2 hours, wait for next scheduled dose (don't double this dose).

What drug does:
Chemically related to marijuana, it probably regulates the vomiting control center in the brain.

Continued next column

OVERDOSE

SYMPTOMS:
Mood changes; confusion and delusions; hallucinations; mental depression; nervousness; breathing difficulty; fast, slow or pounding heartbeat; fainting.
WHAT TO DO:
- **Dial 911 (emergency) or 0 (operator) for an ambulance or medical help. Then give first aid immediately.**
- **If patient is unconscious and not breathing, give mouth-to-mouth breathing. If there is no heartbeat, use cardiac massage and mouth-to-mouth breathing (CPR). Don't try to make patient vomit. If you can't get help quickly, take patient to nearest emergency facility.**
- **See emergency information on inside covers.**

Time lapse before drug works:
2 hours.

Don't take with:
Alcohol or any drug that depresses the central nervous system. See Central Nervous System (CNS) Depressants in the Glossary.

POSSIBLE ADVERSE REACTIONS OR SIDE EFFECTS

SYMPTOMS	WHAT TO DO
Life-threatening: Mood changes; fainting; hallucinations; fast, slow or pounding heartbeat; confusion and delusions; mental depression; nervousness; breathing difficulty.	Seek emergency treatment.
Common: Dry mouth.	Continue. Call doctor when convenient.
Infrequent: Clumsiness, mental changes, drowsiness, headache, false sense of well-being.	Discontinue. Call doctor right away.
Rare: Blurred vision, dizziness on standing, appetite loss, muscle pain.	Discontinue. Call doctor right away.

WARNINGS & PRECAUTIONS

Don't take if:
- You are allergic to nabilone or marijuana.
- You have schizophrenic, manic or depressive states.

Before you start, consult your doctor:
- If you have abused drugs or are dependent on them, including alcohol.
- If you have had high blood pressure or heart disease.
- If you have had impaired liver function.

Over age 60:
Adverse reactions and side effects may be more frequent and severe than in younger persons. You may need smaller doses for shorter periods of time.

Pregnancy:
Decide with your doctor whether drug benefits justify risk to unborn child. Risk category C (see page xxiii).

Breast-feeding:
Drug passes into milk. Avoid drug or discontinue nursing until you finish medicine. Consult doctor for advice on maintaining milk supply.

Infants & children:
Not recommended for children 18 and younger. Use only under doctor's supervision.

Prolonged use:
- Avoid prolonged use. This medicine is intended to be used only during a cycle of cancer chemotherapy.
- Talk to your doctor about the need for follow-up medical examinations or laboratory studies to check blood pressure, heart function.

Skin & sunlight:
No problems expected.

Driving, piloting or hazardous work:
Don't drive or pilot aircraft until you learn how medicine affects you. Don't work around dangerous machinery. Don't climb ladders or work in high places. Danger increases if you drink alcohol or take medicine affecting alertness and reflexes.

Discontinuing:
No problems expected.

Others:
- Blood pressure should be measured regularly.
- Learn to count and recognize changes in your pulse.
- Get up from bed or chair slowly to avoid fainting.

POSSIBLE INTERACTION WITH OTHER DRUGS

GENERIC NAME OR DRUG CLASS	COMBINED EFFECT
Apomorphine	Decreased effect of apomorphine.
Central nervous system (CNS) depressants*, other	Greater depression of the central nervous system.

POSSIBLE INTERACTION WITH OTHER SUBSTANCES

INTERACTS WITH	COMBINED EFFECT
Alcohol:	Dangerous depression of the central nervous system. Avoid.
Beverages:	None expected.
Cocaine:	Decreased nabilone effect. Avoid.
Foods:	None expected.
Marijuana:	None expected.
Tobacco:	None expected.

*See Glossary

NAFARELIN

BRAND NAMES

Synarel

BASIC INFORMATION

Habit forming? No
Prescription needed? Yes
Available as generic? No
Drug class: Gonadotropin inhibitor

 USES

- Treatment for endometriosis to relieve pain and reduce scattered implants of endometrial tissue.
- Treatment for central precocious puberty.

 DOSAGE & USAGE INFORMATION

How to take:
Nasal spray—Follow instructions on package insert provided with your medicine.

When to take:
As directed by your doctor. Usually two times a day.

If you forget a dose:
Take as soon as you remember. Don't double this dose.

What drug does:
Reduces estrogen production by ovaries.

Time lapse before drug works:
May require 6 months for full effect.

Don't take with:
- Birth control pills.
- Nasal sprays to decongest the membranes in the nose.
- Any other medicine without consulting your doctor or pharmacist.

 OVERDOSE

SYMPTOMS:
None expected.
WHAT TO DO:
Overdose unlikely to threaten life. If person takes much larger amount than prescribed, call doctor, poison control center or hospital emergency room for instructions.

 POSSIBLE ADVERSE REACTIONS OR SIDE EFFECTS

SYMPTOMS	WHAT TO DO
Life-threatening: None expected.	
Common: Hot flashes.	No action necessary.
Infrequent: Decreased sexual desire, vaginal dryness, headache, acne, swelling of hands and feet, reduction of breast size, weight gain, itchy scalp with flaking, muscle ache, nasal irritation.	Continue. Call doctor when convenient.
Rare: Insomnia, depression, weight loss.	Continue. Call doctor when convenient.

WARNINGS & PRECAUTIONS

Don't take if:
- You become pregnant.
- You have breast cancer.
- You are allergic to any of the ingredients in nafarelin.
- You have undiagnosed abnormal vaginal bleeding.

Before you start, consult your doctor:
- If you take birth control pills.
- If you have diabetes.
- If you have heart disease.
- If you have epilepsy.
- If you have kidney disease.
- If you have liver disease.
- If you have migraine headaches.
- If you need to use topical nasal decongestants.

Over age 60:
Adverse reactions and side effects may be more frequent and severe than in younger persons.

Pregnancy:
Risk to unborn child outweighs drug benefits. Don't use. Stop if you get pregnant. Consult doctor. Risk category X (see page xxiii).

Breast-feeding:
Unknown whether medicine filters into milk. Consult doctor.

Infants & children:
Not recommended.

Prolonged use:
- Full effect requires prolonged use. Don't discontinue without consulting doctor.
- Talk to your doctor about the need for mammogram, follow-up medical examinations or laboratory studies to check liver function.

Skin & sunlight:
No special problems expected.

Driving, piloting or hazardous work:
No special problems expected.

Discontinuing:
Don't discontinue without consulting doctor. Menstrual periods may be absent for 2 to 3 months after discontinuation.

Others:
- May alter blood sugar levels in diabetic persons.
- Interferes with accuracy of laboratory tests to study pituitary gonadotropic and gonadal functions.
- Experience with nafarelin has been limited to women 18 years of age and older.
- Bone density decreases during treatment phase, but recovers following treatment.

POSSIBLE INTERACTION WITH OTHER DRUGS

GENERIC NAME OR DRUG CLASS	COMBINED EFFECT
Decongestant nasal sprays*	Decreased absorption of nafarelin.

POSSIBLE INTERACTION WITH OTHER SUBSTANCES

INTERACTS WITH	COMBINED EFFECT
Alcohol:	Excessive nervous system depression. Avoid.
Beverages: Caffeine drinks.	Rapid, irregular heartbeat. Avoid.
Cocaine:	May interfere with expected action of nafarelin. Avoid.
Foods:	None expected.
Marijuana:	May interfere with expected action of nafarelin. Avoid.
Tobacco:	Rapid, irregular heartbeat; increased leg cramps. Avoid.

*See Glossary

NALIDIXIC ACID

BRAND NAMES

NegGram

BASIC INFORMATION

Habit forming? No
Prescription needed? Yes
Available as generic? Yes
Drug class: Antimicrobial

 USES

Treatment for urinary tract infections.

 DOSAGE & USAGE INFORMATION

How to take:
• Tablet—Swallow with food or milk to lessen stomach irritation. If you can't swallow whole, crumble tablet and take with liquid or food.
• Liquid—Take with liquid or food.

When to take:
At the same times each day.

If you forget a dose:
Take as soon as you remember up to 2 hours late. If more than 2 hours, wait for next scheduled dose (don't double this dose).

What drug does:
Destroys bacteria susceptible to nalidixic acid.

Time lapse before drug works:
1 to 2 weeks.

Don't take with:
Any other medicine without consulting your doctor or pharmacist.

 OVERDOSE

SYMPTOMS:
Lethargy, stomach upset, behavioral changes, hyperglycemia, psychosis, convulsions and stupor.
WHAT TO DO:
• Dial 911 (emergency) or 0 (operator) for an ambulance or medical help. Then give first aid immediately.
• If patient is unconscious and not breathing, give mouth-to-mouth breathing. If there is no heartbeat, use cardiac massage and mouth-to-mouth breathing (CPR). Don't try to make patient vomit. If you can't get help quickly, take patient to nearest emergency facility.
• See emergency information on inside covers.

 POSSIBLE ADVERSE REACTIONS OR SIDE EFFECTS

SYMPTOMS	WHAT TO DO
Life-threatening: Hives, rash, intense itching, faintness soon after a dose (anaphylaxis).	Seek emergency treatment immediately.
Common: Rash; itchy skin; decreased, blurred or double vision; halos around lights or excess brightness; changes in color vision; nausea; vomiting; diarrhea.	Discontinue. Call doctor right away.
Infrequent: • Dizziness, drowsiness, sensitivity to sun, headache.	Continue. Call doctor when convenient.
• Dark urine, hallucinations, mood changes.	Discontinue. Call doctor right away.
Rare: Paleness, sore throat or fever, severe abdominal pain, pale stool, unusual bleeding or bruising, jaundice, fatigue, weakness, seizures, psychosis, joint pain, numbness or tingling in hands or feet.	Discontinue. Call doctor right away.

WARNINGS & PRECAUTIONS

Don't take if:
- You are allergic to nalidixic acid.
- You have a seizure disorder (epilepsy, convulsions).

Before you start, consult your doctor:
- If you plan to become pregnant within medication period.
- If you have or have had kidney or liver disease.
- If you have impaired circulation of the brain (hardened arteries).
- If you have Parkinson's disease.
- If you have diabetes (drug may affect urine sugar tests).

Over age 60:
Adverse reactions and side effects may be more frequent and severe than in younger persons.

Pregnancy:
Consult doctor. Risk category B (see page xxiii).

Breast-feeding:
Drug passes into milk. Avoid drug or discontinue nursing until you finish medicine. Consult doctor for advice on maintaining milk supply.

Infants & children:
Not recommended.

Prolonged use:
Talk to your doctor about the need for follow-up medical examinations or laboratory studies to check complete blood counts (white blood cell count, platelet count, red blood cell count, hemoglobin, hematocrit), liver function, kidney function.

Skin & sunlight:
May cause rash or intensify sunburn in areas exposed to sun or ultraviolet light (photosensitivity reaction). Avoid overexposure. Notify doctor if reaction occurs.

Driving, piloting or hazardous work:
Avoid if you feel drowsy, dizzy or have vision problems. Otherwise, no problems expected.

Discontinuing:
Don't discontinue without consulting doctor. Dose may require gradual reduction if you have taken drug for a long time. Doses of other drugs may also require adjustment.

Others:
Periodic blood counts and liver and kidney function tests recommended.

POSSIBLE INTERACTION WITH OTHER DRUGS

GENERIC NAME OR DRUG CLASS	COMBINED EFFECT
Antacids*	Decreased absorption of nalidixic acid.
Anticoagulants*, oral	Increased anticoagulant effect.
Calcium supplements*	Decreased effect of nalidixic acid.
Nitrofurantoin	Decreased effect of nalidixic acid.
Probenecid	Decreased effect of nalidixic acid.
Vitamin C (in large doses)	Increased effect of nalidixic acid.

POSSIBLE INTERACTION WITH OTHER SUBSTANCES

INTERACTS WITH	COMBINED EFFECT
Alcohol:	Impaired alertness, judgment and coordination.
Beverages:	None expected.
Cocaine:	Impaired judgment and coordination.
Foods:	None expected.
Marijuana:	Impaired alertness, judgment and coordination.
Tobacco:	None expected.

NALTREXONE

BRAND NAMES

Barr   ReVia

BASIC INFORMATION

Habit forming? No
Prescription needed? Yes
Available as generic? Yes
Drug class: Narcotic antagonist

USES

- Treats detoxified former narcotics addicts. It helps maintain a drug-free state.
- May be used to treat alcoholism (in conjunction with counseling).

DOSAGE & USAGE INFORMATION

How to take:
- *Don't take at all until detoxification has been accomplished.*
- Tablets—Swallow with liquid or food to lessen stomach irritation. If you can't swallow whole, crumble tablet and take with liquid or food.

When to take:
At the same time every day or every other day as directed.

If you forget a dose:
Follow detailed instructions from the one who prescribed for you.

What drug does:
Binds to opioid receptors in the central nervous system and blocks the effects of narcotic drugs.

Time lapse before drug works:
1 hour.

Don't take with:
- Narcotics.
- Any other medicine without consulting your doctor or pharmacist.

OVERDOSE

SYMPTOMS:
Seizures, coma.
WHAT TO DO:
- Dial 911 (emergency) or 0 (operator) for an ambulance or medical help. Then give first aid immediately.
- See emergency information at end of book.

POSSIBLE ADVERSE REACTIONS OR SIDE EFFECTS

SYMPTOMS	WHAT TO DO
Life-threatening: Hallucinations, very fast heartbeat, fainting, breathing difficulties.	Seek emergency treatment immediately.
Common: Skin rash, chills, constipation, appetite loss, irritability, insomnia, anxiety, headache, nausea, vomiting.	Continue. Call doctor when convenient.
Infrequent: • Nosebleeds, joint pain.	Discontinue. Call doctor right away.
• Abdominal pain, blurred vision, confusion, earache, fever, depression, diarrhea, common cold symptoms.	Continue. Call doctor when convenient.
Rare: • Pain, tenderness or color change in feet.	Discontinue. Call doctor right away.
• Ringing in ears, swollen glands, decreased sex drive.	Continue. Call doctor when convenient.

WARNINGS & PRECAUTIONS

Don't take if:
- You don't have close medical supervision.
- You are currently dependent on drugs.
- You have severe liver disease.

Before you start, consult your doctor:
If you have mild liver disease.

Over age 60:
Adverse reactions and side effects may be more frequent and severe than in younger persons. You may need smaller doses for shorter periods of time.

Pregnancy:
Decide with your doctor whether drug benefits justify risk to unborn child. Risk category C (see page xxiii).

Breast-feeding:
Safety not established. Consult doctor.

Infants & children:
Not recommended.

Prolonged use:
- Not recommended.
- Talk to your doctor about the need for follow-up medical examinations or laboratory studies to check kidney function.

Skin & sunlight:
No problems expected.

Driving, piloting or hazardous work:
Don't drive or pilot aircraft until you learn how medicine affects you. Don't work around dangerous machinery. Don't climb ladders or work in high places. Danger increases if you drink alcohol or take medicine affecting alertness and reflexes.

Discontinuing:
Don't discontinue without consulting doctor. Dose may require gradual reduction if you have taken drug for a long time. Doses of other drugs may also require adjustment.

Others:
- Probably not effective in treating people addicted to substances other than opium or morphine derivatives.
- Must be given under close supervision by people experienced in using naltrexone to treat addicts.
- Attempting to use narcotics to overcome effects of naltrexone may lead to coma and death.
- Advise any doctor or dentist whom you consult that you take this medicine.
- Withdraw from medication several days prior to expected surgery.

POSSIBLE INTERACTION WITH OTHER DRUGS

GENERIC NAME OR DRUG CLASS	COMBINED EFFECT
Narcotic medicines* (butorphanol, codeine, heroin, hydrocodone, hydromorphone, levorphanol, morphine, nalbuphine, opium, oxycodone, oxymorphone, paregoric, pentazocine, propoxyphene)	1. Precipitates withdrawal symptoms. May lead to cardiac arrest, coma and death (if naltrexone taken while person is dependent on these drugs). 2. If these drugs are taken while person is taking naltrexone, opioid effect (pain relief) will be blocked.
Isoniazid	Increased risk of liver damage.

POSSIBLE INTERACTION WITH OTHER SUBSTANCES

INTERACTS WITH	COMBINED EFFECT
Alcohol:	Unpredictable effects. Avoid.
Beverages:	None expected.
Cocaine:	Unpredictable effects. Avoid.
Foods:	None expected.
Marijuana:	Unpredictable effects. Avoid.
Tobacco:	None expected.

*See Glossary

NARCOTIC ANALGESICS

GENERIC AND BRAND NAMES

See complete list of generic and brand names in the *Generic and Brand Name Directory*, page 885.

BASIC INFORMATION

Habit forming? Yes
Prescription needed? Yes
Available as generic? Yes
Drug class: Narcotic

 ## USES

Relieves pain and diarrhea; suppresses cough.

 ## DOSAGE & USAGE INFORMATION

How to take:
- Tablet, capsule or extended-release tablet—Swallow with liquid. If you can't swallow whole, crumble tablet or open capsule and take with liquid or food. Do not crush or crumble extended release forms.
- Liquid form of morphine—Mix with fruit juice just before taking to improve taste.
- Syrup—Mix with one-half glass of water (4 oz.) before swallowing.
- Dispersible tablets—Stir into water or fruit juice just before taking each dose.
- Liquid forms—May need to be diluted with water before taking. Follow directions on label.
- Suppositories—Remove wrapper and moisten suppository with water. Gently insert into rectum, small end first.
- Transdermal—follow instructions on prescription.
- Nasal—Follow package instructions.

Continued next column

 ## OVERDOSE

SYMPTOMS:
Deep sleep, slow breathing; slow pulse; respiratory arrest; flushed, warm skin; seizures; constricted pupils.
WHAT TO DO:
- **Dial 911 (emergency) or 0 (operator) for an ambulance or medical help. Then give first aid immediately.**
- **If patient is unconscious and not breathing, give mouth-to-mouth breathing. If there is no heartbeat, use cardiac massage and mouth-to-mouth breathing (CPR). Don't try to make patient vomit. If you can't get help quickly, take patient to nearest emergency facility.**
- **See emergency information on inside covers.**

When to take:
When needed. No more often than every 4 hours.

If you forget a dose:
Take as soon as you remember. Wait 4 hours for next dose.

What drug does:
- Blocks pain messages to brain and spinal cord.
- Reduces sensitivity of brain's cough control center.

Time lapse before drug works:
30 minutes.

Don't take with:
Any other medicine without consulting your doctor or pharmacist.

 ## POSSIBLE ADVERSE REACTIONS OR SIDE EFFECTS

SYMPTOMS	WHAT TO DO
Life-threatening: Irregular or slow heartbeat, difficult breathing, wheezing.	Discontinue. Seek emergency treatment.
Common: Dizziness, drowsiness, tiredness, headache, lightheadedness, nausea or vomiting, stomach cramps, overexcitement.	Continue. Call doctor when convenient.
Infrequent: • Black, tarry stools; bloody or cloudy urine; painful or frequent urination; fast, slow or pounding heartbeat; hallucinations; breathing problems, wheezing; back or side pain; red dots on skin; red or flushed face; ringing or buzzing in ears; skin rash, hives or itching; sore throat; fever; face swelling; decreased urine; trembling; uncontrolled muscle movements; unusual bleeding or bruising; yellow skin or eyes.	Discontinue. Call doctor right away.
• Feeling depressed, pale stools.	Continue. Call doctor when convenient.
Rare: Changes in vision, constipation, dry mouth, loss of appetite, restlessness, nightmares, trouble sleeping.	Discontinue. Call doctor when convenient.

WARNINGS & PRECAUTIONS

Don't take if:
- You are allergic to any narcotic.
- Diarrhea is due to toxic effect of drugs or poisons.

Before you start, consult your doctor:
- If you have impaired liver or kidney function.
- If you will have surgery within 2 months, including dental surgery, requiring general or spinal anesthesia.
- If you have asthma.

Over age 60:
More likely to be drowsy, dizzy, unsteady or constipated. Use only if absolutely necessary.

Pregnancy:
Risk factors vary for drugs in this group. See category list on page xxiii and consult doctor.

Breast-feeding:
Drug filters into milk. May harm child. Avoid.

Infants & children:
Not recommended.

Prolonged use:
- With high doses and long-term use, can cause psychological and physical dependence (addiction).
- May cause chronic constipation.

Skin & sunlight:
No special problems expected.

Driving, piloting or hazardous work:
Don't drive or pilot aircraft until you learn how medicine affects you. Don't work around dangerous machinery. Don't climb ladders or work in high places. Danger increases if you drink alcohol or take medicine affecting alertness and reflexes, such as antihistamines, tranquilizers, sedatives, pain medicine, narcotics and mind-altering drugs.

Discontinuing:
- Discontinue in 2 days if symptoms don't improve. Report to the doctor any symptoms that develop after discontinuing, such as gooseflesh, irritability, insomnia, yawning, weakness, large eye pupils.
- If used for several weeks or more, consult doctor before discontinuing.

Others:
- Some products contain tartrazine dye. Avoid, especially if you are allergic to aspirin.
- Lying down after the first few doses may decrease unwanted effects of nausea, vomiting, lightheadedness or dizziness.

POSSIBLE INTERACTION WITH OTHER DRUGS

GENERIC NAME OR DRUG CLASS	COMBINED EFFECT
Analgesics*, other	Increased analgesic effect.
Anticoagulants*, oral	Possible increased anticoagulant effect.
Anticholinergics*	Increased anticholinergic effect.
Antidepressants*	Increased sedative effect.
Antihistamines*	Increased sedative effect.
Anti-inflammatory drugs, nonsteroidal (NSAIDs)*	Increased narcotic effect.
Butorphanol	Possibly precipitates withdrawal with chronic narcotic use.
Carbamazepine	Increased carbamazepine effect possible with propoxyphene.
Carteolol	Increased narcotic effect. Dangerous sedation.
Cimetidine	Possible increased narcotic effect and toxicity.
Clozapine	Toxic effect on the central nervous system.

Continued on page 924

POSSIBLE INTERACTION WITH OTHER SUBSTANCES

INTERACTS WITH	COMBINED EFFECT
Alcohol:	Increased intoxicating effect of alcohol. Avoid.
Beverages:	None expected.
Cocaine:	Increased toxic effects of cocaine. Avoid.
Foods:	None expected.
Marijuana:	Impaired physical and mental performance. Avoid.
Tobacco:	None expected.

*See Glossary

GENERIC AND BRAND NAMES

See complete list of generic and brand names in the *Generic and Brand Name Directory*, page 886.

BASIC INFORMATION

Habit forming? Yes
Prescription needed? Yes
Available as generic? Yes
Drug class: Narcotic, analgesic, fever reducer

 USES

Relieves pain.

 DOSAGE & USAGE INFORMATION

How to take:
* Tablet or capsule—Swallow with liquid. If you can't swallow whole, crumble tablet or open capsule and take with liquid or food.
* Syrup—Mix with one-half glass of water (4 oz.) before swallowing.
* Liquid forms—May need to be diluted with water before taking. Follow directions on label.

When to take:
When needed. No more often than every 4 hours.

If you forget a dose:
Take as soon as you remember. Wait 4 hours for next dose.

Continued next column

 OVERDOSE

SYMPTOMS:
Stomach upset; irritability; sweating, convulsions; deep sleep; slow breathing; slow pulse; flushed, warm skin; constricted pupils; coma.
WHAT TO DO:
* **Dial 911 (emergency) or 0 (operator) for an ambulance or medical help. Then give first aid immediately.**
* **If patient is unconscious and not breathing, give mouth-to-mouth breathing. If there is no heartbeat, use cardiac massage and mouth-to-mouth breathing (CPR). Don't try to make patient vomit. If you can't get help quickly, take patient to nearest emergency facility.**
* **See emergency information on inside covers.**

What drug does:
* May affect hypothalamus—the part of the brain that helps regulate body heat and receives body's pain messages.
* Blocks pain messages to brain and spinal cord.
* Reduces sensitivity of brain's cough control center.

Time lapse before drug works:
15 to 30 minutes. May last 4 hours.

Don't take with:
* Other drugs with acetaminophen. Too much acetaminophen can damage liver and kidneys.
* Any other medicine without consulting your doctor or pharmacist.

 POSSIBLE ADVERSE REACTIONS OR SIDE EFFECTS

SYMPTOMS	WHAT TO DO
Life-threatening: Irregular or slow heartbeat, difficult breathing, wheezing.	Discontinue. Seek emergency treatment.
Common: Dizziness, drowsiness, tiredness, headache, lightheadedness, nausea or vomiting, stomach cramps, overexcitement.	Continue. Call doctor when convenient.
Infrequent: • Black, tarry stools; bloody or cloudy urine; painful or frequent urination; fast, slow or pounding heartbeat; hallucinations; breathing problems, wheezing; back or side pain; red dots on skin; red or flushed face; ringing or buzzing in ears; skin rash, hives or itching; sore throat; fever; face swelling; decreased urine; trembling; uncontrolled muscle movements; unusual bleeding or bruising; yellow skin or eyes.	Discontinue. Call doctor right away.
• Feeling depressed, pale stools.	Continue. Call doctor when convenient.
Rare: Changes in vision, constipation, dry mouth, loss of appetite, restlessness, nightmares, trouble sleeping.	Discontinue. Call doctor when convenient.

WARNINGS & PRECAUTIONS

Don't take if:
- You are allergic to any narcotic or acetaminophen.
- Your symptoms don't improve after 2 days use. Call your doctor.

Before you start, consult your doctor:
- If you have bronchial asthma, kidney disease or liver damage.
- If you will have surgery within 2 months, including dental surgery, requiring general or spinal anesthesia.

Over age 60:
More likely to be drowsy, dizzy, unsteady or constipated. Don't exceed recommended dose. You can't eliminate drug as efficiently as younger persons. Use only if absolutely necessary.

Pregnancy:
Risk factors vary for drugs in this group. See category list on page xxiii and consult doctor.

Breast-feeding:
Drug filters into milk. May harm child. Avoid.

Infants & children:
Not recommended.

Prolonged use:
- With high doses and long-term use, can cause psychological and physical dependence (addiction).
- May cause chronic constipation.

Skin & sunlight:
No problems expected.

Driving, piloting or hazardous work:
Don't drive or pilot aircraft until you learn how medicine affects you. Don't work around dangerous machinery. Don't climb ladders or work in high places. Danger increases if you drink alcohol or take medicine affecting alertness and reflexes, such as antihistamines, tranquilizers, sedatives, pain medicine, narcotics and mind-altering drugs.

Discontinuing:
- Discontinue in 2 days if symptoms don't improve. Report to your doctor any symptoms that develop after discontinuing, such as gooseflesh, irritability, insomnia, yawning, weakness, large eye pupils.
- If used for several weeks or more, consult doctor before discontinuing.

Others:
Lying down after the first few doses may decrease unwanted effects of nausea, vomiting, lightheadedness or dizziness.

POSSIBLE INTERACTION WITH OTHER DRUGS

GENERIC NAME OR DRUG CLASS	COMBINED EFFECT
Analgesics*, other	Increased analgesic effect.
Anticoagulants*, other	May increase anticoagulant effect. Prothrombin times should be monitored.
Anticholinergics*	Increased anticholinergic effect.
Antidepressants*	Increased sedative effect.
Antihistamines*	Increased sedative effect.
Carteolol	Increased narcotic effect. Dangerous sedation.
Mind-altering drugs*	Increased sedative effect.
Narcotics*, other	Increased narcotic effect.
Nitrates*	Excessive blood pressure drop.
Phenobarbital and other barbiturates*	Quicker elimination and decreased effect of acetaminophen.

Continued on page 924

POSSIBLE INTERACTION WITH OTHER SUBSTANCES

INTERACTS WITH	COMBINED EFFECT
Alcohol:	Increased intoxicating effect of alcohol. Long-term use may cause toxic effect in liver. Avoid.
Beverages:	None expected.
Cocaine:	Increased toxic effects of cocaine. Avoid.
Foods:	None expected.
Marijuana:	Impaired physical and mental performance. Avoid.
Tobacco:	None expected.

*See Glossary

NARCOTIC ANALGESICS & ASPIRIN

GENERIC AND BRAND NAMES

See complete list of generic and brand names in the *Generic and Brand Name Directory*, page 887.

BASIC INFORMATION

Habit forming? Yes
Prescription needed? Yes
Available as generic? Yes
Drug class: Narcotic, analgesic, anti-inflammatory (nonsteroidal)

USES

Reduces pain, fever, inflammation.

DOSAGE & USAGE INFORMATION

How to take:
Tablet or capsule—Swallow with liquid. If you can't swallow whole, crumble tablet or open capsule and take with liquid or food.

When to take:
When needed. No more often than every 4 hours.

If you forget a dose:
Take as soon as you remember. Wait 4 hours for next dose.

Continued next column

OVERDOSE

SYMPTOMS:
Ringing in ears; nausea; vomiting; dizziness; fever; deep sleep; slow breathing; slow pulse; flushed, warm skin; constricted pupils; hallucinations; convulsions; coma.
WHAT TO DO:
- **Dial 911 (emergency) or 0 (operator) for an ambulance or medical help. Then give first aid immediately.**
- **If patient is unconscious and not breathing, give mouth-to-mouth breathing. If there is no heartbeat, use cardiac massage and mouth-to-mouth breathing (CPR). Don't try to make patient vomit. If you can't get help quickly, take patient to nearest emergency facility.**
- **See emergency information on inside covers.**

What drug does:
- Affects hypothalamus, the part of the brain which regulates temperature by dilating small blood vessels in skin.
- Prevents clumping of platelets (small blood cells) so blood vessels remain open.
- Decreases prostaglandin effect.
- Suppresses body's pain messages.
- Reduces sensitivity of brain's cough control center.

Time lapse before drug works:
30 minutes.

Don't take with:
- Tetracyclines. Space doses 1 hour apart.
- Any other medicine without consulting your doctor or pharmacist.

POSSIBLE ADVERSE REACTIONS OR SIDE EFFECTS

SYMPTOMS	WHAT TO DO
Life-threatening: Irregular or slow heartbeat, difficult breathing, wheezing.	Discontinue. Seek emergency treatment.
Common: Dizziness, drowsiness, tiredness, headache, lightheadedness, nausea or vomiting, stomach cramps, overexcitement.	Continue. Call doctor when convenient.
Infrequent: • Black, tarry stools; bloody or cloudy urine; painful or frequent urination; fast, slow or pounding heartbeat; hallucinations; breathing problems, wheezing; back or side pain; red dots on skin; red or flushed face; ringing or buzzing in ears; skin rash, hives or itching; sore throat; fever; face swelling; decreased urine; trembling; uncontrolled muscle movements; unusual bleeding or bruising; yellow skin or eyes.	Discontinue. Call doctor right away.
• Feeling depressed, pale stools.	Continue. Call doctor when convenient.
Rare: Changes in vision, constipation, dry mouth, loss of appetite, restlessness, nightmares, trouble sleeping.	Discontinue. Call doctor when convenient.

WARNINGS & PRECAUTIONS

Don't take if:
- You are allergic to any narcotic or subject to any substance abuse.
- You have a peptic ulcer of stomach or duodenum or a bleeding disorder.

Before you start, consult your doctor:
- If you have impaired liver or kidney function, asthma or nasal polyps.
- If you have had stomach or duodenal ulcers, gout.
- If you will have surgery within 2 months, including dental surgery, requiring general or spinal anesthesia.

Over age 60:
- More likely to be drowsy, dizzy, unsteady or constipated. Use only if absolutely necessary.
- More likely to cause hidden bleeding in stomach or intestines. Watch for dark stools.

Pregnancy:
Risk factors vary for drugs in this group. See category list on page xxiii and consult doctor.

Breast-feeding:
Drug passes into milk and may harm child. Avoid drug or discontinue nursing until you finish medicine. Consult doctor for advice on maintaining milk supply.

Infants & children:
Not recommended.

Prolonged use:
- With high doses and long-term use, can cause psychological and physical dependence (addiction).
- May cause chronic constipation.

Skin & sunlight:
No special problems expected.

Driving, piloting or hazardous work:
Don't drive or pilot aircraft until you learn how medicine affects you. Don't work around dangerous machinery. Don't climb ladders or work in high places. Danger increases if you drink alcohol or take medicine affecting alertness and reflexes, such as antihistamines, tranquilizers, sedatives, pain medicine, narcotics and mind-altering drugs.

Discontinuing:
- Discontinue in 2 to 3 days if symptoms don't improve. Report to your doctor any symptoms that develop after discontinuing, such as gooseflesh, irritability, insomnia, yawning, weakness, large eye pupils.
- If used for several weeks or more, consult doctor before discontinuing.

Others:
- Aspirin can complicate surgery; illness; pregnancy, labor and delivery.
- Urine tests for blood sugar may be inaccurate

- Lying down after the first few doses may decrease unwanted effects of nausea, vomiting, lightheadedness or dizziness.
- Don't use if medicine has a strong vinegar-like odor. This means the aspirin is breaking down.

POSSIBLE INTERACTION WITH OTHER DRUGS

GENERIC NAME OR DRUG CLASS	COMBINED EFFECT
Acebutolol	Decreased anti-hypertensive effect of acebutolol.
Adrenocorticoids, systemic	Increased risk of ulcers. Increased adrenocorticoid effect.
Alendonate	Increased risk of stomach irritation.
Allopurinol	Decreased allopurinol effect.
Angiotensin-converting enzyme (ACE) inhibitors*	Decreased effect of ACE inhibitor.
Antacids*	Decreased aspirin effect.
Anticoagulants*, oral	Increased anticoagulant effect. Abnormal bleeding.
Antidepressants*	Increased sedative effect.
Antidiabetics*, oral	Low blood sugar.

Continued on page 925

POSSIBLE INTERACTION WITH OTHER SUBSTANCES

INTERACTS WITH	COMBINED EFFECT
Alcohol:	Possible stomach irritation and bleeding. Increased intoxicating effect of alcohol. Avoid.
Beverages:	None expected.
Cocaine:	Decreased cocaine toxic effects. Avoid.
Foods:	None expected.
Marijuana:	Impaired physical and mental performance. Avoid.
Tobacco:	None expected.

*See Glossary

NATAMYCIN (Ophthalmic)

BRAND NAMES

Natacyn   Pimaricin

BASIC INFORMATION

Habit forming? No
Prescription needed? Yes
Available as generic? No
Drug class: Antifungal (ophthalmic)

USES

Treats fungus infections of the eye.

DOSAGE & USAGE INFORMATION

How to use:
Eye drops
- Wash hands.
- Apply pressure to inside corner of eye with middle finger.
- Tilt head backward. Pull lower lid away from eye with index finger of the same hand.
- Drop eye drops into pouch and close eye. Don't blink.
- Continue pressure for 1 minute after placing medicine in eye.
- Keep eyes closed for 1 to 2 minutes.
- Don't touch applicator tip to any surface (including the eye). If you accidentally touch tip, clean with warm soap and water.
- Keep container tightly closed.
- Keep drops cool, but don't freeze.
- Wash hands immediately after using.

When to use:
As directed. Usually 1 drop in eye every 1 or 2 hours for 3 or 4 days, then every 3 to 4 hours.

If you forget a dose:
Use as soon as you remember.

What drug does:
Changes cell membrane of fungus causing loss of essential constituents of fungus cell.

Continued next column

OVERDOSE

SYMPTOMS:
None expected.
WHAT TO DO:
Not intended for internal use. If child accidentally swallows, call poison control center.

Time lapse before drug works:
Starts to work immediately. May require 2 weeks or more to cure infection.

Don't use with:
Other eye drops without consulting your eye doctor.

POSSIBLE ADVERSE REACTIONS OR SIDE EFFECTS

SYMPTOMS	WHAT TO DO
Life-threatening: None expected.	
Common: None expected.	
Infrequent: Eye irritation not present before using natamycin.	Discontinue. Call doctor right away.
Rare: None expected.	

WARNINGS & PRECAUTIONS

Don't use if:
You are allergic to natamycin or any antifungal medicine*.

Before you start, consult your doctor:
If you have allergies to any substance.

Over age 60:
No problems expected.

Pregnancy:
Decide with your doctor if drug benefits justify risk to unborn child. Risk category C (see page xxiii).

Breast-feeding:
No problems expected, but check with doctor.

Infants & children:
No problems expected.

Prolonged use:
May cause eye irritation.

Skin & sunlight:
No problems expected.

Driving, piloting or hazardous work:
No problems expected.

Discontinuing:
Don't discontinue without consulting your eye doctor.

Others:
* Keep eye drops cool, but don't freeze.
* Notify doctor if condition doesn't improve within 1 week.

POSSIBLE INTERACTION WITH OTHER DRUGS

GENERIC NAME OR DRUG CLASS	COMBINED EFFECT
Clinically significant interactions with oral or injected medicines unlikely.	

POSSIBLE INTERACTION WITH OTHER SUBSTANCES

INTERACTS WITH	COMBINED EFFECT
Alcohol:	None expected.
Beverages:	None expected.
Cocaine:	None expected.
Foods:	None expected.
Marijuana:	None expected.
Tobacco:	None expected.

*See Glossary

NEDOCROMIL

BRAND NAMES

Tilade

BASIC INFORMATION

Habit forming? No
Prescription needed? Yes
Available as generic? No
**Drug class: Antiasthmatic (anti-
inflammatory)**

 USES

For maintenance treatment of mild to moderate
asthma. Not used to treat an active asthma
attack.

 **DOSAGE & USAGE
INFORMATION**

How to take:
Inhaler—Follow instructions on the metered-dose
inhaler pack.

When to take:
At the same times each day. Initial treatment is
usually 2 inhalations 4 times a day. After
symptoms subside, dosage may be reduced by
your doctor.

If you forget a dose:
Take as soon as you remember up to 2 hours
late. If more than 2 hours, wait for next
scheduled dose (don't double this dose).

What drug does:
Inhibits inflammatory cells associated with
asthma. Inhibits reflex reactions to irritants and to
exercise and cold.

Time lapse before drug works:
2 to 4 days, but may require several weeks to
achieve maximum effectiveness.

Don't take with:
Any other prescription or nonprescription drug
without consulting your doctor.

 OVERDOSE

SYMPTOMS:
None expected.
WHAT TO DO:
Overdose unlikely to threaten life. If person
takes much larger amount than prescribed,
call doctor, poison control center or hospital
emergency room for instructions.

 **POSSIBLE
ADVERSE REACTIONS
OR SIDE EFFECTS**

SYMPTOMS	WHAT TO DO
Life-threatening: None expected.	
Common: Unpleasant taste.	No action necessary.
Infrequent: • Headache, nausea, throat irritation, cough, runny nose or stuffy nose.	Continue. Call doctor when convenient.
• Increased broncho-spasm (increased wheezing, tightness in chest, difficulty in breathing).	Discontinue. Call doctor right away.
Rare: None expected.	

WARNINGS & PRECAUTIONS

Don't take if:
You are allergic to nedocromil.

Before you start, consult your doctor:
No problems expected.

Over age 60:
No problems expected.

Pregnancy:
Decide with your doctor if drug benefits outweigh risks to unborn child. Risk category C (see page xxiii).

Breast-feeding:
Not known if drug passes into milk. Consult with your doctor.

Infants & children:
Give only under close medical supervision, especially to children younger than age 12.

Prolonged use:
No problems expected.

Skin & sunlight:
No problems expected.

Driving, piloting or hazardous work:
No problems expected.

Discontinuing:
No problems expected. Don't discontinue abruptly without talking to your doctor.

Others:
* Advise any doctor or dentist whom you consult that you take this medicine.
* May affect the results in some medical tests.

POSSIBLE INTERACTION WITH OTHER DRUGS

GENERIC NAME OR DRUG CLASS	COMBINED EFFECT
None expected.	

POSSIBLE INTERACTION WITH OTHER SUBSTANCES

INTERACTS WITH	COMBINED EFFECT
Alcohol:	None expected.
Beverages:	None expected.
Cocaine:	None expected.
Foods:	None expected.
Marijuana:	None expected.
Tobacco:	None expected.

NEFAZODONE

BRAND NAMES

Serzone

BASIC INFORMATION

Habit forming? No
Prescription needed? Yes
Available as generic? No
Drug class: Antidepressant
  (phenylpiperazine)

 ## USES

Treats symptoms of mental depression.

 ## DOSAGE & USAGE INFORMATION

How to take:
Tablet—Swallow with liquid. May be taken with or without food.

When to take:
At the same times each day. The prescribed dosage may be increased weekly until maximum benefits are achieved.

If you forget a dose:
Take as soon as you remember up to 2 hours late. If more than 2 hours, wait for the next scheduled dose (don't double this dose).

What drug does:
The exact mechanism is unknown. It appears to block reuptake of serotonin and norepinephrine (stimulating chemicals in the brain that play a role in emotions and psychological disturbances).

Time lapse before drug works:
Will take up to several weeks to relieve the depression.

Don't take with:
Any other medication without consulting your doctor or pharmacist.

 ## OVERDOSE

SYMPTOMS:
Drowsiness, nausea, vomiting, low blood pressure (faintness, weakness, dizziness, lightheadedness) or increased severity of adverse reactions.
WHAT TO DO:
- **Dial 911 (emergency) or 0 (operator) for an ambulance or medical help. Then give first aid immediately.**
- **See emergency information at end of book.**

 ## POSSIBLE ADVERSE REACTIONS OR SIDE EFFECTS

SYMPTOMS	WHAT TO DO
Life-threatening:	
In case of overdose, see previous column.	
Common:	
• Clumsiness or unsteadiness, blurred vision or other vision changes, fainting, lightheadedness, ringing in the ears, skin rash or itching.	Discontinue. Call doctor right away.
• Strange dreams, constipation or diarrhea, dry mouth, heartburn, fever, chills, flushing or feeling warm, headache, increased appetite, insomnia, coughing, tingling or prickly sensations, sore throat, trembling, drowsiness, confusion or agitation, memory lapses.	Continue. Call doctor when convenient.
Infrequent:	
• Tightness in chest; trouble breathing; wheezing; eye pain; combination of nausea, vomiting, diarrhea and stomach pain.	Discontinue. Call doctor right away.
• Joint pain, breast pain, increased thirst.	Continue. Call doctor when convenient.
Rare:	
• Face swelling, hives, muscle pain or stiffness, chest pain, fast heartbeat, mood or mental changes, difficulty speaking, hallucinations, uncontrolled excited behavior, twitching, ear pain, increased hearing sensitivity, bleeding or bruising, irritated red eyes, eyes sensitive to light, pain in back or side, swollen glands, problems with urination.	Discontinue. Call doctor right away.
• Unusual tiredness or weakness, false sense of well-being, menstrual changes, change in sexual desire or function.	Continue. Call doctor when convenient.

WARNINGS & PRECAUTIONS

Don't use if:
You are allergic to nefazodone or trazodone (phenylpiperazine antidepressants).

Before you start, consult your doctor:
- If you have a seizure disorder, heart disease or blood circulation problem or have had a stroke.
- If you are dehydrated.
- If you have a history of drug dependence or drug abuse.
- If you have a history of mood disorders, such as mania, or thoughts of suicide.
- If you are allergic to any medication, food or other substances.

Over age 60:
A lower starting dosage is usually recommended until a response is determined.

Pregnancy:
Decide with your doctor if drug benefits justify risk to unborn child. Risk category C (see page xxiii).

Breast-feeding:
It is unknown if drug passes into milk. Avoid drug or discontinue nursing until you finish medicine. Consult doctor for advice on maintaining milk supply.

Infants & children:
Safety in children under age 18 has not been established.

Prolonged use:
Consult with your doctor on a regular basis while taking this drug to check your progress and to discuss any increase or changes in side effects and the need for continued treatment.

Skin & sunlight:
May cause a rash or intensify sunburn in areas exposed to sun or ultraviolet light (photosensitivity reaction). Avoid excess sun exposure and use sunscreen. Consult doctor if reaction occurs.

Driving, piloting or hazardous work:
Don't drive or pilot aircraft until you learn how medicine affects you. Don't work around dangerous machinery. Don't climb ladders or work in high places. Danger increases if you drink alcohol or take medicine affecting alertness and reflexes.

Discontinuing:
Don't discontinue this drug without consulting doctor. Dosage may require a gradual reduction before stopping.

Others:
- Get up slowly from a sitting or lying position to avoid dizziness, faintness or lightheadedness.
- May affect the results of some medical tests.
- Advise any doctor or dentist whom you consult that you take this medicine.

- Take medicine only as directed. Do not increase or reduce dosage without doctor's approval.

POSSIBLE INTERACTION WITH OTHER DRUGS

GENERIC NAME OR DRUG CLASS	COMBINED EFFECT
Alprazolam	Increased effect of alprazolam.
Antihistamines, nonsedating	Serious heart rhythm problems with astemizole or terfenadine. Avoid.
Antihypertensives*	Possible too-low blood pressure.
Astemizole	Serious heart problems. Avoid.
Central nervous system (CNS) depressants*	Increased sedation. Avoid.
Digoxin	Increased digoxin effect.
Haloperidol	Unknown effect. May need dosage adjustment.
Monoamine oxidase (MAO) inhibitors*	Potentially life-threatening. Allow 14 days between use of 2 drugs.
Propranolol	Unknown effect. May need dosage adjustment of both drugs.
Selective serotonin reuptake inhibitors*	Potentially life-threatening serotonin syndrome (see Glossary). Avoid.

Continued on page 925

POSSIBLE INTERACTION WITH OTHER SUBSTANCES

INTERACTS WITH	COMBINED EFFECT
Alcohol:	Increased sedative affect. Avoid.
Beverages:	None expected.
Cocaine:	Unknown. Avoid.
Foods:	None expected.
Marijuana:	Unknown. Best to avoid.
Tobacco:	None expected.

*See Glossary

NEOMYCIN (Oral)

BRAND NAMES

Mycifradin

BASIC INFORMATION

Habit forming? No
Prescription needed? Yes
Available as generic? Yes
Drug class: Antibacterial

USES

- Clears intestinal tract of germs prior to surgery.
- Treats some causes of diarrhea.
- Lowers blood cholesterol.
- Lessens symptoms of hepatic coma.

DOSAGE & USAGE INFORMATION

How to take:
Tablet—Swallow with liquid or food to lessen stomach irritation. If you can't swallow whole, crumble tablet and take with liquid or food.

When to take:
According to directions on prescription.

If you forget a dose:
Take as soon as you remember up to 2 hours late. If more than 2 hours, wait for next scheduled dose (don't double this dose).

What drug does:
Kills germs susceptible to neomycin.

Time lapse before drug works:
2 to 3 days.

Continued next column

OVERDOSE

SYMPTOMS:
Loss of hearing, difficulty breathing, respiratory paralysis.
WHAT TO DO:
- **Dial 911 (emergency) or 0 (operator) for an ambulance or medical help. Then give first aid immediately.**
- **If patient is unconscious and not breathing, give mouth-to-mouth breathing. If there is no heartbeat, use cardiac massage and mouth-to-mouth breathing (CPR). Don't try to make patient vomit. If you can't get help quickly, take patient to nearest emergency facility.**
- **See emergency information on inside covers.**

Don't take with:
Any other medicine without consulting your doctor or pharmacist.

POSSIBLE ADVERSE REACTIONS OR SIDE EFFECTS

SYMPTOMS	WHAT TO DO
Life-threatening: In case of overdose, see previous column.	
Common: Sore mouth or rectum, nausea, vomiting.	Continue. Call doctor when convenient.
Infrequent: None expected.	
Rare: Clumsiness, dizziness, rash, hearing loss, ringing or noises in ear, frothy stools, gaseousness, decreased frequency of urination, diarrhea.	Discontinue. Call doctor right away.

WARNINGS & PRECAUTIONS

Don't take if:
You are allergic to neomycin or any aminoglycoside*.

Before you start, consult your doctor:
- If you will have surgery within 2 months, including dental surgery, requiring general or spinal anesthesia.
- If you have hearing loss or loss of balance secondary to 8th cranial nerve disease.
- If you have intestinal obstruction.
- If you have myasthenia gravis, Parkinson's disease, kidney disease, ulcers in intestines.

Over age 60:
Adverse reactions and side effects may be more frequent and severe than in younger persons.

Pregnancy:
Risk to unborn child outweighs drug benefits. Don't use. Risk category D (see page xxiii).

Breast-feeding:
Avoid if possible. Effect unknown. Consult doctor.

Infants & children:
Give only under close medical supervision.

Prolonged use:
- Adverse effects more likely.
- Talk to your doctor about the need for follow-up medical examinations or laboratory studies to check hearing, kidney function.

Skin & sunlight:
No problems expected.

Driving, piloting or hazardous work:
No problems expected.

Discontinuing:
May be unnecessary to finish medicine. Follow doctor's instructions.

Others:
No problems expected.

POSSIBLE INTERACTION WITH OTHER DRUGS

GENERIC NAME OR DRUG CLASS	COMBINED EFFECT
Aminoglycosides*	Increased chance of toxic effect on hearing, kidneys, muscles.
Beta carotene	Decreased absorption of beta carotene.
Capreomycin	Increased chance of toxic effects on hearing, kidneys.
Cephalothin	Increased chance of toxic effect on kidneys.
Cisplatin	Increased chance of toxic effects on hearing, kidneys.
Ethacrynic acid	Increased chance of toxic effects on hearing, kidneys.
Furosemide	Increased chance of toxic effects on hearing, kidneys.
Mercaptomerin	Increased chance of toxic effects on hearing, kidneys.
Penicillins*	Decreased antibiotic effect.
Tiopronin	Increased risk of toxicity to kidneys.
Vancomycin	Increased chance of toxic effects on hearing, kidneys.

POSSIBLE INTERACTION WITH OTHER SUBSTANCES

INTERACTS WITH	COMBINED EFFECT
Alcohol:	Increased chance of toxicity. Avoid.
Beverages:	No problems expected.
Cocaine:	Increased chance of toxicity. Avoid.
Foods:	No problems expected.
Marijuana:	Increased chance of toxicity. Avoid.
Tobacco:	No problems expected.

NEOMYCIN (Topical)

BRAND NAMES

Myciguent

BASIC INFORMATION

Habit forming? No
Prescription needed? No
Available as generic? Yes
Drug class: Antibacterial (topical)

 ## USES

Treats skin infections that may accompany burns, superficial boils, insect bites or stings, skin ulcers, minor surgical wounds.

 ## DOSAGE & USAGE INFORMATION

How to take:
- Cream, lotion, ointment—Bathe and dry area before use. Apply small amount and rub gently.
- May cover with gauze or bandage if desired.

When to take:
3 or 4 times daily, or as directed by doctor.

If you forget a dose:
Use as soon as you remember.

What drug does:
Kills susceptible bacteria by interfering with bacterial DNA and RNA.

Time lapse before drug works:
Begins first day. May require treatment for a week or longer to cure infection.

Don't take with:
Any other medicine without consulting your doctor or pharmacist.

 ## OVERDOSE

SYMPTOMS:
None expected.
WHAT TO DO:
- Not for internal use. If child accidentally swallows, call poison control center.
- Dial 911 (emergency) or 0 (operator) for an ambulance or medical help. Then give first aid immediately.
- See emergency information on inside covers.

 ## POSSIBLE ADVERSE REACTIONS OR SIDE EFFECTS

SYMPTOMS	WHAT TO DO
Life-threatening: None expected.	
Common: None expected.	
Infrequent: Itching, swollen, red skin.	Discontinue. Call doctor right away.
Rare: None expected.	

WARNINGS & PRECAUTIONS

Don't take if:
You are allergic to neomycin or any topical medicine.

Before you start, consult your doctor:
If any lesions on the skin are open sores.

Over age 60:
No problems expected.

Pregnancy:
Consult doctor. Risk category C (see page xxiii).

Breast-feeding:
No problems expected, but check with doctor.

Infants & children:
No problems expected, but check with doctor.

Prolonged use:
No problems expected, but check with doctor.

Skin & sunlight:
No special problems expected.

Driving, piloting or hazardous work:
No problems expected, but check with doctor.

Discontinuing:
No problems expected, but check with doctor.

Others:
- Heat and moisture in bathroom medicine cabinet can cause breakdown of medicine. Store someplace else.
- Keep medicine cool, but don't freeze.

POSSIBLE INTERACTION WITH OTHER DRUGS

GENERIC NAME OR DRUG CLASS	COMBINED EFFECT
Any other topical medication	Hypersensitivity reactions more likely to occur.

POSSIBLE INTERACTION WITH OTHER SUBSTANCES

INTERACTS WITH	COMBINED EFFECT
Alcohol:	None expected.
Beverages:	None expected.
Cocaine:	None expected.
Foods:	None expected.
Marijuana:	None expected.
Tobacco:	None expected.

NIACIN
(Vitamin B-3, Nicotinic Acid, Nicotinamide)

BRAND AND GENERIC NAMES

Endur-Acin	Nicotinyl alcohol
Nia-Bid	Papulex
Niac	Roniacol
Niacels	Ronigen
Niacin	Rycotin
Niacor	Slo-Niacin
Nico-400	Span-Niacin
Nicobid	Tega-Span
Nicolar	Tri-B3
Nicotinex	

There are numerous other multiple vitamin-mineral supplements available. Check labels.

BASIC INFORMATION

Habit forming? No
Prescription needed?
  Tablets: No
  Liquid, capsules: Yes
Available as generic? Yes
Drug class: Vitamin supplement, vasodilator, antihyperlipidemic

USES

- Replacement for niacin lost due to inadequate diet.
- Treatment for vertigo (dizziness) and ringing in ears.
- Prevention of premenstrual headache.
- Reduction of blood levels of cholesterol and triglycerides.
- Treatment for pellagra.

OVERDOSE

SYMPTOMS:
Body flush, nausea, vomiting, abdominal cramps, diarrhea, weakness, lightheadedness, fainting, sweating.
WHAT TO DO:
Overdose unlikely to threaten life. If person takes much larger amount than prescribed, call doctor, poison control center or hospital emergency room for instructions.

DOSAGE & USAGE INFORMATION

How to take:
- Tablet, capsule or liquid—Swallow with liquid or food to lessen stomach irritation.
- Extended-release tablets or capsules—Swallow each dose whole.

When to take:
At the same times each day.

If you forget a dose:
Take as soon as you remember. Wait 4 hours for next dose.

What drug does:
- Corrects niacin deficiency.
- Dilates blood vessels.
- In large doses, decreases cholesterol production.

Time lapse before drug works:
15 to 20 minutes.

Don't take with:
Any other medicine without consulting your doctor or pharmacist.

POSSIBLE ADVERSE REACTIONS OR SIDE EFFECTS

SYMPTOMS	WHAT TO DO
Life-threatening:	
None expected.	
Common:	
Dry skin.	Continue. Call doctor when convenient.
Infrequent:	
• Upper abdominal pain, diarrhea.	Discontinue. Call doctor right away.
• Headache, dizziness, faintness, temporary numbness and tingling in hands and feet.	Continue. Call doctor when convenient.
• "Hot" feeling, flush.	No action necessary.
Rare:	
Rash, itching, jaundice, double vision, weakness and faintness when arising from bed or chair.	Discontinue. Call doctor right away.

WARNINGS & PRECAUTIONS

Don't take if:
You are allergic to niacin or any niacin-containing vitamin mixtures.

Before you start, consult your doctor:
- If you have sensitivity to tartrazine dye.
- If you have diabetes.
- If you have gout.
- If you have gallbladder or liver disease.
- If you have impaired liver function.
- If you have active peptic ulcer.

Over age 60:
Response to drug cannot be predicted. Dose must be individualized.

Pregnancy:
Consult doctor. Risk category C (see page xxiii).

Breast-feeding:
Studies inconclusive. Consult doctor.

Infants & children:
- Use only under supervision.
- Keep vitamin-mineral supplements out of children's reach.

Prolonged use:
- May cause impaired liver function.
- Talk to your doctor about the need for follow-up medical examinations or laboratory studies to check liver function, blood sugar.

Skin & sunlight:
No problems expected.

Driving, piloting or hazardous work:
Avoid if you feel dizzy or faint. Otherwise, no problems expected.

Discontinuing:
May be unnecessary to finish medicine. Follow doctor's instructions.

Others:
- A balanced diet should provide all the niacin a healthy person needs and make supplements unnecessary. Best sources are meat, eggs and dairy products.
- Store in original container in cool, dry, dark place. Bathroom medicine chest too moist.
- Obesity reduces effectiveness.
- Some nicotinic acid products contain tartrazine dye. Read labels carefully if sensitive to tartrazine.

POSSIBLE INTERACTION WITH OTHER DRUGS

GENERIC NAME OR DRUG CLASS	COMBINED EFFECT
Antidiabetics*	Decreased antidiabetic effect.
Beta-adrenergic blocking agents*	Excessively low blood pressure.
Dexfenfluramine	May require dosage change as weight loss occurs.
HMG-CoA reductase inhibitors*	Increased risk of muscle or kidney problems.
Mecamylamine	Excessively low blood pressure.
Methyldopa	Excessively low blood pressure.
Probenecid	Decreased effect of probenecid.
Sulfinpyrazone	Decreased effect of sulfinpyrazone.

POSSIBLE INTERACTION WITH OTHER SUBSTANCES

INTERACTS WITH	COMBINED EFFECT
Alcohol:	Excessively low blood pressure. Use caution.
Beverages:	None expected.
Cocaine:	Increased flushing.
Foods:	None expected.
Marijuana:	None expected.
Tobacco:	Decreased niacin effect.

*See Glossary

NICOTINE

BRAND NAMES

Habitrol
Nicoderm
Nicoderm CQ
Nicorette

Nicorette DS
Nicotrol
Nicotrol NS
ProStep

BASIC INFORMATION

Habit Forming? Yes
Prescription needed? No
Available as generic? Yes, for some
Drug class: Antismoking agent

USES

Treatment aid to giving up smoking. Nicotine replacement is to be used in conjunction with a medically supervised, behavioral modification program for smoking cessation.

DOSAGE & USAGE INFORMATION

How to use:
- Skin patch—Apply to clean, nonhairy site on the trunk or upper outer arm. Fold old patch in half (sticky sides together) and dispose of where children and pets cannot get to it.
- Chewing gum—Chew gum pieces slowly and intermittently (chew several times, then place between cheek and gum) for best effect.
- Nasal spray—Spray one or two sprays in each nostril.

When to use:
- Skin patch—Daily. Remove old patch and apply new patch to new location on the skin.
- Chewing gum—When there is an urge to smoke, chew the gum for about 30 minutes.
- Nasal spray—Hourly, or as directed. Dosage adjustments should be made as needed.
- For all—Always follow product's directions.

Continued next column

OVERDOSE

SYMPTOMS:
Early symptoms—Nausea, vomiting, severe diarrhea, increased mouth watering, abdominal pain, cold sweat, severe headache, dizziness, confusion, vision and hearing changes. Late symptoms—Irregular or fast pulse, fainting, breathing difficulty, convulsions.
WHAT TO DO:
- **Dial 911 (emergency) or 0 (operator) for an ambulance or medical help. Then give first aid immediately.**
- **See emergency information on inside covers.**

If you forget a dose:
- Skin patch—Remove old patch and apply new patch as soon as you remember, then return to regular schedule.
- Chewing gum or nasal spray—Use as soon as you remember (don't double dosages).

What drug does:
Delivers a supply of nicotine to the body for relief of smoking withdrawal symptoms (irritability, headache, nervousness, drowsiness, fatigue). Reduces craving for cigarettes.

Time lapse before drug works:
Minutes to hours depending on type of product.

Don't take with:
Other prescription or nonprescription drugs without consulting your doctor or pharmacist.

POSSIBLE ADVERSE REACTIONS OR SIDE EFFECTS

SYMPTOMS	WHAT TO DO
Life-threatening: In case of overdose, see previous column.	
Common: • Skin patch—itching, redness, burning or skin rash at site of patch. • Chewing gum—dental problems, sore mouth or throat, belching, mouth watering. • Nasal spray—runny nose, watering eyes, throat irritation, sneezing and cough.	Continue. Call doctor when convenient.
Infrequent: Diarrhea, dizziness, indigestion, nervousness, strange dreams, muscle aches, nausea, constipation, increased cough, tiredness, irritability, changes in menstruation, insomnia, headache, increase in sweating.	Continue. Call doctor when convenient.
Rare: • Allergic reaction (swelling, hives, rash, itching, vomiting, irregular or fast heartbeat); symptoms of overdose occur (high doses of nicotine can cause toxic effects, even in people who are nicotine tolerant).	Discontinue. Call doctor right away.
• Hiccups or hoarsenss with chewing gum.	Continue. Call doctor when convenient.

WARNINGS & PRECAUTIONS

Don't take if:
You are allergic to nicotine or any of the components in the skin patch.

Before you start, consult your doctor:
- If you are pregnant.
- If you have a skin disorder; mouth, throat, dental or TMJ disorder; long-term nasal disorder (allergy, hay fever, sinusitis, polyps) or asthma.
- If you have cardiovascular or peripheral vascular disease or high blood pressure.
- If you have liver or kidney disease.
- If you have hyperthyroidism, insulin-dependent diabetes, pheochromocytoma, peptic ulcer disease or endocrine disorder.

Over age 60:
Adverse reactions and side effects may be more frequent and severe than in younger persons.

Pregnancy:
Tobacco smoke and nicotine are harmful to the fetus. The specific effects of nicotine from these drugs are unknown. Discuss the risks of both with your doctor. Risk category varies for drugs in this group (see page xxiii).

Breast-feeding:
Drug passes into breast milk. Avoid drug or discontinue nursing until you finish medicine. Consult doctor for advice on maintaining milk supply.

Infants & children:
Not recommended.

Prolonged use:
Treatment may take several months. Nicotine replacement therapy is not intended for long-term use.

Skin & sunlight:
No problems expected.

Driving, piloting or hazardous work:
Avoid if you feel dizzy or lightheaded. Otherwise, no problems expected.

Discontinuing:
Adverse reactions and side effects related to nicotine withdrawal may continue for some time after discontinuing.

Others:
- Advise any doctor or dentist whom you consult that you take this medicine.
- May affect results of some medical tests.
- Keep both the used and unused skin patches out of the reach of children and pets. Dispose of old patches according to directions.
- For full benefit from this treatment and to decrease risk of side effects, stop cigarette smoking as soon as you begin treatment.

 POSSIBLE INTERACTION WITH OTHER DRUGS

GENERIC NAME OR DRUG CLASS	COMBINED EFFECT
Acetaminophen	Increased effect of acetaminophen.
Beta-adrenergic blocking agents*	Increased effect of beta blocker.
Bronchodilators, xanthine* (except dyphylline)	Increased broncho-dilator effect.
Imipramine	Increased effect of imipramine.
Insulin & Insulin lispro	May require insulin dosage adjustment.
Isoproterenol	Decreased effect of isoproterenol.
Oxazepam	Increased effect of oxazepam.
Pentazocine	Increased effect of pentazocine.
Phenylephrine	Decreased effect of phenylephrine.
Propoxyphene	Increased effect of propoxyphene.
Theophylline	Increased effect of theophylline.

 POSSIBLE INTERACTION WITH OTHER SUBSTANCES

INTERACTS WITH	COMBINED EFFECT
Alcohol:	Increased cardiac irritability. Avoid.
Beverages:	None expected.
Cocaine:	Increased cardiac irritability. Avoid.
Foods:	None expected.
Marijuana:	Increased toxic effects. Avoid.
Tobacco:	Increased adverse effects of nicotine. Must avoid.

*See Glossary

NIMODIPINE

BRAND NAMES

Nimotop

BASIC INFORMATION

Habit Forming? No
Prescription needed? Yes
Available as generic? No
Drug class: Calcium channel blocker

USES

Helps repair the damage caused by a ruptured blood vessel in the head (also called ruptured aneurysm or subarachnoid hemorrhage). Note: Unlike other calcium channel blockers, nimodipine is not used for angina or high blood pressure.

DOSAGE & USAGE INFORMATION

How to take:
Capsule—Swallow with liquid.

When to take:
Results are best if you begin taking within 96 hours after bleeding into the brain begins. Continue taking for 21 days or as directed by your physician.

If you forget a dose:
Take as soon as you remember up to 2 hours late. If more than 2 hours, wait for next scheduled dose (don't double this dose).

What drug does:
This is a calcium channel blocking drug that crosses easily from blood vessels into the brain, where it prevents spasms of the brain's arteries.

Continued next column

OVERDOSE

SYMPTOMS:
Unusally fast or unusually slow heartbeat, loss of consciousness, cardiac arrest.
WHAT TO DO:
- **Dial 911 (emergency) or 0 (operator) for an ambulance or medical help. Then give first aid immediately.**
- **If patient is unconscious and not breathing, give mouth-to-mouth breathing. If there is no heartbeat, use cardiac massage and mouth-to-mouth breathing (CPR). Don't try to make patient vomit. If you can't get help quickly, take patient to nearest emergency facility.**
- **See emergency information on inside covers.**

Time lapse before drug works:
1 to 2 hours.

Don't take with:
Any other medicine without consulting your doctor or pharmacist.

POSSIBLE ADVERSE REACTIONS OR SIDE EFFECTS

SYMPTOMS	WHAT TO DO
Life-threatening:	
In case of overdose, see previous column.	
Common:	
Tiredness, flushing, swelling of feet, ankles and abdomen.	Continue. Tell doctor at next visit.
Infrequent:	
• Unusually fast or unusually slow heartbeat, wheezing, cough, shortness of breath.	Discontinue. Call doctor right away.
• Dizziness; numbness or tingling in hands or feet; difficult urination.	Continue. Call doctor when convenient.
• Nausea, constipation.	Continue. Tell doctor at next visit.
Rare:	
• Transient blindness, increased angina, chest pain.	Discontinue. Seek emergency treatment.
• Fainting, fever, rash, jaundice, depression, psychosis.	Discontinue. Call doctor right away.
• Pain and swelling in joints, hair loss, vivid dreams.	Continue. Call doctor when convenient.
• Headache.	Continue. Tell doctor at next visit.

WARNINGS & PRECAUTIONS

Don't take if:
- You are allergic to any calcium channel blocking drug*.
- You have very low blood pressure.

Before you start, consult your doctor:
- If you have kidney or liver disease.
- If you have high blood pressure.
- If you have heart disease other than coronary artery disease.

Over age 60:
Adverse reactions and side effects may be more frequent and severe than in younger persons.

Pregnancy:
Decide with your doctor if drug benefits justify risk to unborn child. Risk category C (see page xxiii).

Breast-feeding:
Safety not established. Avoid if possible. Consult doctor.

Infants & children:
Not recommended.

Prolonged use:
Talk to your doctor about the need for follow-up medical examinations or laboratory studies to check blood pressure, liver function, kidney function, ECG*.

Skin & sunlight:
No special problems expected.

Driving, piloting or hazardous work:
Avoid if you feel dizzy. Otherwise, no problems expected.

Discontinuing:
Don't discontinue without doctor's advice until you complete prescribed dose, even though symptoms diminish or disappear.

Others:
- Learn to check your own pulse rate. If it drops to 50 beats per minute or lower, don't take nimodipine until you consult your doctor.
- Drug may lower blood sugar level if daily dose is more than 60 mg.

 POSSIBLE INTERACTION WITH OTHER DRUGS

GENERIC NAME OR DRUG CLASS	COMBINED EFFECT
Angiotensin-converting enzyme (ACE) inhibitors*	Possible excessive potassium in blood. Dosages may need adjustment.
Antiarrhythmics*	Possible increased effect and toxicity of each drug.
Anticoagulants*, oral	Possible increased anticoagulant effect.
Anticonvulsants, hydantoin*	Increased anticonvulsant effect.
Antihypertensives*	Blood pressure changes. Dosage may need adjustment.
Beta-adrenergic blocking agents* (oral or ophthalmic)	Possible irregular heartbeat. May worsen congestive heart failure.
Betaxolol eye drops	May cause increased effect of nimodipine on heart function.
Calcium (large doses)	Possible decreased nimodipine effect.
Carbamazepine	May increase carbamazepine effect and toxicity.
Cimetidine	Possible increased nimodipine effect and toxicity.
Cyclosporine	Increased cyclosporine toxicity.
Disopyramide	May cause dangerously slow, fast or irregular heartbeat.
Diuretics*	Dangerous blood pressure drop.
Levobutanol eye drops	May cause increased effect of nimodipine on heart function.
Lithium	Possible decreased lithium effect.
Nicardipine	Possible increased effect and toxicity of each drug.
Phenytoin	Possible decreased nimodipine effect.
Quinidine	Increased quinidine effect.
Rifampin	Decreased nimodipine effect.

Continued on page 926

 POSSIBLE INTERACTION WITH OTHER SUBSTANCES

INTERACTS WITH	COMBINED EFFECT
Alcohol:	Dangerously low blood pressure. Avoid.
Beverages:	None expected.
Cocaine:	Possible irregular heartbeat. Avoid.
Foods:	None expected.
Marijuana:	Possible irregular heartbeat. Avoid.
Tobacco:	Possible rapid heartbeat. Avoid.

GENERIC AND BRAND NAMES

See complete list of generic and brand names in the *Generic and Brand Name Directory*, page 887.

BASIC INFORMATION

Habit forming? No
Prescription needed? Yes
Available as generic? Yes
Drug class: Antianginal (nitrate)

USES

- Reduces frequency and severity of angina attacks.
- Treats congestive heart failure.

DOSAGE & USAGE INFORMATION

How to take:
- Extended-release tablets or capsules— Swallow each dose whole with liquid.
- Chewable tablet—Chew tablet at earliest sign of angina, and hold in mouth for 2 minutes.
- Regular tablet or capsule—Swallow whole with liquid. Don't crush, chew or open.
- Buccal tablets (Nitrogard)—Allow to dissolve inside of mouth.
- Translingual spray (Nitrolingual)—Spray under tongue according to instructions enclosed with prescription.
- Ointment—Apply as directed.
- Patches—Apply to skin according to package instructions.
- Sublingual tablets—Place under tongue every 3 to 5 minutes at earliest sign of angina. If you don't have complete relief with 3 or 4 tablets, call doctor.

Continued next column

OVERDOSE

SYMPTOMS:
Dizziness; blue fingernails and lips; feeling of pressure in head, fever, fainting; shortness of breath; weak, fast heartbeat; convulsions.
WHAT TO DO:
- **Dial 911 (emergency) or 0 (operator) for an ambulance or medical help. Then give first aid immediately.**
- **See emergency information on inside covers.**

When to take:
- Swallowed tablets—Take at the same times each day, 1 or 2 hours after meals.
- Sublingual tablets or spray—At onset of angina.
- Ointment—Follow prescription directions.
- Patches—According to physician's instructions.

If you forget a dose:
Take as soon as you remember up to 2 hours late. If more than 2 hours, wait for next scheduled dose (don't double this dose).

What drug does:
Relaxes blood vessels, increasing blood flow to heart muscle.

Time lapse before drug works:
- Sublingual tablets and spray—1 to 3 minutes.
- Other forms—15 to 30 minutes. Will not stop an attack, but may prevent attacks.

Don't take with:
Any other medicine without consulting your doctor or pharmacist.

POSSIBLE ADVERSE REACTIONS OR SIDE EFFECTS

SYMPTOMS	WHAT TO DO
Life-threatening:	
In case of overdose, see previous column.	
Common:	
Headache, flushed face and neck, dry mouth, nausea, vomiting.	Continue. Tell doctor at next visit.
Infrequent:	
• Fainting, rapid heartbeat.	Discontinue. Call doctor right away.
• Restlessness, blurred vision, dizziness.	Continue. Call doctor when convenient.
Rare:	
• Rash.	Discontinue. Call doctor right away.
• Severe irritation, peeling.	Continue. Call doctor when convenient.

WARNINGS & PRECAUTIONS

Don't take if:
You are allergic to nitrates, including nitroglycerin.

Before you start, consult your doctor:
- If you are taking nonprescription drugs.
- If you plan to become pregnant within medication period.
- If you have glaucoma.

- If you have reacted badly to any vasodilator drug.
- If you drink alcoholic beverages or smoke marijuana.

Over age 60:
Adverse reactions and side effects may be more frequent and severe than in younger persons.

Pregnancy:
Decide with your doctor if drug benefits justify risk to unborn child. Risk category C (see page xxiii).

Breast-feeding:
Effect unknown. Consult your doctor.

Infants & children:
Not recommended.

Prolonged use:
- Drug may become less effective and require higher doses.
- Talk to your doctor about the need for follow-up medical examinations or laboratory studies to check blood pressure, heart rate.

Skin & sunlight:
No problems expected.

Driving, piloting or hazardous work:
Don't drive or pilot aircraft until you learn how medicine affects you. Don't work around dangerous machinery. Don't climb ladders or work in high places. Danger increases if you drink alcohol or take medicine affecting alertness and reflexes.

Discontinuing:
Except for sublingual tablets, don't discontinue without doctor's advice until you complete prescribed dose, even though symptoms diminish or disappear.

Others:
- If discomfort is not caused by angina, nitrate medication will not bring relief. Call doctor if discomfort persists.
- Periodic urine and laboratory blood studies of white cell counts recommended if you take nitrates.
- Keep sublingual tablets in original container. Always carry them with you, but keep from body heat if possible.
- Sublingual tablets produce a burning, stinging sensation when placed under the tongue. Replace supply if no burning or stinging is noted.
- To avoid development of tolerance, drug-free intervals of 10 hours are sufficient.

POSSIBLE INTERACTION WITH OTHER DRUGS

GENERIC NAME OR DRUG CLASS	COMBINED EFFECT
Anticholinergics*	Increased internal eye pressure.
Antihypertensives*	Excessive blood pressure drop.
Beta-adrenergic blocking agents*	Excessive blood pressure drop.
Calcium channel blockers*	Decreased blood pressure.
Carteolol	Possible excessive blood pressure drop.
Guanfacine	Increased effects of both drugs.
Narcotics*	Excessive blood pressure drop.
Phenothiazines*	May decrease blood pressure.
Sildenafil	Increased effect of nitrates.
Sympathomimetics*	Possible reduced effects of both medicines.

POSSIBLE INTERACTION WITH OTHER SUBSTANCES

INTERACTS WITH	COMBINED EFFECT
Alcohol:	Excessive blood pressure drop.
Beverages:	None expected.
Cocaine:	Reduced effectiveness of nitrates.
Foods:	None expected.
Marijuana:	Decreased nitrate effect.
Tobacco:	Decreased nitrate effect.

NITROFURANTOIN

BRAND NAMES

Apo-Nitrofurantoin	Nephronex
Cyantin	Nifuran
Furadantin	Nitrex
Furalan	Nitrofan
Furaloid	Nitrofor
Furan	Nitrofuracot
Furanite	Novofuran
Furantoin	Ro-Antoin
Furatine	Sarodant
Furaton	Trantoin
Macrobid	Urotoin
Macrodantin	

BASIC INFORMATION

Habit forming? No
Prescription needed? Yes
Available as generic? Yes
Drug class: Antimicrobial, antibacterial (antibiotic)

USES

Treatment for urinary tract infections.

DOSAGE & USAGE INFORMATION

How to take:
- Tablet or capsule—Swallow with food or milk to lessen stomach irritation. If you can't swallow whole, crumble tablet or open capsule and take with liquid or food.
- Extended-release capsule—Swallow with liquid. Do not open capsule.
- Liquid—Shake well and take with food. Use a measuring spoon to ensure accuracy.

When to take:
At the same times each day.

If you forget a dose:
Take as soon as you remember up to 2 hours late. If more than 2 hours, wait for next scheduled dose (don't double this dose).

Continued next column

OVERDOSE

SYMPTOMS:
Nausea, vomiting, abdominal pain, diarrhea.
WHAT TO DO:
Overdose unlikely to threaten life. If person takes much larger amount than prescribed, call doctor, poison control center or hospital emergency room for instructions.

What drug does:
Prevents susceptible bacteria in the urinary tract from growing and multiplying.

Time lapse before drug works:
1 to 2 weeks.

Don't take with:
Any other medicine without consulting your doctor or pharmacist.

POSSIBLE ADVERSE REACTIONS OR SIDE EFFECTS

SYMPTOMS	WHAT TO DO
Life-threatening:	
Hives, rash, intense itching, faintness soon after a dose (anaphylaxis).	Seek emergency treatment immediately.
Common:	
• Diarrhea, appetite loss, nausea, vomiting, chest pain, cough, difficult breathing, chills or unexplained fever, abdominal pain.	Discontinue. Call doctor right away.
• Rusty-colored or brown urine.	No action necessary.
Infrequent:	
• Rash, itchy skin, numbness, tingling or burning of face or mouth, fatigue, weakness.	Discontinue. Call doctor right away.
• Dizziness, headache, drowsiness, paleness (in children), discolored teeth (from liquid form).	Continue. Call doctor when convenient.
Rare:	
Jaundice.	Discontinue. Call doctor right away.

WARNINGS & PRECAUTIONS

Don't take if:
- You are allergic to nitrofurantoin.
- You have impaired kidney function.
- You drink alcohol.

Before you start, consult your doctor:
- If you are prone to allergic reactions.
- If you are pregnant and within 2 weeks of delivery.
- If you have had kidney disease, lung disease, anemia, nerve damage, or G6PD* deficiency (a metabolic deficiency).
- If you have diabetes. Drug may affect urine sugar tests.

Over age 60:
Adverse reactions and side effects may be more frequent and severe than in younger persons.

Pregnancy:
Consult doctor. Risk category B (see page xxiii).

Breast-feeding:
Drug passes into milk. Avoid drug or discontinue nursing until you finish medicine. Consult doctor for advice on maintaining milk supply.

Infants & children:
Don't give to infants younger than 1 month. Use only under medical supervision for older children.

Prolonged use:
- Chest pain, cough, shortness of breath.
- Talk to your doctor about the need for follow-up medical examinations or laboratory studies to check liver function, lung function.

Skin & sunlight:
No problems expected.

Driving, piloting or hazardous work:
Avoid if you feel dizzy or drowsy. Otherwise, no problems expected.

Discontinuing:
Don't discontinue without consulting doctor. Dose may require gradual reduction if you have taken drug for a long time. Doses of other drugs may also require adjustment.

Others:
Periodic blood counts, liver function tests, and chest x-rays recommended.

POSSIBLE INTERACTION WITH OTHER DRUGS

GENERIC NAME OR DRUG CLASS	COMBINED EFFECT
Antivirals, HIV/AIDS*	Increased risk of pancreatitis and peripheral neuropathy.
Hemolytics*, other	Increased risk of toxicity.
Nalidixic acid	Decreased nitrofurantoin effect.
Neurotoxic medicines*	Increased risk of damage to nerve cells.
Probenecid	Increased nitrofurantoin effect.
Sulfinpyrazone	Possible nitrofurantoin toxicity.

POSSIBLE INTERACTION WITH OTHER SUBSTANCES

INTERACTS WITH	COMBINED EFFECT
Alcohol:	Possible disulfiram reaction*. Avoid.
Beverages:	None expected.
Cocaine:	No proven problems.
Foods:	None expected.
Marijuana:	None expected.
Tobacco:	None expected.

NON-NUCLEOSIDE REVERSE TRANSCRIPTASE INHIBITORS

GENERIC AND BRAND NAMES

DELAVIRDINE
  Rescriptor
EFAVIRENZ
  Sustiva

NEVIRAPINE
  Viramune

BASIC INFORMATION

Habit forming? No
Prescription needed? Yes
Available as generic? No
Drug class: Antiviral, HIV and AIDS

USES

For treatment of HIV and AIDS patients. Used in combination with one or more of the other AIDS drugs.

DOSAGE & USAGE INFORMATION

How to take:
- Oral suspension—Swallow with liquid.
- Tablet—Swallow with liquid. May be taken with or without food.

When to take:
At the same time each day. At the start of treatment, one tablet is taken daily for 2 weeks and then increased to 2 tablets daily. This helps to decrease risk of side effects.

If you forget a dose:
Twice-a-day dose—Take as soon as you remember up to 2 hours late. If more than 2 hours, wait for next scheduled dose (don't double this dose).

What drug does:
The drug interferes with HIV replication. It helps slow the progress of HIV disease, but does not cure it.

Continued next column

OVERDOSE

SYMPTOMS:
Unknown.
WHAT TO DO:
Overdose unlikely to threaten life. If person takes much larger amount than prescribed, call doctor, poison control center or hospital emergency room for instructions.

Time lapse before drug works:
May require several weeks or months before full benefits are apparent.

Don't take with:
Any other prescription or nonprescription drugs without consulting your doctor or pharmacist.

POSSIBLE ADVERSE REACTIONS OR SIDE EFFECTS

SYMPTOMS	WHAT TO DO
Life-threatening:	
Severe skin rash.	Discontinue. Call doctor right away or get emergency help.
Common:	
Mild to moderate skin rash.	Discontinue. Call doctor right away.
Infrequent:	
• Fever, blistering skin, mouth sores, aching joints or muscles, eye inflammation, unusual tiredness.	Discontinue. Call doctor right away.
• Headache, nausea, diarrhea.	Continue. Call doctor when convenient.
Rare:	
• Yellow skin or eyes.	Discontinue. Call doctor right away.
• Any other unusual symptoms that occur (may be due to the illness, this drug or other drugs being taken).	Continue, but call doctor right away.

WARNINGS & PRECAUTIONS

Don't take if:
You are allergic to non-nucleoside reverse transcriptase inhibitors.

Before you start, consult your doctor:
- If you are allergic to any medicine, food or other substance, or have a family history of allergies.
- If you have liver disease.

Over age 60:
Though medical studies are incomplete, the adverse reactions and side effects may be more frequent and severe than in younger persons.

Pregnancy:
Decide with your doctor if drug benefits justify risk to unborn child. Risk category C (see page xxiii).

Breast-feeding:
Drug passes into milk. Avoid drug or discontinue nursing until you finish medicine. Consult doctor for advice on maintaining milk supply.

Infants & children:
Safety and efficacy have not been established. Use only under close medical supervision.

Prolonged use:
- Long-term effects have not been established.
- Talk to your doctor about frequent blood counts and liver function studies.

Skin & sunlight:
No problems expected.

Driving, piloting or hazardous work:
No problems expected.

Discontinuing:
Don't discontinue without doctor's advice until you complete prescribed dose, even though symptoms diminish or disappear.

Others:
- Advise any doctor or dentist whom you consult that you take this medicine.
- Consult your doctor if any signs of infection develop (fever, chills, sore throat, intestinal problems, etc.).
- If a rash does occur when the drug is first started, it is vital to consult your doctor.
- Do not increase dosage without doctor's approval.

POSSIBLE INTERACTION WITH OTHER DRUGS

GENERIC NAME OR DRUG CLASS	COMBINED EFFECT
Contraceptives, oral*	Decreased contraceptive effect. Use alternative birth control method.
Protease inhibitors	May require dosage adjustment of protease inhibitor.
Rifabutin	May require dosage adjustment of rifabutin.
Rifampin	May require dosage adjustment of rifampin.

POSSIBLE INTERACTION WITH OTHER SUBSTANCES

INTERACTS WITH	COMBINED EFFECT
Alcohol:	None expected.
Beverages:	None expected.
Cocaine:	Unknown effect. Best to avoid.
Foods:	None expected.
Marijuana:	Unknown effect. Best to avoid.
Tobacco:	None expected.

NUCLEOSIDE REVERSE TRANSCRIPTASE INHIBITORS

GENERIC AND BRAND NAMES

ABACAVIR
Ziagen
DIDANOSINE (ddI)
Videx
LAMIVUDINE
3TC
Combivir
Epivir
STAVUDINE
d4T
Zerit

ZALCITABINE
ddC
Hivid
ZIDOVUDINE
Apo-Zidovudine
AZT
Combivir
Novo-AZT
Retrovir

BASIC INFORMATION

Habit forming? No
Prescription needed? Yes
Available as generic? No
Drug class: Antiviral

 ## USES

- Treats human immunodeficiency virus (HIV).
- Treats acquired immunodeficiency syndrome (AIDS).

 ## DOSAGE & USAGE INFORMATION

How to take:
- Didanosine tablets—Chew or manually crumble tablet. If crumble tablet, mix with at least 1 oz. of water and swallow immediately.
- Tablets or capsules—Swallow with water.
- Syrup—Measure correct dosage with a specially marked measuring device.
- Buffered didanosine for oral solution—Follow instructions on label. Swallow immediately after mixing.

Continued next column

 ## OVERDOSE

SYMPTOMS:
Seizures, severe nausea and vomiting, extreme tiredness or weakness, increase in bruising or bleeding, loss of coordination, involuntary eye movements.
WHAT TO DO:
- Dial 911 (emergency) or 0 (operator) for an ambulance or medical help. Then give first aid immediately.
- See emergency information on inside covers.

When to take:
At the same time each day, according to instructions on prescription label. Follow directions on label for taking with or without food.

If you forget a dose:
Take as soon as you remember up to 2 hours late. If more than 2 hours, wait for next scheduled dose (don't double this dose).

What drug does:
Suppresses replication of human immunodeficiency virus.

Time lapse before drug works:
Depends on the progress of the disease.

Don't take with:
Any other medicine without consulting your doctor or pharmacist.

 ## POSSIBLE ADVERSE REACTIONS OR SIDE EFFECTS

SYMPTOMS	WHAT TO DO
Life-threatening:	
In case of overdose, see previous column.	
Common:	
• Tingling, numbness and burning in the feet and ankles (peripheral neuropathy).	Discontinue. Call doctor right away.
• Headache, anxiety, restlessness, digestive disturbances, diarrhea.	Continue. Call doctor when convenient.
Infrequent:	
• Unusual tiredness and weakness, fever, chills, sore throat, unusual bleeding or bruising, yellow skin and eyes, skin rash, pale skin, muscle or joint pain, mouth or throat sores, stomach pain, nausea and vomiting.	Discontinue. Call doctor right away.
• Lack of strength or energy, difficulty sleeping, discolored nails.	Continue. Call doctor when convenient.
Rare:	
Seizures, mood or mental changes, confusion.	Discontinue. Call doctor right away.

 ## WARNINGS & PRECAUTIONS

Don't take if:
You are allergic to antivirals for HIV and AIDS.

NUCLEOSIDE REVERSE TRANSCRIPTASE INHIBITORS

Before you start, consult your doctor:
- If you have a history of alcoholism.
- If you have hypertriglyceridemia, anemia, gout, phenylketonuria or pancreatitis.
- If you have any condition requiring sodium restriction.
- If you have liver or kidney disease.
- If you have peripheral neuropathy.

Over age 60:
No special problems expected.

Pregnancy:
Risk factors vary for drugs in this group. See category list on page xxiii and consult doctor.

Breast-feeding:
Unknown effects. Consult doctor.

Infants & children:
May cause depigmentation of the retina. Children should have eye exams every 3 to 6 months to check for vision changes.

Prolonged use:
Talk with your doctor about the need for follow-up medical examination or laboratory studies to check blood serum and uric acid levels.

Skin & sunlight:
No special problems expected.

Driving, piloting or hazardous work:
Don't drive or pilot aircraft until you learn how medicine affects you. Don't work around dangerous machinery. Don't climb ladders or work in high places. Danger increases if you drink alcohol or take medicine affecting alertness and reflexes, such as antihistamines, tranquilizers, sedatives, pain medicines, narcotics and mind-altering drugs.

Discontinuing:
Don't discontinue without consulting doctor. Dose may require gradual reduction if you have taken drug for a long time. Doses of other drugs may require adjustment.

Others:
- Advise any doctor or dentist whom you consult that you take this medicine.
- Avoid sexual intercourse or use condoms to help prevent the transmission of HIV. Don't share needles or equipment for injections with other persons.
- The drugs in this group may be combined for treatment. This increases the risk of side effects such as peripheral neuropathy.
- Numerous medical studies are ongoing concerning the use of these and other anti-HIV drugs. Full safety and effectiveness are still being determined.

POSSIBLE INTERACTION WITH OTHER DRUGS

GENERIC NAME OR DRUG CLASS	COMBINED EFFECT
Antacids*, aluminum- or magnesium-containing	Decreased effect of zalcitabine.
Bone marrow depressants*, other	Drugs may need dosage changes.
Cimetidine	Increased effect of zalcitabine and zidovudino.
Clarithromycin	Decreased effect of zidovudine.
Dapsone	Increased risk of peripheral neuropathy. Reduced absorption of both drugs.
Fluoroquinolones	Decreased antibiotic effect.
Gancyclovir	Increased toxicity of both drugs. Use with caution.
Itraconazole	Decreased absorption of itraconazole.
Ketoconazole	Decreased effect of ketoconazole.
Pancreatitus-associated drugs*	Increased risk of pancreatitus with didanosine.
Peripheral neuropathy-associated drugs*	Increased risk of peripheral neuropathy.

Continued on page 926

POSSIBLE INTERACTION WITH OTHER SUBSTANCES

INTERACTS WITH	COMBINED EFFECT
Alcohol:	Increased chance of pancreatitis or peripheral neuropathy.
Beverages:	No proven problems.
Cocaine:	No proven problems.
Foods:	No proven problems.
Marijuana:	No proven problems.
Tobacco:	No proven problems.

NYSTATIN

BRAND NAMES

Dermacomb	Mykacet II
Myco II	Mytrex
Mycobiotic II	Nadostine
Mycogen II	Nilstat
Mycolog II	Nystaform
Mycostatin	Nystex
Myco-Triacet II	Tristatin II
Mykacet	

BASIC INFORMATION

Habit forming? No
Prescription needed? Yes
Available as generic? Yes
Drug class: Antifungal

 USES

Treatment of fungus infections of the mouth or vagina that are susceptible to nystatin.

 DOSAGE & USAGE INFORMATION

How to take:
- Tablet—Swallow with liquid. If you can't swallow whole, crumble tablet and take with liquid or food.
- Ointment, cream or lotion—Use as directed by doctor and label.
- Liquid—Take as directed. Instruction varies by preparation.
- Lozenges—Take as directed on label.

When to take:
At the same time each day.

If you forget a dose:
Take as soon as you remember up to 2 hours late. If more than 2 hours, wait for next scheduled dose (don't double this dose).

Continued next column

 OVERDOSE

SYMPTOMS:
Mild overdose may cause nausea, vomiting, diarrhea.
WHAT TO DO:
Overdose unlikely to threaten life. If person takes much larger amount than prescribed, call doctor, poison control center or hospital emergency room for instructions.

What drug does:
Prevents growth and reproduction of fungus.

Time lapse before drug works:
Begins immediately. May require 3 weeks for maximum benefit, depending on location and severity of infection.

Don't take with:
Any other medicine without consulting your doctor or pharmacist.

 POSSIBLE ADVERSE REACTIONS OR SIDE EFFECTS

SYMPTOMS	WHAT TO DO
Life-threatening: None expected.	
Common: (at high doses) Nausea, stomach pain, vomiting, diarrhea.	Discontinue. Call doctor right away.
Infrequent: Mild irritation, itch at application site.	Discontinue. Call doctor right away.
Rare: None expected.	

WARNINGS & PRECAUTIONS

Don't take if:
You are allergic to nystatin.

Before you start, consult your doctor:
If you plan to become pregnant within medication period.

Over age 60:
No problems expected.

Pregnancy:
No proven harm to unborn child. Avoid if possible. Consult doctor. Risk category B (see page xxiii).

Breast-feeding:
No proven problems. Consult doctor.

Infants & children:
No problems expected.

Prolonged use:
No problems expected.

Skin & sunlight:
No problems expected.

Driving, piloting or hazardous work:
No problems expected.

Discontinuing:
Don't discontinue without doctor's advice until you complete prescribed dose, even though symptoms diminish or disappear.

Others:
No problems expected.

POSSIBLE INTERACTION WITH OTHER DRUGS

GENERIC NAME OR DRUG CLASS	COMBINED EFFECT
None reported.	

POSSIBLE INTERACTION WITH OTHER SUBSTANCES

INTERACTS WITH	COMBINED EFFECT
Alcohol:	None expected.
Beverages:	None expected.
Cocaine:	None expected.
Foods:	None expected.
Marijuana:	None expected.
Tobacco:	None expected.

OLANZAPINE

BRAND NAMES

Zyprexa

BASIC INFORMATION

Habit forming? No
Prescription needed? Yes
Available as generic? No
Drug class: Antipsychotic

 USES

Treatment for symptoms of schizophrenia and other psychotic disorders.

 DOSAGE & USAGE INFORMATION

How to take:
Tablet—Swallow with liquid. May be taken with or without food.

When to take:
Once a day at the same time each day. The prescribed dosage may be increased over the first few days of use.

If you forget a dose:
Take as soon as you remember. If it is almost time for the next dose, wait for the next scheduled dose (don't double this dose).

What drug does:
The exact mechanism is unknown. It appears to alleviate symptoms of schizophrenia by blocking certain nerve impulses between nerve cells.

Time lapse before drug works:
One to 7 days. Further increases in the dosage amount may be necessary to relieve symptoms for some patients.

Don't take with:
Any other medication without consulting your doctor or pharmacist. All possible drug interactions have not been studied.

 OVERDOSE

SYMPTOMS:
Drowsiness and slurred speech; other symptoms may occur that were not observed in medical studies of the drug.
WHAT TO DO:
If person takes much larger amount than prescribed, call doctor, poison control center or hospital emergency room for instructions.

 POSSIBLE ADVERSE REACTIONS OR SIDE EFFECTS

SYMPTOMS	WHAT TO DO
Life-threatening: High fever, rapid pulse, profuse sweating, muscle rigidity, confusion and irritability, seizures (neuroleptic malignant syndrome - rare).	Discontinue. Seek emergency treatment.
Common: • Dizziness, difficulty in speaking or swallowing, shaking hands and fingers, trembling, vision problems, weakness, lightheadedness when arising from a sitting or lying position.	Continue. Call doctor right away.
• Drowsiness, constipation, weight gain, agitation, insomnia, headache, nervousness, runny nose, anxiety, dry mouth, personality disorder, arm or leg stiffness.	Continue. Call doctor when convenient.
Infrequent: • Jerky or involuntary movements, especially of the face, lips, jaw, tongue; chest pain, fast heartbeat.	Continue. Call doctor right away.
• Fever, flu-like symptoms, twitching, mood or mental changes, speech unclear, swollen feet or ankles, appetite increased, cough, saliva increased, muscle tightness, muscle spasms (face, neck, back), joint pain, nausea or vomiting, sore throat, thirstiness, incontinence, abdominal pain.	Continue. Call doctor when convenient.
Rare: • Breathing difficulty.	Discontinue. Call doctor right away.
• Swollen face, rash, confusion, decreased sex drive, menstrual changes, sluggishness.	Continue. Call doctor when convenient.

WARNINGS & PRECAUTIONS

Don't take if:
You are allergic to olanzapine

Before you start, consult your doctor:
- If you have liver disease, heart disease or a blood vessel disorder.
- If you have Alzheimer's.
- If you have a history of breast cancer.
- If you have intestinal blockage.
- If you are subject to dehydration or low body temperature.
- If you have a history of drug abuse/dependence.
- If you have glaucoma.
- If you have prostate problems.
- If you are allergic to any medication, food or other substance.
- If you have a history of seizures.

Over age 60:
Adverse reactions and side effects may be more severe than in younger persons. A lower starting dosage is usually recommended until a response is determined.

Pregnancy:
Decide with your doctor if drug benefits justify any possible risk to unborn child. Risk category C (see page xxiii).

Breast-feeding:
It is unknown if drug passes into milk. It is not recommended for nursing mothers.

Infants & children:
Safety in children under age 18 has not been established. Use only under close medical supervision.

Prolonged use:
Consult with your doctor on a regular basis while taking this drug to check your progress or to discuss any increase or changes in side effects and the need for continued treatment. Long term effectiveness has not been established.

Skin & sunlight:
- May cause rash or intensify sunburn in areas exposed to sun or ultraviolet light (photosensitivity reaction). Use sunscreen and avoid overexposure. Notify doctor if reaction occurs.
- Hot temperatures, exercise, and hot baths can increase risk of heatstroke. Drug may affect body's ability to maintain normal temperature.

Driving, piloting or hazardous work:
Don't drive or pilot aircraft until you learn how medicine affects you. Don't work around dangerous machinery. Don't climb ladders or work in high places. Danger increases if you drink alcohol or take medicine affecting alertness and reflexes.

Discontinuing:
Don't discontinue this drug without consulting doctor. Dosage may require a gradual reduction before stopping.

Others:
- Get up slowly from a sitting or lying position to avoid any dizziness, faintness or lightheadedness.
- Advise any doctor or dentist whom you consult that you take this medicine.
- Take medicine only as directed. Do not increase or reduce dosage without doctor's approval.
- Doctor may need to monitor enzymes in liver to ensure liver functions are not affected by medication.

POSSIBLE INTERACTION WITH OTHER DRUGS

GENERIC NAME OR DRUG CLASS	COMBINED EFFECT
Anticholinergics*, other	Increased risk of side effects.
Antihypertensives*	Increased effect of antihypertensive.
Carbamazepine	Decreased effect of olanzapine.
Central nervous system (CNS) depressants*, other	Increased sedative effect.
Enzyme inducers*	May decrease olanzapine effect.
Enzyme inhibitors*	May increase olanzapine effect.
Dopamine agonists*	May decrease effect of dopamine agonist.
Hepatotoxics*	Increased risk of liver problems.
Levodopa	May decrease levodopa effect.

POSSIBLE INTERACTION WITH OTHER SUBSTANCES

INTERACTS WITH	COMBINED EFFECT
Alcohol:	Increased sedation and dizziness. Avoid.
Beverages:	None expected.
Cocaine:	Effect not known. Best to avoid.
Foods:	None expected.
Marijuana:	Effect not known. Best to avoid.
Tobacco:	Decreased olanzapine effect. Avoid.

OLSALAZINE

BRAND NAMES

Dipentum

BASIC INFORMATION

Habit forming? No
Prescription needed? Yes
Available as generic? No
Drug class: Inflammatory bowel disease suppressant

 ## USES

To maintain remission of ulcerative colitis. Generally prescribed when intolerance to sulfasalazine exists.

 ## DOSAGE & USAGE INFORMATION

How to take:
Capsule—Swallow with liquid or food to lessen stomach irritation. If you can't swallow whole, open capsule and take with liquid or food.

When to take:
Usually twice a day, or as directed on prescription label.

If you forget a dose:
- Take as soon as possible.
- Skip if it is almost time for next dose.
- Don't double next dose.
- Notify your doctor if there are questions.

What drug does:
Inhibits prostaglandin production in the colon.

Time lapse before drug works:
1 hour.

Don't take with:
Any other medicine without consulting your doctor or pharmacist.

 ## OVERDOSE

SYMPTOMS:
None expected.
WHAT TO DO:
Overdose unlikely to threaten life. If person takes much larger amount than prescribed, call doctor, poison control center or hospital emergency room for instructions.

 ## POSSIBLE ADVERSE REACTIONS OR SIDE EFFECTS

SYMPTOMS	WHAT TO DO
Life-threatening: Fever, sore throat, paleness, unusual bleeding (representing effect on blood, a rare complication).	Seek emergency treatment.
Common: Diarrhea, appetite loss, nausea, vomiting.	Continue. Call doctor when convenient.
Infrequent: Mood changes, sleeplessness, headache.	Continue. Call doctor when convenient.
Rare: Skin eruption (acne-like), muscle aches.	Continue. Call doctor when convenient.

WARNINGS & PRECAUTIONS

Don't take if:
- You are allergic to aspirin or any other salicylate.
- You are allergic to mesalamine.

Before you start, consult your doctor:
- If you have kidney disease.
- If you are taking any other prescription or nonprescription medicine.

Over age 60:
No special problems expected.

Pregnancy:
Decide with your doctor if drug benefits justify risk to unborn child. Risk category C (see page xxiii).

Breast-feeding:
Unknown effects. Consult doctor.

Infants & children:
Effect not documented. Consult your family doctor or pediatrician.

Prolonged use:
Follow through with full prescribed course of treatment.

Skin & sunlight:
No special problems expected.

Driving, piloting or hazardous work:
Don't drive or pilot aircraft until you learn how medicine affects you. Don't work around dangerous machinery. Don't climb ladders or work in high places. Danger increases if you drink alcohol or take medicine affecting alertness and reflexes.

Discontinuing:
Don't discontinue without consulting doctor. Dose may require gradual reduction if you have taken drug for a long time. Doses of other drugs may also require adjustment.

Others:
Request your doctor to check blood counts and kidney function on a regular basis.

POSSIBLE INTERACTION WITH OTHER DRUGS

GENERIC NAME OR DRUG CLASS	COMBINED EFFECT
None expected since olsalazine is not appreciably absorbed from the gastrointestinal tract into the bloodstream.	

POSSIBLE INTERACTION WITH OTHER SUBSTANCES

INTERACTS WITH	COMBINED EFFECT
Alcohol:	Increased risk of gastrointestinal upset and/or bleeding.
Beverages: Highly spiced beverages.	Will irritate underlying condition that olsalazine treats.
Cocaine:	Avoid.
Foods: Highly spiced foods.	Will irritate underlying condition that olsalazine treats.
Marijuana:	Avoid.
Tobacco:	Will irritate underlying condition that olsalazine treats. Avoid.

ORPHENADRINE

BRAND NAMES

Banflex	Myotrol
Blanex	Neocyten
Disipal	Noradex
Flexagin	Norflex
Flexain	O-Flex
Flexoject	Orflagen
Flexon	Orfro
K-Flex	Orphenate
Marflex	Tega-Flex
Myolin	

BASIC INFORMATION

Habit forming? Possibly
Prescription needed?
  U.S.: Yes
  Canada: No
Available as generic? Yes
Drug class: Muscle relaxant, anticholinergic, antihistamine, antiparkinsonism

USES

- Reduces discomfort of muscle strain.
- Relieves symptoms of Parkinson's disease.
- Adjunctive treatment to rest, analgesics and physical therapy for muscle spasms.

DOSAGE & USAGE INFORMATION

How to take:
- Tablet—Swallow with liquid. If you can't swallow whole, crumble tablet and take with liquid or food.
- Extended-release tablet—Swallow whole. Do not crumble.

When to take:
At the same times each day.

Continued next column

OVERDOSE

SYMPTOMS:
Fainting, confusion, blurred vision, difficulty swallowing, difficulty breathing, decreased urination, widely dilated pupils, rapid heartbeat, rapid pulse, paralysis, convulsions, coma.
WHAT TO DO:
- **Dial 911 (emergency) or 0 (operator) for an ambulance or medical help. Then give first aid immediately.**
- **See emergency information on inside covers.**

If you forget a dose:
Take as soon as you remember up to 6 hours late. If more than 6 hours, wait for next scheduled dose (don't double this dose).

What drug does:
Sedative and analgesic effects reduce spasm and pain in skeletal muscles.

Time lapse before drug works:
1 to 2 hours.

Don't take with:
Any other medicine without consulting your doctor or pharmacist.

POSSIBLE ADVERSE REACTIONS OR SIDE EFFECTS

SYMPTOMS	WHAT TO DO
Life-threatening: Extreme weakness; transient paralysis; temporary loss of vision; hives, rash, intense itching, faintness soon after a dose (anaphylaxis).	Seek emergency treatment immediately.
Common: None expected.	
Infrequent: • Weakness, headache, dizziness, agitation, drowsiness, tremor, confusion, rapid or pounding heartbeat, depression, hearing loss.	Discontinue. Call doctor right away.
• Dry mouth, nausea, vomiting, constipation, urinary hesitancy or retention, abdominal pain, muscle weakness.	Continue. Call doctor when convenient.
Rare: Rash, itchy skin, blurred vision, hallucinations.	Discontinue. Call doctor right away.

WARNINGS & PRECAUTIONS

Don't take if:
- You are allergic to orphenadrine.
- You are allergic to tartrazine dye.

Before you start, consult your doctor:
- If you have glaucoma.
- If you have myasthenia gravis.
- If you have difficulty emptying bladder.
- If you have had heart disease or heart rhythm disturbance.
- If you have had a peptic ulcer.
- If you have prostate enlargement.

Over age 60:
Adverse reactions and side effects may be more frequent and severe than in younger persons.

Pregnancy:
Decide with your doctor if drug benefits justify risk to unborn child. Risk category C (see page xxiii).

Breast-feeding:
No proven problems. Consult doctor.

Infants & children:
Not recommended for children younger than 12.

Prolonged use:
* Increased internal eye pressure.
* Talk to your doctor about the need for follow-up medical examinations or laboratory studies to check complete blood counts (white blood cell count, platelet count, red blood cell count, hemoglobin, hematocrit), liver function, kidney function.

Skin & sunlight:
No problems expected.

Driving, piloting or hazardous work:
Don't drive or pilot aircraft until you learn how medicine affects you. Don't work around dangerous machinery. Don't climb ladders or work in high places. Danger increases if you drink alcohol or take medicine affecting alertness and reflexes, such as antihistamines, tranquilizers, sedatives, pain medicine, narcotics and mind-altering drugs.

Discontinuing:
May be unnecessary to finish medicine. Follow doctor's instructions.

Others:
No problems expected.

POSSIBLE INTERACTION WITH OTHER DRUGS

GENERIC NAME OR DRUG CLASS	COMBINED EFFECT
Anticholinergics*	Increased anticholinergic effect.
Antidepressants, tricyclic*	Increased sedation.
Antihistamines*	Increased sedation.
Attapulgite	Decreased orphenadrine effect.
Carteolol	Decreased antihistamine effect.
Chlorpromazine	Hypoglycemia (low blood sugar).
Cisapride	Decreased orphenadrine effect.

Contraceptives, oral*	Decreased contraceptive effect.
Griseofulvin	Decreased griseofulvin effect.
Levodopa	Increased levodopa effect. (Improves effectiveness in treating Parkinson's disease.)
Nabilone	Greater depression of central nervous system.
Nitrates*	Increased internal eye pressure.
Nizatidine	Increased nizatidine effect.
Phenylbutazone	Decreased phenylbutazone effect.
Potassium supplements*	Increased possibility of intestinal ulcers with oral potassium tablets.
Propoxyphene	Possible confusion, nervousness, tremors.

POSSIBLE INTERACTION WITH OTHER SUBSTANCES

INTERACTS WITH	COMBINED EFFECT
Alcohol:	Increased drowsiness. Avoid.
Beverages:	None expected.
Cocaine:	Decreased orphenadrine effect. Avoid.
Foods:	None expected.
Marijuana:	Increased drowsiness, mouth dryness, muscle weakness, fainting.
Tobacco:	None expected.

ORPHENADRINE, ASPIRIN & CAFFEINE

BRAND NAMES

N3 Gesic
N3 Gesic Forte
Norgesic
Norgesic Forte
Norphadrine
Norphadrine Forte
Orphenagesic
Orphenagesic Forte

BASIC INFORMATION

Habit forming? Yes
Prescription needed? Yes
Available as generic? No
Drug class: Stimulant, vasoconstrictor, muscle relaxant, analgesic, anti-inflammatory (nonsteroidal)

USES

- Reduces discomfort of muscle strain.
- Reduces pain, fever, inflammation.
- Relieves swelling, stiffness, joint pain.
- Treats drowsiness and fatigue.

DOSAGE & USAGE INFORMATION

How to take:
Tablet—Swallow with liquid. If you can't swallow whole, crumble and take with liquid or food.

When to take:
At the same times each day.

If you forget a dose:
Take as soon as you remember up to 2 hours late. If more than 2 hours, wait for next scheduled dose (don't double this dose).

What drug does:
- Sedative and analgesic effects reduce spasm and pain in skeletal muscles.
- Affects hypothalamus, the part of the brain which regulates temperature by dilating small blood vessels in skin.

Continued next column

OVERDOSE

SYMPTOMS:
Fainting, confusion, widely dilated pupils, rapid pulse, ringing in ears, nausea, vomiting, dizziness, fever, deep and rapid breathing, excitement, rapid heartbeat, hallucinations, coma.
WHAT TO DO:
- **Dial 911 (emergency) or 0 (operator) for an ambulance or medical help. Then give first aid immediately.**
- **See emergency information on inside covers.**

- Prevents clumping of platelets (small blood cells) so blood vessels remain open.
- Decreases prostaglandin effect.
- Suppresses body's pain messages.
- Constricts blood vessel walls.
- Stimulates central nervous system.

Time lapse before drug works:
1 hour.

Don't take with:
- Tetracyclines. Space doses 1 hour apart.
- Nonprescription drugs without consulting doctor.
- Any other medicine without consulting your doctor or pharmacist.

POSSIBLE ADVERSE REACTIONS OR SIDE EFFECTS

SYMPTOMS	WHAT TO DO
Life-threatening:	
Hives, rash, intense itching, wheezing, faintness soon after a dose (anaphylaxis), convulsions, fever.	Seek emergency treatment immediately.
Common:	
• Nausea, vomiting, abdominal cramps, nervousness, urgent urination, low blood sugar (hunger, anxiety, cold sweats, rapid pulse).	Discontinue. Call doctor right away.
• Ringing in ears, indigestion, heartburn, insomnia.	Continue. Call doctor when convenient.
Infrequent:	
• Weakness, headache, dizziness, drowsiness, agitation, tremor, confusion, irregular heartbeat, hearing loss, diarrhea, hallucinations.	Discontinue. Call doctor right away.
• Dry mouth, constipation.	Continue. Call doctor when convenient.
Rare:	
• Black or bloody vomit.	Discontinue. Seek emergency treatment.
• Change in vision; blurred vision; black, bloody or tarry stool; bloody urine; dilated pupils; uncontrolled movement of hands; sore throat; fever.	Discontinue. Call doctor right away.

WARNINGS & PRECAUTIONS

Don't take if:
- You need to restrict sodium in your diet. Buffered effervescent tablets and sodium salicylate are high in sodium.
- Aspirin has a strong vinegar-like odor, which means it has decomposed.
- You have a peptic ulcer of stomach or duodenum, a bleeding disorder, heart disease.
- You are allergic to any stimulant or orphenadrine.

Before you start, consult your doctor:
- If you have had stomach or duodenal ulcers, gout, heart disease or heart rhythm disturbance, peptic ulcer.
- If you have asthma, nasal polyps, irregular heartbeat, hypoglycemia (low blood sugar), epilepsy, glaucoma, myasthenia gravis, difficulty emptying bladder, prostate enlargement.

Over age 60:
- More likely to cause hidden bleeding in stomach or intestines. Watch for dark stools.
- Adverse reactions and side effects may be more frequent and severe than in younger persons.

Pregnancy:
Risk to unborn child outweighs drug benefits. Don't use. Risk category D (see page xxiii).

Breast-feeding:
Drug passes into milk. Avoid drug or discontinue nursing until you finish medicine. Consult doctor for advice on maintaining milk supply.

Infants & children:
- Overdose frequent and severe. Keep bottles out of children's reach.
- Consult doctor before giving to persons under age 18 who have fever and discomfort of viral illness, especially chicken pox and influenza. Probably increases risk of Reye's syndrome.
- Not recommended for children under 12.

Prolonged use:
- Kidney damage. Periodic kidney function test recommended.
- Stomach ulcers more likely.
- Increased internal eye pressure.
- Talk to your doctor about the need for follow-up medical examinations or laboratory studies to check liver function, complete blood counts (white blood cell count, platelet count, red blood cell count, hemoglobin, hematocrit).

Skin & sunlight:
No special problems expected.

Driving, piloting or hazardous work:
Don't drive or pilot aircraft until you learn how medicine affects you. Don't work around dangerous machinery. Don't climb ladders or work in high places. Danger increases if you drink alcohol or take medicine affecting alertness and reflexes, such as antihistamines, tranquilizers, sedatives, pain medicine, narcotics and mind-altering drugs.

Discontinuing:
- For chronic illness—Don't discontinue without doctor's advice until you complete prescribed dose, even though symptoms diminish or disappear.
- May be unnecessary to finish medicine if you take it for a short-term illness. Follow doctor's instructions.

Others:
- Aspirin can complicate surgery; illness; pregnancy, labor and delivery.
- For arthritis, don't change dose without consulting doctor.
- Urine tests for blood sugar may be inaccurate.
- May produce or aggravate fibrocystic breast disease in women.

POSSIBLE INTERACTION WITH OTHER DRUGS

GENERIC NAME OR DRUG CLASS	COMBINED EFFECT
Acebutolol	Decreased antihypertensive effect of acebutolol.

Continued on page 926

POSSIBLE INTERACTION WITH OTHER SUBSTANCES

INTERACTS WITH	COMBINED EFFECT
Alcohol:	Possible stomach irritation and bleeding, increased drowsiness. Avoid.
Beverages: Caffeine drinks.	Increased caffeine effect.
Cocaine:	Decreased orphenadrine effect. Overstimulation. Avoid.
Foods:	No proven problems.
Marijuana:	Increased effect of drugs. May lead to dangerous, rapid heartbeat. Increased dry mouth. Avoid.
Tobacco:	Increased heartbeat. Avoid.

OXTRIPHYLLINE & GUAIFENESIN

BRAND NAMES

Brondecon   Choledyl
Brondelate   Expectorant

BASIC INFORMATION

Habit forming? No
Prescription needed? Yes
Available as generic? Yes
Drug class: Bronchodilator (xanthine),
  cough/cold preparation

USES

- Treatment for bronchial asthma symptoms.
- Loosens mucus in respiratory passages from allergies and infections.

DOSAGE & USAGE INFORMATION

How to take:
Tablet or elixir—Swallow with liquid. If you can't swallow tablet whole, crumble and take with liquid or food.

When to take:
Most effective taken on empty stomach 1 hour before or 2 hours after eating. However, may take with food to lessen stomach upset.

If you forget a dose:
Take as soon as you remember up to 2 hours late. If more than 2 hours, wait for next scheduled dose (don't double this dose).

What drug does:
- Relaxes and expands bronchial tubes.
- Increases production of watery fluids to thin mucus so it can be coughed out or absorbed.

Time lapse before drug works:
15 to 30 minutes.

Don't take with:
- Any stimulant.
- Any other medicine without consulting your doctor or pharmacist.

OVERDOSE

SYMPTOMS:
Restlessness, irritability, confusion, delirium, convulsions, rapid pulse, nausea, vomiting, coma.
WHAT TO DO:
- **Dial 911 (emergency) or 0 (operator) for an ambulance or medical help. Then give first aid immediately.**
- **See emergency information on inside covers.**

POSSIBLE ADVERSE REACTIONS OR SIDE EFFECTS

SYMPTOMS	WHAT TO DO
Life-threatening:	
Difficult breathing, irregular or fast heartbeat.	Discontinue. Seek emergency treatment.
Common:	
Headache, irritability, nervousness, restlessness, insomnia, nausea, vomiting, abdominal pain, drowsiness.	Continue. Call doctor when convenient.
Infrequent:	
• Hives, rash, red or flushed face, diarrhea, heartburn, muscle twitching.	Discontinue. Call doctor right away.
• Dizziness, lightheadedness, appetite loss.	Continue. Call doctor when convenient.
Rare:	
None expected.	

WARNINGS & PRECAUTIONS

Don't take if:
- You are allergic to any cough or cold preparation containing guaifenesin or any bronchodilator.
- You have an active peptic ulcer.

Before you start, consult your doctor:
- If you have had impaired kidney or liver function.
- If you have gastritis, peptic ulcer, high blood pressure or heart disease.
- If you take medication for gout.

Over age 60:
Adverse reactions and side effects may be more frequent and severe than in younger persons. For drug to work, you must drink 8 to 10 glasses of fluid per day.

Pregnancy:
Decide with your doctor if drug benefits justify risk to unborn child. Risk category C (see page xxiii).

Breast-feeding:
Drug passes into milk. Avoid drug or discontinue nursing until you finish medicine. Consult doctor for advice on maintaining milk supply.

Infants & children:
Use only under medical supervision.

Prolonged use:
- Stomach irritation.
- Talk to your doctor about the need for follow-up medical examinations or laboratory studies to check serum oxtriphylline levels, lung function.

Skin & sunlight:
No problems expected.

Driving, piloting or hazardous work:
Avoid if lightheaded or dizzy. Otherwise, no problems expected.

Discontinuing:
May be unnecessary to finish medicine. Follow doctor's instructions.

Others:
No problems expected.

POSSIBLE INTERACTION WITH OTHER DRUGS

GENERIC NAME OR DRUG CLASS	COMBINED EFFECT
Allopurinol	Decreased allopurinol effect.
Anticoagulants,* oral	Possible risk of bleeding.
Ephedrine	Increased effect of both drugs.
Epinephrine	Increased effect of both drugs.
Erythromycins*	Increased bronchodilator effect.
Furosemide	Increased furosemide effect.
Lincomycins*	Increased bronchodilator effect.
Lithium	Decreased lithium effect.
Probenecid	Decreased effect of both drugs.
Propranolol	Decreased bronchodilator effect.
Rauwolfia alkaloids*	Rapid heartbeat.
Sulfinpyrazone	Decreased sulfinpyrazone effect.
Troleandomycin	Increased bronchodilator effect.

POSSIBLE INTERACTION WITH OTHER SUBSTANCES

INTERACTS WITH	COMBINED EFFECT
Alcohol:	None expected.
Beverages: Caffeine drinks.	Nervousness and insomnia.
Other.	You must drink 8 to 10 glasses of fluid per day for drug to work.
Cocaine:	Excess stimulation. Avoid.
Foods:	None expected.
Marijuana:	Slightly increased antiasthmatic effect of bronchodilator.
Tobacco:	Decreased bronchodilator effect and harmful for all conditions requiring bronchodilator treatment. Avoid.

OXYBUTYNIN

BRAND NAMES

Ditropan

BASIC INFORMATION

Habit forming? No
Prescription needed? Yes
Available as generic? Yes
Drug class: Antispasmodic (urinary tract)

 ## USES

Reduces spasms of urinary bladder and urethra that cause symptoms of frequent urination, urgency, night-time urination and incontinence.

 ## DOSAGE & USAGE INFORMATION

How to take:
Tablets or syrup—Swallow with water.

When to take:
At the same time every day. Do not take with food unless instructed to do so by doctor.

If you forget a dose:
Take as soon as you remember up to 2 hours late. If more than 2 hours, wait for next scheduled dose. Don't double this dose.

What drug does:
Blocks nerve impulses at parasympathetic nerve endings, preventing muscle contractions and gland secretions of organs involved.

Time lapse before drug works:
30 minutes to 1 hour.

Don't take with:
Any other medicine without consulting your doctor or pharmacist.

 ## OVERDOSE

SYMPTOMS:
Unsteadiness, confusion, dizziness, severe drowsiness, fast heartbeat, fever, red face, hallucinations, difficult breathing.
WHAT TO DO:
Overdose unlikely to threaten life. If person takes much larger amount than prescribed, call doctor, poison control center or hospital emergency room for instructions.

 ## POSSIBLE ADVERSE REACTIONS OR SIDE EFFECTS

SYMPTOMS	WHAT TO DO
Life-threatening: In case of overdose, see previous column.	
Common: Constipation; decreased sweating; drowsiness; dryness of mouth, nose and throat.	Continue. Call doctor when convenient.
Infrequent: Difficult swallowing, decreased sexual ability, headache, difficult urination, sensitivity to light, nausea, vomiting, insomnia, tiredness.	Continue. Call doctor when convenient.
Rare: Skin rash, eye pain, blurred vision.	Discontinue. Call doctor right away.

WARNINGS & PRECAUTIONS

Don't take if:
- You are allergic to any anticholinergic.
- You have trouble with stomach bloating.
- You have difficulty emptying your bladder completely.
- You have narrow-angle glaucoma.
- You have severe ulcerative colitis.

Before you start, consult your doctor:
- If you have open-angle glaucoma.
- If you have angina or fast heartbeat.
- If you have chronic bronchitis or asthma.
- If you have hiatal hernia; liver, kidney or thyroid disease; enlarged prostate or myasthenia gravis.
- If you will have surgery within 2 months, including dental surgery, requiring general or spinal anesthesia.

Over age 60:
Adverse reactions and side effects may be more frequent and severe than in younger persons. You may require smaller doses for shorter periods of time.

Pregnancy:
No proven harm to unborn child, but avoid if possible. Consult doctor. Risk category B (see page xxiii).

Breast-feeding:
Unknown effect. Consult doctor.

Infants & children:
Not recommended for children under 5.

Prolonged use:
Side effects more likely.

Skin & sunlight:
No special problems expected.

Driving, piloting or hazardous work:
Don't drive or pilot aircraft until you learn how medicine affects you. Don't work around dangerous machinery. Don't climb ladders or work in high places. Danger increases if you drink alcohol or take medicine affecting alertness and reflexes.

Discontinuing:
May be unnecessary to finish medicine. Follow doctor's instructions.

Others:
Advise any doctor or dentist whom you consult that you take this medicine.

POSSIBLE INTERACTION WITH OTHER DRUGS

GENERIC NAME OR DRUG CLASS	COMBINED EFFECT
Anticholinergics*	Increased effect of oxybutynin.
Central nervous system (CNS) depressants*	Increased sedative effect.

POSSIBLE INTERACTION WITH OTHER SUBSTANCES

INTERACTS WITH	COMBINED EFFECT
Alcohol:	Increased sedative effect.
Beverages:	None expected.
Cocaine:	Excessively rapid heartbeat. Avoid.
Foods:	None expected.
Marijuana:	Drowsiness and dry mouth.
Tobacco:	None expected.

*See Glossary

OXYMETAZOLINE (Nasal)

BRAND NAMES

See complete list of brand names in the *Generic and Brand Name Directory*, page 887.

BASIC INFORMATION

Habit forming? No
Prescription needed? No
Available as generic? Yes
Drug class: Sympathomimetic

USES

Relieves congestion of nose, sinuses and throat from allergies and infections.

DOSAGE & USAGE INFORMATION

How to take:
Nasal solution, nasal spray—Use as directed on label. Avoid contamination. Don't use same container for more than 1 person.

When to take:
When needed, no more often than every 4 hours.

If you forget a dose:
Take as soon as you remember. Wait 4 hours for next dose.

What drug does:
Constricts walls of small arteries in nose, sinuses and eustachian tubes.

Time lapse before drug works:
5 to 30 minutes. May last 8 to 12 hours.

Continued next column

OVERDOSE

SYMPTOMS:
Headache, sweating, anxiety, agitation, rapid and irregular heartbeat (rare occurrence with systemic absorption).
WHAT TO DO:
- **Dial 911 (emergency) or 0 (operator) for an ambulance or medical help. Then give first aid immediately.**
- **If patient is unconscious and not breathing, give mouth-to-mouth breathing. If there is no heartbeat, use cardiac massage and mouth-to-mouth breathing (CPR). If you can't get help quickly, take patient to nearest emergency facility.**
- **See emergency information on inside covers.**

Don't take with:
- Nonprescription drugs for allergy, cough or cold without consulting doctor.
- Any other medicine without consulting your doctor or pharmacist.

POSSIBLE ADVERSE REACTIONS OR SIDE EFFECTS

SYMPTOMS	WHAT TO DO
Life-threatening:	
In case of overdose, see previous column.	
Common:	
None expected.	
Infrequent:	
Burning, dry or stinging nasal passages.	Continue. Call doctor when convenient.
Rare:	
Rebound congestion (increased runny or stuffy nose); headache, insomnia, nervousness (may occur with systemic absorption).	Discontinue. Call doctor right away.

OXYMETAZOLINE (Nasal)

WARNINGS & PRECAUTIONS

Don't take if:
You are allergic to oxymetazoline or other nasal spray.

Before you start, consult your doctor:
- If you have heart disease or high blood pressure.
- If you have diabetes.
- If you have overactive thyroid.
- If you have taken MAO inhibitors in past 2 weeks.
- If you have glaucoma.

Over age 60:
Adverse reactions and side effects may be more frequent and severe than in younger persons.

Pregnancy:
Consult doctor. Risk category C (see page xxiii).

Breast-feeding:
No proven problems. Consult doctor.

Infants & children:
Don't give to children younger than 2.

Prolonged use:
Drug may lose effectiveness, cause increased congestion (rebound effect*) and irritate nasal membranes.

Skin & sunlight:
No problems expected.

Driving, piloting or hazardous work:
No problems expected.

Discontinuing:
May be unnecessary to finish medicine. Follow doctor's instructions.

Others:
Don't use for more than 3 days in a row.

POSSIBLE INTERACTION WITH OTHER DRUGS

GENERIC NAME OR DRUG CLASS	COMBINED EFFECT
Antidepressants, tricyclic*	Possible rise in blood pressure.
Butorphanol	Delays start of butorphanol effect.
Maprotiline	Possible increased blood pressure.

POSSIBLE INTERACTION WITH OTHER SUBSTANCES

INTERACTS WITH	COMBINED EFFECT
Alcohol:	None expected.
Beverages: Caffeine drinks.	Nervousness or insomnia.
Cocaine:	High risk of heartbeat irregularities and high blood pressure.
Foods:	None expected.
Marijuana:	Overstimulation. Avoid.
Tobacco:	None expected.

PACLITAXEL

BRAND NAMES

Taxol

BASIC INFORMATION

Habit forming? No
Prescription needed? Yes
Available as generic? No
Drug class: Antineoplastic

 ## USES

Treats ovarian cancer, breast cancer and some lung cancers.

 ## DOSAGE & USAGE INFORMATION

How to take:
Injection—Administered only by a doctor or under the supervision of a doctor.

When to take:
Your doctor will determine the schedule. Usually the drug is infused over a 24-hour period at 21-day intervals. Other drugs may be given prior to paclitaxel injection to help prevent adverse effects.

If you forget a dose:
Not a concern since drug is administered by a doctor.

What drug does:
Interferes with the growth of cancer cells, which are eventually destroyed.

Time lapse before drug works:
Results may not show for several weeks or months.

Don't take with:
Any other prescription or nonprescription drug without consulting your doctor.

 ## OVERDOSE

SYMPTOMS:
None expected.
WHAT TO DO:
Overdose is unlikely. You will be monitored by medical personnel during the time of the infusion.

 ## POSSIBLE ADVERSE REACTIONS OR SIDE EFFECTS

SYMPTOMS	WHAT TO DO
Life-threatening:	
Anaphylactic reaction soon after an injection (hives, rash, intense itching, faintness, breathing difficulty).	Emergency care will be provided.
Common:	
• Paleness, tiredness, flushing of face, skin rash or itching, shortness of breath, fever, chills, cough or hoarseness, back or side pain, difficult or painful urination, unusual bleeding or bruising, black or tarry stools, blood in stool or urine, pinpoint red spots on skin, bleeding gums, delayed wound healing.	Call doctor right away.
• Pain in joints or muscles; diarrhea; nausea and vomiting; numbness, burning or tingling in hands or feet.	Call doctor when convenient.
• Loss of hair (should regrow after treatment completed).	No action necessary.
Infrequent:	
Heart rhythm disturbances, chest pain.	Call doctor right away.
Rare:	
Pain or redness at injection site, mouth or lip sores.	Call doctor right away.

WARNINGS & PRECAUTIONS

Don't take if:
You are allergic to paclitaxel.

Before you start, consult your doctor:
- If you have an infection or any other medical problem.
- If you have or recently had chickenpox or herpes zoster (shingles).
- If you have heart problems.
- If you are pregnant or if you plan to become pregnant.
- If you have had radiation therapy or previously taken anticancer drugs.

Over age 60:
No problems expected.

Pregnancy:
Animal studies show fetal abnormalities and increased risk of abortion. Discuss with your doctor whether drug benefits justify risk to unborn child. Risk category D (see page xxiii).

Breast-feeding:
Not known if drug passes into milk. Avoid drug or discontinue nursing until you finish medicine. Consult doctor for advice on maintaining milk supply.

Infants & children:
Safety and effectiveness of use in children not established.

Prolonged use:
Not recommended for long-term use.

Skin & sunlight:
No problems expected.

Driving, piloting or hazardous work:
Avoid if you feel side effects such as nausea and vomiting.

Discontinuing:
Your doctor will determine the schedule.

Others:
- Advise any doctor or dentist whom you consult that you take this medicine.
- May affect the results in some medical tests.
- Do not have any immunizations (vaccinations) without doctor's approval. Other household members should not take oral polio vaccine. It could pass the polio virus on to you. Avoid any contact with persons who have taken oral polio vaccine.
- Possible delayed effects (including some types of cancers) may occur months to years after use. Your doctor should discuss with you all risks involving this drug.

- You will have increased risk of infections. Take extra precautions (handwashing), and avoid people with infections. Avoid crowds if possible. Contact your doctor immediately if you develop signs or symptoms of infection.
- Use care in the use of toothbrushes, dental floss and toothpicks. Talk to your medical doctor before you have dental work done.
- Do not touch your eyes or the inside of your nose without carefully washing your hands first.
- Avoid activities (e.g., contact sports) that could cause bruising or injury.
- Avoid cutting yourself when using a safety razor, fingernail or toenail clippers.

POSSIBLE INTERACTION WITH OTHER DRUGS

GENERIC NAME OR DRUG CLASS	COMBINED EFFECT
Blood dyscrasia-causing medicines*	Increased risk of paclitaxel toxicity.
Bone marrow depressants,* (other)	Increased risk of paclitaxel toxicity.

POSSIBLE INTERACTION WITH OTHER SUBSTANCES

INTERACTS WITH	COMBINED EFFECT
Alcohol:	None expected.
Beverages:	None expected.
Cocaine:	None expected.
Foods:	None expected.
Marijuana:	None expected.
Tobacco:	None expected.

PANCREATIN, PEPSIN, BILE SALTS, HYOSCYAMINE, ATROPINE, SCOPOLAMINE & PHENOBARBITAL

BRAND NAMES

Donnazyme

BASIC INFORMATION

Habit forming? Yes
Prescription needed? Yes
Available as generic? No
Drug class: Digestant, sedative, anticholinergic

USES

- Replaces deficient digestive enzymes.
- Sometimes used to relieve indigestion.

DOSAGE & USAGE INFORMATION

How to take:
Tablet—Swallow with liquid or food to lessen stomach irritation. If you can't swallow whole, crumble tablet and take with food or liquid.

When to take:
With or after meals.

If you forget a dose:
Skip it and resume schedule. Don't double dose.

What drug does:
Blocks nerve impulses at parasympathetic nerve endings, preventing smooth muscle contraction and gland secretions.

Time lapse before drug works:
30 to 60 minutes.

Continued next column

OVERDOSE

SYMPTOMS:
Hallucinations, excitement, breathing difficulty, irregular heartbeat (too fast or too slow), fainting, collapse, coma.
WHAT TO DO:
- Dial 911 (emergency) or 0 (operator) for an ambulance or medical help. Then give first aid immediately.
- See emergency information on inside covers.

Don't take with:
Any medicine that will decrease mental alertness or reflexes, such as alcohol, other mind-altering drugs, cough/cold medicines, antihistamines, allergy medicine, sedatives, tranquilizers (sleeping pills or "downers"), barbiturates, seizure medicine, narcotics, other prescription medicine for pain, muscle relaxants, anesthetics.

POSSIBLE ADVERSE REACTIONS OR SIDE EFFECTS

SYMPTOMS	WHAT TO DO
Life-threatening:	
In case of overdose, see previous column.	
Common:	
• Constipation, decreased sweating, headache.	Discontinue. Call doctor right away.
• Drowsiness, dry mouth, frequent urination.	Continue. Call doctor when convenient.
Infrequent:	
• Blurred vision.	Discontinue. Call doctor right away.
• Diminished sex drive, swallowing difficulty, sensitivity to light, insomnia.	Continue. Call doctor when convenient.
Rare:	
• Jaundice; unusual bleeding or bruising; swollen feet and ankles; abdominal pain; sore throat, fever, mouth sores; rash; hives; vomiting; joint pain; eye pain; diarrhea; blood in urine.	Discontinue. Call doctor right away.
• Unusual tiredness.	Continue. Call doctor when convenient.

WARNINGS & PRECAUTIONS

Don't take if:
- You are allergic to any of the drugs in this combination.
- You have trouble with stomach bloating, difficulty emptying your bladder completely, narrow-angle glaucoma, severe ulcerative colitis, porphyria.

PANCREATIN, PEPSIN, BILE SALTS, HYOSCYAMINE, ATROPINE, SCOPOLAMINE & PHENOBARBITAL

Before you start, consult your doctor:
- If you have open-angle glaucoma, angina, chronic bronchitis or asthma, liver disease, hiatal hernia, enlarged prostate, myasthenia gravis, epilepsy, kidney or liver damage, anemia, chronic pain.
- If you will have surgery within 2 months, including dental surgery, requiring general or spinal anesthesia.

Over age 60:
Adverse reactions and side effects may be more frequent and severe than in younger persons

Pregnancy:
Decide with your doctor if drug benefits justify risk to unborn child. Risk category C (see page xxiii).

Breast-feeding:
Drug passes into milk. Avoid drug or discontinue nursing until you finish medicine. Consult doctor for advice on maintaining milk supply.

Infants & children:
Use only under medical supervision.

Prolonged use:
- Chronic constipation, possible fecal impaction.
- May cause addiction, anemia, chronic intoxication.
- May lower body temperature, making exposure to cold temperatures hazardous.

Skin & sunlight:
One or more drugs in this group may cause rash or intensify sunburn in areas exposed to sun or ultraviolet light (photosensitivity reaction). Avoid overexposure. Notify doctor if reaction occurs..

Driving, piloting or hazardous work:
Don't drive or pilot aircraft until you learn how medicine affects you. Don't work around dangerous machinery. Don't climb ladders or work in high places. Danger increases if you drink alcohol or take medicine affecting alertness and reflexes, such as antihistamines, tranquilizers, sedatives, pain medicine, narcotics and mind-altering drugs.

Discontinuing:
- May be unnecessary to finish medicine. Follow doctor's instructions.
- If you develop withdrawal symptoms of hallucinations, agitation or sleeplessness after discontinuing, call doctor right away.

Others:
- Potential for abuse.
- Enzyme deficiencies probably better treated with identified separate substances rather than a mixture of components.

 POSSIBLE INTERACTION WITH OTHER DRUGS

GENERIC NAME OR DRUG CLASS	COMBINED EFFECT
Adrenocorticoids, systemic	Possible glaucoma.
Amantadine	Increased atropine effect.
Antacids*	Decreased absorption of scopolamine.
Anticholinergics*, other	Increased anticholinergic effect.
Anticoagulants*, oral	Decreased anticoagulant effect.
Antidepressants, tricyclic*	Decreased antidepressant effect. Possible dangerous oversedation.
Antidiabetics*, oral	Increased phenobartital effect.
Antihistamines*	Increased atropine effect.
Anti-inflammatory drugs, nonsteroidal (NSAIDs)*	Decreased antiinflammatory effects.

Continued on page 927

 POSSIBLE INTERACTION WITH OTHER SUBSTANCES

INTERACTS WITH	COMBINED EFFECT
Alcohol:	Possible fatal oversedation. Avoid.
Beverages:	None expected.
Cocaine:	Excessively rapid heartbeat. Avoid.
Foods:	None expected.
Marijuana:	Excessive sedation, drowsiness and dry mouth.
Tobacco:	May increase stomach acidity, decreasing the effectiveness of the drug. Avoid.

PANCRELIPASE

BRAND NAMES

Cotazym	Pancrease MT4
Cotazym E.C.S.	Pancrease MT10
Cotazym-65B	Pancrease MT16
Cotazym-S	Protilase
Enzymase-16	Ultrase MT 12
Ilozyme	Ultrase MT 20
Ku-Zyme HP	Ultrase MT 24
Lipancreatin	Viokase
Pancoate	Zymase
Pancrease	

BASIC INFORMATION

Habit forming? No
Prescription needed? Yes
Available as generic? Yes
Drug class: Enzyme (pancreatic)

USES

- Replaces pancreatic enzyme lost due to surgery or disease.
- Treats fatty stools (steatorrhea).

DOSAGE & USAGE INFORMATION

How to take:
- Tablets, capsules or delayed-release capsules—Swallow whole. Do not take with milk or milk products.
- Powder—Sprinkle on liquid or soft food.

When to take:
Before meals.

If you forget a dose:
Take as soon as you remember up to 2 hours late. If more than 2 hours, wait for next scheduled dose (don't double this dose).

What drug does:
Enhances digestion of proteins, carbohydrates and fats.

OVERDOSE

SYMPTOMS:
Shortness of breath, wheezing, diarrhea.
WHAT TO DO:
Overdose unlikely to threaten life. If person takes much larger amount than prescribed, call doctor, poison control center or hospital emergency room for instructions.

Time lapse before drug works:
30 minutes.

Don't take with:
Any other medicine without consulting your doctor or pharmacist.

POSSIBLE ADVERSE REACTIONS OR SIDE EFFECTS

SYMPTOMS	WHAT TO DO
Life-threatening: None expected.	
Common: None expected.	
Infrequent: Diarrhea, asthma.	Discontinue. Call doctor right away.
Rare: • Rash, hives, blood in urine, swollen feet or legs, abdominal cramps.	Discontinue. Call doctor right away.
• Nausea, joint pain.	Continue. Call doctor when convenient.

WARNINGS & PRECAUTIONS

Don't take if:
You are allergic to pancreatin, pancrelipase, or pork.

Before you start, consult your doctor:
If you take any other medicines.

Over age 60:
Adverse reactions and side effects may be more frequent and severe than in younger persons.

Pregnancy:
Decide with your doctor if drug benefits justify risk to unborn child. Risk category C (see page xxiii).

Breast-feeding:
Drug may pass into milk. Avoid drug or discontinue nursing until you finish medicine. Consult doctor for advice on maintaining milk supply.

Infants & children:
Give under close medical supervision only.

Prolonged use:
No additional problems expected.

Skin & sunlight:
No problems expected.

Driving, piloting or hazardous work:
No problems expected.

Discontinuing:
Don't discontinue without consulting doctor. Dose may require gradual reduction if you have taken drug for a long time. Doses of other drugs may also require adjustment.

Others:
If you take powder form, avoid inhaling.

POSSIBLE INTERACTION WITH OTHER DRUGS

GENERIC NAME OR DRUG CLASS	COMBINED EFFECT
Calcium carbonate antacids*	Decreased effect of pancrelipase.
Iron supplements	Decreased iron absorption.
Magnesium hydroxide antacids*	Decreased effect of pancrelipase.

POSSIBLE INTERACTION WITH OTHER SUBSTANCES

INTERACTS WITH	COMBINED EFFECT
Alcohol:	Unknown.
Beverages: Milk.	Decreased effect of pancrelipase.
Cocaine:	Unknown.
Foods: Ice cream, milk products.	Decreased effect of pancrelipase.
Marijuana:	Decreased absorption of pancrelipase.
Tobacco:	Decreased absorption of pancrelipase.

PANTOTHENIC ACID (Vitamin B-5)

BRAND AND GENERIC NAMES

CALCIUM   Dexol T.D.
  PANTOTHENATE

An ingredient in numerous multiple vitamin-mineral supplements. Check labels.

BASIC INFORMATION

Habit forming? No
Prescription needed? No
Available as generic? Yes
Drug class: Vitamin supplement

USES

Prevents and treats vitamin B-5 deficiency.

DOSAGE & USAGE INFORMATION

How to take:
Tablet—Swallow with liquid.

When to take:
At the same times each day.

If you forget a dose:
Take as soon as you remember, then resume regular schedule.

What drug does:
Acts as co-enzyme in carbohydrate, protein and fat metabolism.

Time lapse before drug works:
15 to 20 minutes.

Don't take with:
- Levodopa—Small amounts of pantothenic acid will nullify levodopa effect. Carbidopa-levodopa combination not affected by this interaction.
- Any other medicine without consulting your doctor or pharmacist.

OVERDOSE

SYMPTOMS:
None expected.
WHAT TO DO:
Overdose unlikely to threaten life.

POSSIBLE ADVERSE REACTIONS OR SIDE EFFECTS

SYMPTOMS	WHAT TO DO
Life-threatening: None expected.	
Common: Heartburn.	Discontinue. Seek emergency treatment.
Infrequent: Cramps.	Discontinue Call doctor right away.
Rare: Rash, hives, difficult breathing.	Discontinue. Seek emergency treatment.

PANTOTHENIC ACID (Vitamin B-5)

 WARNINGS & PRECAUTIONS

Don't take if:
You are allergic to pantothenic acid.

Before you start, consult your doctor:
If you have hemophilia.

Over age 60:
No problems expected.

Pregnancy:
Risk factor not designated. See category list on page xxiii and consult doctor.

Breast-feeding:
Don't exceed recommended dose. Consult doctor.

Infants & children:
Don't exceed recommended dose.

Prolonged use:
Large doses for more than 1 month may cause toxicity.

Skin & sunlight:
No problems expected.

Driving, piloting or hazardous work:
No problems expected.

Discontinuing:
No problems expected.

Others:
Regular pantothenic acid supplements are recommended if you take chloramphenicol, cycloserine, ethionamide, hydralazine, immunosuppressants*, isoniazid or penicillamine. These decrease pantothenic acid absorption and can cause anemia or tingling and numbness in hands and feet.

 POSSIBLE INTERACTION WITH OTHER DRUGS

GENERIC NAME OR DRUG CLASS	COMBINED EFFECT
None significant.	

 POSSIBLE INTERACTION WITH OTHER SUBSTANCES

INTERACTS WITH	COMBINED EFFECT
Alcohol:	None expected.
Beverages:	None expected.
Cocaine:	None expected.
Foods:	None expected.
Marijuana:	None expected.
Tobacco:	May decrease pantothenic acid absorption. Decreased pantothenic acid effect.

PAPAVERINE

BRAND NAMES

Cerespan	Pavarine
Genabid	Pavased
Pavabid	Pavatine
Pavabid Plateau Caps	Pavatym
Pavacot	Paverolan
Pavagen	

BASIC INFORMATION

Habit forming? No
Prescription needed? Yes
Available as generic? Yes
Drug class: Vasodilator

USES

- May improve circulation in the extremities or brain.
- Injected into penis to produce erections.

DOSAGE & USAGE INFORMATION

How to take:
- Tablet—Swallow with liquid or food to lessen stomach irritation. If you can't swallow whole, crumble tablet and take with liquid or food.
- Extended-release capsules—Swallow whole with liquid.
- Injections to penis—Follow doctor's instructions.

When to take:
At the same times each day.

If you forget a dose:
Take as soon as you remember up to 2 hours late. If more than 2 hours, wait for next scheduled dose (don't double this dose).

What drug does:
Relaxes and expands blood vessel walls, allowing better distribution of oxygen and nutrients.

Time lapse before drug works:
30 to 60 minutes.

Continued next column

OVERDOSE

SYMPTOMS:
Weakness, fainting, flush, sweating, stupor, irregular heartbeat.
WHAT TO DO:
- **Dial 911 (emergency) or 0 (operator) for an ambulance or medical help. Then give first aid immediately.**
- **See emergency information on inside covers.**

Don't take with:
- Nonprescription drugs without consulting doctor.
- Any other medicine without consulting your doctor or pharmacist.

POSSIBLE ADVERSE REACTIONS OR SIDE EFFECTS

SYMPTOMS	WHAT TO DO
Life-threatening: None expected.	
Common:	
• Drowsiness, dizziness, headache, flushed face, stomach irritation, indigestion, nausea, mild constipation.	Continue. Call doctor when convenient.
• Dry mouth, throat.	Continue. Tell doctor at next visit.
Infrequent: Rash, itchy skin, blurred or double vision, weakness, fast heartbeat.	Discontinue. Call doctor right away.
Rare: Jaundice.	Discontinue. Call doctor right away.

WARNINGS & PRECAUTIONS

Don't take if:
You are allergic to papaverine.

Before you start, consult your doctor:
- If you plan to become pregnant within medication period.
- If you have had a heart attack, heart disease, angina or stroke.
- If you have Parkinson's disease.

Over age 60:
Adverse reactions and side effects may be more frequent and severe than in younger persons.

Pregnancy:
Decide with your doctor if drug benefits justify risk to unborn child. Risk category C (see page xxiii).

Breast-feeding:
Drug may filter into milk. May harm child. Avoid.

Infants & children:
Not recommended.

Prolonged use:
No problems expected.

Skin & sunlight:
No problems expected.

Driving, piloting or hazardous work:
Don't drive or pilot aircraft until you learn how medicine affects you. Don't work around dangerous machinery. Don't climb ladders or work in high places. Danger increases if you drink alcohol or take medicine affecting alertness and reflexes, such as antihistamines, tranquilizers, sedatives, pain medicine, narcotics and mind-altering drugs.

Discontinuing:
May be unnecessary to finish medicine. If drug does not help in 1 to 2 weeks, consult doctor about discontinuing.

Others:
- Periodic liver function tests recommended.
- Internal eye pressure measurements recommended if you have glaucoma.

POSSIBLE INTERACTION WITH OTHER DRUGS

GENERIC NAME OR DRUG CLASS	COMBINED EFFECT
Levodopa	Decreased levodopa effect.
Narcotics*	Increased sedation.
Pain relievers*	Increased sedation.
Pergolide	Decreased pergolide effect.
Sedatives*	Increased sedation.
Sympathomimetics*	Reversal of the effect of papaverine.
Tranquilizers*	Increased sedation.

POSSIBLE INTERACTION WITH OTHER SUBSTANCES

INTERACTS WITH	COMBINED EFFECT
Alcohol:	None expected.
Beverages:	None expected.
Cocaine:	Decreased papaverine effect.
Foods:	None expected.
Marijuana:	None expected.
Tobacco:	Decrease in papaverine's dilation of blood vessels.

*See Glossary

PARALDEHYDE

BRAND NAMES

Paral

BASIC INFORMATION

Habit forming? Yes
Prescription needed? Yes
Available as generic? Yes
Drug class: Anticonvulsant

 ## USES

- Treats convulsions.
- Treats toxic symptoms caused by drugs that may produce convulsions.

 ## DOSAGE & USAGE INFORMATION

How to take:
- Follow doctor's instructions.
- May be given orally, rectally or by injection into a muscle.

When to take:
Follow doctor's instructions.

If you forget a dose:
Take as soon as you remember up to 2 hours late. If more than 2 hours, wait for next scheduled dose (don't double this dose).

What drug does:
Depresses central nervous system.

Time lapse before drug works:
- Oral—30 minutes to 1 hour.
- Rectal—2 to 3 hours.

Don't take with:
Any other medicines (including over-the-counter drugs such as cough and cold medicines, laxatives, antacids, diet pills, caffeine, nose drops or vitamins) without consulting your doctor.

 ## OVERDOSE

SYMPTOMS:
Decreased urination, breathing difficulty, confusion, slow heartbeat, weakness.
WHAT TO DO:
- Dial 911 (emergency) or 0 (operator) for an ambulance or medical help. Then give first aid immediately.
- See emergency information on inside covers.

 ## POSSIBLE ADVERSE REACTIONS OR SIDE EFFECTS

SYMPTOMS	WHAT TO DO
Life-threatening:	
In case of overdose, see previous column.	
Common:	
• Skin rash, jaundice (yellow skin and eyes).	Discontinue. Call doctor right away.
• Drowsiness, nausea, halitosis.	Continue. Call doctor when convenient.
Infrequent:	
Clumsiness, dizziness, headache.	Continue. Call doctor when convenient.
Rare:	
Abdominal cramps.	Continue. Call doctor when convenient.

WARNINGS & PRECAUTIONS

Don't take if:
You know you are allergic to paraldehyde.

Before you start, consult your doctor:
- If you have chronic lung disease.
- If you have history of drug abuse.
- If you have liver disease.
- If you have peptic ulcer.
- If you have colitis.

Over age 60:
No special problems expected.

Pregnancy:
Decide with your doctor if drug benefits justify risk to unborn child. Risk category C (see page xxiii).

Breast-feeding:
Effect not documented. Consult your doctor.

Infants & children:
No special problems expected.

Prolonged use:
- May be habit forming.
- Talk to your doctor about the need for follow-up medical examinations or laboratory studies to check liver function.

Skin & sunlight:
No problems expected.

Driving, piloting or hazardous work:
Avoid if you feel confused, drowsy or dizzy.

Discontinuing:
May develop withdrawal symptoms, such as: convulsions, hallucinations, sweating, muscle cramps, nausea or vomiting, trembling. If you experience any of these, notify your doctor right away.

Others:
- Advise any doctor or dentist whom you consult that you take this medicine.
- May affect results in some medical tests.
- Strong odor of paraldehyde on breath lasts for 24 hours.

POSSIBLE INTERACT WITH OTHER DRUGS

GENERIC NAME OR DRUG CLASS	COMBINED EFFECT
Addictive drugs*	Increased risk of addiction.
Central nervous system (CNS) depressants*, other	Possible oversedation. Avoid simultaneous use.
Disulfiram	Increased paraldehyde effect. Avoid simultaneous use.
Sertraline	Increased depressive effects of both drugs.

POSSIBLE INTERACTION WITH OTHER SUBSTANCES

INTERACTS WITH	COMBINED EFFECT
Alcohol:	Dangerous sedation. Avoid.
Beverages:	No special problems expected.
Cocaine:	No special problems expected.
Foods:	No special problems expected.
Marijuana:	No special problems expected.
Tobacco:	No special problems expected.

PAREGORIC

BRAND NAMES

Brown Mixture
Camphorated Opium
  Tincture

Kapectolin with
  Paregoric
Parapectolin

BASIC INFORMATION

Habit forming? Yes
Prescription needed? Yes
Available as generic? Yes
Drug class: Narcotic, antidiarrheal

USES

Reduces intestinal cramps and diarrhea.

DOSAGE & USAGE INFORMATION

How to take:
Drops or liquid—Dilute dose in beverage before swallowing.

When to take:
As needed for diarrhea, no more often than every 4 hours.

If you forget a dose:
Take as soon as you remember. Wait 4 hours for next dose.

What drug does:
Anesthetizes surface membranes of intestines and blocks nerve impulses.

Time lapse before drug works:
2 to 6 hours.

Don't take with:
Any other medicine without consulting your doctor or pharmacist.

OVERDOSE

SYMPTOMS:
Deep sleep; slow breathing; slow pulse; flushed, warm skin; constricted pupils.
WHAT TO DO:
- **Dial 911 (emergency) or 0 (operator) for an ambulance or medical help. Then give first aid immediately.**
- **If patient is unconscious and not breathing, give mouth-to-mouth breathing. If there is no heartbeat, use cardiac massage and mouth-to-mouth breathing (CPR). Don't try to make patient vomit. If you can't get help quickly, take patient to nearest emergency facility.**
- **See emergency information on inside covers.**

POSSIBLE ADVERSE REACTIONS OR SIDE EFFECTS

SYMPTOMS	WHAT TO DO
Life-threatening:	
In case of overdose, see previous column.	
Common:	
Dizziness, flushed face, unusual tiredness, difficult urination.	Continue. Call doctor when convenient.
Infrequent:	
Severe constipation, abdominal pain, vomiting.	Discontinue. Call doctor right away.
Rare:	
• Hives, rash, itchy skin, slow heartbeat, irregular breathing.	Discontinue. Call doctor right away.
• Depression.	Continue. Call doctor when convenient.

WARNINGS & PRECAUTIONS

Don't take if:
You are allergic to any narcotic*.

Before you start, consult your doctor:
If you have impaired liver or kidney function.

Over age 60:
More likely to be drowsy, dizzy, unsteady or constipated.

Pregnancy:
Risk factor varies with length of pregnancy. See category list on page xxiii and consult doctor.

Breast-feeding:
Drug filters into milk. May depress infant. Avoid.

Infants & children:
Use only under medical supervision.

Prolonged use:
Causes psychological and physical dependence.

Skin & sunlight:
No problems expected.

Driving, piloting or hazardous work:
Don't drive or pilot aircraft until you learn how medicine affects you. Don't work around dangerous machinery. Don't climb ladders or work in high places. Danger increases if you drink alcohol or take medicine affecting alertness and reflexes, such as antihistamines, tranquilizers, sedatives, pain medicine, narcotics and mind-altering drugs.

Discontinuing:
May be unnecessary to finish medicine. Follow doctor's instructions.

Others:
Great potential for abuse.

POSSIBLE INTERACTION WITH OTHER DRUGS

GENERIC NAME OR DRUG CLASS	COMBINED EFFECT
Analgesics*	Increased analgesic effect.
Anticholinergics*	Increased risk of constipation.
Antidepressants*	Increased sedation.
Antidiarrheal preparations*	Increased sedative effect. Avoid.
Antihistamines*	Increased sedation.
Central nervous system (CNS) depressants*	Increased central nerve system depression.
Naloxone	Decreased paregoric effect.
Naltrexone	Decreased paregoric effect.
Narcotics*, other	Increased narcotic effect.

POSSIBLE INTERACTION WITH OTHER SUBSTANCES

INTERACTS WITH	COMBINED EFFECT
Alcohol:	Increases alcohol's intoxicating effect. Avoid.
Beverages:	None expected.
Cocaine:	None expected.
Foods:	None expected.
Marijuana:	Impairs physical and mental performance.
Tobacco:	None expected.

*See Glossary

PAROXETINE

BRAND NAMES

Paxil

BASIC INFORMATION

Habit forming? No
Prescription needed? Yes
Available as generic? No
Drug class: Antidepressant (selective
serotonin reuptake inhibitor)

 USES

- Treats mental depression.
- Treats obsessive-compulsive disorder and panic disorder.

 DOSAGE & USAGE INFORMATION

How to take:
- Oral suspension—Take as directed on label.
- Tablet—Swallow with liquid. May be taken with food to lessen gastric irritation.

When to take:
At the same times each day, usually in the morning.

If you forget a dose:
Take as soon as you remember up to 2 hours late. If more than 2 hours, wait for next scheduled dose (don't double this dose).

What drug does:
Affects serotonin, one of the chemicals in the brain called neurotransmitters, that plays a role in emotions and psychological disturbances.

Time lapse before drug works:
1 to 4 weeks.

Don't take with:
- Any other medication without consulting your doctor or pharmacist.
- Any monoamine oxidase (MAO) inhibitor* or within 14 days of stopping one. To do so may result in a serious or fatal reaction.

 OVERDOSE

SYMPTOMS:
Vomiting, severe drowsiness, heart rhythm disturbances, dilated pupils, severe mouth dryness.
WHAT TO DO:
- **Dial 911 (emergency) or 0 (operator) for an ambulance or medical help. Then give first aid immediately.**
- **See emergency information at end of book.**

 POSSIBLE ADVERSE REACTIONS OR SIDE EFFECTS

SYMPTOMS	WHAT TO DO
Life-threatening: Rash, itchy skin, breathing difficulty (allergic reaction); chest pain.	Seek emergency treatment immediately.
Common: Weakness, sweating, nausea, sleepiness, dry mouth, dizziness, insomnia, tremor, male ejaculatory problems, male genital disorders, constipation, diarrhea, problems urinating, vomiting.	Continue. Call doctor when convenient.
Infrequent: Anxiety, nervousness, decreased or increased appetite, decreased libido, heart palpitations, taste changes, weight loss or gain.	Continue. Call doctor when convenient.
Rare: • Blurred vision.	Continue. Call doctor when convenient.
• Mania* symptoms.	Discontinue. Call doctor right away.

WARNINGS & PRECAUTIONS

Don't take if:
- You are allergic to paroxetine.
- You are taking astemizole, cisapride or terfenadine.
- You currently take (or have taken in the last 2 weeks) a monoamine oxidase (MAO) inhibitor*.

Before you start, consult your doctor:
- If you have a history of seizure disorders.
- If you have thoughts of suicide.
- If you have kidney or liver disease.
- If you have a history of drug abuse or mania.

Over age 60:
Adverse reactions and side effects may be more frequent and severe than in younger persons. You may need smaller dosages for shorter periods of time.

Pregnancy:
Consult doctor. Risk category B (see page xxiii).

Breast-feeding:
Drug passes into milk. Avoid drug or discontinue nursing until you finish medicine. Consult doctor for advice on maintaining milk supply.

Infants & children:
Safety and effectiveness not yet determined.

Prolonged use:
No problems expected. Your doctor should periodically evaluate your response to the drug and adjust the dosage if necessary.

Skin & sunlight:
No problems expected.

Driving, piloting or hazardous work:
Don't drive or pilot aircraft until you learn how medicine affects you. Don't work around dangerous machinery. Don't climb ladders or work in high places. Danger increases if you drink alcohol or take other medicines affecting alertness and reflexes such as antihistamines, tranquilizers, sedatives, pain medicine, narcotics and mind-altering drugs.

Discontinuing:
- Don't discontinue without consulting doctor. Dose may require gradual reduction if you have taken drug for a long time. Doses of other drugs may also require adjustment.
- Consult doctor if the following symptoms appear after you discontinue the drug: dizziness, lightheadedness, agitation, confusion, restlessness, vision changes, insomnia, headache, muscle aches, runny nose, unusual tiredness or weakness, nausea or vomiting.

Others:
Advise any doctor or dentist whom you consult that you take this medicine.

POSSIBLE INTERACTION WITH OTHER DRUGS

GENERIC NAME OR DRUG CLASS	COMBINED EFFECT
Anticoagulants, oral*	Increased risk of bleeding.
Antidepressants*, other	Increased effects of both drugs.
Cimetidine	Increased levels of paroxetine in blood.
Dexfenfluramine	May cause serotonin syndrome*. Avoid.
Digoxin	Decreased digoxin effect.
Lithium	Unknown effect. Consult doctor.
Monoamine oxidase (MAO) inhibitors*	Can cause a life-threatening reaction. Avoid.
Phenytoin	Decreased effect of phenytoin.
Selegiline	Increased risk of adverse effects. May lead to convulsions and hypertensive crisis. Let 14 days elapse between taking the 2 drugs.

POSSIBLE INTERACTION WITH OTHER SUBSTANCES

INTERACTS WITH	COMBINED EFFECT
Alcohol:	Contributes to depression. Avoid.
Beverages:	None expected.
Cocaine:	Effects unknown. Avoid.
Foods:	None expected.
Marijuana:	Effects unknown. Avoid.
Tobacco:	None expected.

*See Glossary

PEDICULICIDES (Topical)

GENERIC AND BRAND NAMES

LINDANE	PYRETHRINS &
GBH	PIPERONYL
G-Well	BUTOXIDE
Kwellada	A-200 Gel
Kwildane	A-200 Shampoo
PMS Lindane	Barc
MALATHION	Blue
Derbac	Lice-Enz Foam And
Ovide	Comb Lice Killing
PERMETHRIN	Shampoo Kit
Acticin	Pyrinyl
Elimite Cream	R&C
Nix Cream Rinse	TISIT
	TISIT Blue
	Triple X

BASIC INFORMATION

Habit forming? No
Prescription needed? Yes
Available as generic? Yes, some
Drug class: Pediculicide, scabicide

USES

- Treats scabies and lice infections of skin or scalp.
- Cream and lotion treats scabies.
- Shampoo treats lice infections.

OVERDOSE

SYMPTOMS:
Rarely (toxic effects from too much absorbed through skin)—Vomiting, muscle cramps, dizziness, seizure, rapid heartbeat.
WHAT TO DO:
- Not for internal use. If child accidentally swallows, call poison control center.
- Dial 911 (emergency) or 0 (operator) for an ambulance or medical help. Then give first aid immediately.
- See emergency information on inside covers.

DOSAGE & USAGE INFORMATION

How to use:
- All household members should be examined for infection and treated if infected.
- Read directions on product for proper application technique and length of time to leave on the body.
- Wear plastic gloves when you apply. Use care not to apply more than directed. Avoid contact with eyes, nose and mouth. Flush eyes with water if product gets in the eyes.
- Bathe before applying. Wash hands after applying.
- Use in well-ventilated room.

When to use:
As directed on package.

If you forget a dose:
Use as soon as you remember.

What drug does:
Absorbed into bodies of lice and scabies organisms, killing them.

Time lapse before drug works:
Cream or lotion requires 8 to 12 hours contact with skin.

Don't use with:
Other medicines for scabies or lice.

POSSIBLE ADVERSE REACTIONS OR SIDE EFFECTS

SYMPTOMS	WHAT TO DO
Life-threatening	
None expected.	
Common	
None expected.	
Infrequent	
None expected.	
Rare	
• Skin irritation or rash.	Discontinue. Call doctor right away.
• Skin itch that continues 1 week to several weeks after treatment.	Call doctor when convenient.

WARNINGS & PRECAUTIONS

Don't use if:
You are allergic to any medicine with lindane, pyrethrins or piperonyl butoxide.

Before you start, consult your doctor:
- If you are allergic to anything that touches your skin.
- If you are using any other medicines, creams, lotions or oils.

Over age 60:
Adverse reactions and side effects may be more frequent and severe than in younger persons. Ask doctor about smaller doses.

Pregnancy:
Risk factors vary for drugs in this group. See category list on page xxiii and consult doctor.

Breast-feeding:
Effect unknown. Avoid if possible. Consult doctor.

Infants & children:
More likely to be toxic. Use only under close medical supervision.

Prolonged use:
Not recommended. Avoid.

Skin & sunlight:
No problems expected, but check with doctor.

Driving, piloting or hazardous work:
No problems expected, but check with doctor.

Discontinuing:
No problems expected, but check with doctor.

Others:
- Don't use on open sores or wounds.
- Put on freshly dry cleaned or washed clothing after treatment.
- After treatment, boil all bed sheets, covers and towels before using.
- Store items that can't be washed or cleaned in plastic bags for 2 weeks.
- Avoid inhaling or swallowing drug.
- Thoroughly clean house.
- Wash combs and hairbrushes in hot soapy water. Don't share with others.
- Even after successful treatment, itching can continue due to remaining inflammation in the skin. This should not be confused with a reinfection. Consult doctor if you are unsure.

POSSIBLE INTERACTION WITH OTHER DRUGS

GENERIC NAME OR DRUG CLASS	COMBINED EFFECT
Antimyasthenics*	Excessive absorption and chance of toxicity (with malathion only).
Cholinesterase inhibitors*	Excessive absorption and chance of toxicity (with malathion only).

POSSIBLE INTERACTION WITH OTHER SUBSTANCES

INTERACTS WITH	COMBINED EFFECT
Alcohol:	None expected.
Beverages:	None expected.
Cocaine:	None expected.
Foods:	None expected.
Marijuana:	None expected.
Tobacco:	None expected.

*See Glossary

PEMOLINE

BRAND NAMES

Cylert   Cylert Chewable

BASIC INFORMATION

Habit forming? Yes
Prescription needed? Yes
Available as generic? No
Drug class: Central nervous system
   stimulant

 USES

Decreases overactivity and lengthens attention
span in children with attention-deficit hyperactivity disorder (ADHD). It is used as part of the
total management plan that includes educational,
social and psychological treatment.

 DOSAGE & USAGE INFORMATION

How to take:
• Tablet—Swallow with liquid or food to lessen
  stomach irritation. If you can't swallow whole,
  crumble tablet and take with liquid or food.
• Chewable tablets—Chew well before
  swallowing.

When to take:
Daily in the morning.

Continued next column

 OVERDOSE

SYMPTOMS:
**Agitation, confusion, fast heartbeat,
hallucinations, severe headache, high fever
with sweating, large pupils, muscle twitching
or trembling, uncontrolled eye or body
movements, vomiting.**
WHAT TO DO:
• **Dial 911 (emergency) or 0 (operator) for an
  ambulance or medical help. Then give first
  aid immediately.**
• **If patient is unconscious and not breathing,
  give mouth-to-mouth breathing. If there is
  no heartbeat, use cardiac massage and
  mouth-to-mouth breathing (CPR). Don't try
  to make patient vomit. If you can't get help
  quickly, take patient to nearest emergency
  facility.**
• **See emergency information at end of book.**

If you forget a dose:
Take as soon as you remember up to 2 hours
late. If more than 2 hours, wait for next
scheduled dose (don't double this dose).

What drug does:
Stimulates brain to improve alertness,
concentration and attention span. Calms the
hyperactive child.

Time lapse before drug works:
• 1 month or more for maximum effect on child.
• 30 minutes to stimulate adults.

Don't take with:
Any other medicine without consulting your
doctor or pharmacist.

 POSSIBLE ADVERSE REACTIONS OR SIDE EFFECTS

SYMPTOMS	WHAT TO DO
Life-threatening:	
In case of overdose, see previous column.	
Common:	
Trouble sleeping, loss of appetite, weight loss.	Continue. Call doctor when convenient.
Infrequent:	
Irritability, depression dizziness, headache, drowsiness, skin rash, stomach ache.	Continue. Call doctor when convenient.
Rare:	
Yellow skin or eyes; symptoms of overdose (agitation, confusion, fast heart-beat, hallucinations, severe headache, high fever with sweating, large pupils, muscle twitching or trembling, uncontrolled eye or body movements, vomiting).	Discontinue. Call doctor right away.

644

WARNINGS & PRECAUTIONS

Don't take if:
You are allergic to pemoline.

Before you start, consult your doctor:
- If you have liver disease.
- If you have kidney disease.
- If patient Is younger than 6 years.
- If there is marked emotional instability.

Over age 60:
Adverse reactions and side effects may be more frequent and severe than in younger persons.

Pregnancy:
No proven harm to unborn child. Avoid if possible. Consult doctor. Risk category B (see page xxiii).

Breast-feeding:
Effect unknown. Consult doctor.

Infants & children:
Use only under close medical supervision.

Prolonged use:
- Rare possibility of physical growth retardation.
- Talk to your doctor about the need for follow-up medical examinations or laboratory studies to check liver function, growth charts.

Skin & sunlight:
No problems expected.

Driving, piloting or hazardous work:
Don't drive or pilot aircraft until you learn how medicine affects you. Don't work around dangerous machinery. Don't climb ladders or work in high places. Danger increases if you drink alcohol or take medicine affecting alertness and reflexes, such as antihistamines, tranquilizers, sedatives, pain medicine, narcotics and mind-altering drugs.

Discontinuing:
- Don't discontinue without consulting doctor. Dose may require gradual reduction if you have taken drug for a long time. Doses of other drugs may also require adjustment.
- If you notice any of the following symptoms after discontinuing, notify your doctor: mental depression (severe), tiredness or weakness.

Others:
- Dose must be carefully adjusted by doctor. Don't give more or less than prescribed dose.
- Be sure you and the doctor discuss benefits and risks of this drug before starting.
- Consult doctor if no improvement is noticed after 1 month of drug use.
- Advise any doctor or dentist whom you consult about the use of this medicine.

 ## POSSIBLE INTERACTION WITH OTHER DRUGS

GENERIC NAME OR DRUG CLASS	COMBINED EFFECT
Anticonvulsants*	Dosage adjustment for anticonvulsant may be necessary.
Central nervous system (CNS) stimulants*, other	May increase toxic effects of both drugs.

 ## POSSIBLE INTERACTION WITH OTHER SUBSTANCES

INTERACTS WITH	COMBINED EFFECT
Alcohol:	More chance of depression. Avoid.
Beverages: Caffeine drinks.	Overstimulation. Avoid.
Cocaine:	Convulsions or excessive nervousness.
Foods:	No problems expected.
Marijuana:	Unknown.
Tobacco:	Unknown.

PENICILLAMINE

BRAND NAMES

Cuprimine   Depen

BASIC INFORMATION

Habit forming? No
Prescription needed? Yes
Available as generic? No
Drug class: Chelating agent, antirheumatic, antidote (heavy metal)

USES

- Treatment for rheumatoid arthritis.
- Prevention of kidney stones.
- Treatment for heavy metal poisoning.

DOSAGE & USAGE INFORMATION

How to take:
Tablets or capsules—With liquid on an empty stomach 1 hour before or 2 hours after eating.

When to take:
At the same times each day.

If you forget a dose:
- 1 dose a day—Take as soon as you remember up to 12 hours late. If more than 12 hours, wait for next scheduled dose (don't double this dose).
- More than 1 dose a day—Take as soon as you remember up to 2 hours late. If more than 2 hours, wait for next scheduled dose (don't double this dose).

Continued next column

OVERDOSE

SYMPTOMS:
Ulcers, sores, convulsions, coughing up blood, coma.
WHAT TO DO:
- **Dial 911 (emergency) or 0 (operator) for an ambulance or medical help. Then give first aid immediately.**
- **See emergency information on inside covers.**

What drug does:
- Combines with heavy metals so kidney can excrete them.
- Combines with cysteine (amino acid found in many foods) to prevent cysteine kidney stones.
- May improve protective function of some white blood cells against rheumatoid arthritis.

Time lapse before drug works:
2 to 3 months.

Don't take with:
Any other medicine without consulting your doctor or pharmacist.

POSSIBLE ADVERSE REACTIONS OR SIDE EFFECTS

SYMPTOMS	WHAT TO DO
Life-threatening: In case of overdose, see previous column.	
Common: Rash, itchy skin, swollen lymph glands, appetite loss, nausea, diarrhea, vomiting, decreased taste.	Discontinue. Call doctor right away.
Infrequent: Sore throat, fever, unusual bruising, swollen feet or legs, bloody or cloudy urine, weight gain, fatigue, weakness, joint pain.	Discontinue. Call doctor right away.
Rare: Double or blurred vision; pain; ringing in ears; ulcers, sores, white spots in mouth; difficult breathing; coughing up blood; jaundice; abdominal pain; skin blisters; peeling skin.	Discontinue. Call doctor right away.

WARNINGS & PRECAUTIONS

Don't take if:
- You are allergic to penicillamine.
- You have severe anemia.

Before you start, consult your doctor:
- If you have kidney disease.
- If you are allergic to any penicillin antibiotic.

Over age 60:
More likely to damage blood cells and kidneys.

Pregnancy:
Decide with your doctor if drug benefits justify risk to unborn child. Risk category C (see page xxiii).

Breast-feeding:
Safety not established. Consult doctor.

Infants & children:
Use only under medical supervision.

Prolonged use:
- May damage blood cells, kidney, liver.
- Talk to your doctor about the need for follow-up medical examinations or laboratory studies to check complete blood counts (white blood cell count, platelet count, red blood cell count, hemoglobin, hematocrit), kidney function, liver function.

Skin & sunlight:
No problems expected.

Driving, piloting or hazardous work:
No problems expected.

Discontinuing:
No problems expected.

Others:
Request laboratory studies on blood and urine every 2 weeks. Kidney and liver function studies recommended every 6 months.

POSSIBLE INTERACTION WITH OTHER DRUGS

GENERIC NAME OR DRUG CLASS	COMBINED EFFECT
Gold compounds*	Damage to blood cells and kidney.
Immuno-suppressants*	Damage to blood cells and kidney.
Iron supplements*	Decreased effect of penicillamine. Wait 2 hours between doses.
Pyridoxine (vitamin B-6)	Increased need for pyridoxine.

POSSIBLE INTERACTION WITH OTHER SUBSTANCES

INTERACTS WITH	COMBINED EFFECT
Alcohol:	Increased side effects of penicillamine.
Beverages:	None expected.
Cocaine:	Increased side effects of penicillamine.
Foods:	Possible decreased penicillamine effect due to decreased absorption.
Marijuana:	Increased side effects of penicillamine.
Tobacco:	None expected.

PENICILLINS

GENERIC AND BRAND NAMES

See complete list of generic and brand names in the *Generic and Brand Name Directory*, page 887.

BASIC INFORMATION

Habit forming? No
Prescription needed? Yes
Available as generic? Yes
Drug class: Antibacterial

USES

Treatment of bacterial infections that are susceptible to penicillin, including lower respiratory tract infections, otitis media, sinusitis, skin and skin structure infections, urinary tract infections, gastrointestinal disorders, ulcers, endocarditis, pharyngitis. Different penicillins treat different kinds of infections.

DOSAGE & USAGE INFORMATION

How to take:
- Tablet or capsule—Swallow with liquid on an empty stomach 1 hour before or 2 hours after eating. You may take amoxicillin, penicillin V, pivampicillin or pivmecillinam on a full stomach.
- Chewable tablet—Chew or crush before swallowing.
- Oral suspension—Measure each dose with an accurate measuring device (not a household teaspoon). Store according to instructions.

When to take:
Follow instructions on prescription label, or take as directed by doctor. The number of doses, the time between doses and the length of treatment will depend on the problem being treated.

If you forget a dose:
Take as soon as you remember, then continue regular schedule. If it is almost time for the next dose, wait for that dose (don't double that dose).

Continued next column

OVERDOSE

SYMPTOMS:
Severe diarrhea, nausea or vomiting.
WHAT TO DO:
Overdose unlikely to threaten life. If person takes much larger amount than prescribed, call doctor, poison control center or hospital emergency room for instructions.

What drug does:
Destroys susceptible bacteria. Does not kill viruses (e.g., colds or influenza), fungi or parasites.

Time lapse before drug works:
May be several days before medicine affects infection.

Don't take with:
Any other medicine without consulting your doctor or pharmacist.

POSSIBLE ADVERSE REACTIONS OR SIDE EFFECTS

SYMPTOMS	WHAT TO DO
Life-threatening: Hives, rash, intense itching, shortness of breath, faintness soon after a dose (anaphylaxis).	Seek emergency treatment immediately.
Common: Nausea, vomiting or diarrhea (all mild); sore mouth or tongue; white patches in mouth or on tongue; vaginal itching or discharge; stomach pain.	Continue. Call doctor when convenient.
Infrequent: None expected.	
Rare: Unexplained bleeding or bruising, weakness, sore throat, fever, severe abdominal cramps, diarrhea (watery and severe), convulsions.	Discontinue. Call doctor right away.

WARNINGS & PRECAUTIONS

Don't take if:
You are allergic to penicillins* or cephalosporins*. A life-threatening reaction may occur.

Before you start, consult your doctor:
• If you are allergic to any substance or drug.
• If you have mononucleosis.
• If you have congestive heart failure.
• If you have high blood pressure or any bleeding disorder.
• If you have cystic fibrosis.
• If you have kidney disease or a stomach or intestinal disorder.

Over age 60:
No special problems expected.

Pregnancy:
Consult doctor. Risk category B (see page xxiii).

Breast-feeding:
Drug passes into milk. Child may become sensitive to penicillins and have allergic reactions to penicillin drugs. Discuss risks and benefits with your doctor.

Infants & children:
No special problems expected.

Prolonged use:
• You may become more susceptible to infections caused by germs not responsive to penicillins.
• Talk to your doctor about the need for follow-up medical examinations or laboratory studies.

Skin & sunlight:
No problems expected.

Driving, piloting or hazardous work:
Usually not dangerous. Most hazardous reactions likely to occur a few minutes after taking penicillin.

Discontinuing:
Don't discontinue without doctor's advice until you complete prescribed dose, even though symptoms diminish or disappear.

Others:
• Urine sugar test for diabetes may show false positive result.
• If your symptoms don't improve within a few days (or if they worsen), call your doctor.
• Don't take medicines for diarrhea without your doctor's approval.
• Birth control pills may not be effective. Use additional birth control methods.

POSSIBLE INTERACTION WITH OTHER DRUGS

GENERIC NAME OR DRUG CLASS	COMBINED EFFECT
Chloramphenicol	Decreased effect of both drugs.
Cholestyramine	May decrease penicillin effect.
Colestipol	May decrease penicillin effect.
Contraceptives, oral*	Impaired contraceptive efficiency.
Erythromycins*	Decreased effect of both drugs.
Methotrexate	Increased risk of methotrexate toxicity.
Probenecid	Increased effect of all penicillins.
Sodium benzoate & sodium phenylacetate	May reduce effect of sodium benzoate & sodium phenylacetate.
Sulfonamides*	Decreased penicillin effect.
Tetracyclines*	Decreased effect of both drugs.

POSSIBLE INTERACTION WITH OTHER SUBSTANCES

INTERACTS WITH	COMBINED EFFECT
Alcohol:	Occasional stomach irritation.
Beverages:	None expected.
Cocaine:	No proven problems.
Foods: Acidic fruits or juices, aged cheese, wines, syrups (if taken with penicillin G).	Decreased antibiotic effect.
Marijuana:	No proven problems.
Tobacco:	None expected.

PENICILLINS & BETA-LACTAMASE INHIBITORS

GENERIC AND BRAND NAMES

AMOXICILLIN & CLAVULANATE	Augmentin Clavulin

BASIC INFORMATION

Habit forming? No
Prescription needed? Yes
Available as generic? No
Drug class: Antibacterial

 USES

Treatment of bacterial infections that are susceptible to penicillin and beta-lactamase inhibitors, including lower respiratory tract infections, otitis media, sinusitis, skin and skin structure infections, urinary tract infections.

 DOSAGE & USAGE INFORMATION

How to take:
- Tablet—Swallow with liquid on a full or empty stomach. Taking with food may lessen any stomach irritation.
- Chewable tablet—Chew or crush before swallowing.
- Oral suspension—Measure each dose with an accurate measuring device (not a household teaspoon).

When to take:
Follow instructions on prescription label, or take as directed by doctor. Normally the drug is taken every 8 hours for 7 to 10 days.

If you forget a dose:
Take as soon as you remember, then continue regular schedule. If it is almost time for the next dose, wait for that dose (don't double it).

Continued next column

 OVERDOSE

SYMPTOMS:
Severe diarrhea, nausea or vomiting.
WHAT TO DO:
Overdose unlikely to threaten life. If person takes much larger amount than prescribed, call doctor, poison control center or hospital emergency room for instructions.

What drug does:
Destroys susceptible bacteria. Does not kill viruses, fungi or parasites. Beta-lactamase inhibitors increase penicillin's effectiveness by inactivating beta-lactamase (a substance in some bacteria which destroys the penicillin).

Time lapse before drug works:
May be several days before medicine affects infection.

Don't take with:
Any other medicine without consulting your doctor or pharmacist.

 POSSIBLE ADVERSE REACTIONS OR SIDE EFFECTS

SYMPTOMS	WHAT TO DO
Life-threatening:	
Hives, rash, intense itching, shortness of breath, faintness soon after a dose (anaphylaxis).	Seek emergency treatment immediately.
Common:	
Nausea, vomiting or diarrhea (all mild); sore mouth or tongue; white patches in mouth or on tongue; vaginal itching or discharge; stomach pain.	Continue. Call doctor when convenient.
Infrequent:	
None expected.	
Rare:	
Unexplained bleeding or bruising, weakness, sore throat, fever, severe abdominal cramps, diarrhea (watery and severe), convulsions.	Discontinue. Call doctor right away.

WARNINGS & PRECAUTIONS

Don't take if:
You are allergic to penicillins or cephalosporins. Life-threatening reaction may occur.

Before you start, consult your doctor:
- If you are allergic to any substance or drug.
- If you have mononucleosis.
- If you have congestive heart failure.
- If you have high blood pressure or any bleeding disorder.
- If you have cystic fibrosis.
- If you have kidney disease or a stomach or intestinal disorder.

Over age 60:
No special problems expected.

Pregnancy:
Consult doctor. Risk category B (see page xxiii).

Breast-feeding:
Drug passes into milk. Child may become sensitive to penicillins and have allergic reactions to penicillin drugs. Avoid penicillin or discontinue nursing until you finish medicine. Consult doctor for advice on maintaining milk supply.

Infants & children:
No special problems expected.

Prolonged use:
- You may become more susceptible to infections caused by germs not responsive to penicillins.
- Talk to your doctor about the need for follow-up medical examinations or laboratory studies to check SGPT*, SGOT*.

Skin & sunlight:
No problems expected.

Driving, piloting or hazardous work:
Usually not dangerous. Most hazardous reactions likely to occur a few minutes after taking.

Discontinuing:
Don't discontinue without doctor's advice until you complete prescribed dose, even though symptoms diminish or disappear.

Others:
- Urine sugar test for diabetes may show false positive result.
- If your symptoms don't improve within a few days (or if they worsen), call your doctor.
- Don't take for diarrhea without your doctor's approval.
- Birth control pills may not be effective. Use additional birth control methods.

POSSIBLE INTERACTION WITH OTHER DRUGS

GENERIC NAME OR DRUG CLASS	COMBINED EFFECT
Chloramphenicol	Decreased effect of both drugs.
Cholestyramine	May decrease penicillin effect.
Colestipol	May decrease penicillin effect.
Contraceptives, oral*	Impaired contraceptive efficiency.
Erythromycins*	Decreased effect of both drugs.
Methotrexate	Increased risk of methotrexate toxicity.
Probenecid	Increased effect of all penicillins.
Sodium benzoate & sodium phenylacetate	May reduce effect of sodium benzoate & sodium phenylacetate.
Tetracyclines*	Decreased effect of both drugs.

POSSIBLE INTERACTION WITH OTHER SUBSTANCES

INTERACTS WITH	COMBINED EFFECT
Alcohol:	Occasional stomach irritation.
Beverages:	None expected.
Cocaine:	No proven problems.
Foods:	None expected.
Marijuana:	No proven problems.
Tobacco:	None expected.

*See Glossary

PENTAMIDINE

BRAND NAMES

NebuPent   Pneumopent
Pentacarinat

BASIC INFORMATION

Habit forming? No
Prescription needed? Yes
Available as generic? No
Drug class: Antiprotozoal

 USES

- Treats pneumocystis carinii, which is common in AIDS patients.
- Treats some tropical diseases such as leishmaniasis, African sleeping sickness and others.

 DOSAGE & USAGE INFORMATION

How to take:
Inhalation—Follow package instructions.

When to take:
According to doctor's instructions.

If you forget a dose:
Not likely to happen.

What drug does:
Interferes with RNA and DNA of infecting organisms.

Time lapse before drug works:
30 minutes to 1 hour.

Don't take with:
Any other medicines (including over-the-counter drugs such as cough and cold medicines, laxatives, antacids, diet pills, caffeine, nose drops or vitamins) without consulting your doctor.

 OVERDOSE

SYMPTOMS:
None expected.
WHAT TO DO:
Overdose unlikely to threaten life. If person takes much larger amount than prescribed, call doctor, poison control center or hospital emergency room for instructions.

 POSSIBLE ADVERSE REACTIONS OR SIDE EFFECTS

SYMPTOMS	WHAT TO DO
Life-threatening: Unconsciousness, rapid pulse, cold sweats.	Seek emergency treatment immediately.
Common: Chest pain or congestion; wheezing; coughing; difficulty in breathing; skin rash; pain, dryness or sensation of lump in throat.	Discontinue. Call doctor right away.
Infrequent: • Abdomen or back pain, nausea, vomiting, anxiety, cold sweats, chills, headache, appetite changes, decreased urination, unusual tiredness.	Discontinue. Call doctor right away.
• Bitter or metallic taste.	No action necessary.
Rare: None expected.	

WARNINGS & PRECAUTIONS

Don't take if:
You know you are allergic to pentamidine.

Before you start, consult your doctor:
If you have asthma.

Over age 60:
Adverse reactions and side effects may be more frequent and severe than in younger persons. You may need smaller doses for shorter periods of time.

Pregnancy:
Decide with your doctor if drug benefits justify risk to unborn child. Risk category C (see page xxiii).

Breast-feeding:
Unknown effects. Not recommended. Consult doctor.

Infants & children:
Unknown effects. Consult doctor.

Prolonged use:
Talk to your doctor about the need for follow-up medical examinations or laboratory studies to check blood sugar; blood pressure; kidney, liver and heart function; complete blood counts (white blood cell count, platelet count, red blood cell count, hemoglobin, hematocrit); ECG* and serum calcium.

Skin & sunlight:
No problems expected.

Driving, piloting or hazardous work:
Avoid if you feel confused, drowsy or dizzy.

Discontinuing:
No special problems expected.

Others:
- Advise any doctor or dentist whom you consult that you take this medicine.
- May affect results in some medical tests.
- Avoid exposure to people who have infectious diseases.
- To help decrease bitter taste in mouth, dissolve a hard candy after taking medicine.
- Consult your doctor for additional information on the injectable form of this drug.

 ## POSSIBLE INTERACTION WITH OTHER DRUGS

GENERIC NAME OR DRUG CLASS	COMBINED EFFECT
None reported with inhalation form of drug.	

 ## POSSIBLE INTERACTION WITH OTHER SUBSTANCES

INTERACTS WITH	COMBINED EFFECT
Alcohol:	Increased likelihood of adverse reactions. Avoid.
Beverages:	No special problems expected.
Cocaine:	Increased likelihood of adverse reactions. Avoid.
Foods:	No special problems expected.
Marijuana:	Increased likelihood of adverse reactions. Avoid.
Tobacco:	Increased likelihood of adverse reactions. Avoid.

PENTOXIFYLLINE

BRAND NAMES

Trental

BASIC INFORMATION

Habit forming? No
Prescription needed? Yes
Available as generic? Yes
Drug class: Hemorrheologic agent

 ## USES

Reduces pain in legs caused by poor circulation.

 ## DOSAGE & USAGE INFORMATION

How to take:
Extended-release tablets—Swallow whole with water and food.

When to take:
At mealtimes. Taking with food decreases the likelihood of irritating the stomach to cause nausea.

If you forget a dose:
Take as soon as you remember up to 3 hours late. If more than 3 hours, wait for next scheduled dose (don't double this dose).

What drug does:
- Reduces "stickiness" of red blood cells and improves flexibility of the red cells.
- Improves blood flow through blood vessels.

Time lapse before drug works:
1 hour. Several weeks for full effect on circulation.

Don't take with:
- Tobacco or medicines to treat hypertension.
- Any other medicine without consulting your doctor or pharmacist.

 ## OVERDOSE

SYMPTOMS:
Drowsiness, flushed face, fainting, nervousness, convulsions, coma.
WHAT TO DO:
- Dial 911 (emergency) or 0 (operator) for an ambulance or medical help. Then give first aid immediately.
- See emergency information on inside covers.

 ## POSSIBLE ADVERSE REACTIONS OR SIDE EFFECTS

SYMPTOMS	WHAT TO DO
Life-threatening:	
Chest pain, irregular heartbeat.	Discontinue. Seek emergency treatment.
Common:	
None expected.	
Infrequent:	
• Dizziness, headache, nausea, vomiting. low blood pressure, nosebleed, swollen feet and ankles, viral-like syndrome, nasal congestion, laryngitis, rash, itchy skin, blurred vision, abdominal pain.	Discontinue. Call doctor right away.
• Insomnia, nervousness, red eyes.	Continue. Call doctor when convenient.
Rare:	
None expected.	

WARNINGS & PRECAUTIONS

Don't take if:
You are allergic to pentoxifylline.

Before you start, consult your doctor:
- If you are allergic to caffeine, theophylline, theobromine, aminophyllin, dyphyllin, oxtriphyllino, thcobromine.
- If you have angina.
- If you have liver or kidney disease.

Over age 60:
Adverse reactions and side effects may be more frequent and severe than in younger persons. Ask doctor about smaller doses.

Pregnancy:
Decide with your doctor if drug benefits justify risk to unborn child. Risk category C (see page xxiii).

Breast-feeding:
Drug passes into milk. Avoid drug or discontinue nursing until you finish medicine. Consult doctor for advice on maintaining milk supply.

Infants & children:
Not recommended.

Prolonged use:
No problems expected.

Skin & sunlight:
No problems expected.

Driving, piloting or hazardous work:
Wait to see if drug causes drowsiness or dizziness. If none, no problems expected.

Discontinuing:
No problems expected.

Others:
Don't smoke.

POSSIBLE INTERACTION WITH OTHER DRUGS

GENERIC NAME OR DRUG CLASS	COMBINED EFFECT
Anticoagulants*, oral	Possible decreased effect of anticoagulant.
Antihypertensives*	Possible increased effect of hypertensive medication.

POSSIBLE INTERACTION WITH OTHER SUBSTANCES

INTERACTS WITH	COMBINED EFFECT
Alcohol:	Unknown. Best to avoid.
Beverages: Coffee, tea or other caffeine-containing beverages.	May decrease effectiveness of pentoxifylline.
Cocaine:	Reduced effect of pentoxifylline.
Foods:	None expected.
Marijuana:	Decreased effect of pentoxifylline.
Tobacco:	Decreased effect of pentoxifylline. Avoid.

PERGOLIDE

BRAND NAMES

Permax

BASIC INFORMATION

Habit forming? No
Prescription needed? Yes
Available as generic? No
Drug class: Antidyskinetic

USES

Treats Parkinson's disease when used together with levodopa or carbidopa.

DOSAGE & USAGE INFORMATION

How to take:
Tablets—Swallow with liquid. If you can't swallow whole, crumble tablet and take with liquid or food. Instructions to take on empty stomach mean 1 hour before or 2 hours after eating.

When to take:
Follow doctor's instructions. Usually 3 times a day.

If you forget a dose:
Take as soon as you remember up to 2 hours late. If more than 2 hours, wait for next scheduled dose (don't double this dose).

What drug does:
- Stimulates dopamine receptors in the central nervous system to make them more active.
- Lowers the required dosage of carbidopa and levodopa.

Time lapse before drug works:
Not documented.

Don't take with:
Any other medicines (including over-the-counter drugs such as cough and cold medicines, laxatives, antacids, diet pills, caffeine, nose drops or vitamins) without consulting your doctor or pharmacist.

OVERDOSE

SYMPTOMS:
None expected.
WHAT TO DO:
Overdose unlikely to threaten life. If person takes much larger amount than prescribed, call doctor, poison control center or hospital emergency room for instructions.

POSSIBLE ADVERSE REACTIONS OR SIDE EFFECTS

SYMPTOMS	WHAT TO DO
Life-threatening: Seizures, chest pain, shortness of breath.	Seek emergency treatment immediately.
Common:	
• Confusion; hallucinations; painful urination; unusual movements of face, head, hands andtongue.	Discontinue. Seek emergency treatment.
• Abdominal pain, constipation, dizziness, nasal stuffiness.	Continue. Call doctor when convenient.
Infrequent: Chills, diarrhea, dry mouth, appetite loss, facial swelling, increased sex drive.	Continue. Call doctor when convenient.
Rare: Weakness, vision changes, fainting, increased sweating, nausea and vomiting.	Discontinue. Seek emergency treatment.

PERGOLIDE

Methyldopa	Decreased pergolide effect.
Metoclopropamide	Decreased pergolide effect.
Molindone	Decreased pergolide effect.
Papaverine	Decreased pergolide effect.
Phenothiazines*	Decreased pergolide effect.
Reserpine	Decreased pergolide effect.
Sertraline	Increased depressive effects of both drugs
Thiothixene	Decreased pergolide effect.

WARNINGS & PRECAUTIONS

Don't take if:
You are allergic to pergolide or any ergot preparation*.

Before you start, consult your doctor:
• If you have heartbeat irregularities.
• It you have hallucinations.

Over age 60:
No special problems expected.

Pregnancy:
Consult doctor. Risk category B (see page xxiii).

Breast-feeding:
Not recommended. Pergolide can prevent lactation. Consult doctor.

Infants & children:
Effect not documented. Consult your doctor.

Prolonged use:
Request frequent blood pressure checks.

Skin & sunlight:
No problems expected.

Driving, piloting or hazardous work:
Don't drive or pilot aircraft until you learn how medicine affects you. Don't work around dangerous machinery. Don't climb ladders or work in high places. Danger increases if you drink alcohol or take medicine affecting alertness and reflexes.

Discontinuing:
No special problems expected.

Others:
• Advise any doctor or dentist whom you consult that you take this medicine.
• May affect results in some medical tests.

POSSIBLE INTERACTION WITH OTHER SUBSTANCES

INTERACTS WITH	COMBINED EFFECT
Alcohol:	Increased likelihood of adverse reactions. Avoid.
Beverages:	No special problems expected.
Cocaine:	Increased likelihood of adverse reactions. Avoid.
Foods:	No special problems expected.
Marijuana:	Increased likelihood of adverse reactions. Avoid.
Tobacco:	No special problems expected.

POSSIBLE INTERACTION WITH OTHER DRUGS

GENERIC NAME OR DRUG CLASS	COMBINED EFFECT
Chlorprothixene	Decreased pergolide effect.
Droperidol	Decreased pergolide effect.
Flupenthixol	Decreased pergolide effect.
Haloperidol	Decreased pergolide effect.
Hypotension-causing drugs*	Increased hypotension effect.
Loxapine	Decreased pergolide effect.

*See Glossary

PERPHENAZINE & AMITRIPTYLINE

BRAND NAMES

Elavil Plus
Etrafon
Etrafon-A
Etrafon-D

Etrafon-F
Etrafon-Forte
PMS Levazine
Triavil

BASIC INFORMATION

Habit forming? No
Prescription needed? Yes
Available as generic? Yes
Drug class: Tranquilizer (phenothiazine),
antidepressant, antipsychotic

 ## USES

- Decreases nausea, vomiting, hiccups.
- Gradually relieves, but doesn't cure, symptoms of depression, anxiety, agitation.
- Pain relief (sometimes).

 ## DOSAGE & USAGE INFORMATION

How to take:
Tablet or liquid—Swallow with liquid.

When to take:
At the same time each day.

If you forget a dose:
Bedtime dose—If you forget your once-a-day bedtime dose, don't take it more than 3 hours late. If more than 3 hours, wait for next scheduled dose (don't double this dose).

Continued next column

 ## OVERDOSE

SYMPTOMS:
Stupor, convulsions, hallucinations, coma.
WHAT TO DO:
- Dial 911 (emergency) or 0 (operator) for an ambulance or medical help. Then give first aid immediately.
- If patient is unconscious and not breathing, give mouth-to-mouth breathing. If there is no heartbeat, use cardiac massage and mouth-to-mouth breathing (CPR). Don't try to make patient vomit. If you can't get help quickly, take patient to nearest emergency facility.
- See emergency information on inside covers.

What drug does:
- Suppresses brain's vomiting center.
- Suppresses brain centers that control abnormal emotions and behavior.
- Probably affects part of brain that controls messages between nerve cells.

Time lapse before drug works:
- Nausea and vomiting—1 hour or less.
- Nervous and mental disorders—4 to 6 weeks.
- Begins in 1 to 2 weeks. May require 4 to 6 weeks for maximum benefit.

Don't take with:
- Antacid or medicine for diarrhea.
- Any other medicine without consulting your doctor or pharmacist.

 ## POSSIBLE ADVERSE REACTIONS OR SIDE EFFECTS

SYMPTOMS	WHAT TO DO
Life-threatening: Seizures; irregular heartbeat; weak pulse; fainting; muscle spasms; uncontrolled muscle movements of tongue, face and other muscles (neuroleptic malignant syndrome*).	Discontinue. Seek emergency treatment.
Common:	
• Headache, nausea, vomiting, irregular heartbeat, drowsiness.	Discontinue. Call doctor right away.
• Insomnia, dry mouth, "sweet tooth," decreased sweating, runny nose, constipation.	Continue. Call doctor when convenient.
Infrequent:	
• Hallucinations, dizziness, tremor, blurred vision, eye pain, inflamed tongue, joint pain, back pain, hiccups.	Discontinue. Call doctor right away.
• Frequent urination, diminished sex drive, breast swelling, menstrual irregularities, nasal congestion.	Continue. Call doctor when convenient.
Rare:	
• Rash; itchy skin; jaundice; change in vision; sore throat, fever, mouth sores; abdominal pain.	Discontinue. Call doctor right away.
• Fatigue, weakness.	Continue. Call doctor when convenient.

WARNINGS & PRECAUTIONS

Don't take if:
- You are allergic to any phenothiazine, tricyclic antidepressant.
- You have a blood or bone marrow disease, glaucoma, prostate trouble.
- You drink alcohol.
- You have had a heart attack within 6 weeks.
- You have taken MAO inhibitors within 2 weeks.
- Patient is younger than 12.

Before you start, consult your doctor:
- If you have asthma, emphysema or other lung disorder.
- If you have an enlarged prostate, heart disease, high blood pressure, stomach or intestinal problems, overactive thyroid, liver disease.
- If you take nonprescription ulcer medicine, asthma medicine or amphetamines.
- If you will have surgery within 2 months, including dental surgery, requiring general or spinal anesthesia.

Over age 60:
Adverse reactions and side effects may be more frequent and severe than in younger persons. More likely to develop involuntary movement of jaws, lips, tongue; chewing; difficult urination. Report this to your doctor immediately. Early treatment can help.

Pregnancy:
Risk to unborn child outweighs drug benefits. Don't use. Risk category D (see page xxiii).

Breast-feeding:
Drug passes into milk. Avoid drug or discontinue nursing until you finish medicine. Consult doctor for advice on maintaining milk supply.

Infants & children:
Don't give to children younger than 12.

Prolonged use:
May lead to tardive dyskinesia (involuntary movement of jaws, lips, tongue; chewing).

Skin & sunlight:
May cause rash or intensify sunburn in areas exposed to sun or ultraviolet light (photosensitivity reaction). Avoid overexposure. Notify doctor if reaction occurs. Skin may remain sensitive for 3 months after discontinuing.

Driving, piloting or hazardous work:
Don't drive or pilot aircraft until you learn how medicine affects you. Don't work around dangerous machinery. Don't climb ladders or work in high places. Danger increases if you drink alcohol or take medicine affecting alertness and reflexes, such as antihistamines, tranquilizers, sedatives, pain medicine, narcotics and mind-altering drugs.

Discontinuing:
- Nervous and mental disorders—Don't discontinue without doctor's advice until you complete prescribed dose, even though symptoms diminish or disappear.
- Dose may require gradual reduction if you have taken drug for a long time. Doses of other drugs may also require adjustment.

Others:
No problems expected.

POSSIBLE INTERACTION WITH OTHER DRUGS

GENERIC NAME OR DRUG CLASS	COMBINED EFFECT
Anticholinergics*	Increased anticholinergic effect, increased sedation.
Anticoagulants*, oral	Increased anticoagulant effect.
Antihistamines*	Increased antihistamine effect.
Appetite suppressants*	Decreased appetite suppressant effect.
Barbiturates*	Decreased antidepressant effect. Increased sedation.
Cimetidine	Possible increased effect and toxicity of perphenazine and amitriptyline.
Clonidine	Possible decreased clonidine effect.

Continued on page 928

POSSIBLE INTERACTION WITH OTHER SUBSTANCES

INTERACTS WITH	COMBINED EFFECT
Alcohol: Beverages or medicines with alcohol.	Excessive intoxication. Avoid.
Beverages: Coffee.	Reduced effectiveness.
Cocaine:	Excessive intoxication. Avoid.
Foods:	None expected.
Marijuana:	Excessive drowsiness. Avoid.
Tobacco:	None expected.

*See Glossary

PHENAZOPYRIDINE

BRAND NAMES

Azo-Cheragan
Azo-Gantrisin
Azo-Standard
Baridium
Eridium
Geridium
Phen-Azo
Phenazodine

Pyrazodine
Pyridiate
Pyridium
Pyronium
Urodine
Urogesic
Viridium

BASIC INFORMATION

Habit forming? No
Prescription needed? Yes
Available as generic? Yes
Drug class: Analgesic (urinary)

 USES

Relieves pain of lower urinary tract irritation, as in cystitis, urethritis or prostatitis. Relieves symptoms only. Phenazopyridine alone does not cure infections.

 DOSAGE & USAGE INFORMATION

How to take:
Tablet—Swallow with liquid or food to lessen stomach irritation.

When to take:
At the same times each day.

If you forget a dose:
Take as soon as you remember up to 2 hours late. If more than 2 hours, wait for next scheduled dose (don't double this dose).

What drug does:
Anesthetizes lower urinary tract. Relieves pain, burning, pressure and urgency to urinate.

Time lapse before drug works:
1 to 2 hours.

 OVERDOSE

SYMPTOMS:
Shortness of breath, weakness.
WHAT TO DO:
Overdose unlikely to threaten life. If person takes much larger amount than prescribed, call doctor, poison control center or hospital emergency room for instructions.

Don't take with:
Any other medicine without consulting your doctor or pharmacist.

 POSSIBLE ADVERSE REACTIONS OR SIDE EFFECTS

SYMPTOMS	WHAT TO DO
Life-threatening:	
In case of overdose, see previous column.	
Common:	
Red-orange urine.	No action necessary.
Infrequent:	
Indigestion, fatigue, weakness, dizziness, abdominal pain.	Continue. Call doctor when convenient.
Rare:	
• Rash, jaundice, bluish skin color.	Discontinue. Call doctor right away.
• Headache.	Continue. Call doctor when convenient.

WARNINGS & PRECAUTIONS

Don't take if:
- You have hepatitis.
- You are allergic to any urinary analgesic.

Before you start, consult your doctor:
If you have kidney or liver disease.

Over age 60:
Adverse reactions and side effects may be more frequent and severe than in younger persons.

Pregnancy:
No proven harm to unborn child. Avoid if possible. Consult doctor. Risk category B (see page xxiii).

Breast-feeding:
Effect unknown. Consult doctor.

Infants & children:
Not recommended.

Prolonged use:
- Orange or yellow skin.
- Anemia. Occasional blood studies recommended.

Skin & sunlight:
No problems expected.

Driving, piloting or hazardous work:
No problems expected.

Discontinuing:
May be unnecessary to finish medicine. Follow doctor's instructions.

Others:
No problems expected.

POSSIBLE INTERACTION WITH OTHER DRUGS

GENERIC NAME OR DRUG CLASS	COMBINED EFFECT
None significant.	

POSSIBLE INTERACTION WITH OTHER SUBSTANCES

INTERACTS WITH	COMBINED EFFECT
Alcohol:	None expected.
Beverages:	None expected.
Cocaine:	None expected.
Foods:	None expected.
Marijuana:	None expected.
Tobacco:	None expected.

PHENOTHIAZINES

GENERIC AND BRAND NAMES

See complete list of generic and brand names in the *Generic and Brand Name Directory*, page 888.

BASIC INFORMATION

Habit forming? No
Prescription needed? Yes
Available as generic? Yes, for some.
Drug class: Tranquilizer, antiemetic (phenothiazine)

 ## USES

- Reduces anxiety, agitation.
- Stops nausea, vomiting, hiccups.

 ## DOSAGE & USAGE INFORMATION

How to take:
- Tablet or extended-release capsule—Swallow with liquid or food to lessen stomach irritation.
- Suppositories—Remove wrapper and moisten suppository with water. Gently insert into rectum, pointed end first.
- Drops or liquid—Dilute dose in beverage.

When to take:
- Nervous and mental disorders—Take at the same times each day.
- For other uses, take as directed by your doctor.

If you forget a dose:
Nervous and mental disorders—Take up to 2 hours late. If more than 2 hours, wait for next scheduled dose (don't double this dose).

What drug does:
- Suppresses brain centers that control abnormal emotions and behavior.
- Suppresses brain's vomiting center.

Continued next column

 ## OVERDOSE

SYMPTOMS:
Stupor, convulsions, coma.
WHAT TO DO:
- **Dial 911 (emergency) or 0 (operator) for an ambulance or medical help. Then give first aid immediately.**
- **See emergency information at end of book.**

Time lapse before drug works:
Some benefit seen within a week; takes 4 to 6 weeks for full effect.

Don't take with:
- Antacid or medicine for diarrhea.
- Nonprescription drug for cough, cold or allergy.
- Any other medicine without consulting your doctor or pharmacist.

 ## POSSIBLE ADVERSE REACTIONS OR SIDE EFFECTS

SYMPTOMS	WHAT TO DO
Life-threatening:	
High fever, rapid pulse, profuse sweating, muscle rigidity, confusion and irritability, seizures.	Discontinue. Seek emergency treatment.
Common:	
Dry mouth, blurred vision, constipation, difficulty urinating; sedation, dizziness, low blood pressure.	Continue. Call doctor when convenient.
Infrequent:	
• Continuous jerky or involuntary movements, especially of the face, lips, jaw, tongue; slow-frequency tremor of head or limbs, especially while moving; muscle rigidity, lack of facial expression and slow, inflexible movements.	Discontinue. Call doctor right away.
• Pacing or restlessness; intermittent spasms of muscles of face, eyes, tongue, jaw, neck, body or limbs; jaundice (yellow skin or eyes).	Continue. Call doctor when convenient.
Rare:	
Other symptoms not listed above.	Continue. Call doctor when convenient.

WARNINGS & PRECAUTIONS

Don't take if:
- You are allergic to any phenothiazine.
- You have a blood or bone marrow disease.

Before you start, consult your doctor:
- If you will have surgery within 2 months, including dental surgery, requiring general or spinal anesthesia.
- If you have asthma, emphysema or other lung disorder; glaucoma; or prostate trouble.
- If you take nonprescription ulcer medicine, asthma medicine or amphetamines.

Over age 60:
Adverse reactions and side effects may be more frequent and severe than in younger persons. More likely to develop involuntary movement of jaws, lips, tongue; chewing. Report this to your doctor immediately. Early treatment can help.

Pregnancy:
Risk factors vary for drugs in this group. See category list on page xxiii and consult doctor.

Breast-feeding:
Drug passes into milk. Avoid drug or discontinue nursing until you finish medicine. Consult doctor for advice on maintaining milk supply.

Infants & children:
- Don't give to children younger than 2.
- Children more likely than adults to develop adverse reactions from these drugs.

Prolonged use:
May lead to tardive dyskinesia (involuntary movement of jaws, lips, tongue; chewing).

Skin & sunlight:
- One or more drugs in this group may cause rash or intensify sunburn in areas exposed to sun or ultraviolet light (photosensitivity reaction). Use sunscreen and avoid over-exposure. Notify doctor if reaction occurs. Sensitivity may remain for 3 months after discontinuing drug.
- Avoid getting overheated or chilled. These drugs affect body temperature and sweating.

Driving, piloting or hazardous work:
Don't drive or pilot aircraft until you learn how medicine affects you. Don't work around dangerous machinery. Don't climb ladders or work in high places. Danger increases if you drink alcohol or take medicine affecting alertness and reflexes.

Discontinuing:
- Nervous and mental disorders—Don't discontinue without doctor's advice until you complete prescribed dose, even though symptoms diminish or disappear.
- Other disorders—Follow doctor's instructions about discontinuing.

- Adverse reactions may occur after drug is discontinued. Consult doctor if new symptoms develop, such as dizziness, nausea, stomach pain, trembling or tardive dyskinesia*.

Others:
- To relieve mouth dryness, chew or suck sugarless gum, candy, or ice.
- Avoid getting the liquid form of the drug on the skin. It may cause a skin rash or irritation.
- Advise any doctor or dentist whom you consult that you take this medicine.

POSSIBLE INTERACTION WITH OTHER DRUGS

GENERIC NAME OR DRUG CLASS	COMBINED EFFECT
Anticholinergics*	Increased phenothiazine effect
Anticonvulsants*	Increased risk of seizures. May need to increase dosage of anticonvulsant.
Antidepressants, tricyclic*	Increased anti-depressant effect.
Antihistamines*	Increased antihistamine effect.
Antihypertensives*	Severe low blood pressure.
Appetite suppressants*	Decreased appetite suppressant effect.
Bupropion	Increased risk of seizures.

Continued on page 928

POSSIBLE INTERACTION WITH OTHER SUBSTANCES

INTERACTS WITH	COMBINED EFFECT
Alcohol:	Dangerous oversedation. Avoid
Beverages:	None expected.
Cocaine:	Decreased phenothiazine effect. Avoid.
Foods:	None expected.
Marijuana:	Drowsiness. May increase antinausea effect.
Tobacco:	None expected.

*See Glossary

PHENYLEPHRINE

BRAND NAMES

See complete list of brand names in the *Generic and Brand Name Directory*, page 888.

BASIC INFORMATION

Habit forming? No
Prescription needed? No
Available as generic? Yes
Drug class: Sympathomimetic, decongestant

 ## USES

- Temporary relief of congestion of nose, sinuses and throat caused by allergies, colds or sinusitis.
- Treats congestion of eustachian tubes caused by middle ear infections.

 ## DOSAGE & USAGE INFORMATION

How to take:
- Nasal drops or spray—Wash hands before use. Blow nose gently, and then use the drops or spray according to instructions on the label.
- Combination drug products—Use according to label directions. Phenylephrine is the decongestant ingredient in many combination cough, cold and hay fever remedies.

When to take:
As needed, no more often than every 4 hours.

If you forget a dose:
Take when you remember. Wait 4 hours for next dose. Never double a dose.

What drug does:
Contracts blood vessel walls of nose, sinus and throat tissues, enlarging airways.

Time lapse before drug works:
5 to 30 minutes.

Continued next column

 ## OVERDOSE

SYMPTOMS:
Headache, heart palpitations, vomiting, blood pressure rise, slow and forceful pulse.
WHAT TO DO:
- Dial 911 (emergency) or 0 (operator) for an ambulance or medical help. Then give first aid immediately.
- See emergency information on inside covers.

Don't take with:
Nonprescription drugs for asthma, cough, cold, allergy, appetite suppressants, sleeping pills or drugs containing caffeine without consulting doctor.

 ## POSSIBLE ADVERSE REACTIONS OR SIDE EFFECTS

SYMPTOMS	WHAT TO DO
Life-threatening: In case of overdose, see previous column.	
Common: Burning, dryness, stinging inside nose; headache.	Continue. Call doctor when convenient.
Infrequent: None expected.	
Rare: Unusual sweating, fast or pounding heartbeat, nervousness, insomnia (all symptoms of too much being absorbed into body).	Discontinue. Call doctor right away.

WARNINGS & PRECAUTIONS

Don't take if:
You are allergic to any sympathomimetic.

Before you start, consult your doctor:
- If you have high blood pressure.
- If you have heart disease.
- If you have diabetes.
- If you have overactive thyroid.
- If you have taken MAO inhibitors in past 2 weeks.

Over age 60:
Adverse reactions and side effects may be more frequent and severe than in younger persons.

Pregnancy:
Decide with your doctor if drug benefits justify risk to unborn child. Risk category C (see page xxiii).

Breast-feeding:
Drug passes into milk. Avoid drug or discontinue nursing until you finish medicine. Consult doctor for advice on maintaining milk supply.

Infants & children:
Use only under close supervision.

Prolonged use:
- Rebound* congestion and chemical irritation of nasal membranes.
- May cause functional dependence.
- Talk to your doctor about the need for follow-up medical examinations or laboratory studies to check blood pressure, ECG*.

Skin & sunlight:
No problems expected.

Driving, piloting or hazardous work:
No problems expected.

Discontinuing:
May be unnecessary to finish medicine. Follow label or doctor's instructions.

Others:
- Call the doctor if symptoms worsen or new symptoms develop with use of this medicine.
- Heed all warnings on the product label.

POSSIBLE INTERACTION WITH OTHER DRUGS

GENERIC NAME OR DRUG CLASS	COMBINED EFFECT
Antidepressants, tricyclic*	Increased phenylephrine effect.
Guanadrel	Heart or blood pressure problems. Avoid.
Guanethidine	Heart or blood pressure problems. Avoid.
Maprotiline	Dangerous blood pressure rise. Don't use within 14 days.
Monoamine oxidase (MAO) inhibitors*	Dangerous blood pressure rise. Don't use within 14 days.
Nicotine	Decreased effect of phenylephrine.

POSSIBLE INTERACTION WITH OTHER SUBSTANCES

INTERACTS WITH	COMBINED EFFECT
Alcohol:	None expected.
Beverages: Caffeine drinks.	Excess brain stimulation.
Cocaine:	Excess brain stimulation.
Foods:	None expected.
Marijuana:	None expected.
Tobacco:	None expected.

*See Glossary

PHENYLEPHRINE (Ophthalmic)

BRAND NAMES

Ak-Dilate	Neofrin
Ak-Nefrin	Neo-Synephrine
Dilatair	Ocugestrin
Dionephrine	Ocu-Phrin
I-Phrine	Phenoptic
Isopto Frin	Prefrin Liquifilm
Minims	Relief Eye Drops
Phenylephrine	for Red Eyes
Mydfrin	Spersaphrine

BASIC INFORMATION

Habit forming? No
Prescription needed? Yes, some strengths
Available as generic? No
Drug class: Mydriatic, decongestant
  (ophthalmic)

 ## USES

- High-concentration drops—Dilates pupils.
- Low-concentration drops (available without prescription)—Relieves minor eye irritations caused by colds, hay fever, dust, wind, swimming, sun, smog, hard contact lenses, eye strain, smoke.

 ## DOSAGE & USAGE INFORMATION

How to use:
Eye drops
- Wash hands.
- Apply pressure to inside corner of eye with middle finger.
- Continue pressure for 1 minute after placing medicine in eye.
- Tilt head backward. Pull lower lid away from eye with index finger of the same hand.
- Drop eye drops into pouch and close eye. Don't blink.
- Keep eyes closed for 1 to 2 minutes.
- Don't touch applicator tip to any surface (including the eye). If you accidentally touch tip, clean with warm soap and water.
- Keep container tightly closed.

Continued next column

 ## OVERDOSE

SYMPTOMS:
None expected.
WHAT TO DO:
Not intended for internal use. If child accidentally swallows, call poison control center.

- Keep cool, but don't freeze.
- Wash hands immediately after using.

When to use:
As directed on label.

If you forget a dose:
Use as soon as you remember.

What drug does:
Acts on small blood vessels to make them constrict.

Time lapse before drug works:
15 to 90 minutes.

Don't use with:
- Other eye drops or ointment without consulting your eye doctor.
- Antidepressants*, guanadrel, guanethidine, maprotiline, pargyline, any monoamine oxidase (MAO) inhibitor*.

 ## POSSIBLE ADVERSE REACTIONS OR SIDE EFFECTS

SYMPTOMS	WHAT TO DO
Life-threatening: None expected, unless you use much more than directed.	Discontinue. Call doctor right away.
Common: None expected.	
Infrequent: Burning or stinging eyes, headache, eyes more sensitive to light, watery eyes, eye irritation not present before.	Continue. Call doctor when convenient.
Rare: None expected, unless too much gets absorbed. If so, symptoms will be paleness, dizziness, tremor, increased sweating, irregular or fast heartbeat.	Discontinue. Call doctor right away.

WARNINGS & PRECAUTIONS

Don't use if:
- You are allergic to phenylephrine.
- You have glaucoma.

Before you start, consult your doctor:
- If you have heart disease with irregular heart-beat, high blood pressure, diabetes.
- If you take antidepressants*, guanadrel, guanethidine, maprotiline, pargyline, any monoamine oxidase (MAO) inhibitor*.

Over age 60:
Adverse reactions and side effects may be more frequent and severe than in younger persons. Ask doctor about smaller doses.

Pregnancy:
Decide with your doctor if drug benefits justify risk to unborn child. Risk category C (see page xxiii).

Breast-feeding:
Safety not established. Consult doctor.

Infants & children:
Use only under close medical supervision.

Prolonged use:
Avoid if possible.

Skin & sunlight:
No special problems expected.

Driving, piloting or hazardous work:
No problems expected.

Discontinuing:
No problems expected.

Others:
- Keep cool, but don't freeze.
- Consult doctor if condition doesn't improve in 3 to 4 days.

POSSIBLE INTERACTION WITH OTHER DRUGS

GENERIC NAME OR DRUG CLASS	COMBINED EFFECT
Clinically significant interactions with oral or injected medicines unlikely.	

POSSIBLE INTERACTION WITH OTHER SUBSTANCES

INTERACTS WITH	COMBINED EFFECT
Alcohol:	None expected.
Beverages:	None expected.
Cocaine:	None expected.
Foods:	None expected.
Marijuana:	None expected.
Tobacco:	None expected.

PHENYLPROPANOLAMINE

BRAND NAMES

See complete list of brand names in the *Generic and Brand Name Directory*, page 889.

BASIC INFORMATION

Habit forming? No
Prescription needed?
  High strength: Yes
  Low strength: No
Available as generic? Yes
Drug class: Sympathomimetic, decongestant

 ## USES

- Relieves bronchial asthma.
- Decreases congestion of breathing passages.
- Suppresses allergic reactions.
- Decreases appetite. Used for obesity.
- Treatment for urinary incontinence.

 ## DOSAGE & USAGE INFORMATION

How to take:
- Tablet—Swallow with liquid. You may chew or crush tablet.
- Extended-release tablet or capsule—Swallow whole with liquid. Do not crush, break or crumble tablet.

When to take:
As needed, no more often than every 4 hours.

If you forget a dose:
Take up to 2 hours late. If more than 2 hours, wait for next dose (don't double this dose).

What drug does:
- Relaxes muscles of bronchial tubes.
- Decreases blood vessel size and blood flow, thus causing decongestion.

Time lapse before drug works:
30 to 60 minutes.

Continued next column

 ## OVERDOSE

SYMPTOMS:
Severe anxiety, confusion, delirium, muscle tremors, rapid and irregular pulse.
WHAT TO DO:
- **Dial 911 (emergency) or 0 (operator) for an ambulance or medical help. Then give first aid immediately.**
- **See emergency information on inside covers.**

Don't take with:
Nonprescription drugs for cough, cold, allergy or asthma without consulting doctor.

 ## POSSIBLE ADVERSE REACTIONS OR SIDE EFFECTS

SYMPTOMS	WHAT TO DO
Life-threatening: In case of overdose, see previous column.	
Common: None expected.	
Infrequent: Dizziness, nausea, nervousness, dry nose or mouth, false sense of well-being, trouble sleeping, mild headache.	Continue. Call doctor when convenient.
Rare: Tightness in chest, severe headache, painful or difficult urination.	Discontinue. Call doctor right away.

 ## WARNINGS & PRECAUTIONS

Don't take if:
You are allergic to any sympathomimetic drug*.

Before you start, consult your doctor:
- If you have high blood pressure, diabetes, overactive thyroid gland, difficulty urinating.
- If you have taken any MAO inhibitors in past 2 weeks.
- If you have taken digitalis preparations in the last 7 days.
- If you will have surgery within 2 months, including dental surgery, requiring general or spinal anesthesia.

Over age 60:
More likely to develop high blood pressure, heart rhythm disturbances and angina and to feel drug's stimulant effects.

Pregnancy:
Decide with your doctor if drug benefits justify risk to unborn child. Risk category C (see page xxiii).

Breast-feeding:
Safety not established. Consult doctor.

Infants & children:
Don't give to children under 6 years old.

Prolonged use:
- Excessive doses—Rare toxic psychosis.
- Men with enlarged prostate gland may have more urination difficulty.
- Talk to your doctor about the need for follow-up medical examinations or laboratory studies.

Skin & sunlight:
No special problems expected.

Driving, piloting or hazardous work:
No restrictions unless you feel dizzy.

Discontinuing:
May be unnecessary to finish medicine. Follow doctor's instructions.

Others:
No problems expected.

POSSIBLE INTERACTION WITH OTHER DRUGS

GENERIC NAME OR DRUG CLASS	COMBINED EFFECT
Anesthetics, general*	Increased phenylpropanolamine effect.
Antidepressants, tricyclic*	Increased phenylpropanolamine effect. Excessive stimulation of heart and blood pressure.
Antihypertensives*	Decreased antihypertensive effect.
Beta-adrenergic blocking agents*	Decreased effect of both drugs.
Central nervous system (CNS) stimulants*	Increased CNS stimulation.
Digitalis preparations*	Serious heart rhythm disturbances.
Diuretics*	Decreased antihypertensive effect of diuretic.
Epinephrine	Increased epinephrine effect.
Guanethidine	Decreased effect of both drugs.
Guanadrel	Decreased effect of both drugs.
Methyldopa	Possible increased blood pressure.
Monoamine oxidase (MAO) inhibitors*	Increased phenypropanolamine effect. Dangerous blood pressure rise.
Phenothiazines*	Possible increased phenypropanolamine toxicity. Possible decreased phenylpropanolamine effect.
Rauwolfia	Decreased rauwolfia effect.
Sympathomimetics*, other	Increased phenypropanolamine effect.
Terazosin	Decreased effectiveness of terazosin.

POSSIBLE INTERACTION WITH OTHER SUBSTANCES

INTERACTS WITH	COMBINED EFFECT
Alcohol:	Increased sedation.
Beverages: Caffeine drinks.	Nervousness or insomnia.
Cocaine:	High risk of heartbeat irregularities and high blood pressure.
Foods:	None expected.
Marijuana:	Rapid heartbeat, possible heart rhythm disturbance. Avoid.
Tobacco:	None expected.

PILOCARPINE

BRAND NAMES

Adsorbocarpine	Pilocar
Akarpine	Pilopine HS
Almocarpine	Piloptic
Isopto Carpine	Pilostat
Minims Pilocarpine	P.V. Carpine
Miocarpine	P.V. Carpine
Ocu-Carpine	Liquifilm
Ocusert Pilo	Salagen

BASIC INFORMATION

Habit forming? No
Prescription needed?
  U.S.: Yes
  Canada: No
Available as generic? Yes
Drug class: Antiglaucoma

 USES

Treatment for glaucoma.

 DOSAGE & USAGE INFORMATION

How to take:
- Drops—Apply to eyes. Close eyes for 1 or 2 minutes to absorb medicine.
- Eye system—Follow label directions.
- Gel—Follow label directions.

Continued next column

 OVERDOSE

SYMPTOMS:
If swallowed—Nausea, vomiting, diarrhea, forceful urination, profuse sweating, rapid pulse, breathing difficulty, loss of consciousness.
WHAT TO DO:
- **Dial 911 (emergency) or 0 (operator) for an ambulance or medical help. Then give first aid immediately.**
- **If patient is unconscious and not breathing, give mouth-to-mouth breathing. If there is no heartbeat, use cardiac massage and mouth-to-mouth breathing (CPR). Don't try to make patient vomit. If you can't get help quickly, take patient to nearest emergency facility.**
- **See emergency information on inside covers.**

When to use:
As directed on label.

If you forget a dose:
Apply as soon as possible, then return to prescribed schedule. Don't double dose.

What drug does:
Reduces internal eye pressure.

Time lapse before drug works:
15 to 30 minutes.

Don't take with:
Any other medicine without consulting your doctor or pharmacist.

 POSSIBLE ADVERSE REACTIONS OR SIDE EFFECTS

SYMPTOMS	WHAT TO DO
Life-threatening:	
In case of overdose, see previous column.	
Common:	
Pain, blurred or altered vision.	Continue. Call doctor when convenient.
Infrequent:	
• Headache, eye irritation or twitching, nausea, vomiting, diarrhea, difficult breathing, muscle tremors.	Discontinue. Call doctor right away.
• Profuse sweating, unusual saliva flow.	Continue. Call doctor when convenient.
Rare:	
None expected.	

WARNINGS & PRECAUTIONS

Don't take if:
You are allergic to pilocarpine.

Before you start, consult your doctor:
- If you take sedatives, sleeping pills, tranquilizers, antidepressants, antihistamines, narcotics or mind-altering drugs.
- If you have asthma.
- If you have conjunctivitis (pink eye).

Over age 60:
Adverse reactions and side effects may be more frequent and severe than in younger persons.

Pregnancy:
Decide with your doctor if drug benefits justify risk to unborn child. Risk category C (see page xxiii).

Breast-feeding:
Effect unknown. Consult doctor.

Infants & children:
Not recommended.

Prolonged use:
- You may develop tolerance for drug, making it ineffective.
- Talk to your doctor about the need for follow-up medical examinations to check eye pressure.

Skin & sunlight:
No problems expected.

Driving, piloting or hazardous work:
Don't drive or pilot aircraft until you learn how medicine affects you. Don't work around dangerous machinery. Don't climb ladders or work in high places. Danger increases if you drink alcohol or take medicine affecting alertness and reflexes, such as antihistamines, tranquilizers, sedatives, pain medicine, narcotics and mind-altering drugs.

Discontinuing:
Doctor may discontinue and substitute another drug to keep treatment effective.

Others:
- Can provoke asthma attack in susceptible individuals.
- Drops may impair vision for 2 to 3 hours.

POSSIBLE INTERACTION WITH OTHER DRUGS

GENERIC NAME OR DRUG CLASS	COMBINED EFFECT
Belladonna (ophthalmic)	Decreased pilocarpine effect.
Cyclopentolate	Decreased pilocarpine effect.

POSSIBLE INTERACTION WITH OTHER SUBSTANCES

INTERACTS WITH	COMBINED EFFECT
Alcohol:	May prolong alcohol's effect on brain.
Beverages:	None expected.
Cocaine:	Decreased pilocarpine effect. Avoid.
Foods:	None expected.
Marijuana (if prescribed):	Used once or twice weekly—May help lower internal eye pressure.
Tobacco:	None expected.

POTASSIUM & SODIUM PHOSPHATES

GENERIC AND BRAND NAMES

POTASSIUM
PHOSPHATES
K-Phos Original
Neutra-Phos K

POTASSIUM &
SODIUM
PHOSPHATES
K-Phos 2
K-Phos M.F.
K-Phos Neutral
Neutra-Phos
Uro-KP-Neutral

BASIC INFORMATION

Habit forming? No
Prescription needed? Yes
Available as generic? Yes
Drug class: Electrolyte replenisher

USES

- Provides supplement of phosphorus for people with diseases which decrease phosphorus absorption from food.
- Treatment of hypercalcemia due to cancer.

DOSAGE & USAGE INFORMATION

How to take:
- Tablets or capsules—Dissolve tablets or open capsules in 3/4 to 1 glass of water. Let tablets soak 2 to 5 minutes, then stir to completely dissolve.
- Oral solution—Take after meals with liquid to decrease stomach irritation.

When to take:
After meals or with food to prevent or lessen stomach irritation or loose stools.

If you forget a dose:
Take within 1 hour, then return to original schedule. If later than 1 hour, skip dose. Don't double dose.

Continued next column

OVERDOSE

SYMPTOMS:
Irregular heartbeat, blood pressure drop with weakness, coma, cardiac arrest.
WHAT TO DO:
- Dial 911 (emergency) or 0 (operator) for an ambulance or medical help. Then give first aid immediately.
- See emergency information on inside covers.

What drug does:
- Provides supplemental phosphates.
- Makes uric acid.

Time lapse before drug works:
30-60 minutes.

Don't take with:
Any other medicine without consulting your doctor or pharmacist.

POSSIBLE ADVERSE REACTIONS OR SIDE EFFECTS

SYMPTOMS	WHAT TO DO
Life-threatening: Irregular heartbeat, difficult breathing, anxiety, weak legs, seizures.	Discontinue. Seek emergency treatment.
Common: None expected.	
Infrequent: Numbness or tingling in hands or feet, diarrhea, nausea, abdominal pain, vomiting, headache, dizziness, muscle cramps, swollen feet and ankles, thirst, weakness.	Discontinue. Call doctor right away.
Rare: Confusion.	Discontinue. Call doctor right away.

WARNINGS & PRECAUTIONS

Don't take if:
You have had allergic reaction to potassium, sodium or phosphates; severe kidney disease; severe burns.

Before you start, consult your doctor:
If you have heart problems, adrenal sufficiency, liver disease, high blood pressure, pregnancy, hypoparathyroidism, chronic kidney disease, osteomalacia, pancreatitis, rickets.

Over age 60:
Adverse reactions and side effects may be more frequent and severe than in younger persons. Ask doctor about smaller doses.

Pregnancy:
Decide with your doctor if drug benefits justify risk to unborn child. Risk category C (see page xxiii).

Breast-feeding:
Effect unknown. Consult doctor.

Infants & children:
Use only under medical supervision.

Prolonged use:
Monitor ECG*, serum calcium, phosphorus and potassium levels.

Skin & sunlight:
No problems expected.

Driving, piloting or hazardous work:
Avoid if medicine causes dizziness or confusion.

Discontinuing:
Don't discontinue without consulting doctor. Dose may require gradual reduction if you have taken drug for a long time. Doses of other drugs may also require adjustment.

Others:
Protect liquid medicine from freezing.

POSSIBLE INTERACTION WITH OTHER DRUGS

GENERIC NAME OR DRUG CLASS	COMBINED EFFECT
Angiotensin-converting enzyme (ACE) inhibitors*	Level of potassium in blood too high.
Antacids*	May decrease potassium absorption.
Calcium	Decreased potassium effect.
Cortisone drugs*	Increased fluid retention.
Digitalis preparations*	Level of potassium in blood too high.
Diuretics* (amiloride, spironolactone, triamterene)	Level of potassium in blood too high.
Male hormones*	Fluid retention.
Potassium supplements*	Level of potassium in blood too high.
Vitamin D (calcifidiol and calcitriol)	Level of phosphorus in blood too high.

POSSIBLE INTERACTION WITH OTHER SUBSTANCES

INTERACTS WITH	COMBINED EFFECT
Alcohol:	None expected.
Beverages: Salty drinks such as tomato juice, commercial thirst quenchers, salt substitutes.	Increased fluid retention.
Cocaine:	May cause irregular heartbeat.
Foods: Salty foods such as canned soups, potato chips, TV dinners, hot dogs, pickles.	Increased fluid retention.
Marijuana:	May cause irregular heartbeat.
Tobacco:	May aggravate irregular heartbeat.

POTASSIUM IODIDE

BRAND NAMES

KI

Pima

SSKI

Thyro-Block

BASIC INFORMATION

Habit forming? No
Prescription needed? Yes
Available as generic? Yes
Drug class: Antihyperthyroid

 ## USES

- Treats overactive thyroid disease.
- Treats iodine deficiency.
- Formerly used to decrease thickness of bronchial secretions.

 ## DOSAGE & USAGE INFORMATION

How to take:
Tablets or syrup—Take in full glass of water, fruit juice, milk or broth.

When to take:
- Take after meals and at bedtime with food or milk.
- Follow your doctor's instructions.

If you forget a dose:
Take as soon as you remember up to 2 hours late. If more than 2 hours, wait for next scheduled dose (don't double this dose).

What drug does:
Decreases release of thyroid hormone.

Time lapse before drug works:
Approximately 10 days.

Don't take with:
Any other medicines (including over-the-counter drugs such as cough and cold medicines, laxatives, antacids, diet pills, caffeine, nose drops or vitamins) without consulting your doctor.

 ## OVERDOSE

SYMPTOMS:
None expected.
WHAT TO DO:
Overdose unlikely to threaten life. If person takes much larger amount than prescribed, call doctor, poison control center or hospital emergency room for instructions.

 ## POSSIBLE ADVERSE REACTIONS OR SIDE EFFECTS

SYMPTOMS	WHAT TO DO
Life-threatening: Black or tarry stools.	Discontinue. Seek emergency treatment.
Common: • Skin rash, swollen salivary glands.	Discontinue. Call doctor right away.
• Diarrhea, nausea, abdominal pain.	Continue. Call doctor when convenient.
Infrequent: Burning mouth, severe headache, increased salivation.	Discontinue. Call doctor right away.
Rare: Confusion, fever, heartbeat irregularities, numbness and tingling of feet and hands, swollen neck, unusual tiredness.	Discontinue. Call doctor right away.

WARNINGS & PRECAUTIONS

Don't take if:
You are intolerant of or allergic to potassium iodide.

Before you start, consult your doctor:
If you have kidney disease.

Over age 60:
No special problems expected.

Pregnancy:
Risk to unborn child outweighs drug benefits. Don't use. Risk category D (see page xxiii).

Breast-feeding:
Drug passes into milk. Avoid drug or discontinue nursing until you finish medicine. Consult doctor for advice on maintaining milk supply.

Infants & children:
Avoid.

Prolonged use:
* Talk to your doctor about the need for follow-up medical examinations or laboratory studies to check serum potassium levels.
* If burning mouth, headache or salivation occur, discontinue and call doctor.

Skin & sunlight:
No problems expected.

Driving, piloting or hazardous work:
Avoid if you feel confused, drowsy or dizzy.

Discontinuing:
No special problems expected.

Others:
* Advise any doctor or dentist whom you consult that you take this medicine.
* Don't use if solution turns yellow.

POSSIBLE INTERACTION WITH OTHER DRUGS

GENERIC NAME OR DRUG CLASS	COMBINED EFFECT
Angiotensin-converting enzyme (ACE) inhibitors*	May raise potassium in blood to toxic levels.
Antithyroid drugs*	Excessive effect of antithyroid drugs.
Diuretics, potassium-sparing	May raise potassium in blood to toxic levels.
Lithium	Increased chance of producing a thyroid goiter.

POSSIBLE INTERACTION WITH OTHER SUBSTANCES

INTERACTS WITH	COMBINED EFFECT
Alcohol:	No special problems expected.
Beverages:	No special problems expected.
Cocaine:	No special problems expected.
Foods: Foods high in iodine.	Too much iodine in blood.
Marijuana:	No special problems expected.
Tobacco:	No special problems expected.

POTASSIUM PHOSPHATES

BRAND NAMES

K-Phos Original   Neutra-Phos K

BASIC INFORMATION

Habit forming? No
Prescription needed? Yes, for some
Available as generic? Yes, for some
Drug class: Electrolyte replenisher

USES

- Provides supplement of phosphorus for people with diseases which decrease phosphorus absorption from food.
- Treatment of hypercalcemia due to cancer.

DOSAGE & USAGE INFORMATION

How to take:
- Tablets—Dissolve tablets in 3/4 to 1 glass of water. Let tablets soak 2 to 5 minutes, then stir to completely dissolve.
- Oral solution—Follow directions on label.

When to take:
After meals or with food to prevent or lessen stomach irritation or loose stools.

If you forget a dose:
Take within 1 hour then return to original schedule. If later than 1 hour, skip dose. Don't double dose.

What drug does:
- Provides supplemental phosphates.
- Makes uric acid.

Time lapse before drug works:
30-60 minutes.

Don't take with:
Any other medicine without consulting your doctor or pharmacist.

OVERDOSE

SYMPTOMS:
Irregular heartbeat, blood pressure drop with weakness, coma, cardiac arrest.
WHAT TO DO:
- **Dial 911 (emergency) or 0 (operator) for an ambulance or medical help. Then give first aid immediately.**
- **See emergency information on inside covers.**

POSSIBLE ADVERSE REACTIONS OR SIDE EFFECTS

SYMPTOMS	WHAT TO DO
Life-threatening: Irregular heartbeat, shortness of breath, seizures.	Discontinue. Seek emergency treatment.
Common: Muscle cramps.	Discontinue. Call doctor right away.
Infrequent: Bone and joint pain, numbness or tingling in hands or feet, unusual tiredness, weakness, diarrhea, nausea, abdominal pain, vomiting, confusion, headache, dizziness.	Discontinue. Call doctor right away.
Rare: Foot and leg swelling.	Discontinue. Call doctor right away.

WARNINGS & PRECAUTIONS

Don't take if:
You have had allergic reaction to potassium, sodium or phosphates; severe kidney disease; severe burns.

Before you start, consult your doctor:
If you have heart problems, adrenal sufficiency, liver disease, high blood pressure, pregnancy, hypoparathyroidism, chronic kidney disease, osteomalacia, pancreatitis, rickets.

Over age 60:
Adverse reactions and side effects may be more frequent and severe than in younger persons. Ask doctor about smaller doses.

Pregnancy:
Decide with your doctor if drug benefits justify risk to unborn child. Risk category C (see page xxiii).

Breast-feeding:
Effect unknown. Consult doctor.

Infants & children:
Use only under medical supervision.

Prolonged use:
Monitor ECG*, serum calcium, phosphorus and potassium levels.

Skin & sunlight:
No problems expected.

Driving, piloting or hazardous work:
Avoid if medicine causes dizziness or confusion.

Discontinuing:
Don't discontinue without consulting doctor. Dose may require gradual reduction if you have taken drug for a long time. Doses of other drugs may also require adjustment.

Others:
Protect liquid medicine from freezing.

POSSIBLE INTERACTION WITH OTHER DRUGS

GENERIC NAME OR DRUG CLASS	COMBINED EFFECT
Angiotensin-converting enzyme (ACE) inhibitors*	Level of potassium in blood too high.
Antacids*	May decrease potassium absorption.
Calcium	Decreased potassium effect.
Cortisone drugs*	Increased fluid retention.
Digitalis preparations*	Level of potassium in blood too high.
Diuretics* (amiloride, spironolactone, triamterene)	Level of potassium in blood too high.
Male hormones*	Fluid retention.
Potassium supplements*	Level of potassium in blood too high.
Vitamin D (calcifidiol and calcitriol)	Level of phosphorus in blood too high.

POSSIBLE INTERACTION WITH OTHER SUBSTANCES

INTERACTS WITH	COMBINED EFFECT
Alcohol:	None expected.
Beverages: Salty drinks such as tomato juice, commercial thirst quenchers, salt substitutes.	Increased fluid retention.
Cocaine:	May cause irregular heartbeat.
Foods: Salty foods such as canned soups, potato chips, TV dinners, hot dogs, pickles.	Increased fluid retention.
Marijuana:	May cause irregular heartbeat.
Tobacco:	May aggravate irregular heartbeat.

POTASSIUM SUPPLEMENTS

GENERIC AND BRAND NAMES

See complete list of generic and brand names in the *Generic and Brand Name Directory*, page 891.

BASIC INFORMATION

Habit forming? No
Prescription needed? Yes
Available as generic? Yes
Drug class: Mineral supplement (potassium)

USES

- Treatment for potassium deficiency due to diuretics, cortisone or digitalis medicines.
- Treatment for low potassium associated with some illnesses.

DOSAGE & USAGE INFORMATION

How to take:
- Tablet or capsule—Swallow with liquid or food to lessen stomach irritation. You may chew or crush tablet.
- Extended-release tablets or capsules—Swallow each dose whole with liquid.
- Effervescent tablets, granules, powder or liquid—Dilute dose in water.

When to take:
At the same time each day, preferably with food or immediately after meals.

If you forget a dose:
Take as soon as you remember. Don't double next dose.

What drug does:
Preserves or restores normal function of nerve cells, heart and skeletal muscle cells and kidneys, as well as stomach juice secretions.

Continued next column

OVERDOSE

SYMPTOMS:
Paralysis of arms and legs, irregular heart-beat, blood pressure drop, convulsions, coma, cardiac arrest.
WHAT TO DO:
- **Dial 911 (emergency) or 0 (operator) for an ambulance or medical help. Then give first aid immediately.**
- **See emergency information on inside covers.**

Time lapse before drug works:
1 to 2 hours. Full benefit may require 12 to 24 hours.

Don't take with:
Any other medicine without consulting your doctor or pharmacist.

POSSIBLE ADVERSE REACTIONS OR SIDE EFFECTS

SYMPTOMS	WHAT TO DO
Life-threatening:	
In case of overdose, see previous column.	
Common:	
None expected.	
Infrequent:	
Diarrhea, nausea, vomiting, skin rash, abdominal pain.	Continue. Call doctor when convenient.
Rare:	
• Confusion; irregular heartbeat; difficult breathing; unusual fatigue; weakness; heaviness of legs; hemorrhage, perforation with enteric-coated tablets (rarely with wax matrix tablets); esophageal ulceration with tablets; bloody stools.	Discontinue. Call doctor right away.
• Numbness or tingling in hands or feet, anxiety.	Continue. Call doctor when convenient.

WARNINGS & PRECAUTIONS

Don't take if:
- You are allergic to any potassium supplement.
- You have acute or chronic kidney disease.

Before you start, consult your doctor:
- If you have Addison's disease or familial periodic paralysis.
- If you have heart disease.
- If you have intestinal blockage.
- If you have a stomach ulcer.
- If you use diuretics.
- If you use heart medicine.
- If you use laxatives or have chronic diarrhea.
- If you use salt substitutes or low-salt milk.

Over age 60:
Observe dose schedule strictly. Potassium balance is critical. Deviation above or below normal can have serious results.

Pregnancy:
Decide with your doctor if drug benefits justify risk to unborn child. Risk category C (see page xxiii).

Breast-feeding:
Studies inconclusive on harm to infant. Consult doctor.

Infants & children:
Use only under doctor's supervision.

Prolonged use:
- Slows absorption of vitamin B-12. May cause anemia.
- Request frequent lab tests to monitor potassium levels in blood, especially if you take digitalis preparations.

Skin & sunlight:
No problems expected.

Driving, piloting or hazardous work:
No problems expected.

Discontinuing:
Don't discontinue without consulting doctor. Dose may require gradual reduction if you have taken drug for a long time. Doses of other drugs may also require adjustment.

Others:
- Overdose or underdose serious. Frequent EKGs and laboratory blood studies to measure serum electrolytes and kidney function recommended.
- Prolonged diarrhea may call for increased dosage of potassium.
- Serious injury may necessitate temporary decrease in potassium.
- Some products contain tartrazine dye. Avoid, especially if you are allergic to aspirin.

POSSIBLE INTERACTION WITH OTHER DRUGS

GENERIC NAME OR DRUG CLASS	COMBINED EFFECT
Adrenocorticoids, systemic	Decreased potassium effect.
Amiloride	Dangerous rise in blood potassium.
Angiotensin-converting enzyme (ACE) inhibitors*	Possible increased potassium effect.
Anticholinergics, other*	Increased possibility of intestinal ulcers, which sometimes occur with oral potassium tablets.
Anti-inflammatory drugs, nonsteroidal (NSAIDs)*	Increased risk of stomach irritation.

Beta-adrenergic blocking agents*	Increased potassium levels.
Digitalis preparations*	Possible irregular heartbeat.
Diuretics, thiazide or loop*	Decreased potassium effect.
Laxatives*	Possible decreased potassium effect.
Losartan	Increased potassium levels.
Potassium-containing drugs*	Increased potassium levels.
Spironolactone	Dangerous rise in blood potassium.
Triamterene	Dangerous rise in blood potassium.
Vitamin B-12	Extended-release tablets may decrease vitamin B-12 absorption and increase vitamin B-12 requirements.

POSSIBLE INTERACTION WITH OTHER SUBSTANCES

INTERACTS WITH	COMBINED EFFECT
Alcohol:	None expected.
Beverages: • Salty drinks such as tomato juice, commercial thirst quenchers.	Increased fluid retention.
• Low-salt milk or salt substitutes.	Increased potassium levels.
Cocaine:	May cause irregular heartbeat.
Foods: Salty foods.	Increased fluid retention.
Marijuana:	May cause irregular heartbeat.
Tobacco:	None expected.

PRIMAQUINE

GENERIC NAMES

PRIMAQUINE

BASIC INFORMATION

Habit forming? No
Prescription needed? Yes
Available as generic? Yes
Drug class: Antiprotozoal (antimalarial)

 ## USES

- Treats some forms of malaria.
- Prevents relapses of some forms of malaria.
- Treats pneumocystis carinii pneumonia (used in combination with clindamycin).

 ## DOSAGE & USAGE INFORMATION

How to take:
Tablets—Take with meals or antacids to minimize stomach irritation.

When to take:
At the same time each day, according to instructions on prescription label.

If you forget a dose:
Take as soon as you remember up to 2 hours late. If more than 2 hours, wait for next scheduled dose. Don't double this dose.

What drug does:
Alters the properties of DNA in malaria organisms to prevent them from multiplying.

Time lapse before drug works:
2 to 3 hours.

Don't take with:
Any other medicine without consulting your doctor or pharmacist.

 ## OVERDOSE

SYMPTOMS:
None expected.
WHAT TO DO:
Overdose unlikely to threaten life. If person takes much larger amount than prescribed, call doctor, poison control center or hospital emergency room for instructions.

 ## POSSIBLE ADVERSE REACTIONS OR SIDE EFFECTS

SYMPTOMS	WHAT TO DO
Life-threatening: None expected.	
Common: None expected.	
Infrequent: Dark urine; back, leg or stomach pain; appetite loss; pale skin; fever.	Discontinue. Call doctor right away.
Rare: Blue fingernails, lips and skin; dizziness; difficult breathing; extraordinary tiredness; sore throat; fever.	Discontinue. Call doctor right away.

WARNINGS & PRECAUTIONS

Don't take if:
- You have G6PD* deficiency.
- You are hypersensitive to primaquine.

Before you start, consult your doctor:
If you are Black, Oriental, Asian or of Mediterranean origin.

Over age 60:
No special problems expected.

Pregnancy:
Decide with your doctor if drug benefits justify risk to unborn child. Risk category C (see page xxiii).

Breast-feeding:
Effect unknown. Consult doctor.

Infants & children:
No special problems expected.

Prolonged use:
No special problems expected.

Skin & sunlight:
No special problems expected.

Driving, piloting or hazardous work:
No special problems expected.

Discontinuing:
No special problems expected.

Others:
- If you are Black, Asian, Oriental or of Mediterranean origin, insist on a test for G6PD* deficiency before taking this medicine.
- Advise any doctor or dentist whom you consult that you take this medicine.

 POSSIBLE INTERACTION WITH OTHER DRUGS

GENERIC NAME OR DRUG CLASS	COMBINED EFFECT
Hemolytics*, other	Increased risk of serious side effects affecting the blood.
Quinacrine	Increased toxic effects of primaquine.

 POSSIBLE INTERACTION WITH OTHER SUBSTANCES

INTERACTS WITH	COMBINED EFFECT
Alcohol:	Possible liver toxicity. Avoid.
Beverages:	None expected.
Cocaine:	None expected.
Foods:	None expected.
Marijuana:	None expected.
Tobacco:	None expected.

PRIMIDONE

BRAND NAMES

Apo-Primidone
Myidone
Mysoline

PMS Primadone
Sertan

BASIC INFORMATION

Habit forming? No
Prescription needed? Yes
Available as generic? Yes
Drug class: Anticonvulsant

USES

Prevents some forms of epileptic seizures.

DOSAGE & USAGE INFORMATION

How to take:
- Tablet—Swallow with liquid. If you can't swallow whole, crumble tablet and take with liquid or food.
- Liquid—If desired, dilute dose in beverage before swallowing.

When to take:
Daily in regularly spaced doses, according to doctor's prescription.

If you forget a dose:
Take as soon as you remember up to 2 hours late. If more than 2 hours, wait for next scheduled dose (don't double this dose).

What drug does:
Probably inhibits repetitious spread of impulses along nerve pathways.

Continued next column

OVERDOSE

SYMPTOMS:
Slow, shallow breathing; weak, rapid pulse; confusion, deep sleep, coma.
WHAT TO DO:
- Dial 911 (emergency) or 0 (operator) for an ambulance or medical help. Then give first aid immediately.
- If patient is unconscious and not breathing, give mouth-to-mouth breathing. If there is no heartbeat, use cardiac massage and mouth-to-mouth breathing (CPR). Don't try to make patient vomit. If you can't get help quickly, take patient to nearest emergency facility.
- See emergency information on inside covers.

Time lapse before drug works:
2 to 3 weeks.

Don't take with:
Any other medicine without consulting your doctor or pharmacist.

POSSIBLE ADVERSE REACTIONS OR SIDE EFFECTS

SYMPTOMS	WHAT TO DO
Life-threatening:	
In case of overdose, see previous column.	
Common:	
• Difficult breathing.	Discontinue. Call doctor right away.
• Confusion, change in vision.	Continue. Call doctor when convenient.
• Clumsiness, dizziness, drowsiness.	Continue. Tell doctor at next visit.
Infrequent:	
• Unusual excitement, particularly in children; nausea; vomiting.	Discontinue. Call doctor right away.
• Headache, fatigue, weakness.	Continue. Call doctor when convenient.
Rare:	
• Rash or hives, appetite loss, acute psychosis, hair loss, fever, joint pain.	Discontinue. Call doctor right away.
• Swollen eyelids or legs.	Continue. Call doctor when convenient.
• Decreased sexual ability.	Continue. Tell doctor at next visit.

WARNINGS & PRECAUTIONS

Don't take if:
- You are allergic to any barbiturate.
- You have had porphyria.

Before you start, consult your doctor:
- If you have had liver, kidney or lung disease or asthma.
- If you have lupus.

Over age 60:
Adverse reactions and side effects may be more frequent and severe than in younger persons.

Pregnancy:
Consult doctor. Risk category D (see page xxiii).

Breast-feeding:
Drug filters into milk. May harm child. Avoid. Consult doctor.

Infants & children:
Use only under medical supervision.

Prolonged use:
- Enlarged lymph and thyroid glands.
- Anemia.
- Rickets in children and osteomalacia (insufficient calcium to bones) in adults.
- Talk to your doctor about the need for follow-up medical examinations or laboratory studies to check complete blood counts (white blood cell count, platelet count, red blood cell count, hemoglobin, hematocrit), liver function, kidney function.

Skin & sunlight:
No special problems expected.

Driving, piloting or hazardous work:
Don't drive or pilot aircraft until you learn how medicine affects you. Don't work around dangerous machinery. Don't climb ladders or work in high places. Danger increases if you drink alcohol or take medicine affecting alertness and reflexes.

Discontinuing:
Don't discontinue abruptly or without doctor's advice until you complete prescribed dose, even though symptoms diminish or disappear.

Others:
- Tell doctor if you become ill or injured and must interrupt dose schedule.
- Periodic laboratory blood tests of drug level recommended.

 POSSIBLE INTERACTION WITH OTHER DRUGS

GENERIC NAME OR DRUG CLASS	COMBINED EFFECT
Adrenocorticoids, systemic	Decreased adreno-corticoid effect.
Anticoagulants*, oral	Decreased primidone effect.
Anticonvulsants*, other	Changed seizure pattern.
Antidepressants*	Increased anti-depressant effect.
Antihistamines*	Increased sedation effect of primidone.
Aspirin	Decreased aspirin effect.
Carbamazepine	Unpredictable increase or decrease of primidone effect.
Carbonic anhydrase inhibitors*	Possible decreased primidone effect.
Central nervous system (CNS) depressants*	Increased CNS depressant effects.

Contraceptives, oral*	Decreased contraceptive effect.
Cyclosporine	Decreased cyclosporine effect.
Digitalis preparations*	Decreased digitalis effect.
Disulfiram	Possible increased primidone effect.
Estrogens*	Decreased estrogen effect.
Griseofulvin	Possible decreased griseofulvin effect.
Isoniazid	Decreased primidone effect.
Lamotrigine	Decreased lamotrigine effect.
Leucovorin (large dose)	May counteract anti-convulsant effect of primidone.
Loxapine	Decreased anti-convulsant effect of primidone.
Metronidazole	Possible decreased metronidazole effect.
Mind-altering drugs*	Increased effect of mind-altering drug.
Monoamine oxidase (MAO) inhibitors*	Increased sedation effect of primidone.
Nabilone	Greater depression of central nervous system.

Continued on page 929

 POSSIBLE INTERACTION WITH OTHER SUBSTANCES

INTERACTS WITH	COMBINED EFFECT
Alcohol:	Dangerous sedative effect. Avoid.
Beverages:	None expected.
Cocaine:	Decreased primidone effect.
Foods:	Possible need for more vitamin D.
Marijuana:	Decreased anti-convulsant effect of primidone. Drowsiness, unsteadiness.
Tobacco:	None expected.

*See Glossary

PROBENECID

BRAND NAMES

Benemid   Probalan
Benuryl

BASIC INFORMATION

Habit forming? No
Prescription needed? Yes
Available as generic? Yes
Drug class: Antigout

 ## USES

- Treats chronic gout.
- Increases blood levels of penicillins and cephalosporins.

 ## DOSAGE & USAGE INFORMATION

How to take:
Tablet—Swallow with liquid or food to lessen stomach irritation. If you can't swallow whole, crumble tablet and take with liquid or food.

When to take:
At the same time each day.

If you forget a dose:
Take as soon as you remember up to 12 hours late. If more than 12 hours, wait for next scheduled dose (don't double this dose).

What drug does:
- Forces kidneys to excrete uric acid.
- Reduces amount of penicillin excreted in urine.

Time lapse before drug works:
May require several months of regular use to prevent acute gout.

Don't take with:
- Nonprescription drugs containing aspirin or caffeine.
- Any other medicine without consulting your doctor or pharmacist.

 ## OVERDOSE

SYMPTOMS:
Breathing difficulty, severe nervous agitation, vomiting, seizures, convulsions, delirium, coma.
WHAT TO DO:
- **Dial 911 (emergency) or 0 (operator) for an ambulance or medical help. Then give first aid immediately.**
- **See emergency information on inside covers.**

 ## POSSIBLE ADVERSE REACTIONS OR SIDE EFFECTS

SYMPTOMS	WHAT TO DO
Life-threatening:	
In case of overdose, see previous column.	
Common:	
Headache, appetite loss, nausea, vomiting.	Continue. Call doctor when convenient.
Infrequent:	
• Blood in urine, low back pain. worsening gout.	Discontinue. Call doctor right away.
• Dizziness, flushed face, itchy skin.	Continue. Call doctor when convenient.
• Painful or frequent urination, sore gums.	Continue. Tell doctor at next visit.
Rare:	
Sore throat, fever and chills; difficult breathing; unusual bleeding or bruising; red, painful joint; jaundice; foot, leg or face swelling.	Discontinue. Call doctor right away.

 ## WARNINGS & PRECAUTIONS

Don't take if:
- You are allergic to any uricosuric*.
- You have acute gout.
- Patient is younger than 2.

Before you start, consult your doctor:
- If you have had kidney stones or kidney disease.
- If you have a peptic ulcer.
- If you have bone marrow or blood cell disease.
- If you are undergoing chemotherapy for cancer.

Over age 60:
Adverse reactions and side effects may be more frequent and severe than in younger persons.

Pregnancy:
Consult doctor. Risk category B (see page xxiii).

Breast-feeding:
Effect unknown. Consult doctor.

Infants & children:
Not recommended.

Prolonged use:
- Possible kidney damage.
- Talk to your doctor about the need for follow-up medical examinations or laboratory studies to check serum uric acid, urine uric acid.

Skin & sunlight:
No problems expected.

Driving, piloting or hazardous work:
Avoid if you feel dizzy. Otherwise, no problems expected.

Discontinuing:
Don't discontinue without consulting doctor. Dose may require gradual reduction if you have taken drug for a long time. Doses of other drugs may also require adjustment.

Others:
If signs of gout attack develop while taking medicine, consult doctor.

 ## POSSIBLE INTERACTION WITH OTHER DRUGS

GENERIC NAME OR DRUG CLASS	COMBINED EFFECT
Allopurinol	Increased effect of each drug.
Anticoagulants*, oral	Increased anti-coagulant effect.
Anti-inflammatory drugs, nonsteroidal (NSAIDs)*	Increased toxic risk.
Aspirin	Decreased probenecid effect.
Bismuth subsalicylate	Decreased probenecid effect.
Cephalosporins*	Increased cephalosporin effect.
Ciprofloxacin	May cause kidney dysfunction.
Dapsone	Increased dapsone effect. Increased toxicity.
Diclofenac	Increased diclofenac effect.
Diuretics, thiazide*	Decreased probenecid effect.
Hypoglycemics, oral*	Increased hypo-glycemic effect.
Indomethacin	Increased adverse effects of indomethacin.
Ketoprofen	Increased risk of ketoprofen toxicity.

Loracarbef	Increased loracarbef effect.
Methotrexate	Increased methotrexate toxicity.
Nitrofurantoin	Incresed effect of nitrofurantoin.
Para-aminosalicylic acid	Increased effect of para-aminosalicylic acid.
Penicillins*	Enhanced penicillin effect.
Pyrazinamide	Decreased probenecid effect.
Salicylates*	Decreased probenecid effect.
Sodium benzoate & sodium phenylacetate	May reduce effect of sodium benzoate & sodium phenylacetate.
Sulfa drugs*	Slows elimination. May cause harmful accumulation of sulfa.
Thioguanine	More likelihood of toxicity of both drugs.
Valacyclovir	Increased valacyclovir effect.
Zidovudine	Increased zidovudine toxicity risk.

 ## POSSIBLE INTERACTION WITH OTHER SUBSTANCES

INTERACTS WITH	COMBINED EFFECT
Alcohol:	Decreased probenecid effect.
Beverages: Caffeine drinks.	Loss of probenecid effectiveness.
Cocaine:	None expected.
Foods:	None expected.
Marijuana:	Daily use— Decreased probenecid effect.
Tobacco:	None expected.

PROBENECID & COLCHICINE

BRAND NAMES

Col Benemid   Proben-C
Col-Probenecid

BASIC INFORMATION

Habit forming? No
Prescription needed? Yes
Available as generic? Yes
Drug class: Antigout

USES

- Increases blood levels of penicillins and cephalosporins.
- Relieves joint pain, inflammation, swelling from gout.
- Also used for familial Mediterranean fever, dermatitis herpetiformis.

DOSAGE & USAGE INFORMATION

How to take:
Tablet—Swallow with liquid or food to lessen stomach irritation. If you can't swallow whole, crumble tablet and take with liquid or food.

When to take:
At the same time each day.

If you forget a dose:
Take as soon as you remember up to 12 hours late. If more than 12 hours, wait for next scheduled dose (don't double this dose).

What drug does:
- Forces kidneys to excrete uric acid.
- Reduces amount of penicillin excreted in urine.
- Decreases acidity of joint tissues and prevents deposits of uric acid crystals.

Time lapse before drug works:
12 to 48 hours.

Continued next column

OVERDOSE

SYMPTOMS:
Breathing difficulty, severe nervous agitation, convulsions, bloody urine, diarrhea, vomiting, muscle weakness, fever, stupor, seizures, delirium, coma.
WHAT TO DO:
- **Dial 911 (emergency) or 0 (operator) for an ambulance or medical help. Then give first aid immediately.**
- **See emergency information on inside covers.**

Don't take with:
- Nonprescription drugs containing aspirin or caffeine.
- Any other medicine without consulting your doctor or pharmacist.

POSSIBLE ADVERSE REACTIONS OR SIDE EFFECTS

SYMPTOMS	WHAT TO DO
Life-threatening: Blood in urine; convulsions; severe muscle weakness; difficult breathing; burning feeling of stomach, throat or skin; worsening gout.	Discontinue. Seek emergency treatment.
Common: Diarrhea, headache, abdominal pain.	Discontinue. Call doctor right away.
Infrequent: • Back pain; painful, difficult urination.	Discontinue. Call doctor right away.
• Dizziness, red or flushed face, urgent urination, sore gums, hair loss.	Continue. Call doctor when convenient.
Rare: Sudden decrease in urine output; nausea; vomiting; mood change; fever; chills; diarrhea; jaundice; numbness or tingling in hands or feet; rash; sore throat, fever, mouth sores; swollen face, feet and ankles; unexplained bleeding or bruising; weight gain or loss; low white or red blood cells.	Discontinue. Call doctor right away.

WARNINGS & PRECAUTIONS

Don't take if:
You are allergic to any uricosuric* or colchicine.

Before you start, consult your doctor:
- If you have had kidney stones, kidney disease, heart or liver disease, peptic ulcers or ulcerative colitis.
- If you have bone marrow or blood cell disease.
- If you will have surgery within 2 months, including dental surgery, requiring general or spinal anesthesia.
- If you are undergoing chemotherapy for cancer.

Over age 60:
Adverse reactions and side effects may be more frequent and severe than in younger persons. Colchicine has a narrow margin of safety for people in this age group.

Pregnancy:
Risk factor varies with length of pregnancy. See category list on page xxiii and consult doctor.

Breast-feeding:
No problems expected, but consult doctor.

Infants & children:
Not recommended.

Prolonged use:
- Possible kidney damage.
- Permanent hair loss.
- Anemia. Request blood counts.
- Numbness or tingling in hands and feet.
- Talk to your doctor about the need for follow-up medical examinations or laboratory studies to check serum uric acid, urine uric acid.

Skin & sunlight:
No problems expected.

Driving, piloting or hazardous work:
Don't drive or pilot aircraft until you learn how medicine affects you. Don't work around dangerous machinery. Don't climb ladders or work in high places. Danger increases if you drink alcohol or take medicine affecting alertness and reflexes, such as antihistamines, tranquilizers, sedatives, pain medicine, narcotics and mind-altering drugs.

Discontinuing:
- May be unnecessary to finish medicine. Follow doctor's instructions.
- Stop taking if severe digestive upsets occur before symptoms are relieved.

Others:
- If signs of gout attack develop while taking medicine, consult doctor.
- Limit each course of treatment to 8 mg. Don't exceed 3 mg per 24 hours.
- May decrease sperm count in males.

POSSIBLE INTERACTION WITH OTHER DRUGS

GENERIC NAME OR DRUG CLASS	COMBINED EFFECT
Acetohexamide	Increased acetohexamide effect.
Allopurinol	Increased effect of each drug.

Anticoagulants*, oral	Irregular effect on anticoagulation, sometimes increased, sometimes decreased. Follow prothrombin times.
Antidepressants*	Oversedation.
Antihistamines*	Oversedation.
Antihypertensives*	Decreased antihypertensive effect.
Anti-inflammatory drugs, nonsteroidal (NSAIDs)*	Increased toxic risk.
Appetite suppressants*	Increased appetite suppressant effect.
Bismuth subsalicylate	Decreased probenecid effect.
Cephalosporins*	Increased cephalosporin effect.
Dapsone	Increased dapsone effect. Increased toxicity.
Diclofenac	Increased diclofenac effect.
Diuretics, thiazide*	Decreased probenecid effect.
Indomethacin	Increased adverse effects of indomethacin.
Ketoprofen	Increased effect of ketoprofen toxicity.

Continued on page 929

POSSIBLE INTERACTION WITH OTHER SUBSTANCES

INTERACTS WITH	COMBINED EFFECT
Alcohol:	Decreased probenecid effect.
Beverages: Caffeine drinks.	Loss of probenecid effectiveness.
Herbal teas.	Increased colchicine effect. Avoid.
Cocaine:	Overstimulation. Avoid.
Foods:	No proven problems.
Marijuana:	Decreased colchicine and probenecid effect.
Tobacco:	No proven problems.

*See Glossary

PROBUCOL

BRAND NAMES

Lorelco

BASIC INFORMATION

Habit forming? No
Prescription needed? Yes
Available as generic? No
Drug class: Antihyperlipidemic

 ## USES

Lowers cholesterol level in blood in persons with type IIa hyperlipoproteinemia.

 ## DOSAGE & USAGE INFORMATION

How to take:
Tablet—Swallow with liquid. If you can't swallow whole, crumble tablet and take with liquid or food.

When to take:
With morning and evening meals.

If you forget a dose:
Take as soon as you remember up to 2 hours late. If more than 2 hours, wait for next scheduled dose (don't double this dose).

What drug does:
Reduces serum cholesterol without reducing liver cholesterol.

Time lapse before drug works:
3 to 4 months.

Don't take with:
Other medicines or vitamins. Separate by 1 to 2 hours.

 ## OVERDOSE

SYMPTOMS:
None reported.
WHAT TO DO:
Overdose unlikely to threaten life. If person takes much larger amount than prescribed, call doctor, poison control center or hospital emergency room for instructions.

 ## POSSIBLE ADVERSE REACTIONS OR SIDE EFFECTS

SYMPTOMS	WHAT TO DO
Life-threatening: None expected.	
Common: Bloating, diarrhea, nausea, vomiting, abdominal pain, flatus.	Continue. Call doctor when convenient.
Infrequent:	
• Dizziness, headache.	Discontinue. Call doctor right away.
• Numbness or tingling in feet, toes, fingers, face.	Continue. Call doctor when convenient.
Rare:	
• Swelling of hands, face, feet, mouth.	Discontinue. Seek emergency treatment.
• Rash.	Discontinue. Call doctor right away.

WARNINGS & PRECAUTIONS

Don't take if:
You are allergic to probucol.

Before you start, consult your doctor:
- If you have liver disease such as cirrhosis.
- If you have heartbeat irregularity.
- If you have congestive heart failure that is not under control.
- If you have gallstones.

Over age 60:
Adverse reactions and side effects may be more frequent and severe than in younger persons.

Pregnancy:
No proven problems. Avoid if possible. Continue using birth control methods for 6 months after discontinuing medicine. Consult doctor. Risk category B (see page xxiii).

Breast-feeding:
Not recommended. Animal studies show drug passes into milk. Studies not available for human beings. Consult doctor.

Infants & children:
Not recommended. Safety and dosage have not been established.

Prolonged use:
Request serum cholesterol and serum triglyceride laboratory studies every 2 to 4 months.

Skin & sunlight:
No problems expected.

Driving, piloting or hazardous work:
If medicine does not cause dizziness, no problems expected.

Discontinuing:
Don't discontinue without consulting doctor. Dose may require gradual reduction if you have taken drug for a long time. Doses of other drugs may also require adjustment.

Others:
- Medicine works best in conjunction with low-fat, low-cholesterol diet and an active, regular exercise program.
- May affect results in some medical tests.

POSSIBLE INTERACTION WITH OTHER DRUGS

GENERIC NAME OR DRUG CLASS	COMBINED EFFECT
Chenodiol	Decreased chenodiol effect.
Clofibrate	Combination no more effective than one drug only, so don't take both.
Dexfenfluramine	May require dosage change as weight loss occurs.
Ursodiol	Decreased ursodiol effect.

POSSIBLE INTERACTION WITH OTHER SUBSTANCES

INTERACTS WITH	COMBINED EFFECT
Alcohol:	May aggravate liver problems. Avoid.
Beverages:	None expected.
Cocaine:	None expected.
Foods:	None expected.
Marijuana:	None expected.
Tobacco:	None expected.

PROCAINAMIDE

BRAND NAMES

Procan SR   Pronestyl
Promine   Pronestyl SR

BASIC INFORMATION

Habit forming? No
Prescription needed? Yes
Available as generic? Yes
Drug class: Antiarrhythmic

USES

Stabilizes irregular heartbeat.

DOSAGE & USAGE INFORMATION

How to take:
- Tablet or capsule—Swallow with liquid.
- Extended-release tablets—Swallow each dose whole. Do not crush them.

When to take:
Best taken on empty stomach, 1 hour before or 2 hours after meals. If necessary, may be taken with food or milk to lessen stomach upset.

If you forget a dose:
Take as soon as you remember up to 2 hours late (4 hours for extended-release tablets). If more than 2 hours, wait for next scheduled dose (don't double this dose).

What drug does:
Slows activity of pacemaker (rhythm control center of heart) and delays transmission of electrical impulses.

Time lapse before drug works:
30 to 60 minutes.

Don't take with:
Any other medicine without consulting your doctor or pharmacist.

OVERDOSE

SYMPTOMS:
Fast and irregular heartbeat, confusion, stupor, decreased blood pressure, fainting, cardiac arrest.
WHAT TO DO:
- **Dial 911 (emergency) or 0 (operator) for an ambulance or medical help. Then give first aid immediately.**
- **See emergency information on inside covers.**

POSSIBLE ADVERSE REACTIONS OR SIDE EFFECTS

SYMPTOMS	WHAT TO DO
Life-threatening: Hives, rash, intense itching, faintness soon after dose (anaphylaxis); convulsions.	Seek emergency treatment immediately.
Common: Diarrhea, appetite loss, nausea, vomiting, bitter taste.	Continue. Call doctor when convenient.
Infrequent: Joint pain, painful breathing, dizziness.	Discontinue. Call doctor right away.
Rare: • Hallucinations, depression, confusion, psychosis, itchy skin, rash, sore throat, fever, jaundice, unusual bleeding or bruising.	Discontinue. Call doctor right away.
• Headache, fatigue.	Continue. Call doctor when convenient.

WARNINGS & PRECAUTIONS

Don't take if:
- You are allergic to procainamide.
- You have myasthenia gravis.

Before you start, consult your doctor:
- If you are allergic to local anesthetics that end in "caine."
- If you have had liver or kidney disease or impaired kidney function.
- If you have had lupus.
- If you take digitalis preparations*.
- If you will have surgery within 2 months, including dental surgery, requiring general or spinal anesthesia.

Over age 60:
Adverse reactions and side effects may be more frequent and severe than in younger persons.

Pregnancy:
Decide with your doctor if drug benefits justify risk to unborn child. Risk category C (see page xxiii).

Breast-feeding:
No proven problems. Consult doctor.

Infants & children:
Not recommended.

Prolonged use:
- May cause lupus*-like illness.
- Talk to your doctor about the need for follow-up medical examinations or laboratory studies to check ANA titers*, blood pressure, complete blood counts (white blood cell count, platelet count, red blood cell count, hemoglobin, hematocrit).

Skin & sunlight:
No problems expected.

Driving, piloting or hazardous work:
Use caution if you feel dizzy or weak. Otherwise, no problems expected.

Discontinuing:
Don't discontinue without doctor's advice until you complete prescribed dose, even though symptoms diminish or disappear.

Others:
- Some products contain tartrazine dye. Avoid, especially if you are allergic to aspirin.
- May affect results of some medical tests.

POSSIBLE INTERACTION WITH OTHER DRUGS

GENERIC NAME OR DRUG CLASS	COMBINED EFFECT
Acetazolamide	Increased procainamide effect.
Ambenonium	Decreased ambenonium effect.
Aminoglycosides*	Possible severe muscle weakness, impaired breathing.
Antiarrhythmics*, other	Increased likelihood of adverse reactions with either drug. Possible increased effect of both drugs.
Anticholinergics*	Increased anti-cholinergic effect.
Antihypertensives*	Increased anti-hypertensive effect.
Antimyasthenics*	Decreased anti-myasthenic effect.
Cimetidine	Increased procainamide effect.
Cisapride	Decreased procainamide effect.
Metformin	Increased metformin effect.

POSSIBLE INTERACTION WITH OTHER SUBSTANCES

INTERACTS WITH	COMBINED EFFECT
Alcohol:	None expected.
Beverages: Caffeine drinks, iced drinks.	Irregular heartbeat.
Cocaine:	Decreased procainamide effect.
Foods:	None expected.
Marijuana:	None expected.
Tobacco:	Decreased procainamide effect.

PROCARBAZINE

BRAND NAMES

Matulane   Natulan

BASIC INFORMATION

Habit forming? No
Prescription needed? Yes
Available as generic? No
Drug class: Antineoplastic

 ## USES

Treatment for some kinds of cancer.

 ## DOSAGE & USAGE INFORMATION

How to take:
Capsule—Swallow with liquid after light meal.
Don't drink fluids with meals. Drink extra fluids
between meals. Avoid sweet or fatty foods.

When to take:
At the same time each day.

If you forget a dose:
Take as soon as you remember. Don't double
dose ever.

What drug does:
Inhibits abnormal cell reproduction. Procarbazine
is an alkylating agent* and an MAO inhibitor.

Time lapse before drug works:
Up to 6 weeks for full effect.

Don't take with:
Any other medicine without consulting your
doctor or pharmacist.

 ## OVERDOSE

SYMPTOMS:
**Restlessness, agitation, fever, convulsions,
bleeding.**
WHAT TO DO:
- **Dial 911 (emergency) or 0 (operator) for an
  ambulance or medical help. Then give first
  aid immediately.**
- **If patient is unconscious and not breathing,
  give mouth-to-mouth breathing. If there is
  no heartbeat, use cardiac massage and
  mouth-to-mouth breathing (CPR). Don't try
  to make patient vomit. If you can't get help
  quickly, take patient to nearest emergency
  facility.**
- **See emergency information on inside
  covers.**

 ## POSSIBLE ADVERSE REACTIONS OR SIDE EFFECTS

SYMPTOMS	WHAT TO DO
Life-threatening:	
In case of overdose, see previous column.	
Common:	
• Nausea, vomiting, decreased urination, numbness or tingling in hands or feet, hair loss, rapid or pounding heartbeat, shortness of breath.	Discontinue. Call doctor right away.
• Fatigue, weakness, confusion.	Continue. Call doctor when convenient.
• Dizziness when changing position, dry mouth, inflamed tongue, constipation, difficult urination.	Continue. Tell doctor at next visit.
Infrequent:	
• Fainting.	Discontinue. Seek emergency treatment.
• Severe headache; abnormal bleeding or bruising; muscle, joint or chest pain, enlarged eye pupils; black, tarry stools; bloody urine.	Discontinue. Call doctor right away.
• Hallucinations, insomnia, nightmares, diarrhea, swollen feet or legs, nervousness, eyes sensitive to light, cough or hoarseness, mouth sores depression.	Continue. Call doctor when convenient.
• Diminished sex drive.	Continue. Tell doctor at next visit.
Rare:	
Rash, stiff neck, jaundice, fever, sore throat, vomiting blood, wheezing.	Discontinue. Call doctor right away.

 ## WARNINGS & PRECAUTIONS

Don't take if:
- You are allergic to any MAO inhibitor.
- You have heart disease, congestive heart
  failure, heart rhythm irregularities or high blood
  pressure.
- You have liver or kidney disease.

Before you start, consult your doctor:
- If you are alcoholic.
- If you have asthma.
- If you have had a stroke.

- If you have diabetes or epilepsy.
- If you have overactive thyroid.
- If you have schizophrenia.
- If you have Parkinson's disease.
- If you have adrenal gland tumor.
- If you will have surgery within 2 months, including dental surgery, requiring general or spinal anesthesia.

Over age 60:
Not recommended.

Pregnancy:
Consult doctor. Risk category D (see page xxiii).

Breast-feeding:
Safety not established. Consult doctor.

Infants & children:
Not recommended.

Prolonged use:
- May be toxic to liver.
- Talk to your doctor about the need for follow-up medical examinations or laboratory studies to check complete blood counts (white blood cell count, platelet count, red blood cell count, hemoglobin, hematocrit), bone marrow, kidney function.

Skin & sunlight:
No special problems expected.

Driving, piloting or hazardous work:
Don't drive or pilot aircraft until you learn how medicine affects you. Don't work around dangerous machinery. Don't climb ladders or work in high places. Danger increases if you drink alcohol or take medicine affecting alertness and reflexes.

Discontinuing:
- Don't discontinue without doctor's advice until you complete prescribed dose, even though symptoms diminish or disappear.
- Follow precautions regarding foods, drinks and other medicines for 2 weeks after discontinuing.

Others:
- May affect blood sugar levels in patients with diabetes.
- Advise any doctor or dentist whom you consult that you take this drug.

POSSIBLE INTERACTION WITH OTHER DRUGS

GENERIC NAME OR DRUG CLASS	COMBINED EFFECT
Amphetamines*	Blood pressure rise to life-threatening level.
Anticonvulsants*, oral	Changed seizure pattern.
Antidepressants, tricyclic*	Blood pressure rise to life-threatening level.
Antidiabetics*, oral and insulin	Excessively low blood sugar.
Antihistamines*	Increased sedation.
Barbiturates*	Increased sedation.
Bone marrow depressants*	Increased toxicity to bone marrow.
Buspirone	Elevated blood pressure.
Caffeine	Irregular heartbeat or high blood pressure.
Carbamazepine	Fever, seizures. Avoid.
Central nervous system (CNS) depressants*	Increased CNS depression.
Clozapine	Toxic effect on bone marrow and central nervous system.
Cyclobenzaprine	Fever, seizures. Avoid.
Dextromethorphan	Fever, hypertension.

Continued on page 929

POSSIBLE INTERACTION WITH OTHER SUBSTANCES

INTERACTS WITH	COMBINED EFFECT
Alcohol:	Increased sedation to dangerous level. Disulfiram-like reaction*.
Beverages: Caffeine drinks.	Irregular heartbeat or high blood pressure.
Drinks containing tyramine*.	Blood pressure rise to life-threatening level.
Cocaine:	Overstimulation. Possibly fatal.
Foods: Foods containing tyramine*.	Blood pressure rise to life-threatening level.
Marijuana:	Overstimulation. Avoid.
Tobacco:	No proven problems.

PROGESTINS

GENERIC AND BRAND NAMES

See complete list of generic and brand names in the *Generic and Brand Names Directory*, page 891.

BASIC INFORMATION

Habit forming? No
Prescription needed? Yes
Available as generic? Yes, for some.
Drug class: Female sex hormone (progestin)

USES

- Treatment for menstrual or uterine disorders caused by progestin imbalance.
- Contraceptive (when combined with estrogens in birth control pills).
- Treatment for cancer of breast and uterus.
- Treatment for toxic sleep apnea.
- Treatment for female hormone imbalance.
- Megestrol is used for treatment of weight loss in AIDS and cancer patients.
- Treatment for female infertility caused by progesterone deficiency.
- Treatment for hyperplasia.

DOSAGE & USAGE INFORMATION

How to take:
- Capsule—Swallow with liquid. Do not crush, chew or break.
- Tablet—Swallow with liquid or food to lessen stomach irritation. You may crumble tablet.
- Injection—Under doctor's supervision.
- Oral suspension—Follow package instructions.

When to take:
At the same time each day.

If you forget a dose:
- Treatment for menstrual disorders—Take up to 2 hours late. If more than 2 hours, wait for next dose (don't double this dose).
- Contraceptive—Consult your doctor. You may need to use another birth control method until next period.

Continued next column

OVERDOSE

SYMPTOMS:
Nausea, vomiting, fluid retention, breast discomfort or enlargement, vaginal bleeding.
WHAT TO DO:
Overdose unlikely to threaten life. If person takes much larger amount than prescribed, call doctor, poison control center or hospital emergency room for instructions.

What drug does:
- Creates a uterine lining similar to that of pregnancy that prevents bleeding.
- Suppresses a pituitary gland hormone responsible for ovulation.
- Stimulates cervical mucus, which stops sperm penetration and prevents pregnancy.
- Mechanism that produces weight gain is unknown. Appears to stimulate appetite and metabolism without fluid retention.

Time lapse before drug works:
- Menstrual disorders—24 to 48 hours.
- Contraception—3 weeks.
- Cancer—May require 2 to 3 months regular use for maximum benefit.

Don't take with:
Any other medicine without consulting your doctor or pharmacist.

POSSIBLE ADVERSE REACTIONS OR SIDE EFFECTS

SYMPTOMS	WHAT TO DO
Life-threatening: Blood clot in leg, brain or lung; hives, rash, intense itching, faintness soon after a dose (anaphylaxis).	Seek emergency treatment immediately.
Common: Appetite or weight changes, swollen feet or ankles, unusual tiredness or weakness, menstrual cycle changes.	Continue. Tell doctor at next visit.
Infrequent: • Prolonged vaginal bleeding, pain in calf. • Depression. • Acne, increased facial or body hair, nausea, tender breasts, headache, enlarged clitoris.	Discontinue. Call doctor right away. Continue. Call doctor when convenient. Continue. Tell doctor at next visit.
Rare: • Rash, stomach or side pain, jaundice, fever, vision changes. • Amenorrhea*, hair loss, insomnia, brown skin spots, voice change.	Discontinue. Call doctor right away. Continue. Call doctor when convenient.

WARNINGS & PRECAUTIONS

Don't take if:
- You are allergic to any progestin hormone.
- You may be pregnant.
- You have liver or gallbladder disease.
- You have had thrombophlebitis, embolism or stroke.
- You have unexplained vaginal bleeding.
- You have had breast or uterine cancer.

Before you start, consult your doctor:
- If you have heart or kidney disease.
- If you have diabetes.
- If you have a seizure disorder.
- If you suffer migraines.
- If you are easily depressed.

Over age 60:
No special problems expected.

Pregnancy:
Risk factors vary for drugs in this group. See category list on page xxiii and consult doctor.

Breast-feeding:
Drug passes into milk. Avoid drug or discontinue nursing until you finish medicine. Consult doctor for advice on maintaining milk supply.

Infants & children:
Use only for female children under medical supervision.

Prolonged use:
No problems expected.

Skin & sunlight:
No problems expected.

Driving, piloting or hazardous work:
No problems expected.

Discontinuing:
Consult doctor. This medicine stays in the body and causes fetal abnormalities. Wait at least 3 months before becoming pregnant.

Others:
- Patients with diabetes must be monitored closely.
- Symptoms of blood clot in leg, brain or lung are: chest, groin, leg pain; sudden, severe headache; loss of coordination; vision change; shortness of breath; slurred speech.
- May affect results in some medical tests.
- Advise any doctor or dentist whom you consult that you take this medicine.

POSSIBLE INTERACTION WITH OTHER DRUGS

GENERIC NAME OR DRUG CLASS	COMBINED EFFECT
Bromocriptine	Decreased bromocriptine effect.
Hypoglycemics, oral*	Decreased oral hypoglycemic effect.
Insulin	Decreased insulin effect.
Phenobarbital	Decreased progestin effect.
Phenothiazines*	Increased phenothiazine effect.
Phenylbutazone	Decreased progestin effect.
Rifampin	Decreased contraceptive effect.

POSSIBLE INTERACTION WITH OTHER SUBSTANCES

INTERACTS WITH	COMBINED EFFECT
Alcohol:	None expected.
Beverages:	None expected.
Cocaine:	Decreased progestin effect.
Foods: Salt.	Fluid retention.
Marijuana:	Possible menstrual irregularities or bleeding between periods.
Tobacco: All forms.	Possible blood clots in lung, brain, legs. Avoid.

PROPAFENONE

BRAND NAMES

Rhythmol

BASIC INFORMATION

Habit forming? No
Prescription needed? Yes
Available as generic? No
Drug class: Antiarrhythmic

 USES

Treats severe heartbeat irregularities (life-threatening ventricular rhythm disturbances).

 DOSAGE & USAGE INFORMATION

How to take:
Tablet—Swallow with liquid or food to lessen stomach irritation. If you can't swallow whole, crumble tablet and take with liquid or food.

When to take:
At the same time each day, according to instructions on prescription label.

If you forget a dose:
Take as soon as you remember up to 2 hours late. If more than 2 hours, wait for next scheduled dose. Don't double this dose.

What drug does:
Slows electrical activity in the heart to decrease the excitability of the heart muscle.

Time lapse before drug works:
3-1/2 hours to 1 week for full effect. Begins working almost immediately.

Don't take with:
Any other medicine (including nonprescription drugs such as cough and cold medicines, nose drops, vitamins, laxatives, antacids, diet pills, or caffeine) without consulting your doctor or pharmacist.

 OVERDOSE

SYMPTOMS:
Very rapid heart rate that is also irregular.
WHAT TO DO:
Overdose unlikely to threaten life. If person takes much larger amount than prescribed, call doctor, poison control center or hospital emergency room for instructions.

 POSSIBLE ADVERSE REACTIONS OR SIDE EFFECTS

SYMPTOMS	WHAT TO DO
Life-threatening:	
Severe chest pain, severe shortness of breath	Seek emergency treatment.
Common:	
• Faster or more irregular heartbeat.	Discontinue. Call doctor right away.
• Taste change, dizziness.	Continue. Call doctor when convenient.
Infrequent:	
• Blurred vision, skin rash.	Discontinue. Call doctor right away.
• Constipation, diarrhea.	Continue. Call doctor when convenient.
• Dry mouth, nausea.	Continue. Tell doctor at next visit.
Rare:	
Fever, chills, trembling, joint pain, slow heartbeat.	Discontinue. Call doctor right away.

WARNINGS & PRECAUTIONS

Don't take if:
You are allergic to propafenone.

Before you start, consult your doctor:
- If you have asthma or bronchospasm.
- If you have congestive heart failure.
- If you have liver disease or kidney disease.
- If you have a recent history of heart attack.
- If you have a pacemaker.

Over age 60:
More likely to have decreased kidney function and require dosage modification.

Pregnancy:
Decide with your doctor if drug benefits justify risk to unborn child. Risk category C (see page xxiii).

Breast-feeding:
No proven problems. Consult doctor.

Infants & children:
Safety and efficacy not established.

Prolonged use:
Don't discontinue without consulting doctor. Dose may require gradual reduction if you have taken drug for a long time. Dosages of other drugs may also require adjustment.

Skin & sunlight:
No special problems expected.

Driving, piloting or hazardous work:
Don't drive or pilot aircraft until you learn how medicine affects you. Don't work around dangerous machinery. Don't climb ladders or work in high places. Danger increases if you drink alcohol or take medicine affecting alertness and reflexes.

Discontinuing:
Don't discontinue without consulting doctor. Dose may require gradual reduction if you have taken drug for a long time. Doses of other drugs may also require adjustment.

Others:
- Advise any doctor or dentist whom you consult that you take this medicine, especially if you are to be anesthetized.
- Report changes in symptoms to your doctor and return for periodic visits to check progress.
- Carry or wear a medical I.D. card or bracelet.

POSSIBLE INTERACTION WITH OTHER DRUGS

GENERIC NAME OR DRUG CLASS	COMBINED EFFECT
Anesthetics, local (e.g., prior to dental procedures)	May increase risk of side effects.
Antiarrhythmics*, other	Increased risk of adverse reactions.
Beta-adrenergic blocking agents*	Increased beta blocker effect.
Digitalis preparations*	Increased digitalis absorption. May require decreased dosage of digitalis preparation.
Doxepin (topical)	Increased risk of toxicity of both drugs.
Warfarin	Increased warfarin effect.

POSSIBLE INTERACTION WITH OTHER SUBSTANCES

INTERACTS WITH	COMBINED EFFECT
Alcohol:	Unpredictable effect on heartbeat. Avoid.
Beverages: Caffeine drinks.	Increased heartbeat irregularity. Avoid.
Cocaine:	Increased heartbeat irregularity. Avoid.
Foods:	None expected.
Marijuana:	Increased heartbeat irregularity. Avoid.
Tobacco:	Increased heartbeat irregularity. Avoid.

*See Glossary

PROPANTHELINE

BRAND NAMES

Pro-Banthine   Propanthel

BASIC INFORMATION

Habit forming? No
Prescription needed?
  High strength: Yes
  Low strength: No
Available as generic? Yes
Drug class: Antispasmodic, anticholinergic

USES

Reduces spasms of digestive system, bladder and urethra.

DOSAGE & USAGE INFORMATION

How to take:
Tablet—Swallow with liquid or food to lessen stomach irritation.

When to take:
30 minutes before meals (unless directed otherwise by doctor).

If you forget a dose:
Take as soon as you remember up to 2 hours late. If more than 2 hours, wait for next scheduled dose (don't double this dose).

What drug does:
Blocks nerve impulses at parasympathetic nerve endings, preventing muscle contractions and gland secretions of organs involved.

Time lapse before drug works:
15 to 30 minutes.

Don't take with:
Any other medicine without consulting your doctor or pharmacist.

OVERDOSE

SYMPTOMS:
Dilated pupils, blurred vision, rapid pulse and breathing, dizziness, fever, hallucinations, confusion, slurred speech, agitation, flushed face, convulsions, coma.
WHAT TO DO:
- **Dial 911 (emergency) or 0 (operator) for an ambulance or medical help. Then give first aid immediately.**
- **See emergency information on inside covers.**

POSSIBLE ADVERSE REACTIONS OR SIDE EFFECTS

SYMPTOMS	WHAT TO DO
Life-threatening: Hives, rash, intense itching, faintness soon after a dose (anaphylaxis).	Seek emergency treatment immediately.
Common:	
• Confusion, delirium, rapid heartbeat.	Discontinue. Call doctor right away.
• Nausea, vomiting, decreased sweating.	Continue. Call doctor when convenient.
• Constipation, loss of taste.	Continue. Tell doctor at next visit.
• Dry ears, nose, throat, mouth.	No action necessary.
Infrequent:	
• Headache, difficult urination, nasal congestion, altered taste, impotence.	Continue. Call doctor when convenient.
• Lightheadedness.	Discontinue. Call doctor right away.
Rare: Rash or hives, eye pain, blurred vision.	Discontinue. Call doctor right away.

WARNINGS & PRECAUTIONS

Don't take if:
- You are allergic to any anticholinergic.
- You have trouble with stomach bloating.
- You have difficulty emptying your bladder completely.
- You have narrow-angle glaucoma.
- You have severe ulcerative colitis.

Before you start, consult your doctor:
- If you have open-angle glaucoma.
- If you have angina.
- If you have chronic bronchitis or asthma.
- If you have hiatal hernia.
- If you have liver, kidney or thyroid disease.
- If you have enlarged prostate.
- If you have myasthenia gravis.
- If you have peptic ulcer.
- If you will have surgery within 2 months, including dental surgery, requiring general or spinal anesthesia.

Over age 60:
Adverse reactions and side effects may be more frequent and severe than in younger persons.

Pregnancy:
Decide with your doctor whether drug benefits justify risk to unborn child. Risk category C (see page xxiii).

Breast-feeding:
Drug passes into milk and decreases milk flow. Avoid drug or discontinue nursing until you finish medicine. Consult doctor for advice on maintaining milk supply.

Infants & children:
Use only under medical supervision.

Prolonged use:
Chronic constipation, possible fecal impaction. Consult doctor immediately.

Skin & sunlight:
No problems expected.

Driving, piloting or hazardous work:
Use disqualifies you for piloting aircraft. Otherwise, no problems expected.

Discontinuing:
May be unnecessary to finish medicine. Follow doctor's instructions.

Others:
Advise any doctor or dentist whom you consult that you take this medicine.

POSSIBLE INTERACTION WITH OTHER DRUGS

GENERIC NAME OR DRUG CLASS	COMBINED EFFECT
Adrenocorticoids, systemic	Possible glaucoma.
Amantadine	Increased propantheline effect.
Antacids*	Decreased propantheline effect.
Anticholinergics*, other	Increased propantheline effect.
Antidepressants, tricyclic*	Increased propantheline effect. Increased sedation.
Antidiarrhea preparations*	Reduced propantheline effect.
Antihistamines*	Increased propantheline effect.
Attapulgite	Decreased propantheline effect.
Buclizine	Increased propantheline effect.
Digitalis preparations*	Possible decreased absorption of digitalis.
Haloperidol	Increased internal eye pressure.
Ketoconazole	Decreased ketoconazole effect.
Meperidine	Increased propantheline effect.
Methylphenidate	Increased propantheline effect.
Molindone	Increased anticholinergic effect.
Monoamine oxidase (MAO) inhibitors*	Increased propantheline effect.
Nitrates*	Increased internal eye pressure.
Nizatidine	Increased nizatidine effect.
Orphenadrine	Increased propantheline effect.
Phenothiazines*	Increased propantheline effect.
Pilocarpine	Loss of pilocarpine effect in glaucoma treatment.
Potassium supplements*	Increased possibility of intestinal ulcers with oral potassium tablets.
Quinidine	Increased propantheline effect.
Sedatives* or central nervous system (CNS) depressants*	Increased sedative effect of both drugs.
Vitamin C	Decreased propantheline effect. Avoid large doses of vitamin C.

POSSIBLE INTERACTION WITH OTHER SUBSTANCES

INTERACTS WITH	COMBINED EFFECT
Alcohol:	None expected.
Beverages:	None expected.
Cocaine:	Excessively rapid heartbeat. Avoid.
Foods:	None expected.
Marijuana:	Drowsiness and dry mouth.
Tobacco:	None expected.

*See Glossary

PROTEASE INHIBITORS

GENERIC AND BRAND NAMES

INDINAVIR
  Crixivan
NELFINAVIR
  Viracept

RITONAVIR
  Norvir
SAQUINAVIR
  Fortovase
  Invirase

BASIC INFORMATION

Habit forming? No
Prescription needed? Yes
Available as generic? No
Drug class: Protease inhibitor

 ## USES

Used in combination with other drugs as a treatment for advanced HIV infection in selected patients. Does not cure HIV infection.

 ## DOSAGE & USAGE INFORMATION

How to take:
* Tablet or capsule—Swallow with liquid. Take with food or meal to enhance drug's absorption. Take indinavir 1 hour before or 2 hours after eating. Your doctor may recommend additional methods to help the body absorb the drug.
* Liquid ritonavir—Swallow with chocolate milk or liquid nutritional supplement to disguise unpleasant taste.

When to take:
At the same times each day, according to instructions on prescription label.

If you forget a dose:
Take as soon as you remember up to 2 hours late. If more than 2 hours, wait for next scheduled dose (don't double this dose).

What drug does:
Blocks an enzyme called protease that is vital to the final stages of HIV replication (reproduction). Blocking protease causes HIV to make copies of itself that can't infect new cells.

Continued next column

 ## OVERDOSE

SYMPTOMS:
Unknown effect.
WHAT TO DO:
Overdose unlikely to threaten life. If person takes much larger amount than prescribed, call doctor, poison control center or hospital emergency room for instructions.

Time lapse before drug works:
It will take weeks to months of treatment with the drug to determine the benefits of this therapy.

Don't take with:
Any other medicine without consulting your doctor or pharmacist. This includes any nonprescription medication.

 ## POSSIBLE ADVERSE REACTIONS OR SIDE EFFECTS

SYMPTOMS	WHAT TO DO
Life-threatening: None expected.	
Common: Diarrhea, abdominal discomfort, nausea, sores on mouth, dizziness, dry mouth, tiredness, appetite loss.	Continue. Call doctor when convenient
Infrequent: Rash, muscle or joint pain, headache, abdominal pain, weakness, back pain, numbness or tingling in hands or feet, tingling around mouth.	Continue. Call doctor when convenient.
Rare: • Confusion, yellow skin or eyes, severe skin reaction, lack of coordination, seizures. Watch for warning signs of hyperglycemia or diabetes (increased thirst and hunger, unexplained weight loss, increased urination, fatigue and dry itchy skin).	Continue, but call doctor right away.
• Other symptoms not listed. They may be drug-associated or infection-associated.	Continue. Call doctor when convenient.

Note: Additional adverse reactions and side effects are often caused by other HIV medications that are used in combination with protease inhibitors.

WARNINGS & PRECAUTIONS

Don't take if:
You are allergic to protease inhibitors.

Before you start, consult your doctor:
- If you have liver or kidney disease
- If you have diabetes or hypertension.
- If you have peripheral neuropathy*.
- If you have any questions or concerns about the drug. Protease Inhibitors are a new class of anti-HIV drugs that are still undergoing medical testing. Ask your doctor about new or additional information regarding adverse reactions, side effects, drug interactions, absorption problems, effectiveness and long-term use.

Over age 60:
No special problems expected.

Pregnancy:
Risk factors vary for drugs in this group. See category list on page xxiii and consult doctor.

Breast-feeding:
It is unknown if drug passes into milk. Breast-feeding not recommended in HIV-infected women.

Infants & children:
Nelfinavir and ritonavir have been approved for use in children 2 to 13.

Prolonged use:
- The effects of long-term use are unknown.
- Medical studies have shown that HIV can become resistant to the effects of these drugs.

Skin & sunlight:
No special problems expected.

Driving, piloting or hazardous work:
Don't drive or pilot aircraft until you learn how medicine affects you. Don't work around dangerous machinery. Don't climb ladders or work in high places. Danger increases if you drink alcohol or take medicine affecting alertness and reflexes.

Discontinuing:
Don't discontinue without consulting doctor.

Others:
- Advise any doctor or dentist whom you consult that you take this medicine.
- These drugs have not been shown to reduce the risk of transmitting HIV to others through sexual contact. Avoid sexual activities or use condoms to help prevent the transmission of HIV. In addition, don't share needles or equipment for injections with other persons.
- These drugs may cause or aggravate diabetes or hypertension.

POSSIBLE INTERACTION WITH OTHER DRUGS

GENERIC NAME OR DRUG CLASS	COMBINED EFFECT
Anticonvulsants*	Decreased effect of ritonavir.
Astemizole	Serious heart rhythm problems. Avoid.
Contraceptives, oral	Decreased contraceptive effect with ritonavir.
Dexamethasone	Decreased effect of ritonavir.
Enzyme inducers*	Decreased effect of protease inhibitor.
Enzyme inhibitors*	Increased effect of enzyme inhibitor.
Non-nucleoside reverse transcriptase inhibitors	May require dosage adjustment of protease inhibitor.
Rifabutin	Decreased effect of protease inhibitor.
Rifampin	Decreased effect of protease inhibitor.
Numerous other drugs	Unknown effect. Consult doctor.

POSSIBLE INTERACTION WITH OTHER SUBSTANCES

INTERACTS WITH	COMBINED EFFECT
Alcohol:	No special problems expected.
Beverages:	No special problems expected.
Cocaine:	Problems not known. Best to avoid.
Foods:	No special problems expected.
Marijuana:	Problems not known. Best to avoid.
Tobacco:	Decreased effect of ritonavir.

*See Glossary

PROTECTANT (Ophthalmic)

GENERIC AND BRAND NAMES

HYDROXYPROPYL
  CELLULOSE
  Lacrisert

HYDROXYPROPYL
  METHYLCELL-
  ULOSE
  Artificial Tears
  Bion Tears
  Eye Lube
  Gonak
  Goniosoft
  Goniosol
  Isopto Alkaline
  Isopto Plain
  Isopto Tears
  Just Tears
  Lacril
  Methocel
  Moisture Drops
  Nature's Tears
  Ocutears
  Tearisol
  Tears Naturale
  Tears Naturale Free
  Tears Naturale II
  Tears Renewed
  Ultra Tears

BASIC INFORMATION

Habit forming? No
Prescription needed? Yes
Available as generic? Yes, for some
Drug class: Protectant (ophthalmic), artificial tears

USES

- Relieves eye dryness and irritation caused by inadequate flow of tears.
- Moistens contact lenses and artificial eyes.

OVERDOSE

SYMPTOMS:
None expected.
WHAT TO DO:
Not intended for internal use. If child accidentally swallows, call poison control center.

DOSAGE & USAGE INFORMATION

How to use:
Eye drops
- Wash hands.
- Apply pressure to inside corner of eye with middle finger.
- Continue pressure for 1 minute after placing medicine in eye.
- Tilt head backward. Pull lower lid away from eye with index finger of the same hand.
- Drop eye drops into pouch and close eye. Don't blink.
- Keep eyes closed for 1 to 2 minutes.
- Don't touch applicator tip to any surface (including the eye). If you accidentally touch tip, clean with warm soap and water.
- Keep container tightly closed.
- Keep cool, but don't freeze.
- Wash hands immediately after using.

When to use:
As directed. Usually every 3 or 4 hours.

If you forget a dose:
Use as soon as you remember.

What drug does:
- Stabilizes and thickens tear film.
- Lubricates and protects eye.

Time lapse before drug works:
2 to 10 minutes.

Don't use with:
Other eye drops without consulting your doctor.

POSSIBLE ADVERSE REACTIONS OR SIDE EFFECTS

SYMPTOMS	WHAT TO DO
Life-threatening None expected.	
Common None expected.	
Infrequent Eye irritation not present before using artificial tears.	Discontinue. Call doctor right away.
Rare None expected.	

WARNINGS & PRECAUTIONS

Don't use if:
You are allergic to any artificial tears.

Before you start, consult your doctor:
If you use any other eye drops.

Over age 60:
No problems expected.

Pregnancy:
Risk factor not designated. See category list on page xxiii and consult doctor.

Breast-feeding:
No problems expected, but check with doctor.

Infants & children:
Don't use.

Prolonged use:
Don't use for more than 3 or 4 days.

Skin & sunlight:
No problems expected.

Driving, piloting or hazardous work:
No problems expected.

Discontinuing:
May not need all the medicine in container. If symptoms disappear, stop using.

Others:
* Keep cool, but don't freeze.
* Check with your doctor if eye irritation continues or becomes worse.

POSSIBLE INTERACTION WITH OTHER DRUGS

GENERIC NAME OR DRUG CLASS	COMBINED EFFECT
Clinically significant interactions with oral or injected medicines unlikely.	

POSSIBLE INTERACTION WITH OTHER SUBSTANCES

INTERACTS WITH	COMBINED EFFECT
Alcohol:	None expected.
Beverages:	None expected
Cocaine:	None expected.
Foods:	None expected.
Marijuana:	None expected.
Tobacco:	None expected.

PROTON PUMP INHIBITORS

GENERIC AND BRAND NAMES

LANSPORAZOLE
  Prevacid
OMEPRAZOLE
  Losec
  Prilosec

PANTOPRAZOLE
  Pantoloc

BASIC INFORMATION

Habit forming? No
Prescription needed? Yes
Available as generic? No
Drug class: Antiulcer agent, proton pump inhibitor

USES

- Treats gastroesophageal reflux (splashing of stomach acid from the stomach up onto the lower end of the esophagus).
- Treats ulcers in the stomach and duodenum.
- Treats any disorder associated with excess production of stomach acid (such as Zollinger-Ellison syndrome).

DOSAGE & USAGE INFORMATION

How to take:
- Delayed-release and extended-release capsules—Swallow whole. Do not crush, chew or break open.
- Tablets (enteric coated)—Swallow with liquid.

When to take:
Once daily, immediately before a meal (preferably breakfast), unless otherwise directed by your doctor. With once-a-day dosing, it is important to take the medicine on schedule.

If you forget a dose:
Take as soon as you remember. If it is almost time for the next dose, wait for next scheduled dose (don't double this dose).

Continued next column

OVERDOSE

SYMPTOMS:
Severe drowsiness, seizures, breathing difficulty, decreased body temperature.
WHAT TO DO:
- **Dial 911 (emergency) or 0 (operator) for an ambulance or medical help. Then give first aid immediately.**
- **See emergency information on inside covers.**

What drug does:
Inhibits secretion of stomach acid.

Time lapse before drug works:
1 to 3 hours.

Don't take with:
Any other medicine without consulting your doctor or pharmacist.

POSSIBLE ADVERSE REACTIONS OR SIDE EFFECTS

SYMPTOMS	WHAT TO DO
Life-threatening: In case of overdose, see previous column.	
Common: Diarrhea, stomach pain.	Continue. Call doctor when convenient.
Infrequent: Nausea, loss of appetite, headache, heartburn, muscle pain, skin rash, drowsiness.	Continue. Call doctor when convenient.
Rare: Weakness or unusual tiredness; sore throat and fever; sores on mouth; unusual bleeding or bruising; cloudy or bloody urine; difficult, frequent or painful urination.	Discontinue. Call doctor right away.

WARNINGS & PRECAUTIONS

Don't take if:
You are allergic to omeprazole or lansoprazole.

Before you start, consult your doctor:
- If you are allergic to any medicines, foods or other substances.
- If you have or have had liver disease.

Over age 60:
No special problems expected.

Pregnancy:
Risk factors may vary for drugs in this group. See category list on page xxiii and consult doctor.

Breast-feeding:
Safety not established. Best to avoid or discontinue nursing until you finish medicine. Consult doctor for advice on maintaining milk supply.

Infants & children:
Safety not established. Consult doctor.

Prolonged use:
The length of treatment can run from 4 to 8 weeks or may be indefinite. Though your symptoms may improve in 1 to 2 weeks, your doctor will determine when healing is complete.

Skin & sunlight:
No special problems expected.

Driving, piloting or hazardous work:
No special problems expected.

Discontinuing:
Don't discontinue without consulting doctor until you complete prescribed dose, even though symptoms diminish or disappear

Others:
- Advise any doctor or dentist whom you consult that you take this medicine.
- If directed by your doctor, it is permissible and sometimes helpful to take with antacids* to relieve upper abdominal pain. Antacids may be used more than once daily if needed.
- May affect results of some medical tests.

POSSIBLE INTERACTION WITH OTHER DRUGS

GENERIC NAME OR DRUG CLASS	COMBINED EFFECT
Anticoagulants* (warfarin, coumadin, indandione derivatives)	Increased anticoagulant effect with omeprazole.
Diazepam	Increased effect of diazepam with omeprazole.
Phenytoin	Increased effect of phenytoin with omeprazole.
Sucralfate	Decreased effect of lansoprazole. Take it 30 minutes before sucralfate.
Theophylline	May require dosage adjustment of theophylline with lansoprazole.

POSSIBLE INTERACTION WITH OTHER SUBSTANCES

INTERACTS WITH	COMBINED EFFECT
Alcohol:	No special problems expected.
Beverages:	No special problems expected.
Cocaine:	No special problems expected.
Foods:	No special problems expected.
Marijuana:	No special problems expected.
Tobacco:	No special problems expected.

*See Glossary

PSEUDOEPHEDRINE

BRAND NAMES

See complete list of brand names in the *Generic and Brand Name Directory*, page 891.

BASIC INFORMATION

Habit forming? No
Prescription needed?
  U.S.: High strength—Yes
        Low strength—No
  Canada: No
Available as generic? Yes
Drug class: Sympathomimetic, decongestant

USES

Reduces congestion of nose, sinuses, eustachian tubes and throat from allergies and infections.

DOSAGE & USAGE INFORMATION

How to take:
- Tablet or capsule—Swallow with liquid. You may chew or crush tablet or open capsule.
- Extended-release tablet or capsule—Swallow each dose whole.
- Syrup—Take as directed on label.
- Drops—Place directly on tongue and swallow.
- Oral solution—Take as direced on label.
- Combination products—Follow instructions on label.

When to take:
- At the same times each day.
- To prevent insomnia, take last dose of day a few hours before bedtime.

If you forget a dose:
Take up to 2 hours late. If more than 2 hours, wait for next dose (don't double this dose).

Continued next column

OVERDOSE

SYMPTOMS:
Nervousness, restlessness, headache, rapid or irregular heartbeat, sweating, nausea, vomiting, anxiety, confusion, delirium, muscle tremors, convulsions, hallucinations.
WHAT TO DO:
- **Dial 911 (emergency) or 0 (operator) for an ambulance or medical help. Then give first aid immediately.**
- **See emergency information on inside covers.**

What drug does:
Decreases blood volume in nasal tissues, shrinking tissues and enlarging airways.

Time lapse before drug works:
15 to 20 minutes.

Don't take with:
- Nonprescription drugs with caffeine without consulting doctor.
- Any other medicine without consulting your doctor or pharmacist.

POSSIBLE ADVERSE REACTIONS OR SIDE EFFECTS

SYMPTOMS	WHAT TO DO
Life-threatening:	
In case of overdose, see previous column.	
Common:	
None expected.	
Infrequent:	
• Nausea or vomiting, irregular or slow heartbeat, difficult breathing, unusually fast or pounding heartbeat, painful or difficult urination, increased sweating, trembling.	Discontinue. Call doctor right away.
• Agitation, insomnia, dizziness, headache, shakiness, weakness, paleness.	Continue. Call doctor when convenient.
Rare:	
Hallucinations, seizures.	Discontinue. Seek emergency treatment.

706

WARNINGS & PRECAUTIONS

Don't take if:
You are allergic to any sympathomimetic drug.

Before you start, consult your doctor:
- If you have overactive thyroid or diabetes.
- If you have taken any monoamine oxidase (MAO) Inhibitor* in past 2 weeks.
- If you take digitalis preparations or have high blood pressure or heart disease.
- If you will have surgery within 2 months, including dental surgery, requiring general or spinal anesthesia.
- If you have urination difficulty.

Over age 60:
Adverse reactions and side effects may be more frequent and severe than in younger persons.

Pregnancy:
No proven harm to unborn child. Avoid if possible. Consult doctor. Risk category B (see page xxiii).

Breast-feeding:
Drug passes into milk. Avoid drug or discontinue nursing until you finish medicine. Consult doctor for advice on maintaining milk supply.

Infants & children:
Keep dose low or avoid.

Prolonged use:
No proven problems.

Skin & sunlight:
No problems expected.

Driving, piloting or hazardous work:
Avoid if you feel dizzy. Otherwise, no problems expected.

Discontinuing:
May be unnecessary to finish medicine. Follow doctor's instructions.

Others:
- Call the doctor if symptoms worsen or new symptoms develop with use of this medicine.
- Heed all warnings on the product label.

POSSIBLE INTERACTION WITH OTHER DRUGS

GENERIC NAME OR DRUG CLASS	COMBINED EFFECT
Antidepressants, tricyclic*	Increased risk of heart toxicity or severe headaches.
Antihypertensives*	Decreased antihypertensive effect.
Beta-adrenergic blocking agents*	Decreased effect of both drugs.
Calcium supplements*	Increased pseudoephedrine effect.
Digitalis preparations*	Irregular heartbeat.
Epinephrine	Increased epinephrine effect. Excessive heart stimulation and blood pressure increase.
Ergot preparations*	Serious blood pressure rise.
Guanadrel	Decreased effect of both drugs.
Guanethidine	Decreased effect of both drugs.
Methyldopa	Possible increased blood pressure.
Monoamine oxidase (MAO) inhibitors*	Increased pseudoephedrine effect.
Nitrates*	Possible decreased effects of both drugs.
Phenothiazines*	Possible increased pseudoephedrine toxicity. Possible decreased pseudoephedrine effect.
Rauwolfia	Decreased rauwolfia effect.
Sympathomimetics*, other	Increased pseudoephedrine effect.
Terazosin	Decreased effectiveness of terazosin.

POSSIBLE INTERACTION WITH OTHER SUBSTANCES

INTERACTS WITH	COMBINED EFFECT
Alcohol:	None expected.
Beverages: Caffeine drinks.	Nervousness or insomnia.
Cocaine:	High risk of heartbeat irregularities and high blood pressure.
Foods:	None expected.
Marijuana:	Rapid heartbeat.
Tobacco:	None expected.

*See Glossary

PSORALENS

GENERIC AND BRAND NAMES

METHOXSALEN
Oxsoralen
Oxsoralen Topical
Oxsoralen Ultra
UltraMOP

TRIOXSALEN
Trisoralen

BASIC INFORMATION

Habit forming? No
Prescription needed? Yes
Available as generic? No
Drug class: Repigmenting agent (psoralen)

USES

- Repigmenting skin affected with vitiligo (absence of skin pigment).
- Treatment for psoriasis, when other treatments haven't helped.
- Treatment for mycosis fungoides.

DOSAGE & USAGE INFORMATION

How to take or apply:
- Tablet or capsule—Swallow with liquid or food to lessen stomach irritation.
- Topical—As directed by doctor.

When to take or apply:
2 to 4 hours before exposure to sunlight or sunlamp.

If you forget a dose:
Take as soon as you remember. Delay sun exposure for at least 2 hours after taking.

What drug does:
Helps pigment cells when used in conjunction with ultraviolet light.

Time lapse before drug works:
- For vitiligo, 6 to 9 months.
- For psoriasis, 10 weeks or longer.
- For tanning, 3 to 4 days.

Don't take with:
Any other medicine that causes skin sensitivity to sun. Ask pharmacist.

OVERDOSE

SYMPTOMS:
Blistering skin, swelling feet and legs.
WHAT TO DO:
Overdose unlikely to threaten life. If person takes much larger amount than prescribed, call doctor, poison control center or hospital emergency room for instructions.

POSSIBLE ADVERSE REACTIONS OR SIDE EFFECTS

SYMPTOMS	WHAT TO DO
Life-threatening: None expected.	
Common:	
• Increased skin sensitivity to sun.	Always protect from overexposure.
• Increased eye sensitivity to sunlight.	Always protect with wrap-around sunglasses.
• Nausea.	Continue. Call doctor when convenient.
Infrequent:	
• Skin red and sore.	Discontinue. Call doctor right away.
• Dizziness, headache, depression, leg cramps, insomnia.	Continue. Call doctor when convenient.
Rare:	
Hepatitis with jaundice, blistering and peeling.	Discontinue. Call doctor right away.

WARNINGS & PRECAUTIONS

Don't take if:
- You are allergic to any other psoralen.
- You are unwilling or unable to remain under close medical supervision.

Before you start, consult your doctor:
- If you have heart or liver disease.
- If you have allergy to sunlight.
- If you have cataracts.
- If you have albinism.
- If you have lupus erythematosis, porphyria, chronic infection, skin cancer or peptic ulcer.
- If you will have surgery within 2 months, including dental surgery, requiring general or spinal anesthesia.
- If you have skin cancer.

Over age 60:
Adverse reactions and side effects may be more frequent and severe than in younger persons.

Pregnancy:
Risk factors vary for drugs in this group. See category list on page xxiii and consult doctor.

Breast-feeding:
Drug may pass into milk. Avoid drug or discontinue nursing until you finish medicine. Consult doctor for advice on maintaining milk supply.

Infants & children:
Not recommended.

Prolonged use:
- Increased chance of toxic effects.
- Talk to your doctor about the need for follow-up medical examinations or laboratory studies to check ANA titers*, complete blood counts (white blood cell count, platelet count, red blood cell count, hemoglobin, hematocrit), liver function, kidney function, eyes.

Skin & sunlight:
- One or more drugs in this group may cause rash or intensify sunburn in areas exposed to sun or ultraviolet light (photosensitivity reaction). Avoid overexposure. Notify doctor if reaction occurs.
- Too much can burn skin. Cover skin for 24 hours before and 8 hours following treatments.

Driving, piloting or hazardous work:
No problems expected. Protect eyes and skin from bright light.

Discontinuing:
Skin may remain sensitive for some time after treatment stops. Use extra protection from sun.

Others:
- Use sunblock on lips.
- Don't use just to make skin tan.
- Don't use hard gelatin capsules interchangeably with soft gelatin capsules.

POSSIBLE INTERACTION WITH OTHER DRUGS

GENERIC NAME OR DRUG CLASS	COMBINED EFFECT
Photosensitizing medications*	Greatly increased likelihood of extreme sensitivity to sunlight.

POSSIBLE INTERACTION WITH OTHER SUBSTANCES

INTERACTS WITH	COMBINED EFFECT
Alcohol:	May increase chance of liver toxicity.
Beverages: Lime drinks.	Avoid—toxic.
Cocaine:	Increased chance of toxicity. Avoid.
Foods: Those containing furocoumarin (limes, parsley, figs, parsnips, carrots, celery, mustard).	May cause toxic reaction to psoralens.
Marijuana:	Increased chance of toxicity. Avoid.
Tobacco:	May cause uneven absorption of medicine. Avoid.

PYRIDOXINE (Vitamin B-6)

BRAND NAMES

Beesix   Rodex
Hexa-Betalin   Vitabec 6
Pyroxine
Numerous other multiple vitamin-mineral
supplements. Check labels.

BASIC INFORMATION

Habit forming? No
Prescription needed?
  High strength: Yes
  Low strength: No
Available as generic? Yes
Drug class: Vitamin supplement

 ## USES

- Prevention and treatment of pyridoxine
  deficiency.
- Treatment of some forms of anemia.
- Treatment of INH (isonicotinic acid hydrozide),
  cycloserine poisoning.

 ## DOSAGE & USAGE INFORMATION

How to take:
- Tablets—Swallow with liquid.
- Extended-release capsules—Swallow each
  dose whole with liquid.

When to take:
At the same times each day.

If you forget a dose:
Take as soon as you remember, then resume
regular schedule.

What drug does:
Acts as co-enzyme in carbohydrate, protein and
fat metabolism.

Time lapse before drug works:
15 to 20 minutes.

Don't take with:
- Levodopa—Small amounts of pyridoxine will
  nullify levodopa effect. Carbidopa-levodopa
  combination not affected by this interaction.
- Any other medicine without consulting your
  doctor or pharmacist.

 ## OVERDOSE

SYMPTOMS:
None expected.
WHAT TO DO:
Overdose unlikely to threaten life.

 ## POSSIBLE ADVERSE REACTIONS OR SIDE EFFECTS

SYMPTOMS	WHAT TO DO
Life-threatening: None expected.	
Common: None expected.	
Infrequent: Nausea, headache.	Discontinue. Call doctor right away.
Rare: Numbness or tingling in hands or feet (large doses).	Discontinue. Call doctor right away.

WARNINGS & PRECAUTIONS

Don't take if:
You are allergic to pyridoxine.

Before you start, consult your doctor:
If you are pregnant or breast-feeding.

Over age 60:
No problems expected.

Pregnancy:
Don't exceed recommended dose. Consult doctor. Risk category A (see page xxiii).

Breast-feeding:
Don't exceed recommended dose. Consult doctor.

Infants & children:
Don't exceed recommended dose.

Prolonged use:
Large doses for more than 1 month may cause toxicity.

Skin & sunlight:
No problems expected.

Driving, piloting or hazardous work:
No problems expected.

Discontinuing:
No problems expected.

Others:
Regular pyridoxine supplements recommended if you take chloramphenicol, cycloserine, ethionamide, hydralazine, immuno-suppressants, isoniazid or penicillamine. These decrease pyridoxine absorption and can cause anemia or tingling and numbness in hands and feet.

POSSIBLE INTERACTION WITH OTHER DRUGS

GENERIC NAME OR DRUG CLASS	COMBINED EFFECT
Contraceptives, oral*	Decreased pyridoxine effect.
Cycloserine	Decreased pyridoxine effect.
Estrogens*	Decreased pyridoxine effect.
Ethionamide	Decreased pyridoxine effect.
Hydralazine	Decreased pyridoxine effect.
Hypnotics, barbiturates*	Decreased hypnotic effect.
Immuno-suppressants*	Decreased pyridoxine effect.
Isoniazid	Decreased pyridoxine effect.
Levodopa	Decreased levodopa effect.
Penicillamine	Decreased pyridoxine effect.
Phenobarbital	Possible decreased phenobarbital effect.
Phenytoin	Decreased phenytoin effect.

POSSIBLE INTERACTION WITH OTHER SUBSTANCES

INTERACTS WITH	COMBINED EFFECT
Alcohol:	None expected.
Beverages:	None expected.
Cocaine:	None expected.
Foods:	None expected.
Marijuana:	None expected.
Tobacco:	May decrease pyridoxine absorption. Decreased pyridoxine effect.

QUETIAPINE

BRAND NAMES

Seroquel

BASIC INFORMATION

Habit forming? No
Prescription needed? Yes
Available as generic? No
Drug class: Antipsychotic

 ## USES

Treatment for symptoms of schizophrenia and other psychotic disorders.

 ## DOSAGE & USAGE INFORMATION

How to take:
Tablet—Swallow with liquid. May be taken with or without food.

When to take:
As directed by your doctor—2 to 3 times a day at the same times each day. The prescribed dosage may be increased over the first few days of use.

If you forget a dose:
Take as soon as you remember. If it is almost time for the next dose, wait for the next scheduled dose (don't double this dose).

What drug does:
The exact mechanism is unknown. It appears to alleviate symptoms of schizophrenia by blocking certain nerve impulses between nerve cells.

Time lapse before drug works:
One to 7 days. Further increases in the dosage amount may be necessary to relieve symptoms for some patients.

Don't take with:
Any other medication without consulting your doctor or pharmacist. All possible drug interactions have not been studied.

 ## OVERDOSE

SYMPTOMS:
Drowsiness and slurred speech; other symptoms may occur that were not observed in medical studies of the drug.
WHAT TO DO:
If person takes much larger amount than prescribed, call doctor, poison control center or hospital emergency room for instructions.

 ## POSSIBLE ADVERSE REACTIONS OR SIDE EFFECTS

SYMPTOMS	WHAT TO DO
Life-threatening:	
High fever, rapid pulse, profuse sweating, muscle rigidity, confusion and irritability, seizures (neuroleptic malignant syndrome —rare).	Discontinue. Seek emergency treatment.
Common:	
• Dizziness, difficulty in speaking or swallowing, shaking hands and fingers, trembling, vision problems, weakness, lightheadedness when arising from a sitting or lying position.	Continue. Call doctor right away.
• Drowsiness, constipation, weight gain, agitation, insomnia, headache, nervousness, runny nose, anxiety, dry mouth, personality disorder, arm or leg stiffness.	Continue. Call doctor when convenient.
Infrequent:	
• Jerky or involuntary movements, especially of the face, lips, jaw, tongue; chest pain, fast heartbeat.	Continue. Call doctor right away.
• Fever, flu-like symptoms, twitching, mood or mental changes, speech unclear, swollen feet or ankles, appetite increased, cough, saliva increased, muscle tightness, muscle spasms (face, neck, back), joint pain, nausea or vomiting, sore throat, thirstiness, incontinence, abdominal pain.	Continue. Call doctor when convenient.
Rare:	
• Breathing difficulty.	Discontinue. Call doctor right away.
• Swollen face, rash, confusion, decreased sex drive, menstrual changes, sluggishness.	Continue. Call doctor when convenient.

WARNINGS & PRECAUTIONS

Don't take if:
You are allergic to quetiapine

Before you start, consult your doctor:
- If you have liver disease, heart disease or a blood vessel disorder.
- If you have Alzheimer's.
- If you have a history of breast cancer.
- If you have intestinal blockage.
- If you are subject to dehydration or low body temperature.
- If you have a history of drug abuse or dependence.
- If you have glaucoma or cataracts.
- If you have prostate problems.
- If you are allergic to any medication, food or other substance.
- If you have a history of seizures.

Over age 60:
Adverse reactions and side effects may be more severe than in younger persons. A lower starting dosage is usually recommended until a response is determined.

Pregnancy:
Decide with your doctor if drug benefits justify any possible risk to unborn child. Risk category C (see page xxiii).

Breast-feeding:
It is unknown if drug passes into milk. It is not recommended for nursing mothers.

Infants & children:
Safety in children under age 18 has not been established. Use only under close medical supervision.

Prolonged use:
- Consult with your doctor on a regular basis while taking this drug to check your progress or to discuss any increase or changes in side effects and the need for continued treatment. Long term effectiveness has not been established.
- Get eyes examined every 6 months.

Skin & sunlight:
- May cause rash or intensify sunburn in areas exposed to sun or ultraviolet light (photosensitivity reaction). Use sunscreen and avoid overexposure. Notify doctor if reaction occurs.
- Hot temperatures, exercise, and hot baths can increase risk of heatstroke. Drug may affect body's ability to maintain normal temperature.

Driving, piloting or hazardous work:
Don't drive or pilot aircraft until you learn how medicine affects you. Don't work around dangerous machinery. Don't climb ladders or work in high places. Danger increases if you drink alcohol or take medicine affecting alertness and reflexes.

Discontinuing:
Don't discontinue this drug without consulting doctor. Dosage may require a gradual reduction before stopping.

Others:
- Get up slowly from a sitting or lying position to avoid any dizziness, faintness or lightheadedness.
- Advise any doctor or dentist whom you consult that you take this medicine.
- Take medicine only as directed. Do not increase or reduce dosage without doctor's approval.

POSSIBLE INTERACTION WITH OTHER DRUGS

GENERIC NAME OR DRUG CLASS	COMBINED EFFECT
Central nervous system (CNS) depressants*, other	Increased sedative effect.
Enzyme inhibitors*	May increase quetiapine effect.
Enzyme inducers*	Decreased quetiapine effect.
Phenytoin	Decreased quetiapine effect.
Thioridazine	Decreased quetiapine effect.

POSSIBLE INTERACTION WITH OTHER SUBSTANCES

INTERACTS WITH	COMBINED EFFECT
Alcohol:	Increased sedation and dizziness. Avoid.
Beverages:	None expected.
Cocaine:	Effect not known. Best to avoid.
Foods:	None expected.
Marijuana:	Effect not known. Best to avoid.
Tobacco:	None expected.

*See Glossary

QUINACRINE

BRAND NAMES

Atabrine

BASIC INFORMATION

Habit forming? No
Prescription needed? Yes
Available as generic? Yes
Drug class: Antiprotozoal

 ## USES

- Treats disease caused by the intestinal parasite *Giardia lamblia*.
- Treats mild to moderate discoid lupus erythematosus.

 ## DOSAGE & USAGE INFORMATION

How to take:
Tablets—Swallow with full glass of water, tea or fruit juice. If you can't swallow whole, crumble tablet and mix with jam or chocolate syrup.

When to take:
After meals.

If you forget a dose:
Take as soon as you remember up to 2 hours late. If more than 2 hours, wait for next scheduled dose (don't double this dose).

What drug does:
Destroys *Giardia lamblia* parasites in the gastrointestinal system.

Continued next column

 ## OVERDOSE

SYMPTOMS:
Severe abdominal cramps, convulsions, severe diarrhea, fainting, irregular heartbeat, restlessness.
WHAT TO DO:
- **Dial 911 (emergency) or 0 (operator) for an ambulance or medical help. Then give first aid immediately.**
- **If patient is unconscious and not breathing, give mouth-to-mouth breathing. If there is no heartbeat, use cardiac massage and mouth-to-mouth breathing (CPR). Don't try to make patient vomit. If you can't get help quickly, take patient to nearest emergency facility.**
- **See emergency information on inside covers.**

Time lapse before drug works:
1 day.

Don't take with:
Any other medicine without consulting your doctor or pharmacist.

 ## POSSIBLE ADVERSE REACTIONS OR SIDE EFFECTS

SYMPTOMS	WHAT TO DO
Life-threatening:	
In case of overdose, see previous column.	
Common:	
• Dizziness, nausea, headache.	Discontinue. Call doctor right away.
• Yellow eyes, skin, urine (due to dye-like characteristics of quinacrine).	Report to doctor, but no action necessary.
Infrequent:	
• Mild abdominal cramps; mild diarrhea; appetite loss; skin rash, itching or peeling.	Discontinue. Call doctor right away.
• Mood changes.	Continue. Call doctor when convenient.
Rare:	
Hallucinations, nightmares.	Discontinue. Call doctor right away.

WARNINGS & PRECAUTIONS

Don't take if:
You are allergic to quinacrine.

Before you start, consult your doctor:
• If you have porphyria.
• If you have had psoriasis.
• If you have a history of severe mental disorders.
• If you are on a low-salt, low-sugar or other special diet.

Over age 60:
No special problems.

Pregnancy:
Decide with your doctor whether drug benefits justify risk to unborn child. Treatment best begun after child has been delivered. Risk category C (see page xxiii).

Breast-feeding:
Effect unknown. Consult doctor.

Infants & children:
Children tolerate quinacrine poorly. Quinacrine may cause vomiting due to bitter taste. Try crushing tablets in jam, honey or chocolate syrup.

Prolonged use:
• Can cause eye problems, liver disease, aplastic anemia. Don't use for more than 5 days.
• Talk to your doctor about the need for follow-up medical examinations or laboratory studies to check stools for giardiasis.

Skin & sunlight:
No problems expected.

Driving, piloting or hazardous work:
Don't drive or pilot aircraft until you learn how medicine affects you. Don't work around dangerous machinery. Don't climb ladders or work in high places. Danger increases if you drink alcohol or take medicine affecting alertness and reflexes, such as antihistamines, tranquilizers, sedatives, pain medicine, narcotics and mind-altering drugs.

Discontinuing:
Don't discontinue before 5 days without consulting doctor.

Others:
Request 3 stool exams several days apart.

POSSIBLE INTERACTION WITH OTHER DRUGS

GENERIC NAME OR DRUG CLASS	COMBINED EFFECT
Primaquine	Decreased effect of primaquine.

POSSIBLE INTERACTION WITH OTHER SUBSTANCES

INTERACTS WITH	COMBINED EFFECT
Alcohol:	Increased adverse effects of both. Avoid.
Beverages:	No special problems expected.
Cocaine:	No special problems expected.
Foods:	No special problems expected.
Marijuana:	No special problems expected.
Tobacco:	No special problems expected.

QUINIDINE

BRAND NAMES

Apo-Quinidine
Cardioquin
Cin-Quin
Duraquin
Novoquinidin

Quinaglute Dura-
   Tabs
Quinalan
Quinate
Quinidex Extentabs
Quinora

BASIC INFORMATION

Habit forming? No
Prescription needed?
  U.S.: Yes
  Canada: No
Available as generic? Yes
Drug class: Antiarrhythmic

 ## USES

- Corrects heart rhythm disorders.
- May be used in treatment of malaria.

 ## DOSAGE & USAGE INFORMATION

How to take:
- Tablet or capsule—Swallow with liquid or food to lessen stomach irritation.
- Extended-release tablets—Swallow each dose whole. Don't crush them.

When to take:
At the same times each day.

If you forget a dose:
Take as soon as you remember up to 2 hours late. If more than 2 hours, wait for next scheduled dose (don't double this dose).

Continued next column

 ## OVERDOSE

SYMPTOMS:
Confusion, severe blood pressure drop, lethargy, breathing difficulty, fainting, seizures, coma.
WHAT TO DO:
- Dial 911 (emergency) or 0 (operator) for an ambulance or medical help. Then give first aid immediately.
- If patient is unconscious and not breathing, give mouth-to-mouth breathing. If there is no heartbeat, use cardiac massage and mouth-to-mouth breathing (CPR). Don't try to make patient vomit. If you can't get help quickly, take patient to nearest emergency facility.
- See emergency information on inside covers.

What drug does:
Delays nerve impulses to the heart to regulate heartbeat.

Time lapse before drug works:
2 to 4 hours.

Don't take with:
Any other medicine without consulting your doctor or pharmacist.

 ## POSSIBLE ADVERSE REACTIONS OR SIDE EFFECTS

SYMPTOMS	WHAT TO DO
Life-threatening:	
Hives, rash, intense itching, faintness soon after a dose (anaphylaxis); wheezing.	Seek emergency treatment immediately.
Common:	
Bitter taste, diarrhea, nausea, vomiting, appetite loss, abdominal pain.	Discontinue. Call doctor right away.
Infrequent:	
• Dizziness, lightheadedness, fainting, headache, confusion, rash, change in vision, difficult breathing, rapid heartbeat.	Discontinue. Call doctor right away.
• Ringing in ears.	Continue. Call doctor when convenient.
Rare:	
• Unusual bleeding or bruising, difficulty or pain on swallowing, fever, joint pain, jaundice, hepatitis.	Discontinue. Call doctor right away.
• Weakness.	Continue. Call doctor when convenient.

 ## WARNINGS & PRECAUTIONS

Don't take if:
- You are allergic to quinidine.
- You have an active infection.

Before you start, consult your doctor:
About any drug you take, including nonprescription drugs.

Over age 60:
Adverse reactions and side effects may be more frequent and severe than in younger persons.

Pregnancy:
Decide with your doctor if drug benefits justify risk to unborn child. Risk category C (see page xxiii).

Breast-feeding:
Drug filters into milk. May harm child. Consult doctor.

Infants & children:
No problems expected.

Prolonged use:
Talk to your doctor about the need for follow-up medical examinations or laboratory studies to check complete blood counts (white blood cell count, platelet count, red blood cell count, hemoglobin, hematocrit), liver function, kidney function, serum potassium levels, ECG*.

Skin & sunlight:
May cause rash or intensify sunburn in areas exposed to sun or ultraviolet light (photosensitivity reaction). Avoid overexposure. Notify doctor if reaction occurs.

Driving, piloting or hazardous work:
Don't drive or pilot aircraft until you learn how medicine affects you. Don't work around dangerous machinery. Don't climb ladders or work in high places. Danger increases if you drink alcohol or take medicine affecting alertness and reflexes, such as antihistamines, tranquilizers, sedatives, pain medicine, narcotics and mind-altering drugs.

Discontinuing:
Don't discontinue without doctor's advice until you complete prescribed dose, even though symptoms diminish or disappear.

Others:
No problems expected.

POSSIBLE INTERACTION WITH OTHER DRUGS

GENERIC NAME OR DRUG CLASS	COMBINED EFFECT
Alkalizers, urinary*	Slows quinidine elimination, increasing its effect and toxicity.
Antiarrhythmics*	May increase or decrease effect or toxicity of quinidine.
Anticholinergics*	Increased anticholinergic effect.
Anticoagulants*, oral	Possible increased anticoagulant effect.
Antihypertensives*	Increased antihypertensive effect.
Beta-adrenergic blocking agents*	May slow heartbeat excessively.
Cholinergics*	Decreased cholinergic effect.
Cimetidine	Increased quinidine effect.
Cisapride	Decreased quinidine effect.

Dapsone	Increased risk of adverse effect on blood cells.
Digitalis preparations*	May slow heartbeat excessively. Dose adjustments may be needed.
Doxepin (topical)	Increased risk of toxicity of both drugs.
Encainide	Increased effect of toxicity on heart muscle.
Flecainide	Possible irregular heartbeat.
Guanfacine	Increased effect of both medicines.
Metformin	Increased metformin effect.
Nicardipine	Possible increased effect and toxicity of each drug.
Nifedipine	Possible decreased quinidine effect.
Nimodipine	Increased quinidine effect.
Phenobarbital	Decreased quinidine effect.
Phenothiazines*	Possible increased quinidine effect.
Phenytoin	Decreased quinidine effect.
Pimozide	Increased risk of heartbeat irregularities.

Continued on page 930

POSSIBLE INTERACTION WITH OTHER SUBSTANCES

INTERACTS WITH	COMBINED EFFECT
Alcohol:	None expected.
Beverages: Caffeine drinks.	Causes rapid heartbeat. Use sparingly.
Cocaine:	Irregular heartbeat. Avoid.
Foods:	None expected.
Marijuana:	Can cause fainting.
Tobacco:	Irregular heartbeat. Avoid.

*See Glossary

QUININE

BRAND NAMES

Legatrin	Quinamm
NovoQuinine	Quindan
Quin-260	Quiphile
Quin-amino	Q-Vel

BASIC INFORMATION

Habit forming? No
Prescription needed?
  High strength: Yes
  Low strength: No
Available as generic? Yes
Drug class: Antiprotozoal

 ## USES

- Treatment or prevention of malaria.
- Relief of muscle cramps.

 ## DOSAGE & USAGE INFORMATION

How to take:
Tablet or capsule—Swallow with liquid or food to lessen stomach irritation.

When to take:
- Prevention—At the same time each day, usually at bedtime.
- Treatment—At the same times each day in evenly spaced doses.

If you forget a dose:
- Prevention—Take as soon as you remember up to 12 hours late. If more than 12 hours, wait for next scheduled dose (don't double this dose).
- Treatment—Take as soon as you remember up to 2 hours late. If more than 2 hours, wait for next scheduled dose (don't double this dose).

Continued next column

 ## OVERDOSE

SYMPTOMS:
Severe impairment of vision and hearing; severe nausea, vomiting, diarrhea; shallow breathing, fast heartbeat; apprehension, confusion, delirium.
WHAT TO DO:
Dial 911 (emergency) or 0 (operator) for an ambulance or medical help. Then give first aid immediately.

What drug does:
- Reduces contractions of skeletal muscles.
- Increases blood flow.
- Interferes with genes in malaria micro-organisms.

Time lapse before drug works:
May require several days or weeks for maximum effect.

Don't take with:
Any other medicine without consulting your doctor or pharmacist.

 ## POSSIBLE ADVERSE REACTIONS OR SIDE EFFECTS

SYMPTOMS	WHAT TO DO
Life-threatening:	
In case of overdose, see previous column.	
Common:	
Blurred vision or change in vision, eyes sensitive to light.	Discontinue. Call doctor right away.
Dizziness, headache, abdominal discomfort, mild nausea, vomiting, diarrhea.	Continue. Call doctor when convenient.
Ringing or buzzing in ears, impaired hearing.	Continue. Tell doctor at next visit.
Infrequent:	
Rash, hives, itchy skin, difficult breathing.	Discontinue. Call doctor right away.
Rare:	
Sore throat, fever, unusual bleeding or bruising, unusual tiredness or weakness, angina.	Discontinue. Call doctor right away.

WARNINGS & PRECAUTIONS

Don't take if:
You are allergic to quinine or quinidine.

Before you start, consult your doctor:
- If you plan to become pregnant within medication period.
- If you have asthma.
- If you have eye disease, hearing problems or ringing in the ears.
- If you have heart disease.
- If you have myasthenia gravis.

Over age 60:
Adverse reactions and side effects may be more frequent and severe than in younger persons.

Pregnancy:
Risk to unborn child outweighs drug benefits. Don't use. Risk category X (see page xxiii).

Breast-feeding:
Drug filters into milk. May harm child. Consult doctor.

Infants & children:
Use only under medical supervision.

Prolonged use:
May develop headache, blurred vision, nausea, temporary hearing loss, but seldom need to discontinue because of these symptoms.

Skin & sunlight:
May cause rash or intensity sunburn in areas exposed to sun or ultraviolet light (photosensitivity reaction). Avoid overexposure. Notify doctor if reaction occurs.

Driving, piloting or hazardous work:
Avoid if you feel dizzy or have blurred vision. Otherwise, no problems expected.

Discontinuing:
Don't discontinue without doctor's advice until you complete prescribed dose, even though symptoms diminish or disappear.

Others:
Don't confuse with quinidine, a medicine for heart rhythm problems.

POSSIBLE INTERACTION WITH OTHER DRUGS

GENERIC NAME OR DRUG CLASS	COMBINED EFFECT
Alkalizers*, urinary	Possible toxic effects of quinine.
Antacids* (with aluminum hydroxide)	Decreased quinine effect.
Anticoagulants*, oral	Increased anticoagulant effect.
Dapsone	Increased risk of adverse effect on blood cells.
Digitalis	Possible increased digitalis effect.
Digoxin	Possible increased digoxin effect.
Mefloquine	Increased risk of heartbeat irregularities.
Metformin	Increased metformin effect.
Quinidine	Possible toxic effects of quinine.

POSSIBLE INTERACTION WITH OTHER SUBSTANCES

INTERACTS WITH	COMBINED EFFECT
Alcohol:	No proven problems.
Beverages:	None expected.
Cocaine:	No proven problems.
Foods:	None expected.
Marijuana:	No proven problems.
Tobacco:	None expected.

RALOXIFENE

BRAND NAMES

Evista

BASIC INFORMATION

Habit forming? No
Prescription needed? Yes
Available as generic? No
Drug class: Osteoporosis postmenopausal, prophylactic

 USES

- Prevents osteoporosis in postmenopausal women.
- Lowers low-density lipoprotein (LDL) cholesterol blood levels.
- Does not treat hot flashes of menopause.

 DOSAGE & USAGE INFORMATION

How to take:
Tablets—Swallow with water, with or without food. If you can't swallow whole, crumble tablet and take with liquid or food.

When to take:
At the same time each day.

If you forget a dose:
Take as soon as you remember up to 12 hours late. If more than 12 hours, wait for next scheduled dose (don't double this dose).

What drug does:
Has estrogen-like effects on bone and increases bone mineral density.

Time lapse before drug works:
Up to twelve months.

Don't take with:
Any other prescription or nonprescription drug without consulting your doctor or pharmacist.

 OVERDOSE

SYMPTOMS:
None reported.
WHAT TO DO:
Overdose unlikely to threaten life. If person takes much larger amount than prescribed, call doctor, poison control center or hospital emergency room for instructions.

 POSSIBLE ADVERSE REACTIONS OR SIDE EFFECTS

SYMPTOMS	WHAT TO DO
Life-threatening:	
Blood clot formation.	Discontinue. Seek emergency treatment immediately.
Common:	
• Chest pain; bloody or cloudy urine; burning or painful urination; frequent urge to urinate; infection; cold- or flu-like symptoms; leg cramping; skin rash; swelling of hands, ankle or feet; vaginal itching.	Discontinue. Call doctor right away.
• Joint or muscle pain, swollen joints, gas, upset stomach, vomiting, hot flashes, insomnia, white vaginal discharge, depression, sweating, unexplained weight gain.	Continue. Call doctor if symptoms persist.
Infrequent:	
Abdominal pain, diarrhea, loss of appetite, nausea, weakness, migraine headache, difficulty breathing, fever, congestion.	Discontinue. Call doctor right away.
Rare:	
None expected.	

WARNINGS & PRECAUTIONS

Don't take if:
- You are allergic to raloxifene.
- You are scheduled for surgery within 72 hours.

Before you start, consult your doctor:
- If you have any other medical problem.
- If you plan to become pregnant within the medication period.
- If you have or have had a history of blood clot formation.
- If you have or have had cancer or tumors.
- If you have liver disease.

Over age 60:
Adverse reactions and side effects in older adults have been similar to those experienced by women who have just undergone menopause.

Pregnancy:
Use of raloxifene is not recommended during pregnancy. Risk category X (see page xxiii).

Breast-feeding:
Unknown whether drug passes into milk and is not recommended during breast-feeding. Presently raloxifene is to be used in post-menopausal women only.

Infants & children:
Not recommended for this age group.

Prolonged use:
No problems expected. Your doctor should periodically evaluate your response to the drug and adjust the dose if necessary.

Skin & sunlight:
No problems expected.

Driving, piloting or hazardous work:
No problems expected.

Discontinuing:
Don't discontinue without consulting doctor.

Others:
- Advise any doctor or dentist whom you consult that you take this medicine.
- In addition to taking the drug, weight-bearing exercise and adequate intake of calcium and vitamin D are essential in preventing bone loss. Periods of prolonged activity may worsen your condition. Daily dietary supplements of elemental calcium and vitamin D may be recommended by your doctor.
- May help lower low-density lipoprotein (LDL) cholesterol levels.

POSSIBLE INTERACTION WITH OTHER DRUGS

GENERIC NAME OR DRUG CLASS	COMBINED EFFECT
Cholestyramine	Lessens the effect of raloxifene.
Estrogens	Not recommended for use with raloxifene.
Protein bound drugs*	Caution is recommended; consult doctor before taking any of these in conjunction with raloxifene.
Warfarin	May lessen the effect of warfarin.

POSSIBLE INTERACTION WITH OTHER SUBSTANCES

INTERACTS WITH	COMBINED EFFECT
Alcohol:	None expected.
Beverages:	None expected.
Cocaine:	Effects unknown. Avoid.
Foods:	None expected.
Marijuana:	Effects unknown. Avoid.
Tobacco:	None expected.

RAUWOLFIA & THIAZIDE DIURETICS

GENERIC AND BRAND NAMES

See complete list of generic and brand names in the *Generic and Brand Name Directory*, page 894.

BASIC INFORMATION

Habit forming? No
Prescription needed? Yes
Available as generic? Yes
Drug class: Antihypertensive, diuretic, tranquilizer

 USES

- Controls, but doesn't cure, high blood pressure.
- Reduces fluid retention (edema).

 DOSAGE & USAGE INFORMATION

How to take:
Tablet—Swallow with liquid. If you can't swallow whole, crumble tablet and take with liquid or food.

When to take:
At the same time each day.

If you forget a dose:
Take as soon as you remember up to 2 hours late. If more than 2 hours, wait for next scheduled dose (don't double this dose).

What drug does:
- Forces sodium and water excretion, reducing body fluid. Reduced body fluid and relaxed arteries lower blood pressure.
- Interferes with nerve impulses and relaxes blood vessel muscles, reducing blood pressure.
- Suppresses brain centers that control emotion.

Continued next column

 OVERDOSE

SYMPTOMS:
Cramps; weakness; drowsiness; pinpoint pupils; slow, weak pulse; slow, shallow breathing; diarrhea; flush; low body temperature; coma.
WHAT TO DO:
- **Dial 911 (emergency) or 0 (operator) for an ambulance or medical help. Then give first aid immediately.**
- **See emergency information on inside covers.**

Time lapse before drug works:
3 weeks continual use required to determine effectiveness.

Don't take with:
Any other prescription or nonprescription drugs without consulting your doctor or pharmacist.

 POSSIBLE ADVERSE REACTIONS OR SIDE EFFECTS

SYMPTOMS	WHAT TO DO
Life-threatening: Irregular heartbeat, weak pulse, hives, black stool, bloody vomit.	Discontinue. Seek emergency treatment.
Common: Lethargy, drowsiness, tremor, depression, red eyes, runny nose, diarrhea, dry mouth.	Continue. Call doctor when convenient.
Infrequent: • Blurred vision, abdominal pain, nausea, vomiting, irregular heartbeat, joint pain.	Discontinue. Call doctor right away.
• Dizziness, mood change, headache, dry mouth, weakness, tiredness, weight gain or loss, foot and leg swelling.	Continue. Call doctor when convenient.
Rare: • Sore throat, fever, mouth sores; jaundice; unexplained bleeding or bruising.	Discontinue. Call doctor right away.
• Rash, painful or difficult urination, tremor, impotence, nightmares.	Continue. Call doctor when convenient.

 WARNINGS & PRECAUTIONS

Don't take if:
- You are allergic to any thiazide diuretic drug or any rauwolfia alkaloid.
- You are depressed.
- You have active peptic ulcer or ulcerative colitis.

Before you start, consult your doctor:
- If you are allergic to any sulfa drug*.
- If you have gout, liver, pancreas or kidney disorder, epilepsy.
- If you have had peptic ulcer, ulcerative colitis or gallstones.
- If you have been depressed.

- If you will have surgery within 2 months, including dental surgery, requiring general or spinal anesthesia.

Over age 60:
Adverse reactions and side effects may be more frequent and severe than in younger persons, especially dizziness and excessive potassium loss.

Pregnancy:
Risk factors vary for drugs in this group. See category list on page xxiii and consult doctor.

Breast-feeding:
Drug passes into milk. Avoid drug or discontinue nursing until you finish medicine. Consult doctor for advice on maintaining milk supply.

Infants & children:
Not recommended.

Prolonged use:
- You may need medicine to treat high blood pressure for the rest of your life.
- Causes cancer in laboratory animals. Consult your doctor if you have a family or personal history of cancer.
- Talk to your doctor about the need for follow-up medical examinations or laboratory studies to check blood pressure.

Skin & sunlight:
One or more drugs in this group may cause rash or intensify sunburn in areas exposed to sun or ultraviolet light (photosensitivity reaction). Avoid overexposure. Notify doctor if reaction occurs.

Driving, piloting or hazardous work:
Don't drive or pilot aircraft until you learn how medicine affects you. Don't work around dangerous machinery. Don't climb ladders or work in high places. Danger increases if you drink alcohol or take medicine affecting alertness and reflexes, such as antihistamines, tranquilizers, sedatives, pain medicine, narcotics and mind-altering drugs.

Discontinuing:
Don't discontinue without consulting doctor. Dose may require gradual reduction if you have taken drug for a long time. Doses of other drugs may also require adjustment.

Others:
- Hot weather and fever may cause dehydration and drop in blood pressure. Dose may require temporary adjustment. Weigh daily and report any unexpected weight decreases to your doctor.
- May cause rise in uric acid, leading to gout.
- May cause blood sugar rise in diabetics.
- Consult your doctor if you do isometric exercises. These raise blood pressure. Drug may intensify blood pressure rise.

 ## POSSIBLE INTERACTION WITH OTHER DRUGS

GENERIC NAME OR DRUG CLASS	COMBINED EFFECT
Anticoagulants*, oral	Unpredictable increased or decreased effect of anticoagulant.
Anticonvulsants*	Serious change in seizure pattern.
Antidepressants, tricyclic*	Dangerous drop in blood pressure. Avoid combination unless under medical supervision.
Antihistamines*	Increased antihistamine effect.
Antihypertensives*	Increased rauwolfia effect.
Aspirin	Decreased aspirin effect.

Continued on page 930

 ## POSSIBLE INTERACTION WITH OTHER SUBSTANCES

INTERACTS WITH	COMBINED EFFECT
Alcohol:	Increased intoxication. Dangerous blood pressure drop. Avoid.
Beverages: Carbonated drinks.	Decreased rauwolfia effect.
Cocaine:	Increased risk of heart block and high blood pressure.
Foods: Spicy foods.	Possible digestive upset.
Licorice.	Excessive potassium loss that causes dangerous heart rhythms.
Marijuana:	Occasional use— Mild drowsiness. Daily use—Moderate drowsiness, low blood pressure, depression.
Tobacco:	No proven problems.

RAUWOLFIA ALKALOIDS

GENERIC AND BRAND NAMES

See complete list of generic and brand names in the *Generic and Brand Name Directory*, page 894.

BASIC INFORMATION

Habit forming? No
Prescription needed? Yes
Available as generic? Yes
Drug class: Antihypertensive, tranquilizer (rauwolfia alkaloid)

USES

- Treatment for high blood pressure.
- Tranquilizer for mental and emotional disturbances.

DOSAGE & USAGE INFORMATION

How to take:
Tablet or timed-release capsule—Swallow with liquid or food to lessen stomach irritation. If you can't swallow whole, crumble tablet or open capsule and take with liquid or food.

When to take:
At the same times each day.

If you forget a dose:
Take as soon as you remember up to 2 hours late. If more than 2 hours, wait for next scheduled dose (don't double this dose).

What drug does:
- Interferes with nerve impulses and relaxes blood vessel muscles, reducing blood pressure.
- Suppresses brain centers that control emotions.

Time lapse before drug works:
3 weeks continual use required to determine effectiveness.

Continued next column

OVERDOSE

SYMPTOMS:
Drowsiness; slow, weak pulse; slow, shallow breathing; diarrhea; coma; flush; low body temperature; pinpoint pupils.
WHAT TO DO:
- **Dial 911 (emergency) or 0 (operator) for an ambulance or medical help. Then give first aid immediately.**
- **See emergency information on inside covers.**

Don't take with:
Any other medicine without consulting your doctor or pharmacist.

POSSIBLE ADVERSE REACTIONS OR SIDE EFFECTS

SYMPTOMS	WHAT TO DO
Life-threatening:	
In case of overdose, see previous column.	
Common:	
• Depression, dizziness.	Continue. Call doctor when convenient.
• Headache, faintness, drowsiness, lethargy, red eyes, stuffy nose, impotence, diminished sex drive, diarrhea, dry mouth.	Continue. Tell doctor at next visit.
Infrequent:	
• Black stool; bloody vomit; chest pain; shortness of breath; irregular or slow heartbeat; stiffness in muscles, bones, joints.	Discontinue. Call doctor right away.
• Trembling hands, foot and leg swelling.	Continue. Call doctor when convenient.
Rare:	
• Rash or itchy skin, sore throat, fever, abdominal pain, nausea, vomiting, unusual bleeding or bruising, jaundice.	Discontinue. Call doctor right away.
• Painful urination, nightmares.	Continue. Call doctor when convenient.

WARNINGS & PRECAUTIONS

Don't take if:
- You are allergic to any rauwolfia alkaloid.
- You are depressed.
- You have active peptic ulcer.
- You have ulcerative colitis.

Before you start, consult your doctor:
- If you have been depressed.
- If you have had peptic ulcer, ulcerative colitis or gallstones.
- If you have epilepsy.
- If you will have surgery within 2 months, including dental surgery, requiring general or spinal anesthesia.

Over age 60:
Adverse reactions and side effects may be more frequent and severe than in younger persons.

Pregnancy:
Decide with your doctor whether drug benefits justify risk to unborn child. Risk category C (see page xxiii).

Breast-feeding:
Drug passes into milk. Avoid drug or discontinue nursing until you finish medicine. Consult doctor for advice on maintaining milk supply.

Infants & children:
Not recommended.

Prolonged use:
- Causes cancer in laboratory animals. Consult your doctor if you have a family or personal history of cancer.
- Talk to your doctor about the need for follow-up medical examinations or laboratory studies.

Skin & sunlight:
No problems expected.

Driving, piloting or hazardous work:
Avoid if you feel drowsy, dizzy or faint. Otherwise, no problems expected.

Discontinuing:
Don't discontinue without consulting doctor. Dose may require gradual reduction if you have taken drug for a long time. Doses of other drugs may also require adjustment.

Others:
Consult your doctor if you do isometric exercises. These raise blood pressure. Drug may intensify blood pressure rise.

POSSIBLE INTERACTION WITH OTHER DRUGS

GENERIC NAME OR DRUG CLASS	COMBINED EFFECT
Anticoagulants*, oral	Unpredictable increased or decreased effect of anticoagulant.
Anticonvulsants*	Serious change in seizure pattern.
Antidepressants*	Increased anti-depressant effect.
Antihistamines*	Increased anti-histamine effect.
Antihypertensives*, other	Increased rauwolfia effect.
Aspirin	Decreased aspirin effect.
Beta-adrenergic blocking agents*	Increased rauwolfia alkaloid effect. Excessive sedation.
Carteolol	Increased anti-hypertensive effect.

Central nervous system (CNS) depressants*	Increased CNS depression.
Clozapine	Toxic effect on the central nervous system.
Digitalis preparations*	Possible irregular heartbeat.
Dronabinol	Increased effects of both drugs. Avoid.
Ethinamate	Dangerous increased effects of ethinamate. Avoid combining.
Fluoxetine	Increased depressant effects of both drugs.
Guanfacine	May increase depressant effects of either medicine.
Leucovorin	High alcohol content of leucovorin may cause adverse effects.
Levodopa	Decreased levodopa effect.

Continued on page 931

POSSIBLE INTERACTION WITH OTHER SUBSTANCES

INTERACTS WITH	COMBINED EFFECT
Alcohol:	Increased intoxication. Use with extreme caution.
Beverages: Carbonated drinks.	Decreased rauwolfia alkaloid effect.
Cocaine:	Increased risk of heart block and high blood pressure.
Foods: Spicy foods.	Possible digestive upset.
Marijuana:	Occasional use—Mild drowsiness. Daily use—Moderate drowsiness, low blood pressure, depression.
Tobacco:	No problems expected.

*See Glossary

RESERPINE, HYDRALAZINE & HYDROCHLOROTHIAZIDE

BRAND NAMES

Cam-Ap-Es
Cherapas
Ser-A-Gen
Seralazide

Ser-Ap-Es
Serpazide
Tri-Hydroserpine
Unipres

BASIC INFORMATION

Habit forming? No
Prescription needed? Yes
Available as generic? Yes
Drug class: Antihypertensive

USES

- Treatment for high blood pressure and congestive heart failure.
- Reduces fluid retention (edema).

DOSAGE & USAGE INFORMATION

How to take:
Tablet—Swallow with liquid. If you can't swallow whole, crumble and take with liquid or food.

When to take:
At the same times each day.

If you forget a dose:
Take as soon as you remember up to 2 hours late. If more than 2 hours, wait for next scheduled dose (don't double this dose).

What drug does:
- Interferes with nerve impulses and relaxes blood vessels, reducing blood pressure.
- Suppresses brain centers that control emotions.
- Forces sodium and water excretion, reducing body fluid. Reduced body fluid and relaxed arteries lower blood pressure.

Time lapse before drug works:
Regular use for several weeks may be necessary to determine drug's effectiveness.

Continued next column

OVERDOSE

SYMPTOMS:
Drowsiness; slow, shallow breathing; pinpoint pupils; diarrhea; flush; low body temperature; rapid, weak heartbeat; fainting; extreme weakness; cold, sweaty skin; cramps, coma.
WHAT TO DO:
- Dial 911 (emergency) or 0 (operator) for an ambulance or medical help. Then give first aid immediately.
- See emergency information on inside covers.

Don't take with:
- Nonprescription drugs containing alcohol without consulting doctor.
- Any other medicine without consulting your doctor or pharmacist.

POSSIBLE ADVERSE REACTIONS OR SIDE EFFECTS

SYMPTOMS	WHAT TO DO
Life-threatening:	
Rapid or irregular heartbeat, weak pulse, fainting, black stool, black or bloody vomit, chest pain.	Discontinue. Seek emergency treatment.
Common:	
• Nausea, vomiting.	Discontinue. Call doctor right away.
• Headache, diarrhea, drowsiness, runny nose, appetite loss.	Continue. Call doctor when convenient.
Infrequent:	
• Blurred vision, chest pain, abdominal pain, rash, hives, joint pain.	Discontinue. Call doctor right away.
• Dizziness; mood change; headache; dry mouth; weakness; tiredness; weight gain or loss; eyes red, watery, irritated; confusion; constipation; red or flushed face; joint stiffness; depression; anxiety; foot and leg swelling.	Continue. Call doctor when convenient.
Rare:	
• Jaundice; unexplained bleeding or bruising; sore throat, fever, mouth sores; weakness and faintness when arising from bed or chair.	Discontinue. Call doctor right away.
• Numbness, tingling, burning feeling in feet and hands; nasal congestion; impotence; nightmares.	Continue. Call doctor when convenient.

WARNINGS & PRECAUTIONS

Don't take if:
- You are allergic to any rauwolfia alkaloid, hydralazine, any thiazide diuretic drug*, or tartrazine dye.
- You are depressed.

- You have active peptic ulcer, ulcerative colitis, history of coronary artery disease or rheumatic heart disease.

Before you start, consult your doctor:
- If you have been depressed.
- If you have had peptic ulcer, ulcerative colitis, gallstones, kidney disease or impaired kidney function, lupus or a stroke.
- If you have epilepsy, gout; liver, pancreas or kidney disorder.
- If you feel pain in chest, neck or arms on physical exertion.
- If you are allergic to any sulfa drug*.
- If you will have surgery within 2 months, including dental surgery, requiring general or spinal anesthesia.

Over age 60:
Adverse reactions and side effects may be more frequent and severe than in younger persons, especially dizziness and excessive potassium loss.

Pregnancy:
Decide with your doctor if drug benefits justify risk to unborn child. Risk category C (see page xxiii).

Breast-feeding:
Drug passes into milk. Avoid drug or discontinue nursing until you finish medicine. Consult doctor.

Infants & children:
Not recommended.

Prolonged use:
- Causes cancer in laboratory animals. Consult your doctor if you have a family or personal history of cancer.
- Possible psychosis.
- May cause lupus; numbness, tingling in hands or feet.
- Talk to your doctor about the need for follow-up medical examinations or laboratory studies.

Skin & sunlight:
One or more drugs in this group may cause rash or intensify sunburn in areas exposed to sun or ultraviolet light (photosensitivity reaction). Avoid overexposure. Notify doctor if reaction occurs.

Driving, piloting or hazardous work:
Don't drive or pilot aircraft until you learn how medicine affects you. Don't work around dangerous machinery. Don't climb ladders or work in high places. Danger increases if you drink alcohol or take medicine affecting alertness and reflexes.

Discontinuing:
Don't discontinue without consulting doctor. Dose may require gradual reduction if you have taken drug for a long time. Doses of other drugs may also require adjustment.

Others:
- Consult your doctor if you do isometric exercises. These raise blood pressure. Drug may intensify blood pressure rise.
- Vitamin B-6 supplement may be advisable. Consult doctor.
- Hot weather and fever may cause dehydration and drop in blood pressure. Dose may require temporary adjustment. Weigh daily and report any unexpected weight decreases to your doctor.
- May cause rise in uric acid, leading to gout.
- May cause blood sugar rise in diabetics.
- Some products contain tartrazine dye. Avoid, especially if you are allergic to aspirin.

POSSIBLE INTERACTION WITH OTHER DRUGS

GENERIC NAME OR DRUG CLASS	COMBINED EFFECT
Acebutolol	Possible increased effects of drugs.

Continued on page 931

POSSIBLE INTERACTION WITH OTHER SUBSTANCES

INTERACTS WITH	COMBINED EFFECT
Alcohol:	Increased intoxication. Avoid.
Beverages: Carbonated drinks.	Decreased rauwolfia alkaloids effect.
Cocaine:	Dangerous blood pressure rise. Avoid.
Foods: Spicy foods.	Possible digestive upset.
Licorice.	Excessive potassium loss that causes dangerous heart rhythms.
Marijuana:	Weakness on standing. May increase blood pressure. Occasional use—Mild drowsiness. Daily use—Moderate drowsiness, low blood pressure, depression.
Tobacco:	Possible angina attacks.

RETINOIDS (Oral)

GENERIC AND BRAND NAMES

ACITRETIN
Soriatane

ETRETINATE
Tegison

BASIC INFORMATION

Habit forming? No
Prescription needed? Yes
Available as generic? No
Drug class: Antipsoriatic

 USES

- Treats psoriasis in patients who don't respond well to standard or usual treatment.
- Treats arthritic symptoms sometimes associated with psoriasis.
- Treats ichthyosis.

 DOSAGE & USAGE INFORMATION

How to take:
Capsules—Swallow with liquid or food to lessen stomach irritation. If you can't swallow whole, open capsule and take with liquid or food.

When to take:
At the same time each day, according to instructions on prescription label.

If you forget a dose:
One dose a day—Take as soon as you remember, up to 12 hours late. If more than 12 hours, wait for next scheduled dose (don't double this dose).

What drug does:
- Mechanism of action on skin is unknown, but positive effects on the disease have been documented. It probably reduces the production of protein in the outer layers of skin. It is chemically related to tretinoin (Retin-A).
- Also functions as an anti-inflammatory agent.

Continued next column

 OVERDOSE

SYMPTOMS:
Unknown. If overdose is suspected, follow instructions below.
WHAT TO DO:
- Dial 911 (emergency) or 0 (operator) for an ambulance or medical help. Then give first aid immediately.
- See emergency information on inside covers.

Time lapse before drug works:
- 2 to 6 hours for effects to begin.
- Prolonged treatment, up to 2 to 4 weeks (sometimes with psoralens, ultraviolet light may be necessary to develop maximum benefit).

Don't take with:
Any other medicine without consulting your doctor or pharmacist.

 POSSIBLE ADVERSE REACTIONS OR SIDE EFFECTS

SYMPTOMS	WHAT TO DO
Life-threatening: None expected.	
Common:	
• Bone and joint pain, stiffness, eye irritation or inflammation, unusual tiredness, muscle cramps, abdominal cramps, unusual bruising.	Discontinue. Call doctor right away.
• Dry skin, irritated or inflamed skin, hair thinning, dry eyes, mild nosebleed, mild headache, contact lens sensitivity, peeling of skin on hands or feet, thirstiness.	Continue. Call doctor when convenient.
Infrequent:	
• Blurred vision, hearing loss or other change in hearing, dark-colored urine, jaundice (yellow skin or eyes).	Discontinue. Call doctor right away.
• Dizziness, dry mouth, mild nausea, hair thinning, nail problems (redness, soreness or loosening), runny nose, lip symptoms (chapped, redness, sore, cracking, swelling), sore tongue.	Continue. Call doctor when convenient.
Rare:	
• Nausea and vomiting, severe and continuing headache.	Discontinue. Call doctor right away.
• Confusion, anxiety, depression, bleeding or inflamed gums.	Discontinue. Call doctor when convenient.

 WARNINGS & PRECAUTIONS

Don't take if:
- If you are pregnant or expect to get pregnant in the future. Fetal abnormalities have

occurred while using and after discontinuing the drug.
- If you are allergic to retinoids or parabens (used as preservative in gelatin capsule).

Before you start, consult your doctor:
- If you have heart or blood vessel disease.
- If you are allergic to any medication, food or other substance.
- If you have high plasma triglycerides.
- If you are an alcoholic.
- If you have diabetes mellitus.
- If you are a female of reproductive age.
- If you have kidney or liver disease.

Over age 60:
Adverse reactions and side effects may be more frequent and severe than in younger persons. You may need smaller doses for shorter periods of time.

Pregnancy:
Risk to unborn child outweighs drug benefits. Retinoids have caused major human fetal abnormalities. Don't use. Risk category X (see page xxiii).

Breast-feeding:
Drug passes into milk. Avoid drug or discontinue nursing until you finish medicine. Consult doctor for advice on maintaining milk supply.

Infants & children:
Don't use.

Prolonged use:
- No problems expected if used for no more than 4 months per treatment session.
- Talk to your doctor about the need for follow-up medical examinations or laboratory studies to check blood lipids, liver function.

Skin & sunlight:
May cause rash or intensify sunburn in areas exposed to sun or ultraviolet light (photosensitivity reaction). Avoid overexposure. Notify doctor if reaction occurs.

Driving, piloting or hazardous work:
Don't drive or pilot aircraft until you learn how medicine affects you. Don't work around dangerous machinery. Don't climb ladders or work in high places. Danger increases if you drink alcohol or take medicine affecting alertness and reflexes.

Discontinuing:
Don't discontinue without consulting doctor. Dose may require gradual reduction if you have taken drug for a long time. Doses of other drugs may also require adjustment.

Others:
- Courses of treatment are usually limited to 4 months, and repeating, if necessary, after a 4-month rest period.
- It is strongly recommended to continue birth control indefinitely after treatment is stopped.

- Certain methods of birth control may fail while using this drug, including tubal ligation and progestin (minipill) preparations. Other birth control methods may be affected also. Use two different methods of birth control.
- Don't donate blood during treatment or for 3 years thereafter.
- May cause problem in controlling blood sugar.
- During early treatment, psoriasis may appear to worsen.
- May cause changes in cholesterol levels in blood. Laboratory blood studies should be obtained prior to and during treatment.
- May cause calcium deposits in tendons and ligaments.
- Women who take etretinate should never plan on pregnancy.

POSSIBLE INTERACTION WITH OTHER DRUGS

GENERIC NAME OR DRUG CLASS	COMBINED EFFECT
Abrasive soaps or cleaners	Excessive drying effect on skin.
Acne preparations*	Excessive drying effect on skin.
Any topical preparation containing alcohol such as after-shave lotions	Excessive drying effect on skin.
Carbamazepine	Decreased retinoid activity.

Continued on page 932

POSSIBLE INTERACTION WITH OTHER SUBSTANCES

INTERACTS WITH	COMBINED EFFECT
Alcohol:	May cause hypertriglyceridemia. Avoid.
Beverages: Milk.	Aids absorption of etretinate.
Cocaine:	None expected.
Foods: High-fat diet or milk products.	Aids absorption of etretinate.
Marijuana:	None expected.
Tobacco:	None expected.

RETINOIDS (Topical)

GENERIC AND BRAND NAMES

ADAPALENE
  Differin
TAZAROTENE
  Tazorac

TRETINOIN
  Avita
  Renova
  Retin-A Cream
  Retin-A Cream
    Regimen Kit
  Retin-A Gel
  Retin-A Gel
    Regimen Kit
  Retin-A Solution
  Retinoic Acid
  Stieva-A Cream
  Stieva-A Cream
    Forte
  Stieva-A Gel
  Stieva-A Solution
  Vesanoid
  Vitamin A Acid
    Cream
  Vitamin A Acid Gel

BASIC INFORMATION

Habit forming? No
Prescription needed? Yes
Available as generic? No
Drug class: Antiacne (topical), antipsoriatic

USES

- Treatment for acne, psoriasis, ichthyosis, keratosis, folliculitis, flat warts.
- Treatment for sun-damaged skin (wrinkles), mottled skin, rough skin and pigmented skin.

DOSAGE & USAGE INFORMATION

How to use:
Wash skin with nonmedicated soap, pat dry, wait 20 minutes before applying.
- Cream or gel—Apply to affected areas with fingertips and rub in gently.

Continued next column

OVERDOSE

SYMPTOMS:
None expected.
WHAT TO DO:
- If person accidentally swallows drug, call doctor, poison control center or hospital emergency room for instructions.
- See emergency information on inside covers.

- Solution—Apply to affected areas with gauze pad or cotton swab. Avoid getting too wet so medicine doesn't drip into eyes or mouth, onto lips or inside nose.
- Follow manufacturer's directions on container.

When to use:
Apply once daily, usually in the evening before going to bed.

If you forget a dose:
Use as soon as you remember if it is still the same day. If more than 12 hours late, wait for the next dose (don't double this dose).

What drug does:
Helps control acne inflammation and prevent new acne outbreaks. Increases skin cell turnover so skin layer peels off more easily.

Time lapse before drug works:
May require 2 to 6 weeks for minimum benefit and 3 to 12 months for full benefit.

Don't use with:
Any other topical medicine without consulting your doctor or pharmacist.

POSSIBLE ADVERSE REACTIONS OR SIDE EFFECTS

SYMPTOMS	WHAT TO DO
Life-threatening: None expected.	
Common: • Mild redness, itching, chapping, dryness of skin during first few weeks of use.	Depending on severity, may reduce frequency of use.
• Worsening of acne or psoriasis during first few weeks of use (due to action of the drug on previous unseen breakouts).	Expected effect. No action necessary.
Infrequent: Painful skin irritation, darkening or lightening of skin where treated.	Discontinue. Call doctor when convenient.
Rare: None expected.	

WARNINGS & PRECAUTIONS

Don't take if:
You are allergic to topical retinoids or any of the components of the gel product.

Before you start, consult your doctor:
*   If you are using any other prescription or nonprescription medicine for the skin.
*   If you are using abrasive skin cleansers or medicated cosmetics.

Over age 60:
No problems expected.

Pregnancy:
*   Adapalene and tretinoin—Discuss with your doctor if benefits outweigh risks to unborn child. Risk category C (see page xxiii).
*   Tazarotene—Risk to unborn child outweighs drug's benefits. Don't use. Risk category X (see page xxiii).

Breast-feeding:
Effect unknown. Consult doctor.

Infants & children:
Not recommended.

Prolonged use:
No problems expected.

Skin & sunlight:
*   May cause rash or intensify sunburn in areas exposed to sun or ultraviolet light. Avoid over-exposure. Notify doctor if reaction occurs.
*   If you are normally exposed to considerable sunlight, use extra caution. Use broad spectrum of sunscreen on treated areas and wear protective clothing (e.g., hat).

Driving, piloting or hazardous work:
No problems expected.

Discontinuing:
*   May be unnecessary to finish medicine. Discontinue when acne improves. For some patients, this medicine may be used indefinitely to control acne.
*   If skin problem doesn't improve after first few weeks of use, consult doctor.

Others:
*   Cold or windy weather may further irritate the skin. Avoid if possible.
*   Products with a drying effect on the skin may cause irritation when used with retinoids. These include cosmetics, abrasive soaps and cleansers, astringents, and topical products that contain alcohol, spices or lime.
*   Don't apply drug to skin area that has cuts, abrasions, a rash or is sunburned.

POSSIBLE INTERACTION WITH OTHER DRUGS

GENERIC NAME OR DRUG CLASS	COMBINED EFFECT
Antiacne topical preparations, other	Excessive skin irritation.
Cosmetics (medicated)	Severe skin irritation.
Skin-peeling agents (salicylic acid, sulfur, resorcinol)	Excessive skin irritation.
Skin preparations with alcohol	Severe skin irritation.
Soaps or cleansers (abrasive)	Severe skin irritation.

POSSIBLE INTERACTION WITH OTHER SUBSTANCES

INTERACTS WITH	COMBINED EFFECT
Alcohol:	None expected.
Beverages:	None expected.
Cocaine:	None expected.
Foods:	None expected.
Marijuana:	None expected.
Tobacco:	None expected.

*See Glossary

RIBAVIRIN

BRAND NAMES

Tribavirin   Virazole
Virazid

BASIC INFORMATION

Habit forming? No
Prescription needed? Yes
Available as generic? No
Drug class: Antiviral

USES

- Treats severe viral pneumonia.
- Treats respiratory syncytial virus (RSV) infections in hospitalized infants or children.
- Treats influenza A and B with some success.
- Does not treat other viruses such as the common cold.

DOSAGE & USAGE INFORMATION

How to take:
By inhalation of a fine mist through mouth. Requires a special sprayer attached to oxygen mask, face mask for infants or hood.

When to take:
As ordered by your doctor.

If you forget a dose:
Use as soon as you remember.

What drug does:
Kills virus or prevents its growth.

Time lapse before drug works:
Begins working in 1 hour. May require treatment for 12 to 18 hours per day for 3 to 7 days.

Don't take with:
Any other medicine without consulting your doctor or pharmacist.

OVERDOSE

SYMPTOMS:
None expected.
WHAT TO DO:
Overdose unlikely to threaten life. If person takes much larger amount than prescribed, call doctor, poison control center or hospital emergency room for instructions.

POSSIBLE ADVERSE REACTIONS OR SIDE EFFECTS

SYMPTOMS	WHAT TO DO
Life-threatening: None expected.	
Common: None expected.	
Infrequent:	
• Unusual tiredness or weakness.	Discontinue. Call doctor right away.
• Headache, insomnia, appetite loss, nausea.	Continue. Call doctor when convenient.
Rare: Skin irritation or rash.	Continue. Call doctor when convenient.

WARNINGS & PRECAUTIONS

Don't take if:
You are allergic to ribavirin.

Before you start, consult your doctor:
- If you are now on low-salt, low-sugar or any special diet.
- If you have severe anemia.

Over age 60:
Adverse reactions and side effects may be more frequent and severe than in younger persons. Ask doctor about smaller doses.

Pregnancy:
Risk to unborn child outweighs drug benefits. Don't use. Risk category X (see page xxlll).

Breast-feeding:
Drug may pass into milk. Avoid drug or discontinue nursing until you finish medicine. Consult doctor for advice on maintaining milk supply.

Infants & children:
Use only under close medical supervision.

Prolonged use:
No problems expected.

Skin & sunlight:
No special problems expected.

Driving, piloting or hazardous work:
Don't drive or pilot aircraft until you learn how medicine affects you. Don't work around dangerous machinery. Don't climb ladders or work in high places. Danger increases if you drink alcohol or take medicine affecting alertness and reflexes, such as antihistamines, tranquilizers, sedatives, pain medicine, narcotics and mind-altering drugs.

Discontinuing:
Don't discontinue without consulting doctor. Dose may require gradual reduction if you have taken drug for a long time. Doses of other drugs may also require adjustment.

Others:
- Ribavirin is indicated for use in treatment of severe viral pneumonia caused by repiratory syncytial virus (RSV) in hospitalized infants and young children.
- Health care workers exposed to ribavirin may experience headache; eye itching, redness or swelling.
- Female health care workers who are pregnant or may become pregnant should avoid exposure to drug.

POSSIBLE INTERACTION WITH OTHER DRUGS

GENERIC NAME OR DRUG CLASS	COMBINED EFFECT
Zidovudine	Decreased effect of ribavirin and zidovudine.

POSSIBLE INTERACTION WITH OTHER SUBSTANCES

INTERACTS WITH	COMBINED EFFECT
Alcohol:	None expected.
Beverages:	None expected.
Cocaine:	None expected.
Foods:	None expected.
Marijuana:	None expected.
Tobacco:	None expected.

RIBOFLAVIN (Vitamin B-2)

BRAND NAMES

Many multivitamin preparations. Check labels.

BASIC INFORMATION

Habit forming? No
Prescription needed? No
Available as generic? Yes
Drug class: Vitamin supplement

 USES

* Dietary supplement to ensure normal growth and health.
* Dietary supplement to treat symptoms caused by deficiency of B-2: sores in mouth, eyes sensitive to light, itching and peeling skin.

 DOSAGE & USAGE INFORMATION

How to take:
Tablet—Swallow with liquid or food to lessen stomach irritation. If you can't swallow whole, crumble tablet and take with liquid or food.

When to take:
At the same times each day.

If you forget a dose:
Take as soon as you remember. Resume regular schedule. Don't double dose.

What drug does:
Promotes normal growth and health.

Time lapse before drug works:
Requires continual intake.

Don't take with:
Any other medicine without consulting your doctor or pharmacist.

 OVERDOSE

SYMPTOMS:
Dark urine, nausea, vomiting.
WHAT TO DO:
Overdose unlikely to threaten life. If person takes much larger amount than prescribed, call doctor, poison control center or hospital emergency room for instructions.

 POSSIBLE ADVERSE REACTIONS OR SIDE EFFECTS

SYMPTOMS	WHAT TO DO
Life-threatening: None expected.	
Common: Urine yellow in color.	No action necessary.
Infrequent: None expected.	
Rare: None expected.	

RIBOFLAVIN (Vitamin B-2)

WARNINGS & PRECAUTIONS

Don't take if:
- You are allergic to any B vitamin.
- You have chronic kidney failure.

Before you start, consult your doctor:
If you are pregnant or plan pregnancy.

Over age 60:
No problems expected.

Pregnancy:
Take within recommended guidelines. Consult doctor. Risk category A (see page xxiii).

Breast-feeding:
Take within recommended guidelines. Consult doctor.

Infants & children:
Consult doctor.

Prolonged use:
No problems expected.

Skin & sunlight:
No problems expected.

Driving, piloting or hazardous work:
No problems expected.

Discontinuing:
No problems expected.

Others:
A balanced diet should provide all the vitamin B-2 a healthy person needs and make supplements unnecessary during periods of good health. Best sources are milk, meats and green leafy vegetables.

POSSIBLE INTERACTION WITH OTHER DRUGS

GENERIC NAME OR DRUG CLASS	COMBINED EFFECT
Anticholinergics*	Possible increased riboflavin absorption.
Antidepressants, tricyclic*	Decreased riboflavin effect.
Phenothiazines*	Decreased riboflavin effect.
Probenecid	Decreased riboflavin effect.

POSSIBLE INTERACTION WITH OTHER SUBSTANCES

INTERACTS WITH	COMBINED EFFECT
Alcohol:	Prevents uptake and absorption of vitamin B-2.
Beverages:	No problems expected.
Cocaine:	No problems expected.
Foods:	No problems expected.
Marijuana:	No problems expected.
Tobacco:	Prevents absorption of vitamin B-2 and other vitamins and nutrients.

RIFAMYCINS

GENERIC AND BRAND NAMES

RIFAMPIN
Rifadin
Rifamate
Rifampicin
Rimactane

RIFAPENTINE
Priftin

BASIC INFORMATION

Habit forming? No
Prescription needed? Yes
Available as generic? Yes
Drug class: Antibacterial, antitubercular

USES

Treatment for tuberculosis and other infections. Used in combination with other antitubercular medications.

DOSAGE & USAGE INFORMATION

How to take:
Capsule or tablet—Swallow with liquid or food. If you can't swallow whole, open capsule or crumble tablet and take with liquid or small amount of food. For child, mix with small amount of applesauce or jelly.

When to take:
1 hour before or 2 hours after a meal.

If you forget a dose:
Take as soon as you remember up to 2 hours late. If more than 2 hours, wait for next scheduled dose (don't double this dose).

What drug does:
Prevents multiplication of tuberculosis germs.

Continued next column

OVERDOSE

SYMPTOMS:
Slow, shallow breathing; weak, rapid pulse; cold, sweaty skin; coma.
WHAT TO DO:
- Dial 911 (emergency) or 0 (operator) for an ambulance or medical help. Then give first aid immediately.
- If patient is unconscious and not breathing, give mouth-to-mouth breathing. If there is no heartbeat, use cardiac massage and mouth-to-mouth breathing (CPR). Don't try to make patient vomit. If you can't get help quickly, take patient to nearest emergency facility.
- See emergency information on inside covers.

Time lapse before drug works:
Usually 2 weeks. May require 1 to 2 years without missed doses for maximum benefit.

Don't take with:
Any other medicine without consulting your doctor or pharmacist.

POSSIBLE ADVERSE REACTIONS OR SIDE EFFECTS

SYMPTOMS	WHAT TO DO
Life-threatening: In case of overdose, see previous column.	
Common:	
• Diarrhea; reddish urine, stool, saliva, sweat and tears.	Continue. Call doctor when convenient.
• Blood in urine, joint pain, back or side pain, swelling of feet or legs.	Continue, but call doctor right away.
Infrequent:	
• Rash; flushed, itchy skin of face and scalp; blurred vision; difficulty breathing; nausea, vomiting; abdominal cramps; tiredness; bleeding or bruising.	Continue, but call doctor right away.
• Dizziness, unsteady gait, confusion, muscle or bone pain, heartburn, flatulence, chills, headache, fever, mood or behavior changes.	Continue. Call doctor when convenient.
Rare:	
• Sore throat, mouth or tongue; jaundice.	Discontinue. Call doctor right away.
• Appetite loss, less urination.	Continue. Call doctor when convenient.

WARNINGS & PRECAUTIONS

Don't take if:
- You are allergic to any of the rifamycins.
- You wear soft contact lenses.

Before you start, consult your doctor:
If you are alcoholic or have liver disease.

Over age 60:
Adverse reactions and side effects may be more frequent and severe than in younger persons.

Pregnancy:
Decide with your doctor if drug benefits justify risk to unborn child. Risk category C (see page xxiii).

Breast-feeding:
Effect unknown. Consult doctor.

Infants & children:
Use only under medical supervision.

Prolonged use:
- You may become more susceptible to infections caused by germs not responsive to rifamycins.
- Talk to your doctor about the need for follow-up medical examinations or laboratory studies to check liver function.

Skin & sunlight:
No problems expected.

Driving, piloting or hazardous work:
Don't drive or pilot aircraft until you learn how medicine affects you. Don't work around dangerous machinery. Don't climb ladders or work in high places. Danger increases if you drink alcohol or take medicine affecting alertness and reflexes, such as antihistamines, tranquilizers, sedatives, pain medicine, narcotics and mind-altering drugs.

Discontinuing:
Don't discontinue without doctor's advice until you complete prescribed dose, even though symptoms diminish or disappear.

Others:
- Reddish tears may discolor soft contact lenses.
- Advise any doctor or dentist you consult that you are using this medication.

 POSSIBLE INTERACTION WITH OTHER DRUGS

GENERIC NAME OR DRUG CLASS	COMBINED EFFECT
Adrenocorticoids, systemic	Decreased adrenocorticoid effect.
Anticoagulants*, oral	Decreased anticoagulant effect.
Antidepressants*, tricyclic	Decreased antidepressant effect.
Antidiabetics*, oral	Decreased antidiabetic effect.
Antifungals*, azole	Decreased antifungal effect.
Barbiturates*	Decreased barbiturate effect.
Calcium channel* blockers	Decreased channel blocker effect.
Chloramphenicol	Decreased effect of both drugs.
Ciproflax	Decreased antibiotic effect.
Clarithromycin	Decreased antibiotic effect.
Clofibrate	Decreased clofibrate effect.
Clozapine	Toxic effect on bone marrow.
Contraceptives, oral*	Decreased contraceptive effect.
Cyclosporine	Decreased effect of both drugs.
Dapsone	Decreased dapsone effect.
Diazepam	Decreased diazepam effect.
Digitalis preparations*	Decreased digitoxin effect.
Disopyramide	Decreased disopyramide effect.
Doxycycline	Decreased antibiotic effect.
Estrogens* (including contraceptive pills)	Decreased effect of both drugs.
Haloperidol	Decreased haloperidol effect.
Hepatotoxics*	Increased risk of liver toxicity.
Isoniazid	Possible toxicity to liver.
Levothyroxine	Decreased levothyroxine effect.
Methadone	Decreased methadone effect.
Mexiletine	Decreased mexiletine effect.
Non-nucleoside reverse transcriptase inhibitors	May require dosage adjustment of rifampin.

Continued on page 932

 POSSIBLE INTERACTION WITH OTHER SUBSTANCES

INTERACTS WITH	COMBINED EFFECT
Alcohol:	Possible toxicity to liver.
Beverages:	None expected.
Cocaine:	No proven problems.
Foods:	None expected.
Marijuana:	No proven problems.
Tobacco:	None expected.

RILUZOLE

BRAND NAMES

Rilutek

BASIC INFORMATION

Habit forming? No
Prescription needed? Yes
Available as generic? No
Drug class: Amyotrophic lateral sclerosis
  therapy agent

 ## USES

Treatment for amyotrophic lateral sclerosis (ALS or Lou Gehrig's disease), a motor neuron disorder that causes weakness and atrophy of the muscles. Riluzole may extend a patient's survival time and delay the need for surgery for complications. It does not cure the disorder.

 ## DOSAGE & USAGE INFORMATION

How to take:
Tablet—Swallow with liquid. Instructions to take on an empty stomach mean 1 hour before or 2 hours after eating.

When to take:
Usually every 12 hours.

If you forget a dose:
Take as soon as you remember up to 6 hours late. If more than 6 hours, wait for the next dose (don't double this dose).

What drug does:
The cause of ALS is unknown and the exact mechanism of how the drug works is also unknown. It appears to decrease production of certain chemicals in the body and may affect some cellular activity that leads to the progressive weakness caused by the disorder.

Time lapse before drug works:
6 to 18 months for maximum benefits.

Don't take with:
Any other medicine without consulting your doctor or pharmacist.

 ## OVERDOSE

SYMPTOMS:
None reported to date.
WHAT TO DO:
If person takes much larger amount than prescribed, call doctor, poison control center or hospital emergency room for instructions.

 ## POSSIBLE ADVERSE REACTIONS OR SIDE EFFECTS

SYMPTOMS	WHAT TO DO
Life-threatening: None expected.	
Common: • Difficulty breathing, abdominal pain, increased coughing, blood pressure increased.	Discontinue. Call doctor right away.
• Mouth has a burning, or tingling feeling, constipation, nausea, vomiting, dizziness, mild weakness, headache, diarrhea.	Continue. Call doctor when convenient.
Infrequent: Skin symptoms (redness, itching, scaling, bruising, oozing or thickening), fever, sore feet or legs, sores in mouth or on lips, fast heartbeat.	Discontinue. Call doctor right away.
Rare: Changes in vision, tightness in chest, wheezing, memory loss, mood changes, severe drowsiness, hallucinations, mental changes, swelling (face, hands, fingers, feet or legs), nosebleed, blood in urine, unusual bleeding, unusual tiredness or weakness, severe headache, pain in various parts of the body, eyes red or irritated, continued or painful penile erection, noisy breathing, loss of bladder control, hives.	Discontinue. Call doctor right away.

WARNINGS & PRECAUTIONS

Don't take if:
You are sensitive to riluzole.

Before you start, consult your doctor:
- If you are allergic to any medicine, food or other substance, or have a family history of allergies.
- If you have liver or kidney disease.

Over age 60:
No problems expected.

Pregnancy:
Decide with your doctor if drug benefits justify risk to unborn child. Risk category C (see page xxiii).

Breast-Feeding:
Not recommended. Consult doctor.

Infants & children:
Not recommended for this age group.

Prolonged use:
Talk to your doctor about the need for follow-up medical examinations or laboratory studies to check liver function.

Skin & sunlight:
No problems expected.

Driving, piloting or hazardous work:
Don't drive or pilot aircraft until you learn how medicine affects you. Don't work around dangerous machinery. Don't climb ladders or work in high places. Danger increases if you drink alcohol or take other medicines affecting alertness and reflexes.

Discontinuing:
No problems expected.

Others:
- May affect the results of some medical tests.
- Use as directed. Don't increase or decrease dosage without doctor's approval.
- Advise any doctor or dentist whom you consult that you take this medicine.
- Call your doctor if you develop a fever.

POSSIBLE INTERACTION WITH OTHER DRUGS

GENERIC NAME OR DRUG CLASS	COMBINED EFFECT
Hepatotoxics*	Increased risk of adverse effects.
Other medications	Complete studies have not been done to evaluate interactions with other drugs, but the potential exists for a variety of possible interactions. Consult doctor.

POSSIBLE INTERACTION WITH OTHER SUBSTANCES

INTERACTS WITH	COMBINED EFFECT
Alcohol:	Increased risk of adverse effects.
Beverages:	None expected.
Cocaine:	Problems not known. Best to avoid.
Foods:	None expected.
Marijuana:	Problems not known. Best to avoid.
Tobacco:	May decrease riluzole effect.

*See Glossary

RISPERIDONE

BRAND NAMES

Risperdal

BASIC INFORMATION

Habit forming? No
Prescription needed? Yes
Available as generic? No
Drug class: Antipsychotic

 USES

Treats nervous, mental and emotional conditions. Helps in managing the signs and symptoms of schizophrenia.

 DOSAGE & USAGE INFORMATION

How to take:
* Tablet—Swallow with liquid. May be taken with or without food.
* Oral solution—Dilute in 3 to 4 ounces of liquid (water, orange juice or low fat milk; don't use cola or tea).

When to take:
At the same times each day. The prescribed dosage will gradually be increased over the first few days of use.

If you forget a dose:
Take as soon as you remember. If it is almost time for the next dose, wait for the next scheduled dose (don't double this dose).

What drug does:
The exact mechanism is unknown. It appears to block certain nerve impulses between nerve cells.

Time lapse before drug works:
One to 7 days. A further increase in the dosage amount may be necessary to relieve symptoms for some patients.

Continued next column

 OVERDOSE

SYMPTOMS:
Extreme drowsiness, rapid heartbeat, faintness, convulsions, excessive sweating, difficulty breathing, loss of muscular control.
WHAT TO DO:
* **Dial 911 (emergency) or 0 (operator) for an ambulance or medical help. Then give first aid immediately.**
* **See emergency information at end of book.**

Don't take with:
Any other medication without consulting your doctor or pharmacist.

 POSSIBLE ADVERSE REACTIONS OR SIDE EFFECTS

SYMPTOMS	WHAT TO DO
Life-threatening: High fever, rapid pulse, profuse sweating, muscle rigidity, confusion and irritability, seizures (malignant neuroleptic syndrome - rare).	Discontinue. Seek emergency treatment.
Common: Anxiety, drowsiness, dizziness, digestive problems, rash, sexual dysfunction.	Continue. Call doctor when convenient.
Infrequent: • Jerky or involuntary movements, especially of the face, lips, jaw, tongue (with higher doses only); slow-frequency tremor of head, face, or limbs, especially while moving; muscle rigidity, lack of facial expression and slow, inflexible movements.	Discontinue. Call doctor right away.
• Dry mouth, blurred vision, constipation, difficulty urinating; sedation, dizziness and low blood pressure; pacing or restlessness, intermittent spasms of muscles of face, eyes, tongue, jaw, neck, body or limbs.	Continue. Call doctor when convenient.
Rare: Other symptoms not listed above.	Continue. Call doctor when convenient.

WARNINGS & PRECAUTIONS

Don't take if:
You are allergic to risperidone.

Before you start, consult your doctor:
* If you have liver or kidney disease or heart disease.
* It you are allergic to any other medications.
* If you have a history of seizures.

Over age 60:
Adverse reactions and side effects may be more severe than in younger persons. A lower starting dosage is usually recommended until a response is determined.

Pregnancy:
Decide with your doctor if drug benefits justify any possible risk to unborn child. Risk category C (see page xxiii).

Breast-feeding:
It is unknown if drug passes into milk. Avoid nursing until you finish medicine. Consult doctor for advice on maintaining milk supply.

Infants & children:
Safety in children under age 12 has not been established. Use only under close medical supervision.

Prolonged use:
Consult with your doctor on a regular basis while taking this drug to check your progress or to discuss any increase or changes in side effects and the need for continued treatment.

Skin & sunlight:
* May cause rash or intensify sunburn in areas exposed to sun or ultraviolet light (photosensitivity reaction). Use sunscreen and avoid overexposure. Notify doctor if reaction occurs.
* Hot temperatures and exercise, hot baths can increase risk of heatstroke. Drug may affect body's ability to maintain normal temperature.

Driving, piloting or hazardous work:
Don't drive or pilot aircraft until you learn how medicine affects you. Don't work around dangerous machinery. Don't climb ladders or work in high places. Danger increases if you drink alcohol or take medicine affecting alertness and reflexes.

Discontinuing:
Don't discontinue this drug without consulting doctor. Dosage may require a gradual reduction before stopping.

Others:
* Get up slowly from a sitting or lying position to avoid any dizziness, faintness or lightheadedness.
* Advise any doctor or dentist whom you consult that you take this medicine.
* Take medicine only as directed. Do not increase or reduce dosage without doctor's approval.

POSSIBLE INTERACTION WITH OTHER DRUGS

GENERIC NAME OR DRUG CLASS	COMBINED EFFECT
Antihypertensives*	Increased antihypertensive effect.
Carbamazepine	Decreased effect of risperidone.
Clozapine	Increased effect of risperidone.
Central nervous system (CNS) depressants*, other	Increased sedative effect.
Levodopa	May decrease levodopa effect.

POSSIBLE INTERACTION WITH OTHER SUBSTANCES

INTERACTS WITH	COMBINED EFFECT
Alcohol:	Increased sedative affect. Avoid.
Beverages:	None expected.
Cocaine:	Effect not known. Best to avoid.
Foods:	None expected.
Marijuana:	Effect not known. Best to avoid.
Tobacco:	None expected.

RITODRINE

BRAND NAMES

Yutopar

BASIC INFORMATION

Habit forming? No
Prescription needed? Yes
Available as generic? Yes
Drug class: Labor inhibitor, beta-adrenergic stimulator

 ## USES

Halts premature labor in pregnancies of 20 or more weeks.

 ## DOSAGE & USAGE INFORMATION

How to take:
Tablet—Swallow with liquid or food to lessen stomach irritation. If you can't swallow whole, crumble tablet and take with liquid or food.

When to take:
Every 4 to 6 hours until term.

If you forget a dose:
Take as soon as you remember up to 2 hours late. If more than 2 hours, wait for next scheduled dose (don't double this dose).

What drug does:
Inhibits contractions of uterus (womb).

Time lapse before drug works:
30 to 60 minutes (oral form). Faster intravenously.

Don't take with:
Any other medicine without consulting your doctor or pharmacist.

 ## OVERDOSE

SYMPTOMS:
Rapid, irregular heartbeat to 120 or more; shortness of breath.
WHAT TO DO:
- **Dial 911 (emergency) or 0 (operator) for an ambulance or medical help. Then give first aid immediately.**
- **If patient is unconscious and not breathing, give mouth-to-mouth breathing. If there is no heartbeat, use cardiac massage and mouth-to-mouth breathing (CPR). Don't try to make patient vomit. If you can't get help quickly, take patient to nearest emergency facility.**
- **See emergency information on inside covers.**

 ## POSSIBLE ADVERSE REACTIONS OR SIDE EFFECTS

SYMPTOMS	WHAT TO DO
Life-threatening:	
Hives, rash, intense itching, faintness soon after a dose (anaphylaxis).	Seek emergency treatment immediately.
Common:	
Irregular heartbeat, fast heartbeat.	Discontinue. Call doctor right away.
Infrequent:	
• Shortness of breath.	Discontinue. Call doctor right away.
• Nervousness, trembling, headache, nausea, vomiting.	Continue. Call doctor when convenient.
Rare:	
Rash, angina, jaundice.	Discontinue. Call doctor right away.

WARNINGS & PRECAUTIONS

Don't take if:
- You have heart disease.
- You have eclampsia.
- You have lung congestion.
- You have infection in the uterus.
- You have an overactive thyroid.
- You have a bleeding disorder.

Before you start, consult your doctor:
- If you have asthma.
- If you have diabetes.
- If you have high blood pressure.
- If you have pre-eclampsia.

Over age 60:
Not used.

Pregnancy:
Ritodrine crosses placenta, but animal studies show that it doesn't affect fetuses. Benefits versus risks must be assessed by you and your doctor. Risk category B (see page xxiii).

Breast-feeding:
Not applicable.

Infants & children:
Not used.

Prolonged use:
Talk to your doctor about the need for follow-up medical examinations or laboratory studies to check blood sugar, ECG*, fluid and electrolytes.

Skin & sunlight:
No problems expected.

Driving, piloting or hazardous work:
Don't drive or pilot aircraft until you learn how medicine affects you. Don't work around dangerous machinery. Don't climb ladders or work in high places. Danger increases if you drink alcohol or take medicine affecting alertness and reflexes, such as antihistamines, tranquilizers, sedatives, pain medicine, narcotics and mind-altering drugs.

Discontinuing:
Don't discontinue without consulting doctor. Dose may require gradual reduction if you have taken drug for a long time. Doses of other drugs may also require adjustment.

Others:
No problems expected.

POSSIBLE INTERACTION WITH OTHER DRUGS

GENERIC NAME OR DRUG CLASS	COMBINED EFFECT
Adrenal corticosteroids*	Increased chance of fluid in lungs of mother. Avoid.
Anesthetics, general*	Possible cardiac arrhythmias or hypotension.
Beta-adrenergic blocking agents*	Decreased effect of ritodrine.
Diazoxide	Possible cardiac arrhythmias or hypotension.
Magnesium sulfate	Possible cardiac arrhythmias or hypotension.
Meperidine	Possible cardiac arrhythmias or hypotension.
Sympathomimetics*	Increased side effects of both.

POSSIBLE INTERACTION WITH OTHER SUBSTANCES

INTERACTS WITH	COMBINED EFFECT
Alcohol:	Increased adverse effects. Avoid.
Beverages:	No problems expected.
Cocaine:	Injury to fetus. Avoid.
Foods:	No problems expected.
Marijuana:	Injury to fetus. Avoid.
Tobacco:	Injury to fetus. Avoid.

SALICYLATES

GENERIC AND BRAND NAMES

See complete list of generic and brand names in the *Generic and Brand Name Directory*, page 894.

BASIC INFORMATION

Habit forming? No
Prescription needed? For some
Available as generic? Yes
Drug class: Analgesic, anti-inflammatory (nonsteroidal)

 USES

- Reduces pain, fever, inflammation.
- Relieves swelling, stiffness, joint pain of arthritis or rheumatism.
- Decreases risk of myocardial infarction (aspirin only).

 DOSAGE & USAGE INFORMATION

How to take:
- Tablet or capsule—Swallow with liquid.
- Extended-release tablets—Swallow each dose whole.
- Suppositories—Remove wrapper and moisten suppository with water. Gently insert into rectum, large end first.

When to take:
Pain, fever, inflammation—As needed, no more often than every 4 hours.

If you forget a dose:
- Pain, fever—Take as soon as you remember. Wait 4 hours for next dose.
- Arthritis—Take as soon as you remember up to 2 hours late. Return to regular schedule.

What drug does:
- Affects hypothalamus, the part of the brain that regulates temperature by dilating small blood vessels in skin.

Continued next column

 OVERDOSE

SYMPTOMS:
Ringing in ears; nausea; vomiting; dizziness; fever; deep, rapid breathing; hallucinations; convulsions; coma.
WHAT TO DO:
- **Dial 911 (emergency) or 0 (operator) for an ambulance or medical help. Then give first aid immediately.**
- **See emergency information on inside covers.**

- Prevents clumping of platelets (small blood cells) so blood vessels remain open.
- Decreases prostaglandin effect.
- Suppresses body's pain messages.

Time lapse before drug works:
30 minutes for pain, fever, arthritis.

Don't take with:
- Tetracyclines. Space doses 1 hour apart.
- Any other medicine without consulting your doctor or pharmacist.

 POSSIBLE ADVERSE REACTIONS OR SIDE EFFECTS

SYMPTOMS	WHAT TO DO
Life-threatening:	
Hives, rash, intense itching, faintness soon after a dose (anaphylaxis); black or bloody vomit; blood in urine.	Seek emergency treatment immediately.
Common:	
• Nausea, vomiting, abdominal pain.	Discontinue. Seek emergency treatment.
• Heartburn, indigestion.	Continue. Call doctor when convenient.
• Ringing in ears.	Continue. Tell doctor at next visit.
Infrequent:	
None expected.	
Rare:	
• Black stools, unexplained fever.	Discontinue. Seek emergency treatment.
• Rash, hives, itchy skin, diminished vision, shortness of breath, wheezing, jaundice.	Discontinue. Call doctor right away.
• Drowsiness, headache.	Continue. Call doctor when convenient.

 WARNINGS & PRECAUTIONS

Don't take if:
- You need to restrict sodium in your diet. Buffered effervescent tablets and sodium salicylate are high in sodium.
- Salicylates have a strong vinegar-like odor, which means they have decomposed.
- You have a peptic ulcer of stomach or duodenum.
- You have a bleeding disorder.

Before you start, consult your doctor:
- If you have had stomach or duodenal ulcers.
- If you have had gout.
- If you have asthma or nasal polyps.

Over age 60:
More likely to cause hidden bleeding in stomach or intestines. Watch for dark stools.

Pregnancy:
Risk factors vary for drugs in this group. See category list on page xxiii and consult doctor.

Breast-feeding:
Drug passes into milk. Avoid drug or discontinue nursing until you finish medicine. Consult doctor for advice on maintaining milk supply.

Infants & children:
- Overdose frequent and severe. Keep bottles out of children's reach.
- Do not give to persons under age 18 who have fever and discomfort of viral illness, especially chicken pox and influenza. Probably increases risk of Reye's syndrome.

Prolonged use:
- Kidney damage. Periodic kidney function test recommended.
- Talk to your doctor about the need for follow-up medical examinations or laboratory studies to check liver function.

Skin & sunlight:
No special problems expected.

Driving, piloting or hazardous work:
No restrictions unless you feel drowsy.

Discontinuing:
For chronic illness—Don't discontinue without doctor's advice until you complete prescribed dose, even though symptoms diminish or disappear.

Others:
- Salicylates can complicate surgery, pregnancy, labor and delivery, and illness.
- For arthritis—Don't change dose without consulting doctor.
- Urine tests for blood sugar may be inaccurate.

POSSIBLE INTERACTION WITH OTHER DRUGS

GENERIC NAME OR DRUG CLASS	COMBINED EFFECT
Acetaminophen	Increased risk of kidney damage (with high, prolonged dose of each).
Adrenocorticoids, systemic	Decreased salicylate effect.
Allopurinol	Decreased allopurinol effect.
Angiotensin-converting enzyme (ACE) inhibitors*	Decreased ACE inhibitor effect.

Antacids*	Decreased salicylate effect.
Anticoagulants*, oral	Increased anti-coagulant effect. Abnormal bleeding.
Antidiabetics*, oral	Low blood sugar.
Anti-inflammatory drugs, nonsteroidal (NSAIDs)*	Risk of stomach bleeding and ulcers
Aspirin, other	Likely salicylate toxicity.
Beta-adrenergic blocking agents*	Decreased anti-hypertensive effect.
Bismuth subsalicylate	Increased risk of salicylate toxicity.
Bumetanide	Decreased diuretic effect.
Calcium supplements*	Increased salicylate effect.
Carteolol	Decreased anti-hypertensive effect of carteolol.
Ethacrynic acid	Decreased diuretic effect.
Furosemide	Possible salicylate toxicity.
Gold compounds*	Increased likelihood of kidney damage.
Indomethacin	Risk of stomach bleeding and ulcers.
Insulin	Decreased blood sugar.

Continued on page 933

POSSIBLE INTERACTION WITH OTHER SUBSTANCES

INTERACTS WITH	COMBINED EFFECT
Alcohol:	Possible stomach irritation and bleeding. Avoid.
Beverages:	None expected.
Cocaine:	None expected.
Foods:	None expected.
Marijuana:	Possible increased pain relief, but marijuana may slow body's recovery. Avoid.
Tobacco:	None expected.

*See Glossary

SCOPOLAMINE (Hyoscine)

BRAND NAMES

See complete list of brand names in the *Generic and Brand Name Directory*, page 894.

BASIC INFORMATION

Habit forming? No
Prescription needed?
 High strength: Yes
 Low strength: No
Available as generic? Yes
Drug class: Antispasmodic, anticholinergic

USES

- Reduces spasms of digestive system, bladder and urethra.
- Relieves painful menstruation.
- Prevents motion sickness.

DOSAGE & USAGE INFORMATION

How to take:
- Tablet or capsule—Swallow with liquid or food to lessen stomach irritation.
- Drops—Dilute dose in beverage.
- Skin discs—Clean application site. Change application sites with each dose.

When to take:
- Motion sickness—Apply disc 30 minutes before departure.
- Other uses—Take 30 minutes before meals (unless directed otherwise by doctor).

If you forget a dose:
Take up to 2 hours late. If more than 2 hours, wait for next dose (don't double this dose).

What drug does:
Blocks nerve impulses at parasympathetic nerve endings, preventing muscle contractions and gland secretions of organs involved.

Continued next column

OVERDOSE

SYMPTOMS:
Dilated pupils, blurred vision, rapid pulse and breathing, dizziness, fever, hallucinations, confusion, slurred speech, agitation, flushed face, convulsions, coma.
WHAT TO DO:
- **Dial 911 (emergency) or 0 (operator) for an ambulance or medical help. Then give first aid immediately.**
- **See emergency information on inside covers.**

Time lapse before drug works:
15 to 30 minutes.

Don't take with:
Any other medicine without consulting your doctor or pharmacist.

POSSIBLE ADVERSE REACTIONS OR SIDE EFFECTS

SYMPTOMS	WHAT TO DO
Life-threatening:	
Hives, rash, intense itching, faintness soon after a dose (anaphylaxis).	Seek emergency treatment immediately.
Common:	
• Confusion, delirium, rapid heartbeat.	Discontinue. Call doctor right away.
• Nausea, vomiting, decreased sweating.	Continue. Call doctor when convenient.
• Constipation, loss of taste.	Continue. Tell doctor at next visit.
• Dryness in ears, nose, throat, mouth.	No action necessary.
Infrequent:	
• Headache, difficult urination, nasal congestion, altered taste.	Continue. Call doctor when convenient.
• Lightheadedness.	Discontinue. Call doctor right away.
Rare:	
Rash or hives, eye pain, blurred vision.	Discontinue. Call doctor right away.

WARNINGS & PRECAUTIONS

Don't take if:
- You are allergic to any anticholinergic.
- You have trouble with stomach bloating.
- You have difficulty emptying your bladder completely.
- You have narrow-angle glaucoma.
- You have severe ulcerative colitis.

Before you start, consult your doctor:
- If you have open-angle glaucoma, angina, chronic bronchitis or asthma, hiatal hernia, liver disease, enlarged prostate, myasthenia gravis, peptic ulcer, kidney or thyroid disease.
- If you will have surgery within 2 months, including dental surgery, requiring general or spinal anesthesia.

Over age 60:
Adverse reactions and side effects may be more frequent and severe than in younger persons.

Pregnancy:
Decide with your doctor whether drug benefits justify risk to unborn child. Risk category C (see page xxiii).

Breast-feeding:
Drug passes into milk and decreases milk flow. Avoid drug or discontinue nursing until you finish medicine. Consult doctor for advice on maintaining milk supply.

Infants & children:
Use only under medical supervision.

Prolonged use:
Chronic constipation, possible fecal impaction. Consult doctor immediately.

Skin & sunlight:
No problems expected.

Driving, piloting or hazardous work:
Use disqualifies you for piloting aircraft. Don't drive until you learn how medicine affects you. Don't work around dangerous machinery. Don't climb ladders or work in high places.

Discontinuing:
May be unnecessary to finish medicine. Follow doctor's instructions.

Others:
Advise any doctor or dentist whom you consult that you take this medicine.

POSSIBLE INTERACTION WITH OTHER DRUGS

GENERIC NAME OR DRUG CLASS	COMBINED EFFECT
Adrenocorticoids, systemic	Possible glaucoma.
Amantadine	Increased scopolamine effect.
Antacids*	Decreased scopolamine effect.
Anticholinergics*, other	Increased scopolamine effect.
Antidepressants, tricyclic*	Increased scopolamine effect. Increased sedation.
Antidiarrheals*	Decreased scopolamine effect.
Antihistamines*	Increased scopolamine effect.
Attapulgite	Decreased scopolamine effect.
Buclizine	Increased scopolamine effect.
Clozapine	Toxic effect on the central nervous system.

Digitalis preparations*	Possible decreased absorption of scopolamine.
Encainide	Increased effect of toxicity on heart muscle.
Ethinamate	Dangerous increased effects of ethinamate. Avoid combining.
Fluoxetine	Increased depressant effects of both drugs.
Guanfacine	May increase depressant effects of either medicine.
Haloperidol	Increased internal eye pressure.
Ketoconazole	Decreased keto-conazole effect.
Leucovorin	High alcohol content of leucovorin may cause adverse effects.
Meperidine	Increased scopolamine effect.
Methylphenidate	Increased scopolamine effect.
Methyprylon	May increase seda-tive effect to danger-ous level. Avoid.
Molindone	Increased anti-cholinergic effect.
Monoamine oxidase (MAO) inhibitors*	Increased scopolamine effect.

Continued on page 933

POSSIBLE INTERACTION WITH OTHER SUBSTANCES

INTERACTS WITH	COMBINED EFFECT
Alcohol:	None expected.
Beverages:	None expected.
Cocaine:	Excessively rapid heartbeat. Avoid.
Foods:	None expected.
Marijuana:	Drowsiness, dry mouth.
Tobacco:	None expected.

*See Glossary

SELEGILINE

BRAND NAMES

Carbex	Juprenil
Eldepryl	Movergan
Jumex	Procythol
Jumexal	SD Deprenyl

BASIC INFORMATION

All the information in this chart applies only when selegiline is given with other drugs that treat Parkinson's disease.

Habit forming? No
Prescription needed? Yes
Available as generic? Yes
Drug class: Antidyskinetic

USES

- Treats Parkinson's disease *(paralysis agitans)* when given with levodopa or the combination of levodopa and carbidopa.
- Treats mental depression when taken alone.

DOSAGE & USAGE INFORMATION

How to take:
Tablets—Swallow with liquid. If you can't swallow whole, crumble tablet and take with liquid or food.

Continued next column

OVERDOSE

SYMPTOMS:
Mouth-opening difficulty; neck and heel muscle spasm; sweating; irregular, fast heartbeat; reflexes hyperactive; cold or clammy skin; chest pain; agitation; fainting; seizures; coma. Symptoms can develop 12 to 48 hours after ingestion.
WHAT TO DO:
- **Dial 911 (emergency) or 0 (operator) for an ambulance or medical help. Then give first aid immediately.**
- **If patient is unconsciousness and not breathing, give mouth-to-mouth breathing. If there is no heartbeat, use cardiac massage and mouth-to-mouth breathing (CPR). Don't try to make patient vomit. If you can't get help quickly, take patient to nearest emergency facility.**
- **See emergency information on inside covers.**

When to take:
Usually taken at breakfast and lunch to minimize nausea or insomnia. Don't take after mid-afternoon.

If you forget a dose:
Take as soon as you remember up to 2 hours late. If more than 2 hours, wait for next scheduled dose (don't double this dose).

What drug does:
Inhibits action of monoamine oxidase Type B (MAO B), a major chemical enzyme in the brain. Doses higher than recommended can cause high blood pressure.

Time lapse before drug works:
2 hours.

Don't take with:
- Any foods containing tyramine, such as cheese; wine; beer; nonalcoholic beer; liqueurs; yeast extracts; bean pods; pickled or smoked fish, meat, chicken, turkey or other poultry; fermented sausage (summer sausage, salami, pepperoni); bologna; overripe fruit; caffeine.
- Any other medicines (including over-the-counter drugs such as cough and cold medicines, laxatives, antacids, diet pills, nose drops or vitamins) without consulting your doctor.

POSSIBLE ADVERSE REACTIONS OR SIDE EFFECTS

SYMPTOMS	WHAT TO DO
Life-threatening:	
In case of overdose, see previous column.	
Severe chest pain, enlarged pupils, heartbeat irregularities, severe nausea and vomiting, stiff neck.	Seek emergency treatment.
Common:	
Mood changes, unusual or uncontrolled body movements, hallucinations, headache, lip smacking, difficult urination.	Discontinue. Call doctor right away.
Abdominal pain, dizziness, dry mouth, insomnia, mild nausea.	Continue. Call doctor when convenient.
Infrequent:	
Chest pain, heartbeat irregularities, wheezing, swollen feet, speech difficulty, bloody or black stools.	Discontinue. Seek emergency treatment.

- Constipation; anxiety; tiredness; eyelid spasm; unpleasant taste; blurred vision; leg pain; ringing ears; chills; skin rash; burning lips or mouth; drowsiness; frequent, decreased urination.

  Continue. Call doctor when convenient.

Rare:

Weight loss, heartburn, jaw clenching or teeth gnashing, impaired memory, uncontrolled body movements.

Continue. Call doctor when convenient.

WARNINGS & PRECAUTIONS

Don't take if:
You are allergic to selegiline.

Before you start, consult your doctor:
If you have a past medical history of peptic ulcer, profound dementia, severe psychosis, tardive dyskinesia, excessive tremor.

Over age 60:
Adverse reactions and side effects may be more frequent and severe than in younger persons. You may need smaller doses for shorter periods of time.

Pregnancy:
Decide with your doctor if drug benefits justify risk to unborn child. Risk category C (see page xxiii).

Breast-feeding:
Unknown if drug passes into milk. Consult doctor.

Infants & children:
Not recommended.

Prolonged use:
Talk to your doctor about the need for follow-up medical examinations or laboratory studies to check complete blood counts (white blood cell count, platelet count, red blood cell count, hemoglobin, hematocrit), stomach x-rays.

Skin & sunlight:
May cause rash or intensify sunburn in areas exposed to sun or ultraviolet light (photo-sensitivity reaction). Avoid overexposure. Notify doctor if reaction occurs.

Driving, piloting or hazardous work:
Don't drive or pilot aircraft until you learn how medicine affects you. Don't work around danger-ous machinery. Don't climb ladders or work in high places. Danger increases if you drink alcohol or take medicine affecting alertness and reflexes.

Discontinuing:
No special problems expected.

Others:
- Avoid sudden rises from lying-down or sitting positions.
- Advise any doctor or dentist whom you consult that you take this medicine.
- May affect results in some medical tests.

POSSIBLE INTERACTION WITH OTHER DRUGS

GENERIC NAME OR DRUG CLASS	COMBINED EFFECT
Caffeine (high doses)	Can cause same symptoms as tyramine-containing foods*. (See "Don't Take With" information block on previous page.)
Fluoxetine	Increased risk of mental status changes.
Levodopa	Increased risk of adverse reactions.
Meperdine	Possibly severe drop in blood pressure. Avoid.
Narcotics*	Severe toxic reaction leading to seizures, coma, and/or death.

Continued on page 934

POSSIBLE INTERACTION WITH OTHER SUBSTANCES

INTERACTS WITH	COMBINED EFFECT
Alcohol:	Can cause severe toxicity. Avoid.
Beverages: Drinks containing large quantities of caffeine.	Can cause severe toxicity. Avoid.
Cocaine:	High blood pressure, rapid heartbeat. Avoid.
Foods: Tyramine-containing*. (See "Don't Take With" information block on previous page.)	Severe toxicity, perhaps leading to death. *Carefully* avoid.
Marijuana:	Rapid heart rate. Avoid.
Tobacco:	Rapid heart rate. Avoid.

SERTRALINE

BRAND NAMES

Zoloft

BASIC INFORMATION

Habit forming? No
Prescription needed? Yes
Available as generic? No
Drug class: Antidepressant (selective serotonin reuptake inhibitor)

 ## USES

- Treats mental depression.
- Treats obsessive-compulsive disorder.

 ## DOSAGE & USAGE INFORMATION

How to take:
Tablets—Swallow with liquid. If you can't swallow whole, crumble tablet and take with liquid or food.

When to take:
Once daily, either in the morning or in the evening as directed by your doctor.

If you forget a dose:
Take as soon as you remember up to 2 hours late. If more than 2 hours, wait for next scheduled dose (don't double this dose).

What drug does:
It affects serotonin, one of the chemicals in the brain called neurotransmitters, that plays a role in emotions and psychological disturbances.

Time lapse before drug works:
1 to 4 weeks.

Don't take with:
- Any monoamine oxidase (MAO) inhibitor* (or within 14 days of discontinuing an MAO inhibitor). To do so may cause serious or even fatal reactions.
- Any other medication without consulting your doctor or pharmacist.

 ## OVERDOSE

SYMPTOMS:
Seizures, agitation, violent vomiting.
WHAT TO DO:
- Dial 911 (emergency) or 0 (operator) for an ambulance or medical help. Then give first aid immediately.
- See emergency information at end of book.

 ## POSSIBLE ADVERSE REACTIONS OR SIDE EFFECTS

SYMPTOMS	WHAT TO DO
Life-threatening: Rash, itchy skin, breathing difficulty (allergic reaction); chest pain.	Seek emergency treatment immediately.
Common: Diarrhea, nervousness, drowsiness, headache, increased sweating, insomnia, anxiety.	Continue. Call doctor when convenient.
Infrequent: • Chills, fever, joint or muscle pain, enlarged lymph glands, unusual excitability, blurred vision, chest pain.	Discontinue. Call doctor right away.
• Nightmares, taste changes, vision changes, decreased sex drive, dry mouth, skin flushing, urinating frequently, painful menstruation, stuffy nose, tremors.	Continue. Call doctor when convenient.
Rare: • Convulsions.	Discontinue. Seek emergency treatment.
• Fast heartbeat; abdominal pain; signs of low blood sugar (anxiety, nervousness, chills, increased sweating, difficulty concentrating).	Discontinue. Call doctor right away.
• Nausea, vomiting, constipation, cough, increased appetite.	Continue. Call doctor when convenient.

WARNINGS & PRECAUTIONS

Don't take if:
- You have epilepsy.
- You have an allergy to sertraline.

Before you start, consult your doctor:
If you have severe liver or kidney disease.

Over age 60:
Adverse reactions may be more frequent and severe than in younger persons. You may need smaller doses for shorter periods of time.

Pregnancy:
Don't take unless essential. Consult doctor. Risk category B (see page xxiii).

Breast-feeding:
Unknown effects. Consult doctor.

Infants & children:
Not recommended.

Prolonged use:
No special problems expected.

Skin & sunlight:
No special problems expected.

Driving, piloting or hazardous work:
Don't drive or pilot aircraft until you learn how medicine affects you. Don't work around dangerous machinery. Don't climb ladders or work in high places. Danger increases if you drink alcohol or take medicine affecting alertness and reflexes.

Discontinuing:
Don't discontinue without consulting doctor. Dose may require gradual reduction if you have taken drug for a long time. Doses of other drugs may also require adjustment.

Others:
- Advise any doctor or dentist whom you consult that you take this medicine.
- May affect results of some medical tests.

POSSIBLE INTERACTION WITH OTHER DRUGS

GENERIC NAME OR DRUG CLASS	COMBINED EFFECT
Antidepressants, tricyclic*	Increased levels of tricyclic antidepressant; possible toxicity.
Central nervous system (CNS) depressants*	Increased depressive effects of both drugs.
Dexfenfluramine	May cause serotonin syndrome*. Avoid.
Lithium	May increase risk of side effects.
Monoamine oxidase (MAO) inhibitors*	Increased risk of adverse effects. May lead to convulsions and hypertensive crisis. Let 14 days elapse between taking the 2 drugs.
Selegiline	Increased risk of adverse effects. May lead to convulsions and hypertensive crisis. Let 14 days elapse between taking the 2 drugs.
Warfarin	Increased anticoagulant effect.

POSSIBLE INTERACTION WITH OTHER SUBSTANCES

INTERACTS WITH	COMBINED EFFECT
Alcohol:	May increase depression.
Beverages:	No proven problems.
Cocaine:	Decreased effect of sertraline.
Foods:	No proven problems.
Marijuana:	Decreased effect of sertraline.
Tobacco:	No proven problems.

SIBUTRAMINE

BRAND NAMES

Meridia

BASIC INFORMATION

Habit forming? Dependence possible
Prescription needed? Yes
Available as generic? No
Drug class: Appetite suppressant

 ## USES

Treatment for obesity and maintenance of weight loss. The drug is to be used in conjunction with a reduced calorie diet and weight management program. Treatment with this drug is not recommended for "cosmetic" weight loss—that is when a person's height-to-weight ratio does not provide a medical reason for weight loss. Your doctor will help determine your body mass index (BMI), a method of measuring for obesity.

 ## DOSAGE & USAGE INFORMATION

How to take:
Capsule–Swallow with liquid. It may be taken with or without food. Read instructions carefully that are provided with the prescription.

When to take:
Once a day usually in the morning.

If you forget a dose:
Take as soon as you remember. If it is almost time for the next dose, then skip the missed dose and wait for your next scheduled dose (don't double this dose).

What drug does:
Allows certain chemicals in the brain to act longer in controlling appetite regulating center.

Time lapse before drug works:
Weight loss should begin within 4 weeks.

Continued next column

 ## OVERDOSE

SYMPTOMS:
It is unknown what symptoms may occur. There is very limited experience with overdose.
WHAT TO DO:
If person takes much larger amount than prescribed, call doctor, poison control center or hospital emergency room for instructions.

Don't take with:
Any other prescription or non-prescription drug without consulting your doctor or pharmacist.

 ## POSSIBLE ADVERSE REACTIONS OR SIDE EFFECTS

SYMPTOMS	WHAT TO DO
Life-threatening: None known.	
Common: Dry mouth, headache, constipation, insomnia (these symptoms usually go away with continued treatment).	Continue. Call doctor when convenient.
Infrequent: • Increase in blood pressure or heart rate.	Discontinue. Call doctor right away.
• Back pain, flu-like symptoms, stomach pain, increased appetite, nausea, heartburn, muscle aches, dizziness, nervousness, anxiety, depression, sore throat, runny nose.	Continue. Call doctor when convenient.
Rare: Chest pain, fainting, swelling of feet or ankles, allergic reaction including skin rash or hives, seizure, any other symptoms you are concerned about.	Discontinue. Call doctor right away.

SIBUTRAMINE

WARNINGS & PRECAUTIONS

Don't take if:
- You are allergic to sibutramine.
- If you have a history of anorexia nervosa.

Before you start, consult your doctor:
- If you have a history of uncontrolled high blood pressure, any heart disorder, coronary artery disease, stroke (or symptoms of a stroke), seizures, or other medical problem.
- If you have any kidney or liver disorder.
- If organic causes of obesity have not been ruled out, such as hypothyroidism.
- If you have glaucoma.
- If you are allergic to any other medication, food or other substance.

Over age 60:
No special problems expected, but a lower starting dosage may be recommended.

Pregnancy:
Sibutramine is not recommended for pregnant women. Risk category C (see page xxiii).

Breast-feeding:
It is unknown if drug passes into milk. Avoid drug or discontinue nursing until you finish medicine. Consult doctor for advice on maintaining milk supply.

Infants & children:
Safety and effectiveness in ages under 16 has not established.

Prolonged use:
- Schedule regular visits to your doctor to determine if drug is continuing to be effective in controlling weight and to monitor your blood pressure.
- The effectiveness and safety of taking this drug beyond one year have not been established.

Skin & sunlight:
No problems expected.

Driving, piloting or hazardous work:
Don't drive or pilot aircraft until you learn how medicine affects you. Don't work around dangerous machinery. Don't climb ladders or work in high places. Danger increases if you drink alcohol or take other medicines affecting alertness and reflexes.

Discontinuing:
Notify your doctor if any new symptoms occur after the drug is stopped.

Others:
- Advise any doctor or dentist whom you consult that you take this medicine.
- Use as directed. Don't increase or decrease dosage without doctor's approval.
- Notify your doctor if you don't lose at least 4 pounds in the first month of treatment.
- Other weight control agents have been associated with heart valve problems and primary pulmonary hypertension.
- Monitor blood pressure.

POSSIBLE INTERACTION WITH OTHER DRUGS

GENERIC NAME OR DRUG CLASS	COMBINED EFFECT
Appetite suppressants*, other	Unknown effect. Avoid.
Decongestants*	May cause increase in blood pressure or heart rate. Avoid.
Central nervous system (CNS) depressants*	Increased sedation. Avoid.
Erythromycin	Increased effect of sibutramine.
Ketoconazole	Increased effect of sibutramine.
Monoamine oxidase, (MAO) inhibitors	Potentially life-threatening. Allow 14 days between use of 2 drugs.
Serotonergic agents*, other	May cause serotonin syndrome*. Avoid.

POSSIBLE INTERACTION WITH OTHER SUBSTANCES

INTERACTS WITH	COMBINED EFFECT
Alcohol:	Increased sedation. Avoid.
Beverages:	None expected.
Cocaine:	Unknown effect. Best to avoid.
Foods:	None expected.
Marijuana:	Unknown effect. Best to avoid.
Tobacco:	None expected.

SILDENAFIL CITRATE

BRAND NAMES

Viagra

BASIC INFORMATION

Habit forming? No
Prescription needed? Yes
Available as generic? No
Drug class: Anti-impotence

 ## USES

Treats male sexual function (erection) problems.

 ## DOSAGE & USAGE INFORMATION

How to take:
Tablets—Swallow with water. If you can't swallow whole, crumble tablet and take with liquid or food.

When to take:
Take one-half hour to four hours before sexual activity. Use only once daily.

If you forget a dose:
Does not apply.

What drug does:
Increases blood flow to the penis, resulting in an erection.

Time lapse before drug works:
One-half hour to one hour.

Don't take with:
Any other prescription or nonprescription drug without consulting your doctor or pharmacist.

 ## OVERDOSE

SYMPTOMS:
Same as those listed under Possible Adverse Reactions or Side Effects, with increased likelihood.
WHAT TO DO:
If person takes much larger amount than prescribed, call doctor, poison control center or hospital emergency room for instructions.

 ## POSSIBLE ADVERSE REACTIONS OR SIDE EFFECTS

SYMPTOMS	WHAT TO DO
Life-threatening:	
Fatalities have been reported when used with nitrate medications.	
Common:	
Headache, flushing, stomach upset, nasal stuffiness.	Continue. Call doctor if symptoms persist.
Infrequent:	
• Pain or other urination problems, blurred vision, changes in color perception, sensitivity to light, skin rash, dizziness, prolonged erection (lasting more than 4 hours).	Discontinue. Call doctor right away.
• Diarrhea.	Continue. Call doctor if symptoms persist.
Rare:	
Chest pain, fainting, foot or ankle swelling.	Discontinue. Call doctor right away.

WARNINGS & PRECAUTIONS

Don't take if:
You are allergic to sildenafil citrate.

Before you start, consult your doctor:
- If you have any other medical problem.
- If you have heart problems.
- If you have a bleeding disorder (e.g., ulcer).
- If you have vision problems.
- If you have any physical abnormalities of the penis.
- If you have or have had liver or kidney disease.

Over age 60:
Adverse reactions and side effects, especially, may be more severe and frequent than in younger patients.

Pregnancy:
Not indicated for use in females. Risk category B (see page xxiii).

Breast-feeding:
Not indicated for use in females.

Infants & children:
Safety and effectiveness of use in children not established. Not recommended.

Prolonged use:
Talk to your doctor about the need for follow-up medical examinations or laboratory studies to determine drug's effectiveness.

Skin & sunlight:
No problems expected.

Driving, piloting or hazardous work:
Avoid if you feel side effects such as nausea and vomiting.

Discontinuing:
Your doctor will determine the schedule.

Others:
- Advise any doctor or dentist whom you consult that you take this medicine.
- Consult doctor if there are any significant changes in your vision.
- Do not combine the drug with any other impotence therapy unless approved by your doctor.
- There are many causes of impotence. Your doctor should perform a complete exam before prescribing this medication.

POSSIBLE INTERACTION WITH OTHER DRUGS

GENERIC NAME OR DRUG CLASS	COMBINED EFFECT
Enzyme inhibitors*	Increased blood level of sildenafil.
Nitrates	Increased effect of nitrates. Do not use.
Rifampin	Decreased effect of sildenafil.

POSSIBLE INTERACTION WITH OTHER SUBSTANCES

INTERACTS WITH	COMBINED EFFECT
Alcohol:	May inhibit the effects of sildenafil.
Beverages:	Grapefruit juice may increase blood levels of sildenafil.
Cocaine:	Effects unknown. Avoid.
Foods:	Grapefruit juice may increase blood levels of sildenafil.
Marijuana:	Effects unknown. Avoid.
Tobacco:	None expected.

*See Glossary

SIMETHICONE

BRAND NAMES

Degas	Maximum Strength
Di-Gel	Gas Relief
Extra Strength Gas-X	Maximum Strength
Extra Strength	Phazyme
Maalox Anti-Gas	Mygel
Extra Strength Maalox	Mylanta Gas
GRF Gas Relief	Mylicon
Formula	Mylicon-80
Gas Relief	Mylicon-125
Gas-X	Ovol
Gelusil	Ovol-40
Imodium Advanced	Ovol-80
Maalox Anti-Gas	Phazyme
Maalox GRF Gas	Phazyme 55
Relief Formula	Phazyme 95
	Riopan Plus

BASIC INFORMATION

Habit forming? No
Prescription needed? No
Available as generic? Yes, for some
Drug class: Antiflatulent

 ## USES

- Treatment for retention of abdominal gas.
- Used prior to x-ray of abdomen to reduce gas shadows.

 ## DOSAGE & USAGE INFORMATION

How to take:
- Tablet or capsule—Swallow with liquid.
- Liquid—Dissolve in water. Drink complete dose.
- Chewable tablets—Chew completely. Don't swallow whole.

When to take:
After meals and at bedtime.

If you forget a dose:
Take when remembered if needed.

What drug does:
Reduces surface tension of gas bubbles in stomach.

Continued next column

 ## OVERDOSE

SYMPTOMS:
None expected.
WHAT TO DO:
Overdose unlikely to threaten life.

Time lapse before drug works:
10 minutes.

Don't take with:
Any other medicine without consulting your doctor or pharmacist.

 ## POSSIBLE ADVERSE REACTIONS OR SIDE EFFECTS

SYMPTOMS	WHAT TO DO
Life-threatening: None expected.	
Common: None expected.	
Infrequent: None expected.	
Rare: None expected.	

WARNINGS & PRECAUTIONS

Don't take if:
You are allergic to simethicone.

Before you start, consult your doctor:
No problems expected.

Over age 60:
No problems expected.

Pregnancy:
Consult doctor. Risk category C (see page xxiii).

Breast-feeding:
No problems expected. Consult doctor.

Infants & children:
Not recommended.

Prolonged use:
No problems expected.

Skin & sunlight:
No problems expected.

Driving, piloting or hazardous work:
No problems expected.

Discontinuing:
May be unnecessary to finish medicine.
Discontinue when symptoms disappear.

Others:
No problems expected.

 POSSIBLE INTERACTION WITH OTHER DRUGS

GENERIC NAME OR DRUG CLASS	COMBINED EFFECT
None significant.	

 POSSIBLE INTERACTION WITH OTHER SUBSTANCES

INTERACTS WITH	COMBINED EFFECT
Alcohol:	None expected.
Beverages:	None expected.
Cocaine:	None expected.
Foods:	None expected.
Marijuana:	None expected.
Tobacco:	None expected.

SODIUM BICARBONATE

BRAND NAMES

Alka-Seltzer
  Effervescent Pain
  Reliever & Antacid
Arm & Hammer Pure
  Baking Soda

Bell/ans
Bromo-Seltzer
Citrocarbonate
Soda Mint

BASIC INFORMATION

Habit forming? No
Prescription needed? No
Available as generic? Yes
Drug class: Alkalizer, antacid

USES

- Treats metobolic acidosis.
- Alkalinizes urine to reduce uric acid kidney stones.
- Treats hyperacidity of the stomach that is present with indigestion, gastroesophageal reflux and peptic ulcer disease.

DOSAGE & USAGE INFORMATION

How to take:
- Tablets—Swallow with liquid. If you can't swallow whole, crumble tablet and take with liquid or food.
- Powder—Mix in a glass of water and drink.
- Effervescent sodium bicarbonate—Mix in a glass of cold water and drink.

When to take:
- For hyperacidity—1 to 3 hours after meals.
- For kidney stones—According to prescription instructions.

If you forget a dose:
Take as soon as you remember up to 2 hours late. If more than 2 hours, wait for next scheduled dose (don't double this dose).

What drug does:
- Buffers acid in the stomach.
- Increases excretion of bicarbonate in the urine to help dissolve uric acid stones.

Continued next column

OVERDOSE

SYMPTOMS:
Excessive swelling of feet and lower legs.
WHAT TO DO:
Overdose unlikely to threaten life. If person takes much larger amount than prescribed, call doctor, poison control center or hospital emergency room for instructions.

Time lapse before drug works:
Works immediately, but the duration of effect is short.

Don't take with:
Nonprescription drugs without consulting doctor.

POSSIBLE ADVERSE REACTIONS OR SIDE EFFECTS

SYMPTOMS	WHAT TO DO
Life-threatening: None expected.	
Common: None expected.	
Infrequent: • Stomach cramps that continue.	Discontinue. Call doctor right away.
• Nausea, headache, appetite loss (with long-term use).	Continue. Call doctor when convenient.
Rare: Muscle pain or twitching, nervousness, breathing difficulty, mild swelling of feet or lower legs (with large doses).	Discontinue. Call doctor right away.

WARNINGS & PRECAUTIONS

Don't take if:
You are allergic to sodium bicarbonate.

Before you start, consult your doctor:
If you have heart disease, kidney disease or toxemia of pregnancy.

Over age 60:
Adverse reactions and side effects may be more frequent and severe than in younger persons.

Pregnancy:
May cause weight gain and swelling of feet and ankles. Avoid if you have high blood pressure. Consult doctor. Risk category C (see page xxiii).

Breast-feeding:
No problems expected, but consult doctor.

Infants & children:
Not recommended. Safety and dosage have not been established.

Prolonged use:
Don't use for longer than prescribed or recommended. May cause sodium overload.

Skin & sunlight:
No special problems expected.

Driving, piloting or hazardous work:
No special problems expected.

Discontinuing:
May be unnecessary to finish medicine. Follow doctor's instructions.

Others:
- Heat and moisture in bathroom medicine cabinet can cause breakdown of medicine. Store someplace else.
- May interfere with the accuracy of some medical tests (especially acidosis and urinalysis tests).

POSSIBLE INTERACTION WITH OTHER DRUGS

GENERIC NAME OR DRUG CLASS	COMBINED EFFECT
Adrenocorticoids*	Sodium overload.
Cortisone	Sodium overload.
Ketoconazole	Decreased absorption of ketoconazole.
Mecamylamine	Increased mecamylamine effect.
Methenamine	Decreased methenamine effect.
Tetracyclines*	Greatly reduced absorption of tetracyclines.
Any other medicine	Decreased absorption of other medicine if taken within 1 to 2 hours oftaking sodium bicarbonate.

POSSIBLE INTERACTION WITH OTHER SUBSTANCES

INTERACTS WITH	COMBINED EFFECT
Alcohol:	Decreased effectiveness of sodium bicarbonate.
Beverages: Milk and milk products (large amounts).	Increased risk of side effects.
Cocaine:	None expected.
Foods:	None expected.
Marijuana:	None expected.
Tobacco:	Decreased effectiveness of sodium bicarbonate.

*See Glossary

SODIUM FLUORIDE

BRAND NAMES

Fluor-A-Day
Fluorident
Fluoritab
Fluorodex
Fluotic
Flura
Karidium

Listermint with
  Fluoride
Luride
Luride-SF
Pediaflor
Pedi-Dent
Solu-Flur

Numerous other multiple vitamin-mineral
supplements. Check labels.

BASIC INFORMATION

Habit forming? No
Prescription needed? Yes, for some
Available as generic? Yes
Drug class: Mineral supplement (fluoride)

USES

- Reduces tooth cavities.
- Treats osteoporosis.

DOSAGE & USAGE INFORMATION

How to take:
- Tablet—Swallow with liquid or crumble tablet and take with liquid (not milk) or food.
- Liquid—Measure with dropper and take directly or with liquid.
- Chewable tablets—Chew slowly and thoroughly before swallowing.

When to take:
Usually at bedtime after teeth are thoroughly brushed.

Continued next column

OVERDOSE

SYMPTOMS:
Stomach cramps or pain, nausea, faintness, vomiting (possibly bloody), diarrhea, black stools, shallow breathing, muscle spasms, seizures, arrhythmias.

WHAT TO DO:
- Dial 911 (emergency) or 0 (operator) for an ambulance or medical help. Then give first aid immediately.
- See emergency information on inside covers.

If you forget a dose:
Take as soon as you remember. Don't double a forgotten dose. Return to schedule.

What drug does:
Provides supplemental fluoride to combat tooth decay.

Time lapse before drug works:
8 weeks to provide maximum effect.

Don't take with:
Any other medicine simultaneously.

POSSIBLE ADVERSE REACTIONS OR SIDE EFFECTS

SYMPTOMS	WHAT TO DO
Life-threatening: In case of overdose, see previous column.	
Common: Constipation, appetite loss.	Continue. Call doctor when convenient.
Infrequent: • Rash.	Discontinue. Call doctor right away.
• Tooth discoloration.	Continue. Call doctor when convenient.
Rare: • Severe upsets (digestive) only with overdose.	Discontinue. Seek emergency treatment.
• Sores in mouth and lips, aching bones, stiffness.	Discontinue. Call doctor right away.

WARNINGS & PRECAUTIONS

Don't take if:
- Your water supply contains 0.7 parts fluoride per million. Too much fluoride stains teeth permanently.
- You are allergic to any fluoride-containing product.
- You have underactive thyroid.

Before you start, consult your doctor:
- If you have kidney disease.
- If you have ulcers.
- If you have joint pain.

Over age 60:
No problems expected.

Pregnancy:
Consult doctor. Risk category C (see page xxiii).

Breast-feeding:
No problems expected. Consult doctor.

Infants & children:
No problems expected except accidental overdose. Keep vitamin-mineral supplements out of children's reach.

Prolonged use:
Excess may cause discolored teeth and decreased calcium in blood.

Skin & sunlight:
No problems expected.

Driving, piloting or hazardous work:
No problems expected.

Discontinuing:
No problems expected.

Others:
- Store in original plastic container. Fluoride decomposes glass.
- Some products contain tartrazine dye. Avoid, especially if you are allergic to aspirin.

POSSIBLE INTERACTION WITH OTHER DRUGS

GENERIC NAME OR DRUG CLASS	COMBINED EFFECT
Calcium supplements*	Decreased effect of calcium and fluoride.

POSSIBLE INTERACTION WITH OTHER SUBSTANCES

INTERACTS WITH	COMBINED EFFECT
Alcohol:	None expected.
Beverages: Milk.	Prevents absorption of fluoride. Space dose 2 hours before or after milk.
Cocaine:	None expected.
Foods:	None expected.
Marijuana:	None expected.
Tobacco:	None expected.

SUCRALFATE

BRAND NAMES

Carafate   Sulcrate Suspension
Sulcrate   Plus

BASIC INFORMATION

Habit forming? No
Prescription needed? Yes
Available as generic? Yes
Drug class: Antiulcer agent

USES

- Treatment for duodenal and gastric ulcers.
- Used to relieve side effects of nonsteroidal anti-inflammatory therapy in rheumatoid arthritis.
- Treatment for gastroesophageal reflux disease (GERD).

DOSAGE & USAGE INFORMATION

How to take:
- Tablet—Take as directed on an empty stomach.
- Oral suspension—Follow instructions on package.

When to take:
1 hour before meals and at bedtime. Allow 2 hours to elapse before taking other prescription medicines.

If you forget a dose:
Take as soon as you remember up to 2 hours late. If more than 2 hours, wait for next scheduled dose (don't double this dose).

What drug does:
Covers ulcer site and protects from acid, enzymes and bile salts.

Time lapse before drug works:
Begins in 30 minutes. May require several days to relieve pain.

Don't take with:
Any other medicine without consulting your doctor or pharmacist.

OVERDOSE

SYMPTOMS:
None expected.
WHAT TO DO:
Overdose unlikely to threaten life. If person takes much larger amount than prescribed, call doctor, poison control center or hospital emergency room for instructions.

POSSIBLE ADVERSE REACTIONS OR SIDE EFFECTS

SYMPTOMS	WHAT TO DO
Life-threatening: None expected.	
Common: Constipation.	Continue. Call doctor when convenient.
Infrequent: Dizziness, sleepiness, rash, itchy skin, abdominal pain, indigestion, vomiting, nausea, dry mouth, diarrhea.	Continue. Call doctor when convenient.
Rare: Back pain.	Continue. Call doctor when convenient.

WARNINGS & PRECAUTIONS

Don't take if:
You are allergic to sucralfate.

Before you start, consult your doctor:
- If you will have surgery within 2 months, including dental surgery, requiring general or spinal anesthesia.
- If you have gastrointestinal or kidney disease.

Over age 60:
Adverse reactions and side effects may be more frequent and severe than in younger persons.

Pregnancy:
No proven harm to unborn child. Avoid if possible. Consult doctor. Risk category B (see page xxiii).

Breast-feeding:
Unknown effects. Consult doctor.

Infants & children:
Safety not established.

Prolonged use:
Request blood counts if medicine needed longer than 8 weeks.

Skin & sunlight:
No problems expected.

Driving, piloting or hazardous work:
Don't drive or pilot aircraft until you learn how medicine affects you. Don't work around dangerous machinery. Don't climb ladders or work in high places. Danger increases if you drink alcohol or take medicine affecting alertness and reflexes, such as antihistamines, tranquilizers, sedatives, pain medicine, narcotics and mind-altering drugs.

Discontinuing:
Don't discontinue without consulting doctor. Dose may require gradual reduction if you have taken drug for a long time. Doses of other drugs may also require adjustment.

Others:
No problems expected.

POSSIBLE INTERACTION WITH OTHER DRUGS

GENERIC NAME OR DRUG CLASS	COMBINED EFFECT
Anagrelide	May interfere with anagrelide absorption.
Antacids*	Take 1/2 hour before or after sucralfate.
Cimetidine	Possible decreased absorption of cimetidine if taken simultaneously.
Ciprofloxacin	Decreased absorption of ciprofloxacin. Take 2 hours before sucralfate.
Digoxin	Decreased absorption of digoxin. Take 2 hours before sucralfate.
Fluoroquinolones	Decreased fluoroquinolone effect.
Ketoconazole	Decreased ketoconazole effect.
Lansoprazole	Decreased effect of lansoprazole. Take it 30 minutes before sucralfate.
Norfloxacin	Decreased absorption of norfloxacin. Take 2 hours before sucralfate.

Ofloxacin	Decreased absorption of ofloxacin. Take 2 hours before sucralfate.
Phenytoin	Possible decreased absorption of phenytoin if taken simultaneously.
Tetracyclines*	Possible decreased absorption of tetracycline if taken simultaneously.
Theophylline	Decreased absorption of theophylline. Take 2 hours before sucralfate.
Vitamins A, D, E, K	Decreased vitamin absorption.

POSSIBLE INTERACTION WITH OTHER SUBSTANCES

INTERACTS WITH	COMBINED EFFECT
Alcohol:	Irritates ulcer. Avoid.
Beverages: Caffeine.	Irritates ulcer. Avoid.
Cocaine:	May make ulcer worse. Avoid.
Foods:	No problems expected.
Marijuana:	May make ulcer worse. Avoid.
Tobacco:	May make ulcer worse. Avoid.

SULFADOXINE AND PYRIMETHAMINE

BRAND NAMES

Fansidar

BASIC INFORMATION

Habit forming? No
Prescription needed? Yes
Available as generic? No
Drug class: Antiprotozoal

USES

- Treats malaria *(plasmodium faciparum)*.
- Helps prevent malaria when traveling to areas where it exists.
- Also used to prevent isosporiasis in patients with acquired immunodeficiency disease.

DOSAGE & USAGE INFORMATION

How to take:
Tablets—Swallow with liquid. If you can't swallow whole, crumble tablet and take with liquid or food. Instructions to take on empty stomach mean 1 hour before or 2 hours after eating.

When to take:
Follow doctor's instructions.

If you forget a dose:
Take as soon as you remember. If close to time for next dose, skip this one and wait for next scheduled dose. Don't double dose.

What drug does:
The sulfa component kills bacteria; the pyrimethamine works to kill malaria organisms in red blood cells or human tisue.

Time lapse before drug works:
2 to 6 hours.

Continued next column

OVERDOSE

SYMPTOMS:
Appetite loss, sore throat and fever, seizure, coma.
WHAT TO DO:
- **Dial 911 (emergency) or 0 (operator) for an ambulance or medical help. Then give first aid immediately.**
- **See emergency information on inside front covers.**

Don't take with:
- Any other medicines (including over-the-counter drugs such as cough and cold medicines, laxatives, antacids, diet pills, caffeine, nose drops or vitamins) without consulting your doctor.
- Mefloquine.

POSSIBLE ADVERSE REACTIONS OR SIDE EFFECTS

SYMPTOMS	WHAT TO DO
Life-threatening:	
In case of overdose, see previous column.	
Common:	
Loss or change of taste; diarrhea; skin rash; pale skin; sore throat; sore, red tongue; mouth ulcers; fever; excessive bleeding; tiredness, light sensitivity.	Discontinue. Call doctor right away.
Infrequent:	
Aching joints, fever, skin blisters or peeling, jaundice (yellow skin and eyes).	Discontinue. Call doctor right away.
Rare:	
Bloody urine, burning on urination, back pain, swollen neck.	Discontinue. Call doctor right away.

SULFADOXINE AND PYRIMETHAMINE

WARNINGS & PRECAUTIONS

Don't take if:
You know you are allergic to sulfa drugs, furosemide, thiazide diuretics, carbonase anhydrase inhibitors.

Before you start, consult your doctor:
- If you have AIDS.
- If you have anemia, seizures, G6PD* deficiency, liver disease, porphyria, kidney disease.
- If you can't tolerate sulfa drugs.

Over age 60:
Adverse reactions and side effects may be more frequent and severe than in younger persons. You may need smaller doses for shorter periods of time.

Pregnancy:
Use birth control so you won't get pregnant while in an endemic malaria area. Should not be taken during pregnancy if it can possibly be avoided. Consult doctor. Risk category C (see page xxiii).

Breast-feeding:
Drug passes into milk. Avoid drug or discontinue nursing until you finish medicine. Consult doctor for advice on maintaining milk supply.

Infants & children:
Don't use in infants under 2 months old.

Prolonged use:
Talk to your doctor about the need for follow-up medical examinations or laboratory studies to check complete blood counts (white blood cell count, platelet count, red blood cell count, hemoglobin, hematocrit) and urinalyses.

Skin & sunlight:
May cause rash or intensify sunburn in areas exposed to sun or ultraviolet light (photosensitivity reaction). Avoid overexposure. Notify doctor if reaction occurs.

Driving, piloting or hazardous work:
Avoid if you feel confused, drowsy or dizzy.

Discontinuing:
Don't discontinue for 4 to 6 weeks after you leave endemic malaria areas.

Others:
- Advise any doctor or dentist whom you consult that you take this medicine.
- May affect results in some medical tests.
- Sleep under mosquito netting while in endemic areas. Wear long-sleeved shirts and long pants.
- Report to your doctor if you develop any symptoms of illness while you take this medicine—even if the symptoms seem minor.

POSSIBLE INTERACTION WITH OTHER DRUGS

GENERIC NAME OR DRUG CLASS	COMBINED EFFECT
Anticoagulants*	Increased risk of toxicity.
Anticonvulsants*	Increased risk of toxicity.
Antidiabetics*	Increased risk of toxicity.
Bone marrow depressants*	Increased risk of bleeding or other toxic symptoms.
Clozapine	Toxic effect on the central nervous system.
Contraceptives, oral*	Reduced reliability of the pill.
Hepatotoxic medicines*	Increased risk of liver toxicity.
Methenamine	Increased risk of kidney toxicity.
Methotrexate	Increased risk of toxicity.
Zidovudine	Increased risk of liver toxicity.

POSSIBLE INTERACTION WITH OTHER SUBSTANCES

INTERACTS WITH	COMBINED EFFECT
Alcohol:	Nausea and vomiting. Avoid.
Beverages:	No special problems expected.
Cocaine:	Increased likelihood of adverse reactions or seizures. Avoid.
Foods:	No special problems expected.
Marijuana:	Increased likelihood of adverse reactions. Avoid.
Tobacco:	No special problems expected.

SULFASALAZINE

BRAND NAMES

Azaline	Salazopyrin
Azulfidine	Salazosulfapyridine
Azulfidine En-Tabs	Salicylazosulfa-
PMS Sulfasalazine	pyridine
PMS Sulfasalazine	S.A.S. Enteric-500
EC	S.A.S.-500

BASIC INFORMATION

Habit forming? No
Prescription needed? Yes
Available as generic? Yes
Drug class: Sulfa (sulfonamide)

 USES

- Treatment for ulceration and bleeding from ulcerative colitis.
- Treatment for rheumatoid arthritis for patients not responding to other treatments.

 DOSAGE & USAGE INFORMATION

How to take:
- Tablet—Swallow with liquid. Instructions to take on empty stomach mean 1 hour before or 2 hours after eating.
- Liquid—Shake carefully before measuring.

When to take:
At the same times each day, evenly spaced.

If you forget a dose:
Take as soon as you remember up to 2 hours late. If more than 2 hours, wait for next scheduled dose (don't double this dose).

What drug does:
Anti-inflammatory action reduces tissue destruction in colon.

Time lapse before drug works:
2 to 5 days.

Don't take with:
Any other medicine without consulting your doctor or pharmacist.

 OVERDOSE

SYMPTOMS:
Less urine, bloody urine, coma.
WHAT TO DO:
- Dial 911 (emergency) or 0 (operator) for an ambulance or medical help. Then give first aid immediately.
- See emergency information on inside covers.

 POSSIBLE ADVERSE REACTIONS OR SIDE EFFECTS

SYMPTOMS	WHAT TO DO
Life-threatening:	
In case of overdose, see previous column.	
Common:	
• Itchy skin, rash.	Discontinue. Call doctor right away.
• Headache, nausea, vomiting, diarrhea, appetite loss, skin sensitive to sun.	Continue. Call doctor when convenient.
• Orange urine or skin.	Continue. Tell doctor at next visit.
Infrequent:	
• Red, peeling or blistering skin; sore throat; fever; swallowing difficulty; unusual bruising; aching joints or muscles; jaundice.	Discontinue. Call doctor right away.
• Dizziness, tiredness, weakness, impotence.	Continue. Call doctor when convenient.
Rare:	
Painful urination; low back pain; numbness, tingling, burning feeling in feet and hands, bloody urine, neck swelling.	Discontinue. Call doctor right away.

 WARNINGS & PRECAUTIONS

Don't take if:
You are allergic to any sulfa drug*.

Before you start, consult your doctor:
- If you are allergic to carbonic anhydrase inhibitors, oral antidiabetics or thiazide or loop diuretics.
- If you are allergic by nature.
- If you have liver or kidney disease.
- If you have porphyria.
- If you have developed anemia from use of any drug.

Over age 60:
Adverse reactions and side effects may be more frequent and severe than in younger persons.

Pregnancy:
Consult doctor. Risk category B (see page xxiii).

Breast-feeding:
Drug passes into milk. Avoid drug or discontinue nursing until you finish medicine. Consult doctor for advice on maintaining milk supply.

Infants & children:
Don't give to infants younger than 2 years.

Prolonged use:
- May enlarge thyroid gland.
- You may become more susceptible to infections caused by germs not responsive to this drug.
- Request frequent blood counts, liver and kidney function studies.

Skin & sunlight:
May cause rash or intensify sunburn in areas exposed to sun or ultraviolet light (photosensitivity reaction). Avoid overexposure. Notify doctor if reaction occurs.

Driving, piloting or hazardous work:
Avoid if you feel dizzy. Otherwise, no problems expected.

Discontinuing:
Don't discontinue without doctor's advice until you complete prescribed dose, even though symptoms diminish or disappear.

Others:
- Drink 2 quarts of liquid each day to prevent adverse reactions.
- If you require surgery, tell anesthetist you take sulfa. Pentothal anesthesia should not be used.

POSSIBLE INTERACTION WITH OTHER DRUGS

GENERIC NAME OR DRUG CLASS	COMBINED EFFECT
Aminobenzoates	Possible decreased sulfa effect.
Antibiotics*	Decreased sulfa effect.
Anticoagulants*, oral	Increased anti-coagulant effect.
Anticonvulsants, hydantoin*	Toxic effect on brain.
Antidiabetics*	Toxic effect on brain.
Aspirin	Increased sulfa effect.
Calcium supplements*	Decreased sulfa effect.
Clozapine	Toxic effect on the central nervous system.
Digoxin	Decreased digoxin effect.

Hepatotoxic agents*	Increased liver toxicity.
Iron supplements*	Decreased sulfa effect.
Isoniazid	Possible anemia.
Mecamylamine	Decreased antibiotic effect.
Methenamine	Possible kidney blockage.
Methotrexate	Increased methotrexate effect.
Oxyphenbutazone	Increased sulfa effect.
Para-aminosalicylic acid	Decreased sulfa effect.
Penicillins*	Decreased penicillin effect.
Phenylbutazone	Increased sulfa effect.
Probenecid	Increased sulfa effect.
Sulfinpyrazone	Increased sulfa effect.
Sulfonureas*	May increase hypo-glycemic action.
Trimethoprim	Increased sulfa effect.
Vitamin C	Possible kidney damage. Avoid large doses of vitamin C.
Zidovudine	Increased risk of toxic effects of zidovudine.

POSSIBLE INTERACTION WITH OTHER SUBSTANCES

INTERACTS WITH	COMBINED EFFECT
Alcohol:	Increased alcohol effect.
Beverages: Less than 2 quarts of fluid daily.	Kidney damage.
Cocaine:	None expected.
Foods:	None expected.
Marijuana:	None expected.
Tobacco:	None expected.

SULFINPYRAZONE

BRAND NAMES

Anturan   Apo-Sulfinpyrazone
Anturane   Novopyrazone

BASIC INFORMATION

Habit forming? No
Prescription needed? Yes
Available as generic? Yes
Drug class: Antigout

USES

- Treatment for chronic gout.
- May be prescribed to reduce the risk of recurrent heart attack.

DOSAGE & USAGE INFORMATION

How to take:
Tablet or capsule—Swallow with liquid or food to lessen stomach irritation. If you can't swallow whole, crumble tablet or open capsule and take with liquid or food.

When to take:
At the same times each day.

If you forget a dose:
Take as soon as you remember up to 2 hours late. If more than 2 hours, wait for next scheduled dose (don't double this dose).

Continued next column

OVERDOSE

SYMPTOMS:
Breathing difficulty, vomiting, imbalance, seizures, convulsions, coma.
WHAT TO DO:
- **Dial 911 (emergency) or 0 (operator) for an ambulance or medical help. Then give first aid immediately.**
- **If patient is unconscious and not breathing, give mouth-to-mouth breathing. If there is no heartbeat, use cardiac massage and mouth-to-mouth breathing (CPR). Don't try to make patient vomit. If you can't get help quickly, take patient to nearest emergency facility.**
- **See emergency information on inside covers.**

What drug does:
Reduces uric acid level in blood and tissues by increasing amount of uric acid secreted in urine by kidneys.

Time lapse before drug works:
May require 6 months to prevent gout attacks.

Don't take with:
Any other medicine without consulting your doctor or pharmacist.

POSSIBLE ADVERSE REACTIONS OR SIDE EFFECTS

SYMPTOMS	WHAT TO DO
Life-threatening: In case of overdose, see previous column.	
Common: None expected.	
Infrequent:	
• Painful or difficult urination, worsening gout.	Discontinue. Call doctor right away.
• Rash, nausea, vomiting, abdominal pain, low back pain.	Continue. Call doctor when convenient.
Rare:	
• Black, bloody or tarry stools.	Discontinue. Seek emergency treatment.
• Sore throat; fever; unusual bleeding or bruising; red, painful joints; blood in urine; fatigue or weakness.	Discontinue. Call doctor right away.

WARNINGS & PRECAUTIONS

Don't take if:
- You are allergic to any uricosuric*.
- You have acute gout.
- You have active ulcers (stomach or duodenal), enteritis or ulcerative colitis.
- You have blood cell disorders.
- You are allergic to oxyphenbutazone or phenylbutazone.

Before you start, consult your doctor:
If you have kidney or blood disease.

Over age 60:
Adverse reactions and side effects may be more frequent and severe than in younger persons. You require lower dose because of decreased kidney function.

Pregnancy:
Decide with your doctor whether drug benefits justify risk to unborn child. Risk category C (see page xxiii).

Breast-feeding:
Effect unknown. Consult doctor.

Infants & children:
Not recommended.

Prolonged use:
• Possible kidney damage.
• Talk to your doctor about the need for follow-up medical examinations or laboratory studies to check complete blood counts (white blood cell count, platelet count, red blood cell count, hemoglobin, hematocrit), kidney function, serum uric acid and urine uric acid.

Skin & sunlight:
No problems expected.

Driving, piloting or hazardous work:
No problems expected.

Discontinuing:
Don't discontinue without consulting doctor. Dose may require gradual reduction if you have taken drug for a long time. Doses of other drugs may also require adjustment.

Others:
• Drink 10 to 12 glasses of water each day you take this medicine.
• Periodic blood and urine laboratory tests recommended.

POSSIBLE INTERACTION WITH OTHER DRUGS

GENERIC NAME OR DRUG CLASS	COMBINED EFFECT
Allopurinol	Increased effect of each drug.
Anticoagulants*, oral	Increased anticoagulant effect.
Antidiabetics*, oral	Increased antidiabetic effect.
Aspirin	Bleeding tendency. Decreased sulfinpyrazone effect.
Bismuth subsalicylate	Decreased sulfinpyrazone effect.
Cephalosporins*	Increased risk of bleeding.
Cholestyramine	Decreased sulfinpyrazone effect.
Contraceptives, oral*	Increased bleeding between menstrual periods.
Diuretics*	Decreased sulfinpyrazone effect.
Nitrofurantoin	Increased risk of toxicity.
Penicillins*	Increased penicillin effect.
Salicylates*	Bleeding tendency. Decreased sulfinpyrazone effect.
Sulfa drugs*	Increased effect of sulfa drugs.
Thioguanine	May need increased dosage of sulfinpyrazone.

POSSIBLE INTERACTION WITH OTHER SUBSTANCES

INTERACTS WITH	COMBINED EFFECT
Alcohol:	Decreased sulfinpyrazone effect.
Beverages: Caffeine drinks.	Decreased sulfinpyrazone effect.
Cocaine:	None expected.
Foods:	None expected.
Marijuana:	Occasional use—None expected. Daily use—May increase blood level of uric acid.
Tobacco:	None expected.

SULFONAMIDES

GENERIC AND BRAND NAMES

See complete list of generic and brand names in the *Generic and Brand Names Directory*, page 894.

BASIC INFORMATION

Habit forming? No
Prescription needed? Yes
Available as generic? Yes, for some
Drug class: Antibacterial (antibiotic), antiprotozoal, sulfa (sulfonamide)

 USES

- Treatment of urinary tract and other infections.
- Sulfamethoxazole in combination with trimethoprim, may be used to treat bronchitis, certain types of pneumonia, skin infections, middle ear infections, intestinal tract infections and urinary tract infections.

 DOSAGE & USAGE INFORMATION

How to take:
- Tablet—Swallow with liquid. Instructions to take on empty stomach mean 1 hour before or 2 hours after eating. Drink an extra amount of water daily so that urine output will be adequate.
- Liquid—Shake carefully before measuring.
- Other forms—Follow label instructions.

When to take:
At the same times each day, evenly spaced.

If you forget a dose:
Take as soon as you remember up to 2 hours late. If more than 2 hours, wait for next scheduled dose (don't double this dose).

What drug does:
Interferes with a nutrient (folic acid) necessary for growth and reproduction of bacteria. Will not attack viruses.

Continued next column

 OVERDOSE

SYMPTOMS:
Less urine, bloody urine, stomach pain, light-headedness, headache, drowsiness, coma.
WHAT TO DO:
- **Dial 911 (emergency) or 0 (operator) for an ambulance or medical help. Then give first aid immediately.**
- **See emergency information on inside covers.**

Time lapse before drug works:
2 to 5 days to affect infection.

Don't take with:
Any other medicine without consulting your doctor or pharmacist.

 POSSIBLE ADVERSE REACTIONS OR SIDE EFFECTS

SYMPTOMS	WHAT TO DO
Life-threatening: In case of overdose, see previous column.	
Common:	
• Itchy skin, rash.	Discontinue. Call doctor right away.
• Headache, nausea, vomiting, diarrhea, appetite loss, skin sensitive to sun, dizziness.	Continue. Call doctor when convenient.
Infrequent:	
• Red, peeling or blistering skin; sore throat; fever; swallowing difficulty; unusual bruising or bleeding; aching joints or muscles; yellow skin or eyes; pale skin.	Discontinue. Call doctor right away.
• Weakness or tiredness.	Continue. Call doctor when convenient.
Rare: Painful urination, low back pain, numbness, stomach pain, bloody diarrhea or urine, neck swelling, mood or behavior changes, increased or decreased urine output, thirst.	Discontinue. Call doctor right away.

 WARNINGS & PRECAUTIONS

Don't take if:
You are allergic to any sulfa drug.

Before you start, consult your doctor:
- If you are allergic to carbonic anhydrase inhibitors, oral antidiabetics or diuretics (thiazide or loop).
- If you are allergic by nature.
- If you have liver or kidney disease.
- If you have glucose 6-phosphate dehydrogenase (G6PD) disease.
- If you have porphyria.
- If you have anemia or other blood problems.

Over age 60:
Adverse reactions and side effects may be more frequent and severe than in younger persons.

Pregnancy:
Decide with your doctor if drug benefits justify risk to unborn child. Risk category C (see page xxiii).

Breast-feeding:
Drug passes into milk. Avoid drug or discontinue nursing until you finish medicine. Consult doctor for advice on maintaining milk supply.

Infants & children:
Don't give to infants younger than 2 months.

Prolonged use:
- You may become more susceptible to infections caused by germs not responsive to this drug.
- Drug may enlarge thyroid gland (rare).
- Talk to your doctor about the need for frequent blood counts, liver and kidney function studies.

Skin & sunlight:
May cause rash or intensify sunburn in areas exposed to sun or ultraviolet light (photosensitivity reaction) Avoid excess exposure. Notify doctor if reaction occurs.

Driving, piloting or hazardous work:
Avoid if you feel dizzy. Otherwise, no problems expected.

Discontinuing:
Don't discontinue without doctor's advice until you complete prescribed dose, even though symptoms diminish or disappear.

Others:
- Drink 2 quarts of liquid each day to prevent side effects or adverse reactions.
- Advise any doctor or dentist whom you consult that you take this medicine.
- If you require surgery, tell anesthetist you take sulfa. Pentothal anesthesia should not be used.

POSSIBLE INTERACTION WITH OTHER DRUGS

GENERIC NAME OR DRUG CLASS	COMBINED EFFECT
Aminobenzoate potassium	Possible decreased sulfonamide effect.
Anticoagulants*, oral	Increased anticoagulant effect.
Anticonvulsants*, hydantoin	Increased anti-convulsant effect.
Antidiabetics*, oral	Increased anti-diabetic effect.

Bone marrow depressants*	Increased risk of side effects.
Contraceptives*, oral estrogen	Decreased contraceptive effect.
Cyclosporine	Decreased cyclosproine effect.
Hemolytics*, other	Increased risk of side effects.
Hepatotoxic agents*	Increased liver toxicity.
Mecamylamine	Decreased antibiotic effect.
Methenamine	Possible kidney blockage.
Methotrexate	Increased methotrexate effect.
Penicillins*	Decreased penicillin effect.
Phenylbutazone	Increased sulfonamide effect.
Probenecid	Increased sulfonamide effect.
Sulfinpyrazone	Increased sulfonamide effect.

POSSIBLE INTERACTION WITH OTHER SUBSTANCES

INTERACTS WITH	COMBINED EFFECT
Alcohol:	No special problems expected.
Beverages: Inadequate fluid intake.	Increased risk of side effects.
Cocaine:	No special problems expected.
Foods:	No special problems expected.
Marijuana:	No special problems expected.
Tobacco:	No special problems expected.

SULFONAMIDES & PHENAZOPYRIDINE

BRAND AND GENERIC NAMES

**SULFAMETHOXA-
ZOLE & PHENAZO-
PYRIDINE**
Azo Gantanol
Azo-
  Sulfamethoxazole

**SULFISOXAZOLE &
PHENAZO-
PYRIDINE**
Azo Gantrisin
Azo-Sulfisoxazol
Azo-Truxazole
Sul-Azo

BASIC INFORMATION

Habit forming? No
Prescription needed? Yes
Available as generic? Yes
Drug class: Analgesic (urinary), sulfonamide

USES

- Treats infections responsive to this drug.
- Relieves pain of lower urinary tract irritation, as in cystitis, urethritis or prostatitis.

DOSAGE & USAGE INFORMATION

How to take:
Tablet—Swallow with liquid. Instructions to take on empty stomach mean 1 hour before or 2 hours after eating.

When to take:
At the same times each day, after meals.

If you forget a dose:
Take as soon as you remember up to 2 hours late. If more than 2 hours, wait for next scheduled dose (don't double this dose).

What drug does:
- Interferes with a nutrient (folic acid) necessary for growth and reproduction of bacteria. Will not attack viruses.
- Anesthetizes lower urinary tract. Relieves pain, burning, pressure and urgency to urinate.

Continued next column

OVERDOSE

SYMPTOMS:
Less urine, bloody urine, shortness of breath, weakness, coma.
WHAT TO DO:
- **Dial 911 (emergency) or 0 (operator) for an ambulance or medical help. Then give first aid immediately.**
- **See emergency information on inside covers.**

Time lapse before drug works:
2 to 5 days to affect infection.

Don't take with:
Any other medicine without consulting your doctor or pharmacist.

POSSIBLE ADVERSE REACTIONS OR SIDE EFFECTS

SYMPTOMS	WHAT TO DO
Life-threatening:	
In case of overdose, see previous column.	
Common:	
• Rash, itchy skin.	Discontinue. Call doctor right away.
• Dizziness, diarrhea, headache, appetite loss, nausea, vomiting, skin sensitive to sun.	Continue. Call doctor when convenient.
Infrequent:	
• Joint pain; swallowing difficulty; pale skin; blistering; peeling of skin; sore throat, fever, mouth sores; unexplained bleeding or bruising; jaundice.	Discontinue. Call doctor right away.
• Abdominal pain, indigestion, weakness, tiredness.	Continue. Call doctor when convenient.
Rare:	
Back pain; neck swelling; numbness, tingling, burning feeling in feet and hands; bloody urine; painful urination.	Discontinue. Call doctor right away.

WARNINGS & PRECAUTIONS

Don't take if:
- You are allergic to any sulfa drug or urinary analgesic.
- You have hepatitis.

Before you start, consult your doctor:
- If you are allergic to carbonic anhydrase inhibitors, oral antidiabetics or thiazide or loop diuretics.
- If you are allergic by nature.
- If you have liver or kidney disease, porphyria.
- If you have developed anemia from use of any drug.
- If you have G6PD* deficiency.

Over age 60:
Adverse reactions and side effects may be more frequent and severe than in younger persons.

Pregnancy:
Risk factors vary for drugs in this group. See category list on page xxiii and consult doctor.

Breast-feeding:
Drug passes into milk. Avoid drug or discontinue nursing until you finish medicine. Consult doctor for advice on maintaining milk supply.

Infants & children:
Don't give to infants younger than 1 month.

Prolonged use:
- May enlarge thyroid gland.
- You may become more susceptible to infections caused by germs not responsive to this drug.
- Request frequent blood counts, liver and kidney function studies.
- Orange or yellow skin.
- Anemia. Occasional blood studies recommended.

Skin & sunlight:
One or more drugs in this group may cause rash or intensify sunburn in areas exposed to sun or ultraviolet light (photosensitivity reaction). Avoid overexposure. Notify doctor if reaction occurs.

Driving, piloting or hazardous work:
Avoid if you feel dizzy. Otherwise, no problems expected.

Discontinuing:
Don't discontinue without doctor's advice until you complete prescribed dose, even though symptoms diminish or disappear.

Others:
- Drink 2 quarts of liquid each day to prevent adverse reactions.
- If you require surgery, tell anesthetist you take sulfa.
- Will probably cause urine to be reddish orange. Requires no action.
- May stain fabrics.

POSSIBLE INTERACTION WITH OTHER DRUGS

GENERIC NAME OR DRUG CLASS	COMBINED EFFECT
Aminobenzoates	Possible decreased sulfa effect.
Anticoagulants*, oral	Increased anticoagulant effect.
Anticonvulsants, hydantoin*	Toxic effect on brain.
Antidiabetics*	Toxic effect on brain.
Aspirin	Increased sulfa effect.
Clozapine	Toxic effect on the central nervous system.
Didanosine	Increased risk of pancreatitis.
Hepatotoxic agents*	Increased liver toxicity.
Isoniazid	Possible anemia.
Mecamylamine	Decreased antibiotic effect.
Methenamine	Possible kidney blockage.
Methotrexate	Increased methotrexate effect.
Oxyphenbutazone	Increased sulfa effect.
Para-aminosalicylic acid	Decreased sulfa effect.
Penicillins*	Decreased penicillin effect.
Phenylbutazone	Increased sulfa effect.
Probenecid	Increased sulfa effect.
Sulfinpyrazone	Increased sulfa effect.
Sulfonureas*	May increase hypoglycemic action.
Trimethoprim	Increased sulfa effect.
Zidovudine	Increased risk of toxic effects of zidovudine.

POSSIBLE INTERACTION WITH OTHER SUBSTANCES

INTERACTS WITH	COMBINED EFFECT
Alcohol:	Increased alcohol effect.
Beverages: Less than 2 quarts of fluid daily.	Kidney damage.
Cocaine:	None expected.
Foods:	None expected.
Marijuana:	None expected.
Tobacco:	None expected.

*See Glossary

TACRINE

BRAND NAMES

Cognex

BASIC INFORMATION

Habit forming? No
Prescription needed? Yes
Available as generic? No
Drug class: Cholinesterase inhibitor

 ## USES

Treatment for symptoms of mild to moderate Alzheimer's disease. May improve memory, reasoning and other cognitive functions slightly in some patients or slow the progress of Alzheimer's disease. It will not reverse the disease.

 ## DOSAGE & USAGE INFORMATION

How to take:
Capsule—Swallow with liquid.

When to take:
At the same times each day. Take 1 hour before or 2 hours after eating. Follow doctor's instructions.

If you forget a dose:
Take as soon as you remember up to 2 hours late. If more than 2 hours, wait for next scheduled dose (don't double this dose).

Continued next column

 ## OVERDOSE

SYMPTOMS:
Severe nausea and vomiting, excessive saliva, sweating, blood pressure decrease, slow heartbeat, collapse, convulsions, muscle weakness (including respiratory muscles, which could lead to death).
WHAT TO DO:
- **Dial 911 (emergency) or 0 (operator) for an ambulance or medical help. Then give first aid immediately.**
- **If patient is unconscious and not breathing, use cardiac massage and mouth-to-mouth breathing (CPR). Don't try to make patient vomit. If you can't get help quickly, take patient to nearest emergency facility.**
- **See emergency information at end of book.**

What drug does:
Slows breakdown of a brain chemical (acetylcholine) that gradually disappears from the brains of people with Alzheimer's disease.

Time lapse before drug works:
May take several months before beneficial results are observed. Dosage is normally increased over a period of time to help prevent adverse reactions.

Don't take with:
Any other medication without consulting your doctor or pharmacist.

 ## POSSIBLE ADVERSE REACTIONS OR SIDE EFFECTS

SYMPTOMS	WHAT TO DO
Life-threatening:	
In case of overdose, see previous column.	
Common:	
Nausea, vomiting, diarrhea, lack of coordination.	Continue. Call doctor when convenient.
Infrequent:	
Rash, indigestion, headache, muscle aches, loss of appetite, stomach pain, nervousness, chills, dizziness, drowsiness, dry or itching eyes, increased sweating, joint pain, runny nose, sore throat, swelling of feet or legs, insomnia, weight loss, unusual tiredness or weakness, flushing of face.	Continue. Call doctor when convenient.
Rare:	
Changes in liver function (yellow skin or eyes; black, very dark or light stool color); lack of coordination, convulsions.	Continue. Call doctor right away.

774

WARNINGS & PRECAUTIONS

Don't take if:
You are allergic to tacrine or acridine derivatives*.

Before you start, consult your doctor:
- If you have heart rhythm problems.
- If you have a history of ulcer disease or are at risk of developing ulcers.
- If you have a history of liver disease.
- If you have epilepsy or seizure disorder.
- If you have a history of asthma.
- If you have had previous treatment with tacrine that caused jaundice (yellow skin and eyes) or elevated bilirubin.

Over age 60:
No problems expected.

Pregnancy:
Unknown effect. Drug is usually not prescribed for women of childbearing age. Risk category C (see page xxiii).

Breast-feeding:
Unknown effect. Not recommended for women of childbearing age.

Infants & children:
Not used in this age group.

Prolonged use:
- Drug may lose its effectiveness.
- Talk to your doctor about the need for follow-up medical examinations or laboratory studies to check blood chemistries and liver function.

Skin & sunlight:
No problems expected.

Driving, piloting or hazardous work:
Don't drive or pilot aircraft until you learn how medicine affects you. Don't work around dangerous machinery. Don't climb ladders or work in high places. Danger increases if you drink alcohol or take other medicines affecting alertness and reflexes such as antihistamines, tranquilizers, sedatives, pain medicine, narcotics and mind-altering drugs.

Discontinuing:
Do not discontinue drug unless advised by doctor. Abrupt decreases in dosage may cause a cognitive decline.

Others:
- Advise any doctor or dentist whom you consult that you take this medicine.
- May affect the results in some medical tests.
- Do not increase dosage without doctor's approval.
- Treatment with tacrine may need to be discontinued or the dosage lowered if weekly blood tests indicate a sensitivity to the drug or liver toxicity develops.

POSSIBLE INTERACTION WITH OTHER DRUGS

GENERIC NAME OR DRUG CLASS	COMBINED EFFECT
Anticholinergics*	Decreased anticholinergic effect.
Cimetidine	Increased tacrine effect, especially adverse effects.
Theophylline	Increased theophylline effect or toxicity.

POSSIBLE INTERACTION WITH OTHER SUBSTANCES

INTERACTS WITH	COMBINED EFFECT
Alcohol:	None expected.
Beverages:	None expected.
Cocaine:	None expected.
Foods:	None expected.
Marijuana:	None expected.
Tobacco:	May decrease tacrine effect.

TAMOXIFEN

BRAND NAMES

Alpha-Tamoxifen	Novo-Tamoxifen
Med Tamoxifen	Tamofen
Nolvadex	Tamone
Nolvadex-D	Tamoplex

BASIC INFORMATION

Habit forming? No
Prescription needed? Yes
Available as generic? No
Drug class: Antineoplastic

 ## USES

• Treats advanced breast cancer.
• Can help prevent breast cancer in those at risk.

 ## DOSAGE & USAGE INFORMATION

How to take:
• Tablets—Swallow with liquid. If you can't swallow whole, crumble tablet and take with liquid or food. Instructions to take on empty stomach mean 1 hour before or 2 hours after eating.
• Enteric-coated tablets—Swallow whole.

When to take:
Follow doctor's instructions.

If you forget a dose:
Skip the missed dose and return to regular schedule. Don't double dose.

What drug does:
Blocks uptake of estradiol and inhibits growth of cancer cells.

Time lapse before drug works:
• 4 to 10 weeks.
• With bone metastases—several months.

Continued next column

 ## OVERDOSE

SYMPTOMS:
None expected.
WHAT TO DO:
Overdose unlikely to threaten life. If person takes much larger amount than prescribed, call doctor, poison control center or hospital emergency room for instructions.

Don't take with:
Any other medicines (including over-the-counter drugs such as cough and cold medicines, laxatives, antacids, diet pills, caffeine, nose drops or vitamins) without consulting your doctor or pharmacist.

 ## POSSIBLE ADVERSE REACTIONS OR SIDE EFFECTS

SYMPTOMS	WHAT TO DO
Life-threatening: Leg pain, shortness of breath.	Seek emergency treatment immediately.
Common: Hot flashes, nausea and vomiting, weight gain.	Continue. Call doctor when convenient.
Infrequent: Headache, dry skin, menstrual irregularities, vaginal itching.	Continue. Call doctor when convenient.
Rare: Blurred vision, confusion, sleepiness.	Discontinue. Call doctor right away.

WARNINGS & PRECAUTIONS

Don't take if:
You are allergic to tamoxifen.

Before you start, consult your doctor:
- If you have cataracts.
- If you have blood disorders.
- If you have high cholesterol.

Over age 60:
Adverse reactions and side effects may be more frequent and severe than in younger persons. You may need smaller doses for shorter periods of time.

Pregnancy:
Consult doctor. Risk category D (see page xxiii).

Breast-feeding:
Effect not documented. Consult your doctor.

Infants & children:
Not intended for use in children.

Prolonged use:
Talk to your doctor about the need for follow-up medical examinations (especially pelvic exams) or laboratory studies to check complete blood counts (white blood cell count, platelet count, red blood cell count, hemoglobin, hematocrit) and serum calcium.

Skin & sunlight:
No problems expected.

Driving, piloting or hazardous work:
Avoid if you feel confused, drowsy or dizzy.

Discontinuing:
No special problems expected.

Others:
- Advise any doctor or dentist whom you consult that you take this medicine.
- May affect results in some medical tests.
- Be sure you and your doctor discuss all aspects of using this drug, and read all instructional materials.
- May make you more fertile. Talk to your doctor about using some type of birth control.

POSSIBLE INTERACTION WITH OTHER DRUGS

GENERIC NAME OR DRUG CLASS	COMBINED EFFECT
Antacids*	Decreased tamoxifen effect. Take 1 to 2 hours apart.
Cimetidine	Decreased tamoxifen effect.
Estrogens*	Decreased tamoxifen effect.
Famotidine	Decreased tamoxifen effect.
H$_2$ antagonist antihistamines*	Decreased tamoxifen effect.
Ranitidine	Decreased tamoxifen effect.

POSSIBLE INTERACTION WITH OTHER SUBSTANCES

INTERACTS WITH	COMBINED EFFECT
Alcohol:	No special problems expected.
Beverages:	No special problems expected.
Cocaine:	No special problems expected.
Foods:	No special problems expected.
Marijuana:	No special problems expected.
Tobacco:	No special problems expected.

*See Glossary

TERPIN HYDRATE

BRAND NAMES

Prunicodeine   Terpin-Dex
Terpin Hydrate and
   Codeine Syrup

BASIC INFORMATION

Habit forming? Yes
Prescription needed? Yes
Available as generic? Yes
Drug class: Expectorant

USES

Decreases cough due to simple bronchial
irritation.

DOSAGE & USAGE INFORMATION

How to take:
Follow each dose with 8 oz. water or food to
decrease gastric distress. Works better in
combination with a cool-air vaporizer.

When to take:
3 to 4 times each day, spaced at least 4 hours
apart.

If you forget a dose:
Take as soon as you remember. Wait 4 hours
for next dose.

What drug does:
Loosens mucus in bronchial tubes to make
mucus easier to cough up.

Time lapse before drug works:
10 to 15 minutes.

Don't take with:
Any other medicine without consulting your
doctor or pharmacist.

OVERDOSE

SYMPTOMS:
Nausea, drowsiness.
WHAT TO DO:
**Overdose unlikely to threaten life. If person
takes much larger amount than prescribed,
call doctor, poison control center or hospital
emergency room for instructions.**

POSSIBLE ADVERSE REACTIONS OR SIDE EFFECTS

SYMPTOMS	WHAT TO DO
Life-threatening: None expected.	
Common: None expected.	
Infrequent: Nausea, vomiting, abdominal pain.	Continue. Call doctor when convenient.
Rare: Symptoms of alcohol intoxication, especially in children.	Discontinue. Call doctor right away.

WARNINGS & PRECAUTIONS

Don't take if:
- You are allergic to terpin hydrate.
- You are a recovering or active alcoholic.

Before you start, consult your doctor:
If you plan to become pregnant within medication period.

Over age 60:
No problems expected.

Pregnancy:
Decide with your doctor if drug benefits justify risk to unborn child. Risk category C (see page xxiii).

Breast-feeding:
Drug filters into milk. May harm child. Avoid.

Infants & children:
Use only under medical supervision.

Prolonged use:
Habit forming.

Skin & sunlight:
No problems expected.

Driving, piloting or hazardous work:
Don't drive or pilot aircraft until you learn how medicine affects you. Don't work around dangerous machinery. Don't climb ladders or work in high places. Danger increases if you drink alcohol or take medicine affecting alertness and reflexes, such as antihistamines, tranquilizers, sedatives, pain medicine, narcotics and mind-altering drugs

Discontinuing:
May be unnecessary to finish medicine. Follow doctor's instructions.

Others:
- Exceeding recommended doses may cause intoxication; drug is 42.5% alcohol.
- Frequently combined with codeine, which increases hazards.

POSSIBLE INTERACTION WITH OTHER DRUGS

GENERIC NAME OR DRUG CLASS	COMBINED EFFECT
Antidepressants*	Increased sedation.
Antihistamines*	Increased sedation
Central nervous system (CNS) depressants*	Increased sedative effect of both.
Disulfiram	Possible disulfiram reaction*.
Muscle relaxants*	Increased sedation.
Narcotics*	Increased sedation.
Sedatives*	Increased sedation.
Sleep inducers*	Increased sedation.
Tranquilizers*	Increased sedation.

POSSIBLE INTERACTION WITH OTHER SUBSTANCES

INTERACTS WITH	COMBINED EFFECT
Alcohol:	Contains alcohol. Increased sedative effect of both drugs. Avoid.
Beverages:	None expected.
Cocaine:	Unpredictable effect on nervous system. Avoid.
Foods:	None expected.
Marijuana:	Unpredictable effect on nervous system. Avoid.
Tobacco:	None expected.

TESTOLACTONE

BRAND NAMES

Teslac

BASIC INFORMATION

Habit forming? No
Prescription needed? Yes
Available as generic? No
Drug class: Antineoplastic

 ## USES

Treats advanced breast cancer.

 ## DOSAGE & USAGE INFORMATION

How to take:
Tablets—Swallow with liquid. If you can't swallow whole, crumble tablet and take with liquid or food. Instructions to take on empty stomach mean 1 hour before or 2 hours after eating.

When to take:
Follow doctor's instructions.

If you forget a dose:
Take as soon as you remember up to 2 hours late. If more than 2 hours, wait for next scheduled dose (don't double this dose).

What drug does:
Inhibits growth of cancer cells.

Time lapse before drug works:
6 to 12 weeks.

Don't take with:
Any other medicines (including over-the-counter drugs such as cough and cold medicines, laxatives, antacids, diet pills, caffeine, nose drops or vitamins) without consulting your doctor.

 ## OVERDOSE

SYMPTOMS:
None expected.
WHAT TO DO:
Overdose unlikely to threaten life. If person takes much larger amount than prescribed, call doctor, poison control center or hospital emergency room for instructions.

 ## POSSIBLE ADVERSE REACTIONS OR SIDE EFFECTS

SYMPTOMS	WHAT TO DO
Life-threatening: None expected.	
Common: Appetite loss.	Continue. Call doctor when convenient.
Infrequent: Diarrhea; swollen feet and legs; numb and tingling fingers, toes, face.	Continue. Call doctor when convenient.
Rare: Red tongue.	Continue. Call doctor when convenient.

WARNINGS & PRECAUTIONS

Don't take if:
You are allergic to testosterone.

Before you start, consult your doctor:
- If you have heart disease.
- If you have kidney disease.

Over age 60:
Adverse reactions and side effects may be more frequent and severe than in younger persons. You may need smaller doses for shorter periods of time.

Pregnancy:
Decide with your doctor if drug benefits justify risk to unborn child. Risk category C (see page xxiii).

Breast-feeding:
Effect not documented. Consult your doctor.

Infants & children:
Not recommended.

Prolonged use:
Talk to your doctor about the need for follow-up medical examinations or laboratory studies to check serum calcium levels.

Skin & sunlight:
No problems expected.

Driving, piloting or hazardous work:
No problems expected.

Discontinuing:
No special problems expected.

Others:
- Advise any doctor or dentist whom you consult that you take this medicine.
- May affect results in some medical tests.

 POSSIBLE INTERACTION WITH OTHER DRUGS

GENERIC NAME OR DRUG CLASS	COMBINED EFFECT
Anticoagulants*, oral	Increased anti-coagulant effect.

 POSSIBLE INTERACTION WITH OTHER SUBSTANCES

INTERACTS WITH	COMBINED EFFECT
Alcohol:	No special problems expected.
Beverages:	No special problems expected.
Cocaine:	No special problems expected.
Foods:	No special problems expected.
Marijuana:	No special problems expected.
Tobacco:	No special problems expected.

TETRACYCLINES

GENERIC AND BRAND NAMES

See complete list of generic and brand names in the *Generic and Brand Name Directory*, page 895.

BASIC INFORMATION

Habit forming? No
Prescription needed? Yes
Available as generic? Yes
Drug class: Antibacterial, antiacne

 ## USES

- Treatment for infections susceptible to any tetracycline. Will not cure virus infections such as colds or flu.
- Treatment for acne.
- Used as diuretic.
- Ulcer treatment.

 ## DOSAGE & USAGE INFORMATION

How to take:
- Tablet or capsule—Take on empty stomach 1 hour before or 2 hours after eating. If you can't swallow whole, crumble tablet or open capsule and take with liquid or food.
- Delayed-release capsules—Swallow whole with liquid (don't take with milk).
- Liquid—Shake well. Take with measuring spoon.

When to take:
At the same times each day, evenly spaced.

If you forget a dose:
Take as soon as you remember up to 2 hours late. If more than 2 hours, wait for next scheduled dose (don't double this dose).

What drug does:
Prevents germ growth and reproduction.

Time lapse before drug works:
- Infections—May require 5 days to affect infection.
- Acne—May require 4 weeks to affect acne.

Don't take with:
Any other medicine without consulting your doctor or pharmacist.

 ## OVERDOSE

SYMPTOMS:
Severe nausea, vomiting, diarrhea.
WHAT TO DO:
Overdose unlikely to threaten life. If person takes much larger amount than prescribed, call doctor, poison control center or hospital emergency room for instructions.

 ## POSSIBLE ADVERSE REACTIONS OR SIDE EFFECTS

SYMPTOMS	WHAT TO DO
Life-threatening:	
Hives, rash, intense itching, faintness soon after a dose (anaphylaxis).	Seek emergency treatment immediately.
Common:	
• Mild stomach cramps, diarrhea, nausea or vomiting; dizziness, lightheadedness or unsteadiness (with minocycline).	Continue. Call doctor when convenient.
• Increased sensitivity to sunlight, tooth discoloration (in children age 8 and under).	Discontinue. Call doctor right away.
Infrequent:	
• Frequent or increased urination, excessive thirst, unusual tiredness or weakness (with demeclocycline); darker color or discoloration of skin and mucous membranes (with minocycline).	Discontinue. Call doctor right away.
• Sore mouth or tongue, rectal or genital itch.	Continue. Call doctor when convenient.
• Darkened tongue (will go away when drug is discontinued).	No action necessary.
Rare:	
Changes in vision, yellow skin or eyes, continued vomiting, severe stomach cramps, loss of appetite, ongoing headache, bulging fontanel (soft spot on head of infant).	Discontinue. Call doctor right away.

 ## WARNINGS & PRECAUTIONS

Don't take if:
You are allergic to any tetracycline antibiotic.

Before you start, consult your doctor:
- If you have kidney or liver disease.
- If you have lupus.
- If you have myasthenia gravis.

Over age 60:
Dosage usually less than in younger adults. More likely to cause itching around rectum. Ask your doctor how to prevent it.

Pregnancy:
Risk to unborn child outweighs drug benefits. Don't use. Risk category D (see page xxiii).

Breast-feeding:
Drug passes into milk. Avoid drug or discontinue nursing until you finish medicine. Consult doctor for advice on maintaining milk supply.

Infants & children:
May cause permanent teeth malformation or discoloration in children less than 8 years old. Don't use.

Prolonged use:
- You may become more susceptible to infections caused by germs not responsive to tetracycline.
- May cause rare problems in liver, kidney or bone marrow. Periodic laboratory blood studies, liver and kidney function tests recommended if you use drug a long time.

Skin & sunlight:
May cause rash or intensify sunburn in areas exposed to sun or ultraviolet light (photosensitivity reaction). Avoid overexposure. Notify doctor if reaction occurs.

Driving, piloting or hazardous work:
No problems expected.

Discontinuing:
Don't discontinue without doctor's advice until you complete prescribed dose, even though symptoms diminish or disappear.

Others:
- Avoid using outdated drug.
- May affect results in some medical tests.
- Birth control pills may not be effective. Use additional birth control method.

POSSIBLE INTERACTION WITH OTHER DRUGS

GENERIC NAME OR DRUG CLASS	COMBINED EFFECT
Antacids*	Decreased tetracycline effect.
Anticoagulants*, oral	Increased anticoagulant effect.
Antivirals, HIV/AIDS*	Decreased antibiotic effect.
Bismuth subsalicylate	Decreased tetracycline absorption.
Calcium supplements*	Decreased tetracycline effect.
Cefixime	Decreased antibiotic effect of cefixime.
Cholestyramine or colestipol	Decreased tetracycline effect.

Contraceptives, oral*	Decreased contraceptive effect.
Desmopressin	Possible decreased desmopressin effect.
Digitalis preparations*	Increased digitalis effect.
Etretinate	Increased chance of adverse reactions of etretinate.
Lithium	Increased lithium effect.
Mineral supplements* (iron, calcium, magnesium, zinc)	Decreased tetracycline absorption. Separate doses by 1 to 2 hours.
Penicillins*	Decreased penicillin effect.
Sodium bicarbonate	Greatly reduced tetracycline absorption.
Tiopronin	Increased risk of toxicity to kidneys (except with doxycycline and minocycline).

Continued on page 934

POSSIBLE INTERACTION WITH OTHER SUBSTANCES

INTERACTS WITH	COMBINED EFFECT
Alcohol:	Possible liver damage. Avoid.
Beverages: Milk.	Decreased tetracycline absorption. Take dose 2 hours after or 1 hour before drinking.
Cocaine:	No proven problems.
Foods: Dairy products.	Decreased tetracycline absorption. Take dose 2 hours after or 1 hour before eating.
Marijuana:	No interactions expected, but marijuana may slow body's recovery. Avoid.
Tobacco:	None expected.

THEOPHYLLINE & GUAIFENESIN

BRAND NAMES

Asbron G	Glyceryl T
Asbron G Inlay Tablets	Mudrane GG2
	Quibron
Bronchial	Quibron 300
Broncomar GG	Slo-Phyllin GG
Ed-Bron G	Syncophylate-GG
Elixophyllin-GG	Theolate
Equibron G	Uni-Bronchial

BASIC INFORMATION

Habit forming? No
Prescription needed? Yes
Available as generic? Yes
Drug class: Bronchodilator, expectorant

USES

- Treatment for bronchial asthma symptoms.
- Loosens mucus in respiratory passages.
- Relieves coughing, wheezing, shortness of breath.

DOSAGE & USAGE INFORMATION

How to take:
Tablet, capsule, elixir or syrup—Swallow with liquid.

When to take:
Most effective taken on empty stomach 1 hour before or 2 hours after eating. However, may take with food to lessen stomach upset.

If you forget a dose:
Take as soon as you remember up to 2 hours late. If more than 2 hours, wait for next scheduled dose (don't double this dose).

Continued next column

OVERDOSE

SYMPTOMS:
Restlessness, irritability, confusion, hallucinations, drowsiness, mild weakness, nausea, vomiting blood, delirium, convulsions, rapid pulse, coma.
WHAT TO DO:
- **Dial 911 (emergency) or 0 (operator) for an ambulance or medical help. Then give first aid immediately.**
- **See emergency information on inside covers.**

What drug does:
- Relaxes and expands bronchial tubes.
- Increases production of watery fluids to thin mucus so it can be coughed out or absorbed.

Time lapse before drug works:
15 to 30 minutes.

Don't take with:
Any other medicine without consulting your doctor or pharmacist.

POSSIBLE ADVERSE REACTIONS OR SIDE EFFECTS

SYMPTOMS	WHAT TO DO
Life-threatening:	
Difficult breathing, uncontrollable heart rate, loss of consciousness.	Discontinue. Seek emergency treatment.
Common:	
• Headache, irritability, nervousness, restlessness, insomnia, drowsiness, nausea, vomiting.	Discontinue. Call doctor right away.
• Dizziness, lightheadedness, diarrhea, abdominal pain, heartburn.	Continue. Call doctor when convenient.
Infrequent:	
Skin rash or hives, red or flushed face, appetite loss, diarrhea.	Discontinue. Call doctor right away.
Rare:	
None expected.	

WARNINGS & PRECAUTIONS

Don't take if:
- You are allergic to any bronchodilator or cough or cold preparation containing guaifenesin.
- You have an active peptic ulcer.

Before you start, consult your doctor:
- If you have had impaired kidney or liver function.
- If you have gastritis, peptic ulcer, high blood pressure or heart disease.
- If you take medication for gout.

Over age 60:
Adverse reactions and side effects may be more frequent and severe than in younger persons. For drug to work, you must drink 8 to 10 glasses of fluid per day.

Pregnancy:
Decide with your doctor if drug benefits justify risk to unborn child. Risk category C (see page xxiii).

Breast-feeding:
Drug passes into milk. Avoid drug or discontinue nursing until you finish medicine. Consult doctor for advice on maintaining milk supply.

Infants & children:
Use only under medical supervision.

Prolonged use:
Stomach irritation.

Skin & sunlight:
No problems expected.

Driving, piloting or hazardous work:
Avoid if lightheaded, drowsy or dizzy. Otherwise, no problems expected.

Discontinuing:
May be unnecessary to finish medicine. Follow doctor's instructions.

Others:
No problems expected.

POSSIBLE INTERACTION WITH OTHER DRUGS

GENERIC NAME OR DRUG CLASS	COMBINED EFFECT
Allopurinol	Decreased allopurinol effect.
Anticoagulants*, oral	Possible risk of bleeding.
Ciprofloxacin	Increased possibility of central nervous system poisoning, such as nausea, vomiting, restlessness, palpitations.
Clarithromycin	Increased concentration of theophylline.
Ephedrine	Increased effect of both drugs.
Epinephrine	Increased effect of both drugs.
Erythromycins*	Increased bronchodilator effect.
Finasteride	Decreased theophylline effect.

Furosemide	Increased furosemide effect.
Lincomycins*	Increased bronchodilator effect.
Lithium	Decreased lithium effect.
Moricizine	Decreased bronchodilator effect.
Nicotine	Increased bronchodilator effect.
Probenecid	Decreased effect of both drugs.
Propranolol	Decreased bronchodilator effect.
Rauwolfia alkaloids*	Rapid heartbeat.
Sulfinpyrazone	Decreased sulfinpyrazone effect.
Ticlopidine	Increased theophylline effect.
Troleandomycin	Increased bronchodilator effect.
Zafirlukast	May increase effect of zafirlukast.
Zileuton	Increased effect of zileuton.

POSSIBLE INTERACTION WITH OTHER SUBSTANCES

INTERACTS WITH	COMBINED EFFECT
Alcohol:	No proven problems.
Beverages:	You must drink 8 to 10 glasses of fluid per day for drug to work.
Caffeine drinks.	Nervousness and insomnia.
Cocaine:	Excess stimulation. Avoid.
Foods:	None expected.
Marijuana:	Slightly increased antiasthmatic effect of bronchodilator.
Tobacco:	Decreased bronchodilator effect. Cigarette smoking worsens all problems that this medicine treats. Avoid.

*See Glossary

THEOPHYLLINE, EPHEDRINE & BARBITURATES

BRAND NAMES

Azma Aid	Tedrigen
Phedral-C.T.	T.E.P.
Primatene "P"	Theodrine
Formula	Theodrine Pediatric
Tedral	Theofed
Tedral SA	Theofedral

BASIC INFORMATION

Habit forming? Yes
Prescription needed? Some yes, others no
Available as generic? Some yes, others no
Drug class: Bronchodilator, barbiturate,
sympathomimetic, sedative

USES

- Treats bronchial asthma symptoms.
- Decreases congestion of breathing passages.
- Suppresses allergic reactions.
- Reduces anxiety or nervous tension (low dose).

DOSAGE & USAGE INFORMATION

How to take:
- Tablet or elixir—Swallow with liquid.
- Extended-release tablets—Swallow each dose whole. If you take regular tablets, you may chew or crush them.

When to take:
Most effective taken on empty stomach 1 hour before or 2 hours after eating. However, may take with food to lessen stomach upset.

Continued next column

OVERDOSE

SYMPTOMS:
Restlessness, irritability, anxiety, confusion, hallucinations, vomiting blood, delirium, muscle tremors, convulsions, rapid and irregular pulse, coma.
WHAT TO DO:
- **Dial 911 (emergency) or 0 (operator) for an ambulance or medical help. Then give first aid immediately.**
- **See emergency information on inside covers.**

If you forget a dose:
Take as soon as you remember up to 2 hours late. If more than 2 hours, wait for next scheduled dose (don't double this dose).

What drug does:
- Relaxes and expands bronchial tubes.
- Prevents cells from releasing allergy-causing chemicals (histamines).
- Decreases blood vessel size and blood flow, thus causing decongestion.
- May partially block nerve impulses at nerve cell connections.

Time lapse before drug works:
15 to 30 minutes.

Don't take with:
- Nonprescription drugs with ephedrine, pseudoephedrine or epinephrine.
- Nonprescription drugs for cough, cold, allergy or asthma without consulting doctor.
- Any other medicine without consulting your doctor or pharmacist.

POSSIBLE ADVERSE REACTIONS OR SIDE EFFECTS

SYMPTOMS	WHAT TO DO
Life-threatening:	
Difficult breathing, uncontrollable rapid heart rate, loss of consciousness.	Discontinue. Seek emergency treatment.
Common:	
• Headache, irritability, nervousness, restlessness, insomnia, nausea, vomiting, abdominal pain, irregular heart-beat, "hangover" effect.	Discontinue. Call doctor right away.
• Dizziness, light-headedness, paleness, heartburn.	Continue. Call doctor when convenient.
Infrequent:	
• Rash; hives; red or flushed face; appetite loss; diarrhea; cough; confusion; slurred speech; eyelid, face, lip swelling; joint pain.	Discontinue. Call doctor right away.
• Frequent urination.	Continue. Call doctor when convenient.
Rare:	
Agitation; sore throat, fever, mouth sores; jaundice.	Discontinue. Call doctor right away.

WARNINGS & PRECAUTIONS

Don't take if:
- You are allergic to any bronchodilator or barbiturate.
- You are allergic to ephedrine or any sympathomimetic drug*.
- You have an active peptic ulcer or porphyria.

Before you start, consult your doctor:
- If you have gastritis, peptic ulcer, high blood pressure or heart disease, diabetes, over-active thyroid gland, difficulty urinating, epilepsy, kidney or liver damage, asthma, anemia, chronic pain.
- If you have taken any MAO inhibitor in past 2 weeks, taken digitalis preparations in the last 7 days.
- If you have had impaired kidney or liver function.
- If you take medication for gout.
- If you will have surgery within 2 months, including dental surgery, requiring general or spinal anesthesia.

Over age 60:
- Adverse reactions and side effects may be more frequent and severe than in younger persons. Use small doses.
- More likely to develop high blood pressure, heart rhythm disturbances and angina and to feel drug's stimulant effects.

Pregnancy:
Risk to unborn child outweighs drug benefits. Don't use. Risk category D (see page xxiii).

Breast-feeding:
Drug passes into milk. Avoid drug or discontinue nursing until you finish medicine.

Infants & children:
Use only under medical supervision.

Prolonged use:
- Stomach irritation.
- Excessive doses—Rare toxic psychosis.
- Men with enlarged prostate gland may have more urination difficulty.
- May cause addiction, anemia, chronic intoxication.
- May lower body temperature, making exposure to cold temperatures hazardous.

Skin & sunlight:
May cause rash or intensity sunburn in areas exposed to sun or ultraviolet light (photosensitivity reaction). Avoid overexposure. Notify doctor if reaction occurs.

Driving, piloting or hazardous work:
Don't drive or pilot aircraft until you learn how medicine affects you. Don't work around dangerous machinery. Don't climb ladders or work in high places. Danger increases if you drink alcohol or take medicine affecting alertness and reflexes.

Discontinuing:
- May be unnecessary to finish medicine. Follow doctor's instructions.
- If you develop withdrawal symptoms of hallucinations, agitation or sleeplessness after discontinuing, call doctor right away.

Others:
Potential for abuse.

POSSIBLE INTERACTION WITH OTHER DRUGS

GENERIC NAME OR DRUG CLASS	COMBINED EFFECT
Adrenocorticoids, systemic	Decreased adreno-corticoid effect.
Allopurinol	Decreased allopurinol effect.
Anticoagulants*, oral	Decreased anti-coagulant effect.
Anticonvulsants*, oral	Changed seizure patterns.
Antidepressants, tricyclic*	Decreased anti-depressant effect. Possible dangerous oversedation.
Antidiabetics*, oral	Increased phenobarbital effect.

Continued on page 934

POSSIBLE INTERACTION WITH OTHER SUBSTANCES

INTERACTS WITH	COMBINED EFFECT
Alcohol:	Possible fatal oversedation. Avoid.
Beverages: Caffeine drinks.	Nervousness or insomnia.
Cocaine:	High risk of heartbeat irregularities and high blood pressure.
Foods:	None expected.
Marijuana:	Rapid heartbeat, possible heart rhythm disturbance.
Tobacco:	Decreased bronchodilator effect.

*See Glossary

THEOPHYLLINE, EPHEDRINE & HYDROXYZINE

BRAND NAMES

Ami Rax	Marax D.F.
Hydrophed	T.E.H. Compound
Marax	Theomax DF

BASIC INFORMATION

Habit forming? No
Prescription needed? Yes
Available as generic? Yes
Drug class: Bronchodilator (xanthine),
sympathomimetic, antihistamine

 USES

- Treatment for symptoms of bronchial asthma, emphysema, chronic bronchitis.
- Relieves wheezing, coughing and shortness of breath.

 DOSAGE & USAGE INFORMATION

How to take:
Tablet or syrup—Swallow with liquid.

When to take:
Most effective taken on empty stomach 1 hour before or 2 hours after eating. However, may take with food to lessen stomach upset.

If you forget a dose:
Take as soon as you remember up to 2 hours late. If more than 2 hours, wait for next scheduled dose (don't double this dose).

Continued next column

 OVERDOSE

SYMPTOMS:
Restlessness, irritability, confusion, hallucinations, severe anxiety, muscle tremors, rapid and irregular pulse, agitation, purposeless movements, vomiting blood, delirium, convulsions, coma.
WHAT TO DO:
- **Dial 911 (emergency) or 0 (operator) for an ambulance or medical help. Then give first aid immediately.**
- **See emergency information on inside covers.**

What drug does:
- Relaxes and expands bronchial tubes.
- Prevents cells from releasing allergy-causing chemicals (histamines).
- Decreases blood vessel size and blood flow, thus causing decongestion.
- May reduce activity in areas of the brain that influence emotional stability.

Time lapse before drug works:
15 to 60 minutes.

Don't take with:
- Nonprescription drugs with ephedrine, pseudoephedrine or epinephrine.
- Nonprescription drugs for cough, cold, allergy or asthma without consulting doctor.

 POSSIBLE ADVERSE REACTIONS OR SIDE EFFECTS

SYMPTOMS	WHAT TO DO
Life-threatening: Difficult breathing, uncontrollable rapid heart rate, loss of consciousness.	Discontinue. Seek emergency treatment.
Common: • Headache, irritability, nervousness, restlessness, insomnia, nausea, vomiting, abdominal pain, irregular heartbeat.	Discontinue. Call doctor right away.
• Dizziness, lightheadedness, paleness, heartburn.	Continue. Call doctor when convenient.
Infrequent: • Skin rash or hives, red or flushed face, appetite loss, diarrhea, abdominal pain.	Discontinue. Call doctor right away.
• Frequent urination.	Continue. Call doctor when convenient.
Rare: Tremor.	Discontinue. Call doctor right away.

WARNINGS & PRECAUTIONS

Don't take if:
- You are allergic to any bronchodilator, ephedrine, any sympathomimetic drug*, or antihistamine.
- You have an active peptic ulcer.

Before you start, consult your doctor:
- If you have had impaired kidney or liver function.
- If you have gastritis, peptic ulcer, high blood pressure, heart disease, diabetes, overactive thyroid gland, difficulty urinating, epilepsy.
- If you take medication for gout or have taken any MAO inhibitor in past 2 weeks, taken digitalis preparations in the last 7 days.
- If you will have surgery within 2 months, including dental surgery, requiring general or spinal anesthesia.

Over age 60:
- Adverse reactions and side effects may be more frequent and severe than in younger persons.
- More likely to develop increased urination difficulty, high blood pressure, heart rhythm disturbances and angina and to feel drug's stimulant effects.

Pregnancy:
Risk factors vary for drugs in this group. See category list on page xxiii and consult doctor.

Breast-feeding:
Drug passes into milk. Avoid drug or discontinue nursing until you finish medicine. Consult doctor for advice on maintaining milk supply.

Infants & children:
Use only under medical supervision.

Prolonged use:
- Stomach irritation.
- Excessive doses—Rare toxic psychosis.
- Men with enlarged prostate gland may have more urination difficulty.
- Tolerance develops and reduces effectiveness.

Skin & sunlight:
No problems expected.

Driving, piloting or hazardous work:
Don't drive or pilot aircraft until you learn how medicine affects you. Don't work around dangerous machinery. Don't climb ladders or work in high places. Danger increases if you drink alcohol or take medicine affecting alertness and reflexes, such as antihistamines, tranquilizers, sedatives, pain medicine, narcotics and mind-altering drugs.

Discontinuing:
Don't discontinue without consulting doctor. Dose may require gradual reduction if you have taken drug for a long time. Doses of other drugs may also require adjustment.

Others:
No problems expected.

POSSIBLE INTERACTION WITH OTHER DRUGS

GENERIC NAME OR DRUG CLASS	COMBINED EFFECT
Allopurinol	Decreased allopurinol offoot.
Antidepressants, tricyclic*	Increased ephedrine effect. Excess stimulation of heart and blood pressure.
Antihistamines*	Increased hydroxyzine effect.
Antihypertensives*	Decreased anti-hypertensive effect.
Beta-adrenergic blocking agents*	Decreased effect of both drugs.

Continued on page 935

POSSIBLE INTERACTION WITH OTHER SUBSTANCES

INTERACTS WITH	COMBINED EFFECT
Alcohol:	Increased sedation and intoxication. Avoid.
Beverages: Caffeine drinks.	Nervousness and insomnia.
Cocaine:	High risk of heartbeat irregularities and high blood pressure.
Foods:	None expected.
Marijuana:	Slightly increased antiasthmatic effect of bronchodilator. Rapid heartbeat, possible heart rhythm disturbance.
Tobacco:	Decreased broncho-dilator effect. Smoking is damaging to all problems this medicine treats. Avoid.

*See Glossary

THEOPHYLLINE, EPHEDRINE, GUAIFENESIN & BARBITURATES

BRAND NAMES

Bronkolixir
Bronkotabs

Guaiphed
Mudrane GG

BASIC INFORMATION

Habit forming? Yes (barbiturates)
Prescription needed? Yes
Available as generic? Yes
Drug class: Bronchodilator (xanthine),
cough/cold preparation,
sympathomimetic, sedative

 ## USES

- Treatment for symptoms of bronchial asthma, emphysema, chronic bronchitis.
- Relieves wheezing, coughing and shortness of breath.

 ## DOSAGE & USAGE INFORMATION

How to take:
Tablet, capsule or elixir—Swallow with liquid.

When to take:
Most effective taken on empty stomach 1 hour before or 2 hours after eating. However, may take with food to lessen stomach upset.

If you forget a dose:
Take as soon as you remember up to 2 hours late. If more than 2 hours, wait for next scheduled dose (don't double this dose).

Continued next column

 ## OVERDOSE

SYMPTOMS:
Restlessness, irritability, confusion, hallucinations, muscle tremors, severe anxiety, rapid and irregular pulse, mild weakness, nausea, vomiting blood, delirium, coma.
WHAT TO DO:
- **Overdose unlikely to threaten life. Depending on severity of symptoms and amount taken, call doctor, poison control center or hospital emergency room for instructions.**
- **Dial 911 (emergency) or 0 (operator) for an ambulance or medical help. Then give first aid immediately.**
- **See emergency information on inside covers.**

What drug does:
- Relaxes and expands bronchial tubes.
- Prevents cells from releasing allergy-causing chemicals (histamines).
- Decreases blood vessel size and blood flow, thus causing decongestion.
- Increases production of watery fluids to thin mucus so it can be coughed out or absorbed.
- May partially block nerve impulses at nerve cell connections.

Time lapse before drug works:
30 to 60 minutes.

Don't take with:
- Nonprescription drugs with ephedrine, pseudoephedrine or epinephrine.
- Nonprescription drugs for cough, cold, allergy or asthma without consulting doctor.

 ## POSSIBLE ADVERSE REACTIONS OR SIDE EFFECTS

SYMPTOMS	WHAT TO DO
Life-threatening: Difficult breathing, uncontrollable rapid heart rate, loss of consciousness.	Discontinue. Seek emergency treatment.
Common: • Headache, irritability, nervousness, restlessness, insomnia, nausea, vomiting, abdominal pain, irregular heartbeat.	Discontinue. Call doctor right away.
• Dizziness, lightheadedness, paleness, heartburn.	Continue. Call doctor when convenient.
Infrequent: • Skin rash or hives, red or flushed face, appetite loss, diarrhea, abdominal pain.	Discontinue. Call doctor right away.
• Frequent urination.	Continue. Call doctor when convenient.
Rare: None expected.	

 ## WARNINGS & PRECAUTIONS

Don't take if:
- You are allergic to any bronchodilator, ephedrine, any sympathomimetic drug*, cough or cold preparation containing guaifenesin.
- You have an active peptic ulcer.

THEOPHYLLINE, EPHEDRINE, GUAIFENESIN & BARBITURATES

Before you start, consult your doctor:
- If you have had impaired kidney or liver function.
- If you have gastritis, peptic ulcer, high blood pressure, heart disease, diabetes, overactive thyroid gland, difficulty urinating, epilepsy, anemia, chronic pain.
- If you take medication for gout or have taken any MAO inhibitor in past 2 weeks, or have taken digitalis preparations in the last 7 days.
- If you will have surgery within 2 months, including dental surgery, requiring general or spinal anesthesia.

Over age 60:
- Adverse reactions and side effects may be more frequent and severe than in younger persons. Use small doses. For drug to work, you must drink 8 to 10 glasses of fluid per day.
- More likely to develop high blood pressure, heart rhythm disturbances and angina and to feel drug's stimulant effects.

Pregnancy:
Risk to unborn child outweighs drug benefits. Don't use. Risk category D (see page xxiii).

Breast-feeding:
Drug passes into milk. Avoid drug or discontinue nursing until you finish medicine. Consult doctor for advice on maintaining milk supply.

Infants & children:
Use only under medical supervision.

Prolonged use:
- Stomach irritation.
- Excessive doses—Rare toxic psychosis.
- Men with enlarged prostate gland may have more urination difficulty.
- May cause addiction, anemia, chronic intoxication.
- May lower body temperature, making exposure to cold temperature hazardous.

Skin & sunlight:
May cause rash or intensify sunburn in areas exposed to sun or ultraviolet light (photosensitivity reaction). Avoid overexposure. Notify doctor if reaction occurs.

Driving, piloting or hazardous work:
Don't drive or pilot aircraft until you learn how medicine affects you. Don't work around dangerous machinery. Don't climb ladders or work in high places. Danger increases if you drink alcohol or take medicine affecting alertness and reflexes, such as antihistamines, tranquilizers, sedatives, pain medicine, narcotics and mind-altering drugs.

Discontinuing:
- May be unnecessary to finish medicine. Follow doctor's instructions.
- If you develop withdrawal symptoms of hallucinations, agitation or sleeplessness after discontinuing, call doctor right away.

Others:
Great potential for abuse.

POSSIBLE INTERACTION WITH OTHER DRUGS

GENERIC NAME OR DRUG CLASS	COMBINED EFFECT
Adrenocorticoids, systemic	Possible glaucoma.
Allopurinol	Decreased allopurinol effect.
Anticonvulsants*, oral	Changed seizure patterns.
Antidepressants, tricyclic*	Decreased antidepressant effect.
Antidiabetics, oral*	Increased phenobarbital effect.
Antihistamines*	Dangerous sedation. Avoid.
Anti-inflammatory drugs, nonsteroidal (NSAIDs)*	Decreased anti-inflammatory effect.

Continued on page 936

POSSIBLE INTERACTION WITH OTHER SUBSTANCES

INTERACTS WITH	COMBINED EFFECT
Alcohol:	Possible fatal oversedation. Avoid.
Beverages:	You must drink 8 to 10 glasses of fluid per day for drug to work.
Caffeine drinks.	Nervousness and insomnia.
Cocaine:	High risk of heartbeat irregularities and high blood pressure.
Foods:	None expected.
Marijuana:	Excessive sedation, rapid heartbeat, possible heart rhythm disturbance. Avoid.
Tobacco:	Decreased bronchodilator effect. Smoking is damaging to all problems this medicine treats. Avoid.

*See Glossary

THIAMINE (Vitamin B-1)

BRAND NAMES

Betalin S   Bewon
Betaxin   Biamine

Numerous other multiple vitamin-mineral supplements. Check labels.

BASIC INFORMATION

Habit forming? No
Prescription needed? No
Available as generic? Yes
Drug class: Vitamin supplement

USES

- Dietary supplement to promote normal growth, development and health.
- Treatment for beri-beri (a thiamine-deficiency disease).
- Dietary supplement for alcoholism, cirrhosis, overactive thyroid, infection, breast-feeding, absorption diseases, pregnancy, prolonged diarrhea, burns.

DOSAGE & USAGE INFORMATION

How to take:
Tablet or liquid—Swallow with beverage or food to lessen stomach irritation.

When to take:
At the same time each day.

If you forget a dose:
Take when remembered, then return to regular schedule.

What drug does:
- Promotes normal growth and development.
- Combines with an enzyme to metabolize carbohydrates.

Time lapse before drug works:
15 minutes.

Don't take with:
Any other medicine without consulting your doctor or pharmacist.

OVERDOSE

SYMPTOMS:
Increased severity of adverse reactions and side effects.
WHAT TO DO:
Overdose unlikely to threaten life. If person takes much larger amount than prescribed, call doctor, poison control center or hospital emergency room for instructions.

POSSIBLE ADVERSE REACTIONS OR SIDE EFFECTS

SYMPTOMS	WHAT TO DO
Life-threatening: Hives, rash, intense itching, faintness soon after a dose (anaphylaxis) (injection only).	Seek emergency treatment immediately.
Common: None expected.	
Infrequent: None expected.	
Rare: • Wheezing.	Discontinue. Seek emergency treatment.
• Rash or itchy skin.	Discontinue. Call doctor right away.

WARNINGS & PRECAUTIONS

Don't take if:
You are allergic to any B vitamin.

Before you start, consult your doctor:
If you have liver or kidney disease.

Over age 60:
No problems expected.

Pregnancy:
Consult doctor. Risk category A (see page xxiii).

Breast-feeding:
No problems expected in meeting child's normal daily requirements. Consult doctor.

Infants & children:
No problems expected.

Prolonged use:
No problems expected.

Skin & sunlight:
No problems expected.

Driving, piloting or hazardous work:
No problems expected.

Discontinuing:
No problems expected.

Others:
A balanced diet should provide enough thiamine for healthy people to make a supplement unnecessary. Best dietary sources of thiamine are whole-grain cereals and meats.

POSSIBLE INTERACTION WITH OTHER DRUGS

GENERIC NAME OR DRUG CLASS	COMBINED EFFECT
Barbiturates*	Decreased thiamine effect.

POSSIBLE INTERACTION WITH OTHER SUBSTANCES

INTERACTS WITH	COMBINED EFFECT
Alcohol:	None expected.
Beverages: Carbonates, citrates (additives listed on many beverage labels).	Decreased thiamine effect.
Cocaine:	None expected.
Foods: Carbonates, citrates (additives listed on many food labels).	Decreased thiamine effect.
Marijuana:	None expected.
Tobacco:	None expected.

THIOGUANINE

BRAND NAMES

Lanvis

BASIC INFORMATION

Habit forming? No
Prescription needed? Yes
Available as generic? Yes
Drug class: Antineoplastic

 USES

Treats some forms of leukemia.

 DOSAGE & USAGE INFORMATION

How to take:
Tablets—Swallow with liquid. If you can't swallow whole, crumble tablet and take with liquid or food. Instructions to take on empty stomach mean 1 hour before or 2 hours after eating.

When to take:
According to doctor's instructions.

If you forget a dose:
Skip the missed dose and return to regular schedule. Don't double dose.

What drug does:
Interferes with growth of cancer cells.

Time lapse before drug works:
Varies greatly among patients.

Don't take with:
Any other medicines (including over-the-counter drugs such as cough and cold medicines, laxatives, antacids, diet pills, caffeine, nose drops or vitamins) without consulting your doctor.

 OVERDOSE

SYMPTOMS:
None expected.
WHAT TO DO:
Overdose unlikely to threaten life. If person takes much larger amount than prescribed, call doctor, poison control center or hospital emergency room for instructions.

 POSSIBLE ADVERSE REACTIONS OR SIDE EFFECTS

SYMPTOMS	WHAT TO DO
Life-threatening: Black, tarry stools.	Discontinue. Seek emergency treatment.
Common: • Appetite loss, diarrhea, skin rash.	Continue. Call doctor when convenient.
• Nausea.	No action necessary.
Infrequent: Bloody urine; hoarseness or cough; fever or chills; lower back or side pain; painful or difficult urination; red spots on skin; unusual bleeding or bruising; joint pain; swollen feet and legs; unsteady gait.	Discontinue. Call doctor right away.
Rare: Mouth and lip sores; jaundice (yellow skin and eyes).	Discontinue. Call doctor right away.

 WARNINGS & PRECAUTIONS

Don't take if:
• You are allergic to thioguanine.
• You have chicken pox or shingles.

Before you start, consult your doctor:
• If you have gout.
• If you have an infection.
• If you have kidney or liver disease.
• If you have had radiation or cancer chemotherapy within 6 weeks.

Over age 60:
Adverse reactions and side effects may be more frequent and severe than in younger persons. You may need smaller doses for shorter periods of time.

Pregnancy:
• Risk to unborn child outweighs drug benefits. Don't use.
• Don't use birth control pills for contraception.
• Risk category D (see page xxiii).

Breast-feeding:
Drug may pass into milk. Avoid drug or discontinue nursing until you finish medicine. Consult doctor for advice on maintaining milk supply.

Infants & children:
No special problems expected.

Prolonged use:
- Increased likelihood of side effects.
- Talk to your doctor about the need for follow-up medical examinations or laboratory studies to check kidney and liver function, serum uric acid, and complete blood counts (white blood cell count, platelet count, red blood cell count, hemoglobin, hematocrit).

Skin & sunlight:
No problems expected.

Driving, piloting or hazardous work:
No problems expected.

Discontinuing:
Report to your doctor any of these symptoms that occur after discontinuing: black, tarry stools; bloody urine; hoarseness or cough; fever or chills; lower back or side pain; painful or difficult urination; red spots on skin; unusual bleeding or bruising.

Others:
- Advise any doctor or dentist whom you consult that you take this medicine.
- May affect results in some medical tests.
- Don't use birth control pills for contraception.

POSSIBLE INTERACTION WITH OTHER DRUGS

GENERIC NAME OR DRUG CLASS	COMBINED EFFECT
Antigout drugs*	May need increased antigout dosage.
Bone marrow depressants*, other	Increased risk of bone marrow depression.
Vaccines, live or killed	Increased risk of toxicity or reduced effectiveness of vaccine.
Zidovudine	More likelihood of toxicity of both drugs.

POSSIBLE INTERACTION WITH OTHER SUBSTANCES

INTERACTS WITH	COMBINED EFFECT
Alcohol:	Increased side effects.
Beverages:	None expected.
Cocaine:	Increased side effects.
Foods:	None expected.
Marijuana:	None expected.
Tobacco:	None expected.

THIOTHIXENE

BRAND NAMES

Navane

Thiothixene HCl
Intensol

BASIC INFORMATION

Habit forming? No
Prescription needed? Yes
Available as generic? Yes
Drug class: Antipsychotic (thioxanthine)

 USES

Reduces anxiety, agitation, psychosis.

 DOSAGE & USAGE INFORMATION

How to take:
- Capsule—Swallow with liquid. If you can't swallow whole, open capsule and take with liquid or food.
- Syrup—Dilute dose in beverage before swallowing.

When to take:
At the same times each day.

If you forget a dose:
Take as soon as you remember up to 2 hours late. If more than 2 hours, wait for next scheduled dose (don't double this dose).

What drug does:
Corrects imbalance of nerve impulses.

Continued next column

 OVERDOSE

SYMPTOMS:
Drowsiness, dizziness, weakness, muscle rigidity, twitching, tremors, confusion, dry mouth, blurred vision, rapid pulse, shallow breathing, low blood pressure, convulsions, coma.
WHAT TO DO:
- **Dial 911 (emergency) or 0 (operator) for an ambulance or medical help. Then give first aid immediately.**
- **If patient is unconscious and not breathing, give mouth-to-mouth breathing. If there is no heartbeat, use cardiac massage and mouth-to-mouth breathing (CPR). Don't try to make patient vomit. If you can't get help quickly, take patient to nearest emergency facility.**
- **See emergency information at end of book.**

Time lapse before drug works:
3 weeks.

Don't take with:
Any other medicine without consulting your doctor or pharmacist.

 POSSIBLE ADVERSE REACTIONS OR SIDE EFFECTS

SYMPTOMS	WHAT TO DO
Life-threatening: High fever, rapid pulse, profuse sweating, muscle rigidity, confusion and irritability, seizures.	Discontinue. Seek emergency treatment.
Common: • Jerky or involuntary movements, especially of the face, lips, jaw, tongue; slow-frequency tremor of head or limbs, especially while moving; muscle rigidity, lack of facial expression and slow, inflexible movements.	Discontinue. Call doctor right away.
• Pacing or restlessness; intermittent spasms of muscles of face, eyes, tongue, jaw, neck, body or limbs; dry mouth, blurred vision, constipation, difficulty urinating.	Continue. Call doctor when convenient.
Infrequent: Sedation, low blood pressure and dizziness.	Continue. Call doctor when convenient.
Infrequent: Other symptoms not listed above.	Continue. Call doctor when convenient.

 WARNINGS & PRECAUTIONS

Don't take if:
- You are allergic to any thioxanthine or phenothiazine tranquilizer.
- You have serious blood disorder.
- You have Parkinson's disease.
- Patient is younger than 12.

Before you start, consult your doctor:
- If you have had liver or kidney disease.
- If you have epilepsy, glaucoma, prostate trouble.
- If you have high blood pressure or heart disease (especially angina).
- If you use alcohol daily.
- If you will have surgery within 2 months, including dental surgery, requiring general or spinal anesthesia.

Over age 60:
Adverse reactions and side effects may be more frequent and severe than in younger persons.

Pregnancy:
Decide with your doctor if drug benefits justify risk to unborn child. Risk category C (see page xxiii).

Breast-feeding:
Studies inconclusive. Consult your doctor.

Infants & children:
Not recommended.

Prolonged use:
- Pigment deposits in lens and retina of eye.
- Involuntary movements of jaws, lips, tongue (tardive dyskinesia).
- Talk to your doctor about the need for follow-up medical examinations or laboratory studies to check complete blood counts (white blood cell count, platelet count, red blood cell count, hemoglobin, hematocrit), liver function, eyes.

Skin & sunlight:
- May cause rash or intensify sunburn in areas exposed to sun or ultraviolet light (photosensitivity reaction). Use sunscreen and avoid overexposure. Notify doctor if reaction occurs.
- Hot temperatures and exercise, hot baths can increase risk of heatstroke. Drug may affect body's ability to maintain normal temperature.

Driving, piloting or hazardous work:
Don't drive or pilot aircraft until you learn how medicine affects you. Don't work around dangerous machinery. Don't climb ladders or work in high places. Danger increases if you drink alcohol or take medicine affecting alertness and reflexes.

Discontinuing:
Don't discontinue without consulting doctor. Dose may require gradual reduction if you have taken drug for a long time. Doses of other drugs may also require adjustment.

Others:
- Advise any doctor or dentist whom you consult that you take this medicine.
- For dry mouth, suck sugarless hard candy or chew sugarless gum. If dry mouth persists, consult your dentist.

 POSSIBLE INTERACTION WITH OTHER DRUGS

GENERIC NAME OR DRUG CLASS	COMBINED EFFECT
Anticonvulsants*	Change in seizure pattern.
Antidepressants, tricyclic*	Increased thiothixene effect. Excessive sedation.
Antihistamines*	Increased thiothixene effect. Excessive sedation.
Antihypertensives*	Excessively low blood pressure.
Barbiturates*	Increased thiothixene effect. Excessive sedation.
Bupropion	Increased risk of seizures.
Epinephrine	Excessively low blood pressure.
Guanethidine	Decreased guanethidine effect.
Levodopa	Decreased levodopa effect.
Mind-altering drugs*	Increased thiothixene effect. Excessive sedation.
Monoamine oxidase (MAO) inhibitors*	Excessive sedation.
Narcotics*	Increased thiothixene effect. Excessive sedation.

Continued on page 937

 POSSIBLE INTERACTION WITH OTHER SUBSTANCES

INTERACTS WITH	COMBINED EFFECT
Alcohol:	Excessive brain depression. Avoid.
Beverages:	None expected.
Cocaine:	Decreased thiothixene effect. Avoid.
Foods:	None expected.
Marijuana:	Daily use—Fainting likely, possible psychosis.
Tobacco:	None expected.

*See Glossary

THYROID HORMONES

GENERIC AND BRAND NAMES

LEVOTHYROXINE
   Eltroxin
   Levo-T
   Levothroid
   Levoxyl
   L-Thyroxine
   Synthroid
LIOTHYRONINE
   Cytomel

LIOTRIX
   Euthoid
   Thyrolar
THYROGLOBULIN
   Proloid
THYROID
   Thyroid Strong

BASIC INFORMATION

Habit forming? No
Prescription needed? Yes
Available as generic? Yes, for some
Drug class: Thyroid hormone

USES

Replacement for thyroid hormones lost due to deficiency.

DOSAGE & USAGE INFORMATION

How to take:
Tablet—Swallow with liquid.

When to take:
At the same time each day before a meal or on awakening.

If you forget a dose:
Take as soon as you remember up to 12 hours late. If more than 12 hours, wait for next scheduled dose (don't double this dose).

What drug does:
Increases cell metabolism rate.

Time lapse before drug works:
48 hours.

Continued next column

OVERDOSE

SYMPTOMS:
"Hot" feeling, heart palpitations, nervousness, sweating, hand tremors, insomnia, rapid and irregular pulse, headache, irritability, diarrhea, weight loss, muscle cramps, angina, congestive heart failure possible.
WHAT TO DO:
Overdose unlikely to threaten life. If person takes much larger amount than prescribed, call doctor, poison control center or hospital emergency room for instructions.

Don't take with:
Any other medicine without consulting your doctor or pharmacist.

POSSIBLE ADVERSE REACTIONS OR SIDE EFFECTS

SYMPTOMS	WHAT TO DO
Life-threatening:	
In case of overdose, see previous column.	
Common:	
Tremor, headache, irritability, insomnia, appetite change, diarrhea, leg cramps, menstrual irregularities, fever, heat sensitivity, unusual sweating, weight loss, nervousness.	Continue. Call doctor when convenient.
Infrequent:	
Hives, rash, vomiting, chest pain, rapid and irregular heartbeat, shortness of breath.	Discontinue. Call doctor right away.
Rare:	
None expected.	

WARNINGS & PRECAUTIONS

Don't take if:
- You have had a heart attack within 6 weeks.
- You have no thyroid deficiency, but want to use this to lose weight.

Before you start, consult your doctor:
- If you have heart disease or high blood pressure.
- If you have diabetes.
- If you have Addison's disease, have had adrenal gland deficiency or use epinephrine, ephedrine or isoproterenol for asthma.

Over age 60:
More sensitive to thyroid hormone. May need smaller doses.

Pregnancy:
Considered safe if for thyroid deficiency only. Consult doctor. Risk category A (see page xxiii).

Breast-feeding:
Present in milk. Consult doctor.

Infants & children:
Use only under medical supervision.

Prolonged use:
- No problems expected if dose is correct.
- Talk to your doctor about the need for follow-up medical examinations or laboratory studies to check thyroid, heart.

Skin & sunlight:
No problems expected.

Driving, piloting or hazardous work:
No problems expected.

Discontinuing:
Don't discontinue without consulting doctor. Dose may require gradual reduction if you have taken drug for a long time. Doses of other drugs may also require adjustment.

Others:
- Digestive upsets, tremors, cramps, nervousness, insomnia or diarrhea may indicate need for dose adjustment.
- Different brands can cause different results. Do not change brands without consulting doctor.
- Advise any doctor or dentist whom you consult that you take this medicine.

POSSIBLE INTERACTION WITH OTHER DRUGS

GENERIC NAME OR DRUG CLASS	COMBINED EFFECT
Adrenocorticoids, systemic	May require thyroid hormone dosage change.
Amphetamines*	Increased amphetamine effect.
Anticoagulants*, oral	Increased anti-coagulant effect.
Antidepressants, tricyclic*	Increased anti-depressant effect. Irregular heartbeat.
Antidiabetics*, oral or insulin	Antidiabetic may require adjustment.
Aspirin (large doses, continuous use)	Increased effect of thyroid hormone.
Barbiturates*	Decreased barbiturate effect.
Beta-adrenergic blocking agents*	Possible decreased effect of beta blocker.
Cholestyramine	Decreased effect of thyroid hormone.
Colestipol	Decreased effect of thyroid hormone.
Contraceptives, oral*	Decreased effect of thyroid hormone.

Digitalis preparations*	Decreased digitalis effect.
Ephedrine	Increased ephedrine effect.
Epinephrine	Increased epinephrine effect.
Estrogens*	Decreased effect of thyroid hormone.
Methylphenidate	Increased methylphenidate effect.
Phenytoin	Possible decreased effect of thyroid hormone.
Sympathomimetics*	Increased risk of rapid or irregular heartbeat.

POSSIBLE INTERACTION WITH OTHER SUBSTANCES

INTERACTS WITH	COMBINED EFFECT
Alcohol:	None expected.
Beverages:	None expected.
Cocaine:	Excess stimulation. Avoid.
Foods:	None expected.
Marijuana:	None expected.
Tobacco:	None expected.

TICLOPIDINE

BRAND NAMES

Ticlid

BASIC INFORMATION

Habit forming? No
Prescription needed? Yes
Available as generic? No
Drug class: Platelet aggregation inhibitor

 ## USES

Decreases the risk of stroke in patients who have warning signs of stroke or who have had strokes caused by blood clots.

 ## DOSAGE & USAGE INFORMATION

How to take:
Tablets—Swallow with liquid. If you can't swallow whole, crumble tablet and take with liquid or food.

When to take:
Twice a day with food or as directed.

If you forget a dose:
Take as soon as you remember up to 2 hours late. If more than 2 hours, wait for next scheduled dose (don't double this dose).

What drug does:
Inhibits the clumping of platelets and thereby prevents blood clotting.

Time lapse before drug works:
2 hours.

Don't take with:
Any other drugs (particularly aspirin) without consulting doctor or pharmacist.

 ## OVERDOSE

SYMPTOMS:
Bloody vomit or excessive bleeding from gums, nose or rectum.
WHAT TO DO:
Dial 911 (emergency) or 0 (operator) for an ambulance or medical help. Then give first aid immediately.

 ## POSSIBLE ADVERSE REACTIONS OR SIDE EFFECTS

SYMPTOMS	WHAT TO DO
Life-threatening: None expected.	
Common:	
• Diarrhea, elevated level of cholesterol in blood.	Continue. Call doctor when convenient.
• Nausea, skin rash, abdominal pain.	Discontinue. Call doctor right away.
Infrequent:	
• Unusual bleeding or bruising.	Discontinue. Seek emergency treatment.
• Headache.	Continue. Call doctor when convenient.
Rare:	
• Sore throat, mouth ulcers, fever, chills.	Discontinue. Seek emergency treatment.
• Dizziness, loss of appetite, gaseousness.	Continue. Call doctor when convenient.

WARNINGS & PRECAUTIONS

Don't take if:
- You are allergic to ticlopidine.
- You have reduced white blood cells (neutropenia).

Before you start, consult your doctor:
- If you have liver disease, kidney disease, peptic ulcers or diverticulitis.
- If you have any bleeding disorder.

Over age 60:
No special problems expected.

Pregnancy:
Use during pregnancy only if clearly needed. Consult doctor. Risk category D (see page xxiii).

Breast-feeding:
Safety not established. Consult doctor.

Infants & children:
Not recommended. Safety has not been established.

Prolonged use:
No special problems expected.

Skin & sunlight:
No special problems expected.

Driving, piloting or hazardous work:
Don't drive or pilot aircraft until you learn how the medicine affects you. Don't work around dangerous machinery. Don't climb ladders or work in high places.

Discontinuing:
No special problems expected.

Others:
- Advise any doctor or dentist whom you consult that you take this medicine. This is particularly important if any surgery is scheduled.
- May affect results of some medical tests.
- Report any unusual bleeding to your doctor.

POSSIBLE INTERACTION WITH OTHER DRUGS

GENERIC NAME OR DRUG CLASS	COMBINED EFFECT
Antacids*	Decreased ticlopidine effect.
Aspirin	Increased effects of both drugs.
Digoxin	Slightly decreased digoxin effect.
Theophylline	Increased theophylline effect.

POSSIBLE INTERACTION WITH OTHER SUBSTANCES

INTERACTS WITH	COMBINED EFFECT
Alcohol:	Increased alcohol in blood. Avoid.
Beverages:	No proven problems.
Cocaine:	No proven problems.
Foods:	Best to take with foods to prevent stomach upset.
Marijuana:	No proven problems.
Tobacco:	No proven problems.

*See Glossary

TIOPRONIN

BRAND NAMES

Capen	Thiola
Captimer	Thiosol
Epatiol	Tioglis
Mucolysin	Vincol
Sutilan	

BASIC INFORMATION

Habit forming? No
Prescription needed? Yes
Available as generic? No
Drug class: Antiurolithic

USES

Prevents the formation of kidney stones when there is too much cystine in the urine.

DOSAGE & USAGE INFORMATION

How to take:
Tablets—Swallow with liquid. If you can't swallow whole, crumble tablet and take with liquid or food. Instructions to take on empty stomach mean 1 hour before or 2 hours after eating.

When to take:
3 times daily (once approximately every 8 hours).

If you forget a dose:
Take as soon as you remember up to 2 hours late. If more than 2 hours, wait for next scheduled dose (don't double this dose).

What drug does:
Removes high levels of cystine from the body.

Time lapse before drug works:
Works immediately.

Continued next column

OVERDOSE

SYMPTOMS:
None expected. If massive overdose is suspected, follow instructions below.
WHAT TO DO:
- **Dial 911 (emergency) or 0 (operator) for an ambulance or medical help. Then give first aid immediately.**
- **See emergency information on inside covers.**

Don't take with:
- Medicines that are known to cause kidney damage or depress bone marrow.
- Any other medicine without consulting your doctor or pharmacist.

POSSIBLE ADVERSE REACTIONS OR SIDE EFFECTS

SYMPTOMS	WHAT TO DO
Life-threatening:	
In case of overdose, see previous column	
Common:	
• Skin rash, itching skin, mouth sores, mouth ulcers.	Discontinue. Call doctor right away.
• Abdominal pain, gaseousness, diarrhea, nausea or vomiting.	Continue. Call doctor when convenient.
Infrequent:	
• Cloudy urine, chills, breathing difficulty, joint pain.	Discontinue. Call doctor right away.
• Impaired smell or taste.	Continue. Call doctor when convenient.
Rare:	
Coughing up blood, fever, unusual tiredness or weakness, double vision, muscle weakness.	Discontinue. Call doctor right away.

WARNINGS & PRECAUTIONS

Don't take if:
You are allergic to tiopronin or penicillamine.

Before you start, consult your doctor:
If you have had any of the following in the past:
* Agranulocytosis*
* Aplastic anemia*
* Thrombocytopenia*
* Impaired kidney function

Over age 60:
May require dosage adjustment if kidney function is impaired due to normal aging.

Pregnancy:
Decide with your doctor if drug benefits justify risk to unborn child. Risk category C (see page xxiii).

Breast-feeding:
Drug passes into milk. Avoid or discontinue nursing until you finish medicine. Consult doctor for advice on maintaining milk supply.

Infants & children:
Safety not established. Consult doctor.

Prolonged use:
No special problems expected.

Skin & sunlight:
No special problems expected.

Driving, piloting or hazardous work:
Don't drive or pilot aircraft until you learn how medicine affects you. Don't work around dangerous machinery. Don't climb ladders or work in high places. Danger increases if you drink alcohol or take medicine affecting alertness and reflexes.

Discontinuing:
No special problems expected.

Others:
* Advise any doctor or dentist whom you consult that you take this medicine.
* May affect results of some medical tests.

POSSIBLE INTERACTION WITH OTHER DRUGS

GENERIC NAME OR DRUG CLASS	COMBINED EFFECT
Bone marrow depressants*	May increase possibility of toxic effects of tiopronin.
Medications toxic to kidneys (nephrotoxins*)	May increase possibility of toxic effects of tiopronin.

POSSIBLE INTERACTION WITH OTHER SUBSTANCES

INTERACTS WITH	COMBINED EFFECT
Alcohol:	None expected.
Beverages: Water.	Enhances effects of tiopronin. Drink 8 to 10 glasses daily.
Cocaine:	None expected.
Foods:	None expected.
Marijuana:	None expected.
Tobacco:	None expected.

TIZANIDINE

BRAND NAMES

Zanaflex

BASIC INFORMATION

Habit forming? No
Prescription needed? Yes
Available as generic? No
Drug class: Antispastic, muscle relaxant

 ## USES

- Relieves muscle spasticity caused by diseases such as multiple sclerosis or injury to the spinal cord. It does not appear to improve muscle weakness.
- Relieves muscle spasticity caused by injury to spinal cord.

 ## DOSAGE & USAGE INFORMATION

How to take:
Tablet—Swallow with liquid. It may be taken with or without food.

When to take:
Up to three times a day or as directed by your doctor.

If you forget a dose:
Take as soon as you remember up to 1 hour late. If more than 1 hour, wait for next scheduled dose (don't double this dose).

What drug does:
Slows nerve impulses that stimulate skeletal muscles, decreasing cramping.

Time lapse before drug works:
Within hours. Dosage may be increased over a several week period to achieve maximum effectiveness.

Don't take with:
Any other medicine without consulting your doctor or pharmacist. All possible drug interactions have not been studied.

 ## OVERDOSE

SYMPTOMS:
Breathing difficulties, heartbeat irregularities; other symptoms may occur that were not observed in medical studies of the drug.
WHAT TO DO:
If person takes much larger amount than prescribed, call doctor, poison control center or hospital emergency room for instructions.

 ## POSSIBLE ADVERSE REACTIONS OR SIDE EFFECTS

SYMPTOMS	WHAT TO DO
Life-threatening:	
In case of overdose, see previous column.	
Common:	
• Nervousness, sensation changes (tingling, burning, prickling), skin sores, anxiety, tiredness or weakness, constipation, back pain, dizziness, dry mouth, depression, drowsiness, heartburn, lightheadedness when getting up from a sitting or lying position, increase in muscle spasm, muscle weakness, sore throat, runny nose, increased sweating.	Continue. Call doctor when convenient.
• Fever, liver problems, (weight loss, nausea, vomiting, yellow skin or eyes), pain or burning when urinating, involuntary movements, diarrhea, vomiting, stomach pain, speech problems.	Discontinue. Call doctor when convenient.
Infrequent:	
• Heartbeat irregularity, black or tarry stools, seizures, bloody vomit, fever and chills, fainting.	Discontinue. Call doctor right away
• Mental changes, mood changes, dry skin, swelling of hands or feet or other areas of the body, difficulty swallowing, migraine, neck pain, trembling or shaking, weight loss, joint or muscle pain, skin rash, feeling of coldness, puffy skin, weight gain, cough, white patches on tongue or in mouth, visual changes or eye pain.	Continue. Call doctor when convenient.
Rare:	
Other symptoms not mentioned above.	Continue. Call doctor when convenient.

WARNINGS & PRECAUTIONS

Don't take if:
You are allergic to tizanidine.

Before you start, consult your doctor:
- If you have liver disease.
- If you have kidney disease.
- If you are allergic to any medication, food or other substance.
- If you are taking an alpha-adrenergic blood pressure medicine.

Over age 60:
Adverse reactions and side effects may be more frequent and severe than in younger persons. Lower dosage may be recommended to start.

Pregnancy:
Decide with your doctor if drug benefits justify risk to unborn child. Risk category C (see page xxiii).

Breast-feeding:
It is unknown if drug passes into milk. Avoid nursing or discontinue until you finish drug. Consult doctor.

Infants & children:
Safety and dosage have not been established.

Prolonged use:
Talk to your doctor about the need for liver function studies while using this drug.

Skin & sunlight:
No special problems expected.

Driving, piloting or hazardous work:
Don't drive or pilot aircraft until you learn how medicine affects you. Don't work around dangerous machinery. Don't climb ladders or work in high places. Danger increases if you drink alcohol or take medicine affecting alertness and reflexes, such as antihistamines, tranquilizers, sedatives, pain medicine, narcotics and mind-altering drugs.

Discontinuing:
Don't discontinue without consulting doctor.

Others:
- May interfere with the results in some medical tests.
- Get up slowly from a sitting or lying position to avoid any dizziness, faintness or lightheadedness.
- Advise any doctor or dentist whom you consult that you take this medicine.
- Take medicine only as directed. Do not increase or reduce dosage without doctor's approval.

POSSIBLE INTERACTION WITH OTHER DRUGS

GENERIC NAME OR DRUG CLASS	COMBINED EFFECT
Central nervous system (CNS) depressants *	Increased sedation.
Contraceptives, oral	Increased effect of tizanidine.
Hypotension-causing drugs*, other	Increased effect of hypotension.

POSSIBLE INTERACTION WITH OTHER SUBSTANCES

INTERACTS WITH	COMBINED EFFECT
Alcohol:	Increased sedation, low blood pressure. Avoid.
Beverages:	No problems expected.
Cocaine:	Increased spasticity. Avoid.
Foods:	No problems expected.
Marijuana:	Increased spasticity or sedation. Avoid.
Tobacco:	May interfere with absorption of medicine.

TOCAINIDE

BRAND NAMES

Tonocard

BASIC INFORMATION

Habit forming? No
Prescription needed? Yes
Available as generic? No
Drug class: Antiarrhythmic

 ## USES

Stabilizes irregular heartbeat, particularly irregular contractions of the ventricles of the heart or a too rapid heart rate.

 ## DOSAGE & USAGE INFORMATION

How to take:
Tablet—Swallow with food, water or milk. Dosage may need to be changed according to individual response.

When to take:
Take at regular times each day. For example, instructions to take 3 times a day means every 8 hours.

If you forget a dose:
Take as soon as you remember up to 4 hours late. If more than 4 hours, wait for next scheduled dose (don't double this dose).

What drug does:
Decreases excitability of cells of heart muscle.

Time lapse before drug works:
30 minutes to 2 hours.

Don't take with:
- Any other medicine without consulting your doctor or pharmacist.
- Wear identification information that states that you take this medicine so during an emergency a physician will know to avoid additional medicines that might be harmful or dangerous.

 ## OVERDOSE

SYMPTOMS:
Convulsions, depressed breathing, cardiac arrest.
WHAT TO DO:
- **Dial 911 (emergency) or 0 (operator) for an ambulance or medical help. Then give first aid immediately.**
- **See emergency information on inside covers.**

 ## POSSIBLE ADVERSE REACTIONS OR SIDE EFFECTS

SYMPTOMS	WHAT TO DO
Life-threatening:	
In case of overdose, see previous column.	
Common:	
• Nausea, vomiting, lightheadedness, dizziness.	Discontinue. Call doctor right away.
• Appetite loss.	Continue. Call doctor when convenient.
Infrequent:	
• Trembling, headache.	Discontinue. Call doctor right away.
• Numbness or tingling in hands or feet.	Continue. Call doctor when convenient.
Rare:	
• Sore throat, unexplained bleeding or bruising, fever, chills, blurred vision, accelerated heart rate or more irregular heartbeat, cough, difficult breathing, wheezing, double vision, disorientation, shakiness, seizures, blisters.	Discontinue. Call doctor right away.
• Rash, swollen feet and ankles, unusual sweating.	Continue. Call doctor when convenient.

WARNINGS & PRECAUTIONS

Don't take if:
- You are allergic to tocainide or anesthetics whose names end in "caine."
- You have myasthenia gravis.

Before you start, consult your doctor:
- If you have congestive heart failure.
- If you are pregnant or plan to become pregnant.
- If you take anticancer drugs, trimethoprim, pyrimethamine, primaquine, phenylbutazone, penicillamine or oxyphenbutazone. These may affect blood cell production in bone marrow.
- If you take any other heart medicine such as digitalis, flucystosine, colchicine, chloramphenicol, beta-adrenergic blockers or azathioprine. These can worsen heartbeat irregularity.
- If you will have surgery within 2 months, including dental surgery, requiring general, local or spinal anesthesia.
- If you have liver or kidney disease.

Over age 60:
Adverse reactions and side effects may be more frequent and severe than in younger persons.

Pregnancy:
Decide with your doctor whether drug benefits justify risk to unborn child. Risk category C (see page xxiii).

Breast-feeding:
Avoid if possible. Consult doctor.

Infants & children:
Not recommended. Safety and dosage have not been established.

Prolonged use:
Request periodic lab studies on blood, liver function, potassium levels, x-ray, ECG*.

Skin & sunlight:
No problems expected.

Driving, piloting or hazardous work:
Use caution if medicine causes you to feel dizzy or weak. Otherwise, no problems expected.

Discontinuing:
Don't discontinue without consulting doctor, even though symptoms diminish or disappear.

Others:
No problems expected.

POSSIBLE INTERACTION WITH OTHER DRUGS

GENERIC NAME OR DRUG CLASS	COMBINED EFFECT
Antiarrhythmics*, others	Increased possibility of adverse reactions from either drug.
Beta-adrenergic blocking agents*	Irregular heartbeat. May worsen congestive heart failure.
Bone marrow depressants*	Decreased production of blood cells in bone marrow.

POSSIBLE INTERACTION WITH OTHER SUBSTANCES

INTERACTS WITH	COMBINED EFFECT
Alcohol:	Possible irregular heartbeat. Avoid.
Beverages: Caffeine drinks, iced drinks.	Possible irregular heartbeat.
Cocaine:	Possible light-headedness, dizziness, quivering, convulsions.
Foods:	None expected.
Marijuana:	None expected.
Tobacco:	Possible irregular heartbeat.

TOLCAPONE

BRAND NAMES

Tasmar

BASIC INFORMATION

Habit forming? No
Prescription needed? Yes
Available as generic? No
Drug class: Antidyskinetic,
antiparkinsonism

 ## USES

Used in combination with levodopa and carbidopa for the treatment of the symptoms of Parkinson's disease.

 ## DOSAGE & USAGE INFORMATION

How to take:
Tablets—Swallow with water, with or without food. If you can't swallow whole, crumble tablet and take with liquid or food.

When to take:
At the same time each day.

If you forget a dose:
Take as soon as possible. If it is almost time for your next dose, skip the missed dose and go back to your regular dosing schedule. Do not double doses.

What drug does:
Increases the blood levels of levodopa and carbidopa to restore the chemical balance necessary for normal nerve impulses.

Time lapse before drug works:
Up to two hours.

Don't take with:
Any other prescription or nonprescription drug without consulting your doctor.

 ## OVERDOSE

SYMPTOMS:
Nausea, vomiting and dizziness.
WHAT TO DO:
Overdose unlikely to threaten life. If person uses much larger amount than prescribed, call doctor, poison control center or hospital emergency room for instructions.

 ## POSSIBLE ADVERSE REACTIONS OR SIDE EFFECTS

SYMPTOMS	WHAT TO DO
Life-threatening: None expected.	
Common: • Abdominal pain, loss of appetite, diarrhea, dizziness, twitching or unusual body movements, hallucinations, headache, fainting, sleeplessness, nausea, drowsiness, fainting, cough, fever, congestion, runny nose, sneezing, sore throat, vomiting.	Discontinue. Call doctor right away.
• Constipation, excessive dreaming, increased sweating, dry mouth.	Continue. Call doctor if symptoms persist.
• Change in urine color to bright yellow.	No action necessary.
Infrequent: • Chest pain, confusion, difficulty breathing, fatigue, falling, blood in urine, hyperactivity, flu-like symptoms, loss of balance control.	Discontinue. Call doctor right away.
• Heartburn, gas.	Continue. Call doctor if symptoms persist.
Rare: Agitation; joint pain; redness or swelling; burning feet; chest discomfort; low blood pressure; difficulty thinking or concentrating; muscle cramps; neck pain; burning, prickling or tingling sensations; sinus congestion; stiffness; bloody or cloudy urine; difficult or painful urination; frequent urge to urinate.	Discontinue. Call doctor right away.

WARNINGS & PRECAUTIONS

Don't take if:
- You have been diagnosed with liver problems.
- You are allergic to tolcapone or any other substances such as food preservatives or dyes.

Before you start, consult your doctor:
- If you have any other medical problem.
- If you suffer from hallucinations.
- If you have ever been diagnosed with kidney problems.
- If you have low blood pressure or are dizzy when getting up suddenly from a sitting or lying position.

Over age 60:
The risk of hallucinations (seeing, hearing or feeling things that are not there) may be increased in patients older than 75 years of age.

Pregnancy:
Decide with your doctor whether drug benefits justify risk to unborn child. Risk category C (see page xxiii).

Breast-feeding:
It is not known if drug passes into milk. Avoid drugs or discontinue nursing until you finish medicine. Consult doctor for advice on maintaining milk supply.

Infants & children:
There is no identified potential use of tolcapone in children.

Prolonged use:
No problems expected.

Skin & sunlight:
No problems expected.

Driving, piloting or hazardous work:
Don't drive or pilot aircraft until you learn how medicine affects you. Don't work around dangerous machinery. Don't climb ladders or work in high places. Danger increases if you drink alcohol or take medicine affecting alertness and reflexes.

Discontinuing:
Because of the risk of liver failure, this drug should be stopped if no improvement in 3 weeks.

Others:
- Tolcapone has been indicated in several life-threatening cases of liver failure. This medication should not be used as a first-line treatment for Parkinson's disease.
- You will need frequent liver-function blood tests while you take this medicine.
- Advise any doctor or dentist whom you consult that you take this medicine.

POSSIBLE INTERACTION WITH OTHER DRUGS

GENERIC NAME OR DRUG CLASS	COMBINED EFFECT
Apomorphine	May require adjustment in dosage of apomorphine.
Desipramine	May increase incidence of adverse effects of tolcapone.
Dobutamine	May require adjustment in dosage of dobutamine.
Isoproterenol	May require adjustment in dosage of isoproterenol.
Methyldopa	May require adjustment in dosage of methyldopa.
Monoamine oxidase (MAO) inhibitor*	May reduce the effectiveness of the MAO inhibitor.
Warfarin	May require adjustment in dosage of warfarin.

POSSIBLE INTERACTION WITH OTHER SUBSTANCES

INTERACTS WITH	COMBINED EFFECT
Alcohol:	May increase incidence of hallucinations. Do not use.
Beverages:	None expected.
Cocaine:	May increase incidence of hallucinations. Do not use.
Foods:	None expected.
Marijuana:	May increase incidence of hallucinations. Do not use.
Tobacco:	None expected.

*See Glossary

TOLTERODINE

BRAND NAMES

Detrol

BASIC INFORMATION

Habit forming? No
Prescription needed? Yes
Available as generic? No
Drug class: Antispasmodic

 USES

Used to treat an overactive bladder with symptoms of urinary frequency, urgency or urge incontinence (inability to control bladder).

 DOSAGE & USAGE INFORMATION

How to take:
Tablets—Swallow with water, with or without food. If you can't swallow whole, crumble tablet and take with liquid or food.

When to take:
At the same times each day.

If you forget a dose:
Take as soon as possible. If it is almost time for your next dose, skip the missed dose and go back to your regular dosing schedule. Do not double doses.

What drug does:
Decreases pressure on the bladder thereby easing the symptoms of overactive bladder.

Time lapse before drug works:
1 to 2 hours.

Don't take with:
Any other prescription or nonprescription drug without consulting your doctor.

 OVERDOSE

SYMPTOMS:
Rapid breathing, dry mouth (anticholinergic effect).
WHAT TO DO:
Overdose unlikely to threaten life. If person uses much larger amount than prescribed, call doctor, poison control center or hospital emergency room for instructions.

 POSSIBLE ADVERSE REACTIONS OR SIDE EFFECTS

SYMPTOMS	WHAT TO DO
Life-threatening:	
None expected.	
Common:	
• Change in vision; difficult, burning or painful urination; frequent urge to urinate; bloody or cloudy urine.	Discontinue. Call doctor right away.
• Chest pain, dizziness, dry mouth, vomiting, abdominal pain, constipation, diarrhea, upset stomach, nausea, headache, flu-like symptoms, drowsiness, dry eyes.	Continue. Call doctor if symptoms persist.
• Flatulence (gas).	No action necessary.
Infrequent:	
Difficult urination, dizziness.	Continue. Call doctor if symptoms persist.
Rare:	
None expected.	

WARNINGS & PRECAUTIONS

Don't take if:
You are allergic to tolterodine.

Before you start, consult your doctor:
- If you have ever been diagnosed with urinary retention.
- If you have gastric retention.
- If you have glaucoma.
- If you have been diagnosed with liver or kidney disease.
- If you have any other medical problem.

Over age 60:
No problems expected.

Pregnancy:
Decide with your doctor whether drug benefits justify risk to unborn child. Risk category C (see page xxiii).

Breast-feeding:
It is unknown if drug passes into milk. Avoid drug or discontinue nursing until you finish medicine. Consult doctor for advice on maintaining milk supply.

Infants & children:
Safety and efficacy have not been established in infants and children.

Prolonged use:
No problems expected.

Skin & sunlight:
No problems expected.

Driving, piloting or hazardous work:
Don't drive, pilot an aircraft or engage in any hazardous activities. Tolterodine can cause blurred vision.

Discontinuing:
Don't discontinue without consulting doctor.

Others:
- Advise any doctor or dentist whom you consult that you are taking this medication.
- Chew sugarless gum or suck on ice chips to relieve a dry mouth. Call your doctor or dentist if the dry mouth lasts longer than 2 weeks.

POSSIBLE INTERACTION WITH OTHER DRUGS

GENERIC NAME OR DRUG CLASS	COMBINED EFFECT
Enzyme inhibitors*	May require adjustment in dosage of tolterodine.

POSSIBLE INTERACTION WITH OTHER SUBSTANCES

INTERACTS WITH	COMBINED EFFECT
Alcohol:	None expected.
Beverages:	None expected.
Cocaine:	Effects unknown. Avoid.
Foods:	None expected.
Marijuana:	Effects unknown. Avoid.
Tobacco:	None expected.

TOREMIFENE

BRAND NAMES

Fareston

BASIC INFORMATION

Habit forming? No
Prescription needed? Yes
Available as generic? No
Drug class: Antineoplastic

 USES

Used to treat breast cancer in postmenopausal women.

 DOSAGE & USAGE INFORMATION

How to take:
Tablets—Swallow with water, with or without food. If you can't swallow whole, crumble tablet and take with liquid or food.

When to take:
At the same time each day.

If you forget a dose:
Take as soon as possible. If it is almost time for your next dose, skip the missed dose and go back to your regular dosing schedule. Do not double doses.

What drug does:
Exact mechanism unknown. Appears to block growth-stimulating effects of estrogen in the tumor.

Time lapse before drug works:
4 to 6 weeks to determine effectiveness.

Don't take with:
Any other prescription or nonprescription drug without consulting your doctor.

 OVERDOSE

SYMPTOMS:
Dizziness, headache, nausea and vomiting.
WHAT TO DO:
Overdose unlikely to threaten life. If person uses much larger amount than prescribed, call doctor, poison control center or hospital emergency room for instructions.

 POSSIBLE ADVERSE REACTIONS OR SIDE EFFECTS

SYMPTOMS	WHAT TO DO
Life-threatening:	
Pain or swelling of feet or lower legs, chest pain, shortness of breath.	Seek emergency treatment immediately.
Common:	
Hot flashes, nausea.	Continue. Call doctor if symptoms persist.
Infrequent:	
• Change in vaginal discharge, pain or feeling of pressure in pelvis, vaginal bleeding, confusion, increased urination, loss of appetite, unusual tiredness, changes in vision.	Continue. Call doctor right away.
• Dizziness, dry eyes, bone pain, vomiting.	Continue. Call doctor if symptoms persist.
Rare:	
None expected.	

812

WARNINGS & PRECAUTIONS

Don't take if:
- You are allergic to toremifene.
- You have a history of blood clots or have been diagnosed with thromboembolic disease.

Before you start, consult your doctor:
- If you have any other medical problem.
- If you have any blood or bleeding disorder.
- If you have ever been diagnosed with endometrial hyperplasia (unusual growth of the lining of the uterus).
- If you have a tumor that has spread to your bone.

Over age 60:
No problems expected.

Pregnancy:
Consult doctor. Risk category D (see page xxiii).

Breast-feeding:
Drug may pass into milk. Avoid drug or discontinue nursing until you finish medicine. Consult doctor about maintaining milk supply.

Infants & children:
There is no identified potential use of toremifene in children.

Prolonged use:
Talk to your doctor about the need for follow-up laboratory studies to check complete blood count, blood calcium concentrations and liver function.

Skin & sunlight:
Avoid prolonged or extended exposure to direct sunlight and/or artificial sunlight while using this medication.

Driving, piloting or hazardous work:
No problems expected.

Discontinuing:
Don't discontinue without consulting doctor.

Others:
- Advise any doctor or dentist you consult that you are taking this medication.
- May interfere with the accuracy of some medical tests.

POSSIBLE INTERACTION WITH OTHER DRUGS

GENERIC NAME OR DRUG CLASS	COMBINED EFFECT
Anticoagulants	May increase time it takes blood to clot.
Diuretics, thiazide	Possible increased calcium.
Enzyme inducers*	May lessen the effect of toremifene.
Enzyme inhibitors*	May increase the effect of toremifene.

POSSIBLE INTERACTION WITH OTHER SUBSTANCES

INTERACTS WITH	COMBINED EFFECT
Alcohol:	None expected.
Beverages:	None expected.
Cocaine:	Effects unknown. Avoid.
Foods:	None expected.
Marijuana:	Effects unknown. Avoid.
Tobacco:	None expected.

TRAMADOL

BRAND NAMES

Ultram

BASIC INFORMATION

Habit forming? No
Prescription needed? Yes
Available as generic? No
Drug class: Analgesic

 ## USES

Treatment for moderate to moderately severe pain.

 ## DOSAGE & USAGE INFORMATION

How to take:
Tablet—Swallow with liquid. May be taken with or without food.

When to take:
Every 4 to 6 hours as needed for pain.

If you forget a dose:
Take as soon as you remember. Wait at least 4 hours before the next dose.

What drug does:
The mode of action is not fully understood. It appears to block pain messages to the brain and spinal cord.

Time lapse before drug works:
Within 60 minutes.

Don't take with:
Any other medication without consulting your doctor or pharmacist.

 ## OVERDOSE

SYMPTOMS:
Breathing difficulty, seizures.
WHAT TO DO:
- **Dial 911 (emergency) or 0 (operator) for an ambulance or medical help. Then give first aid immediately.**
- **See emergency information on inside covers.**

 ## POSSIBLE ADVERSE REACTIONS OR SIDE EFFECTS

SYMPTOMS	WHAT TO DO
Life-threatening: In case of overdose, see previous column.	
Common: Constipation, nausea, headache, drowsiness, clumsiness.	Continue. Call doctor when convenient.
Infrequent: • Constant urge to urinate or inability to urinate, blurred vision.	Discontinue. Call doctor right away.
• Loss of appetite, stomach pain, dry mouth, weakness, confusion, sweating, diarrhea, gas, hot flashes, heartburn, tiredness, flushing or redness of skin, nervousness, trouble sleeping.	Continue. Call doctor when convenient.
Rare: Balancing difficulty, skin reaction (itching, redness and swelling), memory problems, shortness of breath, difficulty performing tasks, hallucinations, dizziness or lightheadedness when getting up from a sitting or lying position, sensations in hands and feet (burning, tingling, pain, weakness, trembling or shaking), faintness, fast heartbeat.	Discontinue. Call doctor right away.

WARNINGS & PRECAUTIONS

Don't take if:
You are allergic to tramadol or narcotic medications.

Before you start, consult your doctor:
- If you have a seizure disorder.
- If you have kidney or liver disease.
- If you have a history of drug dependence or drug abuse, Including alcohol abuse.
- If you have respiratory problems.

Over age 60:
Patients over age 75 usually require a dosage adjustment.

Pregnancy:
Decide with your doctor if drug benefits justify risk to unborn child. Risk category C (see page xxiii).

Breast-feeding:
Drug passes into milk. Avoid drug or discontinue nursing until you finish medicine. Consult doctor for advice on maintaining milk supply.

Infants & children:
Safety in children under age 16 has not been established.

Prolonged use:
- Consult with your doctor on a regular basis while using this drug.
- Can cause drug dependence, addiction and withdrawal symptoms.

Skin & sunlight:
No special problems expected.

Driving, piloting or hazardous work:
Don't drive or pilot aircraft until you learn how medicine affects you. Don't work around dangerous machinery. Don't climb ladders or work in high places. Danger increases if you drink alcohol or take medicine affecting alertness and reflexes.

Discontinuing:
If you have taken this drug for a long time, consult with your doctor before discontinuing.

Others:
- Don't increase dosage or frequency of use without your doctor's approval.
- Advise any doctor or dentist whom you consult that you take this medicine.

POSSIBLE INTERACTION WITH OTHER DRUGS

GENERIC NAME OR DRUG CLASS	COMBINED EFFECT
Carbamazepine	Decreased effect of tramadol.
Central nervous system (CNS) depressants*	Increased sedation.
Monoamine oxidase (MAO) inhibitors*	Increased risk of seizures.
Narcotics*	Increased sedation.
Phenothiazines*	Increased sedation.
Quinidine	Unknown effect. May require dosage adjustment.
Tranquilizers*	Increased sedation.

POSSIBLE INTERACTION WITH OTHER SUBSTANCES

INTERACTS WITH	COMBINED EFFECT
Alcohol:	Increased sedation. Avoid.
Beverages:	No special problems expected.
Cocaine:	Unknown effect. Best to avoid.
Foods:	No special problems expected.
Marijuana:	Unknown effect. Best to avoid.
Tobacco:	No special problems expected.

*See Glossary

TRAZODONE

BRAND NAMES

Desyrel   Trialodine
Trazon

BASIC INFORMATION

Habit forming? No
Prescription needed? Yes
Available as generic? Yes
Drug class: Antidepressant (nontricyclic)

USES

- Treats mental depression.
- Treats anxiety.
- Helps promote sleep.
- Treats some types of chronic pain.

DOSAGE & USAGE INFORMATION

How to take:
Tablet—Swallow with liquid or food to lessen stomach irritation. If you can't swallow whole, crumble tablet and take with liquid or food.

When to take:
According to prescription directions. Bedtime dose usually higher than other doses.

If you forget a dose:
Take as soon as you remember up to 2 hours late. If more than 2 hours, wait for next scheduled dose (don't double this dose).

What drug does:
Inhibits serotonin* uptake in brain cells.

Continued next column

OVERDOSE

SYMPTOMS:
Fainting, irregular heartbeat, respiratory arrest, chest pain, seizures, coma.
WHAT TO DO:
- **Dial 911 (emergency) or 0 (operator) for an ambulance or medical help. Then give first aid immediately.**
- **If patient is unconscious and not breathing, give mouth-to-mouth breathing. If there is no heartbeat, use cardiac massage and mouth-to-mouth breathing (CPR). Don't try to make patient vomit. If you can't get help quickly, take patient to nearest emergency facility.**
- **See emergency information at end of book.**

Time lapse before drug works:
2 to 4 weeks for full effect.

Don't take with:
Any other medicine without consulting your doctor or pharmacist.

POSSIBLE ADVERSE REACTIONS OR SIDE EFFECTS

SYMPTOMS	WHAT TO DO
Life-threatening:	
In case of overdose, see previous column.	
Common:	
Drowsiness.	Continue. Call doctor when convenient.
Infrequent:	
• Prolonged penile erections that may be very painful (priapism).	Seek emergency treatment immediately.
• Tremor, fainting, incoordination, blood pressure rise or drop, rapid heartbeat, shortness of breath.	Discontinue. Call doctor right away.
• Disorientation, confusion, fatigue, dizziness on standing, headache, nervousness, rash, itchy skin, blurred vision, ringing in ears, dry mouth, bad taste, diarrhea, nausea, vomiting, constipation, aching, menstrual changes, diminished sex drive, nightmares, vivid dreams.	Continue. Call doctor when convenient.
Rare:	
Unusual excitement	Discontinue. Call doctor right away.

WARNINGS & PRECAUTIONS

Don't take if:
- You are allergic to trazodone.
- You are thinking about suicide.

Before you start, consult your doctor:
- If you have heart rhythm problem.
- If you have any heart disease.
- If you will have surgery within 2 months, including dental surgery, requiring general or spinal anesthesia.
- If you have bipolar (manic-depressive) disorder.
- If you have liver or kidney disease.

Over age 60:
Adverse reactions and side effects may be more frequent and severe than in younger persons.

Pregnancy:
Decide with your doctor if drug benefits justify risk to unborn child. Risk category C (see page xxiii).

Breast-feeding:
Drug passes into milk. Avoid drug or discontinue nursing until you finish medicine. Consult doctor for advice on maintaining milk supply.

Infants & children:
Not recommended.

Prolonged use:
See your doctor for occasional blood counts, especially if you have fever and sore throat.

Skin & sunlight:
May cause rash or intensity sunburn in areas exposed to sun or ultraviolet light (photo-sensitivity reaction). Use sunscreen and avoid overexposure. Notify doctor if reaction occurs.

Driving, piloting or hazardous work:
Don't drive or pilot aircraft until you learn how medicine affects you. Don't work around dangerous machinery. Don't climb ladders or work in high places. Danger increases if you drink alcohol or take medicine affecting alertness and reflexes, such as antihistamines, tranquilizers, sedatives, pain medicine, narcotics and mind-altering drugs.

Discontinuing:
Don't discontinue without consulting doctor. Dose may require gradual reduction if you have taken drug for a long time. Doses of other drugs may also require adjustment.

Others:
- Electroconvulsive therapy* should be avoided. Combined effect is unknown.
- Advise any doctor or dentist whom you consult that you take this medicine.
- For dry mouth, suck on sugarless hard candy or chew sugarless gum.

POSSIBLE INTERACTION WITH OTHER DRUGS

GENERIC NAME OR DRUG CLASS	COMBINED EFFECT
Antidepressants*, other	Excess drowsiness.
Antihistamines*	Excess drowsiness.
Antihypertensives*	Possible too-low blood pressure. Avoid.
Barbiturates*	Too-low blood pressure and drowsiness. Avoid.
Bupropion	Increased risk of seizures.
Central nervous system (CNS) depressants*	Increased sedation.
Digoxin	Possible increased digitalis level in blood.
Guanabenz	Increased effects of both medicines.
Monoamine oxidase (MAO) inhibitors*	May add to toxic effect of each.
Narcotics*	Excess drowsiness.
Phenytoin	Possible increased phenytoin level in blood.

POSSIBLE INTERACTION WITH OTHER SUBSTANCES

INTERACTS WITH	COMBINED EFFECT
Alcohol:	Excess sedation. Avoid.
Beverages: Caffeine.	May add to heartbeat irregularity. Avoid.
Cocaine:	May add to heartbeat irregularity. Avoid.
Foods:	No problems expected.
Marijuana:	May add to heartbeat irregularity. Avoid.
Tobacco:	May add to heartbeat irregularity. Avoid.

TRIAZOLAM

BRAND NAMES

Apo-Triazo   Novo-Triolam
Halcion   Nu-Triazo

BASIC INFORMATION

Habit forming? Yes
Prescription needed? Yes
Available as generic? Yes
Drug class: Sedative-hypnotic agent

USES

- Treatment for insomnia (short term).
- Prevention or treatment of transient insomnia associated with sudden sleep schedule changes, such as travel across several time zones.

DOSAGE & USAGE INFORMATION

How to take:
Tablet—Swallow with liquid. If you can't swallow whole, crumble tablet and take with liquid or food.

When to take:
At the same time each day, according to instructions on prescription label. You should be in bed when you take your dose.

If you forget a dose:
Take as soon as you remember up to 2 hours late. If more than 2 hours, wait for next scheduled dose (don't double this dose).

Continued next column

OVERDOSE

SYMPTOMS:
Drowsiness, weakness, tremor, stupor, coma.
WHAT TO DO:
- **Dial 911 (emergency) or 0 (operator) for an ambulance or medical help. Then give first aid immediately.**
- **If patient is unconscious and not breathing, give mouth-to-mouth breathing. If there is no heartbeat, use cardiac massage and mouth-to-mouth breathing (CPR). Don't try to make patient vomit. If you can't get help quickly, take patient to nearest emergency facility.**
- **See emergency information at end of book.**

What drug does:
Affects limbic system of brain, the part that controls emotions.

Time lapse before drug works:
Within 30 minutes.

Don't take with:
Any prescription or nonprescription drugs without consulting your doctor or pharmacist.

POSSIBLE ADVERSE REACTIONS OR SIDE EFFECTS

SYMPTOMS	WHAT TO DO
Life-threatening:	
In case of overdose, see previous column.	
Common:	
Clumsiness, drowsiness, dizziness.	Continue. Call doctor when convenient.
Infrequent:	
• Amnesia, hallucinations, confusion, depression, irritability, rash, itch, vision changes, sore throat, fever, chills, dry mouth.	Discontinue. Call doctor right away.
• Constipation or diarrhea, nausea, vomiting, difficult urination, vivid dreams, behavior changes, abdominal pain, headache.	Continue. Call doctor when convenient.
Rare:	
• Slow heartbeat, breathing difficulty.	Discontinue. Seek emergency treatment.
• Mouth, throat ulcers; jaundice.	Discontinue. Call doctor right away.
• Decreased sex drive.	Continue. Call doctor when convenient.

WARNINGS & PRECAUTIONS

Don't take if:
- You are allergic to any benzodiazepine.
- You have myasthenia gravis.
- You are an active or recovering alcoholic.
- Patient is younger than 6 months.

Before you start, consult your doctor:
- If you have liver, kidney or lung disease.
- If you have diabetes, epilepsy or porphyria.
- If you have glaucoma.

Over age 60:
Adverse reactions and side effects may be more frequent and severe than in younger persons. You may need smaller doses for shorter periods of time. You may develop agitation, rage or a "hangover" effect.

Pregnancy:
Risk to unborn child outweighs drug benefits. Don't use. Risk category X (see page xxiii).

Breast-feeding:
Drug may pass into milk. Avoid drug or discontinue nursing until you finish medicine. Consult doctor for advice on maintaining milk supply.

Infants & children:
Not recommended.

Prolonged use:
May impair liver function.

Skin & sunlight:
No problems expected.

Driving, piloting or hazardous work:
Don't drive or pilot aircraft until you learn how medicine affects you. Don't work around dangerous machinery. Don't climb ladders or work in high places. Danger increases if you drink alcohol or take medicine affecting alertness and reflexes.

Discontinuing:
Don't discontinue without consulting doctor. Dose may require gradual reduction if you have taken drug for a long time. Doses of other drugs may also require adjustment.

Others:
- Hot weather, heavy exercise and profuse sweating may reduce excretion and cause overdose.
- Blood sugar may rise in diabetics, requiring insulin adjustment.
- Don't use for insomnia more than 4-7 days.
- Advise any doctor or dentist whom you consult that you take this medicine.
- Triazolam has a very short duration of action in the body.

POSSIBLE INTERACTION WITH OTHER DRUGS

GENERIC NAME OR DRUG CLASS	COMBINED EFFECT
Anticonvulsants*	Change in seizure frequency or severity.
Antidepressants*	Increased sedative effects of both drugs.
Antihistamines*	Increased sedative effects of both drugs.

Antihypertensives*	Excessively low blood pressure.
Central nervous system (CNS) depressants*, other	Increased central nervous system depression.
Cimetidine	Increased triazolam effect. May be dangerous.
Clozapine	Toxic effect on the central nervous system.
Contraceptives, oral*	Increased triazolam effect and toxicity.
Disulfiram	Increased triazolam effect and toxicity.
Erythromycins*	Increased triazolam effect and toxicity.
Isoniazid	Increased triazolam effect and toxicity.
Ketoconazole	Increased triazolam effect and toxicity.
Levodopa	Possible decreased levodopa effect and toxicity.
Molindone	Increased tranquilizer effect.
Monoamine oxidase (MAO) inhibitors*	Convulsions, deep sedation, rage.
Narcotics*	Increased sedative effects of both drugs.
Nefazodone	Increased effects of both drugs.

Continued on page 937

POSSIBLE INTERACTION WITH OTHER SUBSTANCES

INTERACTS WITH	COMBINED EFFECT
Alcohol:	Heavy sedation or amnesia. Avoid.
Beverages: Grapefruit juice	Increased triazolam effect.
Cocaine:	Decreased triazolam effect.
Foods:	None expected.
Marijuana:	Heavy sedation. Avoid.
Tobacco:	Decreased triazolam effect.

*See Glossary

TRILOSTANE

BRAND NAMES

Modrastane

BASIC INFORMATION

Habit forming? No
Prescription needed? Yes
Available as generic? No
Drug class: Antiadrenal

 USES

Temporary treatment of Cushing's syndrome until surgery on adrenals or radiation to pituitary gland can be performed.

 DOSAGE & USAGE INFORMATION

How to take:
Capsules—Swallow with liquid. If you can't swallow whole, open capsule and take with liquid or food. Instructions to take on empty stomach mean 1 hour before or 2 hours after eating.

When to take:
Follow doctor's instructions.

If you forget a dose:
Take as soon as you remember up to 2 hours late. If more than 2 hours, wait for next scheduled dose (don't double this dose).

What drug does:
Decreases function of the adrenal cortex.

Time lapse before drug works:
8 hours.

Don't take with:
Any other medicines (including over-the-counter drugs such as cough and cold medicines, laxatives, antacids, diet pills, caffeine, nose drops or vitamins) without consulting your doctor.

 OVERDOSE

SYMPTOMS:
None expected.
WHAT TO DO:
Overdose unlikely to threaten life. If person takes much larger amount than prescribed, call doctor, poison control center or hospital emergency room for instructions.

 POSSIBLE ADVERSE REACTIONS OR SIDE EFFECTS

SYMPTOMS	WHAT TO DO
Life-threatening: None expected.	
Common: Diarrhea, abdominal pain.	Discontinue. Call doctor right away.
Infrequent: Muscle ache, bloating, watery eyes, nausea, increased salivation, flushing, burning mouth or nose.	Continue. Call doctor when convenient.
Rare: Darkening skin, tiredness, appetite loss, depression, skin rash, vomiting.	Continue. Call doctor when convenient.

WARNINGS & PRECAUTIONS

Don't take if:
You know you are allergic to trilostane.

Before you start, consult your doctor:
- If you have an infection.
- If you will have surgery while taking.
- If you have a head injury.
- If you have kidney disease.

Over age 60:
Adverse reactions and side effects may be more frequent and severe than in younger persons. You may need smaller doses for shorter periods of time.

Pregnancy:
Risk to unborn child outweighs drug benefits. Don't use. Risk category X (see page xxiii).

Breast-feeding:
Safety not established. Consult doctor.

Infants & children:
Effect not documented. Consult your pediatrician.

Prolonged use:
- Not intended for prolonged use.
- Talk to your doctor about the need for follow-up medical examinations or laboratory studies to check serum electrolytes and urinary 17 - hydroxycorticosteroid.

Skin & sunlight:
No problems expected.

Driving, piloting or hazardous work:
Avoid if you feel confused, drowsy or dizzy.

Discontinuing:
No special problems expected.

Others:
- Advise any doctor or dentist whom you consult that you take this medicine.
- May affect results in some medical tests.

POSSIBLE INTERACTION WITH OTHER DRUGS

GENERIC NAME OR DRUG CLASS	COMBINED EFFECT
Aminoglutethimide	Too much decrease in adrenal function.
Mitotane	Too much decrease in adrenal function.

POSSIBLE INTERACTION WITH OTHER SUBSTANCES

INTERACTS WITH	COMBINED EFFECT
Alcohol:	No special problems expected.
Beverages:	No special problems expected.
Cocaine:	No special problems expected.
Foods:	No special problems expected.
Marijuana:	No special problems expected.
Tobacco:	No special problems expected.

TRIMETHOBENZAMIDE

BRAND NAMES

Arrestin	T-Gen
Benzacot	Ticon
Bio-Gan	Tigan
Stemetic	Tiject-20
Tebamide	Triban
Tegamide	Tribenzagan

BASIC INFORMATION

Habit forming? No
Prescription needed? Yes
Available as generic? Yes
Drug class: Antiemetic

USES

Reduces nausea and vomiting.

DOSAGE & USAGE INFORMATION

How to take:
* Capsule—Swallow with liquid. If you can't swallow whole, open capsule and take with liquid or food.
* Suppositories—Remove wrapper and moisten suppository with water. Gently insert larger end into rectum. Push well into rectum with finger.

When to take:
When needed, no more often than label directs.

If you forget a dose:
Take when you remember. Wait as long as label directs for next dose.

Continued next column

OVERDOSE

SYMPTOMS:
Confusion, convulsions, coma.
WHAT TO DO:
* **Dial 911 (emergency) or 0 (operator) for an ambulance or medical help. Then give first aid immediately.**
* **If patient is unconscious and not breathing, give mouth-to-mouth breathing. If there is no heartbeat, use cardiac massage and mouth-to-mouth breathing (CPR). Don't try to make patient vomit. If you can't get help quickly, take patient to nearest emergency facility.**
* **See emergency information on inside covers.**

What drug does:
Exact mechanism unknown. Possibly blocks nerve impulses to brain's vomiting centers.

Time lapse before drug works:
20 to 40 minutes.

Don't take with:
Any other prescription or nonprescription drugs without consulting doctor.

POSSIBLE ADVERSE REACTIONS OR SIDE EFFECTS

SYMPTOMS	WHAT TO DO
Life-threatening: In case of overdose, see previous column.	
Common: Drowsiness.	Continue. Call doctor when convenient.
Infrequent: Rash, blurred vision, diarrhea, dizziness, headache, muscle cramps, unusual tiredness.	Discontinue. Call doctor right away.
Rare: Seizures, tremor, depression, sore throat, fever, repeated vomiting, back pain, yellow skin or eyes, body spasm (head and heels bent backward and body bowed forward).	Discontinue. Call doctor right away.

WARNINGS & PRECAUTIONS

Don't take if:
* You are allergic to trimethobenzamide.
* You are allergic to local anesthetics and have suppository form.

Before you start, consult your doctor:
If you have reacted badly to antihistamines.

Over age 60:
More susceptible to low blood pressure and sedative effects of this drug.

Pregnancy:
Decide with your doctor if drug benefits justify risk to unborn child. Risk category C (see page xxiii).

Breast-feeding:
Effect unknown. Avoid if possible. Consult doctor.

Infants & children:
- Injectable form not recommended.
- Avoid during viral infections. Drug may contribute to Reye's syndrome.

Prolonged use:
- Damages blood cell production of bone marrow.
- Causes Parkinson's-like symptoms of tremors, rigidity.

Skin & sunlight:
No special problems expected.

Driving, piloting or hazardous work:
- Use disqualifies you for piloting aircraft.
- Don't drive until you learn how medicine affects you. Don't work around dangerous machinery. Don't climb ladders or work in high places. Danger increases if you drink alcohol or take medicine affecting alertness and reflexes, such as antihistamines, tranquilizers, sedatives, pain medicine, narcotics and mind-altering drugs.

Discontinuing:
May be unnecessary to finish medicine. Follow doctor's instructions.

Others:
No problems expected.

POSSIBLE INTERACTION WITH OTHER DRUGS

GENERIC NAME OR DRUG CLASS	COMBINED EFFECT
Antidepressants*	Increased sedative effect.
Antihistamines*	Increased sedative effect.
Barbiturates*	Increased effect of both drugs.
Belladonna	Increased effect of both drugs.
Cholinergics*	Increased effect of both drugs.
Clozapine	Toxic effect on the central nervous system.
Ethinamate	Dangerous increased effects of ethinamate. Avoid combining.
Fluoxetine	Increased depressant effects of both drugs.
Guanfacine	May increase depressant effects of either medicine.
Leucovorin	High alcohol content of leucovorin may cause adverse effects.
Methyprylon	May increase sedative effect to dangerous level. Avoid.
Mind-altering drugs*	Increased effect of mind-altering drug.
Nabilone	Greater depression of central nervous system.
Narcotics*	Increased sedative effect.
Ototoxic medications*	May mask the symptoms of ototoxicity.
Phenothiazines*	Increased effect of both drugs.
Sedatives*	Increased sedative effect.
Sertraline	Increased depressive effects of both drugs.
Sleep inducers*	Increased effect of sleep inducer.
Tranquilizers*	Increased sedative effect.

POSSIBLE INTERACTION WITH OTHER SUBSTANCES

INTERACTS WITH	COMBINED EFFECT
Alcohol:	Oversedation. Avoid.
Beverages:	None expected.
Cocaine:	None expected.
Foods:	None expected.
Marijuana:	Increased antinausea effect.
Tobacco:	None expected.

TRIMETHOPRIM

BRAND NAMES

Apo-Sulfatrim
Apo-Sulfatrim DS
Bactrim
Bactrim DS
Bethaprim
Cotrim
Cotrim DS
Novotrimel
Novotrimel DS
Nu-Cotrimox
Nu-Cotrimox DS
Proloprim
Protrin
Roubac
Septra
Septra DS
SMZ-TMP

Sulfamethoprim
Sulfamethoprim DS
Sulfaprim
Sulfaprim DS
Sulfatrim
Sulfatrim DS
Sulfoxaprim
Sulfoxaprim DS
Sulmeprim
Triazole
Triazole DS
Trimeth-Sulfa
Trimpex
Trisulfam
Uroplus DS
Uroplus SS

BASIC INFORMATION

Habit forming? No
Prescription needed? Yes
Available as generic? Yes
Drug class: Antimicrobial (antibacterial)

USES

- Treats urinary tract infections susceptible to trimethoprim.
- Helps prevent recurrent urinary tract infections if taken once a day.
- Treats pneumocystis carinii pneumonia.

DOSAGE & USAGE INFORMATION

How to take:
- Tablet—Swallow with liquid or food to lessen stomach irritation. If can't swallow whole, crush or crumble tablet and take with food or liquid.
- Oral suspension (in combination with sulfamethoxazole)—Follow directions on prescription label.

Continued next column

OVERDOSE

SYMPTOMS:
Nausea, vomiting, diarrhea.
WHAT TO DO:
Overdose unlikely to threaten life. If person takes much larger amount than prescribed, call doctor, poison control center or hospital emergency room for instructions.

When to take:
Space doses evenly in 24 hours to keep constant amount in urine.

If you forget a dose:
Take as soon as possible. Wait 5 to 6 hours before next dose. Then return to regular schedule.

What drug does:
Stops harmful bacterial germs from multiplying. Will not kill viruses.

Time lapse before drug works:
2 to 5 days.

Don't take with:
Any other medicine without consulting your doctor or pharmacist.

POSSIBLE ADVERSE REACTIONS OR SIDE EFFECTS

SYMPTOMS	WHAT TO DO
Life-threatening: None expected.	
Common: None expected.	
Infrequent: Diarrhea, nausea, vomiting, stomach cramps, headache.	Continue. Call doctor when convenient.
Rare: Blue fingernails, lips and skin; difficult breathing; sore throat; fever; anemia; jaundice; unusual bleeding or bruising; unusual tiredness or weakness; skin changes (rash, itch, redness, blisters, peeling or loosening); aching joints or muscles.	Discontinue. Call doctor right away.

WARNINGS & PRECAUTIONS

Don't take if:
- You are allergic to trimethoprim or any sulfa drug*.
- You are anemic due to folic acid deficiency.

Before you start, consult your doctor:
If you have had liver or kidney disease.

Over age 60:
- Reduced liver and kidney function may require reduced dose.
- More likely to have severe anal and genital itch.
- Increased susceptibility to anemia.

Pregnancy:
Decide with your doctor whether drug benefits justify risk to unborn child. Risk category C (see page xxiii).

Breast-feeding:
No proven harm to unborn child. Avoid if possible. Consult doctor.

Infants & children:
Use under medical supervision only.

Prolonged use:
- Anemia.
- Talk to your doctor about the need for follow-up medical examinations or laboratory studies to check complete blood counts (white blood cell count, platelet count, red blood cell count, hemoglobin, hematocrit).

Skin & sunlight:
May cause rash or intensify sunburn in areas exposed to sun or ultraviolet light (photosensitivity reaction). Avoid overexposure. Notify doctor if reaction occurs.

Driving, piloting or hazardous work:
No problems expected.

Discontinuing:
Don't discontinue without doctor's advice until you complete prescribed dose, even though symptoms diminish or disappear.

Others:
No problems expected.

POSSIBLE INTERACTION WITH OTHER DRUGS

GENERIC NAME OR DRUG CLASS	COMBINED EFFECT
Anticonvulsants*	Increased risk of anemia.
Bone marrow depressants*	Increased possibility of bone marrow supression.
Folate antagonists*, other	Increased risk of anemia.
Metformin	Increased metformin effect.
Phenytoin	Increased phenytoin effect.

POSSIBLE INTERACTION WITH OTHER SUBSTANCES

INTERACTS WITH	COMBINED EFFECT
Alcohol:	Increased alcohol effect with Bactrim or Septra.
Beverages:	None expected.
Cocaine:	No proven problems.
Foods:	None expected.
Marijuana:	None expected.
Tobacco:	None expected.

*See Glossary

TRIPTANS

GENERIC AND BRAND NAMES

NARATRIPTAN
Amerge
RIZATRIPTAN
Maxalt

SUMATRIPTAN
Imitrex
ZOLMITRIPTAN
Zomig

BASIC INFORMATION

Habit forming? No
Prescription needed? Yes
Available as generic? No
Drug class: Antimigraine

USES

- Treatment for acute migraine headaches not relieved by other medications (aspirin, acetaminophen and other nonsteroidal anti-inflammatory drugs). Does not prevent migraines.
- Treatment for cluster headaches.

DOSAGE & USAGE INFORMATION

How to take:
- Injection (sumatriptan—self-administered)— Inject under the skin (subcutaneous) of the outer thigh or outer upper arm. Follow your doctor's instructions and written package instructions for proper injection technique and method for disposal of the cartridges.
- Tablets—Swallow whole with liquid. Do not crush, break or chew tablet.
- Wafers (rizatriptan)—Place on tongue to dissolve and be swallowed with saliva.
- Nasal spray (sumatriptan)—One spray into one nostril as a single dose.

When to take:
- At the first sign of a migraine (aura or pain). After you administer, lie down in a quiet, dark room to increase effectiveness of drug.

Continued next column

OVERDOSE

SYMPTOMS:
Convulsions, tremor, swelling of arms and legs, breathing difficulty, chest pain, paralysis, skin and hair loss, scab formation at injection site.
WHAT TO DO:
- **Dial 911 (emergency) or 0 (operator) for an ambulance or medical help. Then give first aid immediately.**
- **See emergency information on inside covers.**

- An additional dose may be helpful if the migraine returns. Do not exceed the prescribed quantity or frequency. Do not use additional dose if first dose does not bring substantial relief.
- Zolmitriptan tablets should not be taken until pain actually begins.
- For cluster headache, follow doctor's directions.

If you forget a dose:
Triptans are not taken on a routine schedule. They should be taken at the onset of your migraine.

What drug does:
Helps relieve headache pain and associated symptoms of migraine (nausea, vomiting, sensitivity to light and sound). It helps constrict dilated blood vessels that may contribute to development of migraines.

Time lapse before drug works:
- Oral dosage (tablets/wafers)—within 30 minutes.
- Injection—usually within 10 minutes for headache pain and within 20 minutes for associated nausea, vomiting and sensitivity to light and sound.

Don't take with:
- Ergotamine-containing medicines. Delay 24 hours.
- Any other medication without consulting your doctor or pharmacist.

POSSIBLE ADVERSE REACTIONS OR SIDE EFFECTS

SYMPTOMS	WHAT TO DO
Life-threatening: In case of overdose, see previous column.	
Common: Burning, pain, or redness at sumatriptan injection site; nausea or vomiting (may be from migraine or from drug); drowsiness or dizziness.	May readminister. Call doctor when convenient.
Infrequent: Sensation of burning, warmth, numbness, cold or tingling; discomfort of jaw, mouth, throat, nose or sinuses; dizziness; drowsiness; flushing; light-headedness; muscle aches, cramps, stiffness or weakness; anxiety; tiredness; vision changes; general feeling of illness.	May readminister. Call doctor when convenient.

Rare:
Pain, pressure or tightness in the chest; difficulty swallowing; irregular heartbeat.

Discontinue. Seek emergency help.

WARNINGS & PRECAUTIONS

Don't take if:
- You are allergic to any triptans.
- You have angina pectoris, a history of myocardial infarction or myocardial ischemia, Prinzmetal's angina, uncontrolled hypertension (high blood pressure).

Before you start, consult your doctor:
- If you have heart rhythm problems or coronary artery disease.
- If you have had a cerebrovascular accident (stroke).
- If you have liver or kidney disease.
- If you have controlled hypertension (high blood pressure).

Over age 60:
No problems expected.

Pregnancy:
Decide with your doctor whether drug benefits justify risk to unborn child. Risk category C (see page xxiii).

Breast-feeding:
Unknown effects. Decide with your doctor whether drug benefits justify possible risk.

Infants & children:
Not recommended for patients under age 18.

Prolonged use:
Long-term effects unknown. As a precaution, do not use sumatriptan more often than every 5-7 days or as directed by your doctor.

Skin & sunlight:
No special problems expected.

Driving, piloting or hazardous work:
Avoid if you feel drowsy or dizzy. Otherwise no problems expected.

Discontinuing:
No problems expected. Talk to your doctor if you have plans to discontinue use of drug.

Others:
- Advise any doctor or dentist whom you consult that you take this medicine.
- May affect results in some medical tests (rare).
- Follow your doctor's recommendation of any additional treatment for prevention of migraines.
- Sensitivity to light is a symptom of migraine and is not drug-related.

POSSIBLE INTERACTION WITH OTHER DRUGS

GENERIC NAME OR DRUG CLASS	COMBINED EFFECT
Antidepressants*	Adverse effects unknown. Avoid.
Dihydroergotamine	Increased vaso-constriction. Delay 24 hours between drugs.
Ergotamine	Increased vaso-constriction. Delay 24 hours between drugs.
Furazolidone	Adverse effects unknown. Avoid.
Lithium	Adverse effects unknown. Avoid.
Monoamine oxidase (MAO) inhibitors*	Adverse effects unknown. Avoid.
Procarbazine	Adverse effects unknown. Avoid.
Selegiline	Adverse effects unknown. Avoid.

POSSIBLE INTERACTION WITH OTHER SUBSTANCES

INTERACTS WITH	COMBINED EFFECT
Alcohol:	No interaction known, but alcohol aggravates migraines. Avoid.
Beverages:	None expected.
Cocaine:	None expected.
Foods:	None expected.
Marijuana:	None expected.
Tobacco:	None expected.

*See Glossary

TROGLITAZONE

BRAND NAMES

Rezulin

BASIC INFORMATION

Habit forming? No
Prescription needed? Yes
Available as generic? No
Drug class: Antidiabetic

 ## USES

Treatment for patients with type II non-insulin-dependent diabetes mellitus (NIDDM). Troglitazone may be used alone, with insulin or with other antidiabetic drugs.

 ## DOSAGE & USAGE INFORMATION

How to take:
Tablet, film-coated—Swallow with liquid. Take at mealtime. If you can't swallow whole, crumble tablet and take with liquid or food.

When to take:
Once a day or as directed by doctor. Dosage may be increased after 2 to 4 weeks.

If you forget a dose:
Wait for your next meal that same day and take dose then. If you forget until the next day, take that day's regular dose on schedule (don't double this dose).

Continued next column

 ## OVERDOSE

SYMPTOMS:
Symptoms of hypoglycemia—stomach pain, anxious feeling, cold sweats, chills, confusion, convulsions, cool pale skin, excessive hunger, nausea or vomiting, rapid heartbeat, nervousness, shakiness, unsteady walk, unusual weakness or tiredness, vision changes, unconsciousness.
WHAT TO DO:
- For mild low blood sugar symptoms, drink or eat something containing sugar right away.
- For more severe symptoms, dial 911 (emergency) or 0 (operator) for an ambulance or medical help. Then give first aid immediately.
- See emergency information on inside covers.

What drug does:
Lowers blood glucose by improving target cell response to insulin. However, troglitazone does not cure diabetes.

Time lapse before drug works:
May take several weeks for full effectiveness.

Don't take with:
Any other prescription or nonprescription drug without consulting your doctor or pharmacist. All possible drug interactions have not been studied.

 ## POSSIBLE ADVERSE REACTIONS OR SIDE EFFECTS

SYMPTOMS	WHAT TO DO
Life-threatening:	
In case of overdose or low blood sugar, see previous column.	
Common:	
• Pain in back or other body part, infection.	Continue. Call doctor right away.
• Headache, dizziness, nausea, unusual tiredness or weakness.	Continue. Call doctor when convenient.
Infrequent:	
Sore throat, runny nose, diarrhea.	Continue. Call doctor when convenient.
Rare:	
• Severe low blood sugar (see symptoms under Overdose).	Discontinue. Call doctor right away or seek emergency help.
• Liver problems including jaundice (yellow skin and eyes) and hepatitis that could lead to liver transplantation or death.	Discontinue. Call doctor right away.

 ## WARNINGS & PRECAUTIONS

Don't take if:
You are allergic to troglitazone.

Before you start, consult your doctor:
- If you have liver disease or any heart disorder.
- If you have any chronic health problem.
- If you have a history of acid in the blood (metabolic acidosis or ketoacidosis).
- If you are allergic to any medication, food or other substance.

Over age 60:
No special problems expected.

Pregnancy:
Decide with your doctor if drug benefits justify risks to unborn child. Risk category B (see page xxiii).

Breast-feeding:
It is unknown if drug passes into milk. It is not recommended for use in nursing mothers.

Infants & children:
Safety and efficacy have not been established. Use only under close medical supervision.

Prolonged use:
- Schedule regular doctor visits to determine if the drug is continuing to be effective in controlling the diabetes and to check for any liver function problems.
- You will most likely require an antidiabetic medicine for the rest of your life.
- You will need to test your blood glucose levels several times a day, or for some, once to several times a week.

Skin & sunlight:
No special problems expected.

Driving, piloting or hazardous work:
No special problems expected.

Discontinuing:
Don't discontinue without consulting your doctor even if you feel well. You can have diabetes without feeling any symptoms. Untreated diabetes can cause serious problems.

Others:
- Use of troglitazone may lead to liver problems. Currently, it is necessary to get liver function studies prior to starting the drug, then every month for 6 months, then every other month for 6 months and periodically thereafter while on the drug.
- Advise any doctor or dentist whom you consult that you take this medicine. It may interfere with the accuracy of some medical tests.
- May cause ovulation to resume in some women with ovarian disorders. Discuss the need for nonhormonal contraception with your doctor.
- Follow any special diet your doctor may prescribe. It can help control diabetes.
- Consult doctor if you become ill with vomiting or diarrhea while taking this drug.
- Use caution when exercising. Ask your doctor about an appropriate exercise program.
- Wear medical identification stating that you have diabetes and take this medication.
- Learn to recognize the symptoms of low blood sugar. You and your family need to know what to do if these symptoms occur.
- Have a glucagon kit and syringe in the event severe low blood sugar occurs.

- High blood sugar (hyperglycemia) may occur with diabetes. Ask your doctor about symptoms to watch for and treatment steps to take.
- Educate yourself about diabetes.

 POSSIBLE INTERACTION WITH OTHER DRUGS

GENERIC NAME OR DRUG CLASS	COMBINED EFFECT
Antidiabetic agents, sulfonylurea	May decrease fasting plasma glucose concentrations.
Cholestyramine	Decreased effect of troglitazone. Avoid.
Contraceptives, oral	Decreased effect of contraceptive.
Cyclosporine	Decreased effect of cyclosporine.
HMG-CoA reductase inhibitors	Decreased effect of HMG-CoA reductase inhibitor.
Tacrolimus	Decreased effect of tacrolimus.

 POSSIBLE INTERACTION WITH OTHER SUBSTANCES

INTERACTS WITH	COMBINED EFFECT
Alcohol:	No special problems. Avoid excessive amounts of alcohol.
Beverages:	No special problems.
Cocaine:	No special problems. Best to avoid.
Foods:	No special problems.
Marijuana:	No special problems. Best to avoid.
Tobacco:	People with diabetes should not smoke.

URSODIOL

BRAND NAMES

Actigall   Ursofalk

BASIC INFORMATION

Habit forming? No
Prescription needed? Yes
Available as generic? No
Drug class: Anticholelithic

 ## USES

- Dissolves cholesterol gallstones in selected patients who either can't tolerate surgery or don't require surgery for other reasons. Not used when surgery is clearly indicated.
- Prevention of gallstone formation during rapid weight loss.
- Treatment for primary biliary cirrhosis.

 ## DOSAGE & USAGE INFORMATION

How to take:
Capsules—Swallow with liquid or food to lessen stomach irritation. If you can't swallow whole, open capsule and take with liquid or food.

When to take:
With meals, 2 or 3 times a day according to your doctor's instructions.

If you forget a dose:
Take as soon as you remember up to 2 hours late. If more than 2 hours, wait for next scheduled time. Don't double this dose.

What drug does:
Decreases secretion of cholesterol into bile by suppressing production and secretion of cholesterol by the liver. Ursodiol will not help gallstone problems unless the gallstones are made of cholesterol. It works best when the stones are small.

Time lapse before drug works:
Unpredictable. Varies among patients.

Continued next column

 ## OVERDOSE

SYMPTOMS:
Severe diarrhea.
WHAT TO DO:
Overdose not expected to threaten life. If person takes much larger amount than prescribed, call doctor, poison control center or hospital emergency room for instructions.

Don't take with:
Any other medicine without consulting your doctor or pharmacist.

 ## POSSIBLE ADVERSE REACTIONS OR SIDE EFFECTS

SYMPTOMS	WHAT TO DO
Life-threatening: None expected.	
Common: None expected.	
Infrequent: None expected.	
Rare: Diarrhea.	Continue. Call doctor when convenient.

WARNINGS & PRECAUTIONS

Don't take if:
You can't tolerate other bile acids.

Before you start, consult your doctor:
- If you have complications of gallstones, such as infection or obstruction of the bile ducts.
- If you have had pancreatitis.
- If you have had chronically impaired liver function.
- If you take any other medicines for any reason.

Over age 60:
No special problems expected.

Pregnancy:
Consult doctor. Risk category B (see page xxiii).

Breast-feeding:
Unknown, but no documented problems. Consult doctor.

Infants & children:
Not recommended. Adequate studies have not been performed.

Prolonged use:
- No special problems expected.
- Talk to your doctor about the need for follow-up medical examinations or laboratory studies to check kidney function.

Skin & sunlight:
No problems expected.

Driving, piloting or hazardous work:
Don't pilot aircraft until you learn how medicine affects you. Don't work around dangerous machinery. Don't climb ladders or work in high places. Danger increases if you drink alcohol or take medicine affecting alertness and reflexes, such as antihistamines, tranquilizers, sedatives, pain medicine, narcotics and mind-altering drugs.

Discontinuing:
Don't discontinue without consulting doctor.

Others:
Plan regular visits to your doctor while you take ursodiol. Have ultrasound and liver function studies done at appropriate intervals. Liver damage is unlikely, but theoretically could happen.

POSSIBLE INTERACTION WITH OTHER DRUGS

GENERIC NAME OR DRUG CLASS	COMBINED EFFECT
Antacids* (aluminum-containing)	Decreased absorption of ursodiol.
Cholestyramine	Decreased absorption of ursodiol.
Clofibrate	Decreased effect of ursodiol.
Colestipol	Decreased absorption of ursodiol.
Estrogens*	Decreased effect of ursodiol.
Progestins	Decreased effect of ursodiol.

POSSIBLE INTERACTION WITH OTHER SUBSTANCES

INTERACTS WITH	COMBINED EFFECT
Alcohol:	None expected, unless you have impaired liver function from alcohol abuse.
Beverages:	None expected.
Cocaine:	None expected.
Foods:	None expected.
Marijuana:	None expected.
Tobacco:	None reported. However, tobacco may possibly impair intestinal absorption from the intestinal tract. Better to avoid.

*See Glossary

VALPROIC ACID

GENERIC AND BRAND NAMES

Depakene   Myproic Acid

BASIC INFORMATION

Habit forming? No
Prescription needed? Yes
Available as generic? Yes
Drug class: Anticonvulsant

USES

- Treatment of various types of epilepsy.
- Treatment for bipolar (manic-depressive) disorder.

DOSAGE & USAGE INFORMATION

How to take:
Capsule or syrup—Swallow with liquid or food to lessen stomach irritation.

When to take:
Once a day.

If you forget a dose:
Take as soon as you remember. Don't ever double dose.

What drug does:
Increases concentration of gamma aminobutyric acid, which inhibits nerve transmission in parts of brain.

Time lapse before drug works:
1 to 4 hours, but full effect may take weeks.

Don't take with:
Any other medicine without consulting your doctor or pharmacist.

OVERDOSE

SYMPTOMS:
Coma
WHAT TO DO:
- Dial 911 (emergency) or 0 (operator) for an ambulance or medical help. Then give first aid immediately.
- If patient is unconscious and not breathing, give mouth-to-mouth breathing. If there is no heartbeat, use cardiac massage and mouth-to-mouth breathing (CPR). Don't try to make patient vomit. If you can't get help quickly, take patient to nearest emergency facility.
- See emergency information at end of book.

POSSIBLE ADVERSE REACTIONS OR SIDE EFFECTS

SYMPTOMS	WHAT TO DO
Life-threatening: In case of overdose, see previous column.	
Common: Loss of appetite, indigestion, nausea, vomiting, abdominal cramps, diarrhea, tremor, unusual weight gain or loss, menstrual changes in girls.	Continue. Call doctor when convenient.
Infrequent: Clumsiness, or unsteadiness, constipation, skin rash, dizziness, drowsiness, unusual excitement or irritability.	Continue. Call doctor when convenient.
Rare: Mood or behavior changes; continued nausea, vomiting and appetite loss; increase in number of seizures; swelling of face, feet or legs; yellow skin or eyes; tiredness or weakness; back-and-forth eye movements (nystagmus); seeing double or seeing spots; severe stomach cramps; unusual bleeding or bruising.	Continue, but call doctor right away.

WARNINGS & PRECAUTIONS

Don't take if:
You are allergic to valproic acid.

Before you start, consult your doctor:
- If you have blood, kidney or liver disease.
- If you will have surgery within 2 months, including dental surgery, requiring general or spinal anesthesia.

Over age 60:
Adverse reactions and side effects may be more frequent and severe than in younger persons.

Pregnancy:
Risk to unborn child exists. Use only if benefits of drug greatly exceed fetal risk. Risk category D (see page xxiii).

Breast-feeding:
Drug passes into milk. Avoid drug or discontinue nursing until you finish medicine. Consult doctor for advice on maintaining milk supply.

Infants & children:
Use under close medical supervision only.

Prolonged use:
Request periodic blood tests, liver and kidney function tests. These tests are necessary for safe and effective use.

Skin & sunlight:
No problems expected.

Driving, piloting or hazardous work:
Don't drive or pilot aircraft until you learn how medicine affects you. Don't work around dangerous machinery. Don't climb ladders or work in high places. Danger increases if you drink alcohol or take medicine affecting alertness and reflexes, such as antihistamines, tranquilizers, sedatives, pain medicine, narcotics and mind-altering drugs.

Discontinuing:
Don't discontinue without consulting doctor. Dose may require gradual reduction if you have taken drug for a long time. Doses of other drugs may also require adjustment.

Others:
Advise any doctor or dentist whom you consult that you take this drug.

POSSIBLE INTERACTION WITH OTHER DRUGS

GENERIC NAME OR DRUG CLASS	COMBINED EFFECT
Anticoagulants*, oral	Increased chance of bleeding.
Anticonvulsants*	Unpredictable. May require increase or decrease in dosage of valproic acid or other anticonvulsant.
Anti-inflammatory drugs, nonsteroidal* (NSAIDs)	Increased risk of bleeding problems.
Antivirals, HIV/AIDS*	Increased risk of pancreatitis.
Carbamazepine	Decreased valproic acid effect.
Central nervous system (CNS) depressants*	Increased sedative effect.
Clonazepam	May prolong seizure.

Felbamate	Increased side effects and adverse reactions of valproic acid.
Hepatotoxics*	Increased risk of liver toxicity.
Lamotrigine	Increased lamotrigine effect. Possibly decrease effect valproic acid.
Levocarnitine	Decreased levocarnitine. Patients taking valproic acid may need to take the supplement levocarnitine.
Phenobarbital	Increased phenobarbital levels; possibly toxic or beneficial effect.
Phenytoin	Unpredictable. Dose may require adjustment.
Primidone	Increased primidone effect. Possible toxicity.
Salicylates*	Increased effect of valproic acid.
Sertraline	Increased depressive effects of both drugs.
Sodium benzoate & sodium phenylacetate	May reduce effect of sodium benzoate & sodium phenylacetate.

Continued on page 937

POSSIBLE INTERACTION WITH OTHER SUBSTANCES

INTERACTS WITH	COMBINED EFFECT
Alcohol:	Deep sedation. Avoid.
Beverages:	No problems expected.
Cocaine:	Increased brain sensitivity. Avoid.
Foods:	No problems expected.
Marijuana:	Increased brain sensitivity. Avoid.
Tobacco:	Decreased valproic acid effect.

*See Glossary

VANCOMYCIN

BRAND NAMES

Vancocin

BASIC INFORMATION

Habit forming? No
Prescription needed? Yes
Available as generic? Yes
Drug class: Antibacterial

 ## USES

- Treats colitis when caused by *clostridium* infections.
- Treats some forms of severe diarrhea.

 ## DOSAGE & USAGE INFORMATION

How to take:
- Capsules—Swallow with liquid. If you can't swallow whole, open capsule and take with liquid or food. Instructions to take on empty stomach mean 1 hour before or 2 hours after eating.
- Oral solution—Use the calibrated measuring device. Swallow with other liquid to prevent nausea.
- There is also an injectable form. This information applies to the oral form only.

When to take:
According to doctor's instructions. Usually every 6 hours.

If you forget a dose:
Take as soon as you remember up to 2 hours late. If more than 2 hours, wait for next scheduled dose (don't double this dose).

What drug does:
Kills bacterial cells.

Time lapse before drug works:
None. Works right away. This medicine is not absorbed to a great extent through the intestinal tract.

Continued next column

 ## OVERDOSE

SYMPTOMS:
None expected.
WHAT TO DO:
Overdose unlikely to threaten life. If person takes much larger amount than prescribed, call doctor, poison control center or hospital emergency room for instructions.

Don't take with:
Any other medicines (including over-the-counter drugs such as cough and cold medicines, laxatives, antacids, diet pills, caffeine, nose drops or vitamins) without consulting your doctor.

 ## POSSIBLE ADVERSE REACTIONS OR SIDE EFFECTS

SYMPTOMS	WHAT TO DO
Life-threatening: None expected.	
Common: Bitter taste.	Continue. Tell doctor at next visit.
Infrequent: Nausea or vomiting.	Continue. Call doctor when convenient.
Rare: Hearing loss, ears ringing or buzzing.	Discontinue. Call doctor right away.

WARNINGS & PRECAUTIONS

Don't take if:
You are allergic to vancomycin.

Before you start, consult your doctor:
- If you have hearing problems.
- If you have severe kidney disease.
- If you have intestinal obstruction.

Over age 60:
Adverse reactions and side effects may be more frequent and severe than in younger persons. You may need smaller doses for shorter periods of time.

Pregnancy:
Consult doctor. Risk category B (see page xxiii).

Breast-feeding:
No special problems expected. Consult doctor.

Infants & children:
No special problems expected.

Prolonged use:
Talk to your doctor about the need for follow-up medical examinations or laboratory studies to check hearing acuity, kidney function, vancomycin serum concentration and urinalyses.

Skin & sunlight:
No problems expected.

Driving, piloting or hazardous work:
No problems expected.

Discontinuing:
No special problems expected.

Others:
- Advise any doctor or dentist whom you consult that you take this medicine.
- May affect results in some medical tests.

POSSIBLE INTERACTION WITH OTHER DRUGS

GENERIC NAME OR DRUG CLASS	COMBINED EFFECT
Cholestyramine	Decreased therapeutic effect of vancomycin.
Colestipol	Decreased therapeutic effect of vancomycin.
Metformin	Increased metformin effect.
Nephrotoxics*	Increased risk of liver toxicity.

POSSIBLE INTERACTION WITH OTHER SUBSTANCES

INTERACTS WITH	COMBINED EFFECT
Alcohol:	No special problems expected.
Beverages:	No special problems expected.
Cocaine:	No special problems expected.
Foods:	No special problems expected.
Marijuana:	No special problems expected.
Tobacco:	No special problems expected.

VENLAFAXINE

BRAND NAMES

Effexor

BASIC INFORMATION

Habit forming? Not known
Prescription needed? Yes
Available as generic? No
Drug class: Antidepressant (bicyclic)

 ## USES

Treats mental depression.

 ## DOSAGE & USAGE INFORMATION

How to use:
- Tablet—Swallow with liquid and take with food to lessen stomach irritation.
- Extended-release capsule—Swallow with liquid and take with food to lessen stomach irritation. Do not open, crush or chew capsule.

When to use:
At the same times each day (usually with meals or with a snack).

If you forget a dose:
Take as soon as you remember up to 2 hours late. If more than 2 hours, wait for the next scheduled dose (don't double this dose).

What drug does:
Increases the amount of certain chemicals in the brain that are required for the transmission of messages between nerve cells.

Time lapse before drug works:
Begins in 1 to 3 weeks, but may take 4 to 6 weeks for maximum benefit.

Don't take with:
Any other medication without consulting your doctor or pharmacist.

 ## OVERDOSE

SYMPTOMS:
May cause no symptoms, or there may be extreme drowsiness, convulsions or rapid heartbeat.
WHAT TO DO:
- **Dial 911 (emergency) or 0 (operator) for an ambulance or medical help. Then give first aid immediately.**
- **See emergency information at end of book.**

 ## POSSIBLE ADVERSE REACTIONS OR SIDE EFFECTS

SYMPTOMS	WHAT TO DO
Life-threatening:	
In case of overdose, see previous column.	
Common:	
• Fast heartbeat, blurred vision, increased blood pressure.	Discontinue. Call doctor right away.
• Stomach pain, gas, insomnia or drowsiness, dizziness, decreased sexual drive, impotence, nausea or vomiting, headache, diarrhea or constipation, dryness of mouth, skin flushing, rash, loss of appetite, unusual tiredness, weakness, strange dreams, sweating, tremors, nervousness, headache.	Continue. Call doctor when convenient.
Infrequent:	
• Lightheadedness or faintness when arising from a sitting or lying position, mood or behavior changes, mental changes, difficulty urinating.	Continue. Call doctor when convenient.
• Weight loss or gain, changes in taste, ringing in ears.	Continue. Tell doctor at next visit.
Rare:	
Seizures.	Discontinue. Seek emergency help.

WARNINGS & PRECAUTIONS

Don't take if:
You are allergic to venlafaxine.

Before you start, consult your doctor:
- If you have liver or kidney disease.
- If you have high blood pressure.
- If you have thoughts about suicide.
- If you are allergic to any other medications.
- If you have a history of seizures.

Over age 60:
Adverse reactions and side effects may be more severe than in younger persons.

Pregnancy:
Decide with your doctor if drug benefits justify any possible risk to unborn child. Risk category C (see page xxiii).

Breast-feeding:
It is unknown if drug passes into milk. Avoid nursing until you finish medicine. Consult doctor for advice on maintaining milk supply.

Infants & children:
Safety in children under age 18 has not been established. Use only under close medical supervision.

Prolonged use:
Consult with your doctor on a regular basis while taking this drug to check your progress, to monitor your blood pressure and to determine the need for continued treatment.

Skin & sunlight:
No special problems expected.

Driving, piloting or hazardous work:
Don't drive or pilot aircraft until you learn how medicine affects you. Don't work around dangerous machinery. Don't climb ladders or work in high places. Danger increases if you drink alcohol or take medicine affecting alertness and reflexes.

Discontinuing:
Don't discontinue this drug without consulting doctor. Dosage may require a gradual reduction before stopping.

Others:
- Get up slowly from a sitting or lying position to avoid any dizziness, faintness or lightheadedness.
- Advise any doctor or dentist whom you consult that you take this medicine.
- Take medicine only as directed. Do not increase or reduce dosage without doctor's approval.

POSSIBLE INTERACTION WITH OTHER DRUGS

GENERIC NAME OR DRUG CLASS	COMBINED EFFECT
Antidepressants*, other	Increased sedative effect. Not recommended.
Central nervous system (CNS) depressants*, other	Increased sedative effect.
Cimetidine	Increased risk of adverse reactions.
Monoamine oxidase (MAO) inhibitors*	Increased risk and severity of adverse reactions. Allow 14 days between use of the two drugs.

POSSIBLE INTERACTION WITH OTHER SUBSTANCES

INTERACTS WITH	COMBINED EFFECT
Alcohol:	Increased sedative affect. Avoid.
Beverages:	None expected.
Cocaine:	Effect not known. Best to avoid.
Foods:	None expected.
Marijuana:	Effect not known. Best to avoid.
Tobacco:	None expected.

*See Glossary

VITAMIN A

BRAND NAMES

Acon   Aquasol A
Afaxin   Dispatabs
Alphalin   Sust-A

Numerous multiple vitamin-mineral
supplements. Check labels.

BASIC INFORMATION

Habit forming? No
Prescription needed? No
Available as generic? Yes
Drug class: Vitamin supplement

 ## USES

- Dietary supplement to ensure normal growth and health, especially of eyes and skin.
- Beta carotene form decreases severity of sun exposure in patients with porphyria.

 ## DOSAGE & USAGE INFORMATION

How to take:
- Drops or capsule—Swallow with liquid. If you can't swallow whole, open capsule and take with liquid or food.
- Oral solution—Swallow with liquid.
- Tablet—Swallow with liquid.

When to take:
At the same time each day.

If you forget a dose:
Take as soon as you remember, then resume regular schedule.

What drug does:
- Prevents night blindness.
- Promotes normal growth and health.

Continued next column

 ## OVERDOSE

SYMPTOMS:
Increased adverse reactions and side effects. Jaundice (rare, but may occur with large doses), malaise, vomiting, irritability, bleeding gums, seizures, double vision, peeling skin.
WHAT TO DO:
If person takes much larger amount than prescribed, call doctor, poison control center or hospital emergency room for instructions.

Time lapse before drug works:
Requires continual intake.

Don't take with:
Any other medicine without consulting your doctor or pharmacist.

 ## POSSIBLE ADVERSE REACTIONS OR SIDE EFFECTS

SYMPTOMS	WHAT TO DO
Life-threatening:	
In case of overdose, see previous column.	
Common:	
None expected.	
Infrequent:	
Confusion; dizziness; drowsiness; headache; irritability; dry, cracked lips; peeling skin; hair loss; sensitvity to light.	Continue. Call doctor when convenient.
Rare:	
• Bulging soft spot on baby's head, double vision, bone or joint pain, abdominal pain, frequent urination, vomiting.	Discontinue. Call doctor right away.
• Diarrhea, appetite loss, nausea.	Continue. Call doctor when convenient.

WARNINGS & PRECAUTIONS

Don't take if:
You have chronic kidney failure.

Before you start, consult your doctor:
If you have any kidney disorder.

Over age 60:
No problems expected.

Pregnancy:
Risk factor determined by length of pregnancy and dosage amount. See category list on page xxiii and consult doctor.

Breast-feeding:
No problems expected. Consult doctor.

Infants & children:
* Avoid large doses.
* Keep vitamin-mineral supplements out of children's reach.

Prolonged use:
No problems expected.

Skin & sunlight:
No special problems expected.

Driving, piloting or hazardous work:
No problems expected.

Discontinuing:
Don't discontinue without doctor's advice until you complete prescribed dose, even though symptoms diminish or disappear.

Others:
* Don't exceed dose. Too much over a long time may be harmful.
* A balanced diet should provide all the vitamin A a healthy person needs and prevent need for supplements. Best sources are liver, yellow-orange fruits and vegetables, dark-green, leafy vegetables, milk, butter and margarine.

POSSIBLE INTERACTION WITH OTHER DRUGS

GENERIC NAME OR DRUG CLASS	COMBINED EFFECT
Anticoagulants*	Increased anticoagulant effect with large doses (over 10,000 I.U.) of vitamin A.
Calcium supplements*	Decreased vitamin effect.
Cholestyramine	Decreased vitamin A absorption.
Colestipol	Decreased vitamin absorption.
Contraceptives, oral*	Increased vitamin A levels.
Etretinate	Increased risk of toxic effects.
Isotretinoin	Increased risk of toxic effect of each.
Mineral oil (long-term)	Decreased vitamin A absorption.
Neomycin	Decreased vitamin absorption.
Vitamin A derivatives, other	Increased toxicity risk.
Vitamin E (excess dose)	Vitamin A depletion.

POSSIBLE INTERACTION WITH OTHER SUBSTANCES

INTERACTS WITH	COMBINED EFFECT
Alcohol:	None expected.
Beverages:	None expected.
Cocaine:	None expected.
Foods:	None expected.
Marijuana:	None expected.
Tobacco:	None expected.

VITAMIN B-12 (Cyanocobalamin)

GENERIC AND BRAND NAMES

CYANOCOBALAMIN
Anocobin
Bedoz
Berubigen
Betalin 12
Cyanabin
Kaybovite
Kaybovite-1000
Redisol
Rubion
Rubramin
Rubramin-PC

HYDROXOCOBAL-AMIN
Acti-B-12
Alpha Redisol
Alphamin
Codroxomin
Droxomin

Numerous other multiple vitamin-mineral supplements.

BASIC INFORMATION

Habit forming? No
Prescription needed? Yes, for some
Available as generic? Yes
Drug class: Vitamin supplement

USES

- Dietary supplement for normal growth, development and health.
- Treatment for nerve damage.
- Treatment for pernicious anemia.
- Treatment and prevention of vitamin B-12 deficiencies in people who have had stomach or intestines surgically removed.
- Prevention of vitamin B-12 deficiency in strict vegetarians and persons with absorption diseases.

DOSAGE & USAGE INFORMATION

How to take:
- Tablets—Swallow with liquid.
- Injection—Follow doctor's directions.

When to take:
- Oral—At the same time each day.
- Injection—Follow doctor's directions.

Continued next column

OVERDOSE

SYMPTOMS:
Increased adverse reactions and side effects.
WHAT TO DO:
Overdose unlikely to threaten life. If person takes much larger amount than prescribed, call doctor, poison control center or hospital emergency room for instructions.

If you forget a dose:
Take when remembered. Don't double next dose. Resume regular schedule.

What drug does:
Acts as enzyme to promote normal fat and carbohydrate metabolism and protein synthesis.

Time lapse before drug works:
15 minutes.

Don't take with:
Any other medicine without consulting your doctor or pharmacist.

POSSIBLE ADVERSE REACTIONS OR SIDE EFFECTS

SYMPTOMS	WHAT TO DO
Life-threatening:	
Hives, rash, intense itching, faintness soon after a dose (anaphylaxis).	Seek emergency treatment immediately.
Common:	
None expected.	
Infrequent:	
None expected.	
Rare:	
• Itchy skin, wheezing.	Discontinue. Call doctor right away.
• Diarrhea.	Continue. Call doctor when convenient.

VITAMIN B-12 (Cyanocobalamin)

WARNINGS & PRECAUTIONS

Don't take if:
You have Leber's disease (optic nerve atrophy).

Before you start, consult your doctor:
- If you have gout.
- If you have heart disease.

Over age 60:
Don't take more than 100 mg per day unless prescribed by your doctor.

Pregnancy:
Risk factor determined by length of pregnancy and dosage amount. See category list on page xxiii and consult doctor.

Breast-feeding:
Effect unknown. Consult doctor.

Infants & children:
No problems expected.

Prolonged use:
No problems expected.

Skin & sunlight:
No problems expected.

Driving, piloting or hazardous work:
No problems expected.

Discontinuing:
Don't discontinue without doctor's advice until you complete prescribed dose, even though symptoms diminish or disappear.

Others:
- A balanced diet should provide all the vitamin B-12 a healthy person needs and make supplements unnecessary. Best sources are meat, fish, egg yolk and cheese.
- Tablets should be used only for diet supplements. All other uses of vitamin B-12 require injections.
- Don't take large doses of vitamin C (1,000 mg or more per day) unless prescribed by your doctor.

POSSIBLE INTERACTION WITH OTHER DRUGS

GENERIC NAME OR DRUG CLASS	COMBINED EFFECT
Anticonvulsants*	Decreased absorption of vitamin B-12.
Chloramphenicol	Decreased vitamin B-12 effect.
Cholestyramine	Decreased absorption of vitamin B-12.
Cimetidine	Decreased absorption of vitamin B-12.
Colchicine	Decreased absorption of vitamin B-12.
Famotidine	Decreased absorption of vitamin B-12.
H₂ antagonists*	Decreased absorption of vitamin B-12.
Neomycin	Decreased absorption of vitamin B-12.
Para-aminosalicylic acid	Decreased effects of para-aminosalicyclic acid.
Potassium (extended-release forms)	Decreased absorption of vitamin B-12.
Ranitidine	Decreased absorption of vitamin B-12.
Vitamin C (ascorbic acid)	Destroys vitamin B-12 if taken at same time. Take 2 hours apart.

POSSIBLE INTERACTION WITH OTHER SUBSTANCES

INTERACTS WITH	COMBINED EFFECT
Alcohol:	Decreased absorption of vitamin B-12.
Beverages:	None expected.
Cocaine:	None expected.
Foods:	None expected.
Marijuana:	None expected.
Tobacco:	None expected.

*See Glossary

VITAMIN C (Ascorbic Acid)

BRAND NAMES

Ascorbicap	Ce-Vi-Sol
Cecon	Cevita
Cemill	C-Span
Cenolate	Flavorcee
Cetane	Redoxon
Cevalin	Sunkist
Cevi-Bid	

Numerous other multiple vitamin-mineral supplements.

BASIC INFORMATION

Habit forming? No
Prescription needed? No
Available as generic? Yes
Drug class: Vitamin supplement

USES

- Prevention and treatment of scurvy and other vitamin C deficiencies.
- Treatment of anemia.
- Maintenance of acid urine.

DOSAGE & USAGE INFORMATION

How to take:
- Tablets, capsules, liquid—Swallow with 8 oz. water.
- Extended-release tablets—Swallow whole.
- Drops—Squirt directly into mouth or mix with liquid or food.
- Chewable tablets—Chew well before swallowing.

When to take:
1, 2 or 3 times per day, as prescribed on label.

If you forget a dose:
Take as soon as you remember, then return to regular schedule.

Continued next column

OVERDOSE

SYMPTOMS:
Diarrhea, vomiting, dizziness.
WHAT TO DO:
Overdose unlikely to threaten life. If person takes much larger amount than prescribed, call doctor, poison control center or hospital emergency room for instructions.

What drug does:
- May help form collagen.
- Increases iron absorption from intestine.
- Contributes to hemoglobin and red blood cell production in bone marrow.

Time lapse before drug works:
1 week.

Don't take with:
Any other medicine without consulting your doctor or pharmacist.

POSSIBLE ADVERSE REACTIONS OR SIDE EFFECTS

SYMPTOMS	WHAT TO DO
Life-threatening: None expected.	
Common: None expected.	
Infrequent:	
• Mild diarrhea, nausea, vomiting.	Discontinue. Call doctor right away.
• Flushed face.	Continue. Call doctor when convenient.
Rare:	
• Kidney stones with high doses, anemia, abdominal pain.	Discontinue. Call doctor right away.
• Headache.	Continue. Tell doctor at next visit.

842

VITAMIN C (Ascorbic Acid)

WARNINGS & PRECAUTIONS

Don't take if:
You are allergic to vitamin C.

Before you start, consult your doctor:
- If you have sickle-cell or other anemia.
- If you have had kidney stones.
- If you have gout.

Over age 60:
Don't take more than 1000 mg per day unless prescribed by your doctor.

Pregnancy:
Risk factor determined by length of pregnancy and dosage amount. See category list on page xxiii and consult doctor.

Breast-feeding:
Avoid large doses. Consult doctor.

Infants & children:
- Avoid large doses.
- Keep vitamin-mineral supplements out of children's reach.

Prolonged use:
Large doses for longer than 2 months may cause kidney stones.

Skin & sunlight:
No problems expected.

Driving, piloting or hazardous work:
No problems expected.

Discontinuing:
No problems expected.

Others:
- Store in cool, dry place.
- May cause inaccurate tests for sugar in urine or blood in stool.
- May cause crisis in patients with sickle-cell anemia.
- A balanced diet should provide all the vitamin C a healthy person needs and make supplements unnecessary. Best sources are citrus, strawberries, cantaloupe and raw peppers.
- Don't take large doses of vitamin C (1,000 mg or more per day) unless prescribed by your doctor.
- Some products contain tartrazine dye. Avoid, if allergic (especially aspirin hypersensitivity).

POSSIBLE INTERACTION WITH OTHER DRUGS

GENERIC NAME OR DRUG CLASS	COMBINED EFFECT
Amphetamines*	Possible decreased amphetamine effect.
Anticholinergics*	Possible decreased anticholinergic effect.
Anticoagulants*, oral	Possible decreased anticoagulant effect.
Antidepressants, tricyclic (TCA)*	Possible decreased antidepressant effect.
Aspirin	Decreased vitamin C effect and salicylate excretion.
Barbiturates*	Decreased vitamin C effect. Increased barbiturate effect.
Cellulose sodium phosphate	Decreased vitamin C effect.
Contraceptives, oral*	Decreased vitamin C effect.
Estrogens*	Increased likelihood of adverse effects from estrogen with 1 g or more of vitamin C per day.
Iron supplements*	Increased iron absorption.
Mexiletine	Possible decreased effectiveness of mexiletine.
Quinidine	Possible decreased quinidine effect.
Salicylates*	Decreased vitamin C effect and salicylate excretion. May lead to salicylate toxicity.
Tranquilizers* (phenothiazine)	May decrease phenothiazine effect if no vitamin C deficiency exists.

POSSIBLE INTERACTION WITH OTHER SUBSTANCES

INTERACTS WITH	COMBINED EFFECT
Alcohol:	None expected.
Beverages:	None expected.
Cocaine:	None expected.
Foods:	None expected.
Marijuana:	None expected.
Tobacco:	Increased requirement for vitamin C.

VITAMIN D

GENERIC AND BRAND NAMES

ALFACALCIDOL
  One-Alpha
CALCIFEDOL
  Calderol
CALCITRIOL
  Calcijex
  Rocaltrol
**DIHYDROTACHY-
  STEROL**
  DHT
  DHT Intensol
  Hytakerol

ERGOCALCIFEROL
  Calciferol
  Drisdol
  Osto Forte
  Radiostol
  Radiostol Forte

BASIC INFORMATION

Habit forming? No
Prescription needed?
  Low strength: No
  High strength: Yes
Available as generic? Yes
Drug class: Vitamin supplement

USES

- Dietary supplement.
- Prevention of rickets (bone disease).
- Treatment for hypocalcemia (low blood calcium) in kidney disease.
- Treatment for postoperative muscle contractions.
- Daily supplement for people who must use sunscreen daily.

DOSAGE & USAGE INFORMATION

How to take:
- Tablet, capsule or liquid—Swallow with liquid.
- Drops—Dilute dose in beverage.
- Injection—Take under doctor's supervision.

Continued next column

OVERDOSE

SYMPTOMS:
Severe stomach pain, nausea, vomiting, weight loss; bone and muscle pain; increased urination, cloudy urine; mood or mental changes (possible psychosis); high blood pressure, irregular heartbeat; eye irritation or light sensitivity; itchy skin.
WHAT TO DO:
Overdose unlikely to threaten life. If person takes much larger amount than prescribed, call doctor, poison control center or hospital emergency room for instructions.

When to take:
As directed, usually once a day at the same time each day.

If you forget a dose:
Take up to 12 hours late. If more than 12 hours, wait for next dose (don't double this dose).

What drug does:
- Maintains growth and health.
- Prevents rickets.
- Essential so body can use calcium and phosphate.

Time lapse before drug works:
2 hours. May require 2 to 3 weeks of continual use for maximum effect.

Don't take with:
Nonprescription drugs or drugs in Interaction column without consulting doctor.

POSSIBLE ADVERSE REACTIONS OR SIDE EFFECTS

SYMPTOMS	WHAT TO DO
Life-threatening:	
In case of overdose, see previous column.	
Common:	
None expected.	
Infrequent:	
Headache, metallic taste in mouth, thirst, dry mouth, constipation, appetite loss, nausea, vomiting, weakness, cloudy urine, sensitivity to light.	Continue. Call doctor when convenient.
Rare:	
• Increased urination, pink eye, psychosis, severe abdominal pain, fever.	Discontinue. Call doctor right away.
• Muscle pain, bone pain, diarrhea.	Continue. Tell doctor when convenient.

WARNINGS & PRECAUTIONS

Don't take if:
You are allergic to medicine containing vitamin D.

Before you start, consult your doctor:
- If you plan to become pregnant while taking vitamin D.
- If you have epilepsy.
- If you have heart or blood-vessel disease.
- If you have kidney disease.

Over age 60:
Adverse reactions and side effects may be more frequent and severe than in younger persons.

Pregnancy:
Risk factor determined by length of pregnancy and dosage amount. See category list on page xxiii and consult doctor.

Breast-feeding:
No problems expected, but consult doctor.

Infants & children:
- Avoid large doses.
- Keep vitamins out of children's reach.

Prolonged use:
- No problems expected.
- Talk to your doctor about the need for follow-up medical examinations or laboratory studies to check kidney function, liver function, serum calcium.

Skin & sunlight:
No special problems expected.

Driving, piloting or hazardous work:
No problems expected.

Discontinuing:
Don't discontinue without doctor's advice until you complete prescribed dose, even though symptoms diminish or disappear.

Others:
- Don't exceed dose. Too much over a long time may be harmful.
- A balanced diet should provide all the vitamin D a healthy person needs and make supplements unnecessary. Best sources are fish and vitamin D-fortified milk and bread.
- Some products contain tartrazine dye. Avoid, if allergic (especially aspirin hypersensitivity).
- Sunscreen prevents the body from manufacturing vitamin D from sunshine. Take supplementary vitamin D if you use sunscreen daily. Ask doctor for dosage.

POSSIBLE INTERACTION WITH OTHER DRUGS

GENERIC NAME OR DRUG CLASS	COMBINED EFFECT
Antacids* (magnesium-containing)	Possible excess magnesium.
Anticonvulsants, hydantoin*	Decreased vitamin D effect.
Calcium (high doses)	Excess calcium in blood.
Calcium channel blockers*	Possible decreased effect of calcium channel blockers.
Calcium supplements*	Excessive absorption of vitamin D.
Cholestyramine	Decreased vitamin D effect.
Colestipol	Decreased vitamin D absorption.
Cortisone	Decreased vitamin D effect.
Digitalis preparations*	Heartbeat irregularities.
Diuretics, thiazide*	Possible increased calcium.
Mineral oil	Decreased vitamin D effect.
Neomycin	Decreased vitamin D absorption.
Nicardipine	Decreased nicardipine effect.
Phenobarbital	Decreased vitamin D effect.
Phosphorus preparations*	Accumulation of excess phosphorus.
Rifampin	Possible decreased vitamin D effect.
Vitamin D, other	Possible toxicity.

POSSIBLE INTERACTION WITH OTHER SUBSTANCES

INTERACTS WITH	COMBINED EFFECT
Alcohol:	None expected.
Beverages:	None expected.
Cocaine:	None expected.
Foods:	None expected.
Marijuana:	None expected.
Tobacco:	None expected.

VITAMIN E

BRAND NAMES

Aquasol E
Chew-E
Eprolin

Epsilan-M
Pheryl-E
Viterra E

Numerous other multiple vitamin-mineral supplements. Check labels.

BASIC INFORMATION

Habit forming? No
Prescription needed? No
Available as generic? Yes
Drug class: Vitamin supplement

 ## USES

- Dietary supplement to promote normal growth, development and health.
- Treatment and prevention of vitamin E deficiency, especially in premature or low-birth-weight infants.
- Treatment for fibrocystic disease of the breast.
- Treatment for circulatory problems to the lower extremities.
- Treatment for sickle-cell anemia.
- Treatment for lung toxicity from air pollution.

 ## DOSAGE & USAGE INFORMATION

How to take:
- Tablet or capsule—Swallow with liquid or food to lessen stomach irritation.
- Drops—Dilute dose in beverage before swallowing or squirt directly into mouth.
- Injection—Take under doctor's supervision.

When to take:
At the same times each day.

If you forget a dose:
Take when you remember. Don't double next dose.

What drug does:
- Promotes normal growth and development.
- Prevents oxidation in body.

Continued next column

 ## OVERDOSE

SYMPTOMS:
Nausea, vomiting, fatigue.
WHAT TO DO:
Overdose unlikely to threaten life. If person takes much larger amount than prescribed, call doctor, poison control center or hospital emergency room for instructions.

Time lapse before drug works:
Not determined.

Don't take with:
Any other medicine without consulting your doctor or pharmacist.

 ## POSSIBLE ADVERSE REACTIONS OR SIDE EFFECTS

SYMPTOMS	WHAT TO DO
Life-threatening: None expected.	
Common: Breast enlargement, dizziness, headache.	Continue. Call doctor when convenient.
Infrequent: Nausea, abdominal pain, muscle aches, pain in lower legs, fever, tiredness, weakness.	Continue. Call doctor when convenient.
Rare: Blurred vision, diarrhea.	Discontinue. Call doctor right away.

WARNINGS & PRECAUTIONS

Don't take if:
You are allergic to vitamin E.

Before you start, consult your doctor:
- If you have had blood clots in leg veins (thrombophlebitis).
- If you have liver disease.

Over age 60:
No problems expected. Avoid excessive doses.

Pregnancy:
No problems expected with normal daily requirements. Don't exceed prescribed dose. Consult doctor.

Breast-feeding:
No problems expected. Consult doctor.

Infants & children:
Use only under medical supervision.

Prolonged use:
Toxic accumulation of vitamin E. Don't exceed recommended dose.

Skin & sunlight:
No problems expected.

Driving, piloting or hazardous work:
No problems expected.

Discontinuing:
No problems expected.

Others:
A balanced diet should provide all the vitamin E a healthy person needs and make supplements unnecessary. Best sources are vegetable oils, whole-grain cereals, liver.

POSSIBLE INTERACTION WITH OTHER DRUGS

GENERIC NAME OR DRUG CLASS	COMBINED EFFECT
Anticoagulants*, oral	Increased anti-coagulant effect.
Cholestyramine	Decreased vitamin E absorption.
Colestipol	Decreased vitamin E absorption.
Iron supplements*	Possible decreased effect of iron supplement in patients with iron-deficiency anemia. Decreased vitamin E effect in healthy persons.
Mineral oil	Decreased vitamin E effect.
Neomycin	Decreased vitamin E absorption.
Vitamin A	Recommended dose of vitamin E—Increased benefit and decreased toxicity of vitamin A. Excess dose of vitamin E—Vitamin A depletion.

POSSIBLE INTERACTION WITH OTHER SUBSTANCES

INTERACTS WITH	COMBINED EFFECT
Alcohol:	None expected.
Beverages:	None expected.
Cocaine:	None expected.
Foods:	None expected.
Marijuana:	None expected.
Tobacco:	None expected.

VITAMIN K

GENERIC AND BRAND NAMES

MENADIOL
  Synkayvite

PHYTONADIONE
  Mephyton

BASIC INFORMATION

Habit forming? No
Prescription needed? No
Available as generic? Yes
Drug class: Vitamin supplement

 USES

- Dietary supplement.
- Treatment for bleeding disorders and malabsorption diseases due to vitamin K deficiency.
- Treatment for hemorrhagic disease of the newborn.
- Treatment for bleeding due to overdose of oral anticoagulants.

 DOSAGE & USAGE INFORMATION

How to take:
- Usually given by injection in hospital or doctor's office.
- Tablet—Swallow with liquid. If you can't swallow whole, crumble tablet and take with liquid or food.

When to take:
At the same time each day.

If you forget a dose:
Take as soon as you remember up to 12 hours late. If more than 12 hours, wait for next scheduled dose (don't double this dose).

What drug does:
- Promotes growth, development and good health.
- Supplies a necessary ingredient for blood clotting.

Continued next column

 OVERDOSE

SYMPTOMS:
Nausea, vomiting.
WHAT TO DO:
Overdose unlikely to threaten life. If person takes much larger amount than prescribed, call doctor, poison control center or hospital emergency room for instructions.

Time lapse before drug works:
15 to 30 minutes to support blood clotting.

Don't take with:
Any other medicine without consulting your doctor or pharmacist.

 POSSIBLE ADVERSE REACTIONS OR SIDE EFFECTS

SYMPTOMS	WHAT TO DO
Life-threatening:	
None expected.	
Common:	
None expected.	
Infrequent:	
Unusual taste, face flushing.	Continue. Call doctor when convenient.
Rare:	
Rash, hives.	Discontinue. Call doctor right away.

WARNINGS & PRECAUTIONS

Don't take if:
- You are allergic to vitamin K.
- You have G6PD* deficiency.
- You have liver disease.

Before you start, consult your doctor:
If you are pregnant.

Over age 60:
No problems expected.

Pregnancy:
Risk factor determined by length of pregnancy and dosage amount. See category list on page xxiii and consult doctor.

Breast-feeding:
No problems expected. Consult doctor.

Infants & children:
Phytonadione is the preferred form for hemorrhagic disease of the newborn.

Prolonged use:
Talk to your doctor about the need for follow-up medical examinations or laboratory studies to check prothrombin time.

Skin & sunlight:
No problems expected.

Driving, piloting or hazardous work:
No problems expected.

Discontinuing:
No problems expected.

Others:
- Tell all doctors and dentists you consult that you take this medicine.
- Don't exceed dose. Too much over a long time may be harmful.
- A balanced diet should provide all the vitamin K a healthy person needs and make supplements unnecessary. Best sources are green, leafy vegetables, meat or dairy products.

POSSIBLE INTERACTION WITH OTHER DRUGS

GENERIC NAME OR DRUG CLASS	COMBINED EFFECT
Anticoagulants*, oral	Decreased anti-coagulant effect.
Cholestyramine	Decreased vitamin K effect.
Colestipol	Decreased vitamin K absorption.
Dapsone	Increased risk of adverse effect on blood cells.
Mineral oil (long-term)	Vitamin K deficiency.
Neomycin	Decreased vitamin K absorption.
Sulfa drugs*	Vitamin K deficiency.

POSSIBLE INTERACTION WITH OTHER SUBSTANCES

INTERACTS WITH	COMBINED EFFECT
Alcohol:	None expected.
Beverages:	None expected.
Cocaine:	None expected.
Foods:	None expected.
Marijuana:	None expected.
Tobacco:	None expected.

VITAMINS & FLUORIDE

GENERIC AND BRAND NAMES

Adeflor	Tri-Vi-Flor
Cari-Tab	Vi-Daylin/F
Mulvidren-F	Vi-Penta F
Poly-Vi-Flor	

Also available in the forms of multiple vitamins & fluoride; vitamins A, D & C & fluoride.

BASIC INFORMATION

Habit forming? No
Prescription needed? Yes
Available as generic? No
Drug class: Vitamins, minerals

 ## USES

- Reduces incidence of tooth cavities (fluoride). Children who need supplements should take until age 16.
- Prevents deficiencies of vitamin included in formula (some contain multiple vitamins whose content varies among products; others contain only vitamins A, D and C).

 ## DOSAGE & USAGE INFORMATION

How to take:
- Chewable tablets—Chew or crush before swallowing.
- Oral liquid—Measure with specially marked dropper. May mix with food, fruit juice, cereal.

When to take:
- Bedtime or with or just after meals.
- If at bedtime, brush teeth first.

Continued next column

 ## OVERDOSE

SYMPTOMS:
Minor overdose—Black, brown or white spots on teeth.
Massive overdose—Shallow breathing, black or tarry stools, bloody vomit.
WHAT TO DO:
- **Dial 911 (emergency) or 0 (operator) for an ambulance or medical help. Then give first aid immediately.**
- **See emergency information on inside covers.**

If you forget a dose:
Take as soon as you remember up to 2 hours late. If more than 2 hours, wait for next scheduled dose (don't double this dose).

What drug does:
Provides supplemental fluoride to combat tooth decay.

Time lapse before drug works:
8 weeks to provide maximum benefit.

Don't take with:
- Other medicine simultaneously.
- Any other medicine without consulting your doctor or pharmacist.

 ## POSSIBLE ADVERSE REACTIONS OR SIDE EFFECTS

SYMPTOMS	WHAT TO DO
Life-threatening: Fainting, bloody vomit, bloody or black stool, breathing difficulty.	Discontinue. Seek emergency treatment.
Common: White, black or brown spots on teeth; nausea; vomiting.	Discontinue. Call doctor right away.
Infrequent: • Drowsiness; abdominal pain; increased salivation; watery eyes; weight loss; sore throat, fever, mouth sores; constipation; bone pain; rash; muscle stiffness; weakness; tremor; agitation.	Discontinue. Call doctor right away.
• Diarrhea.	Continue. Call doctor when convenient.
Rare: None expected.	

WARNINGS & PRECAUTIONS

Don't take if:
- Your water supply contains 0.7 parts fluoride per million. Too much fluoride stains teeth permanently.
- You are allergic to any fluoride-containing product.
- You have underactive thyroid.

Before you start, consult your doctor or dentist:
For proper dosage.

Over age 60:
No problems expected.

Pregnancy:
Risk factor determined by length of pregnancy and dosage amount. See category list on page xxiii and consult doctor.

Breast-feeding:
No problems expected. Consult doctor.

Infants & children:
No problems expected in children over 3 years of age except in case of accidental overdose. Keep vitamin-mineral supplements out of children's reach.

Prolonged use:
Excess may cause discolored teeth and decreased calcium in blood.

Skin & sunlight:
No problems expected.

Driving, piloting or hazardous work:
No problems expected.

Discontinuing:
No problems expected.

Others:
- Store in original plastic container. Fluoride decomposes glass.
- Check with dentist once or twice a year to keep cavities at a minimum. Topical applications of fluoride may also be helpful.
- Fluoride probably not necessary if water contains about 1 part per million of fluoride or more. Check with health department.
- Don't freeze.
- Don't keep outdated medicine.

POSSIBLE INTERACTION WITH OTHER DRUGS

GENERIC NAME OR DRUG CLASS	COMBINED EFFECT
Anticoagulants*	Decreased effect of anticoagulant.
Iron supplements*	Decreased effect of any vitamin E if present in multivitamin product.
Vitamin A	May lead to vitamin A toxicity if vitamin A is in combination.
Vitamin D	May lead to vitamin D toxicity if vitamin D is in combination.

POSSIBLE INTERACTION WITH OTHER SUBSTANCES

INTERACTS WITH	COMBINED EFFECT
Alcohol:	None expected.
Beverages: Milk.	Prevents absorption of fluoride. Space dose 2 hours before or after milk.
Cocaine:	None expected.
Foods:	None expected.
Marijuana:	None expected.
Tobacco:	None expected.

XYLOMETAZOLINE

BRAND NAMES

Chlorohist-LA
Inspire
Neo-Synephrine II
  Long Acting Nasal
  Spray Adult Strength
Neo-Synephrine II
  Long Acting Nose
  Drops Adult Strength
Otrivin Decongestant
  Nose Drops

Otrivin Nasal Drops
Otrivin Nasal Spray
Otrivin Pediatric
  Decongestant Nose
  Drops
Otrivin Pediatric
  Nasal Drops
Otrivin Pediatric
  Nasal Spray
Otrivin with M-D
  Pump

BASIC INFORMATION

Habit forming? No
Prescription needed? No
Available as generic? Yes
Drug class: Sympathomimetic

USES

Relieves congestion of nose, sinuses and throat from allergies and infections.

DOSAGE & USAGE INFORMATION

How to take:
Nasal solution, nasal spray—Use as directed on label. Avoid contamination. Don't use same container for more than 1 person.

When to take:
When needed, no more often than every 4 hours.

Continued next column

OVERDOSE

SYMPTOMS:
Headache, sweating, anxiety, agitation, rapid and irregular heartbeat (rare occurrence with systemic absorption).
WHAT TO DO:
- Dial 911 (emergency) or 0 (operator) for an ambulance or medical help. Then give first aid immediately.
- If patient is unconscious and not breathing, give mouth-to-mouth breathing. If there is no heartbeat, use cardiac massage and mouth-to-mouth breathing (CPR). If you can't get help quickly, take patient to nearest emergency facility.
- See emergency information on inside covers.

If you forget a dose:
Take as soon as you remember. Wait 4 hours for next dose.

What drug does:
Constricts walls of small arteries in nose, sinuses and eustachian tubes.

Time lapse before drug works:
5 to 30 minutes.

Don't take with:
- Nonprescription drugs for allergy, cough or cold without consulting doctor.
- Any other medicine without consulting your doctor or pharmacist.

POSSIBLE ADVERSE REACTIONS OR SIDE EFFECTS

SYMPTOMS	WHAT TO DO
Life-threatening: In case of overdose, see previous column.	
Common: None expected.	
Infrequent: Burning, dry or stinging nasal passages.	Continue. Call doctor when convenient.
Rare: Rebound congestion (increased runny or stuffy nose); headache, insomnia, nervousness (may occur with systemic absorption).	Discontinue. Call doctor when convenient.

WARNINGS & PRECAUTIONS

Don't take if:
You are allergic to any sympathomimetic nasal spray.

Before you start, consult your doctor:
- If you have heart disease or high blood pressure.
- If you have diabetes.
- If you have overactive thyroid.
- If you have taken a monoamine oxidase (MAO) inhibitor* in past 2 weeks.
- If you have glaucoma.

Over age 60:
Adverse reactions and side effects may be more frequent and severe than in younger persons.

Pregnancy:
Decide with your doctor if drug benefits justify risk to unborn child. Risk category C (see page xxiii).

Breast-feeding:
No proven problems. Consult doctor.

Infants & children:
Don't give to children younger than 2.

Prolonged use:
Drug may lose effectiveness, cause increased congestion (rebound effect*) and irritate nasal membranes.

Skin & sunlight:
No problems expected.

Driving, piloting or hazardous work:
No problems expected.

Discontinuing:
May be unnecessary to finish medicine. Follow doctor's instructions.

Others:
No problems expected.

POSSIBLE INTERACTION WITH OTHER DRUGS

GENERIC NAME OR DRUG CLASS	COMBINED EFFECT
Antidepressants, tricyclic*	Possible increased blood pressure.
Maprotiline	Possible increased blood pressure.
Monoamine oxidase (MAO) inhibitors*	Possible increased blood pressure.

POSSIBLE INTERACTION WITH OTHER SUBSTANCES

INTERACTS WITH	COMBINED EFFECT
Alcohol:	None expected.
Beverages: Caffeine drinks.	Nervousness or insomnia.
Cocaine:	High risk of heartbeat irregularities and high blood pressure.
Foods:	None expected.
Marijuana:	Overstimulation. Avoid.
Tobacco:	None expected.

*See Glossary

YOHIMBINE

BRAND NAMES

Actibine	Thybine
Aphrodyne	Yocon
Baron-X	Yohimar
Dayto Himbin	Yohimex
PMS-Yohimbine	Yoman
Prohim	Yovital

BASIC INFORMATION

Habit forming? No
Prescription needed? Yes
Available as generic? Yes
Drug class: Impotence therapy

USES

Treatment for men who are unable to have sexual intercourse (impotent). It may be helpful for some, but not all, men who suffer sexual dysfunction.

DOSAGE & USAGE INFORMATION

How to use:
Tablet—Swallow with liquid. May be taken with or without food.

When to use:
At the same times each day.

If you forget a dose:
Take as soon as you remember up to 4 hours late. If more than 4 hours, wait for next scheduled dose (don't double this dose).

What drug does:
It is unknown exactly how the drug works. It appears to increase the supply of certain body chemicals that can help produce erections.

Time lapse before drug works:
May take 2 to 3 weeks.

Don't take with:
Any other prescription or nonprescription drug without consulting your doctor or pharmacist.

OVERDOSE

SYMPTOMS:
May produce increases in heart rate and blood pressure, lack of coordination, trembling.
WHAT TO DO:
Overdose unlikely to threaten life. If person takes much larger amount than prescribed, call doctor, poison control center or hospital emergency room for instructions.

POSSIBLE ADVERSE REACTIONS OR SIDE EFFECTS

SYMPTOMS	WHAT TO DO
Life-threatening: None expected.	
Common: None expected.	
Infrequent:	
• Rapid heartbeat, increased blood pressure.	Discontinue. Call doctor right away.
• Headache, dizziness, restlessness, irritability, nervousness, anxiety, insomnia, muscle aches.	Continue. Call doctor when convenient.
Rare: Nausea, vomiting, flushed skin, sweating, tremor.	Continue. Call doctor when convenient.

WARNINGS & PRECAUTIONS

Don't take if:
- You have an allergy to yohimbine or any rauwolfia alkaloids*.
- You have angina pectoris.
- You have heart disease or high blood pressure.
- You have impaired kidney function.

Before you start, consult your doctor:
- If you suffer from depression.
- If you have any psychiatric disorder.
- If you have liver disease.
- If you have allergies to any medications, foods or other substances.

Over age 60:
Studies have not shown any specific problems. Discuss possible benefits and risk factors with your doctor.

Pregnancy:
Not used in females.

Breast-feeding:
Not used in females.

Infants & children:
Not used in this age group.

Prolonged use:
Effects of long-term use are unknown. Visit your doctor regularly while using this drug to check its effectiveness, as well as your blood pressure and heart rate.

Skin & sunlight:
No special problems expected.

Driving, piloting or hazardous work:
Avoid if you experience any side effects (especially dizziness).

Discontinuing:
No special problems expected.

Others:
- Follow your doctor's instructions for using this drug. Don't take it more often or increase the dosage without your doctor's approval. It will increase the risk of high blood pressure and rapid heartbeat.
- Advise any doctor or dentist whom you consult that you take this medicine.

POSSIBLE INTERACTION WITH OTHER DRUGS

GENERIC NAME OR DRUG CLASS	COMBINED EFFECT
Antidepressants*	Decreased effect of antidepressant.
Antihypertensives*	Decreased effect of antihypertensive.

POSSIBLE INTERACTION WITH OTHER SUBSTANCES

INTERACTS WITH	COMBINED EFFECT
Alcohol:	Decreased yohimbine effect. Avoid.
Beverages:	None expected.
Cocaine	Effect unknown. Best to avoid.
Foods:	None expected.
Marijuana:	Effect unknown. Best to avoid.
Tobacco:	None expected.

*See Glossary

ZINC SUPPLEMENTS

GENERIC AND BRAND NAMES

ZINC ACETATE
  Galzin
ZINC GLUCONATE
  Orazinc

ZINC SULFATE
  Egozinc
  PMS Egozinc
  Verazinc
  Zinc-220
  Zincate

BASIC INFORMATION

Habit forming? No
Prescription needed? No
Available as generic? Yes
Drug class: Nutritional supplement (mineral)

USES

- Treats zinc deficiency that may lead to growth retardation, appetite loss, changes in taste or smell, skin eruptions, slow wound healing, decreased immune function, diarrhea or impaired night vision.
- In absence of a deficiency, is used to treat burns, eating disorders, liver disorders, prematurity in infants, intestinal diseases, parasitism, kidney disorders, skin disorders and stress.
- May be useful as a supplement for those who are breast-feeding or pregnant (under a doctor's supervision).
- Zinc acetate is used for treatment of Wilson's disease.

DOSAGE & USAGE INFORMATION

How to take:
Tablet or capsule—Swallow with liquid. If you can't swallow whole, crumble tablet or open capsule and take with liquid or food.

When to take:
At the same time each day, according to a doctor's instructions or the package label.

Continued next column

OVERDOSE

SYMPTOMS:
Dizziness, yellow eyes and skin, shortness of breath, chest pain, vomiting.
WHAT TO DO:
- **Have patient drink lots of water.**
- **Dial 911 (emergency) or 0 (operator) for an ambulance or medical help. Then give first aid immediately.**

If you forget a dose:
Take as soon as you remember up to 2 hours late. If more than 2 hours, wait for next scheduled dose (don't double this dose).

What drug does:
Required by the body for the utilization of many enzymes, nucleic acids and proteins and for cell growth.

Time lapse before drug works:
2 hours.

Don't take with:
Any other nonprescription or prescription medicine without consulting doctor or pharmacist.

POSSIBLE ADVERSE REACTIONS OR SIDE EFFECTS

SYMPTOMS	WHAT TO DO
Life-threatening:	
In case of overdose, see previous column.	
Common:	
None expected.	
Infrequent:	
None expected.	
Rare:	
• Indigestion, heartburn, nausea and vomiting (only with large doses).	Continue. Call doctor when convenient.
• Fever, chills, sore throat, ulcers in throat or mouth, unusual tiredness or weakness (only with large doses).	Discontinue. Call doctor right away.

WARNINGS & PRECAUTIONS

Don't take if:
You are allergic to zinc.

Before you start, consult your doctor:
If you are pregnant or breast-feeding.

Over age 60:
No special problems expected. Nutritional supplements may be helpful if the diet is restricted in any way.

Pregnancy:
Adequate zinc intake is important. Risk factor not designated. See category list on page xxiii and consult doctor.

Breast-feeding:
Adequate zinc intake important. Consult a doctor.

Infants & children:
Normal daily requirements vary with age. Consult a doctor.

Prolonged use:
No special problems expected.

Skin & sunlight:
No special problems expected.

Driving, piloting or hazardous work:
No special problems expected.

Discontinuing:
No special problems expected.

Others:
The best natural sources of zinc are red meats, oysters, herring, peas and beans.

POSSIBLE INTERACTION WITH OTHER DRUGS

GENERIC NAME OR DRUG CLASS	COMBINED EFFECT
Copper supplements	Inhibited absorption of copper.
Diuretics, thiazide*	Increased need for zinc.
Folic acid	Increased need for zinc.
Iron supplements*	Increased need for zinc
Tetracyclines*	Decreased absorption of tetracycline if taken within 2 hours of each other.

POSSIBLE INTERACTION WITH OTHER SUBSTANCES

INTERACTS WITH	COMBINED EFFECT
Alcohol:	May increase need for zinc.
Beverages:	No proven problems.
Cocaine:	No proven problems.
Foods: High-fiber.	May decrease zinc absorption.
Marijuana:	No proven problems.
Tobacco:	May increase need for zinc.

ZOLPIDEM

BRAND NAMES

Ambien

BASIC INFORMATION

Habit forming? Yes
Prescription needed? Yes
Available as generic? No
Drug class: Sedative-hypnotic agent

 USES

Short-term (less than 2 weeks) treatment for insomnia.

 DOSAGE & USAGE INFORMATION

How to take:
Tablets—Swallow with liquid.

When to take:
Take immediately before bedtime. For best results, do not take with a meal or immediately after eating a meal.

If you forget a dose:
Take as soon as you remember. Take drug only when you are able to get 7 to 8 hours of sleep before your daily activity begins. Do not exceed prescribed dosage.

What drug does:
Acts as a central nervous system depressant, decreasing sleep problems such as trouble falling asleep, waking up too often during the night and waking up too early in the morning.

Time lapse before drug works:
Within 1 to 2 hours.

Don't take with:
Any other prescription or nonprescription drug without consulting your doctor or pharmacist.

 OVERDOSE

SYMPTOMS:
Drowsiness, weakness, stupor, coma.
WHAT TO DO:
* Dial 911 (emergency) or 0 (operator) for an ambulance or medical help. Then give first aid immediately.
* If patient is unconscious and not breathing, use cardiac massage and mouth-to-mouth breathing (CPR). Don't try to make patient vomit. If you can't get help quickly, take patient to nearest emergency facility.
* See emergency information at end of book.

 POSSIBLE ADVERSE REACTIONS OR SIDE EFFECTS

SYMPTOMS	WHAT TO DO
Life-threatening: In case of overdose, see previous column.	
Common: Daytime drowsiness, lightheadedness, dizziness, clumsiness, headache, diarrhea, nausea.	Continue. Call doctor when convenient.
Infrequent: Dry mouth, muscle aches or pain, tiredness, indigestion, joint pain, memory problems.	Continue. Call doctor when convenient.
Rare: Behavioral changes, agitation, confusion, hallucinations, worsening of depression, bloody or cloudy urine, painful or difficult urination, increased urge to urinate, skin rash or hives, itching.	Discontinue. Call doctor right away.

WARNINGS & PRECAUTIONS

Don't take if:
You are allergic to zolpidem.

Before you start, consult your doctor:
- If you have respiratory problems.
- If you have kidney or liver disease.
- If you suffer from depression.
- If you are an active or recovering alcoholic or substance abuser.

Over age 60:
Adverse reactions and side effects may be more frequent and severe than in younger persons. You may need smaller doses for shorter periods of time.

Pregnancy:
Consult doctor. Risk category B (see page xxiii).

Breast-feeding:
Drug passes into milk. Avoid drug or discontinue nursing until you finish medicine. Consult doctor for advice on maintaining milk supply.

Infants & children:
Not recommended for patients under age 18.

Prolonged use:
Not recommended for long-term usage. Don't take for longer than 1 to 2 weeks unless under doctor's supervision.

Skin & sunlight:
No special problems expected.

Driving, piloting or hazardous work:
Don't drive or pilot aircraft until you learn how medicine affects you. Don't work around dangerous machinery. Don't climb ladders or work in high places. Danger increases if you drink alcohol or take other medicines affecting alertness and reflexes.

Discontinuing:
- Don't discontinue without consulting doctor. Dose may require gradual reduction if you have taken drug for a long time.
- You may have sleeping problems for 1 or 2 nights after stopping drug.

Others:
- Advise any doctor or dentist whom you consult that you take this medicine.
- Don't take drug if you are traveling on an overnight airplane trip of less than 7 or 8 hours. A temporary memory loss may occur (traveler's amnesia).

POSSIBLE INTERACTION WITH OTHER DRUGS

GENERIC NAME OR DRUG CLASS	COMBINED EFFECT
Central nervous system (CNS) depressants*	Increased sedative effect. Avoid.
Chlorpromazine	Increased sedative effect. Avoid.
Imipramine	Increased sedative effect. Avoid.

POSSIBLE INTERACTION WITH OTHER SUBSTANCES

INTERACTS WITH	COMBINED EFFECT
Alcohol:	Increased sedation. Avoid.
Beverages:	None expected.
Cocaine:	None expected.
Foods:	Decreased sedative effect if taken with a meal or right after a meal.
Marijuana:	None expected.
Tobacco:	None expected.

*See Glossary

Generic and Brand Name Directory

How to Read the Lists Below

The following drugs are alphabetized by generic name or drug class name, shown in large capital letters. The generic names and brand names that follow each title in this list are the complete list referred to on the drug chart. Generic names are in all capital letters on these lists; brand names are lower case.

Some main headings, such as *ADRENOCORTICOIDS (Systemic)* (a drug class name on page 14), are followed by generic names, which are numbered, and then by brand names, each of which is followed by a superscript number. By matching numbers, you can determine the generic drug(s) in each brand-name drug. For example, under *ADRENOCORTICOIDS (Systemic)*, the brand-name drug Aristocort[8] contains the generic drug *TRIAMCINOLONE*, which is numbered 8.

Other main heads below, such as *ACETAMINOPHEN*, are simple generic names, followed by brand-name drugs containing that generic drug.

ACETAMINOPHEN
4 Way Cold
Abenol
Acephen
Aceta
Acetaminophen Uniserts
Aclophen
Actamin
Actamin Extra
Actamin Super
Actifed A
Actifed Plus
Actifed Plus Caplets
Actimol
Advanced Formula Dristan Caplets
Alba-Temp 300
Allerest Headache Strength
Allerest No-Drowsiness
Allerest Sinus Pain Formula
All-Nite Cold Formula
Alumadrine
Amaphen
Aminofen
Aminofen Max
Anacin-3
Anacin-3 Extra Strength
Anatuss
Anatuss with Codeine
Anolor 300
Anoquan
Anuphen
Apacet Capsules
Apacet Elixir
Apacet Extra Strength Caplets
Apacet Extra Strength Tablets
Apacet Oral Solution
Apacet Regular Strength Tablets
APAP
Apo-Acetaminophen
Arcet
Aspirin Free Anacin Maximum Strength Caplets
Aspirin Free Anacin Maximum Strength Tablets
Aspirin Free Bayer Select Maximum Strength Headache Plus Caplets
Aspirin-Free Excedrin Caplets
Atasol Caplets
Atasol Drops

Atasol Forte
Atasol Forte Caplets
Atasol Forte Tablets
Atasol Oral Solution
Atasol Tablets
Bancap
Banesin
Bayer Select Chest Cold Tablets
Bayer Select Flu Relief Caplets
Bayer Select Head and Chest Cold Caplets
Bayer Select Head Cold Caplets
Bayer Select Maximum Strength Pain Relief Formula
Bayer Select Maximum Strength Sinus Pain Relief Caplets
Bayer Select Night Time Cold Caplets
Benadryl Allergy/Sinus Headache Caplets
Benadryl Cold
Benadryl Cold Nighttime Liquid
Benadryl Plus
Beta-Phed
BQ Cold
Bromaline Plus
Bromo-Seltzer
Bucet
Calmylin Cough & Cold
Campain
Children's Anacin 3
Children's Panadol
Children's Tylenol Cold
Children's Tylenol Cold Multi-Symptom Plus Cough
Children's Tylenol Suspension Liquid
Children's Ty-Tab
Chlor-Trimeton Sinus Caplets
Co-Apap
Codimal
Coldrine
Colrex Compound
Comtrex
Comtrex A/S Caplets
Comtrex Cough Formula
Comtrex Daytime Caplets
Comtrex Daytime Maximum Strength Cold and Flu Relief
Comtrex Daytime Maximum Strength Cold, Cough and Flu Relief

Comtrex Hot Flu Relief
Comtrex Maximum Strength Liqui-Gels
Comtrex Multi-Symptom Cold Reliever
Comtrex Multi-Symptom Hot Flu Relief
Comtrex Multi-Symptom Non-Drowsy Caplets
Comtrex Nighttime
Comtrex Nighttime Maximum Strength Cold and Flu Relief
Comtrex Nighttime Maximum Strength Cold, Cough and Flu Relief
Conacetol
Conar-A
Conex Plus
Congespirin
Congespirin for Children Cold Tablets
Congespirin for Children Liquid Cold Medicine
Congestant D
Contac Allergy/Sinus Day Caplets
Contac Allergy/Sinus Night Caplets
Contac Jr. Children's Cold Medicine
Contac Maximum Strength Sinus Caplets
Contac Night Caplets
Contac Non-Drowsy Formula Sinus Caplets
Contac Severe Cold Formula
Contac Severe Cold Formula Night Strength
Coricidin D Decongestant
Coricidin D Medilets
Coricidin Demilets
Coricidin Maximum Strength Sinus Headache
CoTylenol Cold Medication
Covangesic
Dapa
Dapacin Cold
Datril Extra Strength
DayCare
DayQuil Liquicaps
DayQuil Non-Drowsy Cold/Flu

DayQuil Non-Drowsy Cold/Flu
  Liquicaps
DayQuil Non-Drowsy Sinus
  Pressure and Pain Relief
  Caplets
Dilotab
Dimetapp Cold and Flu Caplets
Dimetapp Plus Caplets
Dimetapp-A
Dimetapp-A Pediatric
Dolanex
Dolmar
Dorcol Children's Fever and Pain
  Reducer
Drinophen
Dristan AF
Dristan AF Plus
Dristan Cold and Flu
Dristan Cold Caplets
Dristan Cold Maximum Strength
  Caplets
Dristan Cold Multi-Symptom
  Formula
Dristan Juice Mix-in Cold, Flu,
  and Cough
Drixoral Cold and Flu
Drixoral Plus
Drixoral Sinus
Duadacin
Endolor
Esgic
Esgic Plus
Excedrin Caplets
Exdol
Exdol Strong
Ezol
Febridyne
Femcet
Fendol
Feverall Children's
Feverall Infants'
Feverall Junior Strength
Feverall Sprinkle Caps
Fioricet
Genapap
Genapap Children's Elixir
Genapap Children's Tablets
Genapap Extra Strength
Genapap Infants'
Genapap Regular Strength
  Tablets
Gendecon
Gen-D-phen
Genebs
Genebs Extra Strength
Genebs Regular Strength Tablets
Genex
Genite
Halenol
Halenol Extra Strength
Histagesic Modified
Histosal
Hycomine Compound
Improved Sino-Tuss
Infants' Anacin-3
Infants' Apacet
Infants' Genapap
Infants' Panadol
Infants' Tylenol Suspension
  Drops
Isopap
Kolephrin
Kolephrin/DM Caplets

Liquiprin Children's Elixir
Liquiprin Infants' Drops
Mapap Cold Formula
Maximum Strength Tylenol
  Allergy Sinus Caplets
Maximum Strength Tylenol Flu
  Gelcaps
Meda Cap
Meda Tab
Medi-Flu
Medi-Flu Caplets
Medigesic
Myapap Elixir
Naldegesic
ND-Gesic
Neocitrin Colds and Flu Calorie
  Reduced
NeoCitrin Extra Strength Colds
  and Flu
NeoCitrin Extra Strength Sinus
Neopap
Nighttime Pamprin
Norel Plus
NyQuil Hot Therapy
NyQuil Liquicaps
NyQuil Nighttime Colds Medicine
Nytcold Medicine
Nytime Cold Medicine Liquid
Omnicol
Oraphen-PD
Ornex Maximum Strength
  Caplets
Ornex No Drowsiness Caplets
Pacaps
Panadol
Panadol Extra Strength
Panadol Junior Strength Caplets
Panadol Maximum Strength
  Caplets
Panadol Maximum Strength
  Tablets
Panex
Panex 500
Paracetamol
Parafon Forte
Pedric
Pertussin All Night PM
PhenAPAP No. 2
Phenapap Sinus Headache &
  Congestion
Phenaphen
Phrenilin
Phrenilin Forte
Pyrroxate
Redutemp
Remcol Cold
Remcol-C
Repan
Rhinocaps
Rhinogesic
Robigesic
Robitussin Night Relief
Robitussin Night Relief Colds
  Formula Liquid
Rounox
Saleto-CF
Saleto-D
Sedapap
Semcet
Simplet
Sinapils
Sinarest
Sinarest Extra Strength

Sinarest No Drowsiness
Sinarest Sinus
Sine-Aid
Sine-Aid Maximum Strength
Sine-Aid Maximum Strength
  Caplets
Sine-Aid Maximum Strength
  Gelcaps
Sine-Off Maximum Strength
  Allergy/Sinus Formula Caplets
Sine-Off Maximum Strength No
  Drowsiness Formula Caplets
Singlet
Sinubid
Sinulin
Sinus Excedrin Extra Strength
Sinus Excedrin Extra Strength
  Caplets
Sinus Excedrin No Drowsiness
Sinus Excedrin No Drowsiness
  Caplets
Sinus Relief
Sinutab
Sinutab Extra Strength
Sinutab II Maximum Strength
Sinutab Maximum Strength Sinus
  Allergy
Sinutab Maximum Strength Sinus
  Allergy Caplets
Sinutab Maximum Strength
  without Drowsiness
Sinutab Maximum Strength
  without Drowsiness Caplets
Sinutab No Drowsiness
Sinutab No Drowsiness Extra
  Strength
Sinutab Regular
Sinutab SA
Sinutrex Extra Strength
Snaplets-FR
St. Joseph Aspirin Free Fever
  Reducer for Children
St. Joseph Cold Tablets for
  Children
Sudafed Cold & Cough Liquid
  Caps
Sudafed Severe Cold Formula
  Caplets
Sudafed Sinus Maximum
  Strength
Sudafed Sinus Maximum
  Strength Caplets
Summit
Super-Anahist
Suppap
Tapanol
Tapanol Extra Strength
Tapar
Tempra
Tempra Caplets
Tempra Chewable Tablets
Tempra Double Strength
Tempra Drops
Tempra D.S.
Tempra Infants
Tempra Syrup
Tencet
Tenol
TheraFlu Maximum Strength
  Non-Drowsy Formula Flu, Cold
  and Cough Medicine
TheraFlu Nighttime Maximum
  Strength

TheraFlu/Flu & Cold
TheraFlu/Flu, Cold & Cough
Thera-Hist
Triad
Triaminic Sore Throat Formula
Triaminicin Cold, Allergy, Sinus
Triaminicin with Codeine
Triaprin
Tricom Tablets
Two-Dyne
Ty-Cold Cold Formula
Tylenol
Tylenol Allergy Sinus Gelcaps
Tylenol Allergy Sinus NightTime
  Maximum Strength Caplets
Tylenol Arthritis Extended Relief
Tylenol Caplets
Tylenol Children's Chewable
  Tablets
Tylenol Children's Elixir
Tylenol Children's Suspension
  Liquid
Tylenol Cold and Flu
Tylenol Cold and Flu No
  Drowsiness Powder
Tylenol Cold Medication
Tylenol Cold Medication,
  Non-Drowsy
Tylenol Cold Night Time
Tylenol Cold No Drowsiness
  Formula Gelcaps
Tylenol Cough
Tylenol Cough with Decongestant
Tylenol Extra Strength
Tylenol Infants' Drops
Tylenol Junior Strength
Tylenol Junior Strength
  Chewable Tablets
Tylenol Maximum Strength
  Cough
Tylenol Maximum Strength Flu
  Gelcaps
Tylenol Maximum Strength
  Gelcaps
Tylenol Regular Strength Caplets
Tylenol Regular Strength Tablets
Tylenol Sinus Maximum Strength
Tylenol Sinus Maximum Strength
  Caplets
Tylenol Sinus Medication
Tylenol Sinus Medication Extra
  Strength
Ty-Pap
Valadol
Valadol Liquid
Valorin
Valorin Extra
Vicks 44 Cold, Flu and Cough
  Liqui-Caps
Vicks 44M Cough, Cold and Flu
  Relief
Vicks 44M Cough, Cold and Flu
  Relief LiquiCaps
Vicks Formula 44M Multi-
  Symptom Cough Mixture
Vicks NyQuil Multi-Symptom
  Cold/Flu Relief
Vicks NyQuil Multi-Symptom
  LiquiCaps

ACETAMINOPHEN & SALICYLATES

GENERIC NAMES
1. ACETAMINOPHEN & ASPIRIN
2. ACETAMINOPHEN &
   SALICYLAMIDE
3. ACETAMINOPHEN, ASPIRIN &
   SALICYLAMIDE

BRAND NAMES
Buffets II[1]
Duoprin[2]
Duradyne[1]
Excedrin Extra Strength Caplets[1]
Excedrin Extra Strength Tablets[1]
Excedrin Migraine[1]
Gelpirin[1]
Gemnisyn[1]
Goody's Extra Strength Tablet[1]
Goody's Headache Powders[1]
Presalin[3]
Rid-A-Pain Compound[2]
S-A-C[2]
Saleto[3]
Salphenyl[2]
Supac[1]
Tenol Plus[1]
Trigesic[1]
Tri-Pain[3]
Vanquis[1]

ADRENOCORTICOIDS (Systemic)

GENERIC NAMES
1. BETAMETHASONE
2. CORTISONE
3. DEXAMETHASONE
4. HYDROCORTISONE (Cortisol)
5. METHYLPREDNISOLONE
6. PREDNISOLONE
7. PREDNISONE
8. TRIAMCINOLONE

BRAND NAMES
Apo-Prednisone[7]
Aristocort[8]
Betnelan[1]
Betnesol[1]
Celestone[1]
Cortef[4]
Cortenema[4]
Cortifoam[4]
Cortone[2]
Cortone Acetate[2]
Decadron[3]
Delta-Cortef[6]
Deltasone[7]
Deronil[3]
Dexasone[3]
Dexone 0.5[3]
Dexone 0.75[3]
Dexone 1.5[3]
Dexone 4[3]
Hexadrol[3]
Hydeltrasol[6]
Hydeltra-TBA[6]
Hydrocortone[4]
Kenacort[8]
Kenacort Diacetate[8]
Medrol[5]
Meprolonel[5]
Meticorten[7]

Mymethasone[3]
Nor-Pred-TBA[6]
Oradexon[3]
Orasone 1[7]
Orasone 5[7]
Orasone 10[7]
Orasone 20[7]
Orasone 50[7]
Pediapred[6]
Predisone Intensol[7]
Prednicen-M[7]
Prelone[6]
Sterapred DS[7]
Winpred[7]

ADRENOCORTICOIDS (Topical)

GENERIC NAMES
1. ALCLOMETASONE (Topical)
2. AMCINONIDE (Topical)
3. BECLOMETHASONE (Topical)
4. BETAMETHASONE (Topical)
5. CLOBETASOL (Topical)
6. CLOBETASONE (Topical)
7. CLOCORTOLONE (Topical)
8. CORTISOL
9. DESONIDE (Topical)
10. DESOXIMETASONE (Topical)
11. DEXAMETHASONE (Topical)
12. DIFLORASONE (Topical)
13. DIFLUCORTOLONE (Topical)
14. FLUMETHASONE (Topical)
15. FLUOCINOLONE (Topical)
16. FLUOCINONIDE (Topical)
17. FLURANDRENOLIDE (Topical)
18. FLUTICASONE
19. HALCINONIDE (Topical)
20. HALOBETASOL
21. HYDROCORTISONE (Dental)
22. HYDROCORTISONE (Topical)
23. METHYLPREDNISOLONE
24. MOMETASONE (Topical)
25. PREDNICARBATE
26. TRIAMCINOLONE (Dental)
27. TRIAMCINOLONE (Topical)

BRAND NAMES
9-1-1[22]
Aclovate[1]
Acticort-100[22]
Adcortyl[27]
Aeroseb-Dex[11]
Aeroseb-HC[22]
Ala-Cort[22]
Ala-Scalp HP[22]
Allercort[22]
Alphaderm[22]
Alphatrex[4]
Anucort-HC[22]
Anusol-HC[22]
Anusol-HC 2.5%[22]
Aristocort[27]
Aristocort A[27]
Aristocort C[27]
Aristocort D[27]
Aristocort R[27]
Bactine[22]
Barriere-HC[22]
Beben[4]
Beta HC[22]
Betacort Scalp Lotion[4]
Betaderm[4]

Betaderm Scalp Lotion[4]
Betamethacot[4]
Betatrex[4]
Beta-Val[4]
Betnovate[4]
Betnovate 1/2[4]
Bio-Syn[15]
CaldeCORT Anti-Itch[22]
CaldeCORT-Light[22]
Carmol-HC[22]
Celestoderm-V[4]
Celestoderm-V/2[4]
Cetacort[22]
Cloderm[7]
Cordran[17]
Cordran SP[17]
Cormax[5]
Cortacet[22]
Cortaid[22]
Cortaid FastStick[22]
Cortate[22]
Cort-Dome[22]
Cort-Dome High Potency[22]
Cortef[22]
Cortef Feminine Itch[22]
Corticaine[22]
Corticreme[22]
Cortifair[22]
Cortiment-10[22]
Cortiment-40[22]
Cortoderm[22]
Cortril[22]
Cultivate[18]
Cyclocort[2]
Decaderm[11]
Decadron[11]
Decaspray[11]
Delacort[22]
Delta-Tritex[27]
Demarest DriCort[22]
Dermabet[4]
Dermacomb[27]
Dermacort[22]
DermAtop[25]
DermiCort[22]
Dermovate[5]
Dermovate Scalp Application[5]
Dermtex HC[22]
DesOwen[9]
Diprolene[4]
Diprolene AF[4]
Diprosone[4]
Drenison[17]
Drenison-1/4[17]
Ectosone[4]
Ectosone Regular[4]
Ectosone Scalp Lotion[4]
Efcortelan[22]
Elocom[24]
Elocon[24]
Emo-Cort[22]
Emo-Cort Scalp Solution[22]
Epifoam[8]
Eumovate[6]
Florone[12]
Florone E[12]
Fludroxycortide[17]
Fluocet[15]
Fluocin[16]
Fluoderm[15]
Fluolar[15]
Fluonid[15]
Fluonide[15]

Flurosyn[15]
Flutex[27]
Foille Cort[22]
Gly-Cort[22]
Gynecort[22]
Gynecort 10[22]
Halciderm[19]
Halog[19]
Halog E[19]
Hi-Cor 1.0[22]
Hi-Cor 2.5[22]
Hyderm[22]
Hydro-Tex[22]
Hytone[22]
Kenac[27]
Kenalog[27]
Kenalog in Orabase[27]
Kenalog-H[27]
Kenonel[27]
Lacticare-HC[22]
Lanacort[22]
Lanacort 10[22]
Lemoderm[22]
Licon[16]
Lidemol[16]
Lidex[16]
Lidex-E[16]
Locacorten[14]
Locoid[22]
Lotrisone[4]
Lyderm[16]
Maxiflor[12]
Maximum Strength Cortald[22]
Maxivate[4]
Metaderm Mild[4]
Metaderm Regular[4] (Topical)
Metosyn[16]
Metosyn FAPG[16]
My Cort[22]
Nerisone[13]
Nerisone Oily[13]
Novobetamet[4]
Novohydrocort[22]
Nutracort[22]
Orabase HCA[22]
Oracort[27]
Oralone[27]
Pandel[22]
Penecort[22]
Pentacort[22]
Pharma-Cort[22]
Prevex B[4]
Prevex HC[4]
Propaderm[3]
Psorcon[12]
Rederm[22]
Rhulicort[22]
Sarna HC[22]
Sential[22]
S-T Cort[22]
Synacort[22]
Synalar[15]
Synalar HP[15]
Synamol[15]
Synemol[15]
Teladar[4]
Temovate[5]
Temovate E[5]
Temovate Emollient[5]
Temovate Gel[5]
Temovate Scalp Application[5]
Texacort[22]
Topicort[10]

Topicort LP[10]
Topicort Mild[10]
Topilene[4]
Topisone[4]
Topsyn[16]
Triacet[27]
Triaderm[27]
Trianide Mild[27]
Trianide Regular[27]
Triderm[27]
Tridesilon[9]
Trymex[27]
Ultravate[20]
Unicort[22]
Uticort[4]
Valisone[4]
Valisone Reduced Strength[4]
Valisone Scalp Lotion[4]
Valnac[4]
Vioform-Hydrocortisone Lotion[22]
Westcort[22]
Some of these brands are available as oral medicine. Look under specific generic name for each brand.

ANDROGENS

GENERIC NAMES
1. ETHYLESTRENOL
2. FLUOXYMESTERONE
3. METHYLTESTOSTERONE
4. NANDROLONE
5. OXANDROLONE
6. OXYMETHOLONE
7. STANOZOLOL
8. TESTOSTERONE

BRAND NAMES
Anabolin[4]
Anabolin LA 100[4]
Anadral[6]
Anapolon 50[6]
Andro 100[8]
Andro-Cyp 100[8]
Andro-Cyp 200[8]
Androderm[8]
Android-10[3]
Android-25[3]
Android-T[8]
Andro-LA 200[8]
Androlone[4]
Andronaq-50[8]
Andronaq-LA[8]
Andronate 100[8]
Andronate 200[8]
Andropository 100[8]
Andryl 200[8]
Deca-Durabolin[4]
Delatest[8]
Delatestryl[8]
Dep Andro 100[8]
Dep Andro 200[8]
Depotest[8]
Depo-Testosterone[8]
Durabolin[4]
Duratest 100[8]
Duratest-200[8]
Durathate 200[8]
Everone[8]
Halotestin[2]
Histerone-50[8]
Histerone-100[8]

Hybolin Decanoate[4]
Hybolin-Improved[4]
Kabolin[4]
Malogen[8]
Malogex[8]
Maxibolin[4]
Metandren[3]
Nandrobolic[4]
Nandrobolic L.A.[4]
Neo-Durabolic[4]
Ora-Testryl[2]
Oreton[3]
T-Cypionate[8]
Testa-C[8]
Testamone 100[8]
Testaqua[8]
Testex[8]
Testoderm with Adhesive[8]
Testoject-50[8]
Testoject-LA[8]
Testone L.A.[8]
Testred[3]
Testred-Cypionate 200[8]
Testrin P.A.[8]
Virilon[3]
Virolon IM[3]
Winstrol[7]

ANDROGENS & ESTROGENS

GENERIC NAMES
1. CONJUGATED ESTROGENS & METHYLTESTOSTERONE
2. DIETHYLSTILBESTROL (DES) & METHYLTESTOSTERONE
3. ESTERIFIED ESTROGENS & METHYLTESTOSTERONE
4. FLUOXYMESTERONE & ETHINYL ESTRADIOL
5. TESTOSTERONE & ESTRADIOL

BRAND NAMES
Andrest 90-4[5]
Andro-Estro 90-4[5]
Androgyn L.A[5]
Climacteron[5]
De-Comberol[5]
Deladumone[5]
Delatestadiol[5]
Dep-Androgyn[5]
Depo-Testadiol[5]
Depotestogen[5]
Duo-Cyp[5]
Duo-Gen L.A.[5]
Duogex L.A.[5]
Dura-Dumone 90/4[5]
Duratestin[5]
Estratest[3]
Estratest H.S.[3]
Halodrin[4]
Menoject L.A.[5]
Neo-Pause[5]
OB[5]
Premarin with Methyltestosterone[1]
Teev[5]
Tes Est Cyp[5]
Test-Estro Cypionate[5]
Tylosterone[2]
Valertest No. 1[5]
Valertest No. 2[5]

ANESTHETICS (Topical)

GENERIC NAMES
1. BENZOCAINE
2. BENZOCAINE & MENTHOL
3. BUTAMBEN
4. DIBUCAINE
5. LIDOCAINE
6. LIDOCAINE & PRILOCAINE
7. PRAMOXINE
8. TETRACAINE
9. TETRACAINE & MENTHOL

BRAND NAMES
Americaine[1]
Amercaine Topical Anesthetic First Aid Ointment[1]
Amercaine Topical Anesthetic Spray[1]
Benzocol[2]
Butesin Picrate[3]
Butyl Aminobenzoate[2]
Cinchocaine[4]
Dermoplast[2]
Emla [6]
Endocaine[1]
Ethyl Aminobenzoate[1]
Lagol[1]
Lignocaine[5]
Nupercainal Cream[4]
Nupercainal Ointment[4]
Pontocaine Cream[8]
Pontocaine Ointment[9]
Pramegel[7]
Prax[7]
Tronothane[7]
Unguentine[1]
Unguentine Plus[1]
Unguentine Spray[1]
Xylocaine[5]

ANGIOTENSIN-CONVERTING ENZYME (ACE) INHIBITORS

GENERIC NAMES
1. BENAZEPRIL
2. CAPTOPRIL
3. ENALAPRIL
4. FOSINOPRIL
5. LISINOPRIL
6. MOEXIPRIL
7. PERINDOPRIL
8. QUINAPRIL
9. RAMIPRIL
10. TRANDOLAPRIL

BRAND NAMES
Accupril[8]
Aceon[7]
Altace[9]
Apo-Capto[2]
Capoten[2]
Lexxel[3]
Lotensin[1]
Lotrel[1]
Mavik[10]
Monopril[4]
Novo-Captoril[2]
Prinivil[5]
Syn-Captopril[2]
Tarka[10]
Teczem[3]
Uniretic[6]
Univasc[6]
Vasotec[3]
Zestril[5]

ANGIOTENSIN-CONVERTING ENZYME (ACE) INHIBITORS & HYDROCHLORO-THIAZIDE

GENERIC NAMES
1. CAPTOPRIL & HYDROCHLOROTHIAZIDE
2. ENALAPRIL & HYDROCHLOROTHIAZIDE
3. LISINOPRIL & HYDROCHLOROTHIAZIDE

BRAND NAMES
Capozide[1]
Prinzide[3]
Vaseretic[2]
Zestoretic[3]

ANTACIDS

GENERIC NAMES
1. ALUMINA & MAGNESIA
2. ALUMINA & MAGNESIUM CARBONATE
3. ALUMINA & MAGNESIUM TRISILICATE
4. ALUMINA, MAGNESIA, & CALCIUM CARBONATE
5. ALUMINA, MAGNESIA, & SIMETHICONE
6. ALUMINA, MAGNESIUM CARBONATE, & CALCIUM CARBONATE
7. ALUMINA, MAGNESIUM TRISILICATE, & SODIUM BICARBONATE
8. ALUMINUM CARBONATE, BASIC
9. ALUMINUM HYDROXIDE
10. CALCIUM & MAGNESIUM CARBONATES
11. CALCIUM CARBONATE
12. CALCIUM CARBONATE & MAGNESIA
13. CALCIUM CARBONATE & SIMETHICONE
14. CALCIUM CARBONATE, MAGNESIA, & SIMETHICONE
15. CALCIUM, MAGNESIUM CARBONATES & MAGNESIUM OXIDE
16. DIHYDROXYALUMINUM AMINOACETATE
17. DIHYDROXYALUMINUM AMINOACETATE, MAGNESIA, & ALUMINA
18. DIHYDROXYALUMINUM SODIUM CARBONATE
19. MAGALDRATE
20. MAGALDRATE & SIMETHICONE
21. MAGNESIUM CARBONATE & SODIUM BICARBONATE
22. MAGNESIUM HYDROXIDE
23. MAGNESIUM OXIDE
24. MAGNESIUM TRISILICATE, ALUMINA, & MAGNESIA

BRAND NAMES

Advanced Formula Di-Gel[14]
Alamag[1]
Algenic Alka[2]
Algenic Alka Improved[2]
Algicon[9]
Alka-Mints[11]
Alkets[11]
Almacone[5]
Almacone II[5]
Alma-Mag #4 Improved[5]
Alma-Mag Improved[5]
AlternaGEL[9]
Alu-Cap[9]
Aludrox[5]
Alu-Tab[9]
Amitone[12]
Amphojel[9]
Amphojel 500[1]
Amphojel Plus[4]
AntaGel[5]
AntaGel-II[5]
Basaljel[9]
Bisodol[21]
Calglycine[11]
Camalox[4]
Chooz[11]
Creamalin[1]
Dialume[9]
Dicarbosil[11]
Di-Gel[5]
Diovol Ex[1]
Diovol Plus[5]
Duracid[9]
Equilet[11]
Foamicon[3]
Gaviscon[2]
Gaviscon Extra Strength Relief
   Formula[9]
Gaviscon-2[7]
Gelusil[5]
Gelusil Extra-Strength[1]
Gelusil-II[5]
Gelusil-M[5]
Genalac[11]
Glycate[11]
Kudrox Double Strength[5]
Lowsium[19]
Lowsium Plus[20]
Maalox[1]
Maalox No. 1[1]
Maalox No. 2[1]
Maalox Plus[5]
Maalox Plus, Extra Strength[5]
Maalox TC[1]
Magnagel[2]
Magnalox[5]
Magnalox Plus[5]
Magnatril[9]
Mag-Ox 400[23]
Mallamint[11]
Maox[23]
Marblen[10]
Mi-Acid[5]
Mintox[1]
Mintox Plus[5]
Mygel[5]
Mygel II[5]
Mylagen[5]
Mylagen II[5]
Mylanta[5]
Mylanta Calcium-Rich[12]

Mylanta Calcium-Rich Double
   Strength[12]
Mylanta Double Strength[5]
Mylanta Double Strength Plain[5]
Mylanta Gelcaps[10]
Mylanta Plain[5]
Mylanta-2 Extra Strength[5]
Mylanta-II[5]
Nephrox[9]
Neutralca-S[1]
Noralac[10]
Phillips' Milk of Magnesia[22]
Riopan[19]
Riopan Extra Strength[19]
Riopan Plus[20]
Riopan Plus 2[20]
Riopan Plus Extra Strength[20]
Rolaids[12]
Rolaids Calcium Rich[11]
Rolaids Sodium Free[11]
Rulox[1]
Rulox No. 1[1]
Rulox No. 2[1]
Rulox Plus[5]
Silain-Gel[5]
Simaal 2 Gel[5]
Simaal Gel[5]
Spastosed[10]
Tempo[26]
Titracid[11]
Titralac[11]
Titralac Plus[11]
Triconsil[7]
Tums[11]
Tums E-X[11]
Tums Liquid Extra Strength[11]
Tums Liquid Extra Strength
   with Simethicone[13]
Univol[1]
Uro-Mag[23]

ANTIBACTERIALS
(Ophthalmic)

GENERIC NAMES

1. CHLORAMPHENICOL
2. CHLORTETRACYCLINE
3. CIPROFLOXACIN
4. ERYTHROMYCIN (Ophthalmic)
5. GENTAMICIN (Ophthalmic)
6. NEOMYCIN
7. NEOMYCIN, POLYMIXIN B &
   BACITRACIN
8. NEOMYCIN, POLYMIXIN B &
   CORTISOL
9. NEOMYCIN, POLYMIXIN B &
   GRAMICIDIN
10. NEOMYCIN, POLYMIXIN B &
    HYDROCORTISONE
11. NORFLOXACIN (Ophthalmic)
12. OFLOXACIN (Ophthalmic)
13. POLYMYXIN B
14. SULFACETAMIDE
    (Ophthalmic)
15. SULFISOXAZOLE
    (Ophthalmic)
16. SULFONAMIDES
    (Ophthalmic)
17. TETRACYCLINE (Ophthalmic)
18. TOBRAMYCIN (Ophthalmic)

BRAND NAMES
Achromycin[17]
Aerosporin[13]

Ak-Chlor Ophthalmic Ointment[1]
Ak-Chlor Ophthalmic Solution[14]
Ak-Spore[13]
Ak-Sulf[14]
Aktob[18]
Alcomicin[5]
Aureomycin[2]
Bio-Triple[13]
Bleph-10[14]
Cetamide[14]
Chibroxin[11]
Chloracol Ophthalmic Solution
   (Ophthalmic)[1]
Chlorofair Ophthalmic Ointment[1]
Chlorofair Ophthalmic Solution[1]
Chloromycetin Ophthalmic
   Ointment[1]
Chloromycetin Ophthalmic
   Solution[1]
Chloroptic Ophthalmic Solution[1]
Chloroptic S.O.P.[1]
Ciloxan[3]
Cortisporin-Ophthalmic[13]
Econochlor Ophthalmic
   Ointment[1]
Econochlor Ophthalmic Solution[1]
Fenicol Ophthalmic Ointment[1]
Gantrisin[15]
Garamycin[5]
Genoptic[5]
Gentacidin[5]
Gentafair[5]
Gentak[5]
Gentrasul[5]
I-Chlor Ophthalmic Solution[1]
Ilotycin[4]
Isopto Cetamide[14]
I-Sulfacet[14]
Mycitracin[13]
Neociden Ophthalmic Ointment[7]
Neociden Ophthalmic Solution[9]
Neosporin[13]
Neosporin Ophthalmic Solution[13]
Neotal[13]
Neotricin[13]
Ocu-Chlor Ophthalmic Ointment[1]
Ocu-Chlor Ophthalmic Solution[1]
Ocuflox[12]
Ocu-Mycin[13]
Ocu-Spor-B[13]
Ocu-Spor-G[13]
Ocusporin[13]
Ocu-Sul-10[14]
Ocu-Sul-15[14]
Ocu-Sul-30[14]
Ocusulf-10[14]
Ocutricin[13]
Ophthacet[14]
Ophthalmic
Ophthochlor Ophthalmic
   Solution[1]
Ophtho-Chloram Ophthalmic
   Solution[1]
Pentamycetin[10]
Pentamycetin Ophthalmic
   Ointment[10]
Pentamycetin Ophthalmic
   Solution[10]
P.N. Ophthalmic[13]
Regasporin[7]
Sodium Sulamyd[14]
Sopamycetin Ophthalmic
   Ointment[10]

Sopamycetin Ophthalmic
  Solution[10]
Spectro-Chlor Ophthalmic
  Ointment[1]
Spectro-Chlor Ophthalmic
  Solution[1]
Spectro-Genta[5]
Spectro-Sporin[13]
Spectro-Sulf[14]
Steri-Units Sulfacetamide[14]
Sulf-10[14]
Sulfair[14]
Sulfair 10[14]
Sulfair 15[14]
Sulfair Forte[14]
Sulfamide[14]
Sulfex[14]
Sulten-10[14]
Tobrex[18]
Tribiotic[13]
Tri-Ophthalmic[13]
Triple Antibiotic[9]
Tri-Thalmic[13]

ANTICHOLINERGICS

GENERIC NAMES
1. ANISOTROPINE
2. ATROPINE
3. CHLORPHENIRAMINE
   MALEATE
4. HOMATROPINE
5. ISOPROPAMIDE
6. MEPENZOLATE
7. METHANTHELINE
8. METHSCOPOLAMINE
9. OXYPHENCYCLIMINE
10. PIRENZEPINE
11. TRIDIHEXETHYL

BRAND NAMES
AH-Chew[8]
Atrohist Plus[3]
Banthine[7]
Baycodan[4]
Cantil[6]
Codan[4]
D.A. Chewable[3]
Dallergy[3]
Dallergy Caplets[3]
Darbid[5]
Daricon[9]
Dura-Vent/DA[3]
Extendryl[3]
Extendryl JR[3]
Extendryl SR[3]
Gastrozepin[10]
Histor-D Timecelles[3]
Homapin[4]
Hycodan[4]
Hydromet[4]
Hydropane[7]
OMNIhist L.A.[3]
Pamine[8]
Pathilon[11]
Phenahist-TR[3]
Phenchlor SHA[3]
Prehist D[3]
Rhinolar[3]
Ru-Tuss[3]
Stahist[3]
Tussigon[4]
Valpin 50[1]

ANTIDEPRESSANTS, TRICYCLIC

GENERIC NAMES
1. AMITRYPTILINE
2. AMOXAPINE
3. CLOMIPRAMINE
4. DESIPRAMINE
5. DOXEPIN
6. IMIPRAMINE
7. NORTRIPTYLINE
8. PROTRIPTYLINE
9. TRIMIPRAMINE

BRAND NAMES
Adapin[5]
Anafranil[3]
Apo-Amitriptyline[1]
Apo-Imipramine[6]
Apo-Trimip[9]
Asendin[2]
Aventyl[7]
Elavil[1]
Emitrip[1]
Endep[1]
Enovil[1]
Impril[6]
Janimine[6]
Levate[1]
Limbitrol[1]
Limbitrol DS[1]
Norfranil[6]
Norpramin[4]
Novo-Doxepin[5]
Novopramine[6]
Novo-Tripramine[9]
Novotriptyn[1]
Pamelor[7]
Pertofrane[4]
PMS Amitriptyline[1]
PMS Imipramine[6]
Rhotrimine[9]
Sinequan[5]
Surmontil[9]
Tipramine[6]
Tofranil[6]
Tofranil-PM[6]
Triadapin[5]
Triptil[8]
Vivactil[8]

ANTIDIABETIC AGENTS, SULFONYLUREA

GENERIC NAMES
1. ACETOHEXAMIDE
2. CHLORPROPAMIDE
3. GLICLAZIDE
4. GLIMEPIRIDE
5. GLIPIZIDE
6. GLYBURIDE
7. TOLAZAMIDE
8. TOLBUTAMIDE

BRAND NAMES
Albert Glyburide[6]
Amaryl[4]
Apo-Chlorpropamide[2]
Apo-Glyburide[6]
Apo-Tolbutamide[8]
DiaBeta[6]
Diabinese[2]
Diamicron[3]
Dimelor[1]
Dymelor[1]
Euglucon[6]
Gen-Glybe[6]
Glucamide[2]
Glucotrol[5]
Glucotrol XL[5]
Glynase PresTab[3]
Micronase[6]
Novo-Butamide[8]
Novo-Glyburide[5]
Novo-Propamide[2]
Orinase[8]
Tolamide[7]
Tolinase[7]

ANTIDYSKINETICS

GENERIC NAMES
1. BENZTROPINE
2. BIPERIDEN
3. ETHOPROPAZINE
4. PIMOZIDE
5. PRAMIPEXOLE
6. PROCYCLIDINE
7. ROPINIROLE
8. TRIHEXYPHENIDYL

BRAND NAMES
Akineton[2]
Apo-Benztropine[1]
Apo-Trihex[3]
Artane[8]
Artane Sequels[8]
Cogentin[1]
Kemadrin[6]
Mirapex[5]
Orap[4]
Parsidol[3]
Parsitan[3]
PMS Benztropine[1]
PMS Procyclidine[6]
PMS Trihexyphenidyl[8]
Procyclid[6]
Requip[7]
Trihexane[8]
Trihexy[8]

ANTIFUNGALS (Topical)

GENERIC NAMES
1. AMPHOTERICIN B
2. BUTENAFINE
3. CICLOPIROX
4. CLOTRIMAZOLE
5. ECONAZOLE
6. FLUCONAZOLE
7. HALOPROGIN
8. KETOCONAZOLE (Topical)
9. MICONAZOLE
10. NAFTIFINE
11. NYSTATIN
12. OXICONAZOLE (Topical)
13. SULCONAZOLE
14. TERBINAFINE
15. TOLNAFTATE
16. UNDECYLENIC ACID

BRAND NAMES
Aftate for Athlete's Foot Aerosol
  Spray Liquid[15]
Aftate for Athlete's Foot Aerosol
  Spray Powder[15]
Aftate for Athlete's Foot Gel[15]
Aftate for Athlete's Foot Sprinkle
  Powder[15]

Aftate for Jock Itch Aerosol
Spray Powder[15]
Aftate for Jock Itch Gel[15]
Aftate for Jock Itch Sprinkle
Powder[15]
Caldesene Medicated Powder[16]
Canesten Cream[4]
Canesten Solution[4]
Cruex Aerosol Powder[16]
Cruex Antifungal Cream[16]
Cruex Antifungal Powder[16]
Cruex Antifungal Spray Powder[16]
Cruex Cream[16]
Cruex Powder[16]
Decylenes[16]
Decylenes Powder[16]
Desenex Aerosol Powder[16]
Desenex Antifungal Cream[16]
Desenex Antifungal Liquid[16]
Desenex Antifungal Ointment[16]
Desenex Antifungal Penetrating
Foam[16]
Desenex Antifungal Powder[16]
Desenex Antifungal Spray
Powder[16]
Desenex Ointment[16]
Desenex Powder[16]
Desenex Solution[16]
Ecostatin[5]
Exelderm[6]
Fungizone[3]
Genaspore Cream[15]
Gordochom Solution[16]
Halotex[7]
Lamisil[14]
Loprox[3]
Lotriderm[4]
Lotrimin AF[4]
Lotrimin Cream[4]
Lotrimin Lotion[4]
Lotrimin Ointment[4]
Lotrisone[4]
Mentax[2]
Micatin[4]
Monistat-Derm[4]
Mycelex Cream[4]
Mycelex Solution[4]
Myclo Cream[4]
Myclo Solution[4]
Myclo Spray[4]
Mycostatin[11]
Nadostine[11]
Naftin[10]
Nilstat[11]
Nizoral Shampoo[8]
NP-27 Cream[15]
NP-27 Powder[15]
NP-27 Solution[15]
NP-27 Spray Powder[15]
Nyaderm[11]
Nystex[11]
Nystop[11]
Oxistat[12]
Pitrex Cream[15]
Spectazole[5]
Tinactin Aerosol Liquid[15]
Tinactin Aerosol Powder[15]
Tinactin Antifungal Deodorant[15]
Powder Aerosol[15]
Tinactin Cream[15]
Tinactin Jock Itch Aerosol
Powder[15]
Tinactin Jock Itch Cream[15]

Tinactin Jock Itch Spray
Powder[15]
Tinactin Plus Powder[15]
Tinactin Powder[15]
Tinactin Solution[15]
Ting Antifungal Cream[15]
Ting Antifungal Powder[15]
Ting Antifungal Spray Liquid[15]
Ting Antifungal Spray Powder[15]
Zeasorb-AF Powder[15]

ANTIFUNGALS (Vaginal)
GENERIC NAMES
1. BUTOCONAZOLE
2. CLOTRIMAZOLE
3. ECONAZOLE
4. GENTIAN VIOLET
5. MICONAZOLE
6. NYSTATIN
7. TERCONAZOLE
8. TIOCONAZOLE

BRAND NAMES
Canesten[2]
Canesten 1[2]
Canesten 3[2]
Canesten 10%[2]
Ecostatin[3]
FemCare[2]
Femizole Prefil[2]
Femizole-7[2]
Femstat 3[1]
Genapax[4]
Gyne-Lotrimin[2]
Gyne-Lotrimin 3[2]
Gyno-Trosyd[8]
Monistat[5]
Monistat 1[8]
Monistat 3[5]
Monistat 5[5]
Monistat 7[5]
Mycelex-7[2]
Mycelex-G[2]
Myclo[2]
Mycostatin[6]
Nadostine[6]
Nilstat[6]
Nyaderm[6]
Terazol 3[7]
Terazol 7[7]
Vagistat[8]
Vagistat-1[8]

ANTIHISTAMINES
GENERIC NAMES
1. ACRIVASTINE
2. AZATADINE
3. BROMODIPHENHYDRAMINE
4. BROMPHENIRAMINE
5. CARBINOXAMINE
6. CHLORPHENIRAMINE
7. CLEMASTINE FUMARATE
8. CYPROHEPTADINE
9. DEXBROMPHENIRAMINE
10. DEXCHLORPHENIRAMINE
11. DIMENHYDRINATE
12. DIPHENHYDRAMINE
13. DIPHENYLPYRALINE
14. DOXYLAMINE
15. PHENINDAMINE
16. PHENIRAMINE
17. PHENYLTOLOXAMINE

18. PYRILAMINE
19. TRIPELENNAMINE
20. TRIPROLIDINE

BRAND NAMES
4 Way Cold[6]
12-Hour Cold[6]
Aclophen[6]
Actacin[20]
Actagen[20]
Actagen-C Cough[20]
Actidil[18]
Actifed[20]
Actifed 12-Hour[20]
Actifed A[20]
Actifed Allergy Nighttime
Caplets[20]
Actifed DM[20]
Actifed Plus[20]
Actifed Plus Caplets
Actifed with Codeine Cough[20]
AH-Chew[6]
Alamine[6]
Alamine-C Liquid[6]
Alersule[6]
Alka-Seltzer Plus Cold[6]
Alka-Seltzer Plus Cold and
Cough[6]
Alka-Seltzer Plus Maximum
Strength Sinus Allergy
Medicine[6]
Alka-Seltzer Plus Nighttime Cold[6]
Allent[5]
Alleract[18]
Aller-Chlor[6]
Allercon[20]
Allerdryl[12]
Allerest 12 Hour[6]
Allerest 12 Hour Maximum
Strength Caplets[6]
Allerest Children's[6]
Allerest Headache Strength[6]
Allerest Maximum Strength[6]
Allerest Sinus Pain Formula[6]
Allerfrim[20]
Allerfrin[20]
Allerfrin with Codeine[20]
Allergy Cold[20]
Allergy Formula Sinutab[9]
Allergy Relief Medicine[6]
AllerMax Caplets[12]
Aller-med[12]
Allerphed[20]
Allert[6]
All-Nite Cold Formula[14]
Alumadrine[6]
Amaril D[6]
Amaril D Spantab[6]
Ambay Cough[3]
Ambenyl Cough[3]
Ambophen Expectorant[3]
Ami-Drix[9]
Anamine[6]
Anamine HD[6]
Anamine T. D.[6]
Anaplex[6]
Anaplex HD[6]
Anaplex S.R.[6]
Anatuss[5]
Anatuss with Codeine[18]
Apo-Dimenhydrinate[11]
Aprodrine[20]
Aprodrine with Codeine[20]

A.R.M. Maximum Strength Caplets[6]
Atrofed[20]
Atrohist Pediatric[6]
Atrohist Pediatric Suspension Dye Free[6, 18]
Atrohist Plus[6]
Atrohist Sprinkle[6]
Banophen[12]
Banophen Caplets[12]
Bayaminicol[6]
Baydec DM Drops[5]
Bayer Select Night Time Cold Caplets[20]
Bayhistine DH[6]
BC Cold Powder[6]
BC Multi-Symptom Cold Powder[6]
Beldin[12]
Belix[12]
Bena-D 10[12]
Bena-D 50[12]
Benadryl 25[12]
Benadryl Allergy/Sinus Headache Caplets[12]
Benadryl Cold[12]
Benadryl Cold Nighttime Liquid[12]
Benadryl Complete Allergy[12]
Benadryl Decongestant[12]
Benadryl Kapseals[12]
Benadryl Plus[12]
Benahist 10[12]
Benahist 50[12]
Ben-Allergin 50[12]
Benaphen[12]
Benoject-10[12]
Benoject-50[12]
Benylin Cold[12]
Benylin Cough[12]
Benylin Decongestant[12]
Biphetane DC Cough[5]
BQ Cold[6]
Brexin[6]
Brexin-L.A[6].
Brofed[5]
Bromaline[5]
Bromaline Plus[5]
Bromanate[5]
Bromanate DC Cough[5]
Bromanyl[3]
Bromarest DX Cough[5]
Bromatane DX Cough[5]
Bromatap[5]
Bromatapp[5]
Bromfed[5]
Bromfed-AT[5]
Bromfed-DM[5]
Bromfed-PD[5]
Bromophen T.D.[5]
Bromphen[5]
Bromphen DC with Codeine Cough[5]
Bromphen DX Cough[5]
Brompheril[9]
Bronkotuss Expectorant[6]
Brotane DX Cough[5]
Bydramine Cough[12]
Caldomine-DH Forte[16,18]
Caldomine-DH Pediatric[16,18]
Calm X[11]
Calmylin #4[12]
Calmylin with Codeine[10]
Carbinoxamine Compound[5]
Carbiset[5]

Carbiset-TR[5]
Carbodec[5]
Carbodec DM Drops[5]
Carbodec TR[5]
Cardec DM[5]
Cardec DM Drops[5]
Cardec DM Pediatric[5]
Cardec-S[5]
Cenafed Plus[20]
Cerose-DM[6]
Cheracol Plus[5]
Cheracol Sinus[5]
Children's Dramamine[11]
Children's Tylenol Cold[6]
Children's Tylenol Cold Multi-Symptom Plus Cough[6]
Chlo-Amine[6]
Chlor-100[6]
Chlorafed[6]
Chlorafed H.S. Timecelles[6]
Chlorafed Timecelles[6]
Chlorate[6]
Chlorgest-HD[6]
Chlor-Niramine[6]
Chlorphed[3]
Chlorphedrine SR[3]
Chlor-Pro[6]
Chlor-Pro 10[6]
Chlor-Rest[6]
Chlorspan-12[6]
Chlortab-4[6]
Chlortab-8[6]
Chlor-Trimeton[6]
Chlor-Trimeton 4 Hour Relief[6]
Chlor-Trimeton 12 Hour Relief[6]
Chlor-Trimeton Allergy[6]
Chlor-Trimeton Decongestant[6]
Chlor-Trimeton Repetabs[6]
Chlor-Trimeton Sinus Caplets[6]
Chlor-Tripolon[6]
Chlor-Tripolon Decongestant[6]
Chlor-Tripolon Decongestant Extra Strength[6]
Chlor-Tripolon Decongestant Repetabs[6]
Citra Forte[6]
CoActifed[20]
CoActifed Expectorant[20]
Co-Apap[6]
Codehist DH[6]
Codimal[6]
Codimal DH[18]
Codimal DM[6]
Codimal PH[18]
Codimal-A[5]
Codimal-L.A.[6]
Codimal-L.A. Half[6]
Colfed-A[6]
Colrex Compound[6]
Colrex Cough[6]
Coltab Children's[6]
Comhist[6]
Comhist LA[6]
Compoz[12]
Comtrex A/S[6]
Comtrex A/S Caplets[5]
Comtrex Hot Flu Relief[6]
Comtrex Maximum Strength Liqui-Gels[6]
Comtrex Multi-Symptom Cold Reliever[6]
Comtrex Multi-Symptom Hot Flu Relief[6]

Comtrex Nighttime[6]
Comtrex Nighttime Maximum Strength Cold and Flu Relief[6]
Comtrex Nighttime Maximum[6] Strength Cold, Cough and Flu Relief[6]
Condrin LA[6]
Conex D.A.[6]
Conex Plus[6]
Congestant D[6]
Conjec-B[5]
Contac 12-Hour[6]
Contac 12-Hour Allergy[7]
Contac Allergy/Sinus Night Caplets[7]
Contac Maximum Strength 12-Hour Caplets[6]
Contac Night Caplets[12]
Contac Severe Cold Formula[6]
Contac Severe Cold Formula Night Strength[6]
Cophene No. 2[6]
Cophene-B[5]
Cophene-S[6]
Cophene-X[17]
Cophene-XP[5]
Co-Pyronil 2[6]
Coricidin D[6]
Coricidin Demilets[6]
Coricidin Maximum Strength Sinus Headache[6]
Coricidin with Codeine[6]
Corsym[6]
Cotridin[20]
Cotridin Expectorant[20]
CoTylenol Cold Medication[6]
Covangesic[6]
D.A. Chewable[6]
Dallergy[6]
Dallergy Caplets[6]
Dallergy Jr[5].
Dallergy-D[6]
Dapacin Cold[6]
Decohistine DH[6]
Deconamine[6]
Deconamine SR[6]
Decongestabs[6]
Dehist[5]
Demazin[10]
Demazin Repetabs[6]
Dexaphen SA[9]
Dexchlor[10]
Dexophed[9]
Diamine T.D.[5]
Dihistine[5]
Dihistine DH[6]
Dimaphen[5]
Dimaphen S.A.[5]
Dimetabs[11]
Dimetane[5]
Dimetane Decongestant Caplets[5]
Dimetane Expectorant[5]
Dimetane Expectorant-C[5]
Dimetane Expectorant-DC[5]
Dimetane Extentabs[5]
Dimetane-DC Cough[5]
Dimetane-DX Cough[5]
Dimetane-Ten[5]
Dimetapp[5]
Dimetapp 4-Hour Liqui-Gels Maximum Strength[5]
Dimetapp Allergy[5]
Dimetapp Allergy Liqui-Gels[5]

PediaCare Cough-Cold[6]
Pediacof Cough[6]
Pelamine[19]
Periactin[8]
Pertussin All Night PM[14]
Pfeiffer's Allergy[6]
Phanadex[18]
Phenahist-TR[6]
Phenapap Sinus Headache & Congestion[6]
Phenchlor SHA[6]
Phendry[12]
Phendry Children's Allergy Medicine[12]
Phenetron[6]
Phenetron Lanacaps[6]
Phenhist DH with Codeine[6]
Phentox Compound[6]
PMS-Dimenhydrinate[11]
Poladex T.D.[10]
Polaramine[10]
Polaramine Expectorant[10]
Polaramine Repetabs[10]
Poly-Histine-CS[5]
Poly-Histine-D[5]
Poly-Histine-D Ped[5]
Poly-Histine-DM[5]
Prehist[6]
Prehist Cough Mixture 4[6]
Prehist D[6]
Prominicol Cough[16,18]
Promist HD Liquid[6]
Pseudo-Car DM[5]
Pseudo-Chlor[6]
Pseudodine C Cough[20]
Pseudo-gest Plus[6]
P-V-Tussin[6]
Pyribenzamine[19]
Pyrilamine Maleate Tablets[18]
Pyrroxate[6]
Quadra-Hist
Quadra-Hist Pediatric Syrup[6]
Quelidrine Cough[6]
Remcol Cold[6]
Remcol-C[6]
Rentamine Pediatric[6]
Resaid S.R.[6]
Rescon-DM[6]
Rescon-ED[6]
Rescon-JR[6]
Resporal TR[9]
Rhinatate[6]
Rhinogesic[6]
Rhinolar[6]
Rhinolar-EX[6]
Rhinolar-EX 12[6]
Rhinosyn[6]
Rhinosyn-DM[6]
Rhinosyn-PD[6]
Rinade B.I.D.[6]
Robitussin A-C[14]
Robitussin Night Relief[18]
Robitussin Night Relief Colds Formula Liquid[18]
Robitussin with Codeine[16]
Rolatuss Expectorant[6]
Rolatuss Plain[6]
Rolatuss with Hydrocodone[16,18]
Rondamine-DM Drops[5]
Rondec[5]
Rondec Drops[5]
Rondec-DM[5]
Rondec-DM Drops[5]

Rondec-TR[5]
R-Tannamine[6]
R-Tannamine Pediatric[6]
R-Tannate[6]
R-Tannate Pediatric[6]
Ru-Tuss[6]
Ru-Tuss with Hydrocodone Liquid[14,18]
Ryna[6]
Ryna-C Liquid[6]
Rynatan[6]
Rynatan Pediatric[6]
Rynatan-S Pediatric[6]
Rynatuss[6]
Rynatuss Pediatric[6]
Salphenyl[6]
Scot-Tussin DM[6]
Scot-Tussin Original 5-Action Cold Medicine[14]
Semprex-D[1]
Siladryl[12]
Silphen[12]
Simplet[6]
Sinapils[6]
Sinarest[6]
Sinarest Extra Strength[6]
Sinarest Sinus[6]
Sine-Off Maximum Strength Allergy/Sinus Formula Caplets[6]
Sine-Off Sinus Medicine[6]
Singlet[6]
Sinucon Pediatric Drops[6]
Sinulin[6]
Sinutab[6]
Sinutab Extra Strength[6]
Sinutab Regular[6]
Sinutab SA[17]
Sinutrex Extra Strength[6]
Sleep-Eze 3[12]
Snaplets Multi[6]
Snaplets-D[6]
Sominex Formula 2[12]
Stahist[6]
Statuss Green[16,18]
Sudafed Plus[6]
Tamine S.R.[5]
Tanoral[6]
Tavist[7]
Tavist-1[7]
Tavist-D[7]
T-Dry[6]
T-Dry Junior[6]
Tega-Vert[11]
Telachlor[6]
Teldrin[6]
Temazin Cold[6]
TheraFlu Nighttime Maximum Strength[6]
TheraFlu/Flu & Cold[6]
TheraFlu/Flu, Cold & Cough[6]
Thera-Hist[6]
Threamine DM[18]
T-Koff[6]
Touro A&H[5]
Travamine[11]
Triacin C Cough[20]
Triafed[20]
Triafed with Codeine[20]
Triaminic[6]
Triaminic Allergy[6]
Triaminic Chewables[6]
Triaminic Cold[6]
Triaminic DM Expectorant[20]

Triaminic DM Nighttime For Children[6]
Triaminic Expectorant[20]
Triaminic Expectorant DH[20]
Triaminic Nite Light[6]
Triaminic Oral Infant Drops[16,18]
Triaminic TR[16,18]
Triaminic-12[6]
Triaminicin Cold, Allergy, Sinus[6]
Triaminicin with Codeine[16,18]
Triaminicol DM[16,18]
Triaminicol Multi-Symptom Relief[6]
Tricodene Forte[6]
Tricodene NN[6]
Tricodene Sugar Free[6]
Tricom Tablets[6]
Trifed[20]
Trifed-C Cough[20]
Trimedine Liquid[6]
Triminol Cough[6]
Trinalin Repetabs[3]
Trind[6]
Trind DM Liquid[6]
Tri-Nefrin Extra Strength[6]
Trinex[6]
Triofed[20]
Triotann[6]
Triotann Pediatric[6]
Tripalgen Cold[6]
Tri-Phen-Chlor[6]
Tri-Phen-Chlor Pediatric[6]
Tri-Phen-Chlor T.R.[6]
Triphenyl[6]
Triphenyl T.D.[16,18]
Tripodrine[20]
Triposed[20]
Trip-Tone[11]
Tritann Pediatric[6]
Tri-Tannate[6]
Tri-Tannate Plus Pediatric[6]
Trymegen[6]
Tusquelin[6]
Tussafed[5]
Tussafed Drops[5]
Tussaminic C[16,18]
Tussaminic C Pediatric[16,18]
Tussaminic DH Forte[16,18]
Tussaminic DH Pediatric[16,18]
Tussanil DH Tablets[6]
Tussanil Plain[6]
Tussar DM[6]
Tussionex[6]
Tussirex with Codeine Liquid[16]
Tuss-Ornade Spansules[6]
Tusstat[6]
Twilite[12]
Ty-Cold Cold Formula[6]
Tylenol Allergy Sinus Gelcaps[12]
Tylenol Allergy Sinus NightTime Maximum Strength Caplets[12]
Tylenol Cold and Flu[6]
Tylenol Cold Medication[6]
Tylenol Cold Night Time[12]
ULTRAbrom PD[5]
Uni-Bent Cough[12]
Uni-DeCon[6]
Unisom Nighttime Sleep Aid[14]
Unisom SleepGels Maximum Strength[12]
Vanex Forte Caplets[6]
Vanex Forte R[6]
Vanex-HD[6]

Veltane[5]
Veltap[5]
Vertab[11]
Vicks 44 Cold, Flu and Cough
Liquid-Caps[17]
Vicks 44M Cough, Cold and Flu
Relief[6]
Vicks 44M Cough, Cold and Flu
Relief LiquiCaps[6]
Vicks Children's NyQuil
Allergy/Head Cold[6]
Vicks DayQuil 4 Hour Allergy
Relief[5]
Vicks DayQuil 12 Hour Allergy
Relief[5]
Vicks NyQuil Multi-Symptom
Cold/Flu Relief[14]
Vicks NyQuil Multi-Symptom
LiquiCaps[14]
Vicks Pediatric Formula 44M
Multi-Symptom Cough & Cold[6]
Viro-Med[6]
Wehamine[11]
Wehdryl[12]
Wehdryl-10[12]
Wehdryl-50[12]

ANTIHISTAMINES, PHENOTHIAZINE-DERIVATIVE

GENERIC NAMES
1. PROMETHAZINE
2. TRIMEPRAZINE

BRAND NAMES
Anergan 25[1]
Anergan 50[1]
Antinaus 50[1]
Histantil[1]
Mallergan-VC with Codeine[1]
Panectyl[2]
Penazine VC with Cough[1]
Pentazine[1]
Phenameth DM[1]
Phenameth VC with Codeine[1]
Phenazine 25[1]
Phenazine 50[1]
Phencen-50[1]
Phenergan[1]
Phenergan Fortis[1]
Phenergan Plain[1]
Phenergan VC[1]
Phenergan VC with Codeine[1]
Phenergan with Codeine[1]
Phenergan with
Dextromethorphan[1]
Phenoject-50[1]
Pherazine DM[1]
Pherazine VC[1]
Pherazine VC with Codeine[1]
Pherazine with Codeine[1]
PMS Promethazine[1]
Pro-50[1]
Pro-Med 50[1]
Promehist with Codeine[1]
Promerhegan[1]
Promet[1]
Prometh VC with Codeine[1]
Prometh VC Plain[1]
Prometh with Dextromethorphan[1]
Prometh-25[1]
Prometh-50[1]

Promethazine DM[1]
Promethazine VC[1]
Prorex-25[1]
Prorex-50[1]
Prothazine[1]
Prothazine Plain[1]
Shogan[1]
TV-Gan-25[1]
V-Gan-50[1]

ANTI-INFLAMMATORY DRUGS, NON-STEROIDAL (NSAIDs)

GENERIC NAMES
1. CELECOXIB
2. DICLOFENAC
3. DIFLUNISAL
4. ETODOLAC
5. FENOPROFEN
6. FLOCTAFENINE
7. FLURBIPROFEN
8. IBUPROFEN
9. INDOMETHACIN
10. KETOPROFEN
11. KETOROLAC
12. MECLOFENAMATE
13. MEFENAMIC ACID
14. NABUMETONE
15. NAPROXEN
16. OXAPROZIN
17. PHENYLBUTAZONE
18. PIROXICAM
19. SULINDAC
20. TENOXICAM
21. TIAPROFENIC ACID
22. TOLMETIN

BRAND NAMES
Aches-N-Pain[8]
Advil[8]
Advil Caplets[8]
Advil Chewable Tablets[8]
Advil Cold and Sinus Caplets[8]
Advil First[8]
Albert Tiafen[21]
Aleve[15]
Alka-Butazolidin[17]
Alkabutazone[17]
Alka-Phenylbutazone[17]
Alrheumat[10]
Amersol[8]
Anaprox[15]
Anaprox DS[15]
Ansaid[7]
Apo-Diclo[2]
Apo-Diflunisal[3]
Apo-Flurbiprofen[7]
Apo-Ibuprofen[8]
Apo-Indomethacin[9]
Apo-Keto[10]
Apo-Keto-E[10]
Apo-Naproxen[15]
Apo-Phenylbutazone[17]
Apo-Piroxicam[18]
Apsifen[8]
Apsifen-F[8]
Arthrotec[2]
Bayer Select Ibuprofen Caplets[8]
Bayer Select Pain Relief Formula
Caplets[8]
Brufen[8]
Butacote[17]

Butazone[17]
Cataflam[2]
Celebrex[1]
Children's Advil[8]
Children's Motrin[8]
Clinoril[19]
CoAdvil Caplets[8]
Cotybutazone[17]
Cramp End[8]
Daypro[16]
Dimetapp Sinus Caplets[8]
Dolgesic[8]
Dolobid[3]
Dristan Sinus Caplets[8]
EC-Naprosyn[15]
Excedrin-IB Caplets[8]
Excedrin-IB Tablets[8]
Feldene[18]
Fenopron[5]
Froben[7]
Froben SR[7]
Genpril[8]
Genpril Caplets[8]
Haltran[8]
Ibifon-600 Caplets[8]
Ibren[8]
Ibu[8]
Ibu-4[8]
Ibu-6[8]
Ibu-8[8]
Ibu-200[8]
Ibumed[8]
Ibuprin[8]
Ibupro-600[8]
Ibu-Tab[8]
Ibutex[8]
Idarac[6]
Ifen[8]
Imbrilon[4]
Indameth[9]
Indocid[9]
Indocid SR[9]
Indocin SR[9]
Lodine[3]
Lodine XL[3]
Meclofen[12]
Meclomen[12]
Medipren[8]
Medipren Caplets[8]
Midol 200[8]
Midol-IB[8]
Mobiflex[20]
Motrin[8]
Motrin, Children's[8]
Motrin-IB[8]
Motrin-IB Caplets[8]
Motrin-IB Sinus[8]
Motrin-IB Sinus Caplets[8]
Nalfon[5]
Nalfon 200[5]
Naprelan[15]
Naprosyn[15]
Naprosyn-E[15]
Naprosyn-SR[15]
Naxen[15]
Novobutazone[17]
Novo-Keto-EC[10]
Novomethacin[9]
Novonaprox[15]
Novopirocam[18]
Novoprofen[8]
Novo-Sundac[19]
Nu-Indo[9]

Nu-Pirox[18]
Nuprin[8]
Nuprin Caplets[8]
Orudis[10]
Orudis-E[10]
Orudis-KT[10]
Orudis-SR[10]
Oruvail[10]
Pamprin-IB[8]
Paxofen[8]
Pedia[8]
Phenylone Plus[17]
Ponstan[13]
Ponstel[13]
Progesic[5]
Relafen[13]
Rhodis[10]
Rhodis-EC[10]
Ro-Profen[8]
Rufen[8]
Saleto-200[8]
Saleto-400[8]
Saleto-600[8]
Saleto-800[8]
Sine-Aid IB[8]
Surgam[21]
Surgam SR[21]
Synflex[15]
Synflex DS[15]
Telectin DS[22]
Toradol[11]
Trendar[8]
Vicoprofen[7]
Voltaren[2]
Voltaren Rapide[2]
Voltaren SR[2]
Voltaren XR[2]
Voltarol[2]
Voltarol Retard[2]

ANTI-INFLAMMATORY DRUGS, STEROIDAL (Ophthalmic)

GENERIC NAMES
1. BETAMETHASONE
2. DEXAMETHASONE
3. FLUOROMETHOLONE
4. HYDROCORTISONE
5. LOTEPREDNOL
6. MEDRYSONE
7. PREDNISOLONE
8. RIMEXOLONE

BRAND NAMES
Ak-Pred[7]
AK-Tate[7]
Alrex[5]
Baldex[2]
Betnesol[1]
Cortamed[4]
Cortisol[4]
Decadron[2]
Dexair[2]
Dexotic[2]
Dexsone[2]
Diodex[2]
Econopred[7]
Econopred Plus[7]
Eflone[3]
Flarex[3]
Fluor-Op[3]
FML Forte[3]

FML Liquifilm[3]
FML S.O.P.[3]
HMS Liquifilm[6]
Inflamase Forte[7]
Inflamase-Mild[7]
I-Pred[7]
Life-Pred[7]
Lotemax[5]
Maxidex[2]
Ocu-Dex[2]
Ocu-Pred[7]
Ocu-Pred Forte[7]
Ocu-Pred-A[7]
PMS-Dexamethasone Sodium Phosphate[2]
Pred Forte[7]
Pred Mild[7]
Predair[7]
Predair Forte[7]
Predair-A[7]
Spersadex[2]
Storz-Dexa[2]
Ultra Pred[7]
Vexol[8]

ANTISEBORRHEICS (Topical)

GENERIC NAMES
1. CHLOROXINE
2. PYRITHIONE
3. SALICYLIC ACID, SULFUR & COAL TAR
4. SELENIUM SULFIDE

BRAND NAMES
Capitrol[1]
Dan-Gard[2]
DHS Zinc Dandruff Shampoo[2]
Exsel[4]
Glo-Sel[4]
Head & Shoulders[2]
Head & Shoulders Antidandruff Cream Shampoo Normal to Dry Formula[2]
Head & Shoulders Antidandruff Cream Shampoo Normal to Oily Formula[2]
Head & Shoulders Antidandruff Lotion Shampoo 2 in 1 Formula[2]
Head & Shoulders Antidandruff Lotion Shampoo Normal to Dry Formula[2]
Head & Shoulders Antidandruff Lotion Shampoo Normal to Oily Formula[2]
Head & Shoulders Dry Scalp 2 in 1 Formula Lotion Shampoo[2]
Head & Shoulders Dry Scalp Conditioning Formula Lotion Shampoo[2]
Head & Shoulders Dry Scalp Regular Formula Lotion Shampoo[2]
Head & Shoulders Intensive Treatment 2 in 1 Formula Dandruff Lotion Shampoo[4]
Head & Shoulders Intensive Treatment Conditioning Formula Dandruff Lotion Shampoo[4]
Head & Shoulders Intensive Treatment Regular Formula Dandruff Lotion Shampoo[4]

Meted Maximum Strength Anti-Dandruff Shampoo with Conditioners[3]
Sebex-T Tar Shampoo[2]
Sebulex Conditioning Suspension Shampoo[3]
Sebulex Lotion Shampoo[3]
Sebulon[2]
Sebutone[3]
Selsun[4]
Selsun Blue[4]
Selsun Blue Dry Formula[4]
Selsun Blue Extra Conditioning Formula[4]
Selsun Blue Extra Medicated Formula[4]
Selsun Blue Oily Formula[4]
Selsun Blue Regular Formula[4]
Theraplex Z[2]
Vanseb Cream Dandruff Shampoo[3]
Vanseb Lotion Dandruff Shampoo[3]
Vanseb-T[3]
Zincon[2]
ZNP[2]

APPETITE SUPPRESSANTS

GENERIC NAMES
1. BENZPHETAMINE
2. DIETHYLPROPION
3. MAZINDOL
4. PHENDIMETRAZINE
5. PHENTERMINE

BRAND NAMES
Adipex-P[5]
Adipost[4]
Adphen[4]
Anorex SR[4]
Anoxine-AM[5]
Appecon[4]
Bontril PDM[4]
Bontril Slow Release[4]
Dapex-37.5[5]
Didrex[1]
Dital[4]
Dyrexan-OD[4]
Fastin[5]
Ionamin[5]
Mazanor[3]
Melfiat-105 Unicelles[4]
Metra[4]
M-Orexic[2]
Obalan[4]
Obe-Del[4]
Obe-Mar[5]
Obe-Nix[5]
Obephen[5]
Obermine[5]
Obestin-30[5]
Obezine[4]
Oby-Trim[5]
Panrexin M[4]
Panrexin MTP[4]
Panshape[5]
Parzine[4]
Phendiet[4]
Phendimet[4]
Phentercot[5]
Phentra[5]
Phentride[5]

Phentrol[5]
Phenzine[4]
Plegine[4]
Prelu-2[4]
Preludin-Endurets[4]
PT 105[4]
Rexigen[4]
Rexigen Forte[4]
Sanorex[3]
Slynn-LL[4]
Statobex[4]
T-Diet[5]
Tega-Nil[1]
Tenuate[2]
Tenuate Dospan[2]
Tepanil[2]
Tepanil Ten-Tab[2]
Teramin[5]
Trimstat[4]
Trimtabs[4]
Wehless[4]
Wehless Timecelles[4]
Weightrol[4]
X-Trozine[4]
X-Trozine LA[4]
Zantryl[5]

ASPIRIN

8-Hour Bayer Timed Release
217
217 Strong
Acetylsalicylic Acid
Alka-Seltzer Effervescent Pain
  Reliever & Antacid
Alka-Seltzer Plus Cold
Alka-Seltzer Plus Cold and
  Cough
Alka-Seltzer Plus Maximum
  Strength Sinus Allergy
  Medicine
Alka-Seltzer Plus Nighttime Cold
Alpha-Phed
Anacin
APAC Improved
APF Arthritic Pain Formula
Arthrinol
Arthrisin
Arthritis Pain Formula
Artria S.R.
A.S.A.
A.S.A. Enseals
Ascriptin
Ascriptin A/D
Aspergum
Astrin
Axotal
Bayer
Bayer Timed-Release Arthritic
  Pain Formula
BC Cold Powder
BC Cold Powder Non-Drowsy
  Formula
BC Multi-Symptom Cold Powder
Buffaprin
Bufferin
Buffinol
Butalgen
Cama Arthritis Reliever
Coricidin with Codeine
Coricidin D
Coryphen
Dristan

Dristan Formula P
Easprin
Ecotrin
Empirin
Entrophen
Fiorgen PF
Fiorinal
Fiormor
Fortabs
Halfprin
Headstart
Isobutal
Isolin
Isollyl Improved
Laniroif
Lanorinal
Magnaprin
Magnaprin Arthritis Strength
Maprin
Marnal
Measurin
Nervine
Night-Time Effervescent Cold
Norwich Aspirin
Novasen
P-A-C Revised Formula
Rhinocaps
Riphen
Robaxisal
Sal-Adult
Salatin
Saleto
Sal-Infant
Salocol
Sine-Off Sinus Medicine
St. Joseph Adult Chewable
  Aspirin
Supasa
Synalgos-DC
Tecnal
Therapy Bayer
Triaphen
Ursinus Inlay
Vibutal
Viro-Med
Zorprin

BARBITURATES

GENERIC NAMES
1. AMOBARBITAL
2. APROBARBITAL
3. BUTABARBITAL
4. BUTALBITAL
5. MEPHOBARBITAL
6. METHARBITAL
7. PENTOBARBITAL
8. PHENOBARBITAL
9. SECOBARBITAL
10. SECOBARBITAL &
  AMOBARBITAL
11. TALBUTAL

BRAND NAMES
Alurate[2]
Amaphen[4]
Amytal[1]
Ancalixir[8]
Anolor-300[4]
Anoquan[4]
Arcet[4]
Axotal[4]
Bancap[4]
Barbita[8]

Bucet[4]
Busodium[3]
Butace[4]
Butalan[3]
Butalgen[4]
Butisol[3]
Cafergot PB[7]
Dolmar[4]
Endolor[4]
Esgic[4]
Esgic-Plus4[1]
Ezol[4]
Femcet[4]
Fiorgen PF[4]
Fioricet[4]
Fiorinal[4]
Fiormor[4]
Fortabs[4]
G-1[4]
Gemonil[6]
Isobutal[4]
Isocet[4]
Isolin[4]
Isollyl Improved[4]
Isopap[4]
Laniroif[4]
Lanorinal[4]
Luminal[8]
Marnal[4]
Mebaral[5]
Medigesic[4]
Nembutal[7]
Nova Rectal[7]
Novopentobarb[7]
Novosecobarb[9]
Pacaps[4]
Phrenilin[4]
Phrenilin Forte[4]
Repan[4]
Sarisol No. 2[3]
Seconal[9]
Sedapap[4]
Solfoton[8]
Tecnal[4]
Tencet[4]
Triad[4]
Triaprin[4]
Tuinal[10]
Two-Dyne[4]
Vibutal[4]

BARBITURATES,
ASPIRIN & CODEINE
(Also contains caffeine)

GENERIC NAMES
1. BUTALBITAL, ASPIRIN &
  CODEINE
2. PHENOBARBITAL, ASPIRIN &
  CODEINE

BRAND NAMES
Ascomp with Codeine No. 3[1]
B-A-C with Codeine[1]
Butalbital Compound with
  Codeine[1]
Butinal with Codeine No. 3[1]
Fiorgen with Codeine[1]
Fiorinal with Codeine[1]
Fiorinal with Codeine No. 3[1]
Fiorinal-C1/4[1]
Fiorinal-C1/2[1]
Fiormor with Codeine[1]

Idenal with Codeine[1]
Isollyl with Codeine[1]
Phenaphen with Codeine No. 2[2]
Phenaphen with Codeine No. 3[2]
Phenaphen with Codeine No. 4[2]

BELLADONNA ALKALOIDS & BARBITURATES

GENERIC NAMES
1. ATROPINE & PHENOBARBITAL
2. ATROPINE, HYOSCYAMINE, SCOPOLAMINE & BUTABARBITAL
3. ATROPINE, HYOSCYAMINE, SCOPOLAMINE & PHENOBARBITAL
4. BELLADONNA & AMOBARBITAL
5. BELLADONNA & BUTABARBITAL
6. BELLADONNA & PHENOBARBITAL
7. HYOSCYAMINE & PHENOBARBITAL

BRAND NAMES
Antrocol[1]
Barbidonna[3]
Barbidonna 2[3]
Barophen[3]
Belladenal[7]
Belladenal Spacetabs[6]
Belladenal-S[7]
Bellalphen[3]
Butibel[5]
Chardonna-2[6]
Donnamor[3]
Donnapine[3]
Donna-Sed[6]
Donnatal[3]
Donnatal Extentabs[3]
Donnatal No. 2[3]
Donphen[3]
Hyosophen[3]
Kinesed[3]
Levsin with Phenobarbital[6]
Levsinex with Phenobarbital Timecaps[7]
Levsin-PB[7]
Malatal[3]
Pheno-Bella[6]
Relaxadon[3]
Spaslin[3]
Spasmolin[3]
Spasmophen[3]
Spasquid[3]
Susano[3]

BENZODIAZEPINES

GENERIC NAMES
1. ALPRAZOLAN
2. BROMAZEPAM
3. CHLORDIAZEPOXIDE
4. CLONAZEPAM
5. CLORAZEPATE
6. DIAZEPAM
7. ESTAZOLAM
8. FLURAZEPAM
9. HALAZEPAM
10. KETAZOLAM
11. LORAZEPAM
12. MIDAZOLAM
13. NITRAZEPAM
14. OXAZEPAM
15. PRAZEPAM
16. QUAZEPAM
17. TEMAZEPAM

BRAND NAMES
Alprazolam Intensol[1]
Apo-Alpraz[1]
Apo-Chlordiazepoxide[3]
Apo-Clorazepate[5]
Apo-Diazepam[6]
Apo-Flurazepam[8]
Apo-Lorazepam[11]
Apo-Oxazepam[14]
Ativan[17]
Centrax[15]
Clindex[3]
Clinoxide[3]
Dalmane[8]
Diastat[6]
Diazemuls[6]
Diazepam Intensol[6]
Doral[16]
Klonopin[4]
Lectopam[2]
Librax[3]
Libritabs[3]
Librium[3]
Lidoxide[3]
Limbitrol[3]
Limbitrol DS[3]
Lipoxide[3]
Loftran[16]
Lorazepam Intensol[11]
Medilium[3]
Meval[6]
Mogadon[15]
Novo-Alprazol[1]
Novoclopate[5]
Novodipam[6]
Novoflupam[8]
Novolorazem[11]
Novopoxide[3]
Novoxapam[14]
Nu-Alpraz[1]
Nu-Loraz[11]
Paxipam[9]
PMS Diazepam[6]
ProSom[7]
Restoril[17]
Rivotril[4]
Serax[14]
Solium[3]
Somnol[8]
T-Quil[6]
Tranxene[5]
Tranxene T-Tab[5]
Tranxene-SD[5]
Valium[6]
Valrelease[6]
Vivol[6]
Xanax[1]
Zapex[14]
Zebrax[3]
Zetran[6]

BENZOYL PEROXIDE

Acetoxyl 2.5 Gel
Acetoxyl 5 Gel
Acetoxyl 10 Gel
Acetoxyl 20 Gel
Acne-5 Lotion
Acne-10 Lotion
Acne-Aid 10 Cream
Acne-Mask
Acnomel B.P. 5 Lotion
Ben-Aqua 2¹/₂ Gel
Ben-Aqua 2¹/₂ Lotion
Ben-Aqua 5 Gel
Ben-Aqua 5 Lotion
Ben-Aqua 10 Gel
Ben-Aqua 10 Lotion
Ben-Aqua Masque 5
Benoxyl 5 Lotion
Benoxyl 5 Wash
Benoxyl 10 Lotion
Benoxyl 10 Wash
Benoxyl 20 Lotion
Benzac Ac 2¹/₂ Gel
Benzac Ac 5 Gel
Benzac Ac 10 Gel
Benzac W 2¹/₂ Gel
Benzac W 5 Gel
Benzac W 10 Gel
Benzagel 5 Acne Lotion
Benzagel 5 Acne Wash
Benzagel 5 Gel
Benzagel 10 Gel
Benzamycin
BenzaShave 5 Cream
BenzaShave 10 Cream
Brevoxyl 4 Gel
Buf-Oxal 10
Clear By Design 2.5 Gel
Clearasil BP Plus 5 Cream
Clearasil BP Plus 5 Lotion
Clearasil Maximum Strength Medicated Anti-Acne 10 Tinted Cream
Clearasil Maximum Strength Medicated Anti-Acne 10 Vanishing Cream
Clearasil Medicated Anti-Acne 10 Vanishing Lotion
Cuticura Acne 5 Cream
Del-Aqua-5 Gel
Del-Aqua-10 Gel
Del-Ray
Dermoxyl 2.5 Gel
Dermoxyl 5 Gel
Dermoxyl 10 Gel
Dermoxyl 20 Gel
Dermoxyl Aqua
Desquam-E 2.5 Gel
Desquam-E 5 Gel
Desquam-E 10 Gel
Desquam-X 2.5 Gel
Desquam-X 5 Gel
Desquam-X 5 Wash
Desquam-X 10 Gel
Desquam-X 10 Wash
Dry and Clear 5 Lotion
Dry and Clear Double Strength 10 Cream
Dryox 5 Gel
Dryox 10 Gel
Dryox 20 Gel
Dryox Wash 5
Dryox Wash 10
Fostex 5 Gel
Fostex 10 Bar
Fostex 10 Cream

Fostex 10 Gel
Fostex 10 Wash
H_2Oxyl 2.5 Gel
H_2Oxyl 5 Gel
H_2Oxyl 10 Gel
H_2Oxyl 20 Gel
Loroxide 5 Lotion with Flesh
   Tinted Base
Loroxide 5.5 Lotion
Neutrogena Acne Mask 5
Noxzema Clear-Ups Maximum
   Strength 10
Noxzema Clear-Ups On-the-Spot
   10 Lotion
Oxy 5 Tinted Lotion
Oxy 5 Vanishing Formula Lotion
Oxy 5 Vanishing Lotion
Oxy 10
Oxy 10 Daily Face Wash
Oxy 10 Tinted Lotion
Oxy 10 Vanishing Lotion
Oxyderm 5 Lotion
Oxyderm 10 Lotion
Oxyderm 20 Lotion
PanOxyl 5 Bar
PanOxyl 5 Gel
PanOxyl 10 Bar
PanOxyl 10 Gel
PanOxyl 15 Gel
PanOxyl 20 Gel
PanOxyl AQ 2½ Gel
PanOxyl AQ 5 Gel
Persa-Gel 5
Persa-Gel 10
Persa-Gel W 5
Persa-Gel W 10
pHisoAc BP 10
Propa P.H. 10 Acne Cover Stick
Propa P.H. 10 Liquid Acne Soap
Stri-Dex Maximum Strength
   Treatment 10 Cream
Theroxide 5 Lotion
Theroxide 10 Lotion
Theroxide 10 Wash
Topex 5 Lotion
Topex 10 Lotion
Vanoxide 5 Lotion
Xerac BP 5 Gel
Xerac BP 10 Gel
Zeroxin-5 Gel
Zeroxin-10 Gel

BETA-ADRENERGIC BLOCKING AGENTS

GENERIC NAMES
1. ACEBUTOLOL
2. ATENOLOL
3. BETAXOLOL
4. BISOPROLOL
5. CARTEOLOL
6. CARVEDILOL
7. LABETALOL
8. METOPROLOL
9. NADOLOL
10. OXPRENOLOL
11. PENBUTOLOL
12. PINDOLOL
13. PROPRANOLOL
14. SOTALOL
15. TIMOLOL

BRAND NAMES
Apo-Atenolol[2]
Apo-Metoprolol[8]
Apo-Nadol[9]
Apo-Pindol[12]
Apo-Propranolol[13]
Apo-Timol[15]
Betaloc[8]
Betapace[14]
Betimol[15]
Betoptic[3]
Blocadren[15]
Cartrol[5]
Corgard[9]
Detensol[13]
Inderal[13]
Inderal LA[13]
Kerlone[3]
Levatol[11]
Lopressor[8]
Lopressor SR[8]
Monitan[1]
Normodyne[7]
Novo-Atenol[2]
Novometoprol[8]
Novo-Pindol[12]
Novopranol[13]
Novo-Timol[15]
Nu-Atenol[2]
NuMetop[8]
Nu-Pindol[12]
pms Propranolol[13]
Sectral[1]
Slow-Trasicor[10]
Sotacor[14]
Syn-Nadolol[9]
Syn-Pindolol[12]
Tenormin[2]
Toprol[8]
Toprol XL[8]
Trandate[7]
Trasicor[10]
Visken[12]
Zebeta[4]

BETA-ADRENERGIC BLOCKING AGENTS & THIAZIDE DIURETICS

GENERIC NAMES
1. ATENOLOL &
   CHLORTHALIDONE
2. BETAXOLOL &
   CHLORTHALIDONE
3. BISOPROLOL &
   HYDROCHLOROTHIAZIDE
4. LABETALOL &
   HYDROCHLOROTHIAZIDE
5. METOPROLOL &
   HYDROCHLOROTHIAZIDE
6. NADOLOL &
   BENDROFLUMETHIAZIDE
7. PINDOLOL &
   HYDROCHLOROTHIAZIDE
8. PROPRANOLOL &
   HYDROCHLOROTHIAZIDE
9. TIMOLOL &
   HYDROCHLOROTHIAZIDE

BRAND NAMES
Co-Betaloc[5]
Corzide[6]
Inderide[8]
Inderide LA[8]
Kerledex[2]
Lopressor HCT[5]
Normozide[4]
Tenoretic[1]
Timolide[9]
Trandate HCT[4]
Viskazide[7]
Ziac[3]

BRONCHODILATORS, ADRENERGIC

GENERIC NAMES
1. ALBUTEROL
2. BITOLTEROL
3. EPHEDRINE SULFATE
4. EPINEPHRINE
5. ETHYLNOREPINEPHRINE
6. FENOTEROL
7. ISOETHARINE
8. ISOPROTERENOL
9. METAPROTERENOL
10. PIRBUTEROL
11. PROCATEROL
12. RACEPINEPHRINE
13. SALMETEROL
14. TERBUTALINE

BRAND NAMES
Adrenalin[1]
Aerolone[8]
Alupent[9]
Ana-Guard[4]
Arm-a-Med Isoetharine[7]
Arm-a-Med Metaproterenol[9]
AsthmaHaler[4]
AsthmaNefrin[12]
Berotec[6]
Brethaire[14]
Brethine[14]
Bricanyl[14]
Bronitin Mist[4]
Bronkaid Mist[4]
Bronkaid Mist Suspension[4]
Bronkaid Mistometer[4]
Bronkephrine[5]
Bronkometer[7]
Bronkosol[7]
Combivent[1]
Dey-Dose Isoetharine[9]
Dey-Dose Isoetharine S/F[9]
Dey-Dose Isoproterenol[8]
Dey-Dose Metaproterenol[9]
Dey-Dose Racepinephrine[12]
Dey-Lute Isoetharine[7]
Dey-Lute Isoetharine S/F[7]
Dey-Lute Metaproterenol[9]
Dispos-a-Med Isoetharine[7]
Dispos-a-Med Isoptroterenol[8]
Ephed II[3]
EpiPen Auto-Injector[4]
EpiPen Jr. Auto-Injector[4]
Isuprel[8]
Isuprel Glossets[8]
Isuprel Mistometer[8]
Maxair[10]
Medihaler-Epi[4]
Medihaler-Iso[8]
Metaprel[9]
microNEFRIN[12]
Nephron[12]
Norisodrine Aerotrol[8]

875

Novosalmol[1]
Primatene Mist[4]
Primatene Mist Suspension[4]
Pro-Air[11]
Prometa[9]
Proventil[1]
Proventil HFA[1]
Proventil Repetabs[1]
Serevent[13]
Sus-Phrine[4]
Tornalate[2]
Vapo-Iso[8]
Vaponefrin[12]
Ventolin[1]
Ventolin Rotocaps[1]
Volmax[1]

BRONCHODILATORS, XANTHINE

GENERIC NAMES
1. AMINOPHYLLINE
2. DYPHILLINE
3. OXTRIPHYLLINE
4. THEOPHYLLINE

BRAND NAMES
Accurbron[4]
Aerolate III[4]
Aerolate Jr.[4]
Aerolate Sr.[4]
Aerophyllin[1]
Aminophyllin[1]
Apo-Oxtriphylline[3]
Aquaphyllin[4]
Asmalix[4]
Bronkodyl[4]
Choledyl[3]
Choledyl Delayed-Release[3]
Choledyl SA[3]
Constant-T[4]
Corophyllin[1]
Dilor[2]
Dilor-400[2]
Duraphyl[4]
Dyflex 200[2]
Dyflex 400[2]
Elixicon[4]
Elixomin[1]
Elixophyllin[4]
Elixophyllin SR[4]
Lanophyllin[4]
Lixolin[4]
Lufyllin[4]
Lufyllin-400[2]
Neothylline[2]
Novotriphyl[3]
Palaron[1]
Phyllocontin[1]
Phyllocontin-350[1]
PMS Theophylline[4]
Protophylline[2]
Pulmophylline[4]
Quibron-T[4]
Quibron-T Dividose[4]
Quibron-T/SR[4]
Quibron-T/SR Dividose[4]
Respbid[4]
Slo-Bid[4]
Slo-bid Gyrocaps[4]
Slophyllin[4]
Slo-Phyllin[4]
Slo-Phyllin Gyrocaps[4]

Solu-Phyllin[4]
Somophyllin[1]
Somophyllin-12[1]
Somophyllin-CRT[1]
Somophyllin-DF[1]
Somophyllin-T[1]
Sustaire[4]
Synophylate[4]
Theo-24[4]
Theo-250[4]
Theobid Duracaps[4]
Theobid Jr. Duracaps[4]
Theochron[4]
Theoclear L.A. 130 Cenules[4]
Theoclear L.A. 260 Cenules[4]
Theoclear-80[4]
Theocot[4]
Theo-Dur[4]
Theo-Dur Sprinkle[4]
Theolair[4]
Theolair-SR[4]
Theomar[4]
Theon[4]
Theophylline SR[4]
Theo-Sav[4]
Theospan SR[4]
Theo-SR[4]
Theostat[4]
Theostat 80[4]
Theo-Time[4]
Theovent Long-acting[4]
Theox[4]
Thylline[2]
T-Phyl[4]
Truphylline[1]
Truxophyllin[4]
Uniphyl[4]

CAFFEINE

222
282
292
692
Actamin Super
Amaphen
Anacin
Anacin with Codeine
Anolor-300
Anoquan
A.P.C.
Aspirin Free Bayer Select
    Maximum Strength Headache
    Pain Relief Caplets
Aspirin-Free Excedrin Caplets
Cafergot
Cafergot PB
Cafertine
Cafetrate
Caffedrine
Caffefrine Caplets
Citrated Caffeine
Cotanal 65
Darvon-N Compound
Dexitac
Dristan
Dristan AF
Dristan AF Plus
Dristan Formula P
Enerjets
Ercaf
Ergo-Caff
Esgic

Esgic-Plus
Excedrin Caplets
Excedrin Extra Strength Caplets
Excedrin Extra Strength Tablets
Fendol
Fiorinal
Gotamine
Histosal
Keep Alert
Kolephrin
Migergot
Novo-AC and C
Omnicol
P-A-C Revised Formula
Pacaps
PC-Cap
Pep-Back
Propoxyphene Compound-65
Quick Pep
Repan
S-A-C
Salatin
Saleto
Saleto-D
Salocol
Scot-tussin Original 5-Action
    Cold Medicine
Sinapils
Snap Back
Supac
Synalgos-DC
Tirend
Triaminicin with Codeine
Trigesic
Two-Dyne
Vanquish
Vivarin
Wake-Up
Wigraine

CALCIUM CHANNEL BLOCKERS

GENERIC NAMES
1. AMLODIPINE
2. BEPRIDIL
3. DILTIAZEM
4. FELODIPINE
5. FLUNARIZINE
6. ISRADIPINE
7. NICARDIPINE
8. NIFEDIPINE
9. NISOLDIPINE
10. VERAPAMIL

BRAND NAMES
Adalat[8]
Adalat CC[8]
Adalat FT[8]
Adalat P.A.[8]
Apo-Diltiaz[3]
Apo-Nifed[8]
Apo-Verap[10]
Bepadin[2]
Calan[10]
Calan SR[10]
Cardene[7]
Cardene SR[7]
Cardizem[3]
Cardizem CD[3]
Cardizem SR[3]
Chronovera[10]
Dilacor-XR[3]

Dyna Circ[6]
Isoptin[10]
Isoptin SR[10]
Lexxel[4]
Lotrel[1]
Norvasc[1]
Novo-Diltazem[3]
Novo-Nifedin[8]
Novo-Veramil[10]
Nu-Diltiaz[3]
Nu-Nifed[8]
Nu-Verap[10]
Plendil[4]
Procardia[8]
Procardia XL[8]
Renedil[4]
Sibelium[5]
Sular[9]
Syn-Diltiazem[3]
Tarka[10]
Teczam[3]
Tiazac[3]
Vascor[2]
Verelan[10]

CALCIUM SUPPLEMENTS

GENERIC NAMES
1. CALCIUM CARBONATE
2. CALCIUM CITRATE
3. CALCIUM GLUBIONATE
4. CALCIUM GLUCONATE
5. CALCIUM GLYCEROPHOSPHATE & CALCIUM LACTATE
6. CALCIUM LACTATE
7. DIBASIC CALCIUM PHOSPHATE
8. TRIBASIC CALCIUM PHOSPHATE

BRAND NAMES
Apo-Cal[1]
BioCal[1]
Calcarb 600[1]
Calci-Chew[1]
Calciday 667[1]
Calcilac[1]
Calcite 500[1]
Calcium Carbonate/600[1]
Calcium Stanley[4]
Calcium-600[1]
Calcium-Sandoz[3]
Calcium-Sandoz Forte[1,6]
Calglycine[1]
Calphosan[5]
Calsan[1]
Caltrate[1]
Caltrate-300[1]
Caltrate-600[1]
Caltrate Chewable[1]
Chooz[1]
Citracal[2]
Citracal Liquitabs[2]
Dicarbosil[1]
Gencalc 600[1]
Gramcal[1,6]
Mallamint[1]
Neo-Calglucon[3]
Nephro-Calci[1]
Os-Cal[1]
Os-Cal 500[1]
Os-Cal Chewable[1]
Oysco[1]

Oysco 500 Chewable[1]
Oyst-Cal[1]
Oyst-Cal 500 Chewable[1]
Oystercal 500[1]
Posture[8]
Rolaids-Calcium Rich[1]
Titralac[1]
Tums[1]
Tums E-X[1]

COAL TAR (Topical)
Alphosyl
Aquatar
Balnetar
Balnetar Therapeutic Tar Bath
Cutar Water Dispersible Emollient Tar
Denorex
Denorex Extra Strength Medicated Shampoo
Denorex Extra Strength Medicated Shampoo with Conditioners
Denorex Medicated Shampoo
Denorex Medicated Shampoo and Conditioner
Denorex Mountain Fresh Herbal Scent Medicated Shampoo
DHS Tar Gel Shampoo
DHS Tar Shampoo
Doak Oil
Doak Oil Forte
Doak Oil Forte Therapeutic Bath Treatment
Doak Oil Therapeutic Bath Treatment For All-Over Body Care
Doak Tar Lotion
Doak Tar Shampoo
Doctar
Doctar Hair & Scalp Shampoo & Conditioner
Estar
Fototar
Ionil-T Plus
Lavatar
Liquor Carbonis Detergens
Medotar
Pentrax Extra-Strength Therapeutic Tar Shampoo
Pentrax Tar Shampoo
psoriGel
PsoriNail
Tar Doak
Taraphilic
Tarbonis
Tarpaste
Tarpaste Doak
T/Derm Tar Emollient
Tegrin Lotion for Psoriasis
Tegrin Medicated Cream Shampoo
Tegrin Medicated Shampoo Concentrated Gel
Tegrin Medicated Shampoo Extra Conditioning Formula
Tegrin Medicated Shampoo Herbal Formula
Tegrin Medicated Shampoo Original Formula
Tegrin Medicated Soap for Psoriasis

Tegrin Skin Cream for Psoriasis
Tersa-Tar Mild Therapeutic Shampoo with Protein and Conditioner
Tersa-Tar Soapless Tar Shampoo
Tersa-Tar Therapeutic Shampoo
T-Gel
T/Gel Therapeutic Conditioner
T/Gel Therapeutic Shampoo
Theraplex T Shampoo
Zetar
Zetar Emulsion
Zetar Medicated Antiseborrheic Shampoo

CONTRACEPTIVES, ORAL

GENERIC NAMES
1. DESOGESTREL & ETHINYL ESTRADIOL
2. ETHYNODIOL DIACETATE & ETHINYL ESTRADIOL
3. LEVONORGESTREL & ETHINYL ESTRADIOL
4. NORETHINDRONE & ETHINYL ESTRADIOL
5. NORETHINDRONE & MESTRANOL
6. NORETHINDRONE ACETATE & ETHINYL ESTRADIOL
7. NORGESTIMATE & ETHINYL ESTRADIOL
8. NORGESTREL & ETHINYL ESTRADIOL

BRAND NAMES
Alesse[3]
Brevicon[4]
Brevicon 0.5/35[4]
Brevicon 1/35[4]
Cyclen[7]
Demulen 1/35[2]
Demulen 1/50[2]
Demulen 30[2]
Demulen 50[2]
Desogen 28[1]
Desogen Ortho-Cept[1]
Estrostep[4]
Estrostep Fe[4]
GenCept 0.5/35[4]
GenCept 1/35[4]
GenCept 10/11[4]
Genora 0.5/35[4]
Genora 1/35[4]
Genora 1/50[5]
Jenest-28[4]
Levlen[3]
Levlite[3]
Levora[3]
Loestrin 1/20[6]
Loestrin 1.5/30[6]
Lo/Ovral[8]
Marvelon[1]
Minestrin 1/20[6]
Min-Ovral[3]
ModiCon[4]
Necon 0.5/35-21[4]
Necon 0.5/35-28[4]
Necon 1/35-21[4]
Necon 1/35-28[4]
Necon 1/50-21[4]
Necon 1/50-28[4]
Necon 10/11-21[4]

Necon 10/11-28[4]
N.E.E. 1/35[4]
N.E.E. 1/50[4]
Nelova 0.5/35E[4]
Nelova 1/35E[4]
Nelova 1/50M[4]
Nelova 10/11[4]
Nelulen 1/35E[2]
Nelulen 1/50E[2]
Norcept-E 1/35[6]
Nordette[3]
Norethin 1/35E[4]
Norethin 1/50M[5]
Norinyl 1+35[4]
Norinyl 1+50[5]
Norinyl 1/50[5]
Norlestrin 1/50[6]
Norlestrin 2.5/50[6]
Ortho 0.5/35[4]
Ortho 1/35[4]
Ortho 7/7/7[4]
Ortho 10/11[4]
Ortho-Cept[1]
Ortho-Cyclen[7]
Ortho-Novum 0.5[4]
Ortho-Novum 1/35[4]
Ortho-Novum 1/50[5]
Ortho-Novum 1/80[5]
Ortho-Novum 2[4]
Ortho-Novum 7/7/7[4]
Ortho-Novum 10/11[5]
Ortho-Tri-Cyclen 21[5]
Ortho-Tri-Cyclen 28[5]
Ovcon-35[4]
Ovcon-50[4]
Ovral[8]
Symphasic[4]
Tri-Cyclen[7]
Tri-Levlen[3]
Tri-Norinyl[4]
Triphasil[3]
Triquilar[3]
Trivora[3]
Zovia 1/35E[2]
Zovia 1/50E[2]

CONTRACEPTIVES, VAGINAL (Spermicides)

GENERIC NAMES
1. BENZALKONIUM CHLORIDE
2. NONOXYNOL 9
3. OCTOXYNOL 9

BRAND NAMES
Advantage 24[2]
Because[2]
Conceptrol Gel[2]
Conceptrol-Contraceptive
  Inserts[2]
Delfen[2]
Emko[2]
Encare[2]
Gynol II Extra Strength[2]
Gynol II Original Formula[2]
Koromex Cream[2]
Koromex Crystal Gel[2]
Koromex Foam[2]
Koromex Jelly[2]
K-Y Plus[2]
Ortho-Creme[2]
Ortho-Gynol[3]
Pharmatex[1]

Pre-Fil[2]
Ramses Contraceptive Foam[2]
Ramses Contraceptive Vaginal
  Jelly[2]
Ramses Crystal Clear Gel[2]
Semicid[2]
Shur-Seal[2]
Solurex
Solurex LA
VCF[2]

DEXTROMETHORPHAN

2/G-DM Cough
Actifed DM
Alka-Seltzer Plus Cold and
  Cough
Alka-Seltzer Plus Nighttime Cold
All-Nite Cold Formula
Ambenyl-D Decongestant Cough
  Formula
Anatuss
Anatuss DM
Anti-Tuss DM Expectorant
Balminil DM
Bayaminicol
Baydec DM Drops
Bayer Cough Syrup for Children
Bayer Select Chest Cold Tablets
Bayer Select Flu Relief Caplets
Bayer Select Head and Chest
  Cold Caplets
Bayer Select Night Time Cold
  Caplets
Baytussin DM
Benylin DM-D
Benylin DM-D-E
Benylin DM-D-E Extra Strength
Benylin DM-E
Benylin Expectorant Cough
  Formula
Bromarest DX Cough
Bromatane DX Cough
Bromfed-AT
Bromfed-DM
Bromphen DX Cough
Broncho-Grippol-DM
Brotane DX Cough
Calmylin
Calmylin #1
Calmylin #2
Calmylin #3
Calmylin #4
Calmylin Cough & Cold
Calmylin Pediatric
Carbinoxamine Compound
Carbodec DM Drops
Cardec DM
Cardec DM Drops
Cardec DM Pediatric
Cerose-DM
Cheracol D Cough
Cheracol Plus
Children's Benylin DM-D
Children's Formula Cough
Children's Hold
Children's Tylenol Cold Multi-
  Symptom Plus Cough
Co-Apap
Codimal DM
Codistan No. 1
Colrex Cough
Comtrex Cough Formula

Comtrex Daytime Caplets
Comtrex Daytime Maximum
  Strength Cold and Flu Relief
Comtrex Daytime Maximum
  Strength Cold, Cough and Flu
  Relief
Comtrex Hot Flu Relief
Comtrex Maximum Strength
  Liqui-Gels
Comtrex Multi-Symptom Cold
  Reliever
Comtrex Multi-Symptom Hot Flu
  Relief
Comtrex Multi-Symptom Non-
  Drowsy Caplets
Comtrex Nighttime
Comtrex Nighttime Maximum
  Strength Cold and Flu Relief
Comtrex Nighttime Maximum
  Strength Cold, Cough and Flu
  Relief
Conar
Conar Expectorant
Conar-A
Concentrin
Congespirin
Contac Jr. Children's Cold
  Medicine
Contac Night Caplets
Contac Severe Cold Formula
Contac Severe Cold Formula
  Night Strength
Coricidin Cough
CoTylenol Cold Medication
Cough X
Cremacoat 1
Cremacoat 3 Throat Coating
  Cough Medicine
Creo-Terpin
DayCare
DayQuil Liquicaps
DayQuil Non-Drowsy Cold/Flu
DayQuil Non-Drowsy Cold/Flu
  LiquiCaps
Delsym
Diabetic Tussin DM
Dimacol
Dimetane-DX Cough
Dimetapp-DM
Dimetapp-DM Cough and Cold
Dimetapp-DM Elixir
DM Cough
DM Syrup
Donatussin
Dondril
Dorcol Children's Cough
Dorcol DM
Dristan Cold and Flu
Dristan Juice Mix-in Cold, Flu,
  & Cough
Drixoral Cough
Effective Strength Cough
  Formula
Effective Strength Cough
  Formula with Decongestant
Efficol Cough Whip (Cough
  Suppressant/Decongestant)
Efficol Cough Whip (Cough
  Suppressant/Decongestant/
  Antihistamine)
Efficol Cough Whip (Cough
  Suppressant/Expectorant)
Extra Action Cough

Father John's Medicine Plus
Genatuss DM
Genite
Glycotuss-dM
GuiaCough CF
Guiamid D.M. Liquid
Guiatuss CF
Guiatuss-DM
Guiatussin with
  Dextromethorphan
Halls Mentho-Lyptus
  Decongestant Cough Formula
Halotussin-DM Expectorant
Histalet-DM
Hold
Hold (Children's Formula)
Humibid DM Sprinkle
Improved Sino-Tuss
Ipsatol Cough Formula for
  Children
Kiddy Koff
Koffex
Kolephrin GG/DM
Kolephrin NN Liquid
Kolephrin/DM Caplets
Kophane
Kophane Cough and Cold
  Formula
Mapap Cold Formula
Maximum Strength Tylenol Flu
  Gelcaps
Meda Syrup Forte
Medatussin
Medi-Flu
Medi-Flu Caplets
Mediquell
Mediquell Decongestant Formula
Myminicol
Mytussin DM
Naldecon Senior DX
Naldecon-DX
Naldecon-DX Adult Liquid
Naldecon-DX Children's Syrup
Naldecon-DX Pediatric Drops
Naldelate DX Adult
NeoCitran DM Coughs & Colds
Neo-DM
Noratuss II Liquid
Novahistex DM
Novahistine Cough & Cold
  Formula Liquid
Novahistine DMX Liquid
NyQuil Hot Therapy
NyQuil Liquicaps
NyQuil Nighttime Colds Medicine
Nytcold Medicine
Nytime Cold Medicine Liquid
Omnicol
Ornade-DM 10
Ornade-DM 15
Ornade-DM 30
Ornex DM 15
Ornex DM 30
Ornex Severe Cold No
  Drowsiness Caplets
Orthoxicol Cough
Par Glycerol-DM
PediaCare 1
PediaCare Children's Cold Relief
  Night Rest Cough-Cold
  Formula
PediaCare Children's Cough-
  Cold

PediaCare Cough-Cold
Pertussin All Night CS
Pertussin All Night PM
Pertussin Cough Suppressant
Pertussin CS
Pertussin ES
Phanadex
Phanatuss
Phenameth DM
Phenergan with Dextromethorphan
Pherazine DM
Poly-Histine-DM
Primatuss Cough Mixture 4
Primatuss Cough Mixture 4D
Prometh with Dextromethorphan
Promethazine DM
Prominicol Cough
Pseudo-Car DM
Quelidrine Cough
Queltuss
Remcol-C
Rescon-DM
Rhinosyn-DM
Rhinosyn-DMX Expectorant
Rhinosyn-X
Robafen CF
Robafen DM
Robidex
Robitussin Cold and Cough
  Liqui-Gels
Robitussin Cough Calmers
Robitussin Maximum Strength
  Cough and Cold
Robitussin Maximum Strength
  Cough Suppressant
Robitussin Night Relief
Robitussin Night Relief Colds
  Formula Liquid
Robitussin Pediatric Cough &
  Cold
Robitussin-CF
Robitussin-DM
Robitussin-Pediatric
Rondamine-DM Drops
Rondec-DM
Rondec-DM Drops
Ru-Tuss Expectorant
SafeTussin 30
Saleto-CF
Scot-Tussin DM
Sedatuss
Silexin Cough
Snaplets-DM
Snaplets-Multi
St. Joseph Cough Suppressant
  for Children
Sucrets Cough Control
Sudafed Cold & Cough Liquid
  Caps
Sudafed Cough
Sudafed DM
Sudafed Severe Cold Formula
  Caplets
Syracol Liquid
Terphan
Terpin-Dex
TheraFlu Maximum Strength
  Non-Drowsy Formula Flu,
  Cold & Cough Medicine
TheraFlu Nighttime Maximum
  Strength
TheraFlu/Flu, Cold & Cough
Threamine DM

Tolu-Sed DM Cough
Touro DM
Triaminic DM Cough Formula
Triaminic DM Daytime
Triaminic DM Expectorant
Triaminic DM Nighttime for
  Children
Triaminic Nite Light
Triaminic Sore Throat Formula
Triaminicol DM
Triaminicol Multi-Symptom Relief
Tricodene Forte
Tricodene NN
Tricodene Pediatric
Tricodene Sugar Free
Trimedine Liquid
Triminol Cough
Trind DM Liquid
Trocal
Tusquelin
Tussafed
Tussafed Drops
Tussar DM
Tuss-DM
Ty-Cold Cold Formula
Tylenol Cold and Flu
Tylenol Cold and Flu No
  Drowsiness Powder
Tylenol Cold Medication
Tylenol Cold Medication,
  Non-Drowsy
Tylenol Cold Night Time
Tylenol Cold No Drowsiness
  Formula Gelcaps
Tylenol Cough
Tylenol Cough with
  Decongestant
Tylenol Maximum Strength
  Cough
Tylenol Maximum Strength Flu
  Gelcaps
Uni-Tussin DM
Unproco
Vicks 44 Cold, Flu and Cough
  Liqui-Caps
Vicks 44 Cough and Cold Relief
  Liqui-Caps
Vicks 44 Non-Drowsy Cold and
  Cough LiquiCaps
Vicks 44D Dry Hacking Cough
  and Head Congestion
Vicks 44M Cough, Cold and Flu
  Relief
Vicks 44M Cough, Cold and Flu
  Relief LiquiCaps
Vicks Children's Cough
Vicks Formula 44D Decongestant
  Cough Mixture
Vicks Formula 44M Multi-
  Symptom Cough Mixture
Vicks NyQuil Multi-Symptom
  Cold/Flu Relief
Vicks NyQuil Multi-Symptom
  LiquiCaps
Vicks Pediatric Formula 44D
  Cough and Decongestant
Vicks Pediatric Formula 44E
Vicks Pediatric Formula 44M
  Multi-Symptom Cough & Cold
Viro-Med

879

DICYCLOMINE

Antispas
A-Spas
Bentyl
Bentylol
Byclomine
Dibent
Di-Cyclonex
Dilomine
Di-Spaz
Forulex
Lomine
Neoquess
Or-Tyl
Protylol
Spasmoban
Spasmoject
Viscerol

DIURETICS, THIAZIDE

GENERIC NAMES
1. BENDROFLUMETHIAZIDE
2. BENZTHIAZIDE
3. CHLOROTHIAZIDE
4. CHLORTHALIDONE
5. CYCLOTHIAZIDE
6. HYDROCHLOROTHIAZIDE
7. HYDROFLUMETHIAZIDE
8. METHYCLOTHIAZIDE
9. METOLAZONE
10. POLYTHIAZIDE
11. QUINETHAZONE
12. TRICHLORMETHIAZIDE

BRAND NAMES
Anhydron[5]
Apo-Chlorthalidone[4]
Apo-Hydro[6]
Aquatensen[8]
Diucardin[7]
Diuchlor H[6]
Diulo[9]
Diuril[3]
Duretic[8]
Enduron[8]
Esidrix[6]
Exna[2]
Hydrex[2]
Hydro-D[6]
HydroDIURIL[6]
Hydromox[1]
Hygroton[4]
Hyzaar[6]
Metahydrin[2]
Minizide[10]
Mykrox[9]
Naqua[12]
Naturetin[1]
Neo-Codema[6]
Novo-Hydrazide[6]
Novo-Thalidone[4]
Oretic[6]
Renese[10]
Saluron[7]
Thalitone[4]
Uniretic[6]
Uridon[4]
Urozide[6]
Zaroxolyn[9]

EPHEDRINE

Broncholate
Bronkotuss Expectorant
Histatuss Pediatric
KIE
Omni-Tuss
Quelidrine Cough
Rentamine Pediatric
Rynatuss
Rynatuss Pediatric

ERYTHROMYCINS

GENERIC NAMES
1. ERYTHROMYCIN ESTOLATE
2. ERYTHROMYCIN
   ETHYLSUCCINATE
3. ERYTHROMYCIN
   GLUCEPTATE
4. ERYTHROMYCIN
   LACTOBIONATE
5. ERYTHROMYCIN STEARATE
6. ERYTHROMYCIN-BASE

BRAND NAMES
Apo-Erythro[6]
Apo-Erythro E-C[6]
Apo-Erythro ES[2]
Apo-Erythro-S[5]
E-Base[6]
E.E.S.[2]
E/Gel[6]
Emgel[6]
E-Mycin[6]
Erybid[6]
ERYC[6]
EryPed[2]
Ery-Tab[6]
Erythraderm[6]
Erythro[2]
Erythrocin[5]
Erythrocot[5]
Erythromid[6]
Eryzole[6]
Ilosone[1]
Ilotycin[3]
My-E[5]
Novorythro[5]
PCE Dispersatabs[5]
Pediazole[6]
Sulfimycin[6]
Wintrocin[5]

ESTROGENS

GENERIC NAMES
1. CHLOROTRIANISENE
2. CONJUGATED ESTROGENS
3. DIETHYLSTILBESTROL
4. ESTERIFIED ESTROGENS
5. ESTRADIOL
6. ESTROGEN
7. ESTRONE
8. ESTROPIPATE
9. ETHINYL ESTRADIOL
10. QUINESTROL

BRAND NAMES
Alora[5]
Aquest[7]
C.E.S.[2]
Climara[6]
Clinagen LA 40[6]
Congest[2]

Deladiol-40[6]
Delestrogen[6]
depGynogen[5]
Depo Estradiol[5]
Depogen[6]
DES[3]
Dioval 40[6]
Dioval XX[6]
Dura-Estrin[6]
Duragen[6]
Duragen-20[6]
Duragen-40[6]
E-Cypionate[6]
Estinyl[9]
Estrace[6]
Estraderm[6]
Estragen 5[7]
Estragen LA 5[6]
Estra-L[6]
Estratab[4]
Estring[5]
Estro-A[7]
Estro-Cyp[6]
Estrofem[6]
Estroject-L.A.[6]
Estro-L.A.[6]
Estrone 5[7]
Estro-Span[6]
Estrovis[10]
Femogex[6]
Fempatch[5]
Gynogen L.A. 20[6]
Gynogen L.A. 40[6]
Honvol [3]
Kestrone-5[7]
Mannest[2]
Menaval-20[6]
Menest [4]
Neo-Estrone[4]
Ogen[8]
Ogen 1.25[8]
Ogen 2.5[8]
Ogen 6.25[8]
Ortho-Est[8]
Piperazine[8]
Premarin[2]
Premphase[2]
Prempro[2]
Stilphostrol[3]
TACE[6]
Valergen-10[6]
Valergen-20[6]
Valergen-40[6]
Vivelle[6]
Wehgen[7]

GUAIFENESIN

2/G-DM Cough
Adatuss D.C. Expectorant
Alamine Expectorant
Ambenyl-D Decongestant Cough
   Formula
Ami-Tex LA
Amonidrin
Anatuss
Anatuss DM
Anatuss LA
Anatuss with Codeine
Anti-Tuss
Anti-Tuss DM Expectorant
Balminil Expectorant
Banex

Banex Liquid
Banex-LA
Bayaminic Expectorant
Bayer Select Head and Chest
  Cold Caplets
Bayhistine Expectorant
Baytussin AC
Baytussin DM
Benylin DM-D-E
Benylin DM-D-E Extra Strength
Benylin DM-E
Benylin Expectorant Cough
  Formula
Benylin with Codeine
Benylin-E
Breonesin
Brexin
Broncholate
Bronkotuss Expectorant
Brontex
Calmylin
Calmylin #3
Calmylin Cough & Cold
Calmylin with Codeine
Cheracol
Cheracol D Cough
Children's Formula Cough
CoActifed Expectorant
Codegest Expectorant
Codiclear DH
Codimal Expectorant
Codistan No. 1
Colrex Expectorant
Comtrex Cough Formula
Conar Expectorant
Conar-A
Concentrin
Conex
Conex with Codeine Liquid
Congess JR
Congess SR
Congestac Caplets
Contuss
Cophene-XP
Coricidin Cough
Cotridin Expectorant
Cremacoat 2
Cremacoat 3 Throat Coating
  Cough Medicine
C-Tussin Expectorant
DayCare
DayQuil Liquicaps
DayQuil Non-Drowsy Cold/Flu
DayQuil Non-Drowsy Cold/Flu
  LiquiCaps
DayQuil Non-Drowsy Sinus
  Pressure and Congestion Relief
  Caplets
Deconsal II
Deconsal Pediatric
Deconsal Sprinkle
Deproist Expectorant with Codeine
Despec
Detussin Expectorant
Diabetic Tussin DM
Diabetic Tussin EX
Dihistine Expectorant
Dilaudid Cough
Dimacol
Dimetane Expectorant
Dimetane Expectorant-C
Dimetane Expectorant-DC
Donatussin

Donatussin DC
Donatussin Drops
Dorcol Children's Cough
Dorcol DM
Dura-Gest
Duratuss
Duratuss HD
Dura-Vent
Efficol Cough Whip (Cough
  Suppressant/Expectorant)
Endal Expectorant
Enomine
Entex
Entex LA
Entex Liquid
Entex PSE
Entuss Expectorant
Entuss Pediatric Expectorant
Entuss-D
Exgest LA
Extra Action Cough
Father John's Medicine Plus
Fedahist Expectorant
Fedahist Expectorant Pediatric
  Drops
Fendol
Fenesin
Gee-Gee
Genatuss
Genatuss DM
GG-CEN
Glyate
Glycofed
Glycotuss
Glycotuss-dM
Glydeine Cough
Glytuss
GP-500
Guaifed
Guaifed-PD
GuaiMAX-D
Guaipax
Guaitab
GuiaCough CF
GuiaCough PE
Guiamid D.M. Liquid
Guiatuss A.C.
Guiatuss CF
Guiatuss DAC
Guiatuss PE
Guiatuss-DM
Guiatussin DAC
Guiatussin with Codeine Liquid
Guiatussin with
  Dextromethorphan
Halotussin
Halotussin-DM Expectorant
Head & Chest
Histalet X
Humibid Guaifenesin Plus
Humibid L.A.
Humibid Sprinkle
Humibid-DM Sprinkle
Hycotuss Expectorant
Hytuss
Hytuss-2X
Ipsatol Cough Formula for
  Children
Isoclor Expectorant
Kiddy Koff
Kolephrin GG/DM
Kwelcof Liquid
Lanatuss Expectorant

Malotuss
Meda Syrup Forte
Medatussin
Medatussin Plus
Myhistine Expectorant
Myminic Expectorant
Mytussin AC
Mytussin DAC
Mytussin DM
Naldecon
Naldecon Senior DX
Naldecon Senior EX
Naldecon-CX Adult Liquid
Naldecon-DX Adult
Naldecon-DX Adult Liquid
Naldecon-DX Children's Syrup
Naldecon-DX Pediatric Drops
Naldecon-EX
Naldecon-EX Pediatric Drops
Naldelate DX Adult
Nasatab LA
NeoCitrin DM Coughs & Colds
Nolex LA
Noratuss II Liquid
Nortussin
Nortussin with Codeine
Novagest Expectorant with
  Codeine
Novahistex DH Expectorant
Novahistine DH Expectorant
Novahistine DMX Liquid
Novahistine Expectorant
Nucochem Expectorant
Nucochem Pediatric Expectorant
Nucofed Expectorant
Nucofed Pediatric Expectorant
Organidin
Ornade Expectorant
Partuss LA
Pertussin All Night CS
Phanadex
Phanatuss
Phenhist Expectorant
Phenylfenesin L.A.
Pneumomist
Polaramine Expectorant
Poly-Histine Expectorant Plain
Prominic Expectorant
Pseudo-Bid
P-V-Tussin Tablets
Queltuss
Quiess
Rescon-GG
Respaire-60 SR
Respaire-120 SR
Respinol G
Respinol LA
Resyl
Rhinosyn-DMX Expectorant
Rhinosyn-X
Robafen AC Cough
Robafen CF
Robafen DAC
Robafen DM
Robitussin
Robitussin A-C
Robitussin Cold & Cough
  Liqui-Gels
Robitussin Severe Congestion
  Liqui-Gels
Robitussin with Codeine
Robitussin-CF
Robitussin-DAC

Robitussin-DM
Robitussin-PE
Ru-Tuss DE
Ru-Tuss Expectorant
Rymed
Rymed Liquid
Rymed-TR
Ryna-CX Liquid
SafeTussin 30
Scot-Tussin
Silexin Cough
Sinufed Timecelles
Sinumist-SR
Sinupan
SINUvent
Snaplets-EX
SRC Expectorant
Stamoist E
Stamoist LA
Sudafed Cough
Sudafed Expectorant
Threamine Expectorant
T-Moist
Tolu-Sed Cough
Tolu-Sed DM Cough
Touro DM
Touro Ex
Touro LA Caplets
Triaminic DM Daytime
Triaminic DM Expectorant
Triaminic Expectorant
Triaminic Expectorant DH
Triaminic Expectorant with Codeine
Trinex
Triphenyl Expectorant
Tussafin Expectorant
Tussanil DH Tablets
Tussar SF
Tussar-2
Tuss-DM
Tuss-LA
ULR-LA
Uni-Tussin
Uni-Tussin DM
Unproco
Utex-S.R.
Vanex Expectorant
Vanex LA
V-Dec-M
Versacaps
Vicks Children's Cough
Vicks Formula 44D Decongestant
  Cough Mixture
Vicks Formula 44M Multi-
  Symptom Cough Mixture
Vicks Pediatric Formula 44E
Vicodin-Tuss
Viro-Med
Zephrex
Zephrex-LA

INSULIN

Humulin BR
Humulin L
Humulin N
Humulin R
Humulin U
Insulatard NPH
Insulatard NPH Human
Lente
Lente Iletin I
Lente Iletin II

Mixtard
Mixtard Human
Novolin 70/30
Novolin 70/30 PenFill
Novolin 70/30 Prefilled
Novolin ge NPH PenFill
Novolin ge Toronto PenFill
Novolin L
Novolin N
Novolin N PenFill
Novolin N Prefilled
Novolin R
Novolin R PenFill
Novolin R Prefilled
NPH
NPH Iletin I
NPH Iletin II
Protamine Zinc & Iletin
Protamine Zinc & Iletin I
Protamine Zinc & Iletin II
PZI
Regular
Regular (Concentrated) Iletin
Regular (Concentrated) Iletin II,
  U-500
Regular Iletin I
Regular Iletin II
Regular Insulin
Semilente
Semilente Iletin
Semilente Iletin I
Ultralente
Ultralente Iletin I
Velosulin
Velosulin BR
Velosulin Human

IRON SUPPLEMENTS

GENERIC NAMES
1. FERROUS FUMARATE
2. FERROUS GLUCONATE
3. FERROUS SULFATE
4. IRON DEXTRAN
5. IRON POLYSACCHARIDE
6. IRON SORBITOL

BRAND NAMES
Apo-Ferrous Gluconate[2]
Apo-Ferrous Sulfate[3]
Femiron[1]
Feosol[3]
Feostat[1]
Feostat Drops[1]
Fergon[2]
Fer-In-Sol[3]
Fer-In-Sol Drops[3]
Fer-In-Sol Syrup[3]
Fer-Iron[3]
Fero-folic 500[3]
Fero-Grad[3]
Fero-Gradumet[3]
Ferralet[2]
Ferralyn[3]
Ferra-TD[3]
Fertinic[3]
Fumasorb[2]
Fumerin[1]
Geritol Tablets[1]
Hemocyte[1]
Hytinic[5]
Ircon[1]
Jectofer[6]
Mol-Iron[3]

Neo-Fer[1]
Niferex[5]
Niferex-150[5]
Novoferrogluc[5]
Novoferrosulfa[2]
Novofumar[3]
Nu-Iron[1]
Nu-Iron 150[5]
Palafer[1]
Palmiron[1]
PMS Ferrous Sulfate[3]
Simiron[2]
Slow Fe[3]
Span-FF[1]

KERATOLYTICS

GENERIC NAMES
1. RESORCINOL
2. RESORCINOL & SULFUR
3. SALICYLIC ACID
4. SALICYLIC ACID & SULFUR
5. SULFUR (Topical)

BRAND NAMES
Acne-Aid Gel[2]
AcnoAcnomel Cake[2]
Acnomel Cream[2]
Acnomel Vanishing Cream[2]
Acnomel-Acne Cream[2]
Acnotex[4]
Antinea[3]
Aveeno Acne Bar[4]
Aveeno Cleansing Bar[4]
Bensulfoid Cream[2]
Buf-Puf Acne Cleansing Bar with
  Vitamin E[3]
Buf-Puf Medicated Maximum
  Strength Pads[3]
Buf-Puf Medicated Regular
  Strength Pads[3]
Calicylic[3]
Clear Away[3]
Clear by Design Medicated
  Cleansing Pads[3]
Clearasil Adult Care Medicated
  Blemish Cream[2]
Clearasil Adult Care Medicated
  Blemish Stick[2]
Clearasil Clearstick Maximum[3]
  Strength Topical Solution[3]
Clearasil Clearstick Regular
  Strength Topical Solution[3]
Clearasil Double Textured Pads
  Maximum Strength[3]
Clearasil Double Textured Pads
  Regular Strength[3]
Clearasil Medicated Deep[3]
  Cleanser Topical Solution
Compound W Gel[3]
Compound W Liquid[3]
Creamy SS Shampoo[4]
Cuplex Gel[3]
Cuticura Ointment[5]
Diasporal Cream[4]
Duofilm[3]
Duoplant[3]
Duoplant Topical Solution[3]
Finac[5]
Fostex CM[4]
Fostex Medicated Cleansing Bar[4]
Fostex Medicated Cleansing
  Cream[4]

Fostex Medicated Cleansing Liquid[4]
Fostex Regular Strength Medicated Cleansing Bar[4]
Fostex Regular Strength Medicated Cleansing Cream[4]
Fostex Regular Strength Medicated Cover-Up[4]
Fostril Cream[5]
Fostril Lotion[5]
Freezone[3]
Gordofilm[3]
Hydrisalic[3]
Ionax Astringent Skin Cleanser Topical Solution[3]
Ionil Plus Shampoo[3]
Ionil Shampoo[3]
Keralyt[3]
Keratex Gel[3]
Lactisol[3]
Listerex Golden Scrub Lotion[3]
Listerex Herbal Scrub Lotion[3]
Lotio Asulfa[3]
Mediplast[3]
Meted Maximum Strength Anti-Dandruff Shampoo with Conditioners[4]
Night Cast R[4]
Night Cast Regular Formula Mask-Lotion[4]
Night Cast Special Formula Mask-Lotion[2]
Noxzema Anti-Acne Gel[3]
Noxzema Anti-Acne Pads Maximum Strength[3]
Noxzema Anti-Acne Pads Regular Strength[3]
Occlusal Topical Solution[3]
Occlusal-HP Topical Solution[3]
Off-Ezy Topical Solution Corn & Callus Removal Kit[3]
Off-Ezy Topical Solution Wart Removal Kit[3]
Oxy Clean Medicated Cleanser[3]
Oxy Clean Medicated Pads Maximum Strength[3]
Oxy Clean Medicated Pads Sensitive Skin[3]
Oxy Clean Regular Strength[3]
Oxy Clean Regular Strength Medicated Cleanser Topical Solution[3]
Oxy Clean Regular Strength Medicated Pads[3]
Oxy Clean Sensitive Skin Cleanser Topical Solution[3]
Oxy Clean Sensitive Skin Pads[3]
Oxy Night Watch Maximum Strength Lotion[3]
Oxy Night Watch Night Time Acne Medication Extra Strength Lotion[3]
Oxy Night Watch Night Time Acne Medication Regular Strength Lotion[3]
Oxy Night Watch Sensitive Skin Lotion[3]
Oxy Sensitive Skin Vanishing Formula Lotion[3]
P&S[3]
Paplex[3]
Paplex Ultra[3]

Pernox Lemon Medicated Scrub Cleanser[4]
Pernox Lotion Lathering Abradant Scrub Cleanser[4]
Pernox Lotion Lathering Scrub Cleanser[4]
Pernox Regular Medicated Scrub Cleanser[4]
Propa pH Medicated Acne Cream Maximum Strength[3]
Propa pH Medicated Cleansing Pads Maximum Strength[3]
Propa pH Medicated Cleansing Pads Sensitive Skin[3]
Propa pH Perfectly Clear Skin Cleanser Topical Solution Oily Skin[3]
Propa pH Perfectly Clear Skin Cleanser Topical Solution Sensitive Skin Formula[3]
R.A.[1]
Rezamid Lotion[2]
Salac[3]
Salacid[3]
Sal-Acid Plaster[3]
Salactic Film Topical Solution[3]
Sal-Clens Plus Shampoo[3]
Sal-Clens Shampoo[3]
Saligel[3]
Salonil[3]
Sal-Plant Gel Topical Solution[3]
Sastid (AL) Scrub[4]
Sastid Plain[4]
Sastid Plain Shampoo and Acne Wash[4]
Sastid Soap[4]
Sebasorb Liquid[4]
Sebex[4]
Sebucare[3]
Sebulex Antiseborrheic Treatment and Conditioning Shampoo[4]
Sebulex Antiseborrheic Treatment Shampoo[4]
Sebulex Conditioning Shampoo[4]
Sebulex Cream Medicated Shampoo[4]
Sebulex Medicated Dandruff Shampoo with Conditioners[4]
Sebulex Medicated Shampoo[4]
Sebulex Regular Medicated Dandruff Shampoo[4]
Sebulex Shampoo[4]
Stri-Dex[3]
Stri-Dex Dual Textured Pads Maximum Strength[3]
Stri-Dex Dual Textured Pads Regular Strength[3]
Stri-Dex Dual Textured Pads Sensitive Skin[3]
Stri-Dex Maximum Strength Pads[3]
Stri-Dex Regular Strength Pads[3]
Stri-Dex Super Scrub Pads[3]
Sulforcin[2]
Sulsal Soap[4]
Tersac Cleansing Gel[3]
Therac Lotion[4]
Trans-Plantar[3]
Trans-Ver-Sal[3]
Vanseb Cream Dandruff Shampoo[4]
Vanseb Lotion Dandruff Shampoo[4]

Verukan Topical Solution[3]
Verukan-HP Topical Solution[3]
Viranol[3]
Viranol Ultra[3]
Wart-Off Topical Solution[3]
X-Seb[3]

LAXATIVES, BULK-FORMING

GENERIC NAMES
1. CALCIUM POLYCARBOPHIL
2. CARBOXYMETHYLCELLUOSE SODIUM
3. MALT SOUP EXTRACT
4. METHYLCELLULOSE
5. POLYCARBOPHIL
6. PSYLLIUM
7. SENNOSIDES

BRAND NAMES
Cillium[6]
Citrucel Orange Flavor[4]
Citrucel Sugar-Free Orange Flavor[4]
Cologel[4]
Disolan Forte[2]
Disoplex[2]
Effer-syllium[6]
Equalactin[5]
Ex-Lax Natural Source Bulk Laxative[7]
Fiberall[5]
Fibercon[5]
FiberNorm[5]
Fiberpur[6]
Hydrocil Instant[6]
Karacil[6]
Konsyl[5]
Konsyl Easy Mix Formula[6]
Konsyl-D[6]
Konsyl-Orange[6]
Maalox Daily Fiber Therapy[6]
Maalox Daily Fiber Therapy Citrus Flavor[6]
Maalox Daily Fiber Therapy Orange Flavor[6]
Maalox Sugar Free Citrus Flavor[6]
Maalox Sugar Free Orange Flavor[6]
Maltsupex[3]
Metamucil[6]
Metamucil Apple Crisp Fiber Wafers[6]
Metamucil Cinnamon Spice Fiber Wafers[6]
Metamucil Instant Mix, Orange Flavor[6]
Metamucil Smooth Citrus Flavor[6]
Metamucil Smooth Orange Flavor[6]
Metamucil Smooth, Sugar-Free Citrus Flavor[6]
Metamucil Smooth, Sugar-Free Orange Flavor[6]
Metamucil Smooth, Sugar-Free Regular Flavor[6]
Metamucil Sugar Free[6]
Metamucil Sugar Free Citrus Flavor[6]
Metamucil Sugar Free Lemon-Lime Flavor[6]
Metamucil Sugar Free Orange Flavor[6]

883

Mitrolan[5]
Modane Bulk[6]
Mylanta Natural Fiber
  Supplement[6]
Mylanta Sugar Free Natural Fiber
  Supplement[6]
Naturacil[6]
Natural Source Fibre Laxative[6]
Perdiem[6]
Perdiem Fiber[6]
Perdiem Plain[6]
Prodiem[6]
Prodiem Plain[6]
Prodiem Plus[6]
Pro-Lax[6]
Prompt[6]
Reguloid Natural[6]
Reguloid Orange[6]
Reguloid Orange Sugar Free[6]
Serutan[6]
Serutan Toasted Granules[6]
Siblin[6]
Syllact[6]
Syllamalt[3]
Versabran[6]
Vitalax Super Smooth Sugar Free
  Orange Flavor[6]
Vitalax Unflavored[6]
V-Lax[6]

LAXATIVES, OSMOTIC

GENERIC NAMES
1. GLYCERIN
2. LACTULOSE
3. MAGNESIUM CITRATE
4. MAGNESIUM HYDROXIDE
5. MAGNESIUM OXIDE
6. MAGNESIUM SULFATE
7. MILK OF MAGNESIA
8. MINERAL OIL
9. SODIUM BIPHOSPHATE
10. SODIUM PHOSPHATE

BRAND NAMES
Agarol Plain[7]
Agarol Strawberry[8]
Agarol Vanilla[8]
Bilagog[6]
Cholac[2]
Chronula[2]
Citroma[3]
Citro-Mag[3]
Citro-Nesia[3]
Constilac[2]
Constulose[2]
Duphalac[2]
Evalose[2]
Fleet Phospho-Soda[9]
Generlac[2]
Hayley's M-O[7]
Heptalac[2]
Lactulax[2]
Magnolax[7]
Mag-Ox 400[5]
Maox[5]
Phillips' Chewable[4]
Phillips' Concentrated[4]
Phillips' Magnesia Tablets[4]
Phillips' Milk of Magnesia[4]
Portalac[2]

LAXATIVES, SOFTENER/LUBRICANT

GENERIC NAMES
1. CASANTHRANOL &
   DOCUSATE
2. DOCUSATE
3. DOCUSATE CALCIUM
4. DOCUSATE POTASSIUM
5. DOCUSATE SODIUM
6. MINERAL OIL
7. POLOXAMER 188
8. SODIUM PHOSPHATE

BRAND NAMES
Afko-Lube[2]
Afko-Lube Lax[2]
Agarol[6]
Agarol Marshmallow[6]
Agarol Plain[6]
Agarol Raspberry[6]
Alaxin[7]
Bilax[2]
Colace[2]
Colace Microenema[5]
Colax[2]
Correctol[2]
Correctol Caplets[2]
Correctol Extra Gentle[2]
Dialose[2]
Dialose Plus[2]
Diocto[2]
Diocto-C[1]
Diocto-K[2]
Diocto-K Plus[1]
Dioeze[2]
Diosuccin[2]
Dio-Sul[2]
Diothron[1]
Disanthrol[1]
Disolan[2]
Disolan Forte[1]
Disonate[2]
Disoplex[2]
Di-Sosul[2]
Di-Sosul Forte[1]
Docucal-P[2]
Docu-K Plus[1]
DOK[2]
DOK Softgels[2]
Doss[2]
Doss Tablets[2]
Doxidan[2]
Doxidan Liqui-Gels[2]
Doxinate[2]
DSMC Plus[1]
Dulcodos[2]
Duosol[2]
Ex-Lax Light Formula[2]
Extra Gentle Ex-Lax[2]
Feen-a-Mint[2]
Feen-a-Mint Pills[2]
Femilax[2]
Fleet Enema Mineral Oil[7]
Gentlax-S[2]
Kasof[2]
Kondremul[7]
Kondremul with Cascara[7]
Kondremul with
   Phenolphthalein[7]
Kondremul Plain[7]
Lansoyl[7]
Laxinate 100[2]
Liqui-Doss[7]

Milkinol[7]
Modane Plus[2]
Modane Soft[2]
Molatoc[2]
Molatoc-CST[2]
Neo-Cultol[7]
Neolax[2]
Nujol[7]
Peri-Colase[1]
Pertrogalar Plain[7]
Phenolphthalein Petrogalar[7]
Phillips' LaxCaps[2]
PMS-Docusate Calcium[2]
PMS-Docusate Sodium[2]
PMS-Phosphates[9]
Pro-Cal-Sof[2]
Pro-Sof[1]
Pro-Sof Liquid Concentrate[1]
Pro-Sof Plus[1]
Regulace[2]
Regulax SS[2]
Regulex[2]
Regulex-D[2]
Regutol[2]
Senokot-S[2]
Stulex[2]
Sulfolax[2]
Surfak[2]
Therevac Plus[2]
Therevac-SB[2]
Trilax[2]
Unilax[2]
Zymenol[7]

LAXATIVES, STIMULANT

GENERIC NAMES
1. ALOE
2. BISACODYL
3. CASANTHRANOL
4. CASCARA
5. CASTOR OIL
6. DEHYDROCHOLIC ACID
7. PHENOLPHTHALEIN
8. SENNA
9. SENNOSIDES

BRAND NAMES
Afko-Lube Lax[3]
Agarol[7]
Agarol Marshmallow[7]
Agarol Raspberry[7]
Agarol Strawberry[7]
Agarol Vanilla[7]
Alophen[7]
Alphamul[5]
Aromatic Cascara Fluidextract[4]
Bilax[6]
Bisac-Evac[2]
Bisacolax[2]
Bisco-Lax[2]
Black Draught[3]
Black-Draught Lax-Senna[8]
Caroid Laxative[2]
Carter's Little Pills[4]
Cascara Aromatic Fluidextract[4]
Cascara Sagrada[4]
Cholan-HMB[6]
Clysodrast[7]
Colax[7]
Correctol[7]
Correctol Caplets[7]
Dacodyl[2]

884

Decholin[6]
Deficol[2]
Dialose Plus[7]
Diocto-C[3]
Diocto-K Plus[1]
Diothron[3]
Disanthrol[3]
Disolan Forte[3]
Di-Sosul Forte[3]
Docucal-P[7]
Docu-K Plus[3]
Dosaflex[8]
Doxidan[7]
Doxidan Liqui-Gels[7]
Dr. Caldwell Senna Laxative[8]
DSMC Plus[3]
Dulcodos[2]
Dulcolax[2]
Emulsoil[5]
Espotabs[7]
Evac-U-Gen[7]
Evac-U-Lax[7]
Ex-Lax[7]
Ex-Lax Gentle Nature[9]
Ex-Lax Light Formula[7]
Ex-Lax Maximum Relief Formula[7]
Ex-Lax Pills[7]
Extra Gentle Ex-Lax[7]
Feen-a-Mint[7]
Feen-a-Mint Gum[7]
Feen-a-Mint Pills[7]
Femilax[7]
Fleet Bisacodyl[2]
Fleet Bisacodyl Prep[2]
Fleet Flavored Castor Oil[5]
Fleet Laxative[2]
Fletcher's Castoria[8]
Gentlax S[8]
Gentle Nature[9]
Glysennid[9]
Hepahydrin[6]
Herbal Laxative[9]
Kellogg's Castor Oil[5]
Kondremul with Cascara[4]
Kondremul with Phenolphthalein[7]
Laxit[2]
Lax-Pills[7]
Medilax[7]
Modane[7]
Molatoc-CST[3]
Mucinum[7]
Mucinum Herbal[9]
Nature's Remedy[4]
Neolax[6]
Neoloid[5]
Nytilax[9]
Perdiem[8]
Peri-Colace[3]
Phenolax[7]
Phenolphthalein Petrogalar[7]
Phillips' Gelcaps[7]
Phillips' LaxCaps[7]
PMS-Bisacodyl[2]
PMS-Sennosides[9]
Prodiem Plus[8]
Prompt[9]
Pro-Sof Plus[3]
Prulet[7]
Purge[5]
Regulace[3]
Senexon[8]
Senokot[8]

Senokot-S[8]
SenokotXTRA[8]
Senolax[8]
Theralax[2]
Trilax[6]
Unilax[7]
Veracolate[7]
X-Prep Liquid[8]

MEPROBAMATE

Acabamate
Apo-Meprobamate
Equanil
Equanil Wyseals
Medi-Tran
Meprospan 200
Meprospan 400
Miltown
Neuramate
Novomepro
Novo-Mepro
Pax 400
Probate
Sedabamate
Trancot
Tranmep

NARCOTIC ANALGESICS

GENERIC NAMES
1. BUPRENORPHINE
2. CODEINE
3. CODEINE & TERPIN HYDRATE
4. DIHYDROCODEINE
5. FENTANYL
6. HYDROCODONE
7. HYDROCODONE & HOMATROPINE
8. HYDROCODONE & IBUPROFEN
9. HYDROMORPHONE
10. LEVORPHANOL
11. MEPERIDINE
12. METHADONE
13. MORPHINE
14. NALBUPHINE
15. OPIUM
16. OXYCODONE
17. OXYMORPHONE
18. PENTAZOCINE
19. PROPOXYPHENE

BRAND NAMES
642 [14]
Actagen-C Cough[2]
Actifed with Codeine Cough[2]
Adatuss D.C. Expectorant[6]
Allerfrin with Codeine[2]
Ambay Cough[2]
Ambenyl Cough[2]
Ambophen Expectorant[2]
Anamine HD[6]
Anaplex HD[6]
Anatuss with Codeine[2]
Aprodrine with Codeine[2]
Astramorph[13]
Astramorph-PF[13]
Baycodan[7]
Baycomine[6]
Baycomine Pediatric[6]
Bayhistine DH[2]
Bayhistine Expectorant[2]
Baytussin AC[2]

Benylin with Codeine[2]
Biphetane DC Cough[2]
Bromanate DC Cough[2]
Bromanyl[2]
Bromphen DC with Codeine Cough[2]
Brontex[2]
Buprenex[1]
Calcidrine[2]
Caldomine-DH Forte[6]
Caldomine-DH Pediatric[6]
Calmylin with Codeine[2]
Cheracol[2]
Chlorgest-HD[6]
Citra Forte[6]
CoActIfed[2]
CoActifed Expectorant[2]
Codamine [6]
Codamine Pediatric[6]
Codan[7]
Codegest Expectorant[2]
Codehist DH[2]
Codeine Sulfate[2]
Codiclear DH[6]
Codimal DH[6]
Codimal PH[2]
Colrex Compound[2]
Conex with Codeine Liquid[2]
Cophene-S[4]
Cophene-XP[6]
Coricidin with Codeine[2]
Coristex-DH [6]
Coristine-DH[6]
Cotanal-65[18]
Cotridin[2]
Cotridin Expectorant[2]
C-Tussin Expectorant[2]
Darvon[19]
Darvon-N[19]
Decohistine DH[2]
Demerol[11]
Deproist Expectorant with Codeine[2]
De-Tuss[6]
Detussin Expectorant[6]
Detussin Liquid[6]
Dihistine DH[2]
Dihistine Expectorant[2]
Dihydromorphinone[9]
Dilaudid[9]
Dilaudid Cough[9]
Dilaudid-HP[9]
Dimetane Expectorant-C[2]
Dimetane Expectorant-DC [6]
Dimetane-DC Cough[2]
Dimetapp with Codeine[2]
Dolene[19]
Dolophine[12]
Donatussin DC[6]
Doxaphene[19]
Dromoran[10]
Duragesic[5]
Duramorph[13]
Duratuss HD[6]
Endagen-HD[6]
Endal Expectorant[2]
Endal-HD[6]
Endal-HD Plus[6]
Entuss Expectorant[6]
Entuss-D[6]
Epimorph[13]
Expectorant with Codeine[2]
Fortral[18]

885

Glydeine Cough[2]
Guiatuss A.C.[2]
Guiatuss DAC[2]
Guiatussin DAC[2]
Guiatussin with Codeine Liquid[2]
Histafed C[2]
Histussin HC[6]
Hycodan[6]
Hycomine[6]
Hycomine Compound[6]
Hycomine Pediatric[6]
Hycomine-S Pediatric[6]
Hycotuss Expectorant[6]
Hydromet[7]
Hydromine[6]
Hydromine Pediatric[6]
Hydropane[7]
Hydrophen[6]
Hydrostal IR[8]
Isoclor Expectorant[2]
Kadian[13]
Kwelcof Liquid[6]
Laudanum[15]
Levo-Dromoran[10]
Levorphan[10]
Mallergan-VC with Codeine[2]
Methadose[12]
Midahist DH[2]
Morphitec[13]
M.O.S.[13]
M.O.S.-SR[13]
MS Contin[13]
MSIR[13]
MST Continus[13]
Myhydromine[6]
Myhydromine Pediatric[6]
Myphetane DC Cough[2]
Mytussin AC[2]
Mytussin DAC[2]
Naldecon-CX Adult Liquid[2]
Normatane DC[2]
Nortussin with Codeine [2]
Novagest Expectorant with
    Codeine[2]
Novahistex C[2]
Novahistex DH[6]
Novahistex DH Expectorant[6]
Novahistine DH Expectorant[2]
Novahistine DH Liquid[2]
Novahistine Expectorant[2]
Nubain[14]
Nucochem[2]
Nucochem Expectorant[2]
Nucochem Pediatric
    Expectorant[2]
Nucofed[2]
Nucofed Expectorant[2]
Nucofed Pediatric Expectorant[2]
Numorphan[17]
Omni-Tuss[2]
Oramorph[13]
Oramorph-SR[13]
Oxycontin SR[16]
Pantapon[15]
Paveral[2]
Pediacof Cough[2]
Pediatuss Cough[2]
Penazine VC with Cough[2]
Pethidine[11]
Phenameth VC with Codeine[2]
Phenergan VC with Codeine[2]
Phenergan with Codeine[2]
Phenhist DH with Codeine[2]

Phenhist Expectorant[2]
Pherazine VC with Codeine[2]
Pherazine with Codeine[2]
Physeptone[12]
Poly-Histine-CS[2]
Promehist with Codeine[2]
Prometh VC with Codeine[2]
Propoxycon[19]
Prunicodeine[2]
Pseudodine C Cough[2]
P-V-Tussin[6]
RMS Uniserts[13]
Robafen AC Cough[2]
Robafen DAC[2]
Robidone[6]
Robitussin A-C[2]
Robitussin with Codeine[2]
Robitussin-DAC[2]
Rolatuss Expectorant[2]
Rolatuss with Hydrocodone[6]
Roxanol[13]
Roxanol SR[13]
Roxicodone[16]
Ru-Tuss with Hydrocodone
    Liquid[6]
Ryna-C Liquid[2]
Ryna-CX Liquid[2]
SRC Expectorant[6]
Statex[13]
Statuss Expectorant[2]
Statuss Green[6]
Supeudol[16]
Talwin[18]
Talwin-NX[18]
Temgesic[1]
Terpin Hydrate and Codeine
    Syrup[2]
T-Koff[2]
Tolu-Sed Cough[2]
Triacin C Cough[2]
Triafed with Codeine[2]
Triaminic Expectorant DH[6]
Triaminic Expectorant with
    Codeine[2]
Triaminicin with Codeine[2]
Tricodene #1[2]
Trifed-C Cough[2]
Tussafin Expectorant[6]
Tussaminic C[2]
Tussaminic C Pediatric[2]
Tussaminic DH Forte[6]
Tussaminic DH Pediatric[6]
Tussanil DH[6]
Tussar SF[2]
Tussar-2[2]
Tussigon[7]
Tussionex[6]
Tussirex with Codeine Liquid[2]
Tyrodone[6]
Vanex Expectorant[6]
Vanex-HD[6]
Vicodin-Tuss[6]
Vicoprofen[8]

NARCOTIC ANALGESICS & ACETAMINOPHEN

GENERIC NAMES
1. ACETAMINOPHEN & CODEINE
2. DIHYDROCODEINE &
    ACETAMINOPHEN
3. HYDROCODONE &
    ACETAMINOPHEN

4. MEPERIDINE &
    ACETAMINOPHEN
5. OXYCODONE &
    ACETAMINOPHEN
6. PENTAZOCINE &
    ACETAMINOPHEN
7. PROPOXYPHENE &
    ACETAMINOPHEN

BRAND NAMES
Allay[3]
Anexsia[3]
Anolor-DH5[3]
APAP with Codeine [1]
Atasol-8[1]
Atasol-15[1]
Atasol-30[1]
Bancap-HC[3]
Capital with Codeine [1]
Co-Gesic[3]
Compal[3]
Darvocet-N 50[7]
Darvocet-N 100[7]
Demerol-APAP[4]
DHCplus[2]
Dolacet[3]
Dolagesic[3]
Dolene-AP 65[7]
Duocet[3]
E-Lor[7]
Empracet 30[1]
Empracet 60[1]
Emtec[1]
Endocet[5]
Exdol-8[1]
Exdol-15[1]
Exdol-30[1]
EZ III[1]
Hycomed[3]
Hyco-Pap[3]
Hydrocet[2]
Hydrocodone with APAP[3]
Hydrogesic[3]
HY-PHEN[3]
Lenoltec with Codeine No. 1[1]
Lenoltec with Codeine No. 2[1]
Lenoltec with Codeine No. 3[1]
Lenoltec with Codeine No. 4[1]
Lorcet[3]
Lorcet 10/650[3]
Lorcet Plus[3]
Lorcet-HD[3]
Lortab[3]
Lortab 5[3]
Lortab 7[3]
Margesic #3[1]
Margesic-H[3]
Novogesic[1]
Onset[3]
Oxycocet[5]
Panacet 5/500[3]
Panlor[3]
Percocet[5]
Percocet-Demi[5]
Phenaphen with Codeine[1]
Polygesic[3]
Pro Pox with APAP[7]
Propacet 100[7]
Pyregesic-C[1]
Roxicet[5]
Roxilox[5]
Stagesic[3]
Talacen[6]

T-gesic[3]
Tylaprin with Codeine[1]
Tylenol No.1[1]
Tylenol No.1 Forte[1]
Tylenol with Codeine[1]
Tylenol with Codeine No. 1[1]
Tylenol with Codeine No. 2[1]
Tylenol with Codeine No. 3[1]
Tylenol with Codeine No. 4[1]
Tylox[5]
Ugesic[3]
Ultragesic[3]
Vanacet[3]
Vapocet[3]
Veganin[1]
Vendone[3]
Vicodin[3]
Vicodin ES[3]
Wygesic[7]
Zydone[3]

NARCOTIC ANALGESICS & ASPIRIN

GENERIC NAMES
1. ASPIRIN & CODEINE
2. BUFFERED ASPIRIN & CODEINE
3. DIHYDROCODEINE & ASPIRIN
4. HYDROCODONE & ASPIRIN
5. OXYCODONE & ASPIRIN
6. PENTAZOCINE & ASPIRIN
7. PROPOXYPHENE & ASPIRIN

BRAND NAMES
222[1]
282[1]
292[1]
293[1]
692[7]
A.C.&C.[1]
Anacin with Codeine[1]
Azdone[1]
Cotanal 65[7]
Damason-P[4]
Darvon Compound[6]
Darvon Compound 65[6]
Darvon with A.S.A.[6]
Darvon-N Compound[7]
Darvon-N with A.S.A.[7]
Drocade and Aspirin[3]
Emcodeine No. 2[1]
Emcodeine No. 3[1]
Emcodeine No. 4[1]
Empirin with Codeine[1]
Empirin with Codeine No. 3[1]
Empirin with Codeine No. 4[1]
Endodan[5]
Lortab ASA[4]
Novo-AC and C[1]
Oxycodan[5]
Panasal 5/500[4]
PC-Cap[7]
Percodan[5]
Percodan-Demi[5]
Propoxyphene Compound-65[7]
Roxiprin[5]
Synalgos-DC[3]
Talwin Compound[6]
Talwin Compound-50[6]

NITRATES

GENERIC NAMES
1. ERYTHRITYL TETRANITRATE
2. ISOSORBIDE DINITRATE
3. ISOSORBIDE MONONITRATE
4. NITROGLYCERIN (GLYCERYL TRINITRATE)
5. PENTAERYTHRITOL TETRANITRATE

BRAND NAMES
Apo-ISDN[2]
Cardilate[1]
Cedocard-SR[2]
Coradur[2]
Coronex[2]
Deponit[4]
Dilatrate-SR[2]
Duotrate[5]
Glyceryl Trinitrate[4]
IMDUR[3]
ISMO[3]
Iso-Bid[2]
Isonate[2]
Isorbid[2]
Isordil[2]
Isotrate[2]
Klavikordal[4]
Minitran[4]
Monoket[3]
Niong[4]
Nitro-Bid[4]
Nitrocap[4]
Nitrocap T.D.[4]
Nitrocine[4]
Nitrodisc[4]
Nitro-Dur[4]
Nitro-Dur II[4]
Nitrogard-SR[4]
Nitroglyn[4]
Nitrol[4]
Nitrolin[4]
Nitrolingual[4]
Nitronet[4]
Nitrong[4]
Nitrong SR[4]
Nitrospan[4]
Nitrostat[4]
Novosorbide[2]
NTS[4]
Pentritol[5]
Pentylan[5]
Peritrate[5]
Peritrate Forte[5]
Peritrate SA[5]
P.E.T.N.[5]
Sorbitrate[2]
Sorbitrate SA[2]
Transderm-Nitro[4]
Tridil[4]

OXYMETAZOLINE (Nasal)

4-Way Long Acting Nasal Spray
12-Hour Nostrilla Nasal Decongestant
Afrin 12 Hour Nasal Spray
Afrin 12 Hour Nose Drops
Afrin Cherry Scented Nasal Spray
Afrin Children's Strength 12 Hour Nose Drops
Afrin Children's Strength Nose Drops

Afrin Extra Moisturizing Nasal Decongestant Spray
Afrin Menthol Nasal Spray
Afrin Nasal Spray
Afrin Nose Drops
Afrin Sinus
Afrin Spray Pump
Allerest 12 Hour Nasal Spray
Cheracol Nasal Spray
Cheracol Nasal Spray Pump Cherry Scented
Coricidin Nasal Mist
Dristan 12-Hour Nasal Spray
Dristan Long Lasting Menthol Nasal Spray
Dristan Long Lasting Nasal Pump Spray
Dristan Long Lasting Nasal Spray
Dristan Long Lasting Nasal Spray 12 Hour Metered Dose Pump
Dristan Mentholated
Drixoral
Duramist Plus Up To 12 Hours Decongestant Nasal Spray
Duration 12 Hour Nasal Spray Pump
Nasal Decongestant Spray
Nasal Relief
Nasal Spray 12-Hour
Nasal Spray Long Acting
Nasal-12 Hour
Neo-Synephrine 12 Hour Nasal Spray
Neo-Synephrine 12 Hour Nasal Spray Pump
Neo-Synephrine 12 Hour Nose Drops
Neo-Synephrine 12 Hour Vapor Nasal Spray
Nostril Nasal Decongestant Mild
Nostril Nasal Decongestant Regular
NTZ Long Acting Decongestant Nasal Spray
NTZ Long Acting Decongestant Nose Drops
Sinarest 12 Hour Nasal Spray
Vicks Sinex 12-Hour Formula Decongestant Nasal Spray
Vicks Sinex 12-Hour Formula Decongestant Ultra Fine Mist
Vicks Sinex Long-Acting 12 Hour Nasal Spray

PENICILLINS

GENERIC NAMES
1. AMOXICILLIN
2. AMPICILLIN
3. BACAMPICILLIN
4. CARBENICILLIN
5. CLOXACILLIN
6. DICLOXACILLIN
7. FLUCLOXACILLIN
8. NAFCILLIN
9. OXACILLIN
10. PENICILLIN G
11. PENICILLIN V
12. PIVAMPICILLIN
13. PIVMECILLINAM

BRAND NAMES
Amoxil[1]
Apo-Amoxi[1]

Apo-Ampi[2]
Apo-Cloxi[5]
Apo-Pen VK[11]
Bactocill[9]
Beepen-VK[11]
Betapen-VK[11]
Cloxapen[5]
Dycill[6]
Dynapen[6]
Fluclox[7]
Geocillin[4]
Geopen Oral[4]
Ledercillin-VK[11]
Megacillin[10]
Nadopen-V[11]
Nadopen-V 200[11]
Nadopen-V 400[11]
Novamoxin[1]
Novo-Ampicillin[2]
Novo-Cloxin[5]
Novo-Pen VK[11]
Nu-Amoxi[11]
Nu-Ampi[2]
Nu-Cloxi[5]
Nu-Pen-VK[11]
Omnipen[2]
Orbenin[5]
Pathocil[6]
Pen Vee[11]
Pen Vee K[11]
Penbritin[2]
Penglobe[3]
Pentids[10]
Polycillin[2]
Polymox[1]
Pondocillin[12]
Principen[2]
Prostaphlin[9]
PVF[11]
PVF K[11]
Selexid[13]
Spectrobid[3]
Tegopen[5]
Totacillin[2]
Trimox[1]
Unipen[8]
V-Cillin K[11]
Veetids[11]
Wymox[1]

PHENOTHIAZINES

GENERIC NAMES
1. ACETOPHENAZINE
2. CHLORPROMAZINE
3. FLUPHENAZINE
4. MESORIDAZINE
5. METHOTRIMEPRAZINE
6. PERICYAZINE
7. PERPHENAZINE
8. PIPOTIAZINE
9. PROCHLORPERAZINE
10. PROMAZINE
11. THIOPROPAZATE
12. THIOPROPERAZINE
13. THIORIDAZINE
14. TRIFLUOPERAZINE
15. TRIFLUPROMAZINE

BRAND NAMES
Apo-Fluphenazine[3]
Apo-Perphenazine[7]
Apo-Thioridazine[13]

Apo-Trifluoperazine[14]
Chlorpromanyl-5[2]
Chlorpromanyl-20[2]
Chlorpromanyl-40[2]
Compazine[9]
Compazine Spansule[9]
Dartal[11]
Largactil[2]
Largactil Liquid[2]
Largactil Oral Drops[2]
Levoprome[5]
Majeptil[12]
Mellaril[13]
Mellaril Concentrate[13]
Mellaril-S[13]
Modecate[3]
Modecate Concentrate[3]
Moditen Enanthate[3]
Moditen HCl[3]
Moditen HCl-H.P.[3]
Neuleptil[6]
Novo-Chlorpromazine[2]
Novo-Flurazine[14]
Novo-Ridazine[13]
Nozinan[5]
Nozinan Liquid[5]
Nozinan Oral Drops[5]
Permitil[3]
Permitil Concentrate[3]
Piportil L₄[8]
PMS Thioridazine[13]
Prolixin[3]
Prolixin Concentrate[3]
Prolixin Decanoate[3]
Prolixin Enanthate[3]
Prorazin[9]
Prozine [10]
Serentil[4]
Serentil Concentrate[4]
Solazine[14]
Stelazine[14]
Stelazine Concentrate[14]
Stemetil[9]
Stemetil Liquid[9]
Suprazine[14]
Terfluzine[14]
Terfluzine Concentrate[14]
Thorazine[2]
Thorazine Concentrate[2]
Thorazine Spansule[2]
Thor-Prom[2]
Tindal[2]
Trilafon[7]
Trilafon Concentrate[7]
Ultrazine-10[9]
Vesprin[5]

PHENYLEPHRINE

Aclophen
Advanced Formula Dristan
  Caplets
AH-Chew
Alersule
Amaril D
Anamine HD
Anaplex HD
Anatuss
Atrohist Pediatric
Atrohist Pediatric Suspension
  Dye Free
Atrohist Plus
Atrohist Sprinkle

Banex
Banex Liquid
Bromophen T.D.
Cerose-DM
Chlorgest-HD
Citra Forte
Codimal DH
Codimal DM
Codimal PH
Colrex Compound
Colrex Cough
Coltab Children's
Comhist
Comhist LA
Conar
Conar Expectorant
Conar-A
Congespirin for Children Cold
  Tablets
Contuss
Cophene-S
Cophene-X
Cophene-XP
Coristex-DH
Coristine-DH
Covangesic
D.A. Chewable
Dallergy
Dallergy Caplets
Dallergy-D Syrup
Decongestabs
Deconsal Sprinkle
Despec
Dihistine
Dimaphen S.A.
Dimetane Decongestant Caplets
Dimetane Expectorant
Dimetane Expectorant-C
Dimetane Expectorant-DC
Dimetapp
Dimetapp Extentabs
Dimetapp Oral Infant Drops
Dimetap with Codeine
Dimetapp-A
Dimetapp-A Pediatric
Dimetapp-DM
Doktors
Donatussin
Donatussin DC
Donatussin Drops
Dondril
Dristan Cold Multi-Symptom
  Formula
Dristan Formula P
Dristan-AF
Dristan-AF Plus
Dura-Vent/DA
Ed A-Hist
Endagen-HD
Endal-HD
Endal-HD Plus
Enomine
Entex
Entex Liquid
Extendryl
Extendryl JR
Extendryl SR
Father John's Medicine Plus
Fendol
Gendecon
Histagesic Modified
Histalet Forte
Histamic

Histatab Plus
Histatan
Histatuss Pediatric
Hista-Vadrin
Histor-D
Histor-D Timecelles
Histussin HC
Hycomine
Hycomine Compound
Hycomine-S Pediatric
Improved Sino-Tuss
Kolephrin
Mallergan-VC with Codeine
Meda Syrup Forte
Myhistine
Naldecon
Naldecon Pediatric Drops
Naldecon Pediatric Syrup
Naldelate
Naldelate Pediatric Syrup
Nalgest
Nalgest Pediatric
Nasahist
ND-Gesic
Neocitran A
Neocitran Colds & Flu Calorie
 Reduced
NeoCitran DM Coughs & Colds
NeoCitran Extra Strength Colds
 & Flu
NeoCitran Extra Strength Sinus
Neo-Synephrine Nasal Drops
Neo-Synephrine Pediatric Nasal
 Drops
New-Decongest Pediatric
New-Decongest Pediatric Syrup
Normatane
Nostril Spray Pump
Novahistex C
Novahistex DH
Novahistex DH Expectorant
Novahistine
Novahistine DH
Novahistine DH Expectorant
Omnicol
OMNIhist L.A.
Par Decon
Partapp TD
Pediacof Cough
Pediatuss Cough
Phenameth VC
Phenameth VC with Codeine
Phenchlor SHA
Phenergan VC
Phenergan VC with Codeine
Phentox Compound
Pherazine VC
Pherazine VC with Codeine
Prehist
Prehist D
Prometh VC Plain
Prometh VC with Codeine
Promethazine VC
Quadra-Hist
Quadra-Hist Pediatric Syrup
Quelidrine Cough
Rentamine Pediatric
Rescon-GG
Respinol G
Respinol LA
Rhinall
Rhinall Children's Flavored Nose
 Drops

Rhinatate
Rhinogesic
Robitussin Night Relief
Robitussin Night Relief Colds
 Formula Liquid
Rolatuss Expectorant
Rolatuss Plain
Rolatuss with Hydrocodone
R-Tannamine
R-Tannamine Pediatric
R-Tannate
R-Tannate Pediatric
Ru-Tuss
Ru-Tuss with Hydrocodone Liquid
Rymed
Rymed Liquid
Rynatan
Rynatan Pediatric
Rynatan-S Pediatric
Rynatuss
Rynatuss Pediatric
Salphenyl
Scot-Tussin
Scot-Tussin Original 5-Action
 Cold Medicine
Sinucon Pediatric Drops
Sinupan
Stahist
Status Expectorant
Statuss Green
Tamine S.R.
Tanoral
T-Koff
Trimedine Liquid
Triotann
Triotann Pediatric
Tri-Phen-Chlor
Tri-Phen-Chlor Pediatric
Tri-Phen-Chlor T.R.
Tritann Pediatric
Tri-Tannate
Tri-Tannate Plus Pediatric
Tusquelin
Tussanil DH Tablets
Tussanil Plain
Tussirex with Codeine Liquid
Uni-DeCon
Vanex Forte Caplets
Vanex-HD
Veltap
Vicks Sinex

PHENYL-
PROPANOLAMINE

4-Way Cold
12-Hour Cold
Acutrim 16 Hour
Acutrim II Maximum Strength
Acutrim Late Day
Alamine
Alka-Seltzer Plus Cold
Alka-Seltzer Plus Cold and
 Cough
Alka-Seltzer Plus Maximum
 Strength Sinus Allergy
 Medicine
Alka-Seltzer Plus Nighttime Cold
Allerest 12 Hour
Allerest 12 Hour Maximum
 Strength Caplets
Allerest Children's
Allerest Headache Strength

Allerest Sinus Pain Formula
Allergy Relief Medicine
Alumadrine
Amaril D
Amaril D Spantabs
Ami-Tex LA
Anatuss
Anatuss with Codeine
A.R.M. Maximum Strength
 Caplets
Atrohist Plus
Banex
Banex Liquid
Banex-LA
Bayaminic Expectorant
Bayaminicol
Baycomine
Baycomine Pediatric
Bayer Cough Syrup
Bayer Cough Syrup for Children
BC Cold Powder
BC Cold Powder Non-Drowsy
 Formula
BC Multi-Symptom Cold Powder
Biphetane DC Cough
BQ Cold
Bromaline
Bromaline Plus
Bromanate
Bromanate DC Cough
Bromatap
Bromatapp
Bromophen T.D.
Bromphen
Bromphen DC with Codeine Cough
Caldomine-DH Forte
Caldomine-DH Pediatric
Cheracol Plus
Chexit
Chlor-Rest
Chlor-Trimeton Sinus Caplets
Chlor-Tripolon Decongestant
Codamine
Codamine Pediatric
Codegest Expectorant
Codimal Expectorant
Comtrex Maximum Strength
 Liqui-Gels
Comtrex Multi-Symptom Cold
 Reliever
Condrin-LA
Conex
Conex D.A.
Conex Plus
Conex with Codeine Liquid
Congespirin for Children Liquid
 Cold Medicine
Congestant D
Contac 12-Hour
Contac Jr. Children's Cold
 Medicine
Contac Maximum Strength
 12-Hour Caplets
Control
Contuss
Cophene-S
Cophene-X
Cophene-XP
Coricidin Cough
Coricidin D
Coricidin D Decongestant
Coricidin D Medilets
Coricidin Demilets

Coricidin Maximum Strength
  Sinus Headache
Corsym
Covangesic
Dapacin Cold
DayQuil Non-Drowsy Sinus
  Pressure and Congestion Relief
  Caplets
Decongestabs
Dehist
Demazin
Demazin Repetabs
Despec
Dexatrim Maximum Strength
  Caplets
Dexatrim Maximum Strength
  Capsules
Dexatrim Maximum Strength
  Tablets
Diet-Aide Maximum Strength
Dilotab
Dimaphen
Dimaphen S.A.
Dimetane Expectorant
Dimetane Expectorant-C
Dimetane Expectorant-DC
Dimetane-DC Cough
Dimetapp
Dimetapp 4-Hour Liqui-Gels
  Maximum Strength
Dimetapp Cold and Allergy
Dimetapp Cold and Flu Caplets
Dimetapp Extentabs
Dimetapp Maximum Strength
  Liquigels
Dimetapp Oral Infant Drops
Dimetapp Plus Caplets
Dimetapp with Codeine
Dimetapp-A
Dimetapp-A Pediatric
Dimetapp-DM
Dimetapp-DM Cough and Cold
Dimetapp-DM Elixir
Dorcol DM
Drinophen
Dristan
Drize
Duadacin
Dura-Gest
Dura-Vent
Dura-Vent/A
Efed II Yellow
Efficol Cough Whip (Cough
  Suppressant/Decongestant)
Efficol Cough Whip (Cough
  Suppressant/Decongestant/
  Antihistamine)
Endal Expectorant
Enomine
Entex
Entex LA
Entex Liquid
Exgest LA
Genamin
Genatap
Gencold
Genex
Guaipax
GuiaCough CF
Guiatuss CF
Guiatuss DAC
Halls Mentho-Lyptus

Halls Mentho-Lyptus
  Decongestant Cough Formula
Head & Chest
Histabid Duracaps
Histalet Forte
Histamic
Hista-Vadrin
Histosal
Hold (Children's Formula)
Hycomine
Hycomine Pediatric
Hydromine
Hydromine Pediatric
Hydrophen
Ipsatol Cough Formula for
  Children
Kiddy Koff
Kolephrin NN Liquid
Kophane
Kophane Cough and Cold
  Formula
Lanatuss Expectorant
Myhydromine
Myhydromine Pediatric
Myminic Expectorant
Myminicol
Myphetane DC Cough
Myphetapp
Naldecon
Naldecon Pediatric Drops
Naldecon Pediatric Syrup
Naldecon-CX Adult Liquid
Naldecon-DX Adult
Naldecon-DX Adult Liquid
Naldecon-DX Children's Syrup
Naldecon-DX Pediatric Drops
Naldecon-EX
Naldecon-EX Pediatric Drops
Naldelate
Naldelate DX Adult
Naldelate Pediatric Syrup
Nalgest
Nalgest Pediatric
Nasahist
New-Decongest Pediatric
New-Decongest Pediatric Syrup
Night-Time Effervescent Cold
Nolamine
Nolex LA
Noraminic
Norel Plus
Normatane
Normatane DC
Oragest S.R.
Oraminic Spancaps
Ornade
Ornade A.F.
Ornade Expectorant
Ornade-DM
Ornade-DM 10
Ornade-DM 15
Ornade-DM 30
Orthoxicol Cough
Par Decon
Partapp
Partapp TD
Partuss LA
Phanadex
Phenahist-TR
PhenAPAP No. 2
Phenate T.D.
Phena-TR
Phenchlor SHA

Phentox Compound
Phenyldrine
Phenylfenesin L.A.
Poly-Histine-CS
Poly-Histine-D
Poly-Histine-D Ped
Poly-Histine-DM
Prolamine
Prominic Expectorant
Prominicol Cough
Propagest
Pyrroxate
Quadra-Hist
Quadra-Hist Pediatric Syrup
Remcol Cold
Resaid S.R.
Rescaps-D S.R.
Respinol LA
Respinol-G
Rhinocaps
Rhinolar
Rhinolar-EX
Rhinolar-EX 12
Robafen CF
Robitussin-CF
Rolatuss with Hydrocodone
Ru-Tuss
Ru-Tuss with Hydrocodone Liquid
Saleto-CF
Saleto-D
Sinapils
Sinarest
Sinarest Extra Strength
Sine-Off Sinus Medicine
Sinucon Pediatric Drops
Sinulin
Sinutab SA
SINUvent
Snaplets-D
Snaplets-DM
Snaplets-EX
Snaplets-Multi
St. Joseph Cold Tablets for
  Children
Stahist
Stamoist LA
Statuss Green
Syracol Liquid
Tamine S.R.
Tavist-D
Temazin Cold
Threamine DM
Threamine Expectorant
T-Koff
Triaminic
Triaminic Allergy
Triaminic Chewables
Triaminic Cold
Triaminic DM Cough Formula
Triaminic DM Daytime
Triaminic DM Expectorant
Triaminic Expectorant
Triaminic Expectorant DH
Triaminic Expectorant with Codeine
Triaminic Oral Infant Drops
Triaminic TR
Triaminic-12
Triaminicin Cold, Allergy, Sinus
Triaminicin with Codeine
Triaminicol DM
Triaminicol Multi-Symptom Relief
Tricodene Forte
Tricodene NN

Tricodene NN Pediatric
  Medication
Tricodene Pediatric
Trind
Trind DM Liquid
Tri-Nefrin Extra Strength
Tripalgen Cold
Tri-Phen-Chlor
Tri-Phen-Chlor Pediatric
Tri-Phen-Chlor T.R.
Triphenyl
Triphenyl Expectorant
Triphenyl T.D.
Tusquelin
Tuss Allergine Modified T.D.
Tuss-Ade
Tussaminic C
Tussaminic C Pediatric
Tussaminic DH Forte
Tussaminic DH Pediatric
Tussanil DH Tablets
Tussogest
Tuss-Ornade Liquid
Tuss-Ornade Spansules
ULR-LA
Uni-DeCon
Utex-S.R.
Vanex Forte Caplets
Vanex LA
Veltap
Vicks DayQuil 4 Hour Allergy
  Relief
Vicks DayQuil 12 Hour Allergy
  Relief

POTASSIUM
SUPPLEMENTS

GENERIC NAMES
1. POTASSIUM ACETATE
2. POTASSIUM BICARBONATE
3. POTASSIUM BICARBONATE &
   POTASSIUM CHLORIDE
4. POTASSIUM BICARBONATE &
   POTASSIUM CITRATE
5. POTASSIUM CHLORIDE
6. POTASSIUM CHLORIDE,
   POTASSIUM BICARBONATE &
   POTASSIUM CITRATE
7. POTASSIUM GLUCONATE
8. POTASSIUM GLUCONATE &
   POTASSIUM CHLORIDE
9. POTASSIUM GLUCONATE &
   POTASSIUM CITRATE
10. POTASSIUM GLUCONATE,
    POTASSIUM CITRATE &
    AMMONIUM

BRAND NAMES
Apo-K[5]
Cena-K[5]
Gen-K[5]
K+Care[5]
K+Care ET[2]
K-10[5]
Kalium Durules[5]
Kaochlor[5]
Kaochlor S-F[5]
Kaochlor-10[5]
Kaochlor-20[5]
Kaochlor-Eff[5]
Kaon[7]
Kaon-Cl[5]

Kaon-Cl 10[5]
Kaon-Cl 20[5]
Kato[5]
Kay Ciel[5]
Kay Ciel Elixir[5]
Kaylixir[7]
KCL[5]
K-Dur[5]
K-G Elixir[7]
K-Lease[5]
K-Long[5]
K-Lor[5]
Klor-Con 8[5]
Klor-Con 10[5]
Klor-Con Powder[5]
Klor-Con/25[5]
Klor-Con/EF[5]
Klorvess[3]
Klorvess 10% Liquid[5]
Klorvess Effervescent Granules[5]
Klotrix[5]
K-Lyte[2]
K-Lyte DS[4]
K-Lyte/Cl[5]
K-Lyte/Cl 50[3]
K-Lyte/CL Powder[5]
K-Norm[5]
Kolyum[8]
K-Tab[5]
Micro-K[5]
Micro-K 10[5]
Micro-K LS[5]
Neo-K[2]
Potasalan[5]
Potassium-Rougier[7]
Potassium-Sandoz[3]
Roychlor 10%[5]
Roychlor 20%[5]
Royonate[7]
Rum-K[5]
Slow-K[5]
Ten K[5]
Tri-K[5]
Trikates[5]
Twin-K[9]
Twin-K-Cl[9]

PROGESTINS

GENERIC NAMES
1. HYDROXYPROGESTERONE
2. MEDROXYPROGESTERONE
3. MEGESTROL
4. NORETHINDRONE
5. NORGESTREL
6. PROGESTERONE

BRAND NAMES
Amen[3]
Aygestin[5]
Crinone[6]
Curretab[3]
Cycrin[3]
Depo-Provera[3]
Duralutin[1]
Gesterol 50[6]
Gesterol L.A.[1]
Hy/Gestrone[1]
Hylutin[1]
Hyprogest[1]
Hyproval P.A.[1]
Megace[4]
Megace Oral Suspension[4]

Micronor[4]
Norlutate[4]
Norlutin[4]
Nor-Q.D.[4]
Ovrette[5]
Premphase[2]
Prempro[2]
Pro-Depo[1]
Prodrox[1]
Progestaject[6]
Progestilin[6]
Provera[3]

PSEUDOEPHEDRINE

Actacin
Actagen
Actagen-C Cough
Actifed
Actifed 12-Hour
Actifed A
Actifed Allergy Nighttime Caplets
Actifed DM
Actifed Plus
Actifed Plus Caplets
Actifed with Codeine Cough
Advil Cold and Sinus Caplets
Afrinol Repetabs
Alamine Expectorant
Alamine-C Liquid
Allegra D
Allent
Allercon
Allerest Maximum Strength
Allerest No-Drowsiness
Allerfrin
Allerfrin with Codeine
Allergy Cold
Allergy Formula Sinutab
AlleRid
Allerphed
All-Nite Cold Formula
Alpha-Phed
Ambenyl-D Decongestant Cough
  Formula
Ami-Drix
Anamine
Anamine T.D.
Anaplex
Anaplex S.R.
Anatuss DM
Anatuss LA
Aprodrine
Aprodrine with Codeine
Atrofed
Balminil Decongestant
BayCotussend Liquid
Baydec DM Drops
Bayer Select Flu Relief Caplets
Bayer Select Head Cold Caplets
Bayer Select Maximum Strength
  Sinus Pain Relief Caplets
Bayer Select Night Time Cold
  Caplets
Bayhistine DH
Bayhistine Expectorant
Benadryl Allergy/Sinus Headache
  Caplets
Benadryl Cold
Benadryl Cold Nighttime Liquid
Benadryl Decongestant
Benadryl Plus
Benylin Cold

Benylin Decongestant
Benylin DM-D
Benylin DM-D-E
Benylin DM-D-E Extra Strength
Benylin with Codeine
Beta-Phed
Brexin
Brexin-L.A.
Brofed
Bromarest DX Cough
Bromatane DX Cough
Bromfed
Bromfed-AT
Bromfed-DM
Bromfed-PD
Bromphen DX Cough
Brompheril
Brotane DX Cough
Calmylin
Calmylin #2
Calmylin #3
Calmylin Cough & Cold
Calmylin Pediatric
Calmylin with Codeine
Carbinoxamine Compound
Carbiset
Carbiset-TR
Carbodec
Carbodec DM Drops
Carbodec TR
Cardec DM
Cardec DM Drops
Cardec DM Pediatric
Cardec-S
Cenafed
Cenafed Plus
Cheracol Sinus
Children's Benylin DM-D
Children's Sudafed Liquid
Children's Tylenol Cold
Children's Tylenol Cold Multi
  Symptom Plus Cough
Chlorafed
Chlorafed H.S. Timecelles
Chlorafed Timecelles
Chlorphedrine SR
Chlor-Trimeton 4 Hour Relief
Chlor-Trimeton 12 Hour Relief
Chlor-Trimeton Decongestant
Chlor-Trimeton Decongestant
  Repetabs
Chlor-Trimeton Non-Drowsy
  Decongestant 4 Hour
Chlor-Tripolon Decongestant
  Extra Strength
Chlor-Tripolon Decongestant
  Repetabs
Chlor-Tripolon Decongestant
  Tablets
Claritin Extra
Claritin-D
Claritin-D 12 Hour
CoActifed
CoActifed Expectorant
CoAdvil Caplets
Co-Apap
Codehist DH
Codimal
Codimal-L.A.
Codimal-L.A. Half
Coldrine
Colfed-A
Comtrex A/S

Comtrex A/S Caplets
Comtrex Cough Formula
Comtrex Daytime Caplets
Comtrex Daytime Maximum
  Strength Cold and Flu Relief
Comtrex Daytime Maximum
  Strength Cold, Cough and Flu
  Relief
Comtrex Hot Flu Relief
Comtrex Multi-Symptom Hot Flu
  Relief
Comtrex Multi-Symptom Non-
  Drowsy Caplets
Comtrex Nighttime
Comtrex Nighttime Maximum
  Strength Cold & Flu Relief
Comtrex Nighttime Maximum
  Strength Cold, Cough & Flu
  Relief
Concentrin
Congess JR
Congess SR
Congestac Caplets
Contac Allergy/Sinus Day
  Caplets
Contac Allergy/Sinus Night
  Caplets
Contac Maximum Strength Sinus
  Caplets
Contac Night Caplets
Contac Non-Drowsy Formula
  Sinus Caplets
Contac Severe Cold Formula
Contac Severe Cold Formula
  Night Strength
Cophene No. 2
Cophene-XP
Co-Pyronil 2
Cotridin
Cotridin Expectorant
CoTylenol Cold Medication
Cremacoat 3 Throat Coating
  Cough Medicine
C-Tussin Expectorant
Dallergy Jr.
Dallergy-D
DayCare
DayQuil Liquicaps
DayQuil Non-Drowsy Cold/Flu
DayQuil Non-Drowsy Cold/Flu
  LiquiCaps
DayQuil Non-Drowsy Sinus
  Pressure and Pain Relief
  Caplets
Decofed
Decohistine DH
Deconamine
Deconamine SR
Deconsal II
Deconsal Pediatric
DeFed-60
Deproist Expectorant with Codeine
De-Tuss
Detussin Expectorant
Detussin Liquid
Dexaphen SA
Dexophed
Dihistine DH
Dihistine Expectorant
Dimacol
Dimetane-DX Cough
Dimetapp Sinus Caplets
Disobrom

Disophrol
Disophrol Chronotabs
Dorcol Children's Cold Formula
Dorcol Children's Cough
Dorcol Children's Decongestant
Dristan Cold and Flu
Dristan Cold Caplets
Dristan Cold Maximum Strength
  Caplets
Dristan Juice Mix-in Cold, Flu,
  & Cough
Dristan Sinus Caplets
Drixoral
Drixoral Cold & Allergy
Drixoral Cold & Flu
Drixoral Non-Drowsy Formula
Drixoral Plus
Drixoral Sinus
Drixtab
Duralex
Dura-Tap PD
Duratuss
Duratuss HD
Effective Strength Cough
  Formula with Decongestant
Efidec/24
Eltor-120
Endafed
Entex PSE
Entuss Pediatric Expectorant
Entuss-D
Fedahist
Fedahist Decongestant
Fedahist Expectorant
Fedahist Expectorant Pediatric
  Drops
Fedahist Gyrocaps
Fedahist Timecaps
Genac
Genaphed
Genite
Glycofed
GP-500
Guaifed
Guaifed-PD
GuaiMAX-D
Guaitab
GuiaCough PE
Guiatuss PE
Guiatussin DAC
Halofed
Halofed Adult Strength
Hayfebrol
Head & Chest
Histafed C
Histalet
Histalet X
Histalet-DM
Humibid Guaifenesin Plus
Isoclor
Isoclor Expectorant
Isoclor Timesules
Klerist-D
Kolephrin/DM Caplets
Kronofed-A
Kronofed-A Jr.
Lodrane LD
Mapap Cold Formula
Maxenal
Maximum Strength Tylenol
  Allergy Sinus Caplets
Maximum Strength Tylenol Flu
  Gelcaps

Medi-Flu
Medi-Flu Caplets
Mediquell Decongestant Formula
Midahist DH
Motrin-IB Sinus
Motrin-IB Sinus Caplets
Myfed
Myfedrine
Myhistine DH
Myhistine Expectorant
Mytussin DAC
Naldegesic
Nasatab LA
ND Clear T.D.
Neofed
Noratuss II Liquid
Novafed
Novafed A
Novagest Expectorant with
  Codeine
Novahistex
Novahistex DM
Novahistine Cough & Cold
  Formula Liquid
Novahistine DH Liquid
Novahistine DMX Liquid
Novahistine Expectorant
Nucochem
Nucochem Expectorant
Nucochem Pediatric Expectorant
Nucofed
Nucofed Expectorant
Nucofed Pediatric Expectorant
NyQuil Hot Therapy
NyQuil Liquicaps
NyQuil Nighttime Colds Medicine
Nytcold Medicine
Nytime Cold Medicine Liquid
Ornex Maximum Strength
  Caplets
Ornex No Drowsiness Caplets
Ornex Severe Cold No
  Drowsiness Caplets
Par-Drix
PediaCare Children's Cold Relief
  Night Rest Cough-Cold
  Formula
PediaCare Children's Cough-
  Cold Formula
PediaCare Cold Formula
PediaCare Cough-Cold
PediaCare Infants' Oral
  Decongestant Drops
Pertussin All Night PM
Phenapap Sinus Headache &
  Congestion
Phenergan-D
Phenhist DH with Codeine
Phenhist Expectorant
Polaramine Expectorant
Primatuss Cough Mixture 4D
Promist HD Liquid
Pseudo
Pseudo-Bid
Pseudo-Car DM
Pseudo-Chlor
Pseudodine C Cough
Pseudofrin
Pseudogest
Pseudogest Plus
P-V-Tussin
Rescon-DM
Rescon-ED

Rescon-JR
Respaire-60 SR
Respaire-120 SR
Resporal TR
Rhinosyn
Rhinosyn-DM
Rhinosyn-PD
Rhinosyn-X
Rinade B.I.D.
Robafen DAC
Robafen DM
Robidrine
Robitussin Cold and Cough
  Liqui-Gels
Robitussin Maximum Strength
  Cough & Cold
Robitussin Night Relief
Robitussin Pediatric Cough &
  Cold
Robitussin Severe Congestion
  Liqui-Gels
Robitussin-DAC
Robitussin-PE
Rondamine-DM Drops
Rondec
Rondec Drops
Rondec-DM
Rondec-DM Drops
Rondec-TR
Ru-Tuss DE
Ru-Tuss Expectorant
Rymed-TR
Ryna
Ryna-C Liquid
Ryna-CX Liquid
Seldane D
Semprex-D
Simplet
Sinarest No-Drowsiness
Sinarest Sinus
Sine-Aid
Sine-Aid IB
Sine-Aid Maximum Strength
Sine-Aid Maximum Strength
  Allergy/Sinus Formula Caplets
Sine-Aid Maximum Strength
  Gelcaps
Sine-Off Maximum Strength
  Allergy/Sinus Formula Caplets
Sine-Off Maximum Strength No
  Drowsiness Formula Caplets
Singlet
Sinufed Timecelles
Sinus Excedrin Extra Strength
Sinus Excedrin Extra Strength
  Caplets
Sinus Excedrin No Drowsiness
Sinus Excedrin No Drowsiness
  Caplets
Sinus Relief
SinuStat
Sinutab
Sinutab Extra Strength
Sinutab II Maximum Strength
Sinutab Maximum Strength
  without Drowsiness
Sinutab Maximum Strength
  without Drowsiness Caplets
Sinutab No Drowsiness
Sinutab No Drowsiness Extra
  Strength
Sinutab Regular
Sinutrex Extra Strength

SRC Expectorant
Stamoist E
Sudafed
Sudafed 12 Hour
Sudafed 60
Sudafed Cold & Cough Liquid
  Caps
Sudafed Cough
Sudafed DM
Sudafed Expectorant
Sudafed Plus
Sudafed Severe Cold Formula
  Caplets
Sudafed Sinus Maximum
  Strength
Sudafed Sinus Maximum
  Strength Caplets
Sudrin
Sufedrin
Super-Anahist
T-Dry
T-Dry Junior
TheraFlu Maximum Strength
  Non-Drowsy Formula Flu, Cold
  & Cough Medicine
TheraFlu Nighttime Maximum
  Strength
TheraFlu/Flu & Cold
TheraFlu/Flu, Cold & Cough
Thera-Hist
T-Moist
Touro A&H
Touro LA Caplets
Triacin C Cough
Triafed
Triafed with Codeine
Triaminic DM Nighttime for
  Children
Triaminic Nite Light
Triaminic Sore Throat Formula
Tricom Caplets
Trifed
Trifed-C Cough
Triminol Cough
Trinalin Repetabs
Trinex
Triofed
Tripodrine
Triposed
Tussafed
Tussafed Drops
Tussafin Expectorant
Tussar DM
Tussar-2
Tussend
Tussend Expectorant
Tussend Liquid
Tussin
Tuss-LA
Ty-Cold Cold Formula
Tylenol Allergy Sinus Gelcaps
Tylenol Allergy Sinus Night Time
  Maximum Strength Caplets
Tylenol Cold & Flu
Tylenol Cold & Flu No
  Drowsiness Powder
Tylenol Cold Medication
Tylenol Cold Medication,
  Non-Drowsy
Tylenol Cold Night Time
Tylenol Cold No Drowsiness
  Formula Gelcaps
Tylenol Cough

Tylenol Cough with Decongestant
Tylenol Maximum Strength Flu Gelcaps
Tylenol Sinus Maximum Strength
Tylenol Sinus Maximum Strength Caplets
Tylenol Sinus Maximum Strength Gelcaps
Tylenol Sinus Medication
Tylenol Sinus Medication Extra Strength
Tyrodone
ULTRAbrom PD
Ursinus Inlay
Vanex Expectorant
V-Dec-M
Versacaps
Vicks 44 Cough and Cold Relief Liqui-Caps
Vicks 44 Non-Drowsy Cold and Cough Liqui-Caps
Vicks 44D Dry Hacking Cough & Head Congestion
Vicks 44M Cough, Cold and Flu Relief
Vicks 44M Cough, Cold and Flu Relief LiquiCaps
Vicks Children's NyQuil Allergy/Head Cold
Vicks Formula 44D Decongestant Cough Mixture
Vicks Formula 44M Multi-Symptom Cough Mixture
Vicks NyQuil Multi-Symptom Cold/Flu Relief
Vicks NyQuil Multi-Symptom LiquiCaps
Vicks Pediatric Formula 44D Cough and Decongestant
Vicks Pediatric Formula 44M Multi-Symptom Cough & Cold
Viro-Med
Zephrex
Zephrex-LA

RAUWOLFIA & THIAZIDE DIURETICS

GENERIC NAMES
1. DESERPIDINE & HYDROCHLOROTHIAZIDE
2. DESERPIDINE & METHYCLOTHIAZIDE
3. RAUWOLFIA SERPENTINA & BENDROFLUMETHIAZIDE
4. RESERPINE & CHLOROTHIAZIDE
5. RESERPINE & CHLORTHALIDONE
6. RESERPINE & HYDROCHLOROTHIAZIDE
7. RESERPINE & HYDROFLUMETHIAZIDE
8. RESERPINE & METHYCLOTHIAZIDE
9. RESERPINE & POLYTHIAZIDE
10. RESERPINE & QUINETHAZONE
11. RESERPINE & TRICHLORMETHIAZIDE

BRAND NAMES
Demi-Regroton[5]
Diupres[4]
Diurese R[11]
Diurigen with Reserpine[4]
Diutensen-R[8]
Dureticyl[2]
Enduronyl[2]
Enduronyl Forte[2]
Hydropine[7]
Hydropres[6]
Hydrosine[6]
Hydrotensin[6]
Mallopres[6]
Metatensin[11]
Naquival[11]
Oreticyl[1]
Oreticyl Forte[1]
Rauzide[3]
Regroton[5]
Renese-R[9]
Salazide[7]
Salutensin[7]
Salutensin-Demi[7]

RAUWOLFIA ALKALOIDS

GENERIC NAMES
1. DESERPIDINE
2. RAUWOLFIA SERPENTINA
3. RESERPINE

BRAND NAMES
Harmonyl[1]
Hydropine H.P.[3]
Novoreserpine[3]
Raudixin[2]
Rauval[2]
Rauverid[2]
Reserfia[3]
Serpalan[3]
Serpasil[3]
Wolfina[2]

SALICYLATES

GENERIC NAMES
1. CHOLINE MAGNESIUM SALICYLATES
2. CHOLINE SALICYLATE
3. MAGNESIUM SALICYLATE
4. SALICYLAMIDE
5. SALSALATE
6. SODIUM SALICYLATE

BRAND NAMES
Amigesic[5]
Arthropan[2]
Choline Magnesium Trisalicylate[1]
Citra Forte[4]
Diagen[5]
Disalcid[5]
Doan's Pills[3]
Dodd's Pills[6]
Fendol[4]
Improved Sino-Tuss[4]
Kolephrin[4]
Kolephrin NN Liquid[4]
Magan[3]
Mobidin[3]
Mono-Gesic[5]
Omnicol[4]
Rhinogesic[4]
Salcylic Acid[4]

Saleto-D[4]
Salflex[5]
Salgesic[4]
Salsitab[5]
Scot-tussin Original 5-Action Cold Medicine[6]
Tricosal[1]
Trilisate[1]
Tussanil DH Tablets[4]
Tussirex with Codeine Liquid[6]
Uracel[6]

SCOPOLAMINE (Hyoscine)

Atrohist Plus
Barbidonna
Barbidonna 2
Buscopan
Kinesed
Phenahist-TR
Phenchlor SHA
Ru-Tuss
Stahist
Transderm-Scop
Transderm-V

SULFONAMIDES

GENERIC NAMES
1. SULFACYTINE
2. SULFADIAZINE
3. SULFAMETHIZOLE
4. SULFAMETHOXAZOLE
5. SULFISOXAZOLE

BRAND NAMES
Apo-Sulfamethoxazole[4]
Apo-Sulfatrim[4]
Apo-Sulfatrim DS[4]
Apo-Sulfisoxizole[5]
Bactrim[4]
Bactrim DS[4]
Cotrim[4]
Cotrim DS[4]
Co-trimoxazole[4]
Eryzole[5]
Gantanol[4]
Gantrisin[5]
Novo-Soxazole[5]
Novotrimel[4]
Novotrimel DS[4]
Nu-Cotrimox[4]
Nu-Cotrimox DS[4]
Pediazole[5]
Protrin[4]
Renoquid[1]
Roubac[4]
Septra[4]
Septra DS[4]
SMZ-TMP[4]
Sulfamethoprim[4]
Sulfamethoprim DS[4]
Sulfaprim[4]
Sulfaprim DS[4]
Sulfatrim[4]
Sulfatrim DS[4]
Sulfimycin[5]
Sulfizole[5]
Sulfoxaprim[4]
Sulfoxaprim DS[4]
Sulmeprim[4]
Thiosulfil Forte[3]
Triazole[4]

Triazole DS[4]
Trimeth-Sulfa[4]
Trisulfam[4]
Urobak[4]
Uroplus DS[4]
Uroplus SS[4]

TETRACYCLINES

GENERIC NAMES
1. DEMECLOCYCLINE
2. DOXYCYCLINE
3. MINOCYCLINE
4. OXYTETRACYCLINE
5. TETRACYCLINE

BRAND NAMES
Achromycin[5]
Achromycin V[5]
Apo-Doxy[2]
Apo-Tetra[5]
Declomycin[1]
Doryx[2]
Doxy-Caps[2]
Doxycin[2]
Doxy-Tabs[2]
E.P. Mycin[4]
Helidac[5]
Minocin[3]
Monodox[2]
Novodoxlin[2]
Novotetra[5]
Nu-Tetra[5]
Panmycin[5]
Periostat[5]
Robitet[5]
Sumycin[5]
Terramycin[4]
Tetracyn[5]
Tija[4]
Vibramycin[2]

Additional Drug Interactions

The following lists of drugs and their interactions with other drugs are continuations of lists found in the alphabetized drug charts beginning on page 2. These lists are alphabetized by generic name or drug class name, shown in large capital letters. Only those lists too long for the drug charts are included in this section. For complete information about any generic drug, see the alphabetized charts.

GENERIC NAME OR DRUG CLASS	COMBINED EFFECT	GENERIC NAME OR DRUG CLASS	COMBINED EFFECT
ACETAMINOPHEN & SALICYLATES			
Furosemide	Possible salicylate toxicity, decreased furosemide effect.	Rifampin	Increased liver toxicity.
Hepatotoxic drugs*	Increased liver toxicity.	Sotalol	Decreased anti-hypertensive effect of sotalol.
Indomethacin	Risk of stomach bleeding and ulcers.	Spironolactone	Decreased spirono-lactone effect.
Lisinopril	Decreased lisinopril effect.	Sulfinpyrazone	Decreased sulfin-pyrazone effect.
Methotrexate	Increased methotrexate effect.	Terazosin	Decreased effective-ness of terazosin. Causes sodium and fluid retention.
Para-aminosalicylic acid (PAS)	Possible salicylate toxicity.		
Phenobarbital	Decreased effect of acetaminophen and salicylates because of quicker elimination.	Tetracyclines* (effervescent granules or tablets)	May slow tetracycline absorption. Space doses 2 hours apart.
		Vancomycin	Hearing loss.
Phenytoin	Increased phenytoin effect.	Verapamil	Increased risk of toxicity.
Primidone	Increased liver toxicity.	Vitamin C (large doses)	Possible aspirin toxicity.
Probenecid	Decreased probenecid effect.	Urinary alkalizers*	Increased risk of toxicity.
Propranolol	Decreased aspirin effect.	Zidovudine	Increased toxicity of both.
Rauwolfia alkaloids*	Decreased aspirin effect.		

ADRENOCORTICOIDS (Systemic)

Attenuated virus vaccines*	Possible viral infection.	Chloral hydrate	Decreased adreno-corticoid effect.
Barbiturates*	Decreased prednisone effect. Oversedation.	Chlorthalidone	Potassium depletion.
		Cholestyramine	Decreased adreno-corticoid effect.
Carbamazepine	Decreased adreno-corticoid effect.	Cholinergics*	Decreased cholinergic effect.
Carbonic anhydrase inhibitors	Increased loss of calcium.	Colestipol	Decreased adreno-corticoid effect.

*See Glossary

GENERIC NAME OR DRUG CLASS	COMBINED EFFECT	GENERIC NAME OR DRUG CLASS	COMBINED EFFECT

ADRENOCORTICOIDS (Systemic) continued

GENERIC NAME OR DRUG CLASS	COMBINED EFFECT	GENERIC NAME OR DRUG CLASS	COMBINED EFFECT
Contraceptives, oral*	Increased adrenocorticoid effect.	Isoniazid	Decreased isoniazid effect.
Cyclosporine	Decreased adrenocorticoid effect. Increased cyclosporine effect.	Ketoconazole	Decreased ketoconazole effect.
		Mitotane	Decreased adrenocorticoid effect.
Digitalis preparations*	Dangerous potassium depletion. Possible digitalis toxicity.	Phenobarbital	Decreased adrenocorticoid effect.
Diuretics	Potassium depletion.	Phenytoin	Decreased adrenocorticoid effect.
Ephedrine	Decreased adrenocorticoid effect.	Potassium supplements*	Decreased potassium effect.
Estrogens*	Increased adrenocorticoid effect.	Primidone	Decreased adrenocorticoid effect.
Foscarnet	Potassium depletion.	Rifampin	Decreased adrenocorticoid effect.
Glutethimide	Decreased adrenocorticoid effect.	Salicylates*	Decreased salicylate effect.
Insulin	Decreased insulin effect.	Sympathomimetics*	Possible glaucoma.
Insulin lispro	May require increased dosage of insulin.	Thyroid hormones*	May require thyroid hormone dosage change.

ANDROGENS & ESTROGENS

GENERIC NAME OR DRUG CLASS	COMBINED EFFECT	GENERIC NAME OR DRUG CLASS	COMBINED EFFECT
Insulin	Unpredictable increase or decrease in blood sugar.	Primidone	Decreased estrogen and testosterone effect.
Nicotinic acid	Decreased nicotinic acid.	Rifampin	Decreased estrogen and testosterone effect.
Oxyphenbutazone	Decreased androgen and estrogen effect.	Terazosin	Decreased effectiveness of terazosin.
Phenobarbital	Decreased androgen and estrogen effect.	Thyroid hormones*	Decreased thyroid effect.
Phenylbutazone	Decreased estrogen and testosterone effect.	Ursodiol	Decreased ursodiol effect.

ANGIOTENSIN-CONVERTING ENZYME (ACE) INHIBITORS

GENERIC NAME OR DRUG CLASS	COMBINED EFFECT	GENERIC NAME OR DRUG CLASS	COMBINED EFFECT
Potassium supplements*	Possible increased potassium in blood.	Spironolactone	Possible excessive potassium in blood.
Sotalol	Increased antihypertensive effects of both drugs. Dosages may require adjustment.	Terazosin	Decreased effectiveness of terazosin.

*See Glossary

GENERIC NAME OR DRUG CLASS	COMBINED EFFECT	GENERIC NAME OR DRUG CLASS	COMBINED EFFECT

ANGIOTENSIN-CONVERTING ENZYME (ACE) INHIBITORS continued

GENERIC NAME OR DRUG CLASS	COMBINED EFFECT	GENERIC NAME OR DRUG CLASS	COMBINED EFFECT
Tiopronin	Increased risk of toxicity to kidneys.	Triamterene	Possible excessive potassium in blood.

ANGIOTENSIN-CONVERTING ENZYME (ACE) INHIBITORS & HYDROCHLOROTHIAZIDE

GENERIC NAME OR DRUG CLASS	COMBINED EFFECT	GENERIC NAME OR DRUG CLASS	COMBINED EFFECT
Diuretics*	Decreased blood pressure.	Nitrates*	Excessive blood pressure drop.
Lisinopril	Increased antihypertensive effect. Dosage of each may require adjustment.	Potassium supplements*	Excessive potassium in blood.
		Probenecid	Decreased probenecid effect.
Lithium	Increased lithium effect.	Sotalol	Increased antihypertensive effects of both drugs. Dosages may require adjustment.
Monoamine oxidase (MAO) inhibitors*	Increased hydrochlorothiazide effect.		
Nicardipine	Blood pressure drop. Dosages may require adjustment.	Spironolactone	Possible excessive potassium in blood.
Nimodipine	Possible irregular heartbeat. May worsen congestive heart failure.	Triamterene	Possible excessive potassium in blood.

ANTICOAGULANTS (Oral)

GENERIC NAME OR DRUG CLASS	COMBINED EFFECT	GENERIC NAME OR DRUG CLASS	COMBINED EFFECT
Citalopram	May lessen the effect of warfarin.	Estramustine	Decreased effect of anticoagulant.
Clofibrate	Increased effect of anticoagulant.	Estrogens	Decreased effect of anticoagulant.
Colestipol	Decreased effect of anticoagulant.	Fenoprofen	Increased effect of anticoagulant.
Contraceptives, oral*	Decreased effect of anticoagulant.	Fluconazole	Increased effect of anticoagulant.
Danazol	Increased effect of anticoagulant.	Fluoxetine	May cause confusion, agitation, convulsions and high blood pressure. Avoid combining.
Dextrothyroxine	Increased effect of anticoagulant.		
Diclofenac	Increased risk of bleeding.	Fluvoxamine	Increased effect of warfarin.
Diflunisal	Increased effect of anticoagulant.	Gemfibrozil	Increased effect of anticoagulant.
Dipyridamole	Increased risk of hemorrhage.	Glutethimide	Decreased effect of anticoagulant.
Disulfiram	Increased effect of anticoagulant.	Griseofulvin	Decreased effect of anticoagulant.
Erythromycins*	Increased effect of anticoagulant.	Indomethacin	Increased effect of anticoagulant.

*See Glossary

GENERIC NAME OR DRUG CLASS	COMBINED EFFECT	GENERIC NAME OR DRUG CLASS	COMBINED EFFECT
ANTICOAGULANTS (Oral) continued			
Itraconazole	Increased effect of anticoagulant.	Quinidine	Increased effect of anticoagulant.
Leukotriene modifiers	Increased effect of warfarin.	Raloxifene	May lessen effect of warfarin.
Levamisole	Increased risk of bleeding.	Rifampin	Decreased effect of anticoagulant.
Methimazole	Increased effect of anticoagulant.	Salicylates	Increased effect of anticoagulant.
Metronidazole	Increased effect of anticoagulant.	Sulfadoxine and pyrimethamine	Increased risk of toxicity.
Mineral Oil	Decreased absorption of anticoagulant.	Sulindac	Increased effect of anticoagulant.
Nalidixic acid	Increased effect of anticoagulant.	Suprofen	Increased risk of bleeding.
Nicardipine	Possible increased effect of anticoagulant.	Testolactone	Increased effect of anticoagulant.
Nimodipine	Possible increased effect of anticoagulant.	Thyroid hormones*	Increased effect of anticoagulant.
Nizatidine	Increased effect of anticoagulant.	Tolcapone	May require adjustment in dosage of warfarin.
Omeprazole	Increased effect of anticoagulant	Toremifene	May increase time it takes blood to clot.
Paroxetine	Increased effect of anticoagulant.	Vitamin E	Increased risk of bleeding.
Phenylbutazone	Increased effect of anticoagulant.	Vitamin K	Decreased effect of anticoagulant.
Phenytoin	Decreased levels of phenytoin.	Zafirlukast	May increase effect of warfarin.
Plicamycin	Increased effect of anticoagulant.	Zileuton	Increased warfarin effect.
Propafenone	May require adjustment of anticoagulant dosage.	Note: Any medicine	Unpredictable absorption.
Primadone	Decreased effect of anticoagulant.		

ANTICONVULSANTS, HYDANTOIN

GENERIC NAME OR DRUG CLASS	COMBINED EFFECT	GENERIC NAME OR DRUG CLASS	COMBINED EFFECT
Cimetidine	Increased anticonvulsant toxicity.	Disulfiram	Increased anticonvulsant effect.
Contraceptives, oral*	Increased seizures.	Estrogens*	Increased estrogen effect.
Cyclosporine	May decrease cyclosporine effect.	Felbamate	Increased side effects and adverse reactions.
Digitalis preparations*	Decreased digitalis effect.	Fluconazole	Increased anticonvulsant effect.
Disopyramide	Decreased disopyramide effect.		

*See Glossary

899

ANTICONVULSANTS, HYDANTOIN continued

GENERIC NAME OR DRUG CLASS	COMBINED EFFECT	GENERIC NAME OR DRUG CLASS	COMBINED EFFECT
Furosemide	Decreased furosemide effect.	Nizatidine	Increased effect and toxicity of phenytoin.
Gold compounds*	Increased anticonvulsant blood levels. Hydantoin dose may require adjustment.	Omeprazole	Delayed excretion of phenytoin causing increased amount of phenytoin in blood.
Glutethimide	Decreased anticonvulsant effect.	Oxyphenbutazone	Increased anticonvulsant effect.
Griseofulvin	Increased griseofulvin effect.	Para-aminosalicylic acid (PAS)	Increased anticonvulsant effect.
Hypoglycemics, oral*	Possible decreased hypoglycemic effect.	Paroxetine	Decreased anticonvulsant effect.
Hypoglycemics, other*	Possible decreased hypoglycemic effect.	Phenacemide	Increased risk of paranoid symptoms.
Isoniazid	Increased anticonvulsant effect.	Phenothiazines*	Increased anticonvulsant effect.
Itraconazole	Decreased itraconazole effect.	Phenylbutazone	Increased anticonvulsant effect.
Lamotrigine	Decreased lamotrigine effect with phenytoin.	Potassium supplements*	Decreased potassium effect.
Leucovorin	May counteract the effect of phenytoin or any hydantoin anticonvulsant.	Probenecid	Decreased probenecid effect.
		Propafenone	Increased effect of both drugs and increased risk of toxicity.
Leukotriene modifiers	Increased phenytoin effect.		
Loxapine	Decreased anticonvulsant effect of phenytoin or any hydantoin anticonvulsant.	Propranolol	Increased propranolol effect.
		Quetiapine	Decreased quetiapine effect with phenytoin.
Methadone	Decreased methadone effect.	Quinidine	Increased quinidine effect.
Methotrexate	Increased methotrexate effect.	Rifampin	Decreased anticonvulsant effect.
Methylphenidate	Increased anticonvulsant effect.	Sedatives*	Increased sedative effect.
Molindone	Increased phenytoin effect.	Sotalol	Decreased sotalol effect.
Monoamine oxidase (MAO) inhibitors*	Increased polythiazide effect.	Sucralfate	Decreased anticonvulsant effect.
Nicardipine	Increased anticonvulsant effect.	Sulfa drugs*	Increased anticonvulsant effect.
Nimodipine	Increased anticonvulsant effect.	Theophylline	Reduced anticonvulsant effect.
Nitrates*	Excessive blood pressure drop.	Trimethoprim	Increased phenytoin effect.

*See Glossary

GENERIC NAME OR DRUG CLASS	COMBINED EFFECT	GENERIC NAME OR DRUG CLASS	COMBINED EFFECT

ANTICONVULSANTS, HYDANTOIN continued

GENERIC NAME OR DRUG CLASS	COMBINED EFFECT	GENERIC NAME OR DRUG CLASS	COMBINED EFFECT
Valproic acid	Breakthrough seizures.	Zafirlukast	May increase effect of phenytoin.
Xanthines*	Decreased effects of both drugs.		

ANTIDEPRESSANTS, TRICYCLIC

GENERIC NAME OR DRUG CLASS	COMBINED EFFECT	GENERIC NAME OR DRUG CLASS	COMBINED EFFECT
Benzodiazepines*	Increased sedation	Haloperidol	Decreased lamotrigine effect.
Bupropion	Increased risk of seizures.	Leucovorin	High alcohol content of leucovorin may cause adverse effects.
Central nervous system (CNS) depressants*	Excessive sedation.	Levodopa	May increase blood pressure. May decrease levodopa effect.
Cimetidine	Possible increased tricyclic antidepressant effect and toxicity.	Lithium	Possible decreased seizure threshold.
Citalopram	Increased tricyclic antidepressant effect and toxicity.	Methyldopa	Possible decreased methyldopa effect.
Clonidine	Blood pressure increase. Avoid combination.	Methylphenidate	Possible increased tricyclic antidepressant effect and toxicity.
Clozapine	Toxic effect on the central nervous system.	Molindone	Increased molindone effect.
Contraceptives, oral*	Increased depression.	Monoamine oxidase (MAO) inhibitors*	Fever, delirium, convulsions.
Dextrothyroxine	Increased antidepressant effect. Irregular heartbeat.	Narcotics*	Oversedation.
Disulfiram	Delirium.	Nicotine	Increased effect of antidepressant (with imipramine).
Ethchlorvynol	Delirium.		
Fluoxetine	Increased effect of tricyclic antidepressant. Possible toxicity.	Phenothiazines*	Possible increased tricyclic antidepressant effect and toxicity.
Fluvoxamine	Increased antidepressant effect.	Phenytoin	Decreased phenytoin effect.
Furazolidine	Sudden, severe increase in blood pressure.	Procainamide	Possible irregular heartbeat.
Guanabenz	Decreased guanabenz effect.	Quinidine	Possible irregular heartbeat.
Guanadrel	Decreased guanadrel effect.	Sertraline	Increased depressive effects of both drugs.
Guanethidine	Decreased guanethidine effect.	Sympathomimetics*	Increased sympathomimetic effect.
		Thyroid hormones*	Irregular heartbeat.

ADDITIONAL DRUG INTERACTIONS

*See Glossary

GENERIC NAME OR DRUG CLASS	COMBINED EFFECT	GENERIC NAME OR DRUG CLASS	COMBINED EFFECT

ANTIDEPRESSANTS, TRICYCLIC continued

Tolcapone	May increase incidence of adverse effects of tolcapone.	Zolpidem	Increased sedative effect. Avoid.

ANTIDIABETIC AGENTS, SULFONYLUREA

Hemolytics*	Increased risk of adverse effect on blood cells.	Phenyramidol	Increased blood sugar lowering.
Insulin	Increased blood sugar lowering.	Phenytoin	Decreased blood sugar lowering.
Insulin lispro	Increased anti-diabetic effect.	Probenecid	Increased blood sugar lowering.
Isoniazid	Decreased blood sugar lowering.	Pyrazinamide	Decreased blood sugar lowering.
Labetalol	Increased blood sugar lowering, may mask hypoglycemia.	Ranitidine	Increased blood sugar lowering.
Leukotriene modifiers	Increased effect of tolbutamide.	Rifampin	Decreased blood sugar lowering.
MAO inhibitors*	Increased blood sugar lowering.	Sulfa drugs*	Increased blood sugar lowering.
Nicotinic acid	Decreased blood sugar lowering.	Sulfadoxine and pyrimethamine	Increased risk of toxicity.
Oxyphenbutazone	Increased blood sugar lowering.	Sulfaphenazole	Increased blood sugar lowering.
Phenothiazines*	Decreased blood sugar lowering.	Thyroid hormones*	Decreased blood sugar lowering.
Phenylbutazone	Increased blood sugar lowering.	Zafirlukast	May increase effect of tolbutamide.

ANTIDYSKINETICS

Levodopa	Possible increased levodopa effect.	Monoamine oxidase (MAO) inhibitors*	Increased antidyskinetic effect.

ANTIHISTAMINES

Procarbazine	May increase sedation.	Sertraline	Increased depressive effects of both drugs.
QT interval prolongation-causing drugs*	Serious heart rhythm problems with astemizole. Avoid.	Sleep inducers*	Excess sedation. Avoid.
Sedatives*	Excess sedation. Avoid.	Sotalol	Increased antihistamine effect.
		Tranquilizers*	Excess sedation. Avoid.

*See Glossary

GENERIC NAME OR DRUG CLASS	COMBINED EFFECT	GENERIC NAME OR DRUG CLASS	COMBINED EFFECT

ANTIHISTAMINES, PHENOTHIAZINE-DERIVATIVE

GENERIC NAME OR DRUG CLASS	COMBINED EFFECT
Dronabinol	Increased effects of both drugs. Avoid.
Epinephrine	Decreased epinephrine effect.
Ethinamate	Dangerous increased effects of ethinamate. Avoid combining.
Extrapyramidal reaction*-causing medicines	Increased frequency and severity of extra-pyramidal reactions.
Fluoxetine	Increased depressant effects of both drugs.
Guanethidine	Decreased guanethidine effect.
Guanfacine	May increase depressant effects of either medicine.
Leucovorin	High alcohol content of leucovorin may cause adverse effects.
Levodopa	Decreased levodopa effect.
Methyprylon	May increase seda-tive effect to danger-ous level. Avoid.
Metyrosine	Increased likelihood of toxic symptoms of each.
Mind-altering drugs*	Increased effect of mind-altering drugs.
Molindone	Increased sedative and antihistamine effect.
Monoamine oxidase (MAO) inhibitors*	Increased anti-histamine effect.
Nabilone	Greater depression of central nervous system.
Narcotics*	Increased narcotic effect.
Sedatives*	Increased sedative effect.
Sertraline	Increased depres-sive effects of both drugs.
Sotalol	Increased antihista-mine effect.
Tranquilizers*	Increased tranquil-izer effect. Avoid.

ANTI-INFLAMMATORY DRUGS, NONSTEROIDAL (NSAIDs)

GENERIC NAME OR DRUG CLASS	COMBINED EFFECT
Diuretics*	May decrease diuretic effect.
Gold compounds*	Increased risk of kidney toxicity.
Lithium	Increased lithium effect.
Losartan	Decreased antihy-pertensive effect.
Methotrexate	Increased risk of side effects of metho-trexate.
Minoxidil	Decreased minoxidil effect.
Probenecid	Increased pain relief.
Terazosin	Decreased effective-ness of terazosin. Causes sodium and fluid retention.
Thyroid hormones*	Rapid heartbeat, blood pressure rise.
Tiopronin	Increased risk of toxicity to kidneys.
Triamterene	Reduced triamterene effect.

GENERIC NAME OR DRUG CLASS	COMBINED EFFECT	GENERIC NAME OR DRUG CLASS	COMBINED EFFECT

ASPIRIN

GENERIC NAME OR DRUG CLASS	COMBINED EFFECT	GENERIC NAME OR DRUG CLASS	COMBINED EFFECT
Dextrothyroxine (large doses, continuous use)	Increased dextrothyroxine effect.	Phenobarbital	Decreased aspirin effect.
Diclofenac	Increased risk of stomach ulcer.	Phenytoin	Increased phenytoin effect.
Ethacrynic acid	Possible aspirin toxicity.	Probenecid	Decreased probenecid effect.
Furosemide	Possible aspirin toxicity. May decrease furosemide effect.	Propranolol	Decreased aspirin effect.
Gold compounds*	Increased likelihood of kidney damage.	Rauwolfia alkaloids*	Decreased aspirin effect.
Indomethacin	Risk of stomach bleeding and ulcers.	Salicylates*	Likely aspirin toxicity.
Ketoprofen	Increased risk of stomach ulcer.	Sotalol	Decreased anti-hypertensive effect of sotalol.
Levamisole	Increased risk of bleeding.	Spironolactone	Decreased spirono-lactone effect.
Methotrexate	Increased methotrexate effect.	Sulfinpyrazone	Decreased sulfin-pyrazone effect.
Minoxidil	Decreased minoxidil effect.	Terazosin	Decreased effective-ness of terazosin. Causes sodium and fluid retention.
Oxprenolol	Decreased anti-hypertensive effect of oxprenolol.	Ticlopidine	Increased effect of both drugs.
Para-aminosalicylic acid	Possible aspirin toxicity.	Vitamin C (large doses)	Possible aspirin toxicity.
Penicillins*	Increased effect of both drugs.	Valproic acid	May increase valproic acid effect.

ATROPINE, HYOSCYAMINE, METHENAMINE, METHYLENE BLUE, PHENYLSALICYLATE & BENZOIC ACID

GENERIC NAME OR DRUG CLASS	COMBINED EFFECT	GENERIC NAME OR DRUG CLASS	COMBINED EFFECT
Diuretics, thiazide*	Decreased urine acidity.	Meperidine	Increased atropine and hyoscyamine effect.
Furosemide	Possible salicylate toxicity.	Methylphenidate	Increased atropine and hyoscyamine effect.
Gold compounds*	Increased likelihood of kidney damage.	Minoxidil	Decreased minoxidil effect.
Haloperidol	Increased internal eye pressure.	Monoamine oxidase (MAO) inhibitors*	Increased belladonna and atropine effect.
Indomethacin	Risk of stomach bleeding and ulcers.	Orphenadrine	Increased atropine and hyoscyamine effect.
Ketoconazole	Reduced ketoconazole effect.		

*See Glossary

GENERIC NAME OR DRUG CLASS	COMBINED EFFECT	GENERIC NAME OR DRUG CLASS	COMBINED EFFECT

ATROPINE, HYOSCYAMINE, METHENAMINE, METHYLENE BLUE, PHENYLSALICYLATE & BENZOIC ACID continued

GENERIC NAME OR DRUG CLASS	COMBINED EFFECT	GENERIC NAME OR DRUG CLASS	COMBINED EFFECT
Oxprenolol	Decreased anti-hypertensive effect of oxprenolol.	Propranolol	Decreased salicylate effect.
Para-aminosalicylic acid (PAS)	Possible salicylate toxicity.	Rauwolfia alkaloids*	Decreased salicylate effect.
Penicillins*	Increased effect of both drugs.	Salicylates*	Likely salicylate toxicity.
Phenobarbital	Decreased salicylate effect.	Sedatives* or central nervous system (CNS) depressants*	Increased sedative effect of both drugs.
Phenothiazines*	Increased atropine and hyoscyamine effect.	Sodium bicarbonate	Decreased methenamine effect.
Phenytoin	Increased phenytoin effect.	Spironolactone	Decreased spirono-lactone effect.
Pilocarpine	Loss of pilocarpine effect in glaucoma treatment.	Sulfa drugs*	Possible kidney damage.
		Sulfinpyrazone	Decreased sulfin-pyrazone effect.
Potassium supplements*	Possible intestinal ulcers with oral potassium tablets.	Vitamin C (1 to 4 grams per day)	Increased effect of methenamine, contributing to urine acidity; decreased atropine effect; possible salicylate toxicity.
Probenecid	Decreased probenecid effect.		

BARBITURATES

GENERIC NAME OR DRUG CLASS	COMBINED EFFECT	GENERIC NAME OR DRUG CLASS	COMBINED EFFECT
Lamotrigine	Decreased lamotrigine effect.	Narcotics*	Dangerous sedation. Avoid.
Leukotriene modifiers	Decreased montelukast effect.	Sertraline	Increased depressive effects of both drugs.
Mind-altering drugs*	Dangerous sedation. Avoid.	Sotalol	Increased barbiturate effect. Dangerous sedation.
Monoamine oxidase (MAO) inhibitors*	Increased barbiurate effect.	Valproic acid	Increased barbiturate effect.

BARBITURATES, ASPIRIN & CODEINE (Also contains caffeine)

GENERIC NAME OR DRUG CLASS	COMBINED EFFECT	GENERIC NAME OR DRUG CLASS	COMBINED EFFECT
Anticonvulsants*	Changed seizure patterns.	Antidiabetics, oral*	Increased butalbital effect. Low blood sugar.
Antidepressants*	Decreased anti-depressant effect. Possible dangerous oversedation.	Antihistamines*	Dangerous sedation. Avoid.
		Anti-inflammatory drugs, nonsteroidal (NSAIDs)*	Risk of stomach bleeding and ulcers.

GENERIC NAME OR DRUG CLASS	COMBINED EFFECT	GENERIC NAME OR DRUG CLASS	COMBINED EFFECT

BARBITURATES, ASPIRIN & CODEINE (Also contains caffeine) continued

GENERIC NAME OR DRUG CLASS	COMBINED EFFECT	GENERIC NAME OR DRUG CLASS	COMBINED EFFECT
Aspirin, other	Likely aspirin toxicity.	Nitrates*	Excessive blood pressure drop.
Beta-adrenergic blocking agents*	Decreased effect of beta-adrenergic blocker.	Pain relievers*	Dangerous sedation. Avoid.
Carteolol	Increased narcotic effect. Dangerous sedation.	Para-aminosalicylic acid	Possible aspirin toxicity.
Contraceptives, oral*	Decreased contraceptive effect.	Penicillins*	Increased effect of drugs.
Digitoxin	Decreased digitoxin effect.	Phenobarbital	Decreased aspirin effect.
Doxycycline	Decreased doxycycline effect.	Phenothiazines*	Increased phenothiazine effect.
Dronabinol	Increased effect of drugs.	Phenytoin	Increased phenytoin effect.
Furosemide	Possible aspirin toxicity.	Probenecid	Decreased probenecid effect.
Gold compounds*	Increased likelihood of kidney damage.	Propranolol	Decreased aspirin effect.
Griseofulvin	Decreased griseofulvin effect.	Rauwolfia alkaloids*	Decreased aspirin effect.
Indapamide	Increased indapamide effect.	Salicylates*	Likely aspirin toxicity.
Indomethacin	Risk of stomach bleeding and ulcers.	Sedatives*	Dangerous sedation. Avoid.
Lamotrigine	Decreased lamotrigine effect.	Sleep inducers*	Dangerous sedation. Avoid.
Methotrexate	Increased methotrexate effect.	Sotalol	Increased narcotic effect. Dangerous sedation.
Mind-altering drugs*	Dangerous sedation. Avoid.	Spironolactone	Decreased spironolactone effect.
Minoxidil	Decreased minoxidil effect.	Sulfinpyrazone	Decreased sulfinpyrazone effect.
Monoamine oxidase (MAO) inhibitors*	Increased butalbital effect.	Tranquilizers*	Dangerous sedation. Avoid.
Naltrexone	Decreased analgesic effect.	Valproic acid	Increased phenobarbital effect.
Narcotics*	Dangerous sedation. Avoid.	Vitamin C (large doses)	Possible aspirin toxicity.
		Zidovudine	Increased toxicity of both.

BELLADONNA ALKALOIDS & BARBITURATES

GENERIC NAME OR DRUG CLASS	COMBINED EFFECT	GENERIC NAME OR DRUG CLASS	COMBINED EFFECT
Attapulgite	Decreased belladonna effect.	Beta-adrenergic blocking agents*	Decreased effects of beta-adrenergic blocker.

*See Glossary

GENERIC NAME OR DRUG CLASS	COMBINED EFFECT	GENERIC NAME OR DRUG CLASS	COMBINED EFFECT

BELLADONNA ALKALOIDS & BARBITURATES continued

GENERIC NAME OR DRUG CLASS	COMBINED EFFECT	GENERIC NAME OR DRUG CLASS	COMBINED EFFECT
Carteolol	Increased barbiturate effect. Dangerous sedation.	Narcotics*	Dangerous sedation. Avoid.
Central nervous system (CNS) depressants*	Dangerous sedation. Avoid.	Nitrates*	Increased internal eye pressure.
Contraceptives, oral*	Decreased contraceptive effect.	Nizatidine	Increased nizatidine effect.
Digitoxin	Decreased digitoxin effect.	Orphenadrine	Increased belladonna effect.
Doxycycline	Decreased doxycycline effect.	Pain relievers*	Dangerous sedation. Avoid.
Dronabinol	Increased effects of both drugs. Avoid.	Phenothiazines*	Increased belladonna effect. Danger of oversedation.
Furosemide	Possible orthostatic hypotension.	Pilocarpine	Loss of pilocarpine effect in glaucoma treatment.
Griseofulvin	Decreased griseofulvin effect.	Potassium supplements*	Possible intestinal ulcers with oral potassium tablets.
Haloperidol	Increased internal eye pressure.	Quinidine	Increased belladonna effect.
Indapamide	Increased indapamide effect.	Sedatives*	Dangerous sedation. Avoid.
Ketoconazole	Decreased ketoconazole effect.	Sleep inducers*	Dangerous sedation. Avoid.
Meperidine	Increased belladonna effect.	Sotalol	Increased barbiturate effect. Dangerous sedation.
Methylphenidate	Increased belladonna effect.	Tranquilizers*	Dangerous sedation. Avoid.
Metronidazole	Decreased metronidazole effect.	Valproic acid	Increased barbiturate effect.
Mind-altering drugs*	Dangerous sedation. Avoid.	Vitamin C	Decreased belladonna effect. Avoid large doses of vitamin C.
Monoamine oxidase (MAO) inhibitors*	Increased belladonna and barbiturate effect.		

BENZODIAZEPINES

GENERIC NAME OR DRUG CLASS	COMBINED EFFECT	GENERIC NAME OR DRUG CLASS	COMBINED EFFECT
Narcotics*	Increased sedative effect of both drugs.	Omeprazole	Delayed excretion of benzodiazepine causing increased amount of benzodiazepine in blood.
Nefazodone	Increased effect of nefazodone and alprazolam.		
Nicotine	Increased benzodiazepine effect.	Probenecid	Increased benzodiazepine effect.

*See Glossary

GENERIC NAME OR DRUG CLASS	COMBINED EFFECT	GENERIC NAME OR DRUG CLASS	COMBINED EFFECT
BENZODIAZEPINES continued			
Sertraline	Increased depressive effects of both drugs.	Zidovudine	Increased toxicity of zidovudine.

BETA-ADRENERGIC BLOCKING AGENTS

GENERIC NAME OR DRUG CLASS	COMBINED EFFECT	GENERIC NAME OR DRUG CLASS	COMBINED EFFECT
Diazoxide	Additional blood pressure drop.	Nefazodone	Dosages of both drugs may require adjustment.
Digitalis preparations*	Can either increase or decrease heart rate. Improves irregular heartbeat.	Nitrates*	Possible excessive blood pressure drop.
Flecainide	Increased effect of toxicity on heart muscle.	Phenytoin	Decreased beta blocker effect.
Fluvoxamine	Increased beta blocker effect.	Propafenone	Increased beta blocker effect.
Indomethacin	Decreased effect of beta blocker.	Quinidine	Slows heart excessively in some patients.
Insulin	Hypoglycemic effects may be prolonged.	Reserpine	Increased reserpine effect. Excessive sedation and depression. Additional blood pressure drop.
Leukotriene modifiers	Increased beta blocker effect.		
Levobunolol eyedrops	Possible increased beta blocker effect.	Sympathomimetics*	Decreased effects of both drugs.
Miglitol	Decreased effect of propranolol.	Timolol eyedrops	Possible increased beta blocker effect.
Molindone	Increased tranquilizer effect.	Tocainide	May worsen congestive heart failure.
Monoamine oxidase (MAO) inhibitors*	High blood pressure following MAO discontinuation.	Warfarin	Increased warfarin effect.
Narcotics*	Increased narcotic effect. Dangerous sedation.	Xanthines (aminophylline, theophylline)	Decreased effects of both drugs.

BETA-ADRENERGIC BLOCKING AGENTS & THIAZIDE DIURETICS

GENERIC NAME OR DRUG CLASS	COMBINED EFFECT	GENERIC NAME OR DRUG CLASS	COMBINED EFFECT
Antidiabetics*	Increased anti-diabetic effect.	Barbiturates*	Increased barbiturate effect. Dangerous sedation.
Antihistamines*	Decreased anti-histamine effect.	Bumetanide	Increased diuretic effect.
Antihypertensives*	Increased anti-hypertensive effect.	Calcium channel blockers*	Increased antihypertensive effect. Dosages of both drugs may require adjustments.
Anti-inflammatory drugs, nonsteroidal (NSAIDs)*	Decreased anti-inflammatory effect.		

GENERIC NAME OR DRUG CLASS	COMBINED EFFECT	GENERIC NAME OR DRUG CLASS	COMBINED EFFECT

BETA-ADRENERGIC BLOCKING AGENTS & THIAZIDE DIURETICS continued

GENERIC NAME OR DRUG CLASS	COMBINED EFFECT	GENERIC NAME OR DRUG CLASS	COMBINED EFFECT
Cholestyramine	Decreased hydro-chlorthiazide effect.	Monoamine oxidase (MAO) inhibitors*	Increased hydro chlorothiazide effect.
Diclofenac	Decreased anti-hypertensive effect.	Narcotics*	Increased narcotic effect. Dangerous sedation.
Digitalis preparations*	Excessive potassium loss that causes dangerous heart rhythms. Can either increase or decrease heart rate. Improves irregular heartbeat.	Nicardipine	Possible irregular heartbeat and con-gestive heart failure.
		Nicotine	Increased beta blocker effect.
Diuretics, thiazide*	Increased effect of other thiazide diuretics.	Nitrates*	Excessive blood pressure drop.
		Phenytoin	Increased beta adrenergic effect.
Ethacrynic acid	Increased diuretic effect.	Potassium supplements*	Decreased potassium effect.
Furosemide	Increased diuretic effect.	Probenecid	Decreased probenecid effect.
Guanfacine	Increased effect of both drugs.	Propafenone	Increased beta blocker effect.
Hypoglycemics, oral*	Decreased ability to lower blood glucose.	Quinidine	Slows heart excessively.
Indapamide	Increased diuretic effect.	Reserpine	Increased reserpine effect. Excessive sedation and depression.
Insulin	Decreased ability to lower blood glucose.		
Lisinopril	Increased anti-hypertensive effect. Dosage of each may require adjustment.	Sympathomimetics*	Decreased effective-ness of both.
		Theophylline	Decreased effective-ness of both.
Metolazone	Increased diuretic effect.	Tocainide	May worsen conges-tive heart failure.
Miglitol	Decreased effect of propranolol.	Zinc supplements	Increased need for zinc.

BRONCHODILATORS, ADRENERGIC

GENERIC NAME OR DRUG CLASS	COMBINED EFFECT	GENERIC NAME OR DRUG CLASS	COMBINED EFFECT
Rauwolfia	Decreased rauwolfia effect.	Theophylline	Increased gastro-intestinal intolerance.
Sympathomimetics*, other	Increased bro-chodilator effect.	Thyroid hormones*	Increased bron-chodilator effect.
Terazosin	Decreased effective-ness of terazosin.	Tolcapone	May require adjust-ment in dosage.

ADDITIONAL DRUG INTERACTIONS

*See Glossary

BRONCHODILATORS, XANTHINE

GENERIC NAME OR DRUG CLASS	COMBINED EFFECT	GENERIC NAME OR DRUG CLASS	COMBINED EFFECT
Ticlopidine	Increased theophylline effect.	Zafirlukast	May increase effect of zafirlukast.
Troleandomycin	Increased bronchodilator effect.	Zileuton	Increased theophylline effect.

CALCIUM CHANNEL BLOCKERS

GENERIC NAME OR DRUG CLASS	COMBINED EFFECT	GENERIC NAME OR DRUG CLASS	COMBINED EFFECT
Metformin	Increased metformin effect.	Quinidine	Increased quinidine effect.
Nicardipine	Possible increased effect and toxicity of each drug.	Rifampin	Decreased effect of calcium channel blocker.
Nimodipine	Dangerous blood pressure drop.	Theophylline	May increase effect and toxicity of theophylline.
Nitrates*	Reduced angina attacks.	Vitamin D	Decreased effect of calcium channel blocker.
Phenytoin	Possible decreased calcium channel blocker effect.	Zafirlukast	May increase calcium channel blocker effect.
Propafenone	Increased effects of both drugs and increased risk of toxicity.		

CALCIUM SUPPLEMENTS

GENERIC NAME OR DRUG CLASS	COMBINED EFFECT	GENERIC NAME OR DRUG CLASS	COMBINED EFFECT
Sulfa drugs*	Decreased sulfa effect.	Vitamin A	Decreased vitamin effect.
Tetracyclines*	Decreased tetracycline effect.	Vitamin D	Increased vitamin absorption, sometimes excessively.

CARBAMAZEPINE

GENERIC NAME OR DRUG CLASS	COMBINED EFFECT	GENERIC NAME OR DRUG CLASS	COMBINED EFFECT
Clozapine	Toxic effect on bone marrow and central nervous system.	Doxycycline	Decreased doxycycline effect.
Contraceptives, oral*	Reduced contraceptive protection. Use barrier birth control method.	Estrogens*	Decreased estrogen effect.
		Erythromycins*	Increased carbamazepine effect.
Desmopressin	May increase desmopressin effect.	Ethinamate	Dangerous increased effects of ethinamate. Avoid combining.
Digitalis preparations*	Excessive slowing of heart.	Felbamate	Increased side effects and adverse reactions.
Diltiazem	Increased effect of carbamzepine.		
Doxepin (topical)	Increased risk of toxicity of both drugs.	Fluoxetine	Increased carbamazepine effect.

*See Glossary

GENERIC NAME OR DRUG CLASS	COMBINED EFFECT	GENERIC NAME OR DRUG CLASS	COMBINED EFFECT
CARBAMAZEPINE continued			
Fluvoxamine	Possible toxicity of carbamazepine.	**Nizatidine**	Increased carbamazepine effect and toxicity.
Guanfacine	May increase depressant effects of either drug.	**Olanzapine**	Decreased effect of olanzapine.
Isoniazid	Increased risk of liver damage.	**Phenytoin**	Decreased carbamazepine effect.
Itraconazole	Decreased itraconazole effect.	**Phenobarbital**	Decreased carbamazepine effect.
Lamotrigine	Decreased lamotrigine effect. Increased risk of side effects.	**Primidone**	Decreased carbamazepine effect.
Leucovorin	High alcohol content of leucovorin may cause adverse effects.	**Propoxyphene (Darvon)**	Increased toxicity of both. Avoid.
		Risperidone	Decreased risperidone effect.
Leukotriene modifiers	Increased effect of carbamazepine.	**Sertraline**	Increased depressive effects of both drugs.
Mebendazole	Decreased effect of mebendazole.	**Tiopronin**	Increased risk of toxicity to bone marrow.
Monoamine oxidase (MAO) Inhibitors*	Dangerous over-stimulation. Avoid.	**Tramadol**	Decreased tramadol effect.
Nicardipine	May increase carbamazepine effect and toxicity.	**Verapamil**	Possible increased carbamazepine effect.
Nimodipine	May increase carbamazepine effect and toxicity.	**Zafirlukast**	May increase effect of carbamazepine.

CHLORPROTHIXENE

GENERIC NAME OR DRUG CLASS	COMBINED EFFECT	GENERIC NAME OR DRUG CLASS	COMBINED EFFECT
Sleep inducers*	Increased chlorprothixene effect. Excessive sedation.	**Tranquilizers***	Increased chlorprothixene effect. Excessive sedation.

CHLORZOXAZONE & ACETAMINOPHEN

GENERIC NAME OR DRUG CLASS	COMBINED EFFECT	GENERIC NAME OR DRUG CLASS	COMBINED EFFECT
Tranquilizers*	Increased sedation.	**Zidovudine**	Increased toxicity of zidovudine.

CLONIDINE & CHLORTHALIDONE

GENERIC NAME OR DRUG CLASS	COMBINED EFFECT	GENERIC NAME OR DRUG CLASS	COMBINED EFFECT
Fenfluramine	Possible increased clonidine effect.	**Monoamine oxidase (MAO) inhibitors***	Increased chlorthalidone effect.
Guanfacine	Impaired blood pressure control.	**Nabilone**	Greater depression of central nervous system.
Indapamide	Increased diuretic effect.	**Nicardipine**	Blood pressure drop. Dosage may require adjustment.
Lithium	Increased lithium effect.		

*See Glossary

ADDITIONAL DRUG INTERACTIONS

GENERIC NAME OR DRUG CLASS	COMBINED EFFECT	GENERIC NAME OR DRUG CLASS	COMBINED EFFECT

CLONIDINE & CHLORTHALIDONE continued

GENERIC NAME OR DRUG CLASS	COMBINED EFFECT	GENERIC NAME OR DRUG CLASS	COMBINED EFFECT
Nitrates*	Possible excessive blood pressure drop.	Sedatives* or central nervous system (CNS) depressants*	Increased sedative effect of both drugs.
Potassium supplements*	Decreased potassium effect.	Sotalol	Decreased anti-hypertensive effect.
Probenecid	Decreased probenecid effect.	Terazosin	Decreased terazosin effect.

CONTRACEPTIVES, ORAL

GENERIC NAME OR DRUG CLASS	COMBINED EFFECT	GENERIC NAME OR DRUG CLASS	COMBINED EFFECT
Meprobamate	Decreased contraceptive effect.	Sulfadoxine and pyrimethamine	Reduced reliability of the pill.
Mineral oil	Decreased contraceptive effect.	Terazosin	Decreases terazosin effect.
Non-nucleoside reverse transcriptase inhibitors	Decreased contraceptive effect. Use alternative birth control method.	Tetracyclines*	Decreased contraceptive effect.
		Ursodiol	Decreased ursodiol effect.
Phenothiazines*	Increased phenothiazine effect.	Vitamin A	Vitamin A excess.
Rifampin	Decreased contraceptive effect.	Vitamin C	Possible increased contraceptive effect.

CYCLOSPORINE

GENERIC NAME OR DRUG CLASS	COMBINED EFFECT	GENERIC NAME OR DRUG CLASS	COMBINED EFFECT
Rifampin	Decreased effect of cyclosporine.	Vancomycin	Increased chance of hearing loss or kidney damage.
Terbinafine (oral)	Decreased effect of cyclosporine.	Virus vaccines	Increased adverse reactions to vaccine.
Tiopronin	Increased risk of toxicity to kidneys.	Zafirlukast	May increase effect of cyclosporine.
Troglitazone	Decreased effect of cyclosporine.		

DIFENOXIN & ATROPINE

GENERIC NAME OR DRUG CLASS	COMBINED EFFECT	GENERIC NAME OR DRUG CLASS	COMBINED EFFECT
Nitrates*	Increased internal eye pressure.	Potassium supplements*	Possible intestinal ulcers with oral potassium tablets.
Orphenadrine	Increased atropine effect.	Procainamide	Increased atropine effect.
Phenothiazines*	Increased atropine effect.	Sertraline	Increased depressive effects of both drugs.
Pilocarpine	Loss of pilocarpine effect in glaucoma treatment.	Vitamin C	Decreased atropine effect. Avoid large doses of vitamin C.

DIGITALIS PREPARATIONS (Digitalis Glycosides)

GENERIC NAME OR DRUG CLASS	COMBINED EFFECT	GENERIC NAME OR DRUG CLASS	COMBINED EFFECT
Metoclopramide	Decreased digitalis absorption.	Rauwolfia alkaloids*	Increased digitalis effect.
Mineral Oil	Decreased digitalis effect.	Rifampin	Possible decreased digitalis effect.
Nefazodone	Increased effect of digoxin.	Sotalol	Can either increase or decrease heart rate. Improves irregular heartbeat.
Nicardipine	Increased digitalis effect. May need to reduce dose.	Spironolactone	Increased digitalis effect. May require digitalis dosage reduction.
Nizatidine	Increased digitalis effect.		
Oxyphenbutazone	Decreased digitalis effect.	Sulfasalazine	Decreased digitalis absorption.
Paroxetine	Increased levels of paroxetine in blood.	Sympathomimetics*	Increased risk of heartbeat irregularities.
Phenobarbital	Decreased digitalis effect.	Tetracycline	May increase digitalis absorption.
Phenylbutazone	Decreased digitalis effect.	Thyroid hormones*	Digitalis toxicity.
Potassium supplements*	Overdose of either drug may cause severe heartbeat irregularity.	Ticlopidine	Slightly decreased digitalis effect (digoxin only).
Propafenone	Increased digitalis absorption. May require decreased digitalis dosage.	Trazodone	Possible increased digitalis toxicity.
		Triamterene	Possible decreased digitalis effect.
PTU/Metronidazole	Decreased digitalis effect.	Verapamil	Increased digitalis effect.
Quinidine	Increased digitalis effect.		

DIURETICS, LOOP

GENERIC NAME OR DRUG CLASS	COMBINED EFFECT	GENERIC NAME OR DRUG CLASS	COMBINED EFFECT
Nephrotoxics*	Increased risk of toxicity.	Potassium supplements*	Decreased potassium effect.
Nimodipine	Dangerous blood pressure drop.	Probenecid	Decreased probenecid effect.
Nitrates*	Excessive blood pressure drop.	Salicylates* (including aspirin)	Dangerous salicylate retention.
Phenytoin	Decreased diuretic effect.	Sedatives*	Increased diuretic effect.

DIURETICS, POTASSIUM-SPARING & HYDROCHLOROTHIAZIDE

GENERIC NAME OR DRUG CLASS	COMBINED EFFECT	GENERIC NAME OR DRUG CLASS	COMBINED EFFECT
Colestipol	Decreased diuretic effect. Take 1 hour before diuretic.	Cyclosporine	Increased potassium levels.

ADDITIONAL DRUG INTERACTIONS

GENERIC NAME OR DRUG CLASS	COMBINED EFFECT	GENERIC NAME OR DRUG CLASS	COMBINED EFFECT

DIURETICS, POTASSIUM-SPARING & HYDROCHLOROTHIAZIDE continued

GENERIC NAME OR DRUG CLASS	COMBINED EFFECT	GENERIC NAME OR DRUG CLASS	COMBINED EFFECT
Digitalis preparations*	Increased digitalis effect.	Lithium	Possible lithium toxicity.
Diuretics*, other	Increased effect of both drugs.	Metformin	Increased metformin effect.
Folic acid	Decreased effect of folic acid.	Potassium-containing medications	Increased potassium levels.

DIURETICS, THIAZIDE

GENERIC NAME OR DRUG CLASS	COMBINED EFFECT	GENERIC NAME OR DRUG CLASS	COMBINED EFFECT
Indapamide	Increased diuretic effect.	Opiates*	Dizziness or weakness when standing up after sitting or lying down.
Indomethacin	Decreased anti-hypertensive effect.		
Lithium	Increased effect of lithium.	Pentoxifylline	Increased anti-hypertensive effect.
Monoamine oxidase (MAO) inhibitors*	Increased anti-hypertensive effect.	Potassium supplements*	Decreased potassium effect.
Nicardipine	Blood pressure drop. Dosages may require adjustment.	Probenecid	Decreased probenecid effect.
		Sotalol	Increased anti-hypertensive effect.
Nimodipine	Dangerous blood pressure drop.	Terazosin	Decreased terazosin effect.
Nitrates*	Excessive blood pressure drop.	Toremifene	Possible increased calcium.
		Zinc supplements	Increased need for zinc.

ERGOTAMINE, BELLADONNA & PHENOBARBITAL

GENERIC NAME OR DRUG CLASS	COMBINED EFFECT	GENERIC NAME OR DRUG CLASS	COMBINED EFFECT
Ephedrine	Dangerous blood pressure rise.	Metoclopramide	May decrease metoclopramide effect.
Epinephrine	Dangerous blood pressure rise.	Mind-altering drugs*	Dangerous sedation. Avoid.
Erythromycin	Decreased ergotamine effect.	Monoamine oxidase (MAO) inhibitors*	Increased belladonna and phenobarbital effect.
Griseofulvin	Decreased griseofulvin effect.	Narcotics*	Dangerous sedation. Avoid.
Guanethidine	Decreased belladonna effect.	Nitrates*	Increased internal eye pressure.
Haloperidol	Increased internal eye pressure.		
Indapamide	Increased indapamide effect.	Nitroglycerin	Decreased nitro-glycerin effect.
Meperidine	Increased belladonna effect.	Orphenadrine	Increased belladonna effect.
Methylphenidate	Increased belladonna effect.	Pain relievers*	Dangerous sedation. Avoid.

*See Glossary

GENERIC NAME OR DRUG CLASS	COMBINED EFFECT	GENERIC NAME OR DRUG CLASS	COMBINED EFFECT

ERGOTAMINE, BELLADONNA & PHENOBARBITAL continued

GENERIC NAME OR DRUG CLASS	COMBINED EFFECT	GENERIC NAME OR DRUG CLASS	COMBINED EFFECT
Phenothiazines*	Increased belladonna effect.	Sleep inducers*	Dangerous sedation. Avoid.
Pilocarpine	Loss of pilocarpine effect in glaucoma treatment.	Sumatriptan	Increased vasoconstriction. Delay 24 hours between drugs.
Potassium supplements*	Possible intestinal ulcers with oral potassium tablets.	Tranquilizers*	Dangerous sedation. Avoid.
Quinidine	Increased belladonna effect.	Troleandomycin	Increased adverse reactions of ergotamine.
Reserpine	Decreased belladonna effect.	Valproic acid	Increased phenobarbital effect.
Sedatives*	Dangerous sedation. Avoid.	Vitamin C	Decreased belladonna effect. Avoid large doses of vitamin C.

ESTROGENS

GENERIC NAME OR DRUG CLASS	COMBINED EFFECT	GENERIC NAME OR DRUG CLASS	COMBINED EFFECT
Insulin lispro	May need increased dosage of insulin.	Rifampin	Decreased estrogen effect.
Meprobamate	Increased estrogen effect.	Tamoxifen	Decreased tamoxifen effect.
Phenobarbital	Decreased estrogen effect.	Thyroid hormones*	Decreased thyroid effect.
Primidone	Decreased estrogen effect.	Ursodiol	Decreased effect of ursodiol.
Pyridoxine (vitamin B-6)	Decreased pyridoxine effect.	Vitamin C	Possible increased estrogen effect.
Raloxifene	Not recommended for use with estrogen.		

FLUOROQUINOLONES

GENERIC NAME OR DRUG CLASS	COMBINED EFFECT	GENERIC NAME OR DRUG CLASS	COMBINED EFFECT
Theophylline	Increased risk of theophylline toxicity.	Zinc	Decreased fluoroquinolone effect.
Warfarin	Increased warfarin effect.		

FLUVOXAMINE

GENERIC NAME OR DRUG CLASS	COMBINED EFFECT	GENERIC NAME OR DRUG CLASS	COMBINED EFFECT
Monoamine oxidase (MAO) inhibitors*	Potentially life-threatening. Allow 14 days between use of 2 drugs.	Selegiline	Increased risk of adverse effects. May lead to convulsions and hypertensive crisis. Let 14 days elapse between taking the 2 drugs.
		Theophylline	Increased theophylline effect.

*See Glossary

GENERIC NAME OR DRUG CLASS	COMBINED EFFECT	GENERIC NAME OR DRUG CLASS	COMBINED EFFECT

GUANETHIDINE

GENERIC NAME OR DRUG CLASS	COMBINED EFFECT	GENERIC NAME OR DRUG CLASS	COMBINED EFFECT
Rauwolfia alkaloids*	Excessively slow heartbeat. Weakness and faintness upon rising from chair or bed.	Terazosin	Decreased effectiveness of terazosin.
		Thioxanthenes*	Decreased guanethidine effect.
Sotalol	Increased antihypertensive effect.	Trimeprazine	Decreased guanethidine effect.

GUANETHIDINE & HYDROCHLOROTHIAZIDE

GENERIC NAME OR DRUG CLASS	COMBINED EFFECT	GENERIC NAME OR DRUG CLASS	COMBINED EFFECT
Digitalis preparations*	Excessive potassium loss that causes dangerous heart rhythms.	Monoamine oxidase (MAO) inhibitors*	Increased hydrochlorothiazide effect.
Diuretics, thiazide*	Increased thiazide and guanethidine effects.	Nicardipine	Blood pressure drop. Dosages may require adjustment.
Haloperidol	Decreased guanethidine effect.	Nimodipine	Dangerous blood pressure drop.
Indapamide	Possible increased effects of both drugs. When monitored carefully, combination may be beneficial in controlling hypertension.	Nitrates*	Excessive blood pressure drop.
		Oxprenolol	Increased antihypertensive effects. Dosages of both drugs may require adjustments.
Insulin	Increased insulin effect.	Phenothiazines*	Decreased guanethidine effect.
Lithium	Increased lithium effect.	Potassium supplements*	Decreased potassium effect.
Minoxidil	Dosage adjustments may be necessary to keep blood pressure at proper level.	Probenecid	Decreased probenecid effect.
		Sotalol	Increased antihypertensive effect.
		Terazosin	Decreased effectiveness of terazosin.

GUANFACINE

GENERIC NAME OR DRUG CLASS	COMBINED EFFECT	GENERIC NAME OR DRUG CLASS	COMBINED EFFECT
Sympathomimetics*	May decrease antihypertensive effects of guanfacine.	Terazosin	Decreased effectiveness of terazosin.

HALOPERIDOL

GENERIC NAME OR DRUG CLASS	COMBINED EFFECT	GENERIC NAME OR DRUG CLASS	COMBINED EFFECT
Fluoxetine	Increased depressant effects of both drugs.	Leucovorin	High alcohol content of leucovorin may cause adverse effects.
Guanethidine	Decreased guanethidine effect.	Levodopa	Decreased levodopa effect.
Guanfacine	May increase depressant effects of either drug.	Lithium	Increased toxicity.

*See Glossary

GENERIC NAME OR DRUG CLASS	COMBINED EFFECT	GENERIC NAME OR DRUG CLASS	COMBINED EFFECT

HALOPERIDOL continued

GENERIC NAME OR DRUG CLASS	COMBINED EFFECT	GENERIC NAME OR DRUG CLASS	COMBINED EFFECT
Loxapine	May increase toxic effects of both drugs.	Pergolide	Decreased pergolide effect.
Methyldopa	Possible psychosis.	Procarbazine	Increased sedation.
Narcotics*	Excessive sedation.	Sertraline	Increased depressive effects of both drugs.
Nefazodone	Unknown effect. May require dosage adjustment.		

HISTAMINE H$_2$ RECEPTOR ANTAGONISTS

GENERIC NAME OR DRUG CLASS	COMBINED EFFECT	GENERIC NAME OR DRUG CLASS	COMBINED EFFECT
Digitalis preparations*	Increased digitalis effect.	Morphine	Increased effect and toxicity of morphine.
Encainide	Increased effect of histamine H$_2$ receptor antagonist.	Nicardipine	Possible increased effect and toxicity of nicardipine.
Flurazepam	Increased effect and toxicity of flurazepam.	Nimodipine	Possible increased effect and toxicity of nimodipine.
Glipizide	Increased effect and toxicity of glipizide.	Paroxetine	Increased levels of paroxetine in blood.
Itraconazole	Decreased absorption of itraconazole.	Phenytoin	Increased effect and toxicity of phenytoin
Ketoconazole	Decreased ketoconazole absorption.	Propafenone	Increased effect of both drugs and increased risk of toxicity.
Labetalol	Increased antihypertensive effects.		
Metformin	Increased metformin effect.	Propranolol	Possible increased propranolol effect.
Metoclopramide	Decreased absorption of histamine H$_2$ receptor antagonist.	Quinidine	Increased quinidine effect.
Methadone	Increased effect and toxicity of methadone.	Tacrine	Increased tacrine effect.
Metoclopramide	Decreased absorption of histamine H$_2$ receptor antagonist.	Tamoxifen	Decreased tamoxifen effect.
Methadone	Increased effect and toxicity of methadone.	Terbinafine (oral)	Increased effect of terbinafine with cimetidine.
Metoprolol	Increased effect and toxicity of metoprolol.	Theophylline	Increases theophylline effect.
Metronidazole	Increased effect and toxicity of metronidazole.	Triazolam	Increased effect and toxicity of triazolam.
Miglitol	Decreased effect of ranitidine.	Venlafaxine	With cimetidine— Increased risk of adverse reactions.
Moricizine	Increased concentration of H$_2$ receptor antagonist in the blood.	Verapamil	Increased effect and toxicity of verapamil.

ADDITIONAL DRUG INTERACTIONS

GENERIC NAME OR DRUG CLASS	COMBINED EFFECT	GENERIC NAME OR DRUG CLASS	COMBINED EFFECT

HYDRALAZINE

Sotalol	Increased anti-hypertensive effect.	Terazosin	Decreased effectiveness of terazosin.

HYDRALAZINE & HYDROCHLOROTHIAZIDE

Antihypertensives*, other	Increased anti-hypertensive effect.	Diuretics*, oral	Increased effect of both drugs. When monitored carefully, combination may be beneficial in controlling hypertension.
Antivirals, HIV/AIDS*	Increased risk of peripheral neuropathy.		
Barbiturates*	Increased hydrochlorothiazide effect.	Indapamide	Increased diuretic effect.
Carteolol	Decreased anti-hypertensive effect.	Lithium	Increased lithium effect.
Cholestyramine	Decreased hydrochlorothiazide effect.	Monoamine oxidase (MAO) inhibitors*	Increased effect of drugs.
		Nimodipine	Dangerous blood pressure drop.
Cortisone drugs*	Excessive potassium loss that causes dangerous heart rhythms.	Nitrates*	Excessive blood pressure drop.
Diazoxide	Increased anti-hypertensive effect.	Potassium supplements*	Decreased potassium effect.
Digitalis preparations*	Excessive potassium loss that causes dangerous heart rhythms.	Probenecid	Decreased probenecid effect.

INDAPAMIDE

Opiates*	Weakness and faintness when arising from bed or chair.	Sotalol	Increased anti-hypertensive effect.
Probenecid	Decreased probenecid effect.	Terazosin	Decreased effectiveness of terazosin.

KAOLIN, PECTIN, BELLADONNA & OPIUM

Ketoconazole	Decreased ketoconazole effect.	Mind-altering drugs*	Increased sedative effect.
Lincomycins*	Decreased absorption of lincomycin. Separate doses by at least 2 hours.	Narcotics, other*	Increased narcotic effect.
		Nitrates*	Increased internal eye pressure.
MAO inhibitors*	Increased belladonna effect.	Orphenadrine	Increased belladonna effect.
Meperidine	Increased belladonna effect.	Phenothiazines*	Increased sedative effect of paregoric.
Methylphenidate	Increased belladonna effect.		

*See Glossary

GENERIC NAME OR DRUG CLASS	COMBINED EFFECT	GENERIC NAME OR DRUG CLASS	COMBINED EFFECT

KAOLIN, PECTIN, BELLADONNA & OPIUM continued

GENERIC NAME OR DRUG CLASS	COMBINED EFFECT	GENERIC NAME OR DRUG CLASS	COMBINED EFFECT
Pilocarpine	Loss of pilocarpine effect in glaucoma treatment.	Tranquilizers*	Increased tranquilizer effect.
Potassium supplements*	Possible intestinal ulcers with oral potassium tablets.	Vitamin C	Decreased belladonna effect. Avoid large doses of vitamin C.
Sedatives*	Excessive sedation.	All other oral medicines	Decreased absorption of other medicines. Separate doses by at least 2 hours.
Sleep inducers*	Increased effect of sleep inducers.		
Sotalol	Increased narcotic effect. Dangerous sedation.		

LITHIUM

GENERIC NAME OR DRUG CLASS	COMBINED EFFECT	GENERIC NAME OR DRUG CLASS	COMBINED EFFECT
Fluvoxamine	Increased risk of seizure.	Phenothiazines*	Decreased lithium effect.
Haloperidol	Increased toxicity of both drugs.	Phenylbutazone	Increased lithium effect.
Indomethacin	Increased lithium effect.	Phenytoin	Increased lithium effect.
Iodide salts	Increased lithium effects on thyroid function.	Potassium iodide	Increased potassium iodide effect.
Ketoprofen	May increase lithium in blood.	Sodium bicarbonate	Decreased lithium effect.
Methyldopa	Increased lithium effect.	Sumatriptan	Adverse effects unknown. Avoid.
Molindone	Brain changes.	Theophylline	Decreased lithium effect.
Oxyphenbutazone	Increased lithium effect.	Tiopronin	Increased risk of toxicity to kidneys.

LOXAPINE

GENERIC NAME OR DRUG CLASS	COMBINED EFFECT	GENERIC NAME OR DRUG CLASS	COMBINED EFFECT
Rauwolfia	May increase toxic effects of both drugs.	Thioxanthenes*	May increase toxic effects of both drugs
Sertraline	Increased depressive effects of both drugs.		

MAPROTILINE

GENERIC NAME OR DRUG CLASS	COMBINED EFFECT	GENERIC NAME OR DRUG CLASS	COMBINED EFFECT
Guanethidine	Decreased guanethidine effect.	Leucovorin	High alcohol content of leucovorin may cause adverse effects.
Guanfacine	May increase depressant effects of either drug.	Levodopa	Decreased levodopa effect.

ADDITIONAL DRUG INTERACTIONS

MAPROTILINE continued

GENERIC NAME OR DRUG CLASS	COMBINED EFFECT	GENERIC NAME OR DRUG CLASS	COMBINED EFFECT
Lithium	Possible decreased seizure threshold.	Phenothiazines*	Possible increased antidepressant effect and toxicity.
Methyldopa	Decreased methyldopa effect.	Phenytoin	Decreased phenytoin effect.
Methylphenidate	Possible increased antidepressant effect and toxicity.	Quinidine	Irregular heartbeat.
Molindone	Increased tranquilizer effect.	Selegiline	Fever, delirium, convulsions.
Monoamine oxidase (MAO) inhibitors*	Fever, delirium, convulsions.	Sertraline	Increased depressive effects of both drugs.
Narcotics*	Dangerous oversedation.	Sympathomimetics*	Increased sympathomimetic effect.
		Thyroid hormones*	Irregular heartbeat.

MEPROBAMATE & ASPIRIN

GENERIC NAME OR DRUG CLASS	COMBINED EFFECT	GENERIC NAME OR DRUG CLASS	COMBINED EFFECT
Ethacrynic acid	Possible aspirin toxicity.	Phenobarbital	Decreased aspirin effect.
Furosemide	Possible aspirin toxicity. May decrease furosemide effect.	Phenytoin	Increased phenytoin effect.
Gold compounds*	Increased likelihood of kidney damage.	Probenecid	Decreased probenecid effect.
Indomethacin	Risk of stomach bleeding and ulcers.	Propranolol	Decreased aspirin effect.
Methotrexate	Increased methotrexate effect.	Rauwolfia alkaloids*	Decreased aspirin effect.
Minoxidil	Decreased minoxidil effect.	Salicylates, other*	Likely aspirin toxicity.
Monoamine oxidase (MAO) inhibitors*	Increased meprobamate effect.	Sedatives*	Increased sedative effect.
Narcotics*	Increased narcotic effect.	Sleep inducers*	Increased effect of sleep inducer.
Oxprenolol	Decreased antihypertensive effect of oxprenolol.	Spironolactone	Decreased spironolactone effect.
Para-aminosalicylic acid (PAS)	Possible aspirin toxicity.	Sulfinpyrazone	Decreased sulfinpyrazone effect.
Penicillins*	Increased effect of both drugs.	Tranquilizers*	Increased tranquilizer effect.
		Vancomycin	Increased chance of hearing loss.
		Vitamin C (large doses)	Possible aspirin toxicity.

METFORMIN

GENERIC NAME OR DRUG CLASS	COMBINED EFFECT	GENERIC NAME OR DRUG CLASS	COMBINED EFFECT
Trimethoprim	Increased metformin effect.	Vancomycin	Increased metformin effect.

*See Glossary

METHOTREXATE

GENERIC NAME OR DRUG CLASS	COMBINED EFFECT	GENERIC NAME OR DRUG CLASS	COMBINED EFFECT
Sulfa drugs*	Possible methotrexate toxicity.	Tiopronin	Increased risk of toxicity to bone marrow and kidneys.
Sulfadoxine and pyrimethamine	Increased risk of toxicity.	Vaccines, live or killed	Increased risk of toxicity or reduced effectiveness of vaccine.
Tetracyclines*	Possible methotrexate toxicity.		

METHYLDOPA

GENERIC NAME OR DRUG CLASS	COMBINED EFFECT	GENERIC NAME OR DRUG CLASS	COMBINED EFFECT
Methyprylon	Increased sedative effect, perhaps to dangerous level. Avoid.	Salicylates* (including aspirin)	Possible methotrexate toxicity.
		Phenoxybenzamine	Urinary retention.
Monoamine oxidase (MAO) inhibitors*	Dangerous blood pressure rise.	Phenylephrine	Decreased methyl-dopa effect.
Nabilone	Greater depression of central nervous system.	Phenylpropanolamine	Decreased methyl-dopa effect.
Nicardipine	Blood pressure drop. Dosages may require adjustment.	Propranolol	Increased blood pressure (rarely).
Nimodipine	Dangerous blood pressure drop.	Sertraline	Increased depressive effects of both drugs.
Norepinephrine	Decreased methyl-dopa effect.	Sotalol	Increased anti-hypertensive effect.
Pergolide	Decreased pergolide effect.	Sympathomimetic drugs*	Increased risk of heart block and high blood pressure.
Phenytoin	Possible increased methotrexate toxicity.	Terazosin	Decreased effective-ness of terazosin.
Probenecid	Possible methotrexate toxicity.	Tolbutamide	Increased tolbutamide effect.
Pyrimethamine	Increased toxic effect of methotrexate.	Tolcapone	May require adjust-ment in dosage of methyldopa.

METHYLDOPA & THIAZIDE DIURETICS

GENERIC NAME OR DRUG CLASS	COMBINED EFFECT	GENERIC NAME OR DRUG CLASS	COMBINED EFFECT
Antihypertensives*	Increased anti-hypertensive effect.	Dapsone	Increased risk of adverse effect on blood cells.
Barbiturates*	Increased hydro-chlorothiazide effect.	Didanosine	Increased risk of pancreatitis.
Carteolol	Increased anti-hypertensive effect.	Digitalis preparations*	Excessive potassium loss that causes dan-gerous heart rhythms.
Cholestyramine	Decreased hydro-chlorothiazide effect.		
Cortisone drugs*	Excessive potassium loss that causes dangerous heart rhythms.	Diuretics, thiazide*	Increased effect of both drugs.
		Haloperidol	Increased sedation, possibly dementia.

*See Glossary

ADDITIONAL DRUG INTERACTIONS

METHYLDOPA & THIAZIDE DIURETICS continued

GENERIC NAME OR DRUG CLASS	COMBINED EFFECT	GENERIC NAME OR DRUG CLASS	COMBINED EFFECT
Indapamide	Increased diuretic effect.	Phenoxybenzanine	Urinary retention.
Levodopa	Increased effect of both drugs.	Phenylephrine	Decreased methyldopa effect.
Lithium	Increased lithium effect.	Phenylpropanolamine	Decreased methyldopa effect.
Monoamine oxidase (MAO) inhibitors*	Dangerous blood pressure changes.	Potassium supplements*	Decreased potassium effect.
Nabilone	Greater depression of central nervous system.	Propranolol	Increased blood pressure (rarely).
Nicardipine	Blood pressure drop. Dosages may require adjustment.	Sertraline	Increased depressive effects of both drugs.
Nimodipine	Dangerous blood pressure drop.	Sotalol	Increased antihypertensive effect.
Nitrates*	Excessive blood pressure drop.	Terazosin	Decreased terazosin effect.
Norepinephrine	Decreased methyldopa effect.	Tolbutamide	Increased tolbutamide effect.
		Zinc supplements	Increased need for zinc.

METOCLOPRAMIDE

GENERIC NAME OR DRUG CLASS	COMBINED EFFECT	GENERIC NAME OR DRUG CLASS	COMBINED EFFECT
Narcotics*	Decreased metoclopramide effect.	Sertraline	Increased depressive effects of both drugs.
Nizatidine	Decreased nizatidine absorption.	Tetracyclines*	Slow stomach emptying.
Pergolide	Decreased pergolide effect.	Thiothixines*	Increased chance of muscle spasm and trembling.
Phenothiazines*	Increased chance of muscle spasm and trembling.		

MOLINDONE

GENERIC NAME OR DRUG CLASS	COMBINED EFFECT	GENERIC NAME OR DRUG CLASS	COMBINED EFFECT
Narcotics*	Increased narcotic effect.	Sertraline	Increased depressive effects of both drugs.
Phenytoin	Increased or decreased phenytoin effect.	Sotalol	Increased tranquilizer effect. Increased sotalol effect.

MONOAMINE OXIDASE (MAO) INHIBITORS

GENERIC NAME OR DRUG CLASS	COMBINED EFFECT	GENERIC NAME OR DRUG CLASS	COMBINED EFFECT
Central nervous system (CNS) depressants*	Excessive depressant action.	Citalopram	Can cause a life-threatening reaction. Avoid.

*See Glossary

MONOAMINE OXIDASE (MAO) INHIBITORS continued

GENERIC NAME OR DRUG CLASS	COMBINED EFFECT	GENERIC NAME OR DRUG CLASS	COMBINED EFFECT
Clozapine	Toxic effect on the central nervous system	Methyldopa	Sudden, severe blood pressure rise.
Doxepin (topical)	Potentially life-threatening. Allow 14 days between use of the 2 drugs.	Methylphenidate	Increased blood pressure.
Dexfenfluramine	Potentially life-threatening. Allow 14 days between use of 2 drugs.	Mirtazapine	Potentially life-threatening. Allow 14 days between use of 2 drugs.
Dextromethorphan	Very high blood pressure.	Monoamine oxidase (MAO) inhibitors (others, when taken together)	High fever, convulsions, death
Diuretics*	Excessively low blood pressure.	Narcotics*	Severe high blood pressure.
Ephedrine	Increased blood pressure.	Nefazodone	Potentially life-threatening. Allow 14 days between use of the 2 drugs.
Fluoxetine	Serotonin syndrome (muscle rigidity, confusion, high fever). Avoid. Increased risk and severity of side effects. Allow 4 weeks between use of the 2 drugs.	Paroxetine	Can cause a life-threatening reaction. Avoid. Increased risk and severity of side effects. Allow 4 weeks between use of the 2 drugs.
Fluvoxamine	Potentially life-threatening. Allow 14 days between use of the 2 drugs.	Phenothiazines*	Possible increased phenothiazine toxicity.
Furazolidine	Sudden, severe increase in blood pressure.	Phenylpropanolamine	Increased blood pressure.
Guanadrel	High blood pressure.	Pseudoephedrine	Increased blood pressure.
Guanethidine	Blood pressure rise.	Sertraline	Serotonin syndrome (muscle rigidity, confusion, high fever). Avoid. Increased risk and severity of side effects. Allow 4 weeks between use of the 2 drugs.
Guanfacine	May increase depressant effects of either drug.		
Indapamide	Increased indapamide effect.		
Insulin	Increased hypoglycemic effect.	Sympathomimetics*	Blood pressure rise to life-threatening level.
Leucovorin	High alcohol content of leucovorin may cause adverse effects.	Tolcapone	May reduce effectiveness of MAO inhibitor.
Levodopa	Sudden, severe blood pressure rise.	Tramadol	Increased risk of seizures.
Maprotiline	Dangerous blood pressure rise.		

ADDITIONAL DRUG INTERACTIONS

GENERIC NAME OR DRUG CLASS	COMBINED EFFECT	GENERIC NAME OR DRUG CLASS	COMBINED EFFECT

MONOAMINE OXIDASE (MAO) INHIBITORS continued

Trazodone	Increased risk of mental status changes.	Venlafaxine	Increased risk and severity of side effects. Allow 4 weeks between use of the 2 drugs.

NARCOTIC ANALGESICS

Ethinamate	Dangerous increased effects of ethinamate. Avoid combining.	Narcotics*, other	Increased narcotic effect.
Fluoxetine	Increased depressant effects of both drugs.	Nicotine	Increased effect of pentazocine and propoxyphene.
Guanfacine	May increase depressant effects of either drug.	Nitrates*	Excessive blood pressure drop.
Leucovorin	High alcohol content of leucovorin may cause adverse effects.	Pentazocine	Possibly precipitates withdrawal with chronic narcotic use.
Methyprylon	Increased sedative effect, perhaps to dangerous level. Avoid.	Phenothiazines*	Increased sedative effect.
		Phenytoin	Possible decreased narcotic effect.
Metformin	Increased effect of metformin with morphine.	Rifampin	Possible decreased narcotic effect.
Mind-altering drugs*	Increased sedative effect.	Sedatives*	Increased sedative effect.
Molindone	Increased narcotic effect.	Selegiline	Severe toxicity characterized by breathing difficulties, seizures, coma.
Monoamine oxidase (MAO) inhibitors*	Serious toxicity (including death).		
Nabilone	Greater depression of central nervous system.	Sertraline	Increased depressive effects of both drugs.
		Sleep inducers*	Increased sedative effect.
Nalbuphine	Possibly precipitates withdrawal with chronic narcotic use.	Sotalol	Increased narcotic effect. Dangerous sedation.
Naltrexone	Precipitates withdrawal symptoms. May lead to respiratory arrest, coma and death.	Tramadol	Increased sedation.
		Tranquilizers*	Increased sedative effect.

NARCOTIC ANALGESICS & ACETAMINOPHEN

Phenothiazines*	Increased phenothiazine effect.	Sedatives*	Increased sedative effect.

*See Glossary

GENERIC NAME OR DRUG CLASS	COMBINED EFFECT	GENERIC NAME OR DRUG CLASS	COMBINED EFFECT

NARCOTIC ANALGESICS & ACETAMINOPHEN continued

GENERIC NAME OR DRUG CLASS	COMBINED EFFECT	GENERIC NAME OR DRUG CLASS	COMBINED EFFECT
Selegiline	Severe toxicity characterized by breathing difficulty, seizures, coma.	Tetracyclines*	May slow tetracycline absorption. Space doses 2 hours apart.
Sertraline	Increased depressive effects of both drugs.	Tramadol	Increased sedation.
		Tranquilizers*	Increased sedative effect.
Sleep inducers*	Increased sedative effect.	Zidovudine	Increased toxicity of zidovudine.
Sotalol	Increased narcotic effect. Dangerous sedation.		

NARCOTIC ANALGESICS & ASPIRIN

GENERIC NAME OR DRUG CLASS	COMBINED EFFECT	GENERIC NAME OR DRUG CLASS	COMBINED EFFECT
Anti-inflammatory drugs, nonsteroidal (NSAIDs)*	Risk of stomach bleeding and ulcers.	Rauwolfia alkaloids*	Decreased aspirin effect.
		Salicylates, other*	Likely aspirin toxicity.
Aspirin, other	Likely aspirin toxicity.	Sedatives*	Increased sedative effect.
Bumetanide	Possible aspirin toxicity.	Selegiline	Severe toxicity characterized by breathing difficulties, seizures, coma.
Carteolol	Increased narcotic effect. Dangerous sedation.		
Ethacrynic acid	Possible aspirin toxicity.	Sleep inducers*	Increased sedative effect.
Furosemide	Possible aspirin toxicity. May decrease furosemide effect.	Sotalol	Increased narcotic effect. Dangerous sedation.
Gold compounds*	Increased likelihood of kidney damage.	Spironolactone	Decreased spironolactone effect.
Indomethacin	Risk of stomach bleeding and ulcers.	Sulfinpyrazone	Decreased sulfinpyrazone effect.
Methotrexate	Increased methotrexate effect.	Ticlopidine	Decreased effects of both drugs.
Minoxidil	Decreased minoxidil effect.	Tramadol	Increased sedation.
Narcotics*, other	Increased narcotic effect.	Tranquilizers*	Increased sedative effect.
Nitrates*	Excessive blood pressure drop.	Valproic acid	May increase valproic acid effect.
Propranolol	Decreased aspirin effect.	Vitamin C (large doses)	Possible aspirin toxicity.

NEFAZODONE

GENERIC NAME OR DRUG CLASS	COMBINED EFFECT
Triazolam	Increased effects of both drugs.

ADDITIONAL DRUG INTERACTIONS

GENERIC NAME OR DRUG CLASS	COMBINED EFFECT	GENERIC NAME OR DRUG CLASS	COMBINED EFFECT

NIMODIPINE

Theophylline	May increase theophylline effect and toxicity.	Tocainide	Increased likelihood of adverse reaction from either drug.
Timolol eye drops	May cause increased effect of nimodipine on heart function.	Vitamin D (large doses)	Decreased nimodipine effect.

NUCLEOSIDE REVERSE TRANSCRIPTASE INHIBITORS

Probenecid	Increased effect of zalcitabine and zidovudine.	Rifampin	Decreased zidovudine effect.
		Tetracyclines	Decreased antibiotic effect.

ORPHENADRINE, ASPIRIN & CAFFEINE

Adrenocorticoids, systemic	Increased risk of ulcers. Increased adrenocorticoid effect.	Indomethacin	Risk of stomach bleeding and ulcers.
		Isoniazid	Increased caffeine effect.
Allopurinol	Decreased allopurinol effect.	Levodopa	Increased levodopa effect. (Improves effectiveness in treating Parkinson's disease.)
Antacids*	Decreased aspirin effect.		
Anticholinergics*	Increased anticholinergic effect.		
Anticoagulants*	Increased anticoagulant effect. Abnormal bleeding.	Methotrexate	Increased methotrexate effect.
Antidepressants, tricyclic*	Increased sedation.	Minoxidil	Decreased minoxidil effect.
		Monoamine oxidase (MAO) inhibitors*	Dangerous blood pressure rise.
Antidiabetics, oral*	Low blood sugar.	Nitrates*	Increased internal eye pressure.
Anti-inflammatory drugs, nonsteroidal (NSAIDs)*	Risk of stomach bleeding and ulcers.	Para-aminosalicylic acid (PAS)	Possible aspirin toxicity.
Aspirin, other	Likely aspirin toxicity.	Penicillins*	Increased effect of drugs.
Chlorpromazine	Hypoglycemia (low blood sugar).		
Contraceptives, oral*	Increased caffeine effect.	Phenobarbital	Decreased aspirin effect.
Furosemide	Possible aspirin toxicity.	Potassium supplements*	Increased possibility of intestinal ulcers with oral potassium tablets.
Gold compounds*	Increased likelihood of kidney damage.		
Griseofulvin	Decreased griseofulvin effect.	Probenecid	Decreased probenecid effect.

*See Glossary

GENERIC NAME OR DRUG CLASS	COMBINED EFFECT	GENERIC NAME OR DRUG CLASS	COMBINED EFFECT

ORPHENADRINE, ASPIRIN & CAFFEINE continued

GENERIC NAME OR DRUG CLASS	COMBINED EFFECT	GENERIC NAME OR DRUG CLASS	COMBINED EFFECT
Propoxyphene	Possible confusion, nervousness, tremors.	Spironolactone	Decreased spirono-lactone effect.
Propranolol	Decreased aspirin effect.	Sulfinpyrazone	Decreased sulfin-pyrazone effect.
Rauwolfia alkaloids*	Decreased aspirin effect.	Sympathomimetics*	Overstimulation.
		Thyroid hormones*	Increased thyroid effect.
Salicylates, other*	Likely aspirin toxicity.	Tranquilizers*	Decreased tranquilizer effect.
Sedatives*	Decreased sedative effect.	Valproic acid	May increase valproic acid effect.
Sleep inducers*	Decreased sedative effect.	Vitamin C (large doses)	Possible aspirin toxicity.

PANCREATIN, PEPSIN, BILE SALTS, HYOSCYAMINE, ATROPINE, SCOPOLAMINE & PHENOBARBITAL

GENERIC NAME OR DRUG CLASS	COMBINED EFFECT	GENERIC NAME OR DRUG CLASS	COMBINED EFFECT
Aspirin	Decreased aspirin effect.	Meperidine	Increased atropine effect.
Attapulgite	Decreased anticholinergic effect.	Methylphenidate	Increased atropine effect.
Beta-adrenergic blocking agents*	Decreased effect of beta-adrenergic blocker.	Mind-altering drugs*	Dangerous sedation. Avoid.
Buclizine	Increased scopolamine effect.	Monoamine oxidase (MAO) inhibitors*	Increased atropine effect.
Central nervous system (CNS) depressants*	Increased CNS depression.	Narcotics*	Dangerous sedation. Avoid.
Contraceptives, oral*	Decreased contraceptive effect.	Nitrates*	Increased internal eye pressure.
Digitalis	Possible decreased absorption of digitalis.	Nizatidine	Increased nizatidine effect.
Disopyramide	Increased atropine effect.	Orphenadrine	Increased atropine effect.
Dronabinol	Increased phenobarbital effect.	Phenothiazines*	Increased atropine effect.
Griseofulvin	Decreased griseofulvin effect.	Pilocarpine	Loss of pilocarpine effect in glaucoma treatment.
Haloperidol	Increased internal eye pressure.	Potassium supplements*	Possible intestinal ulcers with oral potassium tablets.
Indapamide	Increased indapamide effect.	Quinidine	Increased quinidine and scopolamine effect.
Ketoconazole	Decreased ketoconazole effect.	Sedatives*	Dangerous sedation. Avoid.

GENERIC NAME OR DRUG CLASS	COMBINED EFFECT	GENERIC NAME OR DRUG CLASS	COMBINED EFFECT

PANCREATIN, PEPSIN, BILE SALTS, HYOSCYAMINE, ATROPINE, SCOPOLAMINE & PHENOBARBITAL continued

GENERIC NAME OR DRUG CLASS	COMBINED EFFECT	GENERIC NAME OR DRUG CLASS	COMBINED EFFECT
Sleep inducers*	Dangerous sedation. Avoid.	Valproic acid	Increased phenobarbital effect.
Tranquilizers*	Dangerous sedation. Avoid.	Vitamin C	Decreased atropine effect. Avoid large doses of vitamin C.

PERPHENAZINE & AMITRIPTYLINE

GENERIC NAME OR DRUG CLASS	COMBINED EFFECT	GENERIC NAME OR DRUG CLASS	COMBINED EFFECT
Dronabinol	Increased effect of both drugs.	Narcotics*	Increased narcotic effect and dangerous sedation.
Ethchlorvynol	Delirium.		
Guanabenz	Possible decreased guanabenz effect.	Phenothiazines*	Possible increased antidepressant effect.
Guanethidine	Decreased guanethidine effect.	Procainamide	Possible irregular heartbeat.
Guanfacine	Possible decreased guanfacine effect.	Procarbazine	Increased sedation.
Levodopa	Decreased levodopa effect.	Quinidine	Impaired heart function. Dangerous mixture.
Lithium	Possible decreased seizure threshold.		
Methyldopa	Possible decreased methyldopa effect.	Sedatives*	Dangerous oversedation.
Methylphenidate	Possible increased antidepressant effect.	Sympathomimetics*	Increased sympatho-mimetics effect.
		Thyroid hormones*	Irregular heartbeat.
Mind-altering drugs*	Increased effect of mind-altering drugs.	Tranquilizers*, other	Increased tranquilizer effect.
Monoamine oxidase (MAO) inhibitors*	Fever, delirium, convulsions.	Thyroid hormones*	Increased thyroid effect.
Nabilone	Greater depression of central nervous system.	Tranquilizers*	Decreased tranquilizer effect.
		Valproic acid	May increase valproic acid effect.
		Vitamin C (large doses)	Possible aspirin toxicity.

PHENOTHIAZINES

GENERIC NAME OR DRUG CLASS	COMBINED EFFECT	GENERIC NAME OR DRUG CLASS	COMBINED EFFECT
Clozapine	Toxic effect on the central nervous system.	Levodopa	Decreased levodopa effect.
		Lithium	Decreased lithium effect.
Doxepin (topical)	Increased risk of toxicity of both drugs.	Mind-altering drugs*	Increased effect of mind-altering drug.
Guanethidine	Increased guanethidine effect.	Molindone	Increased tranquilizer effect.
Isoniazid	Increased risk of liver damage.		

*See Glossary

GENERIC NAME OR DRUG CLASS	COMBINED EFFECT	GENERIC NAME OR DRUG CLASS	COMBINED EFFECT

PHENOTHIAZINES continued

GENERIC NAME OR DRUG CLASS	COMBINED EFFECT	GENERIC NAME OR DRUG CLASS	COMBINED EFFECT
Narcotics*	Increased narcotic effect.	Tramadol	Increased sedation.
Procarbazine	Increased sedation.	Zolpidem	Increased sedation. Avoid.
Quetiapine	Decreased quetiapine effect with thioridazine.		

PRIMIDONE

GENERIC NAME OR DRUG CLASS	COMBINED EFFECT	GENERIC NAME OR DRUG CLASS	COMBINED EFFECT
Narcotics*	Increased narcotic effect.	Sedatives*	Increased sedative effect.
Oxyphenbutazone	Decreased oxyphenbutazone effect.	Sertraline	Increased depressive effects of both drugs.
Phenylbutazone	Decreased phenylbutazone effect.	Sleep inducers*	Increased effect of sleep inducer.
Phenytoin	Possible increased primidone toxicity.	Tranquilizers*	Increased tranquilizer effect.
Rifampin	Possible decreased primidone effect.		

PROBENECID & COLCHICINE

GENERIC NAME OR DRUG CLASS	COMBINED EFFECT	GENERIC NAME OR DRUG CLASS	COMBINED EFFECT
Methotrexate	Increased methotrexate effect.	Salicylates*	Decreased probenecid effect.
Mind-altering drugs*	Oversedation.	Sedatives*	Oversedation.
Narcotics*	Oversedation.	Sleep inducers*	Oversedation.
Nitrofurantoin	Increased nitrofurantoin effect.	Sulfa drugs*	Slows elimination. May cause harmful accumulation of sulfa.
Para-aminosalicylic acid (PAS)	Increased effect of para-aminosalicylic acid.	Thioguanine	More likelihood of toxicity of both drugs.
Penicillins*	Enhanced penicillin effect.	Tranquilizers*	Oversedation.
Phenylbutazone	Decreased antigout effect of colchicine.	Valacyclovir	Increased valacyclovir effect.
Pyrazinamide	Decreased probenecid effect.	Vitamin B-12	Decreased absorption of vitamin B-12.
		Zidovudine	Increased risk of zidovudine toxicity.

PROCARBAZINE

GENERIC NAME OR DRUG CLASS	COMBINED EFFECT	GENERIC NAME OR DRUG CLASS	COMBINED EFFECT
Diuretics*	Excessively low blood pressure.	Ethinamate	Dangerous increased effects of ethinamate. Avoid combining.
Doxapam	Increased blood pressure.		

GENERIC NAME OR DRUG CLASS	COMBINED EFFECT	GENERIC NAME OR DRUG CLASS	COMBINED EFFECT
PROCARBAZINE continued			
Fluoxetine	Increased depressant effects of both drugs.	Monoamine oxidase (MAO) inhibitors, other*	High fever, convulsions, death.
Guanethidine	Blood pressure rise to life-threatening level.	Nabilone	Greater depression of central nervous system.
Guanfacine	May increase depressant effects of either medicine.	Narcotics*	Increased sedation.
		Phenothiazines*	Increased sedation.
Leucovorin	High alcohol content of leucovorin may cause adverse effects.	Rauwolfia alkaloids*	Very high blood pressure.
		Reserpine	Increased blood pressure, excitation.
Levamisole	Increased risk of bone marrow depression.	Sertraline	Increased depressive effects of both drugs.
Levodopa	Sudden, severe blood pressure rise.	Sumatriptan	Adverse effects unknown. Avoid.
Methyldopa	Severe high blood pressure.	Sympathomimetics*	Heartbeat abnormalities, severe high blood pressure.
Methylphenidate	Excessive high blood pressure.	Tiopronin	Increased risk of toxicity to bone marrow.
Methyprylon	May increase sedative effect to dangerous level. Avoid.		

QUINIDINE

GENERIC NAME OR DRUG CLASS	COMBINED EFFECT	GENERIC NAME OR DRUG CLASS	COMBINED EFFECT
Propafenone	Increased effect of both drugs and increased risk of toxicity.	Tocainide	Increased possibility of adverse reactions from either drug.
Rauwolfia alkaloids*	Possibly disturbs heart rhythms.	Tramadol	May require dosage adjustment.
Rifampin	Decreased quinidine effect.	Venlafaxine	Increased risk of venlafaxine toxicity.
		Verapamil	Hypotension.

RAUWOLFIA & THIAZIDE DIURETICS

GENERIC NAME OR DRUG CLASS	COMBINED EFFECT	GENERIC NAME OR DRUG CLASS	COMBINED EFFECT
Barbiturates*	Increased hydrochlorothiazide effect.	Cortisone drugs*	Excessive potassium loss that causes dangerous heart rhythms.
Beta-adrenergic blocking agents*	Increased effect of rauwolfia alkaloids. Excessive sedation.	Digitalis preparations*	Excessive potassium loss that causes dangerous heart rhythms.
Carteolol	Increased antihypertensive effect.	Diuretics, thiazide*	Increased effect of other thiazide diuretics.
Cholestyramine	Decreased hydrochlorothiazide effect.	Dronabinol	Increased effect of both drugs. Avoid.

GENERIC NAME OR DRUG CLASS	COMBINED EFFECT	GENERIC NAME OR DRUG CLASS	COMBINED EFFECT

RAUWOLFIA & THIAZIDE DIURETICS continued

GENERIC NAME OR DRUG CLASS	COMBINED EFFECT	GENERIC NAME OR DRUG CLASS	COMBINED EFFECT
Indapamide	Increased diuretic effect.	Nitrates*	Excessive blood pressure drop.
Levodopa	Decreased levodopa effect.	Oxprenolol	Increased anti-hypertensive effect. Dosages of both drugs may require adjustments.
Lisinopril	Increased anti-hypertensive effect. Dosage of each may require adjustment.	Pergolide	Decreased pergolide effect.
Lithium	Increased effect of lithium.	Potassium supplements*	Decreased potassium effect.
Mind-altering drugs*	Excessive sedation.	Probenecid	Decreased probenecid effect.
Monoamine oxidase (MAO) inhibitors*	Increased hydro-chlorothiazide effect. Severe depression.	Sotalol	Decreased anti-hypertensive effect.
Nicardipine	Blood pressure drop. Dosages may require adjustment.	Terazosin	Decreased effective-ness of terazosin.

RAUWOLFIA ALKALOIDS

GENERIC NAME OR DRUG CLASS	COMBINED EFFECT	GENERIC NAME OR DRUG CLASS	COMBINED EFFECT
Lisinopril	Increased anti-hypertensive effect. Dosage of each may require adjustment.	Nicardipine	Blood pressure drop. Dosages may require adjustment.
Loxapine	May increase toxic effects of both drugs.	Nimodipine	Dangerous blood pressure drop.
Methyprylon	May increase seda-tive effect to danger-ous level. Avoid.	Pergolide	Decreased pergolide effect.
Mind-altering drugs*	Excessive sedation.	Sertraline	Increased depres-sive effects of both drugs.
Monoamine oxidase (MAO) inhibitors*	Severe depression.	Sotalol	Decreased anti-hypertensive effect.
Nabilone	Greater depression of central nervous system.	Terazosin	Decreased effective-ness of terazosin.

RESERPINE, HYDRALAZINE & HYDROCHLOROTHIAZIDE

GENERIC NAME OR DRUG CLASS	COMBINED EFFECT	GENERIC NAME OR DRUG CLASS	COMBINED EFFECT
Allopurinol	Decreased allopurinol effect.	Antidepressants, tricyclic*	Dangerous drop in blood pressure. Avoid combination unless under medical supervision.
Amphetamines*	Decreased hydralazine effect.	Antihistamines*	Increased anti-histamine effect.
Anticoagulants*, oral	Unpredictable increased or decreased effect of anticoagulant.	Antihypertensives, other*	Increased anti-hypertensive effect.
Anticonvulsants*	Serious change in seizure pattern.		

ADDITIONAL DRUG INTERACTIONS

GENERIC NAME OR DRUG CLASS	COMBINED EFFECT	GENERIC NAME OR DRUG CLASS	COMBINED EFFECT

RESERPINE, HYDRALAZINE & HYDROCHLOROTHIAZIDE continued

GENERIC NAME OR DRUG CLASS	COMBINED EFFECT	GENERIC NAME OR DRUG CLASS	COMBINED EFFECT
Anti-inflammatory drugs, nonsteroidal (NSAIDs)*	Decreased hydralazine effect.	Levodopa	Decreased levodopa effect.
Aspirin	Decreased aspirin effect.	Lisinopril	Increased anti-hypertensive effect. Dosage of each may require adjustment.
Barbiturates*	Increased hydro-chlorothiazide effect.	Lithium	Increased lithium effect.
Beta-adrenergic blocking agents*	Increased effect of rauwolfia alkaloids. Excessive sedation.	Mind-altering drugs*	Excessive sedation.
Carteolol	Increased anti-hypertensive effect.	Monoamine oxidase (MAO) inhibitors*	Increased effects of both drugs. Severe depression.
Cholestyramine	Decreased hydro-chlorothiazide effect.	Nicardipine	Blood pressure drop. Dosages may require adjustment.
Cortisone drugs*	Excessive potassium loss that causes dangerous heart rhythms.	Nimodipine	Dangerous blood pressure drop.
Diazoxide	Increased anti-hypertensive effect.	Nitrates*	Excessive blood pressure drop.
Digitalis preparations*	Excessive potassium loss that causes dangerous heart rhythms.	Oxprenolol	Increased anti-hypertensive effect. Dosages of drugs may require adjustments.
Diuretics, oral*	Increased effects of drugs. When monitored carefully, combination may be beneficial in control-ling hypertension.	Pergolide	Decreased pergolide effect.
		Potassium supplements*	Decreased potassium effect.
Dronabinol	Increased effects of drugs.	Probenecid	Decreased probenecid effect.
Indapamide	Increased diuretic effect.	Sotalol	Decreased anti-hypertensive effect.
		Terazosin	Decreased effective-ness of terazosin.

RETINOIDS (Oral)

GENERIC NAME OR DRUG CLASS	COMBINED EFFECT	GENERIC NAME OR DRUG CLASS	COMBINED EFFECT
Isotretinoin	Increased toxicity.	Tretinoin	Increased toxicity.
Medicated cosmetics	Excessive drying effect on skin.	Vitamin A	Increased toxicity. Avoid.
Methotrexate	Increased toxicity to liver.	Warfarin	Increased warfarin effect.

RIFAMYCINS

GENERIC NAME OR DRUG CLASS	COMBINED EFFECT	GENERIC NAME OR DRUG CLASS	COMBINED EFFECT
Phenytoin	Decreased phenytoin effect.	Protease inhibitors	Decreased protease inhibitor effect.
Probenecid	Possible toxicity to liver.	Quinidine	Decreased effect of both drugs.

*See Glossary

GENERIC NAME OR DRUG CLASS	COMBINED EFFECT	GENERIC NAME OR DRUG CLASS	COMBINED EFFECT

RIFAMYCINS continued

Quinine	Decreased quinine effect.	Tocainide	Possible decreased blood cell production in bone marrow.
Sildenafil	Decreased sildenafil effect.	Trimethoprim	Decreased trimethoprim effect.
Tacrolimus	Decreased tacrolimus effect.	Zidovudine	Decreased zidovudine effect.
Theophyllines*	Decreased theophylline effect.		

SALICYLATES

Insulin lispro	May need decreased dosage of insulin.	Sotalol	Decreased anti hypertensive effect of sotalol.
Ketoconazole	With buffered salicylates—Decreased ketoconazole effect.	Spironolactone	Decreased spironolactone effect.
Methotrexate	Increased methotrexate effect and toxicity.	Sulfinpyrazone	Decreased sulfinpyrazone effect.
Para-aminosalicylic acid	Possible salicylate toxicity.	Terazosin	Decreased effectiveness of terazosin. Causes sodium and fluid retention.
Penicillins*	Increased effect of both drugs.	Urinary acidifiers*	Decreased excretion. Increased salicylate effect.
Phenobarbital	Decreased salicylate effect.		
Phenytoin	Increased phenytoin effect.	Urinary alkalizers*	Increased excretion. Decreased salicylate effect.
Probenecid	Decreased probenecid effect.	Valproic acid	Possible increased valproic acid toxicity.
Rauwolfia alkaloids*	Decreased salicylate effect.	Vitamin C (large doses)	Possible salicylate toxicity.
Salicylates*, other	Likely salicylate toxicity.	Zidovudine	increased zidovudine effect.

SCOPOLAMINE (Hyoscine)

Nabilone	Greater depression of central nervous system.	Pilocarpine	Loss of pilocarpine effect in glaucoma treatment.
Nitrates*	Increased internal eye pressure.	Potassium supplements*	Possible intestinal ulcers with oral potassium tablets.
Nizatidine	Increased nizatidine effect.	Quinidine	Increased scopolamine effect.
Orphenadrine	Increased scopolamine effect.	Sedatives* or central nervous system (CNS) depressants*	Increased sedative effect of both drugs.
Phenothiazines*	Increased scopolamine effect.		

ADDITIONAL DRUG INTERACTIONS

GENERIC NAME OR DRUG CLASS	COMBINED EFFECT	GENERIC NAME OR DRUG CLASS	COMBINED EFFECT

SCOPOLAMINE (Hyoscine) continued

Sertraline	Increased depressive effects of both drugs.	Vitamin C	Decreased scopolamine effect. Avoid large doses of vitamin C.

SELEGILINE

Sertraline	Increased depressive effects of both drugs.	Sumatriptan	Adverse effects unknown. Avoid.

TETRACYCLINES

Vitamin A	Increased risk of intracranial hypertension.	Zinc supplements	Decreased tetracycline absorption if taken within 2 hours of each other.

THEOPHYLLINE, EPHEDRINE & BARBITURATES

Antihistamines*	Dangerous sedation. Avoid.	Dronabinol	Increased effect of drugs. Avoid.
Antihypertensives*	Decreased anti-hypertensive effect.	Ephedrine	Increased effect of drugs.
Anti-inflammatory drugs, nonsteroidal (NSAIDs)*	Decreased anti-inflammatory effect.	Epinephrine	Increased effect of drugs.
Aspirin	Decreased aspirin effect.	Ergot preparations*	Serious blood pressure rise.
Beta-adrenergic blocking agents*	Decreased effect of drugs.	Erythromycins*	Increased bronchodilator effect.
Carteolol	Increased barbiturate effect. Dangerous sedation.	Finasteride	Decreased theophylline effect.
Ciprofloxacin	Increased possibility of central nervous system poisoning, such as nausea, vomiting, restlessness, palpitations.	Furosemide	Increased furosemide effect.
		Griseofulvin	Decreased griseofulvin effect.
		Guanethidine	Decreased effect of drugs.
Clarithromycin	Increased concentration of theophylline.	Indapamide	Increased indapamide effect.
Contraceptives, oral*	Decreased contraceptive effect.	Lincomycins*	Increased bronchodilator effect.
Digitalis preparations*	Serious heart rhythm disturbances.	Lithium	Decreased lithium effect.
Doxycycline	Decreased doxycycline effect.	Mind-altering drugs*	Dangerous sedation. Avoid.

*See Glossary

THEOPHYLLINE, EPHEDRINE & BARBITURATES continued

GENERIC NAME OR DRUG CLASS	COMBINED EFFECT	GENERIC NAME OR DRUG CLASS	COMBINED EFFECT
Monoamine oxidase (MAO) inhibitors*	Increased ephedrine effect. Dangerous blood pressure rise.	Rauwolfia alkaloids*	Rapid heartbeat.
		Sotalol	Increased barbiturate effect. Dangerous sedation.
Narcotics*	Dangerous sedation. Avoid.	Sulfinpyrazone	Decreased sulfin-pyrazone effect.
Nicardipine	May increase theophylline effect and toxiclty.	Terazosin	Decreased terazosin effect.
Nicotine	Increased bronchodilator effect.	Ticlopidine	Increased theophylline effect.
Nitrates*	Possible decreased effect of drugs.	Troleandomycin	Increased bronchodilator effect.
Probenecid	Decreased effect of drugs.	Valproic acid	Increased barbiturate effect.
Propranolol	Decreased bronchodilator effect.	Zafirlukast	May increase effect of zafirlukast.
Pseudoephedrine	Increased pseudo-ephedrine effect.	Zileuton	Increased theophylline effect.

THEOPHYLLINE, EPHEDRINE & HYDROXYZINE

GENERIC NAME OR DRUG CLASS	COMBINED EFFECT	GENERIC NAME OR DRUG CLASS	COMBINED EFFECT
Carteolol	Decreased antihistamine effect.	Lithium	Decreased lithium effect.
Ciprofloxacin	May cause kidney dysfunction.	Monoamine oxidase (MAO) inhibitors*	Increased ephedrine effect. Dangerous blood pressure rise.
Clarithromycin	Increased concentration of theophylline.	Moricizine	Decreased antihistamine effect.
Digitalis preparations*	Serious heart rhythm disturbances.	Nabilone	Greater depression of central nervous system.
Dronabinol	Increased effect of drugs.	Nicardipine	May increase theophylline effect and toxicity.
Ephedrine	Increased effect of drugs.		
Epinephrine	Increased effect of drugs.	Nicotine	Increased bronchodilator effect.
Ergot preparations*	Serious blood pressure rise.	Nitrates*	Possible decreased effect of drugs.
Erythromycins*	Increased bronchodilator effect.	Pain relievers*	Increased effect of drugs.
Finasteride	Decreased theophylline effect.	Probenecid	Decreased effect of drugs.
Furosemide	Increased furosemide effect.	Propranolol	Decreased bronchodilator effect.
Guanethidine	Decreased effect of drugs.	Pseudoephedrine	Increased pseudo-ephedrine effect.
Lincomycins*	Increased bronchodilator effect.	Rauwolfia alkaloids*	Rapid heartbeat.

*See Glossary

935

ADDITIONAL DRUG INTERACTIONS

GENERIC NAME OR DRUG CLASS	COMBINED EFFECT	GENERIC NAME OR DRUG CLASS	COMBINED EFFECT

THEOPHYLLINE, EPHEDRINE & HYDROXYZINE continued

GENERIC NAME OR DRUG CLASS	COMBINED EFFECT	GENERIC NAME OR DRUG CLASS	COMBINED EFFECT
Sotalol	Decreased antihistamine effect.	Tranquilizers*	Increased effect of drugs.
Sulfinpyrazone	Decreased sulfinpyrazone effect.	Troleandomycin	Increased bronchodilator effect.
Terazosin	Decreased effect of terazosin.	Zafirlukast	May increase effect of zafirlukast.
Ticlopidine	Increased theophylline effect.	Zileuton	Increased effect of zileuton.

THEOPHYLLINE, EPHEDRINE, GUAIFENESIN & BARBITURATES

GENERIC NAME OR DRUG CLASS	COMBINED EFFECT	GENERIC NAME OR DRUG CLASS	COMBINED EFFECT
Aspirin, other	Decreased aspirin effect.	Griseofulvin	Decreased griseofulvin effect.
Beta-adrenergic blocking agents*	Decreased effect of drugs.	Guanethidine	Decreased effect of drugs.
Carteolol	Increased barbiturate effect. Dangerous sedation.	Indapamide	Increased indapamide effect.
Clarithromycin	Increased concentration of theophylline.	Lincomycins*	Increased bronchodilator effect.
Ciprofloxacin	Increased possibility of central nervous system poisoning, such as nausea, vomiting, restlessness, palpitations	Lithium	Decreased lithium effect.
		Mind-altering drugs*	Dangerous sedation. Avoid.
		Monoamine oxidase (MAO) inhibitors*	Increased phenobarbital effect.
Contraceptives, oral*	Decreased contraceptive effect	Narcotics*	Dangerous sedation. Avoid.
Digitalis preparations*	Serious heart rhythm disturbances.	Nicardipine	May increase theophylline effect and toxicity.
Digitoxin	Decreased digitoxin effect.	Nicotine	Increased bronchodilator effect.
Doxycycline	Decreased doxycycline effect.	Nitrates*	Possible decreased effect of drugs.
Dronabinol	Increased effect of drugs.	Pain relievers*	Dangerous sedation. Avoid.
Ephedrine	Increased effect of drugs.	Probenecid	Decreased effect of drugs.
Ergot preparations*	Serious blood pressure rise.	Propranolol	Decreased bronchodilator effect.
Erythromycins*	Increased bronchodilator effect.	Pseudoephedrine	Increased pseudoephedrine effect.
Finasteride	Decreased theophylline effect.	Rauwolfia alkaloids*	Rapid heartbeat.
Furosemide	Increased furosemide effect.	Sedatives*	Dangerous sedation. Avoid.

*See Glossary

GENERIC NAME OR DRUG CLASS	COMBINED EFFECT	GENERIC NAME OR DRUG CLASS	COMBINED EFFECT

THEOPHYLLINE, EPHEDRINE, GUAIFENESIN & BARBITURATES continued

GENERIC NAME OR DRUG CLASS	COMBINED EFFECT	GENERIC NAME OR DRUG CLASS	COMBINED EFFECT
Sleep inducers*	Dangerous sedation. Avoid.	Troleandomycin	Increased bronchodilator effect.
Sulfinpyrazone	Decreased sulfinpyrazone effect.	Valproic acid	Increased phenobarbital effect.
Terazosin	Decreased terazosin effect.	Zafirlukast	May increase effect of zafirlukast.
Ticlopidine	Increased theophylline effect.	Zileuton	Increased effect of theophylline.
Tranquilizers*	Dangerous sedation. Avoid.		

THIOTHIXENE

GENERIC NAME OR DRUG CLASS	COMBINED EFFECT	GENERIC NAME OR DRUG CLASS	COMBINED EFFECT
Pergolide	Decreased pergolide effect.	Sertraline	Increased depressive effects of both drugs.
Quinidine	Increased risk of heartbeat irregularities.	Tranquilizers*	Increased thiothixene effect. Excessive sedation.

TRIAZOLAM

GENERIC NAME OR DRUG CLASS	COMBINED EFFECT	GENERIC NAME OR DRUG CLASS	COMBINED EFFECT
Omeprazole	Delayed excretion of triazolam causing increased amount of triazolam in blood.	Probenecid	Increased triazolam effect.
		Zidovudine	Increased toxicity of zidovudine.

VALPROIC ACID

GENERIC NAME OR DRUG CLASS	COMBINED EFFECT	GENERIC NAME OR DRUG CLASS	COMBINED EFFECT
Sulfinpyrazone	Increased chance of bleeding.	Tocainide	Possible decreased blood cell production in bone marrow.

ADDITIONAL DRUG INTERACTIONS

Glossary

The following medical terms are found in the drug charts. Where drug names are listed, the generic or drug class is first, with brand names following in parentheses.

A

ACE Inhibitors—See Angiotensin-Converting Enzyme (ACE) Inhibitors.

Acne Preparations—Creams, lotions and liquids applied to the skin to treat acne. These include adapalene; alcohol and acetone; alcohol and sulfur; azelaic acid; benzoyl peroxide; clindamycin; erythromycin; erythromycin and benzoyl peroxide; isotretinoin; meclocycline; resorcinol; resorcinol and sulfur; salicylic acid gel USP; salicylic acid lotion; salicylic acid ointment; salicylic acid pads; salicylic acid soap; salicylic acid and sulfur bar soap; salicylic acid and sulfur cleansing lotion; salicylic acid and sulfur cleansing suspension; salicylic acid and sulfur lotion; sulfurated lime; sulfur bar soap; sulfur cream; sulfur lotion; tetracycline, oral; tetracycline hydrochloride for topical solution; tretinoin.

Acridine Derivatives—Dyes or stains (usually yellow or orange) used for some medical tests and as antiseptic agents.

Acute—Having a short and relatively severe course.

Addiction—Psychological or physiological dependence upon a drug.

Addictive Drugs—Any drug that can lead to physiological dependence on the drug. These include alcohol, cocaine, marijuana, nicotine, opium, morphine, codeine, heroin (and other narcotics) and others.

Addison's Disease—Changes in the body caused by a deficiency of hormones manufactured by the adrenal gland. Usually fatal if untreated.

Adrenal Cortex—Center of the adrenal gland.

Adrenal Gland—Gland next to the kidney that produces cortisone and epinephrine (adrenalin).

Agranulocytosis—A symptom complex characterized by (1) a sharply decreased number of granulocytes (one of the types of white blood cells), (2) lesions of the throat and other mucous membranes, (3) lesions of the gastrointestinal tract and (4) lesions of the skin. Sometimes also called granulocytopenia.

Alkalizers—These drugs neutralize acidic properties of the blood and urine by making them more alkaline (or basic). Systemic alkalizers include potassium citrate and citric acid, sodium bicarbonate, sodium citrate and citric acid, and tricitrates. Urinary alkalizers include potassium citrate, potassium citrate and citric acid, potassium citrate and sodium citrate, sodium citrate and citric acid.

Alkylating Agent—Chemical used to treat malignant diseases.

Allergy—Excessive sensitivity to a substance that is ordinarily harmless. Reactions include sneezing, stuffy nose, hives, itching.

Alpha-Adrenergic Blocking Agents—A group of drugs used to treat hypertension. These drugs include prazosin, terazosin, doxazosin and labetalol (an alpha-adrenergic and beta-adrenergic combination drug). Also included are other drugs that produce an alpha-adrenergic blocking action such as haloperidol, loxapine, phenothiazines, thioxanthenes.

Amebiasis—Infection with amoebas, one-celled organisms. Causes diarrhea, fever and abdominal cramps.

Amenorrhea—Abnormal absence of menstrual periods.

Aminoglycosides—A family of antibiotics used for serious infections. Their usefulness is limited because of their relative toxicity compared to some other antibiotics. These drugs include amikacin, gentamicin, kanamycin, neomycin, netilmicin, streptomycin, tobramycin.

Amphetamines—A family of drugs that stimulates the central nervous system, prescribed to treat attention-deficit disorders in children and also for narcolepsy. They are habit-forming, are controlled under U.S. law and are no longer prescribed as appetite suppressants. These drugs include amphetamine, dextroamphetamine, methamphetamine. They may be ingredients of several combination drugs.

ANA Titers—A test to evaluate the immune system and to detect antinuclear antibodies (ANAs), substances that appear in the blood of some patients with autoimmune disease.

Analgesics—Agents that reduce pain without reducing consciousness.

Anaphylaxis—Severe allergic response to a substance. Symptoms are wheezing, itching, hives, nasal congestion, intense burning of hands and feet, collapse, loss of consciousness and cardiac arrest. Symptoms appear within a few seconds or minutes after exposure. Anaphylaxis is a severe medical emergency. Without appropriate treatment, it can cause death. Instructions for home treatment for anaphylaxis are on the front inside cover.

Androgens—Male hormones, including fluoxymesterone, methyltestosterone, testosterone, DHEA.

Anemia—Not enough healthy red blood cells in the bloodstream or too little hemoglobin in the red blood cells. Anemia is caused by an imbalance between blood loss and blood production.

Anemia, Aplastic—A form of anemia in which the bone marrow is unable to manufacture adequate numbers of blood cells of all types—red cells, white cells, and platelets.

Anemia, Hemolytic—Anemia caused by a shortened lifespan of red blood cells. The body can't manufacture new cells fast enough to replace old cells.

Anemia, Iron-Deficiency—Anemia caused when iron necessary to manufacture red blood cells is not available.

Anemia, Pernicious—Anemia caused by a vitamin B-12 deficiency. Symptoms include weakness, fatigue, numbness and tingling of the hands or feet and degeneration of the central nervous system.

Anemia, Sickle-Cell—Anemia caused by defective hemoglobin that deprives red blood cells of oxygen, making them sickle-shaped.

Anesthesias, General—Gases that are used in surgery to render patients unconscious and able to withstand the pain of surgical cutting and manipulation. They include enflurane, etomidate, fentanyl, halothane, isoflurane, ketamine, methohexital, methoxyflurane, nitrous oxide, propofol, thiamylal, thiopental, alfentanil, amobarbital, butabarbital, butorphanol, chloral hydrate, etomidate, fentanyl, tentanyl, hydroxyzine, ketamine, levorphanol, meperidine, midazolam, morphine parenteral, nalbuphine, oxymorphone, pentazocine, pentobarbital, phenobarbital, promethazine, propiomazine, scopolamine, secobarbital, sufentanil.

Anesthetics—Drugs that eliminate the sensation of pain.

Angina (Angina Pectoris)—Chest pain with a sensation of suffocation and impending death. Caused by a temporary reduction in the amount of oxygen to the heart muscle through diseased coronary arteries. The pain may also occur in the left shoulder, jaw or arm.

Angiotensin-Converting Enzyme (ACE) Inhibitors—A family of drugs used to treat hypertension and congestive heart failure. Inhibitors decrease the rate of conversion of angiotensin I into angiotensin II, which is the normal process for the angiotensin-converting enzyme. These drugs include benazepril, captopril, enalapril, fosinopril, lisinopril, moexipril, ramipril.

Antacids—A large family of drugs prescribed to treat hyperacidity, peptic ulcer, esophageal reflux and other conditions. These drugs include alumina and magnesia; alumina, magnesia and calcium carbonate; alumina, magnesia and simethicone; alumina and magnesium carbonate; alumina and magnesium trisilicate; alumina, magnesium trisilicate and sodium bicarbonate; aluminum carbonate; aluminum hydroxide; bismuth subsalicylate; calcium carbonate; calcium carbonate and magnesia; calcium carbonate, magnesia and simethicone; calcium and magnesium carbonates; calcium and magnesium carbonates and magnesium oxide; calcium carbonate and simethicone; dihydroxyaluminum aminoacetate; dihydroxyaluminum sodium carbonate; magaldrate; magaldrate and simethicone; magnesium carbonate and sodium bicarbonate; magnesium hydroxide; magnesium oxide; magnesium trisilicate, alumina and magnesia; simethicone, alumina, calcium carbonate and magnesia; simethicone, alumina, magnesium carbonate and magnesia; sodium bicarbonate.

Antacids, Calcium Carbonate—These antacids include calcium carbonate and magnesium, calcium carbonate and simethicone, calcium carbonate and magnesium carbonates.

Antacids, Magnesium-Containing—These antacids include magnesium carbonate, magnesium hydroxide, magnesium oxide and magnesium trisilicate. All these medicines are designed to treat excess stomach acidity. In addition to being an effective antacid, magnesium can sometimes cause unpleasant side effects and drug interactions. Look for the presence of magnesium in nonprescription drugs.

Anthelmintics—A family of drugs used to treat intestinal parasites. Names of these drugs include niclosamide, piperazine, pyrantel, pyrvinium, quinacrine, mebendazole, metronidazole, oxamniquine, praziquantel, thiabendazole.

Antiacne Topical Preparations—See Acne Preparations.

Antiadrenals—Medicines or drugs that prevent the effects of the hormones produced by the adrenal glands.

Antianginals—A group of drugs used to treat angina pectoris (chest pain that comes and goes, caused by coronary artery disease). These drugs include acebutolol, amlodipine, amyl nitrite, atenolol, bepridril, carteolol, diltiazem, erythrityl, felodipine, isosorbide dinitrate, labetalol, metoprolol, nadolol, nicardipine, nifedipine, nitroglycerin, oxprenolol, penbutolol, pentaerythritol, pindolol, propranolol, sotalol, timolol, verapamil.

Antianxiety Drugs—A group of drugs prescribed to treat anxiety. These drugs include alprazolam, bromazepam, buspirone, chlordiazepoxide, chlorpromazine, clomipramine, clorazepate, diazepam, halazepam, hydroxyzine, imipramine, ketazolam, lorazepam, meprobamate, oxazepam, prazepam, prochlorperazine, thioridazine, trifluoperazine.

Antiarrhythmics—A group of drugs used to treat heartbeat irregularities (arrhythmias). These drugs include acebutolol, amiodarone, atenolol, atropine, bretylium, deslanoside, digitalis, digitoxin, diltiazem, disopyramide, edrophonium, encainide, esmolol, flecainide, glycopyrrolate, hyoscyamine, lidocaine, methoxamine, metoprolol, mexiletine, moricizine, nadolol, oxprenolol, phenytoin, procainamide, propafenone, propranolol, quinidine, scopolamine, sotalol, timolol, tocainide, verapamil.

Antiasthmatics—Medicines used to treat asthma, which may be tablets, liquids or aerosols (to be inhaled to get directly to the bronchial tubes rather than through the bloodstream). These medicines include adrenocorticoids, glucocorticoid; albuterol; aminophylline; astemizole; beclomethasone; bitolterol; budesonide; cetirizine; corticotropin; cromolyn; dexamethasone; dyphylline; ephedrine; epinephrine; ethylnorepinephrine; fenoterol; flunisolide; fluticasone; ipratropium, isoetharine; isoproterenol; isoproterenol and phenylephrine; loratadine; metaproterenol; oxtriphylline; oxtriphylline and guaifenesin; pirbuterol; racepinephrine; terbutaline; terfenadine; theophylline; theophylline and guaifenesin; triamcinolone.

Antibacterials (Antibiotics)—A group of drugs prescribed to treat infections. These drugs include aminocillin, amikacin, amoxicillin, amoxicillin and clavulanate, ampicillin, azlocillin, aztreonam, bacampicillin, carbenicillin, cefaclor, cefadroxil, cefamandole, cefazolin, cefonicid, cefoperazone, ceforanide, cefotaxime, cefotetan, cefoxitin, ceftazidime, ceftibuten, ceftizoxime, ceftriaxone, cefuroxime, cephalexin, cephalothin, cephapirin, cephradine, chloramphenicol, cinoxacine, clindamycin, cloxacillin, cyclacillin, cycloserine, demeclocycline, dicloxacillin, doxycycline, erythromycin, erythromycin and sulfisoxazole, flucloxacillin, fusidic acid, gentamicin, imipenem and cilastatin, kanamycin, lincomycin, methacycline, methenamine, methicillin, metronidazole, mezlocillin, minocycline, moxalactam, nafcillin, nalidixic acid, netilmicin, nitrofurantoin, norfloxacin, oxacillin, oxytetracycline, penicillin G, penicillin V, piperacillin, pivampicillin, rifabutin, rifampin, spectinomycin, streptomycin, sulfacytine, sulfadiazine and trimethoprim, sulfamethoxazole, sulfamethoxazole and trimethoprim, sulfisoxazole, tetracycline, ticarcillin, ticarcillin and clavulanate, tobramycin, trimethoprim, vancomycin.

Antibiotics—Chemicals that inhibit the growth of or kill germs. See Antibacterials.

Anticholinergics—Drugs that work against acetylcholine, a chemical found in many locations in the body, including connections between nerve cells and connections between muscle and nerve cells. Anticholinergic drugs include anisotropine, atropine, belladonna, clidinium, dicyclomine, glycopyrrolate, homatropine, hyoscyamine, ipratropium, isopropamide, mepenzolate, methantheline, methscopolamine, pirenzepine, propantheline, scopolamine.

Anticoagulants—A family of drugs prescribed to slow the rate of blood clotting. These drugs include acenocoumarol, anisindione, dicumarol, dihydroergotamine and heparin, heparin, warfarin.

Anticonvulsants—A group of drugs prescribed to treat or prevent seizures (convulsions). These drugs include these families: barbiturates, carbonic anhydrase inhibitors, diones, hydantoins and succinamides. These are the names of the generic drugs in these families: acetazolamide, amobarbital, carbamazepine, carbonic anhydrase inhibitors, clonazepam, clorazepate, diazepam, dichlorphenamide, divalproex, ethosuximide, ethotoin, felbamate, gabapentin, lamotrigine, lorazepam, magnesium sulfate, mephenytoin, mephobarbital, metharbital, methazolamide, methsuximide, metocurine, nitrazepam, paraldehyde, paramethadione, pentobarbital, phenobarbital, phensuximide, phenytoin, primidone, secobarbital, trimethadione, tubocurarine, valproic acid.

Antidepressants—A group of medicines prescribed to treat mental depression. These drugs include amitriptyline, amoxapine, bupropion, clomipramine, desipramine, doxepin, fluoxetine, fluvoxamine, imipramine, isocarboxazid, maprotiline, mirtazapine, moclobemide, nefazodone, nortriptyline, paroxetine, phenelzine, protriptyline, sertraline, tranylcypromine, trazodone, trimipramine, venlafaxine.

Antidepressants, MAO (Monoamine Oxidase) Inhibitors—A special group of drugs prescribed for mental depression. These are not as popular as in years past because of a relatively high incidence of adverse effects. These drugs include isocarboxazid (Marplan), phenelzine (Nardil), tranylcypromine (Parnate).

Antidepressants, Tricyclic (TCAs)—A group of medicines with similar chemical structure and pharmacologic activity used to treat mental depression. These drugs include amitriptyline, amoxapine, clomipramine, desipramine, doxepin, imipramine, nortriptyline, protriptyline, trimipramine.

Antidiabetic Agents—A group of drugs used in the treatment of diabetes mellitus. These medicines all reduce blood sugar. These drugs include acetohexamide, chlorpropamide, glipizide, glyburide, insulin, metformin, tolazamide, tolbutamide.

Antidiarrheal Preparations—Medicines that treat diarrhea symptoms. Most do not cure the cause. Oral medicines include aluminum hydroxide; charcoal, activated; kaolin and pectin; loperamide; polycarbophil; psyllium hydrophilic mucilloid. Systemic medicines include carbohydrates; codeine; difenoxin and atropine; diphenoxylate and atropine; glucose and electrolytes; glycopyrrolate; kaolin, pectin, belladonna alkaloids and opium; kaolin, pectin and paregoric; opium tincture; paregoric.

Antidyskinetics—A group of drugs used for treatment of Parkinsonism (paralysis agitans) and drug-induced extrapyramidal reactions (see elsewhere in Glossary). These drugs include amantadine, benztropine, biperiden, bromocriptine, carbidopa and levodopa, diphenhydramine, ethopropazine, levodopa, levodopa and benserazide, procyclidine, selegiline, trihexyphenidyl.

Antiemetics—A group of drugs used to treat nausea and vomiting. These drugs include buclizine, cyclizine, chlorpromazine, dimenhydrinate, diphenhydramine, diphenidol, domperidone, dronabinol, haloperidol, hydroxyzine, meclizine, metoclopramide, nabilone, ondansetron, perphenazine, prochlorperazine, promethazine, scopolamine, thiethylperazine, triflupromazine, trimethobenzamide.

Antifibronyltic Drugs—Drugs that are used to treat serious bleeding. These drugs include aminocaproic acid and tranexamic acid.

Antifungals—A group of drugs used to treat fungus infections. Those listed as systemic are taken orally or given by injection. Those listed as topical are applied directly to the skin and include liquids, powders, creams, ointments and liniments. Those listed as vaginal are used topically inside the vagina and sometimes on the vaginal lips. These drugs include: Systemic—amphotericin B, miconazole, fluconazole, flucytosine, griseofulvin, itraconazole, ketoconazole, potassium iodide. Topical—amphotericin B; carbol-fuchsin; ciclopirox; clioquinol; clotrimazole; econazole; haloprogin; ketoconzaole; mafenide; miconazole; naftifine; nystatin; oxiconazole; salicylic acid; silver sulfadiazine; sulconazole; sulfur and coal; terbinafine; tioconazole; tolnaftate; undecylenic

acid. Vaginal—butoconazole, clotrimazole, econazole, gentian violet, miconazole, nystatin, terconazole, tioconazole.

Antifungals, Azole—Drugs used to treat certain types of fungal infections. These drugs include fluconazole, itraconazole, ketoconazole, miconazole.

Antiglaucoma Drugs—Medicines used to treat glaucoma. Those listed as systemic are taken orally or given by injection. Those listed as ophthalmic are used as eye drops. These drugs include: Systemic—acetazolamide, dichlorphenamide, glycerin, mannitol, methazolamide, timolol, urea. Ophthalmic—betaxolol, carbachol ophthalmic solution, demecarium, dipivefrin, dorzolamide, echothiophate, epinephrine, epinephrine bitartrate, epinephryl borate, isoflurophate, levobunolol, metipranolol, physostigmine, pilocarpine, timolol.

Antigout Drugs—Drugs to treat the metabolic disease called gout. Gout causes recurrent attacks of joint pain caused by deposits of uric acid in the joints. Antigout drugs include allopurinol, carprofen, colchicine, fenoprofen, ibuprofen, indomethacin, ketoprofen, naproxen, phenylbutazone, piroxicam, probenecid, probenecid and colchicine, sulfinpyrazone, sulindac.

Antihistamines—A family of drugs used to treat allergic conditions, such as hay fever, allergic conjunctivitis, itching, sneezing, runny nose, motion sickness, dizziness, sedation, insomnia and others. These drugs include astemizole, azatadine, brompheniramine, carbinoxamine, cetirizine, chlorpheniramine, clemastine, cyproheptadine, dexchlorpheniramine, dimenhydrinate, diphenhydramine, diphenylpyraline, doxylamine, fexofenadine, hydroxyzine, loratadine, phenindamine, promethazine, pyrilamine, terfenadine, trimeprazine, tripelennamine, triprolidine.

Antihyperammonemias—Medications that decrease the amount of ammonia in the blood. The ones with this pharmacological property that are available in the United States are lactulose, sodium benzoate and sodium phenylacetate.

Antihyperlipidemics—A group of drugs used to treat hyperlipidemia (high levels of lipids in the blood). These include cholestyramine, clofibrate, colestipol, fluvastatin, gemfibrozil, lovastatin, niacin, pravastatin, probucol, simvastatin, sodium dichloroacetate.

Antihypertensives—Drugs used to help lower high blood pressure. These medicines can be used singly or in combination with other drugs. They work best if accompanied by a low-salt, low-fat diet plus an active exercise program. These drugs include acebutolol, amiloride,

amiloride and hydrochlorothiazide, amlodipine, atenolol, atenolol and chlorthalidone, benazepril, bendroflumethiazide, benzthiazide, betaxolol, bisoprolol, bumetanide, captopril, captopril and hydrochlorothiazide, carteolol, carvedilol, chlorothiazide, chlorthalidone, clonidine, clonidine and chlorthalidone, cyclothiazide, debrisoquine, deserpidine, deserpidine and hydrochlorothiazide, deserpidine and methyclothiazide, diazoxide, diltiazem, doxazosin, enalapril, enalapril and hydrochlorothiazide, ethacrynic acid, felodipine, fosinopril, furosemide, guanabenz, guanadrel, guanethidine, guanethidine and hydrochlorothiazide, guanfacine, hydralazine, hydralazine and hydrochlorothiazide, hydrochlorothiazide, hydroflumethiazide, indapamide, isradipine, labetalol, labetalol and hydrochlorothiazide, lisinopril, lisinopril and hydrochlorothiazide, losartan, losartan and hydrochlorothiazide, mecamylamine, methyclothiazide, methyldopa, methyldopa and chlorothiazide, methyldopa and hydrochlorothiazide, metolazone, metoprolol, metoprolol and hydrochlorothiazide, minoxidil, moexipril, nadolol, nadolol and bendroflumethiazide, nicardipine, nifedipine, nitroglycerin, nitroprusside, oxprenolol, penbutolol, pindolol, pindolol and hydrochlorothiazide, polythiazide, prazosin, prazosin and polythiazide, propranolol, propranolol and hydrochlorothiazide, quinapril, quinethazone, ramipril, rauwolfia serpentina, rauwolfia serpentina and bendroflumethazide, reserpine, reserpine and chlorothiazide, reserpine and chlorthalidone, reserpine and hydralazine, reserpine, hydralazine and hydrochlorothiazide, reserpine and hydrochlorothiazide, reserpine and hydroflumethiazide, reserpine and methyclothiazide, reserpine and polythiazide, reserpine and quinethazone, reserpine and trichlormethiazide, sotalol, spironolactone, spironolactone and hydrochlorothiazide, terazosin, timolol, timolol and hydrochlorothiazide, trandolapril, triamterene, triamterene and hydrochlorothiazide, trichlormethiazide, trimethaphan, verapamil.

Anti-Inflammatory Drugs, Nonsteroidal (NSAIDs)—A family of drugs not related to cortisone or other steroids that decrease inflammation wherever it occurs in the body. Used for treatment of pain, fever, arthritis, gout, menstrual cramps and vascular headaches. These drugs include aspirin; aspirin, alumina and magnesia tablets; buffered aspirin; bufexamac; celecoxib; choline salicylate; choline and magnesium salicylates; diclofenac, diflunisal; fenoprofen; flurbiprofen, ibuprofen;

indomethacin; ketoprofen; magnesium salicylate; meclofenamate; naproxen; piroxicam; salsalate; sodium salicylate; sulindac; tolmetin.

Anti-Inflammatory Drugs, Steroidal—A family of drugs with pharmacologic characteristics similar to those of cortisone and cortisone-like drugs. They are used for many purposes to help the body deal with inflammation no matter what the cause. Steroidal drugs may be taken orally or by injection (systemic) or applied locally (topical) for the skin, eyes, ears, bronchial tubes and others. These drugs include: Nasal— beclomethasone, budesonide, dexamethasone, flunisolide, fluticasone, triamcinolone.
Ophthalmic (eyes)—betamethasone, dexamethasone, fluorometholone, hydrocortisone, medrysone, prednisolone, rimexolone. Otic (ears)—betamethasone, desonide and acetic acid, dexamethasone, hydrocortisone, hydrocortisone and acetic acid, prednisolone. Systemic—betamethasone, corticotroprin, cortisone, dexamethasone, hydrocortisone, methylprednisolone, paramethasone, prednisolone, prednisone, triamcinolone. Topical—alclometasone; amcinonide; beclomethasone; betamethasone; clobetasol; clobetasone; clocortolone; desonide; desoximetasone; dexamethasone; diflorasone; diflucortolone; flumethasone; fluocinolone; fluocinonide; fluocinonide; flurandrenolide; fluticasone; halcinonide; halobetasol; mometasone; procinonide and ciprocinonide; flurandrenolid; halcinonide; hydrocortisone; methylprednisolone; mometasone; triamcinolone.

Antimalarials (also called Antiprotozoals)—A group of drugs used to treat malaria. The choice depends on the precise type of malaria organism and its developmental state. These drugs include amphotericin B, chloroquine, dapsone, demeclocycline, doxycycline, halofantrine; hydroxychloroquine, iodoquinol, methacycline, mefloquine, metronidazole, minocycline, oxytetracycline, pentamidine, primaquine, pyrimethamine, quinacrine, quinidine, quinine, sulfadoxine and pyrimethamine, sulfamethoxazole, sulfamethoxazole and trimethoprim, sulfisoxazole, tetracycline.

Antimuscarines—Drugs that block the muscarinic action of acetylcholine and therefore decrease spasms of the smooth muscles. They are prescribed for peptic ulcers, dysmenorrhea, dizziness, seasickness, bedwetting, slow heart rate, toxicity from pesticides made from organophosphates and other medical problems. These drugs include anisotropine, atropine, belladonna, clidinium dicyclomine, glycopyrrolate, homatropine, hyoscyamine, hyoscyamine and scopolamine, isopropamide, mepenzolate, methantheline, methscopolamine, oxyphencyclimine, pirenzepine, propantheline, scopolamine, tridihexethyl.

Antimyasthenics—Medicines to treat myasthenia gravis, a muscle disorder (especially of the face and head) with increasing fatigue and weakness as muscles tire from use. These medicines include ambenonium, neostigmine, pyridostigmine.

Antineoplastics—Potent drugs used for malignant disease. Some of these are not described in this book, but they are listed here for completeness. These drugs include: Systemic—aminoglutethimide, amsacrine, antithyroid agents, asparaginase, azathioprine, bleomycin, busulfan, carboplatin, carmustine, chlorambucil, chloramphenicol, chlorotrianisene, chromic phosphate, cisplatin, colchicine, cyclophosphamide, cyclosporine, cyproterone, cytarabine, dacarbazine, dactinomycin, daunorubicin, deferoxamine, diethylstilbestrol, doxorubicin, dromostanolone, epirubicin, estradiol, estradiol valerate, estramustine, estrogens (conjugated and esterified), estrone, ethinyl estradiol, etoposide, floxuridine, flucytosine, fluorouracil, flutamide, fluoxymesterone, gold compounds, hexamethylmelamine, hydroxyprogesterone, hydroxyurea, interferon alfa-2a and alfa-2b (recombinant), ketoconazole, leuprolide, levamisole, levothyroxine, liothyronine, liotrix, lithium, lomustine, masoprocol, mechlorethamine, medroxyprogesterone, megestrol, melphalan, methyltestosterone, mercaptopurine, methotrexate, mitomycin, mitotane, mitoxantrone, nandrolone, paclitaxel, phenpropionate, penicillamine, plicamycin, procarbazine, sodium iodide I 131, sodium phosphate P 32, streptozocin, tamoxifen, teniposide, testolactone, testosterone, thioguanine, thiotepa, thyroglobulin, thyroid, thyrotropin, uracil mustard, vinblastine, vincristine, vindesine, zidovudine. Topical—fluorouracil, mechlorethamine.

Antiparkisonism Drugs—Drugs used to treat Parkinson's disease. A disease of the central nervous system in older adults, it is characterized by gradual progressive muscle rigidity, tremors and clumsiness. These drugs include amantadine, benztropine, biperiden, bromocriptine, carbidopa and levodopa, diphenhydramine, ethopropazine, levodopa, levodopa and benserazide, orphenadrine, pergolide, procyclidine, seliginine, trihexyphenidyl.

Antipsychotic Drugs—A group of drugs used to treat the mental disease of psychosis, including such variants as schizophrenia, manic-depressive illness, anxiety states, severe behavior problems and others. These drugs include acetophenazine, carbamazepine, chlorpromazine, chlorprothixene, fluphenazine, flupenthixol, fluspirilene, haloperidol, loxapine, mesoridazine, methotrimeprazine, molindone, pericyazine, perphenazine, pimozide, pipotiazine, prochlorperazine, promazine, risperidone, thioproperazine, thioridazine, thiothixene, trifluoperazine, triflupromazine.

Antithyroid Drugs—Drugs that decrease the amount of thyroid hormone produced by the thyroid gland.

Antitussives—A group of drugs used to suppress coughs. These drugs include benzonatate, chlophedianol, codeine (oral), dextromethorphan, diphenhydramine syrup, hydrocodone, hydromorphone, methadone, morphine.

Antiulcer Drugs—A group of medicines used to treat peptic ulcer in the stomach, duodenum or the lower end of the esophagus. These drugs include amitriptyline, antacids, anticholinergics, antispasmotics, bismuth subsalicylate, cimetidine, doxepin, famotidine, lansoprazole, misoprostol, nizatidine, omeprazole, ranitidine, sucralfate, trimipramine.

Antiurolithics—Medicines that prevent the formation of kidney stones.

Antiviral Drugs—A group of drugs used to treat viral infections. These drugs include: Ophthalmic (eye)—idoxuridine, trifluridine, vidarabine. Systemic—acyclovir, amantadine, didanosine, famciclovir, foscarnet, ganciclovir, ribavirin, rimantadine, stavudine, zalcitabine, zidovudine. Topical—acyclovir.

Antivirals, HIV/AIDS—A group of drugs used to treat human immunodeficiency virus (HIV) and acquired immune deficiency syndrome (AIDS). They work by suppressing the replication of HIV. These drugs include didanosine, efavirenz, lamivudine, stavudine, zalcitabine, zidovudine.

Appendicitis—Inflammation or infection of the appendix. Symptoms include loss of appetite, nausea, low-grade fever and tenderness in the lower right of the abdomen.

Appetite Suppressants—A group of drugs used to decrease the appetite as part of an overall treatment for obesity. These drugs include amphetamine and dextroamphetamine, benzphetamine, diethylpropion, fenfluramine, mazindol, phendimetrazine, phentermine, phenylpropanolamine, sibutramine.

Artery—Blood vessel carrying blood away from the heart.

Asthma—Recurrent attacks of breathing difficulty due to spasms and contractions of the bronchial tubes.

Attentuated Virus Vaccines—Liquid products of killed germs used for injections to prevent certain diseases.

B

Bacteria—Microscopic organisms. Some bacteria contribute to health; others (germs) cause disease.

Barbiturates—Powerful drugs used for sedation, to help induce sleep and sometimes to prevent seizures. Except for use in seizures (phenobarbital), barbiturates are being used less and less because there are better, less hazardous drugs that produce the same or better effects. These drugs include amobarbital, aprobarbital, butabarbital, mephobarbital, metharbital, pentobarbital, phenobarbital, secobarbital, secobarbital and amobarbital, talbutal.

Basal Area of Brain—Part of the brain that regulates muscle control and tone.

Benzethonium Chloride—A compound used as a preservative in some drug preparations. It is also used in various concentrations for cleaning cooking and eating utensils and as a disinfectant.

Benzodiazepines—A family of drugs prescribed to treat anxiety and alcohol withdrawal and sometimes prescribed for sedation. These drugs include alprazolam, bromazepam, chlordiazepoxide, clonazepam, clorazepate, diazepam, estazolam, flurazepam, halazepam, ketazolam, lorazepam, nitrazepam, oxazepam, prazepam, quazepam, triazolam.

Beta Agonists—A group of drugs that act directly on cells in the body (beta-adrenergic receptors) to relieve spasms of the bronchial tubes and other organs consisting of smooth muscles. These drugs include albuterol, bitolerol, isoetharine, isoproterenol, methproterenol, terbutaline.

Beta-Adrenergic Blocking Agents—A family of drugs with similar pharmacological actions with some variations. These drugs are prescribed for angina, heartbeat irregularities (arrhythmias), high blood pressure, hypertrophic subaortic stenosis, vascular headaches (as a preventative, not to treat once the pain begins) and others. Timolol is prescribed for treatment of open-angle glaucoma. These drugs include acebutolol, atenolol, betaxolol, bisoprolol, carteolol, labetalol, metoprolol, nadolol, oxprenolol, penbutolol, pindolol, propranolol, sotalol, timolol.

Bile Acids—Components of bile that are derived from cholesterol and formed in the liver. Bile acids aid the digestion of fat.

Blood Count—Laboratory studies to count white blood cells, red blood cells, platelets and other elements of the blood.

Blood Dyscrasia-Causing Medicines—Drugs which cause unpredictable damaging effects to human bone marrow. These effects occur in a small minority of patients and are not dependent upon dosage. These medicines include the following (some of which are not described in this book): ACE inhibitors, aminopyrine, amodiaquine, anticonvulsants (dione, hydantoin, succinimide), antidepressants (tricyclic), antidiabetic agents (sulfonurea), anti-inflammatory analgesics, antithyroid agents, carbamazepine, chloramphenicol, clozapine, dapsone, divalproex, felbamate, flecainide acetate, foscarnet, gold compounds, levamisole, loxapine, maprotiline, methsuximide, mirtazapine, penicillins (some), penicillamine, pentamidine, phenacemide, phenothiazines, phensuximide, phenytoin, pimozide, primaquine, primidone, procainamide, propafenone, pyrimethamine (large doses), rifampin, sulfamethoxazole and trimethoprim, sulfasalazine, sulfonamides, thioxanthenes, ticlopidine, tiopronin, tocainide, trimethobenzamide, trimethoprim, valproic acid.

Blood Pressure, Diastolic—Pressure (usually recorded in millimeters of mercury) in the large arteries of the body when the heart muscle is relaxed and filling for the next contraction.

Blood Pressure, Systolic—Pressure (usually recorded in millimeters of mercury) in the large arteries of the body at the instant the heart muscle contracts.

Blood Sugar (Blood Glucose)—Necessary element in the blood to sustain life.

Bone Marrow Depressants—Medicines that affect the bone marrow to depress its normal function of forming blood cells. These medicines include the following (some of which are not described in this book): aldesleukin, altretamine, amophotericin B (systemic), anticancer drugs, anthithyroid drugs, azathioprine, busulfan, carboplatin, carmustine, chlorambucil, chloramphenicol, chromic phosphate, cisplatin, clozapine, colchicine, cyclophosphamide, cytarabine, dacarbazine, dactinomycin, daunorubicin, didanosine, docetaxel, doxorubicin, eflornithine, etoposide, floxuridine, flucytosine, fludarabine, fluorouracil, ganciclovir, hydroxyurea, idarubicin, ifosfamide, interferon, lomustine, mechlorethamine, melphalan, mercaptopurine, methotrexate, mitomycin, mitoxantrone, paclitaxel, pentostatin, plicamycin, procarbazine, streptozocin, sulfa drugs, thioguanine, thiotepa, trimetrexate, uracil mustard, vidarabine (large doses), vinblastine, vincristine, vinorelbine, zidovudine.

Bone Marrow Depression—Reduction of the blood-producing capacity of human bone marrow. Can be caused by many drugs taken for long periods of time in high doses.

Brain Depressants—Any drug that depresses brain function, such as tranquilizers, narcotics, alcohol and barbiturates.

Bronchodilators—A group of drugs used to dilate the bronchial tubes to treat such problems as asthma, emphysema, bronchitis, bronchiectasis, allergies and others. These drugs include albuterol, aminophylline, bitolterol, dyphylline, ephedrine, epinephrine, ethylnorepinephrine, fenoterol, ipratropium, isoetharine, isoproterenol, metaproterenol, oxtriphylline, oxtriphylline and guaifenesin, pirbuterol, procaterol, salmeterol, terbutaline, theophylline and guaifenesin.

Bronchodilators, Xanthine-Derivative—Drugs of similar chemical structure and pharmacological activity that are prescribed to dilate bronchial tubes in disorders such as asthma, bronchitis, emphysema and other chronic lung diseases. These drugs include aminophylline, dyphylline, oxtriphylline, theophylline.

BUN—Abbreviation for blood urea nitrogen. A test often used as a measurement of kidney function.

C

Calcium Channel Blockers—A group of drugs used to treat angina and heartbeat irregularities. These drugs include bepridril, diltiazem, felodipine, flunarizine, isradipine, nicardipine, nifedipine, nimodipine, verapamil.

Calcium Supplements—Supplements used to increase the calcium concentration in the blood in an attempt to make bones denser (as in osteoporosis). These supplements include calcium citrate, calcium glubionate, calcium gluconate, calcium glycerophosphate and calcium lactate, calcium lactate, dibasic calcium phosphate, tribasic calcium phosphate.

Carbamates—A group of drugs derived from carbamic acid and used for anxiety or as sedatives. They include meprobamate and ethinamate.

Carbonic Anhydrase Inhibitors—Drugs used to treat glaucoma and seizures and to prevent high altitude sickness. They include acetazolamide, dichlorphenamide, methazolamid.

Cataract—Loss of transparency in the lens of the eye.

Catecholamines—A group of drugs, also found naturally in the body, used to treat low blood pressure or shock. These drugs include dopamine, norepinephrine and epinephrine.

Cell—Unit of protoplasm, the essential living matter of all plants and animals.

Central Nervous System (CNS) Depressants—These drugs cause sedation or otherwise diminish brain activity and other parts of the nervous system. These drugs include alcohol, aminoglutethimide, anesthetics (general and injection-local), anticonvulsants, antidepressants (MAO inhibitors, tricyclic), antidyskinetics (except amantadine), antihistamines,

apomorphine, azelastine, baclofen, barbiturates, benzodiazepines, beta-adrenergic blocking agents, buclizine, carbamazepine, chlophedianol, chloral hydrate, chlorzoxazone, clonidine, clozapine, cyclizine, difenoxin and atropine, diphenoxylate and atropine, disulfiram, dronabinol, ethchlorvynol, ethinamate, etomidate, fenfluramine, fluoxetine, glutethimide, guanabenz, guanfacine, haloperidol, hydroxyzine, interferon, loxapine, magnesium sulfate (injection), maprotiline, meclizine, meprobamate, methyldopa, methyprylon, metoclopramide, metyrosine, mirtazapine, mitotane, molindone, nabilone, nefazodone, olanzapine, opioid (narcotic) analgesics, oxybutynin, paraldehyde, paregoric, pargyline, paroxetine, phenothiazines, pimozide, procarbazine, promethazine, propiomazine, rauwolfia alkaloids, risperidone, scopolamine, sertraline, skeletal muscle relaxants (centrally acting), thioxanthenes, trazodone, trimeprazine, trimethobenzamide, zolpidem.

Central Nervous System (CNS) Stimulants—Drugs that cause excitation, anxiety and nervousness or otherwise stimulate the brain and other parts of the central nervous system. These drugs include amantadine, amphetamines, anesthetics (local), appetite suppressants (except fenfluramine), bronchodilators (xanthine-derivative), bupropion, caffeine, chlophedianol, cocaine, dextroamphetamine, doxapram, dronabinol, ephedrine (oral), fluoxetine, methamphetamine, methylphenidate, nabilone, paroxetine, pemoline, selegiline, sertraline, sympathomimetics, tranylcypromine.

Cephalosporins—Antibiotics that kill many bacterial germs that penicillin and sulfa drugs can't destroy.

Cholinergics (Parasympathomimetics)—Chemicals that facilitate passage of nerve impulses through the parasympathetic nervous system.

Cholinesterase Inhibitors—Drugs that prevent the action of cholinesterase (an enzyme that breaks down acetylcholine in the body).

Chronic—Long-term, continuing. Chronic illnesses may not be curable, but they can often be prevented from becoming worse. Symptoms usually can be alleviated or controlled.

Cirrhosis—Disease that scars and destroys liver tissue resulting in abnormal function.

Citrates—Medicines taken orally to make urine more acid. Citrates include potassium citrate, potassium citrate and citric acid, potassium citrate and sodium citrate, sodium citrate and acid, tricitrates.

Coal Tar Preparations—Creams, ointments and lotions used on the skin for various skin ailments.

Cold Urticaria—Hives that appear in areas of the

body exposed to the cold.

Colitis, Ulcerative—Chronic, recurring ulcers of the colon for unknown reasons.

Collagen—Support tissue of skin, tendon, bone, cartilage and connective tissue.

Colostomy—Surgical opening from the colon, the large intestine, to the outside of the body.

Coma—A sleeplike state from which a person cannot be aroused.

Compliance—The extent to which a person follows medical advice.

Congestive—Characterized by excess accumulation of fluid. In congestive heart failure, congestion occurs in the lungs, liver, kidneys and other parts of the body to cause shortness of breath, swelling of the ankles and feet, rapid heartbeat and other symptoms.

Constriction—Tightness or pressure.

Contraceptives, Oral (Birth Control Pills)—A group of hormones used to prevent ovulation, therefore preventing pregnancy. These hormones include ethynodiol diacetate and ethinyl estradiol, ethynodiol diacetate and mestranol, levonorgestrel and ethinyl estradiol, medroxyprogesterone, norethindrone tablets, norethindrone acetate and ethinyl estradiol, norethindrone and ethinyl estradiol, norethindrone and mestranol, norethynodrel and mestranol, norgestrel, norgestrel and ethinyl estradiol.

Contraceptives, Vaginal—Topical medications or devices applied inside the vagina to prevent pregnancy.

Convulsions—Violent, uncontrollable contractions of the voluntary muscles.

Corticosteroids (Adrenocorticosteroids)—Steroid hormones produced by the body's adrenal cortex or their synthetic equivalents.

Cortisone (Adrenocorticoids, Glucocorticoids) and Other Adrenal Steroids—Medicines that mimic the action of the steroid hormone cortisone, manufactured in the cortex of the adrenal gland. These drugs decrease the effects of inflammation within the body. They are available for injection, oral use, topical use for the skin, eyes and nose and inhalation for the bronchial tubes. These drugs include alclometasone; amcinonide; beclomethasone; benzyl benzoate; betamethasone; bismuth; clobetasol; clobetasone 17-butyrate; clocortolone; cortisone; desonide; desoximetasone; desoxycorticosterone; dexamethasone; diflorasone; diflucortolone; fludrocortisone; flumethasone; flunisolide; fluocinonide; fluocinonide, procinonide and ciprocinonide; fluorometholone; fluprednisolone, flurandrenolide; halcinonide; hydrocortisone; medrysone; methylprednisolone; mometasone; paramethasone; peruvian balsam; prednisolone;

prednisone; triamcinolone; zinc oxide.

Cyclopegics—Eye drops that prevent the pupils from accommodating to varying degrees of light.

Cystitis—Inflammation of the urinary bladder.

D

Decongestants—Drugs used to open nasal passages by shrinking swollen membranes lining the nose. These drugs include: Cough-suppressing—phenylephrine and dextromethorphan, phenylpropanolamine and caramiphen, phenylpropanolamine and dextromethorphan, phenylpropanolamine and hydrocodone, pseudoephedrine and codeine, pseudoephedrine and dextromethorphan, pseudoephedrine and hydrocodone. Cough-suppressing and pain-relieving—phenyl-propanolamine, dextromethorphan and acetaminophen. Cough-suppressing and sputum-thinning—phenylephrine, dextromethorphan and guaifenesin; phenylephrine, hydrocodone and guaifenesin; phenylpropanolamine, codeine and guaifenesin; phenylpropanolamine, dextromethorphan and guaifenesin; pseudoephedrine, codeine and guaifenesin; pseudoephedrine, dextromethorphan and guaifenesin; pseudoephedrine, hydrocodone and guaifenesin; phenylephrine, dextromethorphan, guaifenesin and acetaminophen; pseudoephedrine, dextromethorphan, guaifenesin and acetaminophen. Sputum-thinning—ephedrine and guaifenesin; ephedrine and potassium iodide; phenylephrine, phenylpropanolamine and guaifenesin; phenylpropanolamine and guaifenesin; pseudoephedrine and guaifenesin. Nasal—ephedrine (oral), phenylpropanolamine, pseudoephedrine. Ophthalmic (eye)—naphazoline, oxymetazoline, phenylephrine. Topical—oxymetazoline, phenylephrine, xylometazoline.

Delirium—Temporary mental disturbance characterized by hallucinations, agitation and incoherence.

Diabetes—Metabolic disorder in which the body can't use carbohydrates efficiently. This leads to a dangerously high level of glucose (a carbohydrate) in the blood.

Dialysis—Procedure to filter waste products from the bloodstream of patients with kidney failure.

Digitalis Preparations (Digitalis Glycosides)—Important drugs to treat heart disease, such as congestive heart failure, heartbeat irregularities and cardiogenic shock. These drugs include digitoxin, digoxin.

Digoxin—One of the digitalis drugs used to treat heart disease. All digitalis products were originally derived from the foxglove plant.

Dilation—Enlargement.

Disulfiram Reaction—Disulfiram (Antabuse) is a drug to treat alcoholism. When alcohol in the bloodstream interacts with disulfiram, it causes a flushed face, severe headache, chest pains, shortness of breath, nausea, vomiting, sweating and weakness. Severe reactions may cause death. A disulfiram reaction is the interaction of any drug with alcohol or another drug to produce these symptoms.

Diuretics—Drugs that act on the kidneys to prevent reabsorption of electrolytes, especially chlorides. They are used to treat edema, high blood pressure, congestive heart failure, kidney and liver failure and others. These drugs include amiloride, amiloride and hydrochlorothiazide, bendroflumethiazide, benzthiazide, bumetanide, chlorothiazide, chlorthalidone, cyclothiazide, ethacrynic acid, furosemide, glycerin, hydrochlorothiazide, hydroflumethiazide, indapamide, mannitol, methyclothiazide, metolazone, polythiazide, quinethazone, spironolactone, sprionolactone and hydrochlorothiazide, triamterene, triamterene and hydrochlorothiazide, trichlormethiazide, urea.

Diuretics, Loop—Drugs that act on the kidneys to prevent reabsorption of electrolytes, especially sodium. They are used to treat edema, high blood pressure, congestive heart failure, kidney and liver failure and others. These drugs include bumetanide, ethacrynic acid, furosemide.

Diuretics, Potassium-Sparing—Drugs that act on the kidneys to prevent reabsorption of electrolytes, especially sodium. They are used to treat edema, high blood pressure, congestive heart failure, kidney and liver failure and others. This particular group of diuretics does not allow the unwanted side effect of low potassium in the blood to occur. These drugs include amiloride, spironolactone, triamterene.

Diuretics, Thiazide—Drugs that act on the kidneys to prevent reabsorption of electrolytes, especially chlorides. They are used to treat edema, high blood pressure, congestive heart failure, kidney and liver failure and others. These drugs include bendroflumethiazide, benzthiazide, chlorothiazide, chlorthalidone, cyclothiazide, hydrochlorothiazide, hydroflumethiazide, methyclothiazide, metolazone, polythiazide, quinethazone, trichlormethiazide.

Dopamine Agonists—Drugs that stimulate activity of dopamine (a brain chemical that helps control movement). These include bromocriptine, cabergoline, pergolide, ropinirole.

Dopamine Antagonists—Drugs that interfere with dopamine production (brain chemical that helps control movement). These drugs include haloperidol, metoclopramide, phenothiazines, thioxanthenes.

Duodenum—The first 12 inches of the small intestine.

E

ECG (or EKG)—Abbreviation for electrocardiogram or electrocardiograph. An ECG is a graphic tracing representing the electrical current produced by impulses passing through the heart muscle. This is a useful test in the diagnosis of heart disease, but used alone it usually can't make a complete diagnosis. An ECG is most useful in two areas: (1) demonstrating heart rhythm disturbances and (2) demonstrating changes when there is a myocardial infarction (heart attack). It will detect enlargement of either heart chamber, but will not establish a diagnosis of heart failure or disease of the heart valves.

Eczema—Disorder of the skin with redness, itching, blisters, weeping and abnormal pigmentation.

EEG—Electroencephalogram or electro-encephalograph. An EEG is a graphic recording of electrical activity generated spontaneously from nerve cells in the brain. This test is useful in the diagnosis of brain dysfunction, particularly in studying seizure disorders.

Electrolytes—Substances that can transmit electrical impulses when dissolved in body fluids. These include sodium, potassium, chloride and carbon dioxide.

Embolism—Sudden blockage of an artery by a clot or foreign material in the blood.

Emphysema—An irreversible disease in which the lung's air sacs lose elasticity and air accumulates in the lungs.

Endometriosis—Condition in which uterus tissue is found outside the uterus. Can cause pain, abnormal menstruation and infertility.

Enzyme Inducers—Drugs that increase the metabolism of another drug in the liver, resulting in a decrease of that drug's effect. These drugs include alcohol (chronic use), barbiturates (especially phenobarbital), carbamazepine, glutethimide, griseofulvin, phenylbutazone, phenytoin, primadone, rifabutin, rifampin, saquinavir, troglitazone.

Enzyme Inhibitors—Drugs that decrease the metabolism of another drug in the liver, resulting in an increase of that drug's effect. These drugs include alcohol (high doses), allopurinol, azole antifungals, chloramphenicol, cimetidine, clarithromycin, clotrimazole, cyclosporine, danazol, diltiazem, disulfiram, divalproex, erythromycins, fluoroquinolones, fluoxatine, fluvoxamine, isoniazid, itraconazole, ketoconazole, metoprolol, mibefradil, miconazole, monoamine oxidase (MAO) inhibitors, nefazodone, omeprazole, oral estrogen contraceptives, paroxetine, phenylbutazone, propranolol, quinidine, troleandomycin, valproic acid, venlafaxine, verapamil.

Enzymes—Protein chemicals that can accelerate chemical reactions in the body.

Epilepsy—Episodes of brain disturbance that cause convulsions and loss of consciousness.

Ergot Preparations—Medicines used to treat migraine and other types of throbbing headaches. Also used after delivery of babies to make the uterus clamp down and reduce excessive bleeding.

Erythromycins—A group of drugs with similar structure used to treat infections. These drugs include erythromycin, erythromycin estolate, erythromycin ethylsuccinate, erthromycin gluceptate, erythromycin lactobionate, erythromycin stearate.

Esophagitis—Inflammation of the lower part of the esophagus, the tube connecting the throat and the stomach.

Estrogens—Female hormones used to replenish the body's stores after the ovaries have been removed or become nonfunctional after menopause. Also used with progesterone in some birth control pills and for other purposes. These drugs include: Systemic—chlorotrianisene, diethylstilbestrol, estradiol, estrogens (conjugated and esterified), estrone, estropipate, ethinyl estradiol, quinestrol. Vaginal—dienestrol, estradiol, estrogens (conjugated), estrone, estropipate.

Eustachian Tube—Small passage from the middle ear to the sinuses and nasal passages.

Extrapyramidal Reactions—Abnormal reactions in the power and coordination of posture and muscular movements. Movements are not under voluntary control. Some drugs associated with producing extrapyramidal reactions include amoxapine, antidepressants (tricyclic), droperidol, haloperidol, loxapine, metoclopramide, metyrosine, molindone, olanzapine, paroxetine, phenothiazines, pimozide, rauwolfia alkaloids, risperidone, tacrine, thioxanthenes.

Extremity—Arm, leg, hand or foot.

F

Fecal Impaction—Condition in which feces become firmly wedged in the rectum.

Fibrocystic Breast Disease—Overgrowth of fibrous tissue in the breast, producing non-malignant cysts.

Fibroid Tumors—Non-malignant tumors of the muscular layer of the uterus.

Flu (Influenza)—A virus infection of the respiratory tract that lasts three to ten days. Symptoms include headache, fever, runny nose, cough, tiredness and muscle aches.

Fluoroquinolones—A class of drugs used to treat bacterial infections, such as urinary tract infections and some types of bronchitis. These drugs include ciprofloxacin, enoxacin, lomefloxacin, norfloxacin, ofloxacin.

Folate Antagonists—Drugs that impair the body's utilization of folic acid, which is necessary for cell growth. These drugs include dione anticonvulsants, hydantoin anticonvulsants, succinimide anticonvulsants, divalproex, methotrexate, phenobarbital (long-term use), pyrimethamine, sulfonamides, triamterene, trimethoprim, trimetrexate, valproic acid.

Folliculitis—Inflammation of a follicle.

Functional Dependence—The development of dependence on a drug for a normal body function. The primary example is the use of laxatives for a prolonged period so that there is a dependence on the laxative for normal bowel action.

G

G6PD—Deficiency of glucose 6-phosphate, which is necessary for glucose metabolism.

Ganglionic Blockers—Medicines that block the passage of nerve impulses through a part of the nerve cell called a ganglion. Ganglionic blockers are used to treat urinary retention and other medical problems. Bethanechol is one of the best ganglionic blockers.

Gastritis—Inflammation of the stomach.

Gastrointestinal—Of the stomach and intestinal tract.

Gland—Organ that manufactures and excretes materials not required for its own metabolic needs.

Glaucoma—Eye disease in which increased pressure inside the eye damages the optic nerve, causes pain and changes vision.

Glucagon—Injectable drug that immediately elevates blood sugar by mobilizing glycogen from the liver.

Gold Compounds—Medicines which use gold as their base and are usually used to treat joint or arthritic disorders. These medicines include auranofin, aurothioglucose, gold sodium thiomalate.

H

H$_2$ Antagonists—Antihistamines that work against H$_2$ histamine. H$_2$ histamine may be liberated at any point in the body, but most often in the gastrointestinal tract.

Hangover Effect—The same feelings as a "hangover" after too much alcohol consumption. Symptoms include headache, irritability and nausea.

Hemochromatosis—Disorder of iron metabolism in which excessive iron is deposited in and damages body tissues, particularly of the liver and pancreas.

Hemoglobin—Pigment that carries oxygen in red blood cells.

Hemolytics—Drugs that can destroy red blood cells and separate hemoglobin from the blood cells. These include acetohydroxamic acid, antidiabetic agents (sulfonylurea), doxapram, furazolidone, mefenamic acid, menadiol, methyldopa, nitrofurans, primaquine, procainamide, quinidine, quinine, sulfonamides (systemic), sulfones, vitamin K.

Hemorrhage—Heavy bleeding.

Hemorrheologic Agents—Medicines to help control bleeding.

Hemosiderosis—Increase of iron deposits in body tissues without tissue damage.

Hepatitis—Inflammation of liver cells, usually accompanied by jaundice.

Hepatotoxics—Medications that can possibly cause toxicity or decreased normal function of the liver. These drugs include the following (some of which are not described in this book): acetaminophen (with long-term use); alcohol; amiodarone; anabolic steroids; androgens; angiotensin-converting enzyme (ACE) inhibitors; anti-inflammatory drugs, nonsteroidal (NSAIDs); antithyroid agents; asparaginase; azlocillin; carbamazepine; carmustine; dantrolene; dapsone; daunorubicin; disulfiram; divalproex; erythromycins; estrogens; ethionamide; etretinate; felbamate; fluconazole; flutamide; gold compounds; halothane; HMG-CoA reductase inhibitors; isoniazid; itraconazole; ketoconazole (oral); labetalol; mercaptopurine; methotrexate; methyldopa; naltrexone; niacin (high doses); nitrofurans; pemoline; phenothiazines; phenytoin, piperacillin, plicamycin, pravastatin; rifampin; sulfamethoxazole and trimethoprim; sulfonamides; tacrine; testosterone; tizanidine; valproic acid; zidovudine.

Hiatal Hernia—Section of the stomach that protrudes into the chest cavity.

Histamine—Chemical in body tissues that dilates the smallest blood vessels, constricts the smooth muscle surrounding the bronchial tubes and stimulates stomach secretions.

History—Past medical events in a patient's life.

Hives—Elevated patches on the skin that are redder or paler than surrounding skin and often itch severely.

Hoarseness—Husky, gruff, weak voice.

Hormone Replacement Therapy—A medication (estrogen) or combination of medications (estrogen and progestin or estrogen and androgen) used for treatment of premenopausal and menopausal symptoms and for prevention of diseases that affect women in their later years

Hormones—Chemical substances produced in the body to regulate other body functions.

Hypercalcemia—Too much calcium in the blood.

This happens with some malignancies and in calcium overdose.

Hyperglycemia-Causing Medications—A group of drugs that may contribute to hyperglycemia (high blood sugar). These include oral estrogen-containing contraceptives, corticosteroids, estrogens, isoniazid, nicotinic acid, phenothiazines, phenytoin, sympathomimetics, thyroid hormones, thiazide diuretics.

Hyperkalemia-Causing Medications—Medicines that cause too much potassium in the bloodstream. These include ACE inhibitors; anti-inflammatory drugs, nonsteroidal (NSAIDs); cyclosporine; digitalis glycosides; diuretics (potassium-sparing); pentamidine; succinylcholine chloride; tacrolimus; possibly any medicine that is combined with potassium.

Hypersensitivity—Serious reactions to many medications. The effects of hypersensitivity may be characterized by wheezing, shortness of breath, rapid heart rate, severe itching, faintness, unconsciousness and severe drop in blood pressure.

Hypertension—High blood pressure.

Hypervitaminosis—A condition due to an excess of one or more vitamins. Symptoms may include weakness, fatigue, loss of hair and changes in the skin.

Hypnotics—Drugs used to induce a sleeping state. See Barbiturates.

Hypocalcemia—Abnormally low level of calcium in the blood.

Hypoglycemia—Low blood sugar (blood glucose). A critically low blood sugar level will interfere with normal brain function and can damage the brain permanently.

Hypoglycemia-Causing Medications—A group of drugs that may contribute to hypoglycemia (low blood sugar). These include clofibrate, monoamine oxidase (MAO) inhibitors, probenecid, propanolol, rifabutin, rifampicin, salicylates, sulfonamides (long-acting), sulfonylureas.

Hypoglycemics—Drugs that reduce blood sugar. These include acetohexamide, chlorpropamide, gliclazide, glipizide, glyburide, insulin, metformin, tolazamide, tolbutamide.

Hypokalemia-Causing Medications—Medicines that cause a depletion of potassium in the bloodstream. These include adrenocorticoids (systemic), alcohol, amphotericin B (systemic), bronchodilators (adrenergic), carbonic anhydrase inhibitors, diuretics (loop and thiazide), edetate (long-term use), foscarnet, indapamide, insulin, insulin lispro, laxatives (if dependent on), penicillins (some), salicylates, sodium bicarbonate, urea, vitamin D (overdose of).

Hypotension—Blood pressure decrease below normal. Symptoms may include weakness, lightheadedness and dizziness.

Hypotension-Causing Drugs—Medications that might cause hypotension (low blood pressure). These include alcohol, alprostadil, amantadine, anesthetics (general), angiotensin-converting enzyme inhibitors (ACE inhibitors), antidepressants (MAO inhibitors, tricyclic), antihypertensives, benzodiazepines used as preanesthetics, beta-adrenergic blocking agents, bromocriptine, calcium channel-blocking agents, carbidopa and levodopa, clozapine, diuretics, edetate calcium disodium, edetate disodium, haloperidol, hydralazine, levodopa, lidocaine (systemic), loxapine, maprotiline, molindone, nabilone (high doses), nefazodone, nitrates, olanzapine, opioid analgesics (including fentanil, fentanyl and sufentanil), paclitaxel, pentamidine, phenothiazines, pimozide, procainamide, quinidine, radiopaques (materials used in x-ray studies), risperidone, thioxanthenes, tizanidine, tocainide, trazodone, venlafaxine. If you take any of these medications, be sure to tell a dentist, anesthesiologist or anyone else who intends to give you an anesthetic to put you to sleep.

Hypothermia-Causing Medications—Medicines that can cause a significant lowering of body temperature. These drugs include alcohol, alpha-adrenergic blocking agents (dihydroergotamine, ergotamine, labetol, phenoxybenzamine, phentolamine, prazosin, tolazoline), barbiturates (large amounts), beta-adrenergic blocking agents, clonidine, insulin, minoxidil, narcotic analgesics (with overdose), vasodilators.

I

Ichthyosis—Skin disorder with dryness, scaling and roughness.

Ileitis—Inflammation of the ileum, the last section of the small intestine.

Ileostomy—Surgical opening from the ileum, the end of the small intestine, to the outside of the body.

Immunosuppressants—Powerful drugs that suppress the immune system. Immunosuppressants are used in patients who have had organ transplants or severe disease associated with the immune system. These drugs include the following (some of which are not described in this book): azathioprine, betamethasone, chlorambucil, corticotropin, cortisone, cyclophosphamide, cyclosporine, dexamethasone, hydrocortisone, mercaptopurine, methylprednisolone, muromonab, muromonab-CD3, mycophenolate, prednisone, tacrolimus, thalidomide, triamcinolone.

Impotence—Male's inability to achieve or sustain erection of the penis for sexual intercourse.

Insomnia—Sleeplessness.

Interaction—Change in the body's response to one drug when another is taken. Interaction may decrease the effect of one or both drugs, increase the effect of one or both drugs or cause toxicity.

Iron Supplements—Products that contain iron in a form that can be absorbed from the intestinal tract. Supplements include ferrous fumarate, ferrous gluconate, ferrous sulfate, iron dextran, iron-polysaccharide.

J

Jaundice—Symptoms of liver damage, bile obstruction or destruction of red blood cells. Symptoms include yellowed whites of the eyes, yellow skin, dark urine and light stool.

K

Keratosis—Growth that is an accumulation of cells from the outer skin layers.

Kidney Stones—Small, solid stones made from calcium, cholesterol, cysteine and other body chemicals.

L

Laxatives—Medicines prescribed to treat constipation. These medicines include bisacodyl; bisacodyl and docusate; casanthranol; casanthranol and docusate; cascara sagrada; cascara sagrada and aloe; cascara sagrada and phenolphthalein; castor oil; danthron; danthron and docusate; danthron and poloxamer 188; dehydrocholic acid; dehydrocholic acid and docusate; docusate; docusate and phenolphthalein; docusate and mineral oil; docusate and phenolphthalein; docusate, carboxymethylcellulose and casanthranol; glycerin; lactulose; magnesium citrate; magnesium hydroxide; magnesium hydroxide and mineral oil; magnesium oxide; magnesium sulfate; malt soup extract; malt soup extract and psyllium; methylcellulose; mineral oil; mineral oil and cascara sagrada; mineral oil and phenolphthalein; mineral oil, glycerin and phenolphthalein; phenolphthalein; poloxamer; polycarbophil; potassium bitartrate and sodium bicarbonate; psyllium; psyllium and senna; psyllium hydrophilic mucilloid; psyllium hydrophilic mucilloid and carboxymethyl-cellulose; psyllium hydrophilic mucilloid and sennosides; psyllium hydrophilic musilloid and senna; senna; senna and docusate; sennosides; sodium phosphate.

LDH—Abbreviation for lactate dehydrogenase. It is a measurement of cardiac enzymes used to confirm some heart conditions.

Lincomycins—A family of antibiotics used to treat certain infections.

Low-Purine Diet—A diet that avoids high-purine foods, such as liver, sweetbreads, kidneys, sardines, oysters and others. If you need a low-purine diet, request instructions from your doctor.

Lupus—Serious disorder of connective tissue that primarily affects women. Varies in severity with skin eruptions, joint inflammation, low white blood cell count and damage to internal organs, especially the kidneys.

Lymph Glands—Glands in the lymph vessels throughout the body that trap foreign and infectious matter and protect the bloodstream from infection.

M

Macrolides—A class of antibiotic (antibacterial) drugs. They include dirithromycin, erythromycin, lincomycin and vancomycin.

Male Hormones—Chemical substances secreted by the testicles, ovaries and adrenal glands in humans. Some male hormones used by humans are derived synthetically. Male hormones include testosterone cypionate and estradiol cypionate, testosterone enanthate and estradiol valerate.

Mania—A mood disturbance characterized by euphoria, agitation, elation, irritability, rapid and confused speech and excessive activity. Mania usually occurs as part of bipolar (manic-depressive) disorder.

Manic-Depressive Illness—Psychosis with alternating cycles of excessive enthusiasm and depression.

MAO Inhibitors—See Monoamine Oxidase (MAO) Inhibitors.

Mast Cell—Connective tissue cell.

Menopause—The end of menstruation in the female, often accompanied by irritability, hot flashes, changes in the skin and bones and vaginal dryness.

Metabolism—Process of using nutrients and energy to build and break down wastes.

Migraine Headaches—Periodic headaches caused by constriction of arteries to the skull. Symptoms include severe pain, vision disturbances, nausea, vomiting and sensitivity to light.

Mind-Altering Drugs—Any drugs that decrease alertness, perception, concentration, contact with reality or muscular coordination.

Mineral Supplements—Mineral substances added to the diet to treat or prevent mineral deficiencies. They include iron, copper, magnesium, calcium, etc.

Monoamine Oxidase (MAO) Inhibitors—Drugs that prevent the activity of the enzyme monoamine oxidase (MAO) in brain tissue, thus affecting mood. MAO inhibitors include anti-depressants, the use of which is frequently restricted because of severe side effects. These side effects may be interactions with other drugs (such as ephedrine or amphetamine) or foods containing tyramine (such as cheese) and may produce a sudden increase in blood pressure. MAOs include isocarboxazid, phenelzine, tranylcypromine.

Muscle Blockers—Same as muscle relaxants or skeletal muscle relaxants.

Muscle Relaxants—Medicines used to lessen painful contractions and spasms of muscles. These include atracurium, carisoprodol, chlorphenesin, chlorzoxazone, cyclobenzaprine, metaxalone, methcarbamol, metocurine, orphenadrine citrate, orphenadrine hydrochloride, pancuronium, phenytoin, succinylcholine, tubocurarine, vecuronium.

Myasthenia Gravis—Disease of the muscles characterized by fatigue and progressive paralysis. It is usually confined to muscles of the face, lips, tongue and neck.

Mydriatics—Eye drops that cause the pupils to dilate (become larger) to a marked degree.

N

Narcotics—A group of habit-forming, addicting drugs used for treatment of pain, diarrhea, cough, acute pulmonary edema and others. They are all dervied from opium, a milky exudate in capsules of *papaver somniferum*. Law requires licensed physicians to dispense by prescription. These drugs include alfentanil, buprenorphine, butorphanol, codeine, fentanyl, hydrocodone, hydromorphone, levorphanol, meperidine, methadone, morphine, nalbuphine, opium, oxycodone, oxymorphone, paregoric, pentazocine, propoxyphene, sufetanil.

Nephrotoxic (Kidney-Poisoning) Medications—Under some circumstances, these medicines can be toxic to the kidneys. These medicines include acetaminophen (in high doses); acyclovir (injection of); aminoglycosides; amphotericin B (given internally); analgesic combinations containing acetaminophen and aspirin or other salicylates (with chronic high-dose use); anti-inflammatory analgesics (nonsteroidal); bacitracin (injection of); capreomycin; carmustine; cidofovir; ciprofloxacin; cisplatin; cyclosporine; deferoxamine (long-term use); edetate calcium disodium (with high doses); edetate disodium (with high dose); foscarnet; gold compounds; ifosfamide; lithium; methotrexate (with high dose therapy); methoxyflurane; neomycin (oral); penicillamine; pentamidine; phenacetin; plicamycin; polymyxins (injection of); radiopaques (materials used for special x-ray examinations); rifampin; streptozocin; sulfonamides; tacrolimus; tetracyclines (except doxycycline and minocycline); tiopronin; vancomycin (injection of).

Neuroleptic Malignant Syndrome—Ceaseless

951

involuntary, jerky movements of the tongue, facial muscles and hands.

Neuromuscular Blocking Agents—A group of drugs prescribed to relax skeletal muscles. They are all given by injection, and descriptions are not included in this book. These drugs include atracurium, edrohponium, gallamine, neostigmine, metocurine, pancuronium, pyridostigmine, succinylcholine, tubocurarine, vecuronium.

Neurotoxic Medications—Medicines that cause toxicity to the nerve tissues in the body. These drugs include anticonvulsants (hydantoin), capreomycin, carbamazepine, chloramphenicol (oral), chloroquine, ciprofloxacin, cisplatin, cycloserine, cytarabine, didanosine, disulfiram, ethambutol, ethionamide, fludarabine, hydroxychloroquine, interferon, isoniazid, lincomycins, lindane (topical), lithium, metronidazole, mexiletine, nitrofurantoin, pemoline, pyridoxine (large amounts), quinacrine, quinidine, quinine, stavudine, tacrolimus, tetracyclines, vincristine, zalcitabine.

Nitrates—Medicines made from a chemical with a nitrogen base. Nitrates include erythrityl tetranitrate, isosorbide dinitrate, nitroglycerin, pentaerythritol tetranitrate.

Nonsteroidal Anti-Inflammatory Drugs (NSAIDs)—See Anti-Inflammatory Drugs, Nonsteroidal.

Nutritional Supplements—Substances used to treat and prevent deficiencies when the body is unable to absorb them by eating a well-balanced, nutritional diet. These supplements include: Vitamins—ascorbic acid, ascorbic acid and sodium ascorbate, calcifediol, calcitriol, calcium pantothenate, cyanocobalamin, dihydrotachysterol, ergocalciferol, folate sodium, folic acid, hydroxocobalamin, niacin, niacinamide, pantothenic, pyridoxine, riboflavin, sodium ascorbate, thiamine, vitamin A, vitamin E. Minerals—calcium carbonate, calcium citrate, calcium glubionate, calcium gluconate, calcium lactate, calcium phosphate (dibasic and tribasic), sodium fluoride. Other—levocarnitine, omega-3 polyunsaturated fatty acids.

O

Opiates—See Narcotics.

Orthostaic Hypotension—Excess drop in blood pressure when arising from a sitting or lying postion.

Osteoporosis—Softening of bones caused by a loss of calcium usually found in bone. Bones become brittle and fracture easily.

Ototoxic Medications—These medicines may possibly cause hearing damage. They include aminoglycosides, 4-aminoquinolines, anti-inflammatory analgesics (nonsteroidal), bumetanide (injected), capreomycin, chloroquine, cisplatin, deferoxamine, erythromycins, ethacrynic acid, furosemide, hydroxychloroquine, quinidine, quinine, salicylates, vancomycin (injected).

Ovary—Female sexual gland where eggs mature and ripen for fertilization.

P

Pain Relievers—Non-narcotic medicines used to treat pain.

Palpitations—Rapid, forceful or throbbing heartbeat noticeable to the patient.

Pancreatitis—Serious inflammation or infection of the pancreas that causes upper abdominal pain.

Pancreatitis-associated Drugs—Medications associated with the development of pancreatitus. These include alcohol, asparaginase, azithioprine, didanosine, estrogens, furosemide, methyldopa, nitrofurantoin, sulfonamides, tetracyclines, thiazide diuretics, valproic acid.

Parkinson's Disease or Parkinson's Syndrome—Disease of the central nervous system. Characteristics are a fixed, emotionless expression of the face, tremor, slower muscle movements, weakness, changed gait and a peculiar posture.

Pellagra—Disease caused by a deficiency of the water-soluble vitamin thiamine (vitamin B-1). Symptoms include brain disturbance, diarrhea and skin inflammation.

Penicillin—Chemical substance (antibiotic) originally discovered as a product of mold, that can kill some bacterial germs.

Peripheral Neuropathy (Peripheral Neuritis)—Inflammation and degeneration of the nerve endings or of the terminal nerves. It most often occurs in the nerve tissue of the muscles of the extremities (arms and legs). Symptoms include pain of varying intensity and sensations of numbness, tingling and burning in the hands and feet. It can be caused by certain medications or chemicals, infections, chonic inflammation or nutritive disease.

Peripheral-neuropathy Associated Drugs—Medications that are associated with the development of peripheral neuropathy. These include chloramphenicol, cisplatin, dapsone, didanosine, ethambutol, ethionamide, hydralazine, isoniazid, lithium, metronidazole, nitrofurantoin, nitrous oxide, phenytoin, stavudine, vincristine, zalcitabine.

Phenothiazines—Drugs used to treat mental, nervous and emotional conditions. These drugs include acetophenazine, chlorpromazine, fluphenazine, mesoridazine, methotrimeprazine, pericyazine, perphenazine, prochlorperazine, promazine, thiopropazate, thioproperazine, thioridazine, trifluoperazine, triflupromazine.

Pheochromocytoma—A tumor of the adrenal

gland that produces chemicals that cause high blood pressure, headache, nervousness and other symptoms.

Phlegm—Thick mucus secreted by glands in the respiratory tract.

Photophobia—Increased sensitivity to light as perceived by the human eye. Drugs that can cause photophobia include antidiabetic drugs, atropine, belladonna, bromides, chloraquine, ciprofloxacin, chlordiazepoxide, clidinium, clomiphene, dicyclomine, digitalis drugs, doxepin, ethambutol, ethionamide, ethosuximide, etretinate, glycopyrrolate, hydroxychloroquine, hydroxyzine, hyoscyamine, mephenytoin, methenamine, methsuximide, monoamine oxidase (MAO) inhibitors, nalidixic acid, norfloxacin, oral contraceptives, orphenadrine, paramethadione, phenothiazines, propantheline, quinidine, quinine, scopolamine, sopropamide, tetracyclines, tridihexethyl, trimethadione.

Photosensitizing Medications—Medicines that can cause abnormally heightened skin reactions to the effects of sunlight and ultraviolet light. These medicines include acetazolamide, acetohexamide, alprazolam, amantadine, amiloride, amiodarone, amitriptyline, amoxapine, antidiabetic agents (oral), barbiturates, bendroflumethiazide, benzocaine, benzoyl peroxide, benzthiazide, captopril, carbamazepine, chlordiazepoxide, chloroquine, chlorothiazide, chlorpromazine, chlorpropamide, chlortetracycline, chlorthalidone, ciprofloxacin, clindamycin, clofazimine, clofibrate, clomipramine, coal tar, contraceptives (estrogen-containing), cyproheptadine, dacarbazine, dapsone, demeclocycline, desipramine, desoximetasone, diethylstilbestrol, diflunisal, diltiazem, diphenhydramine, disopyramide, doxepin, doxycycline, enoxacin, estrogens, etretinate, flucytosine, fluorescein, fluorouracil, fluphenazine, flutamide, furosemide, glipizide, glyburide, gold preparations, griseofulvin, haloperidol, hexachlorophene, hydrocholothiazide, hydroflumethiazide, ibuprofen, imipramine, indomethacin, isotretinoin, ketoprofen, lincomycin, lomefloxacin, maprotiline, mesoridazine, methacycline, methotrexate, methoxsalen, methylclothiazide, methyldopa, metolazone, minocycline, minoxidil, nabumetone, nalidixic acid, naproxen, nifedipine, norfloxacin, nortriptyline, ofloxacin, oral contraceptives, oxyphenbutazone, oxytetracycline, perphenazine, phenelzine, phenobarbital, phenylbutazone, phenytoin, piroxicam, polythiazide, prochlorperazine, promazine, promethazine, protriptyline, pyrazinamide, quinidine, quinine, sulfonamides, sulindac, tetracycline, thiabendazole, thioridazine, thiothixene, tolazamide, tolbutamide, tranylcypromine, trazodone, tretinoin, triamterene, trichlormethiazide, trifluoperazine, triflupromazine, trimeprazine, trimethoprim, trimipramine, triprolidine, vinblastine.

Pinworms—Common intestinal parasites that cause rectal itching and irritation.

Pituitary Gland—Gland at the base of the brain that secretes hormones to stimulate growth and other glands to produce hormones.

Platelet—Disc-shaped element of the blood, smaller than a red or white blood cell, necessary for blood clotting.

Polymixins—A family of antibiotics that kill bacteria.

Polyp—Growth on a mucous membrane.

Porphyria—Inherited metabolic disorder characterized by changes in the nervous system and kidneys.

Post-Partum—Following delivery of a baby.

Potassium—Important chemical found in body cells.

Potassium Foods—Foods high in potassium content, including dried apricots and peaches, lentils, raisins, citrus and whole-grain cereals.

Potassium Supplements—Medicines needed by people who don't have enough potassium in their diets or by those who develop a deficiency due to illness or taking diuretics and other medicines. These supplements include chloride; potassium acetate; potassium bicarbonate; potassium bicarbonate and potassium chloride; potassium bicarbonate and potassium citrate; potassium chloride; potassium chloride, potassium bicarbonate and potassium citrate; potassium gluconate; potassium gluconate and potassium chloride; potassium gluconate and potassium citrate; potassium gluconate, potassium citrate and ammonium; trikates.

Prostaglandins—A group of drugs used for a variety of therapeutic purposes. These drugs include alprostadil (treats newborns with congenital heart disease), carboprost and dinoprost (both used to induce labor) and dinoprostone (used to induce labor or to induce a late abortion).

Prostate—Gland in the male that surrounds the neck of the bladder and the urethra.

Protein Bound Drugs—Drugs that are firmly bound to protein in the blood serum, including clofibrate, diazepam, diazoxide, ibuprofen, indomethacin and naproxen.

Prothrombin—Blood substance essential in clotting.

Prothrombin Time (Pro Time)—Laboratory study used to follow prothrombin activity and keep coagulation safe.

Psoriasis—Chronic inherited skin disease.

Symptoms are lesions with silvery scales on the edges.

Psychosis—Mental disorder characterized by deranged personality, loss of contact with reality and possible delusions, hallucinations or illusions.

Purine Foods—Foods that are metabolized into uric acid. Foods high in purines include anchovies, liver, brains, sweetbreads, sardines, kidneys, oysters, gravy and meat extracts.

Q

QT Interval Prolongation-Causing Drugs—A group of drugs that can cause serious heart rhythm problems. These drugs include amiodarone, astemizole, calcium channel blockers (especially bepridil), cisapride, disopyramide, erythromycin, maprotiline, pentamidine, phenothiazines, pimozide, procainamide, quinidine, tricyclic antidepressants.

R

Rauwolfia Alkaloids—Drugs that belong to the family of antihypertensives (drugs that lower blood pressure). Rauwolfia alkaloids are not used as extensively as in years past. They include alseroxylon, deserpidine, rauwolfia serpentina, reserpine.

RDA—Recommended daily allowance of a vitamin or mineral.

Rebound Effect—Return of a condition, often with increased severity, once the prescribed drug is withdrawn.

Renal—Pertaining to the kidney.

Retina—Innermost covering of the eyeball on which the image is formed.

Retinoids—A group of drugs that are synthetic vitamin A-like compounds used to treat skin conditions. These drugs include etretinate, isotretinoin and retinoic acid.

Retroperitoneal Imaging—Special x-rays or CT scans of the organs attached to the abdominal wall behind the peritoneum (the covering of the intestinal tract and lining of the walls of the abdominal and pelvic cavities).

Reye's Syndrome—Rare, sometimes fatal, disease of children that causes brain and liver damage.

Rickets—Bone disease caused by vitamin D deficiency. Bones become bent and distorted during infancy or childhood.

S

Salicylates—Medicines to relieve pain and reduce fever. These include aspirin, aspirin and caffeine, buffered aspirin, choline salicylate, choline and magnesium salicylates, magnesium salicylate, salicylamide, salsalate, sodium salicylate.

Sedatives—Drugs that reduce excitement or anxiety. They are used to produce sedation (calmness). These include alprazolam, amobarbital, aprobarbital, bromazepam, butalbital, chloral hydrate, chlorazepate, chlordiazepoxide, diazepam, diphenhydramine, doxylamine, estazolam, ethchlorvynol, ethinamate, flurazepam, glutethimide, halazepam, hydroxyzine, ketazolam, lorazepam, methotrimeprazine, midazolam, nitrazepam, oxazepam, pentobarbital, phenobarbital, prazepam, promethazine, propiomazine, propofol, quazepam, secobarbital, temazepam, triazolam, trimeprazine, zolpidem, zopiclone.

Seizure—Brain disorder causing changes of consciousness or convulsions.

Selective Serotonin Reuptake Inhibitors (SSRIs)—Medications used for treatment of depression that work by increasing the serotonin levels in the brain. Serotonin is a neuro-transmitter (brain chemical) having to do with mood and behavior. These drugs include fluoxetine, fluvoxamine, paroxetine, sertraline. More information can be found on the individual drug chart for each drug.

Serotonergics—Medications or drugs that affect the levels of serotonin (a brain chemical) concerned with conscious processes. These drugs include clomipramine, fluoxetine, fluvoxamine, moclobemide, MAO inhibitors, nefazodone, paroxetine, sertraline, tryptophan, venlafaxine and some drugs of abuse.

Serotonin Syndrome—A potentially very serious interaction between certain drugs. Symptoms include confusion, irritability, muscle rigidity, chills, high fever, poor coordination, restlessness, sweating, trembling or shaking, twitching.

SGOT—Abbreviation for serum glutamic-oxaloacetic transaminase. Measuring the level in the blood helps demonstrate liver disorders and diagnose recent heart damage.

SGPT—Abbreviation for a laboratory study measuring the blood level of serum glutamic-pyruvic transaminase. Deviations from a normal level may indicate liver disease.

Sick Sinus Syndrome—A complicated, serious heartbeat rhythm disturbance characterized by a slow heart rate alternating with a fast or slow heart rate with heart block.

Sinusitis—Inflammation or infection of the sinus cavities in the skull.

Skeletal Muscle Relaxants (same as Skeletal Muscle Blockers)—A group of drugs prescribed to treat spasms of the skeletal muscles. These drugs include carisoprodol, chlorphenesin, chlorzoxazone, cyclobenzaprine, diazepam, lorazepam, metaxalone, methocarbamol, orphenadrine, phenytoin.

Sleep Inducers—Night-time sedatives to aid in falling asleep. See Benzodiazepines.

Streptococci—A bacteria that can cause infections in the throat, respiratory system and skin. Improperly treated, can lead to disease in the heart, joints and kidneys.

Stroke—Sudden, severe attack, usually sudden paralysis, from injury to the brain or spinal cord caused by a blood clot or hemorrhage in the brain.

Stupor—Near unconsciousness.

Sublingual—Under the tongue. Some drugs are absorbed almost as quickly this way as by injection.

Sulfa Drugs—Shorthand for sulfonamide drugs, which are used to treat infections.

Sulfonamides—Sulfa drugs prescribed to treat infections. They include sulfacytine, sulfamethoxazole, sulfamethoxazole and trimethoprin, sulfasalazine, sulfisoxazole.

Sulfonureas—A family of drugs that lower blood sugar (hypoglycemic agents). Used in the treatment of some forms of diabetes.

Sympatholytics—A group of drugs that blocks the action of the sympathetic nervous system. These drugs include beta-blockers, guanethidine, hydralazine and prazosin.

Sympathomimetics—A large group of drugs that mimic the effects of stimulation of the sympathetic part of the autonomic nervous system. These drugs include albuterol, amphetamine, benzphetamine, bioterol, cocaine, dextroamphetamine, diethylpropion, dobutamine, ephedrine, epinephrine, ethylnorepinephrine, fenfluramine, ipratropium, isoproterenol, isotharine, mazindol, mephentermine, metaproterenol, metaraminol, methoxamine, norepinephrine, phendimetrazine, phentermine, phenylephrine, phenylpropanolamine, pirbuterol, pseudoephedrine, ritodrine, terbutaline.

T

Tardive Dyskinesia—Slow, involuntary movements of the jaw, lips and tongue caused by an unpredictable drug reaction. Drugs that can cause this include haloperidol, phenothiazines, thiothixene.

Tartrazine Dye—A dye used in foods and medicine preparations that may cause an allergic reaction in some people.

Tetracyclines—A group of medicines with similar chemical structure used to treat infections. These drugs include demeclocycline, doxycycline, methacycline, minocycline, oxytetracycline, tetracycline.

Thiazides—A group of chemicals that cause diuresis (loss of water through the kidneys). Frequently used to treat high blood pressure and congestive heart failure. Thiazides include bendroflumethiazide, benzthiazide, chlorothiazide, chlorthalidone, cyclothiazide, hydrochlorothiazide, hydroflumethiazide, methyclothiazide, metolazone, polythiazide, quinethazone, trichlormethiazide.

Thiothixines—See Thioxanthenes.

Thioxanthenes—Drugs used to treat emotional, mental and nervous conditions. These drugs include chlorprothixene, fluphenthixol, thiothixene.

Thrombocytopenias—Diseases characterized by inadequate numbers of blood platelets circulating in the bloodstream.

Thrombolytic Agents—Drugs that help to dissolve blood clots. They include alteplase, anistreplase, streptokinase, urokinase.

Thrombophlebitis—Inflammation of a vein caused by a blood clot in the vein.

Thyroid—Gland in the neck that manufactures and secretes several hormones.

Thyroid Hormones—Medications that mimic the action of the thyroid hormone made in the thyroid gland. They include dextrothyroxine, levothyroxine, liothyronine, liotrix, thyroglobulin, thyroid.

Tic Douloureux—Painful condition caused by inflammation of a nerve in the face.

Tolerance—A decreasing response to repeated constant doses of a drug or a need to increase doses to produce the same physical or mental response.

Toxicity—Poisonous reaction to a drug that impairs body functions or damages cells.

Tranquilizers—Drugs that calm a person without clouding consciousness.

Transdermal Patches—Medicated patches that stick to the skin. There are more and more medications in this form. If you are using this form, follow these instructions: Choose an area of skin without cuts, scars or hair, such as the upper arm, chest or behind the ear. Thoroughly clean area where patch is to be applied. If patch gets wet and loose, cover with an additional piece of plastic. Apply a fresh patch if the first one falls off. Apply each dose to a different area of skin if possible.

Tremor—Involuntary trembling.

Trichomoniasis—Infestation of the vagina by *trichomonas*, an infectious organism. The infection causes itching, vaginal discharge and irritation.

Triglyceride—Fatty chemical manufactured from carbohydrates for storage in fat cells.

Tyramine—Normal chemical component of the body that helps sustain blood pressure. Can rise to fatal levels in combination with some drugs. Tyramine is found in many foods:

  Beverages—Alcohol beverages, especially

Chianti or robust red wines, vermouth, ale, beer.

Breads—Homemade bread with a lot of yeast and breads or crackers containing cheese.

Fats—Sour cream.

Fruits—Bananas, red plums, avocados, figs, raisins, raspberries.

Meats and meat substitutes—Aged game, liver (if not fresh), canned meats, salami, sausage, aged cheese, salted dried fish, pickled herring, meat tenderizers.

Vegetables—Italian broad beans, green bean pods, eggplant.

Miscellaneous—Yeast concentrates or extracts, marmite, soup cubes, commercial gravy, soy sauce, any protein food that has been stored improperly or is spoiled.

U

Ulcer, Peptic—Open sore on the mucous membrane of the esophagus, stomach or duodenum caused by stomach acid.

Urethra—Hollow tube through which urine (and semen in men) is discharged.

Urethritis—Inflammation or infection of the urethra.

Uricosurics—A group of drugs that promotes excretion of uric acid in the urine. These drugs include probenecid and sulfinpyrazone.

Urinary Acidifiers—Medications that cause urine to become acid. These include ascorbic acid, potassium phosphate, potassium and sodium phosphates, racemethionine.

Urinary Alkalizers—Medications that cause urine to become alkaline. These include potassium citrate, potassium citrate and citric acid, potassium citrate and sodium citrate, sodium bicarbonate, sodium citrate and citric acid, tricitrate.

Uterus—Also called the womb. A hollow muscular organ in the female in which the embryo develops into a fetus.

V

Vascular—Pertaining to blood vessels.

Vascular Headache Preventatives—Medicines prescribed to prevent the occurrence of or reduce the frequency and severity of vascular headaches such as migraines. These drugs include atenolol; clonidine; ergotamine, belladonna alkaloids and phenobarbital; fenoprofen; flunarizine; ibuprofen; indomethacin; isocarboxazid, lithium; mefenamic acid; methysergide; metoprolol; nadolol; naproxen; phenelzine; pizotyline; propranolol; timolol, tranylcypromine, verapamil.

Vascular Headache Treatment—Medicine prescribed to treat vascular headaches such as migraines. These drugs include butalbital (combined with acetaminophen, aspirin, caffeine or codeine); cyproheptadine; diclofenac; diflunisal; dihydroergotamine; ergotamine; ergotamine and caffeine; ergotamine, caffeine, belladonna alkaloids and pentobarbital; etodolac; fenoprofen; ibuprofen; indomethacin (capsules, oral suspension, rectal); isometheptene, dichloralphenazone and acetaminophen; ketoprofen; meclofenamate; mefenamic acid; metoclopramide; naproxen; phenobarbital; sumatriptan.

Vertigo—A sensation of motion, usually dizziness or whirling either of oneself or one's surroundings.

Virus—Infectious organism that reproduces in the cells of the infected host.

X

Xanthines—Substances that stimulate muscle tissue, especially that of the heart. Types of xanthines include aminophylline, caffeine, dyphylline, oxtriphylline, theophylline.

Y

Yeast—A single-cell organism that can cause infections of the mouth, vagina, skin and parts of the gastrointestinal system.

GUIDE TO INDEX

Alphabetical entries in the index include three categories—generic names, brand names and drug-class names.

1. Generic names appear in capital letters, followed by their chart page number:

ASPIRIN 132

2. Brand names appear in **bold italic**, followed by their generic ingredient and chart page number:

Bayer - See ASPIRIN 132

Some brand names contain two or more generic ingredients. These generic ingredients are listed in capital letters, following the brand name:

Anacin - See
ASPIRIN 132
CAFFEINE 186

3. Drug-class names appear in regular type, capital and lower-case letters. All generic drug names in this book that fall into a drug class are listed after the class name:

Anticonvulsant - See
BARBITURATES 148
BENZODIAZEPINES 156
CARBAMAZEPINE 200
DIVALPROEX 326
FELBAMATE 360
GABAPENTIN 386
LAMOTRIGINE 468
PARALDEHYDE 636
PRIMIDONE 682
VALPROIC ACID 832

Aceon - See ANGIOTENSIN-CONVERTING
ENZYME (ACE) INHIBITORS 50
Acephen - See ACETAMINOPHEN 4
Aceta - See ACETAMINOPHEN 4
ACETAMINOPHEN 4
ACETAMINOPHEN & ASPIRIN - See
ACETAMINOPHEN & SALICYLATES 6
ACETAMINOPHEN & CODEINE - See
NARCOTIC ANALGESICS &
ACETAMINOPHEN 582
ACETAMINOPHEN & SALICYLAMIDE - See
ACETAMINOPHEN & SALICYLATES 6
ACETAMINOPHEN & SALICYLATES 6
ACETAMINOPHEN, ASPIRIN &
SALICYLAMIDE - See ACETAMINOPHEN
& SALICYLATES 6
Acetaminophen Uniserts - See
ACETAMINOPHEN 4
Acetasol HC - See ANTIBACTERIALS (Otic) 70
Acetazolam - See CARBONIC ANHYDRASE
INHIBITORS 206
ACETAZOLAMIDE - See CARBONIC
ANHYDRASE INHIBITORS 206
ACETOHEXAMIDE - See ANTIDIABETIC
AGENTS, SULFONYLUREA 84
ACETOHYDROXAMIC ACID (AHA) 8
ACETOPHENAZINE - See PHENOTHIAZINES
662
Acetoxyl 2.5 Gel - See BENZOYL PEROXIDE
158
Acetoxyl 5 Gel - See BENZOYL PEROXIDE 158
Acetoxyl 10 Gel - See BENZOYL PEROXIDE 158
Acetoxyl 20 Gel - See BENZOYL PEROXIDE 158
Acetylsalicylic Acid - See ASPIRIN 132
Aches-N-Pain - See ANTI-INFLAMMATORY
DRUGS, NONSTEROIDAL (NSAIDs) 104
Achromycin - See
ANTIBACTERIALS FOR ACNE (Topical) 66
ANTIBACTERIALS (Ophthalmic) 68
TETRACYCLINES 782
Achromycin V - See TETRACYCLINES 782
ACITRETIN - See RETINOIDS (Oral) 728
Aclophen - See
ACETAMINOPHEN 4
ANTIHISTAMINES 98
PHENYLEPHRINE 664
Aclovate - See ADRENOCORTICOIDS
(Topical) 16
Acne-5 Lotion - See BENZOYL PEROXIDE 158
Acne-10 Lotion - See BENZOYL PEROXIDE 158
Acne-Aid 10 Cream - See BENZOYL
PEROXIDE 158
Acne-Aid Gel - See KERATOLYTICS 464
Acne-Mask - See BENZOYL PEROXIDE 158
AcnoAcnomel Cake - See KERATOLYTICS 464
Acnomel B.P. 5 Lotion - See BENZOYL
PEROXIDE 158
Acnomel Cream - See KERATOLYTICS 464
Acnomel Vanishing Cream - See
KERATOLYTICS 464

Acnomel-Acne Cream - See KERATOLYTICS
464
Acnotex - See KERATOLYTICS 464
Acon - See VITAMIN A 838
ACRIVASTINE - See ANTIHISTAMINES 98
Acta-Char - See CHARCOAL, ACTIVATED 212
Acta-Char Liquid - See CHARCOAL,
ACTIVATED 212
Actacin - See
ANTIHISTAMINES 98
PSEUDOEPHEDRINE 706
Actagen - See
ANTIHISTAMINES 98
PSEUDOEPHEDRINE 706
Actagen-C Cough - See
ANTIHISTAMINES 98
NARCOTIC ANALGESICS 580
PSEUDOEPHEDRINE 706
Actamin - See ACETAMINOPHEN 4
Actamin Extra - See ACETAMINOPHEN 4
Actamin Super - See
ACETAMINOPHEN 4
CAFFEINE 186
Acti-B-12 - See VITAMIN B-12
(Cyanocobalamin) 840
Actibine - See YOHIMBINE 854
Acticin - See PEDICULICIDES (Topical) 642
Acticort-100 - See ADRENOCORTICOIDS
(Topical) 16
Actidil - See ANTIHISTAMINES 98
Actidose with Sorbitol - See CHARCOAL,
ACTIVATED 212
Actidose-Aqua - See CHARCOAL, ACTIVATED
212
Actifed - See
ANTIHISTAMINES 98
PSEUDOEPHEDRINE 706
Actifed 12-Hour - See
ANTIHISTAMINES 98
PSEUDOEPHEDRINE 706
Actifed A - See
ACETAMINOPHEN 4
ANTIHISTAMINES 98
PSEUDOEPHEDRINE 706
Actifed Allergy Nighttime Caplets - See
ANTIHISTAMINES 98
PSEUDOEPHEDRINE 706
Actifed DM - See
ANTIHISTAMINES 98
DEXTROMETHORPHAN 296
PSEUDOEPHEDRINE 706
Actifed Plus - See
ACETAMINOPHEN 4
ANTIHISTAMINES 98
PSEUDOEPHEDRINE 706
Actifed Plus Caplets - See
ACETAMINOPHEN 4
ANTIHISTAMINES 98
PSEUDOEPHEDRINE 706
Actifed with Codeine Cough - See
ANTIHISTAMINES 98

INDEX

AlleRid - See PSEUDOEPHEDRINE 706
AllerMax Caplets - See ANTIHISTAMINES 98
Aller-med - See ANTIHISTAMINES 98
Allerphed - See
   ANTIHISTAMINES 98
   PSEUDOEPHEDRINE 706
Allert - See ANTIHISTAMINES 98
All-Nite Cold Formula - See
   ACETAMINOPHEN 4
   ANTIHISTAMINES 98
   DEXTROMETHORPHAN 296
   PSEUDOEPHEDRINE 706
Alloprin - See ALLOPURINOL 20
ALLOPURINOL 20
Almacone - See ANTACIDS 54
Almacone II - See ANTACIDS 54
Alma-Mag #4 Improved - See ANTACIDS 54
Alma-Mag Improved - See ANTACIDS 54
Almocarpine - See PILOCARPINE 670
ALOE - See LAXATIVES, STIMULANT 476
Alomide - See ANTIALLERGIC AGENTS
   (Ophthalmic) 62
Alophen - See LAXATIVES, STIMULANT 476
Alora - See ESTROGENS 350
ALPHA ADRENERGIC RECEPTOR
   BLOCKERS 22
Alpha Redisol - See VITAMIN B-12
   (Cyanocobalamin) 840
Alphaderm - See ADRENOCORTICOIDS
   (Topical) 16
Alphalin - See VITAMIN A 838
Alphamin - See VITAMIN B-12
   (Cyanocobalamin) 840
Alphamul - See LAXATIVES, STIMULANT 476
Alpha-Phed - See
   ASPIRIN 132
   PSEUDOEPHEDRINE 706
Alpha-Tamoxifen - See TAMOXIFEN 776
Alphatrex - See ADRENOCORTICOIDS
   (Topical) 16
Alphosyl - See COAL TAR (Topical) 254
Alprazolam Intensol - See
   BENZODIAZEPINES 156
ALPRAZOLAN - See BENZODIAZEPINES 156
ALPROSTADIL 24
Alrex - See ANTI-INFLAMMATORY DRUGS,
   STEROIDAL (Ophthalmic) 108
Alrheumat - See ANTI-INFLAMMATORY
   DRUGS, NONSTEROIDAL (NSAIDs) 104
Altace - See ANGIOTENSIN-CONVERTING
   ENZYME (ACE) INHIBITORS 50
Alti-Bromocriptine - See BROMOCRIPTINE 172
AlternaGEL - See ANTACIDS 54
Alu-Cap - See ANTACIDS 54
Aludrox - See ANTACIDS 54
Alumadrine - See
   ACETAMINOPHEN 4
   ANTIHISTAMINES 98
   PHENYLPROPANOLAMINE 668
ALUMINA & MAGNESIA - See ANTACIDS 54

ALUMINA & MAGNESIUM CARBONATE - See
   ANTACIDS 54
ALUMINA & MAGNESIUM TRISILICATE - See
   ANTACIDS 54
ALUMINA, MAGNESIA, & CALCIUM
   CARBONATE - See ANTACIDS 54
ALUMINA, MAGNESIA, & SIMETHICONE - See
   ANTACIDS 54
ALUMINA, MAGNESIUM CARBONATE, &
   CALCIUM CARBONATE - See ANTACIDS 54
ALUMINA, MAGNESIUM TRISILICATE, &
   SODIUM BICARBONATE - See ANTACIDS
   54
ALUMINUM CARBONATE, BASIC - See
   ANTACIDS 54
ALUMINUM HYDROXIDE - See ANTACIDS 54
Alupent - See BRONCHODILATORS,
   ADRENERGIC 174
Alurate - See BARBITURATES 148
Alu-Tab - See ANTACIDS 54
AMANTIDINE - See ANTIVIRALS FOR
   INFLUENZA 124
Amaphen - See
   ACETAMINOPHEN 4
   BARBITURATES 148
   CAFFEINE 186
Amaril D - See
   ANTIHISTAMINES 98
   PHENYLEPHRINE 664
   PHENYLPROPANOLAMINE 668
Amaril D Spantab - See
   ANTIHISTAMINES 98
   PHENYLPROPANOLAMINE 668
Amaryl - See ANTIDIABETIC AGENTS,
   SULFONYLUREA 84
Ambay Cough - See
   ANTIHISTAMINES 98
   NARCOTIC ANALGESICS 580
AMBENONIUM - See ANTIMYASTHENICS 114
Ambenyl Cough - See
   ANTIHISTAMINES 98
   NARCOTIC ANALGESICS 580
Ambenyl-D Decongestant Cough Formula - See
   DEXTROMETHORPHAN 296
   GUAIFENESIN 398
   PSEUDOEPHEDRINE 706
Ambien - See ZOLPIDEM 858
Ambophen Expectorant - See
   ANTIHISTAMINES 98
   NARCOTIC ANALGESICS 580
AMCINONIDE (Topical) - See
   ADRENOCORTICOIDS (Topical) 16
Amen - See PROGESTINS 694
Amerge - See TRIPTANS 826
Americaine - See ANESTHETICS (Topical) 46
Americaine Hemorrhoidal - See
   ANESTHETICS (Rectal) 44
*Americaine Topical Anesthetic First Aid
   Ointment* - See ANESTHETICS (Topical)
   46

INDEX

Anamine T.D. - See
ANTIHISTAMINES 98
PSEUDOEPHEDRINE 706
Anaplex - See
ANTIHISTAMINES 98
PSEUDOEPHEDRINE 706
Anaplex HD - See
ANTIHISTAMINES 98
NARCOTIC ANALGESICS 580
PHENYLEPHRINE 664
Anaplex S.R. - See
ANTIHISTAMINES 98
PSEUDOEPHEDRINE 706
Anapolon 50 - See ANDROGENS 38
Anaprox - See ANTI-INFLAMMATORY DRUGS,
NONSTEROIDAL (NSAIDs) 104
Anaprox DS - See ANTI-INFLAMMATORY
DRUGS, NONSTEROIDAL (NSAIDs) 104
Anaspaz - See HYOSCYAMINE 428
Anaspaz PB - See HYOSCYAMINE 428
Anatuss - See
ACETAMINOPHEN 4
ANTIHISTAMINES 98
DEXTROMETHORPHAN 296
GUAIFENESIN 398
PHENYLEPHRINE 664
PHENYLPROPANOLAMINE 668
Anatuss DM - See
DEXTROMETHORPHAN 296
GUAIFENESIN 398
PSEUDOEPHEDRINE 706
Anatuss LA - See
GUAIFENESIN 398
PSEUDOEPHEDRINE 706
Anatuss with Codeine - See
ACETAMINOPHEN 4
ANTIHISTAMINES 98
GUAIFENESIN 398
NARCOTIC ANALGESICS 580
PHENYLPROPANOLAMINE 668
Anbesol Baby Gel - See ANESTHETICS
(Mucosal-Local) 42
Anbesol Gel - See ANESTHETICS (Mucosal-
Local) 42
Anbesol Liquid - See ANESTHETICS
(Mucosal-Local) 42
Anbesol Maximum Strength Gel - See
ANESTHETICS (Mucosal-Local) 42
Anbesol Maximum Strength Liquid - See
ANESTHETICS (Mucosal-Local) 42
Anbesol Regular Strength Gel - See
ANESTHETICS (Mucosal-Local) 42
Anbesol Regular Strength Liquid - See
ANESTHETICS (Mucosal-Local) 42
Ancalixir - See BARBITURATES 148
Andrest 90-4 - See ANDROGENS &
ESTROGENS 40
Andro 100 - See ANDROGENS 38
Andro-Cyp 100 - See ANDROGENS 38
Andro-Cyp 200 - See ANDROGENS 38

Androderm - See ANDROGENS 38
Andro-Estro 90-4 - See ANDROGENS &
ESTROGENS 40
Androgen - See ANDROGENS 38
ANDROGENS 38
ANDROGENS & ESTROGENS 40
Androgens-estrogens - See ANDROGENS &
ESTROGENS 40
Androgyn L.A - See ANDROGENS &
ESTROGENS 40
Android-10 - See ANDROGENS 38
Android-25 - See ANDROGENS 38
Android-T - See ANDROGENS 38
Andro-LA 200 - See ANDROGENS 38
Androlone - See ANDROGENS 38
Andronaq-50 - See ANDROGENS 38
Andronaq-LA - See ANDROGENS 38
Andronate 100 - See ANDROGENS 38
Andronate 200 - See ANDROGENS 38
Andropository 100 - See ANDROGENS 38
Andryl 200 - See ANDROGENS 38
Anergan 25 - See ANTIHISTAMINES,
PHENOTHIAZINE-DERIVATIVE 102
Anergan 50 - See ANTIHISTAMINES,
PHENOTHIAZINE-DERIVATIVE 102
Anesthetic - See ANTIPYRINE & BENZOCAINE
(Topical-Otic) 116
Anesthetic (rectal) - See
ANESTHETICS (Rectal) 44
HYDROCORTISONE (Rectal) 420
Anesthetic (topical) - See
ANESTHETICS (Mucosal-Local) 42
ANESTHETICS (Topical) 46
ANESTHETICS (Mucosal-Local) 42
ANESTHETICS (Rectal) 44
ANESTHETICS (Topical) 46
Anexsia - See NARCOTIC ANALGESICS &
ACETAMINOPHEN 582
ANGIOTENSIN II RECEPTOR ANTAGONISTS
48
ANGIOTENSIN-COVERTING ENZYME (ACE)
INHIBITORS 50
ANGIOTENSIN-COVERTING ENZYME (ACE)
INHIBITORS & HYDROCHLOROTHIAZIDE
52
Anhydron - See DIURETICS, THIAZIDE 324
ANISINDIONE - See ANTICOAGULANTS (Oral)
76
ANISOTROPINE - See ANTICHOLINERGICS 74
Anocobin - See VITAMIN B-12
(Cyanocobalamin) 840
Anolor 300 - See
ACETAMINOPHEN 4
BARBITURATES 148
CAFFEINE 186
Anolor-DH5 - See NARCOTIC ANALGESICS &
ACETAMINOPHEN 582
Anoquan - See
ACETAMINOPHEN 4
BARBITURATES 148
CAFFEINE 186

965

INDEX

INDEX

Ascorbicap - See VITAMIN C (Ascorbic Acid) 842

Ascriptin - See ASPIRIN 132

Ascriptin A/D - See ASPIRIN 132

Asendin - See ANTIDEPRESSANTS, TRICYCLIC 82

Asmalix - See BRONCHODILATORS, XANTHINE 176

A-Spas - See DICYCLOMINE 300

Aspergum - See ASPIRIN 132

ASPIRIN 132

ASPIRIN & CODEINE - See NARCOTIC ANALGESICS & ASPIRIN 584

Aspirin Free Anacin Maximum Strength Caplets - See ACETAMINOPHEN 4

Aspirin Free Anacin Maximum Strength Tablets - See ACETAMINOPHEN 4

Aspirin Free Bayer Select Maximum Strength Headache Pain Relief Caplets - See CAFFEINE 186

Aspirin Free Bayer Select Maximum Strength Headache Plus Caplets - See ACETAMINOPHEN 4

Aspirin-Free Excedrin Caplets - See ACETAMINOPHEN 4
CAFFEINE 186

Astelin - See AZELASTINE 144

ASTEMIZOLE - See ANTIHISTAMINES, NONSEDATING 100

AsthmaHaler - See BRONCHODILATORS, ADRENERGIC 174

AsthmaNefrin - See BRONCHODILATORS, ADRENERGIC 174

Astramorph - See NARCOTIC ANALGESICS 580

Astramorph-PF - See NARCOTIC ANALGESICS 580

Astrin - See ASPIRIN 132

Atabrine - See QUINACRINE 714

Atacand - See ANGIOTENSIN II RECEPTOR ANTAGONISTS 48

Atarax - See HYDROXYZINE 426

Atasol Caplets - See ACETAMINOPHEN 4

Atasol Drops - See ACETAMINOPHEN 4

Atasol Forte - See ACETAMINOPHEN 4

Atasol Forte Caplets - See ACETAMINOPHEN 4

Atasol Forte Tablets - See ACETAMINOPHEN 4

Atasol Oral Solution - See ACETAMINOPHEN 4

Atasol Tablets - See ACETAMINOPHEN 4

Atasol-8 - See NARCOTIC ANALGESICS & ACETAMINOPHEN 582

Atasol-15 - See NARCOTIC ANALGESICS & ACETAMINOPHEN 582

Atasol-30 - See NARCOTIC ANALGESICS & ACETAMINOPHEN 582

ATENOLOL - See BETA-ADRENERGIC BLOCKING AGENTS 162

ATENOLOL & CHLORTHALIDONE - See BETA-ADRENERGIC BLOCKING AGENTS & THIAZIDE DIURETICS 164

Ativan - See BENZODIAZEPINES 156

ATORVASTATIN - See HMG-CoA REDUCTASE INHIBITORS 414

ATOVAQUONE 134

Atrofed - See
ANTIHISTAMINES 98
PSEUDOEPHEDRINE 706

Atrohist Pediatric - See
ANTIHISTAMINES 98
PHENYLEPHRINE 664

Atrohist Pediatric Suspension Dye Free - See
ANTIHISTAMINES 98
PHENYLEPHRINE 664

Atrohist Plus - See
ANTICHOLINERGICS 74
ANTIHISTAMINES 98
HYOSCYAMINE 428
PHENYLEPHRINE 664
PHENYLPROPANOLAMINE 668
SCOPOLAMINE (Hyoscine) 746

Atrohist Sprinkle - See
ANTIHISTAMINES 98
PHENYLEPHRINE 664

Atromid-S - See FIBRATES 362

Atropair - See CYCLOPLEGIC, MYDRIATIC (Ophthalmic) 278

ATROPINE - See
ANTICHOLINERGICS 74
CYCLOPLEGIC, MYDRIATIC (Ophthalmic) 278

ATROPINE & PHENOBARBITAL - See BELLADONNA ALKALOIDS & BARBITURATES 154

Atropine Care Eye Drops and Ointment - See CYCLOPLEGIC, MYDRIATIC (Ophthalmic) 278

ATROPINE, HYOSCYAMINE, METHENAMINE, METHYLENE BLUE, PHENYLSALICYLATE & BENZOIC ACID 136

ATROPINE, HYOSCYAMINE, SCOPOLAMINE & BUTABARBITAL - See BELLADONNA ALKALOIDS & BARBITURATES 154

ATROPINE, HYOSCYAMINE, SCOPOLAMINE & PHENOBARBITAL - See BELLADONNA ALKALOIDS & BARBITURATES 154

Atropine Sulfate S.O.P. - See CYCLOPLEGIC, MYDRIATIC (Ophthalmic) 278

Atropisol - See CYCLOPLEGIC, MYDRIATIC (Ophthalmic) 278

Atrosept - See ATROPINE, HYOSCYAMINE, METHENAMINE, METHYLENE BLUE, PHENYLSALICYLATE & BENZOIC ACID 136

Atrosulf - See CYCLOPLEGIC, MYDRIATIC (Ophthalmic) 278

Atrovent - See IPRATROPIUM 442

A/T/S - See ANTIBACTERIALS FOR ACNE (Topical) 66

ATTAPULGITE 138

Augmentin - See PENICILLINS & BETA-LACTAMASE INHIBITORS 650

Banophen Caplets - See ANTIHISTAMINES 98
Banthine - See ANTICHOLINERGICS 74
Barbidonna - See
  BELLADONNA ALKALOIDS &
    BARBITURATES 154
  HYOSCYAMINE 428
  SCOPOLAMINE (Hyoscine) 746
Barbidonna 2 - See
  BELLADONNA ALKALOIDS &
    BARBITURATES 154
  HYOSCYAMINE 428
  SCOPOLAMINE (Hyoscine) 746
Barbita - See BARBITURATES 148
Barbiturate - See THEOPHYLLINE,
  EPHEDRINE & BARBITURATES 786
BARBITURATES 148
BARBITURATES, ASPIRIN & CODEINE (Also
  contains caffeine) 150
Barc - See PEDICULICIDES (Topical) 642
Baridium - See PHENAZOPYRIDINE 660
Baron-X - See YOHIMBINE 854
Barophen - See BELLADONNA ALKALOIDS &
  BARBITURATES 154
Barr - See NALTREXONE 578
Barriere-HC - See ADRENOCORTICOIDS
  (Topical) 16
Basaljel - See ANTACIDS 54
Bayaminic Expectorant - See
  GUAIFENESIN 398
  PHENYLPROPANOLAMINE 668
Bayaminicol - See
  ANTIHISTAMINES 98
  DEXTROMETHORPHAN 296
  PHENYLPROPANOLAMINE 668
Baycodan - See
  ANTICHOLINERGICS 74
  NARCOTIC ANALGESICS 580
Baycol - See HMG-CoA REDUCTASE
  INHIBITORS 414
Baycomine - See
  NARCOTIC ANALGESICS 580
  PHENYLPROPANOLAMINE 668
Baycomine Pediatric - See
  NARCOTIC ANALGESICS 580
  PHENYLPROPANOLAMINE 668
BayCotussend Liquid - See
    PSEUDOEPHEDRINE 706
Baydec DM Drops - See
  ANTIHISTAMINES 98
  DEXTROMETHORPHAN 296
  PSEUDOEPHEDRINE 706
Bayer - See ASPIRIN 132
Bayer Cough Syrup - See
    PHENYLPROPANOLAMINE 668
Bayer Cough Syrup for Children - See
  DEXTROMETHORPHAN 296
  PHENYLPROPANOLAMINE 668
Bayer Select Chest Cold Tablets - See
  ACETAMINOPHEN 4
  DEXTROMETHORPHAN 296

Bayer Select Flu Relief Caplets - See
  ACETAMINOPHEN 4
  DEXTROMETHORPHAN 296
  PSEUDOEPHEDRINE 706
Bayer Select Head and Chest Cold Caplets -
  See
  ACETAMINOPHEN 4
  DEXTROMETHORPHAN 296
  GUAIFENESIN 398
Bayer Select Head Cold Caplets - See
  ACETAMINOPHEN 4
  PSEUDOEPHEDRINE 706
Bayer Select Ibuprofen Caplets - See ANTI-
  INFLAMMATORY DRUGS,
  NONSTEROIDAL (NSAIDs) 104
Bayer Select Maximum Strength Pain Relief
  Formula - See ACETAMINOPHEN 4
Bayer Select Maximum Strength Sinus Pain
  Relief Caplets - See
  ACETAMINOPHEN 4
  PSEUDOEPHEDRINE 706
Bayer Select Night Time Cold Caplets - See
  ACETAMINOPHEN 4
  ANTIHISTAMINES 98
  DEXTROMETHORPHAN 296
  PSEUDOEPHEDRINE 706
Bayer Select Pain Relief Formula Caplets -
  See ANTI-INFLAMMATORY DRUGS,
  NONSTEROIDAL (NSAIDs) 104
Bayer Timed-Release Arthritic Pain Formula -
  See ASPIRIN 132
Bayhistine DH - See
  ANTIHISTAMINES 98
  NARCOTIC ANALGESICS 580
  PSEUDOEPHEDRINE 706
Bayhistine Expectorant - See
  GUAIFENESIN 398
  NARCOTIC ANALGESICS 580
  PSEUDOEPHEDRINE 706
Baytussin AC - See
  GUAIFENESIN 398
  NARCOTIC ANALGESICS 580
Baytussin DM - See
  DEXTROMETHORPHAN 296
  GUAIFENESIN 398
BC Cold Powder - See
  ANTIHISTAMINES 98
  ASPIRIN 132
  PHENYLPROPANOLAMINE 668
BC Cold Powder Non-Drowsy Formula - See
  ASPIRIN 132
  PHENYLPROPANOLAMINE 668
BC Multi-Symptom Cold Powder - See
  ANTIHISTAMINES 98
  ASPIRIN 132
  PHENYLPROPANOLAMINE 668
Beben - See ADRENOCORTICOIDS (Topical) 16
BECAPLERMIN 152
Because - See CONTRACEPTIVES, VAGINAL
  (Spermicides) 264

INDEX

Benylin Cold - See
ANTIHISTAMINES 98
PSEUDOEPHEDRINE 706
Benylin Cough - See ANTIHISTAMINES 98
Benylin Decongestant - See
ANTIHISTAMINES 98
PSEUDOEPHEDRINE 706
Benylin DM-D - See
DEXTROMETHORPHAN 296
PSEUDOEPHEDRINE 706
Benylin DM-D-E - See
DEXTROMETHORPHAN 296
GUAIFENESIN 398
PSEUDOEPHEDRINE 706
Benylin DM-D-E Extra Strength - See
DEXTROMETHORPHAN 296
GUAIFENESIN 398
PSEUDOEPHEDRINE 706
Benylin DM-E - See
DEXTROMETHORPHAN 296
GUAIFENESIN 398
Benylin Expectorant Cough Formula - See
DEXTROMETHORPHAN 296
GUAIFENESIN 398
Benylin with Codeine - See
GUAIFENESIN 398
NARCOTIC ANALGESICS 580
PSEUDOEPHEDRINE 706
Benylin-E - See GUAIFENESIN 398
Benzac Ac 21/2 Gel - See BENZOYL
PEROXIDE 158
Benzac Ac 5 Gel - See BENZOYL PEROXIDE
158
Benzac Ac 10 Gel - See BENZOYL PEROXIDE
158
Benzac W 21/2 Gel - See BENZOYL
PEROXIDE 158
Benzac W 5 Gel - See BENZOYL PEROXIDE
158
Benzac W 10 Gel - See BENZOYL PEROXIDE
158
Benzacot - See TRIMETHOBENZAMIDE 822
Benzagel 5 Acne Lotion - See BENZOYL
PEROXIDE 158
Benzagel 5 Acne Wash - See BENZOYL
PEROXIDE 158
Benzagel 5 Gel - See BENZOYL PEROXIDE 158
Benzagel 10 Gel - See BENZOYL PEROXIDE
158
BENZALKONIUM CHLORIDE - See
CONTRACEPTIVES, VAGINAL
(Spermicides) 264
Benzamycin - See
ANTIBACTERIALS FOR ACNE (Topical) 66
BENZOYL PEROXIDE 158
BenzaShave 5 Cream - See BENZOYL
PEROXIDE 158
BenzaShave 10 Cream - See BENZOYL
PEROXIDE 158

BENZOCAINE - See
ANESTHETICS (Mucosal-Local) 42
ANESTHETICS (Rectal) 44
ANESTHETICS (Topical) 46
BENZOCAINE & MENTHOL - See
ANESTHETICS (Mucosal-Local) 42
ANESTHETICS (Topical) 46
BENZOCAINE & PHENOL - See
ANESTHETICS (Mucosal-Local) 42
Benzocol - See ANESTHETICS (Topical) 46
Benzodent - See ANESTHETICS (Mucosal-
Local) 42
BENZODIAZEPINES 156
BENZOYL PEROXIDE 158
BENZPHETAMINE - See APPETITE
SUPPRESSANTS 130
BENZTHIAZIDE - See DIURETICS, THIAZIDE
324
BENZTROPINE - See ANTIDYSKINETICS 86
Bepadin - See CALCIUM CHANNEL
BLOCKERS 192
BEPRIDIL - See CALCIUM CHANNEL
BLOCKERS 192
Berotec - See BRONCHODILATORS,
ADRENERGIC 174
Berubigen - See VITAMIN B-12
(Cyanocobalamin) 840
BETA CAROTENE 160
Beta HC - See ADRENOCORTICOIDS (Topical)
16
Beta-adrenergic blocker - See BETA-
ADRENERGIC BLOCKING AGENTS &
THIAZIDE DIURETICS 164
BETA-ADRENERGIC BLOCKING AGENTS 162
BETA-ADRENERGIC BLOCKING AGENTS &
THIAZIDE DIURETICS 164
BETA-ADRENERGIC BLOCKING AGENTS
(Ophthalmic) 166
Beta-adrenergic stimulator - See RITODRINE
742
Betacort Scalp Lotion - See
ADRENOCORTICOIDS (Topical) 16
Betaderm - See ADRENOCORTICOIDS
(Topical) 16
Betaderm Scalp Lotion - See
ADRENOCORTICOIDS (Topical) 16
Betagen C Cap B.I.D. - See BETA-
ADRENERGIC BLOCKING AGENTS
(Ophthalmic) 166
Betagen C Cap Q.D. - See BETA-
ADRENERGIC BLOCKING AGENTS
(Ophthalmic) 166
Betagen Standard Cap - See BETA-
ADRENERGIC BLOCKING AGENTS
(Ophthalmic) 166
Betalin 12 - See VITAMIN B-12
(Cyanocobalamin) 840
Betalin S - See THIAMINE (Vitamin B-1) 792
Betaloc - See BETA-ADRENERGIC BLOCKING
AGENTS 162

INDEX

Brexin - See
  ANTIHISTAMINES 98
  GUAIFENESIN 398
  PSEUDOEPHEDRINE 706
Brexin-L.A. - See
  ANTIHISTAMINES 98
  PSEUDOEPHEDRINE 706
Bricanyl - See BRONCHODILATORS,
  ADRENERGIC 174
BRINZOLAMIDE - See CARBONIC
  ANHYDRASE INHIBITORS 206
Brofed - See
  ANTIHISTAMINES 98
  PSEUDOEPHEDRINE 706
Bromaline - See
  ANTIHISTAMINES 98
  PHENYLPROPANOLAMINE 668
Bromaline Plus - See
  ACETAMINOPHEN 4
  ANTIHISTAMINES 98
  PHENYLPROPANOLAMINE 668
Bromanate - See
  ANTIHISTAMINES 98
  PHENYLPROPANOLAMINE 668
Bromanate DC Cough - See
  ANTIHISTAMINES 98
  NARCOTIC ANALGESICS 580
  PHENYLPROPANOLAMINE 668
Bromanyl - See
  ANTIHISTAMINES 98
  NARCOTIC ANALGESICS 580
Bromarest DX Cough - See
  ANTIHISTAMINES 98
  DEXTROMETHORPHAN 296
  PSEUDOEPHEDRINE 706
Bromatane DX Cough - See
  ANTIHISTAMINES 98
  DEXTROMETHORPHAN 296
  PSEUDOEPHEDRINE 706
Bromatap - See
  ANTIHISTAMINES 98
  PHENYLPROPANOLAMINE 668
Bromatapp - See
  ANTIHISTAMINES 98
  PHENYLPROPANOLAMINE 668
BROMAZEPAM - See BENZODIAZEPINES 156
Bromfed - See
  ANTIHISTAMINES 98
  PSEUDOEPHEDRINE 706
Bromfed-AT - See
  ANTIHISTAMINES 98
  DEXTROMETHORPHAN 296
  PSEUDOEPHEDRINE 706
Bromfed-DM - See
  ANTIHISTAMINES 98
  DEXTROMETHORPHAN 296
  PSEUDOEPHEDRINE 706
Bromfed-PD - See
  ANTIHISTAMINES 98
  PSEUDOEPHEDRINE 706

BROMOCRIPTINE 172
BROMODIPHENHYDRAMINE - See
  ANTIHISTAMINES 98
Bromophen T.D. - See
  ANTIHISTAMINES 98
  PHENYLEPHRINE 664
  PHENYLPROPANOLAMINE 668
Bromo-Seltzer - See
  ACETAMINOPHEN 4
  SODIUM BICARBONATE 758
Bromphen - See
  ANTIHISTAMINES 98
  PHENYLPROPANOLAMINE 668
Bromphen DC with Codeine Cough - See
  ANTIHISTAMINES 98
  NARCOTIC ANALGESICS 580
  PHENYLPROPANOLAMINE 668
Bromphen DX Cough - See
  ANTIHISTAMINES 98
  DEXTROMETHORPHAN 296
  PSEUDOEPHEDRINE 706
BROMPHENIRAMINE - See ANTIHISTAMINES
  98
Brompheril - See
  ANTIHISTAMINES 98
  PSEUDOEPHEDRINE 706
Bronalide - See ADRENOCORTICOIDS (Oral
  Inhalation) 12
Bronchial - See THEOPHYLLINE &
  GUAIFENESIN 784
Bronchodilator - See
  IPRATROPIUM 442
  ISOPROTERENOL & PHENYLEPHRINE 450
  THEOPHYLLINE & GUAIFENESIN 784
  THEOPHYLLINE, EPHEDRINE &
    BARBITURATES 786
Bronchodilator (xanthine) - See
  BRONCHODILATORS, XANTHINE 176
  OXTRIPHYLLINE & GUAIFENESIN 620
  THEOPHYLLINE, EPHEDRINE &
    HYDROXYZINE 788
  THEOPHYLLINE, EPHEDRINE,
    GUAIFENESIN & BARBITURATES 790
BRONCHODILATORS, ADRENERGIC 174
BRONCHODILATORS, XANTHINE 176
Broncho-Grippol-DM - See
  DEXTROMETHORPHAN 296
Broncholate - See
  EPHEDRINE 336
  GUAIFENESIN 398
Broncomar GG - See THEOPHYLLINE &
  GUAIFENESIN 784
Brondecon - See OXTRIPHYLLINE &
  GUAIFENESIN 620
Brondelate - See OXTRIPHYLLINE &
  GUAIFENESIN 620
Bronitin Mist - See BRONCHODILATORS,
  ADRENERGIC 174
Bronkaid Mist - See BRONCHODILATORS,
  ADRENERGIC 174

Calcarb 600 - See CALCIUM SUPPLEMENTS 194

Calcibind - See CELLULOSE SODIUM PHOSPHATE 208

Calci-Chew - See CALCIUM SUPPLEMENTS 194

Calciday 667 - See CALCIUM SUPPLEMENTS 194

Calcidrine - See NARCOTIC ANALGESICS 580

CALCIFEDOL - See VITAMIN D 844

Calciferol - See VITAMIN D 844

Calcijex - See VITAMIN D 844

Calcilac - See CALCIUM SUPPLEMENTS 194

CALCIPOTRIENE 188

Calcite 500 - See CALCIUM SUPPLEMENTS 194

CALCITONIN 190

CALCITRIOL - See VITAMIN D 844

CALCIUM & MAGNESIUM CARBONATES - See ANTACIDS 54

CALCIUM CARBONATE - See
   ANTACIDS 54
   CALCIUM SUPPLEMENTS 194

CALCIUM CARBONATE & MAGNESIA - See ANTACIDS 54

CALCIUM CARBONATE & SIMETHICONE - See ANTACIDS 54

CALCIUM CARBONATE, MAGNESIA, & SIMETHICONE - See ANTACIDS 54

Calcium Carbonate/600 - See CALCIUM SUPPLEMENTS 194

Calcium channel blocker - See
   CALCIUM CHANNEL BLOCKERS 192
   NIMODIPINE 600

CALCIUM CHANNEL BLOCKERS 192

CALCIUM CITRATE - See CALCIUM SUPPLEMENTS 194

CALCIUM GLUBIONATE - See CALCIUM SUPPLEMENTS 194

CALCIUM GLUCONATE - See CALCIUM SUPPLEMENTS 194

CALCIUM GLYCEROPHOSPHATE & CALCIUM LACTATE - See CALCIUM SUPPLEMENTS 194

CALCIUM LACTATE - See CALCIUM SUPPLEMENTS 194

CALCIUM, MAGNESIUM CARBONATES & MAGNESIUM OXIDE - See ANTACIDS 54

CALCIUM PANTOTHENATE - See PANTOTHENIC ACID (Vitamin B-5) 632

CALCIUM POLYCARBOPHIL - See LAXATIVES, BULK-FORMING 470

Calcium Stanley - See CALCIUM SUPPLEMENTS 194

CALCIUM SUPPLEMENTS 194

Calcium-600 - See CALCIUM SUPPLEMENTS 194

Calcium-Sandoz - See CALCIUM SUPPLEMENTS 194

Calcium-Sandoz Forte - See CALCIUM SUPPLEMENTS 194

CaldeCORT Anti-Itch - See ADRENOCORTICOIDS (Topical) 16

CaldeCORT-Light - See ADRENOCORTICOIDS (Topical) 16

Calderol - See VITAMIN D 844

Caldesene Medicated Powder - See ANTIFUNGALS (Topical) 90

Caldomine-DH Forte - See
   ANTIHISTAMINES 98
   NARCOTIC ANALGESICS 580
   PHENYLPROPANOLAMINE 668

Caldomine-DH Pediatric - See
   ANTIHISTAMINES 98
   NARCOTIC ANALGESICS 580
   PHENYLPROPANOLAMINE 668

Calglycine - See
   ANTACIDS 54
   CALCIUM SUPPLEMENTS 194

Calicylic - See KERATOLYTICS 464

Calm X - See ANTIHISTAMINES 98

Calmylin - See
   DEXTROMETHORPHAN 296
   GUAIFENESIN 398
   PSEUDOEPHEDRINE 706

Calmylin #1 - See DEXTROMETHORPHAN 296

Calmylin #2 - See
   DEXTROMETHORPHAN 296
   PSEUDOEPHEDRINE 706

Calmylin #3 - See
   DEXTROMETHORPHAN 296
   GUAIFENESIN 398
   PSEUDOEPHEDRINE 706

Calmylin #4 - See
   ANTIHISTAMINES 98
   DEXTROMETHORPHAN 296

Calmylin Cough & Cold - See
   ACETAMINOPHEN 4
   DEXTROMETHORPHAN 296
   GUAIFENESIN 398
   PSEUDOEPHEDRINE 706

Calmylin Pediatric - See
   DEXTROMETHORPHAN 296
   PSEUDOEPHEDRINE 706

Calmylin with Codeine - See
   ANTIHISTAMINES 98
   GUAIFENESIN 398
   NARCOTIC ANALGESICS 580
   PSEUDOEPHEDRINE 706

Calphosan - See CALCIUM SUPPLEMENTS 194

Calsan - See CALCIUM SUPPLEMENTS 194

Caltrate - See CALCIUM SUPPLEMENTS 194

Caltrate Chewable - See CALCIUM SUPPLEMENTS 194

Caltrate-300 - See CALCIUM SUPPLEMENTS 194

Caltrate-600 - See CALCIUM SUPPLEMENTS 194

Cama Arthritis Reliever - See ASPIRIN 132

INDEX

Carter's Little Pills - See LAXATIVES, STIMULANT 476

Cartrol - See BETA-ADRENERGIC BLOCKING AGENTS 162

CARVEDILOL - See BETA-ADRENERGIC BLOCKING AGENTS 162

CASANTHRANOL - See LAXATIVES, STIMULANT 476

CASANTHRANOL & DOCUSATE - See LAXATIVES, SOFTENER/LUBRICANT 474

CASCARA - See LAXATIVES, STIMULANT 476

Cascara Aromatic Fluidextract - See LAXATIVES, STIMULANT 476

Cascara Sagrada - See LAXATIVES, STIMULANT 476

CASTOR OIL - See LAXATIVES, STIMULANT 476

Cataflam - See ANTI-INFLAMMATORY DRUGS, NONSTEROIDAL (NSAIDs) 104

Catapres - See CLONIDINE 246

Catapres-TTS - See CLONIDINE 246

Caverject - See ALPROSTADIL 24

CCNU - See LOMUSTINE 494

Ceclor - See CEPHALOSPORINS 210

Cecon - See VITAMIN C (Ascorbic Acid) 842

Cedocard-SR - See NITRATES 602

CeeNU - See LOMUSTINE 494

CEFACLOR - See CEPHALOSPORINS 210

CEFADROXIL - See CEPHALOSPORINS 210

Cefanex - See CEPHALOSPORINS 210

CEFDINIR - See CEPHALOSPORINS 210

CEFIXIME - See CEPHALOSPORINS 210

Cefotan - See CEPHALOSPORINS 210

CEFOTETAN - See CEPHALOSPORINS 210

CEFPODOXIME - See CEPHALOSPORINS 210

CEFPROZIL - See CEPHALOSPORINS 210

Ceftin - See CEPHALOSPORINS 210

CEFUROXIME - See CEPHALOSPORINS 210

Cefzil - See CEPHALOSPORINS 210

Celebrex - See ANTI-INFLAMMATORY DRUGS, NONSTEROIDAL (NSAIDs) 104

CELECOXIB - See ANTI-INFLAMMATORY DRUGS, NONSTEROIDAL (NSAIDs) 104

Celestoderm-V - See ADRENOCORTICOIDS (Topical) 16

Celestoderm-V/2 - See ADRENOCORTICOIDS (Topical) 16

Celestone - See ADRENOCORTICOIDS (Systemic) 14

Celexa - See CITALOPRAM 236

CellCept - See IMMUNOSUPPRESSIVE AGENTS 430

CELLULOSE SODIUM PHOSPHATE 208

Celontin - See ANTICONVULSANTS, SUCCINIMIDE 80

Cemill - See VITAMIN C (Ascorbic Acid) 842

Cenafed - See PSEUDOEPHEDRINE 706

Cenafed Plus - See
ANTIHISTAMINES 98
PSEUDOEPHEDRINE 706

Cena-K - See POTASSIUM SUPPLEMENTS 678

Cenolate - See VITAMIN C (Ascorbic Acid) 842

Central nervous system stimulant - See
AMPHETAMINES 34
METHYLPHENIDATE 538
PEMOLINE 644

Centrax - See BENZODIAZEPINES 156

CEPHALEXIN - See CEPHALOSPORINS 210

CEPHALOSPORINS 210

CEPHRADINE - See CEPHALOSPORINS 210

Ceporex - See CEPHALOSPORINS 210

Cerespan - See PAPAVERINE 634

CERIVASTATIN - See HMG-CoA REDUCTASE INHIBITORS 414

Cerose-DM - See
ANTIHISTAMINES 98
DEXTROMETHORPHAN 296
PHENYLEPHRINE 664

C.E.S. - See ESTROGENS 350

Cesamet - See NABILONE 572

Cetacort - See ADRENOCORTICOIDS (Topical) 16

Cetamide - See ANTIBACTERIALS (Ophthalmic) 68

Cetane - See VITAMIN C (Ascorbic Acid) 842

CETIRIZINE - See ANTIHISTAMINES, NONSEDATING 100

Cevalin - See VITAMIN C (Ascorbic Acid) 842

Cevi-Bid - See VITAMIN C (Ascorbic Acid) 842

Ce-Vi-Sol - See VITAMIN C (Ascorbic Acid) 842

Cevita - See VITAMIN C (Ascorbic Acid) 842

Charac-50 - See CHARCOAL, ACTIVATED 212

Charac-tol 50 - See CHARCOAL, ACTIVATED 212

Charcoaid - See CHARCOAL, ACTIVATED 212

CHARCOAL, ACTIVATED 212

Charcocaps - See CHARCOAL, ACTIVATED 212

Charcodote - See CHARCOAL, ACTIVATED 212

Charcodote TFS - See CHARCOAL, ACTIVATED 212

Chardonna-2 - See BELLADONNA ALKALOIDS & BARBITURATES 154

Chelating agent - See PENICILLAMINE 646

Cheracol - See
GUAIFENESIN 398
NARCOTIC ANALGESICS 580

Cheracol D Cough - See
DEXTROMETHORPHAN 296
GUAIFENESIN 398

Cheracol Nasal Spray - See OXYMETAZOLINE (Nasal) 624

Cheracol Nasal Spray Pump Cherry Scented - See OXYMETAZOLINE (Nasal) 624

Cheracol Plus - See
ANTIHISTAMINES 98
DEXTROMETHORPHAN 296
PHENYLPROPANOLAMINE 668

Cheracol Sinus - See
ANTIHISTAMINES 98
PSEUDOEPHEDRINE 706

INDEX

INDEX

985

INDEX

Conex Plus - See
  ACETAMINOPHEN 4
  ANTIHISTAMINES 98
  PHENYLPROPANOLAMINE 668
Conex with Codeine Liquid - See
  GUAIFENESIN 398
  NARCOTIC ANALGESICS 580
  PHENYLPROPANOLAMINE 668
Congespirin - See
  ACETAMINOPHEN 4
  DEXTROMETHORPHAN 296
Congespirin for Children Cold Tablets - See
  ACETAMINOPHEN 4
  PHENYLEPHRINE 664
Congespirin for Children Liquid Cold
    Medicine - See
  ACETAMINOPHEN 4
  PHENYLPROPANOLAMINE 668
Congess JR - See
  GUAIFENESIN 398
  PSEUDOEPHEDRINE 706
Congess SR - See
  GUAIFENESIN 398
  PSEUDOEPHEDRINE 706
Congest - See ESTROGENS 350
Congestac Caplets - See
  GUAIFENESIN 398
  PSEUDOEPHEDRINE 706
Congestant D - See
  ACETAMINOPHEN 4
  ANTIHISTAMINES 98
  PHENYLPROPANOLAMINE 668
Conjec-B - See ANTIHISTAMINES 98
CONJUGATED ESTROGENS - See
    ESTROGENS 350
CONJUGATED ESTROGENS &
    METHYLTESTOSTERONE - See
    ANDROGENS & ESTROGENS 40
Constant-T - See BRONCHODILATORS,
    XANTHINE 176
Constilac - See LAXATIVES, OSMOTIC 472
Constulose - See LAXATIVES, OSMOTIC 472
Contac 12-Hour - See
  ANTIHISTAMINES 98
  PHENYLPROPANOLAMINE 668
Contac 12-Hour Allergy - See
  ANTIHISTAMINES 98
Contac Allergy/Sinus Day Caplets - See
  ACETAMINOPHEN 4
  PSEUDOEPHEDRINE 706
Contac Allergy/Sinus Night Caplets - See
  ACETAMINOPHEN 4
  ANTIHISTAMINES 98
  PSEUDOEPHEDRINE 706
Contac Jr. Children's Cold Medicine - See
  ACETAMINOPHEN 4
  DEXTROMETHORPHAN 296
  PHENYLPROPANOLAMINE 668
Contac Maximum Strength 12-Hour Caplets -
    See
  ANTIHISTAMINES 98

PHENYLPROPANOLAMINE 668
Contac Maximum Strength Sinus Caplets - See
  ACETAMINOPHEN 4
  PSEUDOEPHEDRINE 706
Contac Night Caplets - See
  ACETAMINOPHEN 4
  ANTIHISTAMINES 98
  DEXTROMETHORPHAN 296
  PSEUDOEPHEDRINE 706
Contac Non-Drowsy Formula Sinus Caplets -
    See
  ACETAMINOPHEN 4
  PSEUDOEPHEDRINE 706
Contac Severe Cold Formula - See
  ACETAMINOPHEN 4
  ANTIHISTAMINES 98
  DEXTROMETHORPHAN 296
  PSEUDOEPHEDRINE 706
Contac Severe Cold Formula Night Strength -
    See
  ACETAMINOPHEN 4
  ANTIHISTAMINES 98
  DEXTROMETHORPHAN 296
  PSEUDOEPHEDRINE 706
Contraceptive (oral) - See CONTRACEPTIVES,
    ORAL 262
Contraceptive (vaginal) - See
    CONTRACEPTIVES, VAGINAL
    (Spermicides) 264
CONTRACEPTIVES, ORAL 262
CONTRACEPTIVES, VAGINAL (Spermicides)
    264
Control - See PHENYLPROPANOLAMINE 668
Contuss - See
  GUAIFENESIN 398
  PHENYLEPHRINE 664
  PHENYLPROPANOLAMINE 668
Cophene No. 2 - See
  ANTIHISTAMINES 98
  PSEUDOEPHEDRINE 706
Cophene-B - See ANTIHISTAMINES 98
Cophene-S - See
  ANTIHISTAMINES 98
  NARCOTIC ANALGESICS 580
  PHENYLEPHRINE 664
  PHENYLPROPANOLAMINE 668
Cophene-X - See
  ANTIHISTAMINES 98
  PHENYLEPHRINE 664
  PHENYLPROPANOLAMINE 668
Cophene-XP - See
  ANTIHISTAMINES 98
  GUAIFENESIN 398
  NARCOTIC ANALGESICS 580
  PHENYLEPHRINE 664
  PHENYLPROPANOLAMINE 668
  PSEUDOEPHEDRINE 706
Co-Pyronil 2 - See
  ANTIHISTAMINES 98
  PSEUDOEPHEDRINE 706
Coradur - See NITRATES 602

INDEX

991

DESOGESTREL & ETHINYL ESTRADIOL - See
    CONTRACEPTIVES, ORAL 262
DESONIDE (Topical) - See
    ADRENOCORTICOIDS (Topical) 16
DesOwen - See ADRENOCORTICOIDS
    (Topical) 16
DESOXIMETASONE (Topical) - See
    ADRENOCORTICOIDS (Topical) 16
Desoxyn - See AMPHETAMINES 34
Desoxyn Gradumet - See AMPHETAMINES 34
Despec - See
    GUAIFENESIN 398
    PHENYLEPHRINE 664
    PHENYLPROPANOLAMINE 668
Desquam-E 2.5 Gel - See BENZOYL
    PEROXIDE 158
Desquam-E 5 Gel - See BENZOYL PEROXIDE
    158
Desquam-E 10 Gel - See BENZOYL
    PEROXIDE 158
Desquam-X 2.5 Gel - See BENZOYL
    PEROXIDE 158
Desquam-X 5 Gel - See BENZOYL PEROXIDE
    158
Desquam-X 5 Wash - See BENZOYL
    PEROXIDE 158
Desquam-X 10 Gel - See BENZOYL
    PEROXIDE 158
Desquam-X 10 Wash - See BENZOYL
    PEROXIDE 158
Desyrel - See TRAZODONE 816
Detensol - See BETA-ADRENERGIC
    BLOCKING AGENTS 162
Detrol - See TOLTERODINE 810
De-Tuss - See
    NARCOTIC ANALGESICS 580
    PSEUDOEPHEDRINE 706
Detussin Expectorant - See
    GUAIFENESIN 398
    NARCOTIC ANALGESICS 580
    PSEUDOEPHEDRINE 706
Detussin Liquid - See
    NARCOTIC ANALGESICS 580
    PSEUDOEPHEDRINE 706
Devonex - See CALCIPOTRIENE 188
Dexacort Turbinaire - See
    ADRENOCORTICOIDS (Nasal Inhalation) 10
Dexair - See ANTI-INFLAMMATORY DRUGS,
    STEROIDAL (Ophthalmic) 108
DEXAMETHASONE - See
    ADRENOCORTICOIDS (Systemic) 14
    ANTI-INFLAMMATORY DRUGS, STEROIDAL
    (Ophthalmic) 108
DEXAMETHASONE (Nasal) - See
    ADRENOCORTICOIDS (Nasal Inhalation) 10
DEXAMETHASONE (Oral Inhalation) - See
    ADRENOCORTICOIDS (Oral Inhalation) 12
DEXAMETHASONE (otic) - See ANTI-
    INFLAMMATORY DRUGS, STEROIDAL
    (Otic) 110

DEXAMETHASONE (Topical) - See
    ADRENOCORTICOIDS (Topical) 16
Dexaphen SA - See
    ANTIHISTAMINES 98
    PSEUDOEPHEDRINE 706
Dexasone - See ADRENOCORTICOIDS
    (Systemic) 14
Dexatrim Maximum Strength Caplets - See
    PHENYLPROPANOLAMINE 668
Dexatrim Maximum Strength Capsules - See
    PHENYLPROPANOLAMINE 668
Dexatrim Maximum Strength Tablets - See
    PHENYLPROPANOLAMINE 668
DEXBROMPHENIRAMINE - See
    ANTIHISTAMINES 98
Dexchlor - See ANTIHISTAMINES 98
DEXCHLORPHENIRAMINE - See
    ANTIHISTAMINES 98
Dexedrine - See AMPHETAMINES 34
Dexedrine Spansule - See AMPHETAMINES 34
Dexitac - See CAFFEINE 186
Dexol T.D. - See PANTOTHENIC ACID (Vitamin
    B-5) 632
Dexone 0.5 - See ADRENOCORTICOIDS
    (Systemic) 14
Dexone 0.75 - See ADRENOCORTICOIDS
    (Systemic) 14
Dexone 1.5 - See ADRENOCORTICOIDS
    (Systemic) 14
Dexone 4 - See ADRENOCORTICOIDS
    (Systemic) 14
Dexophed - See
    ANTIHISTAMINES 98
    PSEUDOEPHEDRINE 706
Dexotic - See ANTI-INFLAMMATORY DRUGS,
    STEROIDAL (Ophthalmic) 108
Dexsone - See ANTI-INFLAMMATORY
    DRUGS, STEROIDAL (Ophthalmic) 108
DEXTROAMPHETAMINE - See
    AMPHETAMINES 34
DEXTROMETHORPHAN 296
DEXTROTHYROXINE 298
Dey-Dose Isoetharine - See
    BRONCHODILATORS, ADRENERGIC 174
Dey-Dose Isoetharine S/F - See
    BRONCHODILATORS, ADRENERGIC 174
Dey-Dose Isoproterenol - See
    BRONCHODILATORS, ADRENERGIC 174
Dey-Dose Metaproterenol - See
    BRONCHODILATORS, ADRENERGIC 174
Dey-Dose Racepinephrine - See
    BRONCHODILATORS, ADRENERGIC 174
Dey-Lute Isoetharine - See
    BRONCHODILATORS, ADRENERGIC 174
Dey-Lute Isoetharine S/F - See
    BRONCHODILATORS, ADRENERGIC 174
Dey-Lute Metaproterenol - See
    BRONCHODILATORS, ADRENERGIC 174
DHCplus - See NARCOTIC ANALGESICS &
    ACETAMINOPHEN 582

DHEA - See DEHYDROEPIANDROSTERONE
(DHEA) 292

DHS Tar Gel Shampoo - See COAL TAR
(Topical) 254

DHS Tar Shampoo - See COAL TAR (Topical)
254

DHS Zinc Dandruff Shampoo - See
ANTISEBORRHEICS (Topical) 118

DHT - See VITAMIN D 844

DHT Intensol - See VITAMIN D 844

DiaBeta - See ANTIDIABETIC AGENTS,
SULFONYLUREA 84

Diabetic Tussin DM - See
DEXTROMETHORPHAN 296
GUAIFENESIN 398

Diabetic Tussin EX - See GUAIFENESIN 398

Diabinese - See ANTIDIABETIC AGENTS,
SULFONYLUREA 84

Diagen - See SALICYLATES 744

Diagnostic aid - See GLUCAGON 390

Dialose - See LAXATIVES, SOFTENER/
LUBRICANT 474

Dialose Plus - See
LAXATIVES, SOFTENER/LUBRICANT 474
LAXATIVES, STIMULANT 476

Dialume - See ANTACIDS 54

Diamicron - See ANTIDIABETIC AGENTS,
SULFONYLUREA 84

Diamine T.D. - See ANTIHISTAMINES 98

Diamox - See CARBONIC ANHYDRASE
INHIBITORS 206

Diar-Aid - See ATTAPULGITE 138

Diasorb - See ATTAPULGITE 138

Diasporal Cream - See KERATOLYTICS 464

Diastat - See BENZODIAZEPINES 156

Diazemuls - See BENZODIAZEPINES 156

DIAZEPAM - See BENZODIAZEPINES 156

Diazepam Intensol - See BENZODIAZEPINES
156

Diazide - See DIURETICS, POTASSIUM-
SPARING & HYDROCHLOROTHIAZIDE 322

DIBASIC CALCIUM PHOSPHATE - See
CALCIUM SUPPLEMENTS 194

Dibent - See DICYCLOMINE 300

DIBUCAINE - See
ANESTHETICS (Rectal) 44
ANESTHETICS (Topical) 46

Dicarbosil - See
ANTACIDS 54
CALCIUM SUPPLEMENTS 194

DICHLORPHENAMIDE - See CARBONIC
ANHYDRASE INHIBITORS 206

DICLOFENAC - See
ANTI-INFLAMMATORY DRUGS,
NONSTEROIDAL (NSAIDs) 104
ANTI-INFLAMMATORY DRUGS,
NONSTEROIDAL (NSAIDs) (Ophthalmic) 106

DICLOXACILLIN - See PENICILLINS 648

DICYCLOMINE 300

Di-Cyclonex - See DICYCLOMINE 300

DIDANOSINE (ddl) - See NUCLEOSIDE
REVERSE TRANSCRIPTASE INHIBITORS
608

Didrex - See APPETITE SUPPRESSANTS 130

Didronel - See ETIDRONATE 356

Diet-Aide Maximum Strength - See
PHENYLPROPANOLAMINE 668

Dietary replacement - See CALCIUM
SUPPLEMENTS 194

DIETHYLPROPION - See APPETITE
SUPPRESSANTS 130

DIETHYLSTILBESTROL - See ESTROGENS
350

DIETHYLSTILBESTROL (DES) &
METHYLTESTOSTERONE - See
ANDROGENS & ESTROGENS 40

DIFENOXIN & ATROPINE 302

Differin - See RETINOIDS (Topical) 730

DIFLORASONE (Topical) - See
ADRENOCORTICOIDS (Topical) 16

Diflucan - See FLUCONAZOLE 370

DIFLUCORTOLONE (Topical) - See
ADRENOCORTICOIDS (Topical) 16

DIFLUNISAL - See ANTI-INFLAMMATORY
DRUGS, NONSTEROIDAL (NSAIDs) 104

Di-Gel - See
ANTACIDS 54
SIMETHICONE 756

Digestant - See PANCREATIN, PEPSIN, BILE
SALTS, HYOSCYAMINE, ATROPINE,
SCOPOLAMINE & PHENOBARBITAL 628

Digitalis preparation - See DIGITALIS
PREPARATIONS (Digitalis Glycosides) 304

DIGITALIS PREPARATIONS (Digitalis
Glycosides) 304

DIGITOXIN - See DIGITALIS PREPARATIONS
(Digitalis Glycosides) 304

DIGOXIN - See DIGITALIS PREPARATIONS
(Digitalis Glycosides) 304

Dihistine - See
ANTIHISTAMINES 98
PHENYLEPHRINE 664

Dihistine DH - See
ANTIHISTAMINES 98
NARCOTIC ANALGESICS 580
PSEUDOEPHEDRINE 706

Dihistine Expectorant - See
GUAIFENESIN 398
NARCOTIC ANALGESICS 580
PSEUDOEPHEDRINE 706

DIHYDROCODEINE - See NARCOTIC
ANALGESICS 580

Dihydromorphinone - See NARCOTIC
ANALGESICS 580

DIHYDROTACHYSTEROL - See VITAMIN D 844

Dihydrotestosterone inhibitor - See
FINASTERIDE 364

DIHYDROXYALUMINUM AMINOACETATE - See
ANTACIDS 54

DIHYDROXYALUMINUM AMINOACETATE, MAGNESIA, & ALUMINA - See ANTACIDS 54

DIHYDROXYALUMINUM SODIUM CARBONATE - See ANTACIDS 54

Diiodohydroxyquin - See IODOQUINOL 438

Dilacor-XR - See CALCIUM CHANNEL BLOCKERS 192

Dilantin - See ANTICONVULSANTS, HYDANTOIN 78

Dilantin 30 - See ANTICONVULSANTS, HYDANTOIN 78

Dilantin 125 - See ANTICONVULSANTS, HYDANTOIN 78

Dilantin Infatabs - See ANTICONVULSANTS, HYDANTOIN 78

Dilantin Kapseals - See ANTICONVULSANTS, HYDANTOIN 78

Dilatair - See PHENYLEPHRINE (Ophthalmic) 666

Dilatrate-SR - See NITRATES 602

Dilaudid - See NARCOTIC ANALGESICS 580

Dilaudid Cough - See
GUAIFENESIN 398
NARCOTIC ANALGESICS 580

Dilaudid-HP - See NARCOTIC ANALGESICS 580

Dilomine - See DICYCLOMINE 300

Dilor - See BRONCHODILATORS, XANTHINE 176

Dilor-400 - See BRONCHODILATORS, XANTHINE 176

Dilotab - See
ACETAMINOPHEN 4
PHENYLPROPANOLAMINE 668

DILTIAZEM - See CALCIUM CHANNEL BLOCKERS 192

Dimacol - See
DEXTROMETHORPHAN 296
GUAIFENESIN 398
PSEUDOEPHEDRINE 706

Dimaphen - See
ANTIHISTAMINES 98
PHENYLPROPANOLAMINE 668

Dimaphen S.A. - See
ANTIHISTAMINES 98
PHENYLEPHRINE 664
PHENYLPROPANOLAMINE 668

Dimelor - See ANTIDIABETIC AGENTS, SULFONYLUREA 84

DIMENHYDRINATE - See ANTIHISTAMINES 98

Dimetabs - See ANTIHISTAMINES 98

Dimetane - See ANTIHISTAMINES 98

Dimetane Decongestant Caplets - See
ANTIHISTAMINES 98
PHENYLEPHRINE 664

Dimetane Expectorant - See
ANTIHISTAMINES 98
GUAIFENESIN 398
PHENYLEPHRINE 664
PHENYLPROPANOLAMINE 668

Dimetane Expectorant-C - See
ANTIHISTAMINES 98
GUAIFENESIN 398
NARCOTIC ANALGESICS 580
PHENYLEPHRINE 664
PHENYLPROPANOLAMINE 668

Dimetane Expectorant-DC - See
ANTIHISTAMINES 98
GUAIFENESIN 398
NARCOTIC ANALGESICS 580
PHENYLEPHRINE 664
PHENYLPROPANOLAMINE 668

Dimetane Extentabs - See ANTIHISTAMINES 98

Dimetane-DC Cough - See
ANTIHISTAMINES 98
NARCOTIC ANALGESICS 580
PHENYLPROPANOLAMINE 668

Dimetane-DX Cough - See
ANTIHISTAMINES 98
DEXTROMETHORPHAN 296
PSEUDOEPHEDRINE 706

Dimetane-Ten - See ANTIHISTAMINES 98

Dimetapp - See
ANTIHISTAMINES 98
PHENYLEPHRINE 664
PHENYLPROPANOLAMINE 668

Dimetapp 4-Hour Liqui-Gels Maximum Strength - See
ANTIHISTAMINES 98
PHENYLPROPANOLAMINE 668

Dimetapp Allergy - See ANTIHISTAMINES 98

Dimetapp Allergy Liqui-Gels - See
ANTIHISTAMINES 98

Dimetapp Cold and Allergy - See
ANTIHISTAMINES 98
PHENYLPROPANOLAMINE 668

Dimetapp Cold and Flu Caplets - See
ACETAMINOPHEN 4
ANTIHISTAMINES 98
PHENYLPROPANOLAMINE 668

Dimetapp Extentabs - See
ANTIHISTAMINES 98
PHENYLEPHRINE 664
PHENYLPROPANOLAMINE 668

Dimetapp Maximum Strength Liquigels - See
ANTIHISTAMINES 98
PHENYLPROPANOLAMINE 668

Dimetapp Oral Infant Drops - See
ANTIHISTAMINES 98
PHENYLEPHRINE 664
PHENYLPROPANOLAMINE 668

Dimetapp Plus Caplets - See
ACETAMINOPHEN 4
ANTIHISTAMINES 98
PHENYLPROPANOLAMINE 668

Dimetapp Sinus Caplets - See
ANTI-INFLAMMATORY DRUGS, NONSTEROIDAL (NSAIDs) 104
PSEUDOEPHEDRINE 706

INDEX

Efed II Yellow - See
PHENYLPROPANOLAMINE 668
Effective Strength Cough Formula - See
ANTIHISTAMINES 98
DEXTROMETHORPHAN 296
**Effective Strength Cough Formula with
Decongestant** - See
DEXTROMETHORPHAN 296
PSEUDOEPHEDRINE 706
Effer-syllium - See LAXATIVES, BULK-
FORMING 470
Effexor - See VENLAFAXINE 836
**Efficol Cough Whip (Cough Suppressant/
Decongestant)** - See
DEXTROMETHORPHAN 296
PHENYLPROPANOLAMINE 668
**Efficol Cough Whip (Cough Suppressant/
Decongestant/Antihistamine)** - See
ANTIHISTAMINES 98
DEXTROMETHORPHAN 296
PHENYLPROPANOLAMINE 668
**Efficol Cough Whip (Cough Suppressant/
Expectorant)** - See
DEXTROMETHORPHAN 296
GUAIFENESIN 398
Efidac 24 Chlorpheniramine - See
ANTIHISTAMINES 98
Efidec/24 - See PSEUDOEPHEDRINE 706
Eflone - See ANTI-INFLAMMATORY DRUGS,
STEROIDAL (Ophthalmic) 108
Efudex - See FLUOROURACIL (Topical) 374
E/Gel - See ERYTHROMYCINS 346
Egozinc - See ZINC SUPPLEMENTS 856
EHDP - See ETIDRONATE 356
Elavil - See ANTIDEPRESSANTS, TRICYCLIC
82
Elavil Plus - See PERPHENAZINE &
AMITRIPTYLINE 658
Eldepryl - See SELEGILINE 748
Electrolyte replenisher - See
CARBOHYDRATES & ELECTROLYTES 204
POTASSIUM & SODIUM PHOSPHATES 672
POTASSIUM PHOSPHATES 676
Elimite Cream - See PEDICULICIDES (Topical)
642
Elixicon - See BRONCHODILATORS,
XANTHINE 176
Elixomin - See BRONCHODILATORS,
XANTHINE 176
Elixophyllin - See BRONCHODILATORS,
XANTHINE 176
Elixophyllin SR - See BRONCHODILATORS,
XANTHINE 176
Elixophyllin-GG - See THEOPHYLLINE &
GUAIFENESIN 784
Elocom - See ADRENOCORTICOIDS (Topical)
16
Elocon - See ADRENOCORTICOIDS (Topical)
16

E-Lor - See NARCOTIC ANALGESICS &
ACETAMINOPHEN 582
Eltor-120 - See PSEUDOEPHEDRINE 706
Eltroxin - See THYROID HORMONES 798
Emadine - See ANTIALLERGIC AGENTS
(Ophthalmic) 62
EMEDASTINE - See ANTIALLERGIC AGENTS
(Ophthalmic) 62
Emcodeine No. 2 - See NARCOTIC
ANALGESICS & ASPIRIN 584
Emcodeine No. 3 - See NARCOTIC
ANALGESICS & ASPIRIN 584
Emcodeine No. 4 - See NARCOTIC
ANALGESICS & ASPIRIN 584
Emcyt - See ESTRAMUSTINE 348
Emetic - See IPECAC 440
Emex - See METOCLOPRAMIDE 542
Emgel - See ERYTHROMYCINS 346
Emitrip - See ANTIDEPRESSANTS,
TRICYCLIC 82
Emko - See CONTRACEPTIVES, VAGINAL
(Spermicides) 264
Emla - See ANESTHETICS (Topical) 46
Emo-Cort - See ADRENOCORTICOIDS
(Topical) 16
Emo-Cort Scalp Solution - See
ADRENOCORTICOIDS (Topical) 16
Empirin - See ASPIRIN 132
Empirin with Codeine - See NARCOTIC
ANALGESICS & ASPIRIN 584
Empirin with Codeine No. 3 - See NARCOTIC
ANALGESICS & ASPIRIN 584
Empirin with Codeine No. 4 - See NARCOTIC
ANALGESICS & ASPIRIN 584
Empracet 30 - See NARCOTIC ANALGESICS &
ACETAMINOPHEN 582
Empracet 60 - See NARCOTIC ANALGESICS &
ACETAMINOPHEN 582
Emtec - See NARCOTIC ANALGESICS &
ACETAMINOPHEN 582
Emulsoil - See LAXATIVES, STIMULANT 476
E-Mycin - See ERYTHROMYCINS 346
ENALAPRIL - See ANGIOTENSIN-
CONVERTING ENZYME (ACE)
INHIBITORS 50
ENALAPRIL & HYDROCHLOROTHIAZIDE - See
ANGIOTENSIN-CONVERTING ENZYME
(ACE) INHIBITORS &
HYDROCHLOROTHIAZIDE 52
Encare - See CONTRACEPTIVES, VAGINAL
(Spermicides) 264
Endafed - See
ANTIHISTAMINES 98
PSEUDOEPHEDRINE 706
Endagen-HD - See
ANTIHISTAMINES 98
NARCOTIC ANALGESICS 580
PHENYLEPHRINE 664
Endal Expectorant - See
GUAIFENESIN 398

INDEX

Ergomar - See ERGOTAMINE 342
Ergometrine - See ERGONOVINE 340
ERGONOVINE 340
Ergostat - See ERGOTAMINE 342
Ergot preparation - See
   ERGOLOID MESYLATES 338
   ERGOTAMINE 342
Ergot preparation (uterine stimulant) - See
   ERGONOVINE 340
   METHYLERGONOVINE 536
ERGOTAMINE 342
ERGOTAMINE, BELLADONNA &
   PHENOBARBITAL 344
Ergotrate - See ERGONOVINE 340
Ergotrate Maleate - See ERGONOVINE 340
Eridium - See PHENAZOPYRIDINE 660
Erybid - See ERYTHROMYCINS 346
ERYC - See ERYTHROMYCINS 346
Erycette - See ANTIBACTERIALS FOR ACNE
   (Topical) 66
EryDerm - See ANTIBACTERIALS FOR ACNE
   (Topical) 66
EryGel - See ANTIBACTERIALS FOR ACNE
   (Topical) 66
EryMax - See ANTIBACTERIALS FOR ACNE
   (Topical) 66
EryPed - See ERYTHROMYCINS 346
ErySol - See ANTIBACTERIALS FOR ACNE
   (Topical) 66
Ery-Tab - See ERYTHROMYCINS 346
Erythraderm - See ERYTHROMYCINS 346
ERYTHRITYL TETRANITRATE - See
   NITRATES 602
Erythro - See ERYTHROMYCINS 346
Erythrocin - See ERYTHROMYCINS 346
Erythrocot - See ERYTHROMYCINS 346
Erythromid - See ERYTHROMYCINS 346
ERYTHROMYCIN ESTOLATE - See
   ERYTHROMYCINS 346
ERYTHROMYCIN ETHYLSUCCINATE - See
   ERYTHROMYCINS 346
ERYTHROMYCIN GLUCEPTATE - See
   ERYTHROMYCINS 346
ERYTHROMYCIN LACTOBIONATE - See
   ERYTHROMYCINS 346
ERYTHROMYCIN (Ophthalmic) - See
   ANTIBACTERIALS (Ophthalmic) 68
ERYTHROMYCIN STEARATE - See
   ERYTHROMYCINS 346
ERYTHROMYCIN (Topical) - See
   ANTIBACTERIALS FOR ACNE (Topical) 66
ERYTHROMYCIN-BASE - See
   ERYTHROMYCINS 346
ERYTHROMYCINS 346
Erythro-statin - See ANTIBACTERIALS FOR
   ACNE (Topical) 66
Eryzole - See
   ERYTHROMYCINS 346
   SULFONAMIDES 770

Eserine - See ANTIGLAUCOMA, SHORT-
   ACTING (Ophthalmic) 96
Esgic - See
   ACETAMINOPHEN 4
   BARBITURATES 148
   CAFFEINE 186
Esgic Plus - See
   ACETAMINOPHEN 4
   BARBITURATES 148
   CAFFEINE 186
Esidrix - See DIURETICS, THIAZIDE 324
Esimil - See GUANETHIDINE &
   HYDROCHLOROTHIAZIDE 406
Eskalith - See LITHIUM 492
Eskalith CR - See LITHIUM 492
Espotabs - See LAXATIVES, STIMULANT 476
Estar - See COAL TAR (Topical) 254
ESTAZOLAM - See BENZODIAZEPINES 156
ESTERIFIED ESTROGENS - See ESTROGENS
   350
ESTERIFIED ESTROGENS &
   METHYLTESTOSTERONE - See
   ANDROGENS & ESTROGENS 40
Estinyl - See ESTROGENS 350
Estivin II - See DECONGESTANTS
   (Ophthalmic) 290
Estrace - See ESTROGENS 350
Estraderm - See ESTROGENS 350
ESTRADIOL - See ESTROGENS 350
Estragen 5 - See ESTROGENS 350
Estragen LA 5 - See ESTROGENS 350
Estra-L - See ESTROGENS 350
ESTRAMUSTINE 348
Estratab - See ESTROGENS 350
Estratest - See ANDROGENS & ESTROGENS
   40
Estratest H.S. - See ANDROGENS &
   ESTROGENS 40
Estring - See ESTROGENS 350
Estro-A - See ESTROGENS 350
Estro-Cyp - See ESTROGENS 350
Estrofem - See ESTROGENS 350
ESTROGEN - See ESTROGENS 350
ESTROGENS 350
Estroject-L.A. - See ESTROGENS 350
Estro-L.A. - See ESTROGENS 350
ESTRONE - See ESTROGENS 350
Estrone 5 - See ESTROGENS 350
ESTROPIPATE - See ESTROGENS 350
Estro-Span - See ESTROGENS 350
Estrostep - See CONTRACEPTIVES, ORAL 262
Estrostep Fe - See CONTRACEPTIVES, ORAL
   262
Estrovis - See ESTROGENS 350
ETHACRYNIC ACID - See DIURETICS, LOOP
   318
ETHCHLORVYNOL 352
ETHINYL ESTRADIOL - See ESTROGENS 350
ETHIONAMIDE 354
Ethmozine - See MORICIZINE 568

INDEX

1005

F

FAMCICLOVIR - See ANTIVIRALS FOR
   HERPES VIRUS 122
FAMOTIDINE - See HISTAMINE H$_2$
   RECEPTOR ANTAGONISTS 412
Famvir - See ANTIVIRALS FOR HERPES
   VIRUS 122
Fansidar - See SULFADOXINE AND
   PYRIMETHAMINE 764
Fareston - See TOREMIFENE 812
Fastin - See APPETITE SUPPRESSANTS 130
Father John's Medicine Plus - See
   ANTIHISTAMINES 98
   DEXTROMETHORPHAN 296
   GUAIFENESIN 398
   PHENYLEPHRINE 664
FBM - See FELBAMATE 360
Febridyne - See ACETAMINOPHEN 4
Fedahist - See
   ANTIHISTAMINES 98
   PSEUDOEPHEDRINE 706
Fedahist Decongestant - See
   ANTIHISTAMINES 98
   PSEUDOEPHEDRINE 706
Fedahist Expectorant - See
   GUAIFENESIN 398
   PSEUDOEPHEDRINE 706
Fedahist Expectorant Pediatric Drops - See
   GUAIFENESIN 398
   PSEUDOEPHEDRINE 706
Fedahist Gyrocaps - See
   ANTIHISTAMINES 98
   PSEUDOEPHEDRINE 706
Fedahist Timecaps - See
   ANTIHISTAMINES 98
   PSEUDOEPHEDRINE 706
Feen-a-Mint - See
   LAXATIVES, SOFTENER/LUBRICANT 474
   LAXATIVES, STIMULANT 476
Feen-a-Mint Gum - See LAXATIVES,
   STIMULANT 476
Feen-a-Mint Pills - See
   LAXATIVES, SOFTENER/LUBRICANT 474
   LAXATIVES, STIMULANT 476
FELBAMATE 360
Felbatol - See FELBAMATE 360
Feldene - See ANTI-INFLAMMATORY DRUGS,
   NONSTEROIDAL (NSAIDs) 104
FELODIPINE - See CALCIUM CHANNEL
   BLOCKERS 192
Female sex hormone - See
   CONTRACEPTIVES, ORAL 262
Female sex hormone (estrogen) - See
   ESTROGENS 350
Female sex hormone (progestin) - See
   LEVONORGESTREL 488
   PROGESTINS 694
FemCare - See ANTIFUNGALS (Vaginal) 92
Femcet - See
   ACETAMINOPHEN 4

BARBITURATES 148
Femilax - See
   LAXATIVES, SOFTENER/LUBRICANT 474
   LAXATIVES, STIMULANT 476
Femiron - See IRON SUPPLEMENTS 444
Femizole Prefil - See ANTIFUNGALS (Vaginal)
   92
Femizole-7 - See ANTIFUNGALS (Vaginal) 92
Femogex - See ESTROGENS 350
Fempatch - See ESTROGENS 350
Femstat 3 - See ANTIFUNGALS (Vaginal) 92
Fendol - See
   ACETAMINOPHEN 4
   CAFFEINE 186
   GUAIFENESIN 398
   PHENYLEPHRINE 664
   SALICYLATES 744
Fenesin - See GUAIFENESIN 398
Fenicol Ophthalmic Ointment - See
   ANTIBACTERIALS (Ophthalmic) 68
FENOFIBRATE - See FIBRATES 362
FENOPROFEN - See ANTI-INFLAMMATORY
   DRUGS, NONSTEROIDAL (NSAIDs) 104
Fenopron - See ANTI-INFLAMMATORY
   DRUGS, NONSTEROIDAL (NSAIDs) 104
FENOTEROL - See BRONCHODILATORS,
   ADRENERGIC 174
FENTANYL - See NARCOTIC ANALGESICS 580
Fenylhist - See ANTIHISTAMINES 98
Feosol - See IRON SUPPLEMENTS 444
Feostat - See IRON SUPPLEMENTS 444
Feostat Drops - See IRON SUPPLEMENTS 444
Fergon - See IRON SUPPLEMENTS 444
Fer-In-Sol - See IRON SUPPLEMENTS 444
Fer-In-Sol Drops - See IRON SUPPLEMENTS
   444
Fer-In-Sol Syrup - See IRON SUPPLEMENTS
   444
Fer-Iron - See IRON SUPPLEMENTS 444
Fero-folic 500 - See IRON SUPPLEMENTS 444
Fero-Grad - See IRON SUPPLEMENTS 444
Fero-Gradumet - See IRON SUPPLEMENTS
   444
Ferralet - See IRON SUPPLEMENTS 444
Ferralyn - See IRON SUPPLEMENTS 444
Ferra-TD - See IRON SUPPLEMENTS 444
FERROUS FUMARATE - See IRON
   SUPPLEMENTS 444
FERROUS GLUCONATE - See IRON
   SUPPLEMENTS 444
FERROUS SULFATE - See IRON
   SUPPLEMENTS 444
Fertinic - See IRON SUPPLEMENTS 444
Fever reducer - See
   ACETAMINOPHEN 4
   ACETAMINOPHEN & SALICYLATES 6
   ANTI-INFLAMMATORY DRUGS,
      NONSTEROIDAL (NSAIDs) 104
   CHLORZOXAZONE & ACETAMINOPHEN 228
   NARCOTIC ANALGESICS &
      ACETAMINOPHEN 582

INDEX

INDEX

Gentacidin - See ANTIBACTERIALS
(Ophthalmic) 68
Gentafair - See ANTIBACTERIALS
(Ophthalmic) 68
Gentak - See ANTIBACTERIALS (Ophthalmic) 68
Gentamar - See ANTIBACTERIALS (Topical) 72
GENTAMICIN - See ANTIBACTERIALS
(Topical) 72
GENTAMICIN (Ophthalmic) - See
ANTIBACTERIALS (Ophthalmic) 68
GENTAMICIN (Otic) - See ANTIBACTERIALS
(Otic) 70
GENTIAN VIOLET - See ANTIFUNGALS
(Vaginal) 92
Gen-Timolol - See BETA-ADRENERGIC
BLOCKING AGENTS (Ophthalmic) 166
Gentlax-S - See
LAXATIVES, SOFTENER/LUBRICANT 474
LAXATIVES, STIMULANT 476
Gentle Nature - See LAXATIVES, STIMULANT
476
Gentrasul - See ANTIBACTERIALS
(Ophthalmic) 68
Geocillin - See PENICILLINS 648
Geopen Oral - See PENICILLINS 648
Geridium - See PHENAZOPYRIDINE 660
Gerimal - See ERGOLOID MESYLATES 338
Geritol Tablets - See IRON SUPPLEMENTS
444
Gesterol 50 - See PROGESTINS 694
Gesterol L.A. - See PROGESTINS 694
GG-CEN - See GUAIFENESIN 398
Glaucon - See ANTIGLAUCOMA, SHORT-
ACTING (Ophthalmic) 96
GLICLAZIDE - See ANTIDIABETIC AGENTS,
SULFONYLUREA 84
GLIMEPIRIDE - See ANTIDIABETIC AGENTS,
SULFONYLUREA 84
GLIPIZIDE - See ANTIDIABETIC AGENTS,
SULFONYLUREA 84
Glo-Sel - See ANTISEBORRHEICS (Topical) 118
GLUCAGON 390
Glucagon for Injection - See GLUCAGON 390
Glucamide - See ANTIDIABETIC AGENTS,
SULFONYLUREA 84
Glucophage - See METFORMIN 526
Glucotrol - See ANTIDIABETIC AGENTS,
SULFONYLUREA 84
Glucotrol XL - See ANTIDIABETIC AGENTS,
SULFONYLUREA 84
Glyate - See GUAIFENESIN 398
GLYBURIDE - See ANTIDIABETIC AGENTS,
SULFONYLUREA 84
Glycate - See ANTACIDS 54
GLYCERIN - See LAXATIVES, OSMOTIC 472
Glyceryl T - See THEOPHYLLINE &
GUAIFENESIN 784
Glyceryl Trinitrate - See NITRATES 602
Glycofed - See
GUAIFENESIN 398
PSEUDOEPHEDRINE 706

GLYCOPYRROLATE 392
Gly-Cort - See ADRENOCORTICOIDS (Topical)
16
Glycotuss - See GUAIFENESIN 398
Glycotuss-dM - See
DEXTROMETHORPHAN 296
GUAIFENESIN 398
Glydeine Cough - See
GUAIFENESIN 398
NARCOTIC ANALGESICS 580
Glynase PresTab - See ANTIDIABETIC
AGENTS, SULFONYLUREA 84
Glysennid - See LAXATIVES, STIMULANT 476
Glyset - See MIGLITOL 552
Glytuss - See GUAIFENESIN 398
G-Myticin Antibiotic - See ANTIBACTERIALS
(Topical) 72
GOLD COMPOUNDS 394
Gold compounds - See GOLD COMPOUNDS
394
GOLD SODIUM THIOMOLATE - See GOLD
COMPOUNDS 394
Gonad stimulant - See CLOMIPHENE 244
Gonadotropin inhibitor - See
DANAZOL 284
NAFARELIN 574
Gonak - See PROTECTANT (Ophthalmic) 702
Goniosoft - See PROTECTANT (Ophthalmic)
702
Goniosol - See PROTECTANT (Ophthalmic)
702
Goody's Extra Strength Tablet - See
ACETAMINOPHEN & SALICYLATES 6
Goody's Headache Powders - See
ACETAMINOPHEN & SALICYLATES 6
Gordochom Solution - See ANTIFUNGALS
(Topical) 90
Gordofilm - See KERATOLYTICS 464
Gotamine - See
CAFFEINE 186
ERGOTAMINE 342
GP-500 - See
GUAIFENESIN 398
PSEUDOEPHEDRINE 706
Gramcal - See CALCIUM SUPPLEMENTS 194
Gravol - See ANTIHISTAMINES 98
Gravol L/A - See ANTIHISTAMINES 98
GREPAFLOXACIN - See
FLUOROQUINOLONES 372
Grifulvin V - See GRISEOFULVIN 396
Grisactin - See GRISEOFULVIN 396
Grisactin Ultra - See GRISEOFULVIN 396
GRISEOFULVIN 396
Grisovin-FP - See GRISEOFULVIN 396
Gris-PEG - See GRISEOFULVIN 396
Guaifed - See
GUAIFENESIN 398
PSEUDOEPHEDRINE 706
Guaifed-PD - See
GUAIFENESIN 398
PSEUDOEPHEDRINE 706

GUAIFENESIN 398
GuaiMAX-D - See
  GUAIFENESIN 398
  PSEUDOEPHEDRINE 706
Guaipax - See
  GUAIFENESIN 398
  PHENYLPROPANOLAMINE 668
Guaiphed - See THEOPHYLLINE,
  EPHEDRINE, GUAIFENESIN &
  BARBITURATES 790
Guaitab - See
  GUAIFENESIN 398
  PSEUDOEPHEDRINE 706
GUANABENZ 400
GUANADREL 402
GUANETHIDINE 404
GUANETHIDINE & HYDROCHLOROTHIAZIDE
  406
GUANFACINE 408
GuiaCough CF - See
  DEXTROMETHORPHAN 296
  GUAIFENESIN 398
  PHENYLPROPANOLAMINE 668
GuiaCough PE - See
  GUAIFENESIN 398
  PSEUDOEPHEDRINE 706
Guiamid D.M. Liquid - See
  DEXTROMETHORPHAN 296
  GUAIFENESIN 398
Guiatuss A.C. - See
  GUAIFENESIN 398
  NARCOTIC ANALGESICS 580
Guiatuss CF - See
  DEXTROMETHORPHAN 296
  GUAIFENESIN 398
  PHENYLPROPANOLAMINE 668
Guiatuss DAC - See
  GUAIFENESIN 398
  NARCOTIC ANALGESICS 580
  PHENYLPROPANOLAMINE 668
Guiatuss PE - See
  GUAIFENESIN 398
  PSEUDOEPHEDRINE 706
Guiatuss-DM - See
  DEXTROMETHORPHAN 296
  GUAIFENESIN 398
Guiatussin DAC - See
  GUAIFENESIN 398
  NARCOTIC ANALGESICS 580
  PSEUDOEPHEDRINE 706
Guiatussin with Codeine Liquid - See
  GUAIFENESIN 398
  NARCOTIC ANALGESICS 580
Guiatussin with Dextromethorphan - See
  DEXTROMETHORPHAN 296
  GUAIFENESIN 398
G-Well - See PEDICULICIDES (Topical) 642
Gynecort - See ADRENOCORTICOIDS
  (Topical) 16
Gynecort 10 - See ADRENOCORTICOIDS
  (Topical) 16

Gyne-Lotrimin - See ANTIFUNGALS (Vaginal)
  92
Gyne-Lotrimin 3 - See ANTIFUNGALS
  (Vaginal) 92
Gynergen - See ERGOTAMINE 342
Gyno-Trosyd - See ANTIFUNGALS (Vaginal) 92
Gynogen L.A. 20 - See ESTROGENS 350
Gynogen L.A. 40 - See ESTROGENS 350
Gynol II Extra Strength - See
  CONTRACEPTIVES, VAGINAL
  (Spermicides) 264
Gynol II Original Formula - See
  CONTRACEPTIVES, VAGINAL
  (Spermicides) 264

H

H₂Oxyl 2.5 Gel - See BENZOYL PEROXIDE 158
H₂Oxyl 5 Gel - See BENZOYL PEROXIDE 158
H₂Oxyl 10 Gel - See BENZOYL PEROXIDE 158
H₂Oxyl 20 Gel - See BENZOYL PEROXIDE 158
Habitrol - See NICOTINE 598
Hair growth stimulant - See MINOXIDIL (Topical)
  556
HALAZEPAM - See BENZODIAZEPINES 156
Halciderm - See ADRENOCORTICOIDS
  (Topical) 16
HALCINONIDE (Topical) - See
  ADRENOCORTICOIDS (Topical) 16
Halcion - See TRIAZOLAM 818
Haldol - See HALOPERIDOL 410
Haldol Decanoate - See HALOPERIDOL 410
Haldol LA - See HALOPERIDOL 410
Halenol - See ACETAMINOPHEN 4
Halenol Extra Strength - See
  ACETAMINOPHEN 4
Halfan - See ANTIMALARIAL 112
Halfprin - See ASPIRIN 132
Halls Mentho-Lyptus - See
  PHENYLPROPANOLAMINE 668
*Halls Mentho-Lyptus Decongestant Cough
  Formula* - See
  DEXTROMETHORPHAN 296
  PHENYLPROPANOLAMINE 668
HALOBETASOL - See ADRENOCORTICOIDS
  (Topical) 16
Halodrin - See ANDROGENS & ESTROGENS
  40
HALOFANTRINE - See ANTIMALARIAL 112
Halofed - See PSEUDOEPHEDRINE 706
Halofed Adult Strength - See
  PSEUDOEPHEDRINE 706
Halog - See ADRENOCORTICOIDS (Topical) 16
Halog E - See ADRENOCORTICOIDS (Topical)
  16
HALOPERIDOL 410
HALOPROGIN - See ANTIFUNGALS (Topical)
  90
Halotestin - See ANDROGENS 38
Halotex - See ANTIFUNGALS (Topical) 90
Halotussin - See GUAIFENESIN 398

Halotussin-DM Expectorant - See
 DEXTROMETHORPHAN 296
 GUAIFENESIN 398
Halperon - See HALOPERIDOL 410
Haltran - See ANTI-INFLAMMATORY DRUGS,
 NONSTEROIDAL (NSAIDs) 104
Harmonyl - See RAUWOLFIA ALKALOIDS 724
Hayfebrol - See
 ANTIHISTAMINES 98
 PSEUDOEPHEDRINE 706
Hayley's M-O - See LAXATIVES, OSMOTIC 472
Head & Chest - See
 GUAIFENESIN 398
 PHENYLPROPANOLAMINE 668
 PSEUDOEPHEDRINE 706
Head & Shoulders - See ANTISEBORRHEICS
 (Topical) 118
**Head & Shoulders Antidandruff Cream
 Shampoo Normal to Dry Formula** - See
 ANTISEBORRHEICS (Topical) 118
**Head & Shoulders Antidandruff Cream
 Shampoo Normal to Oily Formula** - See
 ANTISEBORRHEICS (Topical) 118
**Head & Shoulders Antidandruff Lotion
 Shampoo 2 in 1 Formula** - See
 ANTISEBORRHEICS (Topical) 118
**Head & Shoulders Antidandruff Lotion
 Shampoo Normal to Dry Formula** - See
 ANTISEBORRHEICS (Topical) 118
**Head & Shoulders Antidandruff Lotion
 Shampoo Normal to Oily Formula** - See
 ANTISEBORRHEICS (Topical) 118
**Head & Shoulders Dry Scalp 2 in 1 Formula
 Lotion Shampoo** - See
 ANTISEBORRHEICS (Topical) 118
**Head & Shoulders Dry Scalp Conditioning
 Formula Lotion Shampoo** - See
 ANTISEBORRHEICS (Topical) 118
**Head & Shoulders Dry Scalp Regular
 Formula Lotion Shampoo** - See
 ANTISEBORRHEICS (Topical) 118
**Head & Shoulders Intensive Treatment 2 in 1
 Formula Dandruff Lotion Shampoo** - See
 ANTISEBORRHEICS (Topical) 118
**Head & Shoulders Intensive Treatment
 Conditioning Formula Dandruff Lotion
 Shampoo** - See ANTISEBORRHEICS
 (Topical) 118
**Head & Shoulders Intensive Treatment
 Regular Formula Dandruff Lotion
 Shampoo** - See ANTISEBORRHEICS
 (Topical) 118
Headstart - See ASPIRIN 132
Helidac - See
 BISMUTH SUBSALICYLATE 170
 METRONIDAZOLE 544
 TETRACYCLINES 782
Helmex - See ANTHELMINTICS 56
Hemocyte - See IRON SUPPLEMENTS 444

Hemorrheologic agent - See PENTOXIFYLLINE
 654
Hemril-HC - See HYDROCORTISONE (Rectal)
 420
Hepahydrin - See LAXATIVES, STIMULANT 476
Heptalac - See LAXATIVES, OSMOTIC 472
Heptogesic - See MEPROBAMATE & ASPIRIN
 520
Herbal Laxative - See LAXATIVES,
 STIMULANT 476
Herplex Eye Drops - See ANTIVIRALS
 (Ophthalmic) 126
Hexa-Betalin - See PYRIDOXINE (Vitamin B-6)
 710
Hexadrol - See ADRENOCORTICOIDS
 (Systemic) 14
Hexalol - See ATROPINE, HYOSCYAMINE,
 METHENAMINE, METHYLENE BLUE,
 PHENYLSALICYLATE & BENZOIC ACID 136
HHistafed C - See ANTIHISTAMINES 98
Hi-Cor 1.0 - See ADRENOCORTICOIDS
 (Topical) 16
Hi-Cor 2.5 - See ADRENOCORTICOIDS
 (Topical) 16
Hiprex - See METHENAMINE 528
Hip-Rex - See METHENAMINE 528
Hismanal - See ANTIHISTAMINES,
 NONSEDATING 100
Histabid Duracaps - See
 ANTIHISTAMINES 98
 PHENYLPROPANOLAMINE 668
Histafed C - See
 NARCOTIC ANALGESICS 580
 PSEUDOEPHEDRINE 706
Histagesic Modified - See
 ANTIHISTAMINES 98
 PHENYLEPHRINE 664
Histagesic Modified - See ACETAMINOPHEN 4
Histaject Modified - See ANTIHISTAMINES 98
Histalet - See
 ANTIHISTAMINES 98
 PSEUDOEPHEDRINE 706
Histalet Forte - See
 ANTIHISTAMINES 98
 PHENYLEPHRINE 664
 PHENYLPROPANOLAMINE 668
Histalet X - See
 GUAIFENESIN 398
 PSEUDOEPHEDRINE 706
Histalet-DM - See
 ANTIHISTAMINES 98
 DEXTROMETHORPHAN 296
 PSEUDOEPHEDRINE 706
Histamic - See
 ANTIHISTAMINES 98
 PHENYLEPHRINE 664
 PHENYLPROPANOLAMINE 668
Histamine H_2 antagonist - See HISTAMINE H_2
 RECEPTOR ANTAGONISTS 412
HISTAMINE H_2 RECEPTOR ANTAGONISTS 412

INDEX

HYDROCHLOROTHIAZIDE - See DIURETICS, THIAZIDE 324

Hydrocil Instant - See LAXATIVES, BULK-FORMING 470

HYDROCODONE - See NARCOTIC ANALGESICS 580

HYDROCODONE & ACETAMINOPHEN - See NARCOTIC ANALGESICS & ACETAMINOPHEN 582

HYDROCODONE & ASPIRIN - See NARCOTIC ANALGESICS & ASPIRIN 584

HYDROCODONE & HOMATROPINE - See NARCOTIC ANALGESICS 580

HYDROCODONE & IBUPROFEN - See NARCOTIC ANALGESICS 580

Hydrocodone with APAP - See NARCOTIC ANALGESICS & ACETAMINOPHEN 582

HYDROCORTISONE - See ANTI-INFLAMMATORY DRUGS, STEROIDAL (Ophthalmic) 108

HYDROCORTISONE & ACETIC ACID - See ANTIBACTERIALS (Otic) 70

HYDROCORTISONE (Cortisol) - See ADRENOCORTICOIDS (Systemic) 14

HYDROCORTISONE (Dental) - See ADRENOCORTICOIDS (Topical) 16

HYDROCORTISONE (otic) - See ANTI-INFLAMMATORY DRUGS, STEROIDAL (Otic) 110

HYDROCORTISONE (Rectal) 420

HYDROCORTISONE (Topical) - See ADRENOCORTICOIDS (Topical) 16

Hydrocortone - See ADRENOCORTICOIDS (Systemic) 14

Hydro-D - See DIURETICS, THIAZIDE 324

HydroDIURIL - See DIURETICS, THIAZIDE 324

HYDROFLUMETHIAZIDE - See DIURETICS, THIAZIDE 324

Hydrogesic - See NARCOTIC ANALGESICS & ACETAMINOPHEN 582

Hydromet - See
  ANTICHOLINERGICS 74
  NARCOTIC ANALGESICS 580

Hydromine - See
  NARCOTIC ANALGESICS 580
  PHENYLPROPANOLAMINE 668

Hydromine Pediatric - See
  NARCOTIC ANALGESICS 580
  PHENYLPROPANOLAMINE 668

HYDROMORPHONE - See NARCOTIC ANALGESICS 580

Hydromox - See DIURETICS, THIAZIDE 324

Hydropane - See
  ANTICHOLINERGICS 74
  NARCOTIC ANALGESICS 580

Hydrophed - See THEOPHYLLINE, EPHEDRINE & HYDROXYZINE 788

Hydrophen - See
  NARCOTIC ANALGESICS 580
  PHENYLPROPANOLAMINE 668

Hydropine - See RAUWOLFIA & THIAZIDE DIURETICS 722

Hydropine H.P. - See RAUWOLFIA ALKALOIDS 724

Hydropres - See RAUWOLFIA & THIAZIDE DIURETICS 722

Hydrosine - See RAUWOLFIA & THIAZIDE DIURETICS 722

Hydrostal IR - See NARCOTIC ANALGESICS 580

Hydrotensin - See RAUWOLFIA & THIAZIDE DIURETICS 722

Hydro-Tex - See ADRENOCORTICOIDS (Topical) 16

HYDROXOCOBALAMIN - See VITAMIN B-12 (Cyanocobalamin) 840

HYDROXYCHLOROQUINE 422

HYDROXYPROGESTERONE - See PROGESTINS 694

HYDROXYPROPYL CELLULOSE - See PROTECTANT (Ophthalmic) 702

HYDROXYPROPYL METHYLCELLULOSE - See PROTECTANT (Ophthalmic) 702

HYDROXYUREA 424

HYDROXYZINE 426

Hy/Gestrone - See PROGESTINS 694

Hygroton - See DIURETICS, THIAZIDE 324

Hylorel - See GUANADREL 402

Hylutin - See PROGESTINS 694

HYOSCYAMINE 428

HYOSCYAMINE & PHENOBARBITAL - See BELLADONNA ALKALOIDS & BARBITURATES 154

Hyosophen - See BELLADONNA ALKALOIDS & BARBITURATES 154

Hyperosmotic - See LAXATIVES, OSMOTIC 472

HY-PHEN - See NARCOTIC ANALGESICS & ACETAMINOPHEN 582

Hypopigmentation agent - See AZELAIC ACID 142

Hyprogest - See PROGESTINS 694

Hyproval P.A. - See PROGESTINS 694

Hyrexin-50 - See ANTIHISTAMINES 98

Hytakerol - See VITAMIN D 844

Hytinic - See IRON SUPPLEMENTS 444

Hytone - See ADRENOCORTICOIDS (Topical) 16

Hytrin - See ALPHA ADRENERGIC RECEPTOR BLOCKERS 22

Hytuss - See GUAIFENESIN 398

Hytuss-2X - See GUAIFENESIN 398

Hyzaar - See
  ANGIOTENSIN II RECEPTOR ANTAGONISTS 48
  DIURETICS, THIAZIDE 324

I

Ibifon-600 Caplets - See ANTI-INFLAMMATORY DRUGS, NONSTEROIDAL (NSAIDs) 104

Inflamase Forte - See ANTI-INFLAMMATORY DRUGS, STEROIDAL (Ophthalmic) 108
Inflamase-Mild - See ANTI-INFLAMMATORY DRUGS, STEROIDAL (Ophthalmic) 108
Inflammatory bowel disease suppressant - See OLSALAZINE 614
INH - See ISONIAZID 448
Insomnal - See ANTIHISTAMINES 98
Inspire - See XYLOMETAZOLINE 852
Insta-Char - See CHARCOAL, ACTIVATED 212
Insulatard NPH - See INSULIN 434
Insulatard NPH Human - See INSULIN 434
INSULIN 434
INSULIN LISPRO 436
Intal - See CROMOLYN 266
Inversine - See MECAMYLAMINE 508
Invirase - See PROTEASE INHIBITORS 700
IODOQUINOL 438
Ionamin - See APPETITE SUPPRESSANTS 130
Ionax Astringent Skin Cleanser Topical Solution - See KERATOLYTICS 464
Ionil Plus Shampoo - See KERATOLYTICS 464
Ionil Shampoo - See KERATOLYTICS 464
Ionil-T Plus - See COAL TAR (Topical) 254
IPECAC 440
Ipecac Syrup - See IPECAC 440
I-Pentolate - See CYCLOPENTOLATE (Ophthalmic) 274
I-Phrine - See PHENYLEPHRINE (Ophthalmic) 666
IPRATROPIUM 442
I-Pred - See ANTI-INFLAMMATORY DRUGS, STEROIDAL (Ophthalmic) 108
Ipsatol Cough Formula for Children - See DEXTROMETHORPHAN 296
GUAIFENESIN 398
PHENYLPROPANOLAMINE 668
IRBESARTAN - See ANGIOTENSIN II RECEPTOR ANTAGONISTS 48
Ircon - See IRON SUPPLEMENTS 444
IRON DEXTRAN - See IRON SUPPLEMENTS 444
IRON POLYSACCHARIDE - See IRON SUPPLEMENTS 444
IRON SORBITOL - See IRON SUPPLEMENTS 444
IRON SUPPLEMENTS 444
Ismelin - See GUANETHIDINE 404
Ismelin-Esidrix - See GUANETHIDINE & HYDROCHLOROTHIAZIDE 406
ISMO - See NITRATES 602
Iso-Acetazone - See ISOMETHEPTENE, DICHLORALPHENAZONE & ACETAMINOPHEN 446
Iso-Bid - See NITRATES 602
Isobutal - See
ASPIRIN 132
BARBITURATES 148
Isocet - See BARBITURATES 148
Isoclor - See
ANTIHISTAMINES 98
PSEUDOEPHEDRINE 706
Isoclor Expectorant - See
GUAIFENESIN 398
NARCOTIC ANALGESICS 580
PSEUDOEPHEDRINE 706
Isoclor Timesules - See ANTIHISTAMINES 98
Isoclor TimesulesKlerist-D - See
PSEUDOEPHEDRINE 706
Isocom - See ISOMETHEPTENE, DICHLORALPHENAZONE & ACETAMINOPHEN 446
ISOETHARINE - See BRONCHODILATORS, ADRENERGIC 174
ISOFLUROPHATE - See ANTIGLAUCOMA, LONG-ACTING (Ophthalmic) 94
Isolin - See
ASPIRIN 132
BARBITURATES 148
Isollyl Improved - See
ASPIRIN 132
BARBITURATES 148
Isollyl with Codeine - See BARBITURATES, ASPIRIN & CODEINE (Also contains caffeine) 150
ISOMETHEPTENE, DICHLORALPHENAZONE & ACETAMINOPHEN 446
Isonate - See NITRATES 602
ISONIAZID 448
Isopap - See
ACETAMINOPHEN 4
BARBITURATES 148
ISOPROPAMIDE - See ANTICHOLINERGICS 74
ISOPROTERENOL - See
BRONCHODILATORS, ADRENERGIC 174
ISOPROTERENOL & PHENYLEPHRINE 450
Isoptin - See CALCIUM CHANNEL BLOCKERS 192
Isoptin SR - See CALCIUM CHANNEL BLOCKERS 192
Isopto Alkaline - See PROTECTANT (Ophthalmic) 702
Isopto Atropine - See CYCLOPLEGIC, MYDRIATIC (Ophthalmic) 278
Isopto Carbachol - See ANTIGLAUCOMA, SHORT-ACTING (Ophthalmic) 96
Isopto Carpine - See PILOCARPINE 670
Isopto Cetamide - See ANTIBACTERIALS (Ophthalmic) 68
Isopto Eserine - See ANTIGLAUCOMA, SHORT-ACTING (Ophthalmic) 96
Isopto Frin - See PHENYLEPHRINE (Ophthalmic) 666
Isopto Homatropine - See CYCLOPLEGIC, MYDRIATIC (Ophthalmic) 278
Isopto Hyoscine - See CYCLOPLEGIC, MYDRIATIC (Ophthalmic) 278
Isopto Plain - See PROTECTANT (Ophthalmic) 702
Isopto Tears - See PROTECTANT (Ophthalmic) 702
Isorbid - See NITRATES 602

INDEX

INDEX

Lenoltec with Codeine No. 1 - See NARCOTIC ANALGESICS & ACETAMINOPHEN 582

Lenoltec with Codeine No. 2 - See NARCOTIC ANALGESICS & ACETAMINOPHEN 582

Lenoltec with Codeine No. 3 - See NARCOTIC ANALGESICS & ACETAMINOPHEN 582

Lenoltec with Codeine No. 4 - See NARCOTIC ANALGESICS & ACETAMINOPHEN 582

Lente - See INSULIN 434

Lente Iletin I - See INSULIN 434

Lente Iletin II - See INSULIN 434

Leponex - See CLOZAPINE 252

Lescol - See HMG-CoA REDUCTASE INHIBITORS 414

LEUCOVORIN 478

Leukeran - See CHLORAMBUCIL 218

LEUKOTRIENE MODIFIERS 480

LEVAMISOLE 482

Levaquin - See FLUOROQUINOLONES 372

Levate - See ANTIDEPRESSANTS, TRICYCLIC 82

Levatol - See BETA-ADRENERGIC BLOCKING AGENTS 162

Levbid - See HYOSCYAMINE 428

Levlen - See CONTRACEPTIVES, ORAL 262

Levlite - See CONTRACEPTIVES, ORAL 262

LEVOBUNOLOL (ophthalmic) - See BETA-ADRENERGIC BLOCKING AGENTS (Ophthalmic) 166

LEVOCABASTINE - See ANTIALLERGIC AGENTS (Ophthalmic) 62

LEVOCARNITINE 484

LEVODOPA 486

Levo-Dromoran - See NARCOTIC ANALGESICS 580

LEVOFLOXACIN - See FLUOROQUINOLONES 372

LEVONORGESTREL 488

LEVONORGESTREL & ETHINYL ESTRADIOL - See CONTRACEPTIVES, ORAL 262

Levoprome - See PHENOTHIAZINES 662

Levora - See CONTRACEPTIVES, ORAL 262

Levorphan - See NARCOTIC ANALGESICS 580

LEVORPHANOL - See NARCOTIC ANALGESICS 580

Levo-T - See THYROID HORMONES 798

Levothroid - See THYROID HORMONES 798

LEVOTHYROXINE - See THYROID HORMONES 798

Levoxyl - See THYROID HORMONES 798

Levsin - See HYOSCYAMINE 428

Levsin S/L - See HYOSCYAMINE 428

Levsin with Phenobarbital - See BELLADONNA ALKALOIDS & BARBITURATES 154

Levsinex - See HYOSCYAMINE 428

Levsinex Timecaps - See HYOSCYAMINE 428

Levsinex with Phenobarbital Timecaps - See BELLADONNA ALKALOIDS & BARBITURATES 154

Levsin-PB - See BELLADONNA ALKALOIDS & BARBITURATES 154

Lexxel - See
ANGIOTENSIN-COVERTING ENZYME (ACE) INHIBITORS 50
CALCIUM CHANNEL BLOCKERS 192

Librax - See
BENZODIAZEPINES 156
CLIDINIUM 240

Libritabs - See BENZODIAZEPINES 156

Librium - See BENZODIAZEPINES 156

Lice-Enz Foam And Comb Lice Killing Shampoo Kit - See PEDICULICIDES (Topical) 642

Licon - See ADRENOCORTICOIDS (Topical) 16

Lidemol - See ADRENOCORTICOIDS (Topical) 16

Lidex - See ADRENOCORTICOIDS (Topical) 16

Lidex-E - See ADRENOCORTICOIDS (Topical) 16

LIDOCAINE - See
ANESTHETICS (Mucosal-Local) 42
ANESTHETICS (Topical) 46

LIDOCAINE & PRILOCAINE - See ANESTHETICS (Topical) 46

Lidox - See CLIDINIUM 240

Lidoxide - See BENZODIAZEPINES 156

Life-Pred - See ANTI-INFLAMMATORY DRUGS, STEROIDAL (Ophthalmic) 108

Lignocaine - See ANESTHETICS (Topical) 46

Limbitrol - See
ANTIDEPRESSANTS, TRICYCLIC 82
BENZODIAZEPINES 156

Limbitrol DS - See
ANTIDEPRESSANTS, TRICYCLIC 82
BENZODIAZEPINES 156

Lincocin - See LINCOMYCIN 490

LINCOMYCIN 490

LINDANE - See PEDICULICIDES (Topical) 642

Lioresal - See BACLOFEN 146

LIOTHYRONINE - See THYROID HORMONES 798

LIOTRIX - See THYROID HORMONES 798

Lipancreatin - See PANCRELIPASE 630

Lipidil - See FIBRATES 362

Lipitor - See HMG-CoA REDUCTASE INHIBITORS 414

Lipoxide - See BENZODIAZEPINES 156

Liqui-Char - See CHARCOAL, ACTIVATED 212

Liqui-Doss - See LAXATIVES, SOFTENER/ LUBRICANT 474

Liquimat - See ANTIACNE, CLEANSING (Topical) 60

Liquiprin Children's Elixir - See ACETAMINOPHEN 4

Liquiprin Infants' Drops - See ACETAMINOPHEN 4

Liquor Carbonis Detergens - See COAL TAR (Topical) 254

INDEX

INDEX

1023

Medipren Caplets - See ANTI-
    INFLAMMATORY DRUGS,
    NONSTEROIDAL (NSAIDs) 104
Mediquell - See DEXTROMETHORPHAN 296
Mediquell Decongestant Formula - See
    DEXTROMETHORPHAN 296
    PSEUDOEPHEDRINE 706
Medi-Tran - See MEPROBAMATE 518
Medotar - See COAL TAR (Topical) 254
Medrol - See ADRENOCORTICOIDS
    (Systemic) 14
MEDROXYPROGESTERONE - See
    PROGESTINS 694
MEDRYSONE - See ANTI-INFLAMMATORY
    DRUGS, STEROIDAL (Ophthalmic) 108
MEFENAMIC ACID - See ANTI-
    INFLAMMATORY DRUGS,
    NONSTEROIDAL (NSAIDs) 104
MEFLOQUINE - See ANTIMALARIAL 112
Megace - See PROGESTINS 694
Megace Oral Suspension - See PROGESTINS
    694
Megacillin - See PENICILLINS 648
MEGESTROL - See PROGESTINS 694
MELATONIN 514
Melfiat-105 Unicelles - See APPETITE
    SUPPRESSANTS 130
Mellaril - See PHENOTHIAZINES 662
Mellaril Concentrate - See PHENOTHIAZINES
    662
Mellaril-S - See PHENOTHIAZINES 662
MELPHALAN 516
MENADIOL - See VITAMIN K 848
Menaval-20 - See ESTROGENS 350
Menest 4 - See ESTROGENS 350
Meni-D - See MECLIZINE 512
Menoject L.A. - See ANDROGENS &
    ESTROGENS 40
Mentax - See ANTIFUNGALS (Topical) 90
MEPENZOLATE - See ANTICHOLINERGICS 74
MEPERIDINE - See NARCOTIC ANALGESICS
    580
MEPERIDINE & ACETAMINOPHEN - See
    NARCOTIC ANALGESICS &
    ACETAMINOPHEN 582
MEPHENYTOIN - See ANTICONVULSANTS,
    HYDANTOIN 78
MEPHOBARBITAL - See BARBITURATES 148
Mephyton - See VITAMIN K 848
Mepro Analgesic - See MEPROBAMATE &
    ASPIRIN 520
MEPROBAMATE 518
MEPROBAMATE & ASPIRIN 520
Meprogese - See MEPROBAMATE & ASPIRIN
    520
Meprogesic - See MEPROBAMATE & ASPIRIN
    520
Meprogesic Q - See MEPROBAMATE &
    ASPIRIN 520

Meprolonel - See ADRENOCORTICOIDS
    (Systemic) 14
Mepron - See ATOVAQUONE 134
Meprospan 200 - See MEPROBAMATE 518
Meprospan 400 - See MEPROBAMATE 518
MERCAPTOPURINE 522
Meridia - See SIBUTRAMINE 752
MESALAMINE 524
Mesalazine - See MESALAMINE 524
Mesantoin - See ANTICONVULSANTS,
    HYDANTOIN 78
MESORIDAZINE - See PHENOTHIAZINES 662
Mestinon - See ANTIMYASTHENICS 114
Mestinon Timespans - See
    ANTIMYASTHENICS 114
Metaderm Mild - See ADRENOCORTICOIDS
    (Topical) 16
Metaderm Regular (Topical) - See
    ADRENOCORTICOIDS (Topical) 16
Metahydrin - See DIURETICS, THIAZIDE 324
Metamucil - See LAXATIVES, BULK-FORMING
    470
Metamucil Apple Crisp Fiber Wafers - See
    LAXATIVES, BULK-FORMING 470
Metamucil Cinnamon Spice Fiber Wafers -
    See LAXATIVES, BULK-FORMING 470
Metamucil Instant Mix, Orange Flavor - See
    LAXATIVES, BULK-FORMING 470
Metamucil Smooth Citrus Flavor - See
    LAXATIVES, BULK-FORMING 470
Metamucil Smooth Orange Flavor - See
    LAXATIVES, BULK-FORMING 470
Metamucil Smooth, Sugar-Free Citrus Flavor
    - See LAXATIVES, BULK-FORMING 470
Metamucil Smooth, Sugar-Free Orange
    Flavor - See LAXATIVES, BULK-FORMING
    470
Metamucil Smooth, Sugar-Free Regular
    Flavor - See LAXATIVES, BULK-FORMING
    470
Metamucil Sugar Free - See LAXATIVES,
    BULK-FORMING 470
Metamucil Sugar Free Citrus Flavor - See
    LAXATIVES, BULK-FORMING 470
Metamucil Sugar Free Lemon-Lime Flavor -
    See LAXATIVES, BULK-FORMING 470
Metamucil Sugar Free Orange Flavor - See
    LAXATIVES, BULK-FORMING 470
Metandren - See ANDROGENS 38
Metaprel - See BRONCHODILATORS,
    ADRENERGIC 174
METAPROTERENOL - See
    BRONCHODILATORS, ADRENERGIC 174
Metatensin - See RAUWOLFIA & THIAZIDE
    DIURETICS 722
METAXALONE - See MUSCLE RELAXANTS,
    SKELETAL 570
Meted Maximum Strength Anti-Dandruff
    Shampoo with Conditioners - See
    ANTISEBORRHEICS (Topical) 118
    KERATOLYTICS 464

Midol 200 - See ANTI-INFLAMMATORY
DRUGS, NONSTEROIDAL (NSAIDs) 104
Midol-IB - See ANTI-INFLAMMATORY DRUGS,
NONSTEROIDAL (NSAIDs) 104
Midquin - See ISOMETHEPTENE,
DICHLORALPHENAZONE &
ACETAMINOPHEN 446
Midrin - See ISOMETHEPTENE,
DICHLORALPHENAZONE &
ACETAMINOPHEN 446
Migergot - See
CAFFEINE 186
ERGOTAMINE 342
MIGLITOL 552
Migquin - See ISOMETHEPTENE,
DICHLORALPHENAZONE &
ACETAMINOPHEN 446
Migrapap - See ISOMETHEPTENE,
DICHLORALPHENAZONE &
ACETAMINOPHEN 446
Migratine - See ISOMETHEPTENE,
DICHLORALPHENAZONE &
ACETAMINOPHEN 446
Migrazone - See ISOMETHEPTENE,
DICHLORALPHENAZONE &
ACETAMINOPHEN 446
Migrend - See ISOMETHEPTENE,
DICHLORALPHENAZONE &
ACETAMINOPHEN 446
Migrex - See ISOMETHEPTENE,
DICHLORALPHENAZONE &
ACETAMINOPHEN 446
MILK OF MAGNESIA - See LAXATIVES,
OSMOTIC 472
Milkinol - See LAXATIVES, SOFTENER/
LUBRICANT 474
Milophene - See CLOMIPHENE 244
Miltown - See MEPROBAMATE 518
MINERAL OIL - See
LAXATIVES, OSMOTIC 472
LAXATIVES, SOFTENER/LUBRICANT 474
Mineral supplement (fluoride) - See SODIUM
FLUORIDE 760
Mineral supplement (iron) - See IRON
SUPPLEMENTS 444
Mineral supplement (potassium) - See
POTASSIUM SUPPLEMENTS 678
Minestrin 1/20 - See CONTRACEPTIVES,
ORAL 262
Minims Atropine - See CYCLOPLEGIC,
MYDRIATIC (Ophthalmic) 278
Minims Cyclopentolate - See
CYCLOPENTOLATE (Ophthalmic) 274
Minims Homatropine - See CYCLOPLEGIC,
MYDRIATIC (Ophthalmic) 278
Minims Phenylephrine - See
PHENYLEPHRINE (Ophthalmic) 666
Minims Pilocarpine - See PILOCARPINE 670
Minipress - See ALPHA ADRENERGIC
RECEPTOR BLOCKERS 22

Minitran - See NITRATES 602
Minizide - See
ALPHA ADRENERGIC RECEPTOR
BLOCKERS 22
DIURETICS, THIAZIDE 324
Minocin - See TETRACYCLINES 782
MINOCYCLINE - See TETRACYCLINES 782
Min-Ovral - See CONTRACEPTIVES, ORAL 262
MINOXIDIL 554
MINOXIDIL (Topical) 556
Mintezol - See ANTHELMINTICS 56
Mintezol Topical - See ANTHELMINTICS 56
Mintox - See ANTACIDS 54
Mintox Plus - See ANTACIDS 54
Minzolum - See ANTHELMINTICS 56
Miocarpine - See PILOCARPINE 670
Miostat - See ANTIGLAUCOMA, SHORT-
ACTING (Ophthalmic) 96
Miradon - See ANTICOAGULANTS (Oral) 76
Mirapex - See ANTIDYSKINETICS 86
MIRTAZAPINE 558
MISOPROSTOL 560
MITOTANE 562
Mitride - See ISOMETHEPTENE,
DICHLORALPHENAZONE &
ACETAMINOPHEN 446
Mitrolan - See LAXATIVES, BULK-FORMING
470
Mixtard - See INSULIN 434
Mixtard Human - See INSULIN 434
Moban - See MOLINDONE 564
Moban Concentrate - See MOLINDONE 564
Mobidin - See SALICYLATES 744
Mobiflex - See ANTI-INFLAMMATORY DRUGS,
NONSTEROIDAL (NSAIDs) 104
Modane - See LAXATIVES, STIMULANT 476
Modane Bulk - See LAXATIVES, BULK-
FORMING 470
Modane Plus - See LAXATIVES, SOFTENER/
LUBRICANT 474
Modane Soft - See LAXATIVES, SOFTENER/
LUBRICANT 474
Modecate - See PHENOTHIAZINES 662
Modecate Concentrate - See
PHENOTHIAZINES 662
ModiCon - See CONTRACEPTIVES, ORAL 262
Modified Shohl's Solution - See CITRATES
238
Moditen Enanthate - See PHENOTHIAZINES
662
Moditen HCl - See PHENOTHIAZINES 662
Moditen HCl-H.P - See PHENOTHIAZINES 662
Modrastane - See TRILOSTANE 820
Moduret - See DIURETICS, POTASSIUM-
SPARING & HYDROCHLOROTHIAZIDE 322
Moduretic - See DIURETICS, POTASSIUM-
SPARING & HYDROCHLOROTHIAZIDE 322
MOEXIPRIL - See ANGIOTENSIN-
CONVERTING ENZYME (ACE)
INHIBITORS 50

INDEX

1027

Mycolog II - See NYSTATIN 610
MYCOPHENOLATE - See
   IMMUNOSUPPRESSIVE AGENTS 430
Mycostatin - See
  ANTIFUNGALS (Topical) 90
  ANTIFUNGALS (Vaginal) 92
  NYSTATIN 610
Myco-Triacet II - See NYSTATIN 610
Mydfrin - See PHENYLEPHRINE (Ophthalmic)
  666
Mydriatic - See
  CYCLOPENTOLATE (Ophthalmic) 274
  CYCLOPLEGIC, MYDRIATIC (Ophthalmic) 278
  PHENYLEPHRINE (Ophthalmic) 666
My-E - See ERYTHROMYCINS 346
Myfed - See
  ANTIHISTAMINES 98
  PSEUDOEPHEDRINE 706
Myfedrine - See PSEUDOEPHEDRINE 706
Mygel - See
  ANTACIDS 54
  SIMETHICONE 756
Mygel II - See ANTACIDS 54
Myhistine - See
  ANTIHISTAMINES 98
  PHENYLEPHRINE 664
Myhistine DH - See
  ANTIHISTAMINES 98
  PSEUDOEPHEDRINE 706
Myhistine Expectorant - See
  GUAIFENESIN 398
  PSEUDOEPHEDRINE 706
Myhydromine - See
  NARCOTIC ANALGESICS 580
  PHENYLPROPANOLAMINE 668
Myhydromine Pediatric - See
  NARCOTIC ANALGESICS 580
  PHENYLPROPANOLAMINE 668
Myidil - See ANTIHISTAMINES 98
Myidone - See PRIMIDONE 682
Mykacet - See NYSTATIN 610
Mykacet II - See NYSTATIN 610
Mykrox - See DIURETICS, THIAZIDE 324
Mylagen - See ANTACIDS 54
Mylagen II - See ANTACIDS 54
Mylanta - See ANTACIDS 54
Mylanta Calcium-Rich - See ANTACIDS 54
Mylanta Calcium-Rich Double Strength - See
  ANTACIDS 54
Mylanta Double Strength - See ANTACIDS 54
Mylanta Double Strength Plain - See
  ANTACIDS 54
Mylanta Gas - See SIMETHICONE 756
Mylanta Gelcaps - See ANTACIDS 54
Mylanta Natural Fiber Supplement - See
  LAXATIVES, BULK-FORMING 470
Mylanta Plain - See ANTACIDS 54
**Mylanta Sugar Free Natural Fiber
  Supplement** - See LAXATIVES, BULK-
  FORMING 470

Mylanta-2 Extra Strength - See ANTACIDS 54
Mylanta-AR - See HISTAMINE H$_2$ RECEPTOR
  ANTAGONISTS 412
Mylanta-II - See ANTACIDS 54
Myleran - See BUSULFAN 182
Mylicon - See SIMETHICONE 756
Mylicon-80 - See SIMETHICONE 756
Mylicon-125 - See SIMETHICONE 756
Mymethasone - See ADRENOCORTICOIDS
  (Systemic) 14
Myminic Expectorant - See
  GUAIFENESIN 398
  PHENYLPROPANOLAMINE 668
Myminicol - See
  ANTIHISTAMINES 98
  DEXTROMETHORPHAN 296
  PHENYLPROPANOLAMINE 668
Myocrisin - See GOLD COMPOUNDS 394
Myolin - See ORPHENADRINE 616
Myotrol - See ORPHENADRINE 616
Myphetane DC Cough - See
  ANTIHISTAMINES 98
  NARCOTIC ANALGESICS 580
  PHENYLPROPANOLAMINE 668
Myphetapp - See
  ANTIHISTAMINES 98
  PHENYLPROPANOLAMINE 668
Myproic Acid - See VALPROIC ACID 832
Myrosemide - See DIURETICS, LOOP 318
Mysoline - See PRIMIDONE 682
Mytelase Caplets - See ANTIMYASTHENICS
  114
Mytrex - See NYSTATIN 610
Mytussin AC - See
  GUAIFENESIN 398
  NARCOTIC ANALGESICS 580
Mytussin DAC - See
  GUAIFENESIN 398
  NARCOTIC ANALGESICS 580
  PSEUDOEPHEDRINE 706
Mytussin DM - See
  DEXTROMETHORPHAN 296
  GUAIFENESIN 398
MZM - See CARBONIC ANHYDRASE
  INHIBITORS 206

N

N3 Gesic - See ORPHENADRINE, ASPIRIN &
  CAFFEINE 618
N3 Gesic Forte - See ORPHENADRINE,
  ASPIRIN & CAFFEINE 618
NABILONE 572
NABUMETONE - See ANTI-INFLAMMATORY
  DRUGS, NONSTEROIDAL (NSAIDs) 104
NADOLOL - See BETA-ADRENERGIC
  BLOCKING AGENTS 162
NADOLOL & BENDROFLUMETHIAZIDE - See
  BETA-ADRENERGIC BLOCKING AGENTS
  & THIAZIDE DIURETICS 164
Nadopen-V - See PENICILLINS 648

INDEX

Narcotic - See
BARBITURATES, ASPIRIN & CODEINE (Also
contains caffeine) 150
KAOLIN, PECTIN, BELLADONNA & OPIUM
462
NARCOTIC ANALGESICS 580
NARCOTIC ANALGESICS &
ACETAMINOPHEN 582
NARCOTIC ANALGESICS & ASPIRIN 584
PAREGORIC 638
Narcotic analgesic - See BUTORPHANOL 184
NARCOTIC ANALGESICS 580
NARCOTIC ANALGESICS &
ACETAMINOPHEN 582
NARCOTIC ANALGESICS & ASPIRIN 584
Narcotic antagonist - See NALTREXONE 578
Nardil - See MONOAMINE OXIDASE (MAO)
INHIBITORS 566
Nasacort - See ADRENOCORTICOIDS (Nasal
Inhalation) 10
Nasacort AQ - See ADRENOCORTICOIDS
(Nasal Inhalation) 10
Nasahist - See
ANTIHISTAMINES 98
PHENYLEPHRINE 664
PHENYLPROPANOLAMINE 668
Nasahist B - See ANTIHISTAMINES 98
Nasal decongestant - See CROMOLYN 266
Nasal Decongestant Spray - See
OXYMETAZOLINE (Nasal) 624
Nasal Relief - See OXYMETAZOLINE (Nasal)
624
Nasal Spray 12-Hour - See OXYMETAZOLINE
(Nasal) 624
Nasal Spray Long Acting - See
OXYMETAZOLINE (Nasal) 624
Nasal-12 Hour - See OXYMETAZOLINE (Nasal)
624
Nasalcrom - See CROMOLYN 266
Nasalide - See ADRENOCORTICOIDS (Nasal
Inhalation) 10
Nasarel - See ADRENOCORTICOIDS (Nasal
Inhalation) 10
Nasatab LA - See
GUAIFENESIN 398
PSEUDOEPHEDRINE 706
Nasonex - See ADRENOCORTICOIDS (Nasal
Inhalation) 10
Natacyn - See NATAMYCIN (Ophthalmic) 586
NATAMYCIN (Ophthalmic) 586
Natulan - See PROCARBAZINE 692
Naturacil - See LAXATIVES, BULK-FORMING
470
Natural Source Fibre Laxative - See
LAXATIVES, BULK-FORMING 470
Nature's Remedy - See LAXATIVES,
STIMULANT 476
Nature's Tears - See PROTECTANT
(Ophthalmic) 702
Naturetin - See DIURETICS, THIAZIDE 324
Nauseatol - See ANTIHISTAMINES 98

Navane - See THIOTHIXENE 796
Naxen - See ANTI-INFLAMMATORY DRUGS,
NONSTEROIDAL (NSAIDs) 104
ND Clear T.D. - See
ANTIHISTAMINES 98
PSEUDOEPHEDRINE 706
ND Stat Revised - See ANTIHISTAMINES 98
ND-Gesic - See
ACETAMINOPHEN 4
ANTIHISTAMINES 98
PHENYLEPHRINE 664
NebuPent - See PENTAMIDINE 652
Necon 0.5/35-21 - See CONTRACEPTIVES,
ORAL 262
Necon 0.5/35-28 - See CONTRACEPTIVES,
ORAL 262
Necon 1/35-21 - See CONTRACEPTIVES,
ORAL 262
Necon 1/35-28 - See CONTRACEPTIVES,
ORAL 262
Necon 1/50-21 - See CONTRACEPTIVES,
ORAL 262
Necon 1/50-28 - See CONTRACEPTIVES,
ORAL 262
Necon 10/11-21 - See CONTRACEPTIVES,
ORAL 262
Necon 10/11-28 - See CONTRACEPTIVES,
ORAL 262
NEDOCROMIL 588
N.E.E. 1/35 - See CONTRACEPTIVES, ORAL
262
N.E.E. 1/50 - See CONTRACEPTIVES, ORAL
262
NEFAZODONE 590
NegGram - See NALIDIXIC ACID 576
NELFINAVIR - See PROTEASE INHIBITORS
700
Nelova 0.5/35E - See CONTRACEPTIVES,
ORAL 262
Nelova 1/35E - See CONTRACEPTIVES, ORAL
262
Nelova 1/50M - See CONTRACEPTIVES, ORAL
262
Nelova 10/11 - See CONTRACEPTIVES, ORAL
262
Nelulen 1/35E - See CONTRACEPTIVES,
ORAL 262
Nelulen 1/50E - See CONTRACEPTIVES,
ORAL 262
Nemasole - See ANTHELMINTICS 56
Nembutal - See BARBITURATES 148
Neo-Calglucon - See CALCIUM
SUPPLEMENTS 194
Neociden Ophthalmic Ointment - See
ANTIBACTERIALS (Ophthalmic) 68
Neociden Ophthalmic Solution - See
ANTIBACTERIALS (Ophthalmic) 68
NeoCitran A - See
ANTIHISTAMINES 98
PHENYLEPHRINE 664

NEVIRAPINE - See NON-NUCLEOSIDE
   REVERSE TRANSCRIPTASE INHIBITORS
   606
New-Decongest Pediatric - See
   ANTIHISTAMINES 98
   PHENYLEPHRINE 664
   PHENYLPROPANOLAMINE 668
New-Decongest Pediatric Syrup - See
   ANTIHISTAMINES 98
   PHENYLEPHRINE 664
   PHENYLPROPANOLAMINE 668
Nia-Bid - See NIACIN (Vitamin B-3, Nicotinic
   Acid, Nicotinamide) 596
Niac - See NIACIN (Vitamin B-3, Nicotinic Acid,
   Nicotinamide) 596
Niacels - See NIACIN (Vitamin B-3, Nicotinic
   Acid, Nicotinamide) 596
Niacin - See NIACIN (Vitamin B-3, Nicotinic
   Acid, Nicotinamide) 596
NIACIN (Vitamin B-3, Nicotinic Acid,
   Nicotinamide) 596
Niacor - See NIACIN (Vitamin B-3, Nicotinic
   Acid, Nicotinamide) 596
NICARDIPINE - See CALCIUM CHANNEL
   BLOCKERS 192
Nico-400 - See NIACIN (Vitamin B-3, Nicotinic
   Acid, Nicotinamide) 596
Nicobid - See NIACIN (Vitamin B-3, Nicotinic
   Acid, Nicotinamide) 596
Nicoderm - See NICOTINE 598
Nicoderm CQ - See NICOTINE 598
Nicolar - See NIACIN (Vitamin B-3, Nicotinic
   Acid, Nicotinamide) 596
Nicorette - See NICOTINE 598
Nicorette DS - See NICOTINE 598
Nicotinamide - See NIACIN (Vitamin B-3,
   Nicotinic Acid, Nicotinamide) 596
NICOTINE 598
Nicotinex - See NIACIN (Vitamin B-3, Nicotinic
   Acid, Nicotinamide) 596
Nicotinic Acid - See NIACIN (Vitamin B-3,
   Nicotinic Acid, Nicotinamide) 596
Nicotinyl alcohol - See NIACIN (Vitamin B-3,
   Nicotinic Acid, Nicotinamide) 596
Nicotrol - See NICOTINE 598
Nicotrol NS - See NICOTINE 598
Nico-Vert - See ANTIHISTAMINES 98
Nidryl - See ANTIHISTAMINES 98
NIFEDIPINE - See CALCIUM CHANNEL
   BLOCKERS 192
Niferex - See IRON SUPPLEMENTS 444
Niferex-150 - See IRON SUPPLEMENTS 444
Nifuran - See NITROFURANTOIN 604
Night Cast R - See KERATOLYTICS 464
Night Cast Regular Formula Mask-Lotion - See
   KERATOLYTICS 464
Night Cast Special Formula Mask-Lotion - See
   KERATOLYTICS 464
Night-Time Effervescent Cold - See
   ANTIHISTAMINES 98

ASPIRIN 132
   PHENYLPROPANOLAMINE 668
Nighttime Pamprin - See ACETAMINOPHEN 4
Niloric - See ERGOLOID MESYLATES 338
Nilstat - See
   ANTIFUNGALS (Topical) 90
   ANTIFUNGALS (Vaginal) 92
   NYSTATIN 610
NIMODIPINE 600
Nimotop - See NIMODIPINE 600
Niong - See NITRATES 602
Nisaval - See ANTIHISTAMINES 98
NISOLDIPINE - See CALCIUM CHANNEL
   BLOCKERS 192
NITRATES 602
NITRAZEPAM - See BENZODIAZEPINES 156
Nitrex - See NITROFURANTOIN 604
Nitro-Bid - See NITRATES 602
Nitrocap - See NITRATES 602
Nitrocap T.D. - See NITRATES 602
Nitrocine - See NITRATES 602
Nitrodisc - See NITRATES 602
Nitro-Dur - See NITRATES 602
Nitro-Dur II - See NITRATES 602
Nitrofan - See NITROFURANTOIN 604
Nitrofor - See NITROFURANTOIN 604
Nitrofuracot - See NITROFURANTOIN 604
NITROFURANTOIN 604
Nitrogard-SR - See NITRATES 602
NITROGLYCERIN (GLYCERYL TRINITRATE) -
   See NITRATES 602
Nitroglyn - See NITRATES 602
Nitrol - See NITRATES 602
Nitrolin - See NITRATES 602
Nitrolingual - See NITRATES 602
Nitronet - See NITRATES 602
Nitrong - See NITRATES 602
Nitrong SR - See NITRATES 602
Nitrospan - See NITRATES 602
Nitrostat - See NITRATES 602
Nix Cream Rinse - See PEDICULICIDES
   (Topical) 642
NIZATIDINE - See HISTAMINE H_2 RECEPTOR
   ANTAGONISTS 412
Nizoral - See KETOCONAZOLE 466
Nizoral Shampoo - See ANTIFUNGALS
   (Topical) 90
Noctec - See CHLORAL HYDRATE 216
Nolahist - See ANTIHISTAMINES 98
Nolamine - See
   ANTIHISTAMINES 98
   PHENYLPROPANOLAMINE 668
Nolex LA - See
   GUAIFENESIN 398
   PHENYLPROPANOLAMINE 668
Nolvadex - See TAMOXIFEN 776
Nolvadex-D - See TAMOXIFEN 776
NON-NUCLEOSIDE REVERSE
   TRANSCRIPTASE INHIBITORS 606

INDEX

Nucochem Expectorant - See
GUAIFENESIN 398
NARCOTIC ANALGESICS 580
PSEUDOEPHEDRINE 706
Nucochem Pediatric Expectorant - See
GUAIFENESIN 398
NARCOTIC ANALGESICS 580
PSEUDOEPHEDRINE 706
Nucofed - See
NARCOTIC ANALGESICS 580
PSEUDOEPHEDRINE 706
Nucofed Expectorant - See
GUAIFENESIN 398
NARCOTIC ANALGESICS 580
PSEUDOEPHEDRINE 706
Nucofed Pediatric Expectorant - See
GUAIFENESIN 398
NARCOTIC ANALGESICS 580
PSEUDOEPHEDRINE 706
Nu-Cotrimox - See
SULFONAMIDES 770
TRIMETHOPRIM 824
Nu-Cotrimox DS - See
SULFONAMIDES 770
TRIMETHOPRIM 824
Nu-Diltiaz - See CALCIUM CHANNEL
BLOCKERS 192
Nu-Indo - See ANTI-INFLAMMATORY DRUGS,
NONSTEROIDAL (NSAIDs) 104
Nu-Iron - See IRON SUPPLEMENTS 444
Nu-Iron 150 - See IRON SUPPLEMENTS 444
Nujol - See LAXATIVES, SOFTENER/
LUBRICANT 474
Nu-Loraz - See BENZODIAZEPINES 156
Nu-Medopa - See METHYLDOPA 532
NuMetop - See BETA-ADRENERGIC
BLOCKING AGENTS 162
Numorphan - See NARCOTIC ANALGESICS
580
Numzident - See ANESTHETICS (Mucosal-
Local) 42
Num-Zit Gel - See ANESTHETICS (Mucosal-
Local) 42
Num-Zit Lotion - See ANESTHETICS (Mucosal-
Local) 42
Nu-Nifed - See CALCIUM CHANNEL
BLOCKERS 192
Nu-Pen-VK - See PENICILLINS 648
Nupercainal - See ANESTHETICS (Rectal) 44
Nupercainal Cream - See ANESTHETICS
(Topical) 46
Nupercainal Ointment - See ANESTHETICS
(Topical) 46
Nu-Pirox - See ANTI-INFLAMMATORY
DRUGS, NONSTEROIDAL (NSAIDs) 104
Nuprin - See ANTI-INFLAMMATORY DRUGS,
NONSTEROIDAL (NSAIDs) 104
Nuprin Caplets - See ANTI-INFLAMMATORY
DRUGS, NONSTEROIDAL (NSAIDs) 104
Nu-Tetra - See TETRACYCLINES 782

Nu-Timolol - See BETA-ADRENERGIC
BLOCKING AGENTS (Ophthalmic) 166
Nutracort - See ADRENOCORTICOIDS
(Topical) 16
Nu-Triazo - See TRIAZOLAM 818
Nutritional supplement - See
BETA CAROTENE 160
LEVOCARNITINE 484
Nutritional supplement (mineral) - See ZINC
SUPPLEMENTS 856
Nu-Verap - See CALCIUM CHANNEL
BLOCKERS 192
Nyaderm - See
ANTIFUNGALS (Topical) 90
ANTIFUNGALS (Vaginal) 92
Nydrazid - See ISONIAZID 448
NyQuil Hot Therapy - See
ACETAMINOPHEN 4
DEXTROMETHORPHAN 296
PSEUDOEPHEDRINE 706
NyQuil Liquicaps - See
ACETAMINOPHEN 4
ANTIHISTAMINES 98
DEXTROMETHORPHAN 296
PSEUDOEPHEDRINE 706
NyQuil Nighttime Colds Medicine - See
ACETAMINOPHEN 4
ANTIHISTAMINES 98
DEXTROMETHORPHAN 296
PSEUDOEPHEDRINE 706
Nystaform - See NYSTATIN 610
NYSTATIN 610
NYSTATIN - See
ANTIFUNGALS (Topical) 90
ANTIFUNGALS (Vaginal) 92
Nystex - See
ANTIFUNGALS (Topical) 90
NYSTATIN 610
Nystop - See ANTIFUNGALS (Topical) 90
Nytcold Medicine - See
ACETAMINOPHEN 4
DEXTROMETHORPHAN 296
PSEUDOEPHEDRINE 706
Nytilax - See LAXATIVES, STIMULANT 476
Nytime Cold Medicine Liquid - See
ACETAMINOPHEN 4
ANTIHISTAMINES 98
DEXTROMETHORPHAN 296
PSEUDOEPHEDRINE 706
Nytol Maximum Strength - See
ANTIHISTAMINES 98
Nytol with DPH - See ANTIHISTAMINES 98

O

OB - See ANDROGENS & ESTROGENS 40
Obalan - See APPETITE SUPPRESSANTS 130
Obe-Del - See APPETITE SUPPRESSANTS 130
Obe-Mar - See APPETITE SUPPRESSANTS 130
Obe-Nix - See APPETITE SUPPRESSANTS 130

INDEX

Ophtho-Chloram Ophthalmic Solution - See
ANTIBACTERIALS (Ophthalmic) 68
Ophtho-Dipivefrin - See ANTIGLAUCOMA,
SHORT-ACTING (Ophthalmic) 96
OPIUM - See NARCOTIC ANALGESICS 580
Opticrom - See CROMOLYN 266
Optimine - See ANTIHISTAMINES 98
OptiPranolol - See BETA-ADRENERGIC
BLOCKING AGENTS (Ophthalmic) 166
Orabase HCA - See ADRENOCORTICOIDS
(Topical) 16
Orabase-B with Benzocaine - See
ANESTHETICS (Mucosal-Local) 42
Oracit - See CITRATES 238
Oracort - See ADRENOCORTICOIDS (Topical)
16
Oradexon - See ADRENOCORTICOIDS
(Systemic) 14
Oragest S.R. - See
ANTIHISTAMINES 98
PHENYLPROPANOLAMINE 668
Orajel Extra Strength - See ANESTHETICS
(Mucosal-Local) 42
Orajel Liquid - See ANESTHETICS (Mucosal-
Local) 42
Orajel Maximum Strength - See
ANESTHETICS (Mucosal-Local) 42
Oral rehydration salts - See
CARBOHYDRATES & ELECTROLYTES 204
Oralone - See ADRENOCORTICOIDS (Topical)
16
Oraminic II - See ANTIHISTAMINES 98
Oraminic Spancaps - See
ANTIHISTAMINES 98
PHENYLPROPANOLAMINE 668
Oramorph - See NARCOTIC ANALGESICS 580
Oramorph-SR - See NARCOTIC ANALGESICS
580
Orap - See ANTIDYSKINETICS 86
Oraphen-PD - See ACETAMINOPHEN 4
Orasone 1 - See ADRENOCORTICOIDS
(Systemic) 14
Orasone 5 - See ADRENOCORTICOIDS
(Systemic) 14
Orasone 10 - See ADRENOCORTICOIDS
(Systemic) 14
Orasone 20 - See ADRENOCORTICOIDS
(Systemic) 14
Orasone 50 - See ADRENOCORTICOIDS
(Systemic) 14
Oratect Gel - See ANESTHETICS (Mucosal-
Local) 42
Ora-Testryl - See ANDROGENS 38
Orazinc - See ZINC SUPPLEMENTS 856
Orbenin - See PENICILLINS 648
Oretic - See DIURETICS, THIAZIDE 324
Oreticyl - See RAUWOLFIA & THIAZIDE
DIURETICS 722
Oreticyl Forte - See RAUWOLFIA & THIAZIDE
DIURETICS 722

Oreton - See ANDROGENS 38
Orflagen - See ORPHENADRINE 616
Orfro - See ORPHENADRINE 616
Organidin - See GUAIFENESIN 398
Orinase - See ANTIDIABETIC AGENTS,
SULFONYLUREA 84
Ornade - See
ANTIHISTAMINES 98
PHENYLPROPANOLAMINE 668
Ornade A.F. - See
ANTIHISTAMINES 98
PHENYLPROPANOLAMINE 668
Ornade Expectorant - See
ANTIHISTAMINES 98
GUAIFENESIN 398
PHENYLPROPANOLAMINE 668
Ornade Spansules - See ANTIHISTAMINES 98
Ornade-DM - See PHENYLPROPANOLAMINE
668
Ornade-DM 10 - See
ANTIHISTAMINES 98
DEXTROMETHORPHAN 296
PHENYLPROPANOLAMINE 668
Ornade-DM 15 - See
ANTIHISTAMINES 98
DEXTROMETHORPHAN 296
PHENYLPROPANOLAMINE 668
Ornade-DM 30 - See
ANTIHISTAMINES 98
DEXTROMETHORPHAN 296
PHENYLPROPANOLAMINE 668
Ornex DM 15 - See DEXTROMETHORPHAN
296
Ornex DM 30 - See DEXTROMETHORPHAN
296
Ornex Maximum Strength Caplets - See
ACETAMINOPHEN 4
PSEUDOEPHEDRINE 706
Ornex No Drowsiness Caplets - See
ACETAMINOPHEN 4
PSEUDOEPHEDRINE 706
Ornex Severe Cold No Drowsiness Caplets -
See
DEXTROMETHORPHAN 296
PSEUDOEPHEDRINE 706
ORPHENADRINE 616
ORPHENADRINE, ASPIRIN & CAFFEINE 618
Orphenagesic - See ORPHENADRINE,
ASPIRIN & CAFFEINE 618
Orphenagesic Forte - See ORPHENADRINE,
ASPIRIN & CAFFEINE 618
Orphenate - See ORPHENADRINE 616
ORS-bicarbonate - See CARBOHYDRATES &
ELECTROLYTES 204
ORS-citrate - See CARBOHYDRATES &
ELECTROLYTES 204
Ortega Otic-M - See ANTIBACTERIALS (Otic)
70
Ortho 0.5/35 - See CONTRACEPTIVES, ORAL
262

INDEX

Pediacof Cough - See
  ANTIHISTAMINES 98
  NARCOTIC ANALGESICS 580
  PHENYLEPHRINE 664
Pediaflor - See SODIUM FLUORIDE 760
Pedialyte - See CARBOHYDRATES &
  ELECTROLYTES 204
Pedialyte Freezer Pops - See
  CARBOHYDRATES & ELECTROLYTES 204
Pediapred - See ADRENOCORTICOIDS
  (Systemic) 14
Pediatric Aqueous Charcodote - See
  CHARCOAL, ACTIVATED 212
Pediatric Charcodote - See CHARCOAL,
  ACTIVATED 212
Pediatuss Cough - See
  NARCOTIC ANALGESICS 580
  PHENYLEPHRINE 664
Pediazole - See
  ERYTHROMYCINS 346
  SULFONAMIDES 770
Pediculicide - See PEDICULICIDES (Topical)
  642
PEDICULICIDES (Topical) 642
Pedi-Dent - See SODIUM FLUORIDE 760
Pediotic - See ANTIBACTERIALS (Otic) 70
Pedric - See ACETAMINOPHEN 4
Peganone - See ANTICONVULSANTS,
  HYDANTOIN 78
Pelamine - See ANTIHISTAMINES 98
PEMOLINE 644
Pen Vee - See PENICILLINS 648
Pen Vee K - See PENICILLINS 648
Penazine VC with Cough - See
  ANTIHISTAMINES, PHENOTHIAZINE-
  DERIVATIVE 102
  NARCOTIC ANALGESICS 580
Penbritin - See PENICILLINS 648
PENBUTOLOL - See BETA-ADRENERGIC
  BLOCKING AGENTS 162
PENCICLOVIR - See ANTIVIRALS (Topical) 128
Penecort - See ADRENOCORTICOIDS
  (Topical) 16
Penetrex - See FLUOROQUINOLONES 372
Penglobe - See PENICILLINS 648
PENICILLAMINE 646
PENICILLIN G - See PENICILLINS 648
PENICILLIN V - See PENICILLINS 648
PENICILLINS 648
PENICILLINS & BETA-LACTAMASE
  INHIBITORS 650
Pentacarinat - See PENTAMIDINE 652
Pentacort - See ADRENOCORTICOIDS
  (Topical) 16
PENTAERYTHRITOL TETRANITRATE - See
  NITRATES 602
PENTAMIDINE 652
Pentamycetin - See ANTIBACTERIALS
  (Ophthalmic) 68
Pentamycetin Ophthalmic Ointment - See
  ANTIBACTERIALS (Ophthalmic) 68

Pentamycetin Ophthalmic Solution - See
  ANTIBACTERIALS (Ophthalmic) 68
Pentasa - See MESALAMINE 524
Pentazine - See ANTIHISTAMINES,
  PHENOTHIAZINE-DERIVATIVE 102
PENTAZOCINE - See NARCOTIC
  ANALGESICS 580
PENTAZOCINE & ACETAMINOPHEN - See
  NARCOTIC ANALGESICS &
  ACETAMINOPHEN 582
PENTAZOCINE & ASPIRIN - See NARCOTIC
  ANALGESICS & ASPIRIN 584
Pentids - See PENICILLINS 648
PENTOBARBITAL - See BARBITURATES 148
Pentolair - See CYCLOPENTOLATE
  (Ophthalmic) 274
PENTOXIFYLLINE 654
**Pentrax Extra-Strength Therapeutic Tar
  Shampoo** - See COAL TAR (Topical) 254
Pentrax Tar Shampoo - See COAL TAR
  (Topical) 254
Pentritol - See NITRATES 602
Pentylan - See NITRATES 602
Pep-Back - See CAFFEINE 186
Pepcid - See HISTAMINE H_2 RECEPTOR
  ANTAGONISTS 412
Pepcid AC - See HISTAMINE H_2 RECEPTOR
  ANTAGONISTS 412
Pepto Diarrhea Control - See LOPERAMIDE
  496
Pepto-Bismol - See BISMUTH
  SUBSALICYLATE 170
Peptol - See HISTAMINE H_2 RECEPTOR
  ANTAGONISTS 412
Percocet - See NARCOTIC ANALGESICS &
  ACETAMINOPHEN 582
Percocet-Demi - See NARCOTIC
  ANALGESICS & ACETAMINOPHEN 582
Percodan - See NARCOTIC ANALGESICS &
  ASPIRIN 584
Percodan-Demi - See NARCOTIC
  ANALGESICS & ASPIRIN 584
Perdiem - See
  LAXATIVES, BULK-FORMING 470
  LAXATIVES, STIMULANT 476
Perdiem Fiber - See LAXATIVES, BULK-
  FORMING 470
Perdiem Plain - See LAXATIVES, BULK-
  FORMING 470
PERGOLIDE 656
Periactin - See ANTIHISTAMINES 98
Peri-Colace - See LAXATIVES, STIMULANT 476
Peri-Colase - See LAXATIVES, SOFTENER/
  LUBRICANT 474
PERICYAZINE - See PHENOTHIAZINES 662
Peridex - See CHLORHEXIDINE 222
Peridol - See HALOPERIDOL 410
PERINDOPRIL - See ANGIOTENSIN-
  CONVERTING ENZYME (ACE)
  INHIBITORS 50
Periochip - See CHLORHEXIDINE 222

Pneumomist - See GUAIFENESIN 398
Pneumopent - See PENTAMIDINE 652
PODOFILOX - See CONDYLOMA
    ACUMINATUM AGENTS 260
Podofin - See CONDYLOMA ACUMINATUM
    AGENTS 260
PODOPHYLLUM - See CONDYLOMA
    ACUMINATUM AGENTS 260
Poladex T.D. - See ANTIHISTAMINES 98
Polaramine - See ANTIHISTAMINES 98
Polaramine Expectorant - See
    ANTIHISTAMINES 98
    GUAIFENESIN 398
    PSEUDOEPHEDRINE 706
Polaramine Repetabs - See ANTIHISTAMINES
    98
POLOXAMER 188 - See LAXATIVES,
    SOFTENER/LUBRICANT 474
POLYCARBOPHIL - See LAXATIVES, BULK-
    FORMING 470
Polycillin - See PENICILLINS 648
Polycitra - See CITRATES 238
Polycitra LC - See CITRATES 238
Polycitra-K - See CITRATES 238
Polygesic - See NARCOTIC ANALGESICS &
    ACETAMINOPHEN 582
Poly-Histine Expectorant Plain - See
    GUAIFENESIN 398
Poly-Histine-CS - See
    ANTIHISTAMINES 98
    NARCOTIC ANALGESICS 580
    PHENYLPROPANOLAMINE 668
Poly-Histine-D - See
    ANTIHISTAMINES 98
    PHENYLPROPANOLAMINE 668
Poly-Histine-D Ped - See
    ANTIHISTAMINES 98
    PHENYLPROPANOLAMINE 668
Poly-Histine-DM - See
    ANTIHISTAMINES 98
    DEXTROMETHORPHAN 296
    PHENYLPROPANOLAMINE 668
Polymox - See PENICILLINS 648
POLYMYXIN B - See ANTIBACTERIALS
    (Ophthalmic) 68
POLYTHIAZIDE - See DIURETICS, THIAZIDE
    324
Poly-Vi-Flor - See VITAMINS & FLUORIDE 850
Pondocillin - See PENICILLINS 648
Ponstan - See ANTI-INFLAMMATORY DRUGS,
    NONSTEROIDAL (NSAIDs) 104
Ponstel - See ANTI-INFLAMMATORY DRUGS,
    NONSTEROIDAL (NSAIDs) 104
Pontocaine Cream - See
    ANESTHETICS (Rectal) 44
    ANESTHETICS (Topical) 46
Pontocaine Ointment - See
    ANESTHETICS (Rectal) 44
    ANESTHETICS (Topical) 46
Portalac - See LAXATIVES, OSMOTIC 472

Postacne - See ANTIACNE, CLEANSING
    (Topical) 60
Posture - See CALCIUM SUPPLEMENTS 194
Potaba - See AMINOBENZOATE POTASSIUM
    26
Potaba Envules - See AMINOBENZOATE
    POTASSIUM 26
Potaba Powder - See AMINOBENZOATE
    POTASSIUM 26
Potasalan - See POTASSIUM SUPPLEMENTS
    678
POTASSIUM & SODIUM PHOSPHATES 672
POTASSIUM ACETATE - See POTASSIUM
    SUPPLEMENTS 678
Potassium Aminobenzoate - See
    AMINOBENZOATE POTASSIUM 26
POTASSIUM BICARBONATE - See
    POTASSIUM SUPPLEMENTS 678
POTASSIUM BICARBONATE & POTASSIUM
    CHLORIDE - See POTASSIUM
    SUPPLEMENTS 678
POTASSIUM BICARBONATE & POTASSIUM
    CITRATE - See POTASSIUM
    SUPPLEMENTS 678
POTASSIUM CHLORIDE - See POTASSIUM
    SUPPLEMENTS 678
POTASSIUM CHLORIDE, POTASSIUM
    BICARBONATE & POTASSIUM CITRATE -
    See POTASSIUM SUPPLEMENTS 678
POTASSIUM CITRATE - See CITRATES 238
POTASSIUM CITRATE & CITRIC ACID - See
    CITRATES 238
POTASSIUM CITRATE & SODIUM CITRATE -
    See CITRATES 238
POTASSIUM GLUCONATE - See POTASSIUM
    SUPPLEMENTS 678
POTASSIUM GLUCONATE & POTASSIUM
    CHLORIDE - See POTASSIUM
    SUPPLEMENTS 678
POTASSIUM GLUCONATE & POTASSIUM
    CITRATE - See POTASSIUM
    SUPPLEMENTS 678
POTASSIUM GLUCONATE, POTASSIUM
    CITRATE & AMMONIUM - See
    POTASSIUM SUPPLEMENTS 678
POTASSIUM IODIDE 674
Potassium Para-aminobenzoate - See
    AMINOBENZOATE POTASSIUM 26
POTASSIUM PHOSPHATES 676
POTASSIUM PHOSPHATES - See
    POTASSIUM & SODIUM PHOSPHATES
    672
POTASSIUM SUPPLEMENTS 678
Potassium-Rougier - See POTASSIUM
    SUPPLEMENTS 678
Potassium-Sandoz - See POTASSIUM
    SUPPLEMENTS 678
Pramegel - See ANESTHETICS (Topical) 46
PRAMIPEXOLE - See ANTIDYSKINETICS 86

INDEX

Proctofoam - See ANESTHETICS (Rectal) 44
Procyclid - See ANTIDYSKINETICS 86
PROCYCLIDINE - See ANTIDYSKINETICS 86
Procythol - See SELEGILINE 748
Procytox - See CYCLOPHOSPHAMIDE 276
Pro-Depo - See PROGESTINS 694
Prodiem - See LAXATIVES, BULK-FORMING 470
Prodiem Plain - See LAXATIVES, BULK-FORMING 470
Prodiem Plus - See
  LAXATIVES, BULK-FORMING 470
  LAXATIVES, STIMULANT 476
Prodrox - See PROGESTINS 694
Profenal - See ANTI-INFLAMMATORY DRUGS, NONSTEROIDAL (NSAIDs) (Ophthalmic) 106
Progesic - See ANTI-INFLAMMATORY DRUGS, NONSTEROIDAL (NSAIDs) 104
Progestaject - See PROGESTINS 694
PROGESTERONE - See PROGESTINS 694
Progestilin - See PROGESTINS 694
PROGESTINS 694
Prograf - See IMMUNOSUPPRESSIVE AGENTS 430
Prohim - See YOHIMBINE 854
Prolamine - See PHENYLPROPANOLAMINE 668
Pro-Lax - See LAXATIVES, BULK-FORMING 470
Prolixin - See PHENOTHIAZINES 662
Prolixin Concentrate - See PHENOTHIAZINES 662
Prolixin Decanoate - See PHENOTHIAZINES 662
Prolixin Enanthate - See PHENOTHIAZINES 662
Proloid - See THYROID HORMONES 798
Proloprim - See TRIMETHOPRIM 824
PROMAZINE - See PHENOTHIAZINES 662
Pro-Med 50 - See ANTIHISTAMINES, PHENOTHIAZINE-DERIVATIVE 102
Promehist with Codeine - See
  ANTIHISTAMINES, PHENOTHIAZINE-DERIVATIVE 102
  NARCOTIC ANALGESICS 580
Promerhegan - See ANTIHISTAMINES, PHENOTHIAZINE-DERIVATIVE 102
Promet - See ANTIHISTAMINES, PHENOTHIAZINE-DERIVATIVE 102
Prometa - See BRONCHODILATORS, ADRENERGIC 174
Prometh VC Plain - See
  ANTIHISTAMINES, PHENOTHIAZINE-DERIVATIVE 102
  PHENYLEPHRINE 664
Prometh VC with Codeine - See
  ANTIHISTAMINES, PHENOTHIAZINE-DERIVATIVE 102
  NARCOTIC ANALGESICS 580
  PHENYLEPHRINE 664

Prometh with Dextromethorphan - See
  ANTIHISTAMINES, PHENOTHIAZINE-DERIVATIVE 102
  DEXTROMETHORPHAN 296
Prometh-25 - See ANTIHISTAMINES, PHENOTHIAZINE-DERIVATIVE 102
Prometh-50 - See ANTIHISTAMINES, PHENOTHIAZINE-DERIVATIVE 102
PROMETHAZINE - See ANTIHISTAMINES, PHENOTHIAZINE-DERIVATIVE 102
Promethazine DM - See
  ANTIHISTAMINES, PHENOTHIAZINE-DERIVATIVE 102
  DEXTROMETHORPHAN 296
Promethazine VC - See
  ANTIHISTAMINES, PHENOTHIAZINE-DERIVATIVE 102
  PHENYLEPHRINE 664
Promine - See PROCAINAMIDE 690
Prominic Expectorant - See
  GUAIFENESIN 398
  PHENYLPROPANOLAMINE 668
Prominicol Cough - See
  ANTIHISTAMINES 98
  DEXTROMETHORPHAN 296
  PHENYLPROPANOLAMINE 668
Promist HD Liquid - See
  ANTIHISTAMINES 98
  PSEUDOEPHEDRINE 706
Prompt - See
  LAXATIVES, BULK-FORMING 470
  LAXATIVES, STIMULANT 476
Pronestyl - See PROCAINAMIDE 690
Pronestyl SR - See PROCAINAMIDE 690
Propa P.H. 10 Acne Cover Stick - See BENZOYL PEROXIDE 158
Propa P.H. 10 Liquid Acne Soap - See BENZOYL PEROXIDE 158
Propa pH Medicated Acne Cream Maximum Strength - See KERATOLYTICS 464
Propa pH Medicated Cleansing Pads Maximum Strength - See KERATOLYTICS 464
Propa pH Medicated Cleansing Pads Sensitive Skin - See KERATOLYTICS 464
Propa pH Perfectly Clear Skin Cleanser Topical Solution Oily Skin - See KERATOLYTICS 464
Propa pH Perfectly Clear Skin Cleanser Topical Solution Sensitive Skin Formula - See KERATOLYTICS 464
Propacet 100 - See NARCOTIC ANALGESICS & ACETAMINOPHEN 582
Propaderm - See ADRENOCORTICOIDS (Topical) 16
PROPAFENONE 696
Propagest - See PHENYLPROPANOLAMINE 668
Propanthel - See PROPANTHELINE 698
PROPANTHELINE 698
Propecia - See FINASTERIDE 364

INDEX

Purinol - See ALLOPURINOL 20
P.V. Carpine - See PILOCARPINE 670
P.V. Carpine Liquifilm - See PILOCARPINE 670
PVF - See PENICILLINS 648
PVF K - See PENICILLINS 648
P-V-Tussin - See
  ANTIHISTAMINES 98
  NARCOTIC ANALGESICS 580
  PSEUDOEPHEDRINE 706
P-V-Tussin Tablets - See GUAIFENESIN 398
PYRANTEL - See ANTHELMINTICS 56
Pyrazodine - See PHENAZOPYRIDINE 660
Pyregesic-C - See NARCOTIC ANALGESICS &
  ACETAMINOPHEN 582
PYRETHRINS & PIPERONYL BUTOXIDE - See
  PEDICULICIDES (Topical) 642
Pyribenzamine - See ANTIHISTAMINES 98
Pyridamole - See DIPYRIDAMOLE 312
Pyridiate - See PHENAZOPYRIDINE 660
Pyridium - See PHENAZOPYRIDINE 660
PYRIDOSTIGMINE - See ANTIMYASTHENICS
  114
PYRIDOXINE (Vitamin B-6) 710
PYRILAMINE - See ANTIHISTAMINES 98
Pyrilamine Maleate Tablets - See
  ANTIHISTAMINES 98
Pyrinyl - See PEDICULICIDES (Topical) 642
PYRITHIONE - See ANTISEBORRHEICS
  (Topical) 118
Pyronium - See PHENAZOPYRIDINE 660
Pyroxine - See PYRIDOXINE (Vitamin B-6) 710
Pyrroxate - See
  ACETAMINOPHEN 4
  ANTIHISTAMINES 98
  PHENYLPROPANOLAMINE 668
PYRVINIUM - See ANTHELMINTICS 56
PZI - See INSULIN 434

Q

Q-gesic - See MEPROBAMATE & ASPIRIN 520
Quadra-Hist - See
  ANTIHISTAMINES 98
  PHENYLEPHRINE 664
  PHENYLPROPANOLAMINE 668
Quadra-Hist Pediatric Syrup - See
  ANTIHISTAMINES 98
  PHENYLEPHRINE 664
  PHENYLPROPANOLAMINE 668
Quarzan - See CLIDINIUM 240
QUAZEPAM - See BENZODIAZEPINES 156
Quelidrine Cough - See
  ANTIHISTAMINES 98
  DEXTROMETHORPHAN 296
  EPHEDRINE 336
  IPECAC 440
  PHENYLEPHRINE 664
Queltuss - See
  DEXTROMETHORPHAN 296
  GUAIFENESIN 398
Questran - See CHOLESTYRAMINE 230
Questran Light - See CHOLESTYRAMINE 230

QUETIAPINE 712
Quiagel PG - See KAOLIN, PECTIN,
  BELLADONNA & OPIUM 462
Quibron - See THEOPHYLLINE &
  GUAIFENESIN 784
Quibron 300 - See THEOPHYLLINE &
  GUAIFENESIN 784
Quibron-T - See BRONCHODILATORS,
  XANTHINE 176
Quibron-T Dividose - See
  BRONCHODILATORS, XANTHINE 176
Quibron-T/SR - See BRONCHODILATORS,
  XANTHINE 176
Quibron-T/SR Dividose - See
  BRONCHODILATORS, XANTHINE 176
Quick Pep - See CAFFEINE 186
Quiess - See GUAIFENESIN 398
Quin-260 - See QUININE 718
QUINACRINE 714
Quinaglute Dura-Tabs - See QUINIDINE 716
Quinalan - See QUINIDINE 716
Quin-amino - See QUININE 718
Quinamm - See QUININE 718
QUINAPRIL - See ANGIOTENSIN-
  CONVERTING ENZYME (ACE)
  INHIBITORS 50
Quinate - See QUINIDINE 716
Quindan - See QUININE 718
QUINESTROL - See ESTROGENS 350
QUINETHAZONE - See DIURETICS, THIAZIDE
  324
Quinidex Extentabs - See QUINIDINE 716
QUINIDINE 716
QUININE 718
Quinora - See QUINIDINE 716
Quiphile - See QUININE 718
Q-Vel - See QUININE 718

R

R&C - See PEDICULICIDES (Topical) 642
R.A. - See KERATOLYTICS 464
RACEPINEPHRINE - See
  BRONCHODILATORS, ADRENERGIC 174
Radiostol - See VITAMIN D 844
Radiostol Forte - See VITAMIN D 844
RALOXIFENE 720
RAMIPRIL - See ANGIOTENSIN-CONVERTING
  ENZYME (ACE) INHIBITORS 50
Ramses Contraceptive Foam - See
  CONTRACEPTIVES, VAGINAL
  (Spermicides) 264
Ramses Contraceptive Vaginal Jelly - See
  CONTRACEPTIVES, VAGINAL
  (Spermicides) 264
Ramses Crystal Clear Gel - See
  CONTRACEPTIVES, VAGINAL
  (Spermicides) 264
RANITIDINE - See HISTAMINE H$_2$ RECEPTOR
  ANTAGONISTS 412
Rapolyte - See CARBOHYDRATES &
  ELECTROLYTES 204

INDEX

1051

RESERPINE & HYDROFLUMETHIAZIDE - See
   RAUWOLFIA & THIAZIDE DIURETICS 722
RESERPINE & METHYCLOTHIAZIDE - See
   RAUWOLFIA & THIAZIDE DIURETICS 722
RESERPINE & POLYTHIAZIDE - See
   RAUWOLFIA & THIAZIDE DIURETICS 722
RESERPINE & QUINETHAZONE - See
   RAUWOLFIA & THIAZIDE DIURETICS 722
RESERPINE & TRICHLORMETHIAZIDE - See
   RAUWOLFIA & THIAZIDE DIURETICS 722
RESERPINE, HYDRALAZINE &
   HYDROCHLOROTHIAZIDE 726
Resol - See CARBOHYDRATES &
   ELECTROLYTES 204
RESORCINOL - See KERATOLYTICS 464
RESORCINOL & SULFUR - See
   KERATOLYTICS 464
Respaire-60 SR - See
  GUAIFENESIN 398
  PSEUDOEPHEDRINE 706
Respaire-120 SR - See
  GUAIFENESIN 398
  PSEUDOEPHEDRINE 706
Respbid - See BRONCHODILATORS,
   XANTHINE 176
Respinol G - See
  GUAIFENESIN 398
  PHENYLEPHRINE 664
  PHENYLPROPANOLAMINE 668
Respinol LA - See
  GUAIFENESIN 398
  PHENYLEPHRINE 664
  PHENYLPROPANOLAMINE 668
Resporal TR - See
  ANTIHISTAMINES 98
  PSEUDOEPHEDRINE 706
Restoril - See BENZODIAZEPINES 156
Resyl - See GUAIFENESIN 398
Retin-A Cream - See RETINOIDS (Topical) 730
Retin-A Cream Regimen Kit - See RETINOIDS
  (Topical) 730
Retin-A Gel - See RETINOIDS (Topical) 730
Retin-A Gel Regimen Kit - See RETINOIDS
  (Topical) 730
Retin-A Solution - See RETINOIDS (Topical) 730
Retinoic Acid - See RETINOIDS (Topical) 730
RETINOIDS (Oral) 728
RETINOIDS (Topical) 730
Retrovir - See NUCLEOSIDE REVERSE
   TRANSCRIPTASE INHIBITORS 608
ReVia - See NALTREXONE 578
Rexigen - See APPETITE SUPPRESSANTS 130
Rexigen Forte - See APPETITE
  SUPPRESSANTS 130
Rezamid Lotion - See KERATOLYTICS 464
Rezulin - See TROGLITAZONE 828
Rheaban - See ATTAPULGITE 138
Rheumatrex - See METHOTREXATE 530
Rhinalar - See ADRENOCORTICOIDS (Nasal
  Inhalation) 10
Rhinall - See PHENYLEPHRINE 664

Rhinall Children's Flavored Nose Drops - See
  PHENYLEPHRINE 664
Rhinatate - See
  ANTIHISTAMINES 98
  PHENYLEPHRINE 664
Rhinocaps - See
  ACETAMINOPHEN 4
  ASPIRIN 132
  PHENYLPROPANOLAMINE 668
Rhinocort Aqua - See ADRENOCORTICOIDS
  (Nasal Inhalation) 10
Rhinocort Nasal Inhaler - See
  ADRENOCORTICOIDS (Nasal Inhalation) 10
Rhinocort Turbuhaler - See
  ADRENOCORTICOIDS (Nasal Inhalation) 10
Rhinogesic - See
  ACETAMINOPHEN 4
  ANTIHISTAMINES 98
  PHENYLEPHRINE 664
  SALICYLATES 744
Rhinolar - See
  ANTICHOLINERGICS 74
  ANTIHISTAMINES 98
  PHENYLPROPANOLAMINE 668
Rhinolar-EX - See
  ANTIHISTAMINES 98
  PHENYLPROPANOLAMINE 668
Rhinolar-EX 12 - See
  ANTIHISTAMINES 98
  PHENYLPROPANOLAMINE 668
Rhinosyn - See
  ANTIHISTAMINES 98
  PSEUDOEPHEDRINE 706
Rhinosyn-DM - See
  ANTIHISTAMINES 98
  DEXTROMETHORPHAN 296
  PSEUDOEPHEDRINE 706
Rhinosyn-DMX Expectorant - See
  DEXTROMETHORPHAN 296
  GUAIFENESIN 398
Rhinosyn-PD - See
  ANTIHISTAMINES 98
  PSEUDOEPHEDRINE 706
Rhinosyn-X - See
  DEXTROMETHORPHAN 296
  GUAIFENESIN 398
  PSEUDOEPHEDRINE 706
Rhodis - See ANTI-INFLAMMATORY DRUGS,
  NONSTEROIDAL (NSAIDs) 104
Rhodis-EC - See ANTI-INFLAMMATORY
  DRUGS, NONSTEROIDAL (NSAIDs) 104
Rhotrimine - See ANTIDEPRESSANTS,
  TRICYCLIC 82
Rhulicort - See ADRENOCORTICOIDS
  (Topical) 16
Rhythmol - See PROPAFENONE 696
RIBAVIRIN 732
RIBOFLAVIN (Vitamin B-2) 734
Ricelyte - See CARBOHYDRATES &
  ELECTROLYTES 204

INDEX

Robitussin-DM - See
  DEXTROMETHORPHAN 296
  GUAIFENESIN 398
Robitussin-PE - See
  GUAIFENESIN 398
  PSEUDOEPHEDRINE 706
Robitussin-Pediatric - See
  DEXTROMETHORPHAN 296
Robomol - See MUSCLE RELAXANTS,
  SKELETAL 570
Rocaltrol - See VITAMIN D 844
Rodex - See PYRIDOXINE (Vitamin B-6) 710
Rogaine - See MINOXIDIL (Topical) 556
Rogaine Extra Strength for Men - See
  MINOXIDIL (Topical) 556
Rogaine for Men - See MINOXIDIL (Topical) 556
Rogaine for Women - See MINOXIDIL (Topical)
  556
Rolaids - See ANTACIDS 54
Rolaids Calcium Rich - See
  ANTACIDS 54
  CALCIUM SUPPLEMENTS 194
Rolaids Sodium Free - See ANTACIDS 54
Rolatuss Expectorant - See
  ANTIHISTAMINES 98
  NARCOTIC ANALGESICS 580
  PHENYLEPHRINE 664
Rolatuss Plain - See
  ANTIHISTAMINES 98
  PHENYLEPHRINE 664
Rolatuss with Hydrocodone - See
  ANTIHISTAMINES 98
  NARCOTIC ANALGESICS 580
  PHENYLEPHRINE 664
  PHENYLPROPANOLAMINE 668
Rondamine-DM Drops - See
  ANTIHISTAMINES 98
  DEXTROMETHORPHAN 296
  PSEUDOEPHEDRINE 706
Rondec - See
  ANTIHISTAMINES 98
  PSEUDOEPHEDRINE 706
Rondec Drops - See
  ANTIHISTAMINES 98
  PSEUDOEPHEDRINE 706
Rondec-DM - See
  ANTIHISTAMINES 98
  DEXTROMETHORPHAN 296
  PSEUDOEPHEDRINE 706
Rondec-DM Drops - See
  ANTIHISTAMINES 98
  DEXTROMETHORPHAN 296
  PSEUDOEPHEDRINE 706
Rondec-TR - See
  ANTIHISTAMINES 98
  PSEUDOEPHEDRINE 706
Roniacol - See NIACIN (Vitamin B-3, Nicotinic
  Acid, Nicotinamide) 596
Ronigen - See NIACIN (Vitamin B-3, Nicotinic
  Acid, Nicotinamide) 596
ROPINIROLE - See ANTIDYSKINETICS 86

Ro-Profen - See ANTI-INFLAMMATORY
  DRUGS, NONSTEROIDAL (NSAIDs) 104
Roubac - See
  SULFONAMIDES 770
  TRIMETHOPRIM 824
Rounox - See ACETAMINOPHEN 4
Rowasa - See MESALAMINE 524
Roxanol - See NARCOTIC ANALGESICS 580
Roxanol SR - See NARCOTIC ANALGESICS 580
Roxicet - See NARCOTIC ANALGESICS &
  ACETAMINOPHEN 582
Roxicodone - See NARCOTIC ANALGESICS
  580
Roxilox - See NARCOTIC ANALGESICS &
  ACETAMINOPHEN 582
Roxiprin - See NARCOTIC ANALGESICS &
  ASPIRIN 584
Roychlor 10% - See POTASSIUM
  SUPPLEMENTS 678
Roychlor 20% - See POTASSIUM
  SUPPLEMENTS 678
Royonate - See POTASSIUM SUPPLEMENTS
  678
R-Tannamine - See
  ANTIHISTAMINES 98
  PHENYLEPHRINE 664
R-Tannamine Pediatric - See
  ANTIHISTAMINES 98
  PHENYLEPHRINE 664
R-Tannate - See
  ANTIHISTAMINES 98
  PHENYLEPHRINE 664
R-Tannate Pediatric - See
  ANTIHISTAMINES 98
  PHENYLEPHRINE 664
Rubion - See VITAMIN B-12 (Cyanocobalamin)
  840
Rubramin - See VITAMIN B-12
  (Cyanocobalamin) 840
Rubramin-PC - See VITAMIN B-12
  (Cyanocobalamin) 840
Rufen - See ANTI-INFLAMMATORY DRUGS,
  NONSTEROIDAL (NSAIDs) 104
Rulox - See ANTACIDS 54
Rulox No. 1 - See ANTACIDS 54
Rulox No. 2 - See ANTACIDS 54
Rulox Plus - See ANTACIDS 54
Rum-K - See POTASSIUM SUPPLEMENTS 678
Ru-Tuss - See
  ANTICHOLINERGICS 74
  ANTIHISTAMINES 98
  HYOSCYAMINE 428
  PHENYLEPHRINE 664
  PHENYLPROPANOLAMINE 668
  SCOPOLAMINE (Hyoscine) 746
Ru-Tuss DE - See
  GUAIFENESIN 398
  PSEUDOEPHEDRINE 706
Ru-Tuss Expectorant - See
  DEXTROMETHORPHAN 296
  GUAIFENESIN 398

PSEUDOEPHEDRINE 706
Ru-Tuss with Hydrocodone Liquid - See
   ANTIHISTAMINES 98
   NARCOTIC ANALGESICS 580
   PHENYLEPHRINE 664
   PHENYLPROPANOLAMINE 668
Ru-Vert-M - See MECLIZINE 512
Rycotin - See NIACIN (Vitamin B-3, Nicotinic
   Acid, Nicotinamide) 596
Rymed - See
   GUAIFENESIN 398
   PHENYLEPHRINE 664
Rymed Liquid - See
   GUAIFENESIN 398
   PHENYLEPHRINE 664
Rymed-TR - See
   GUAIFENESIN 398
   PSEUDOEPHEDRINE 706
Ryna - See
   ANTIHISTAMINES 98
   PSEUDOEPHEDRINE 706
Ryna-C Liquid - See
   ANTIHISTAMINES 98
   NARCOTIC ANALGESICS 580
   PSEUDOEPHEDRINE 706
Ryna-CX Liquid - See
   GUAIFENESIN 398
   NARCOTIC ANALGESICS 580
   PSEUDOEPHEDRINE 706
Rynacrom - See CROMOLYN 266
Rynatan - See
   ANTIHISTAMINES 98
   PHENYLEPHRINE 664
Rynatan Pediatric - See
   ANTIHISTAMINES 98
   PHENYLEPHRINE 664
Rynatan-S Pediatric - See
   ANTIHISTAMINES 98
   PHENYLEPHRINE 664
Rynatuss - See
   ANTIHISTAMINES 98
   EPHEDRINE 336
   PHENYLEPHRINE 664
Rynatuss Pediatric - See
   ANTIHISTAMINES 98
   EPHEDRINE 336
   PHENYLEPHRINE 664
Rythmodan - See DISOPYRAMIDE 314
Rythmodan-LA - See DISOPYRAMIDE 314

S

S-A-C - See
   ACETAMINOPHEN & SALICYLATES 6
   CAFFEINE 186
SafeTussin 30 - See
   DEXTROMETHORPHAN 296
   GUAIFENESIN 398
Salac - See KERATOLYTICS 464
Salacid - See KERATOLYTICS 464
Sal-Acid Plaster - See KERATOLYTICS 464

Salactic Film Topical Solution - See
   KERATOLYTICS 464
Sal-Adult - See ASPIRIN 132
Salagen - See PILOCARPINE 670
Salatin - See
   ASPIRIN 132
   CAFFEINE 186
Salazide - See RAUWOLFIA & THIAZIDE
   DIURETICS 722
Salazopyrin - See SULFASALAZINE 766
Salazosulfapyridine - See SULFASALAZINE 766
Sal-Clens Plus Shampoo - See
   KERATOLYTICS 464
Sal-Clens Shampoo - See KERATOLYTICS 464
Salcylic Acid - See SALICYLATES 744
Saleto - See
   ACETAMINOPHEN & SALICYLATES 6
   ASPIRIN 132
   CAFFEINE 186
Saleto-200 - See ANTI-INFLAMMATORY
   DRUGS, NONSTEROIDAL (NSAIDs) 104
Saleto-400 - See ANTI-INFLAMMATORY
   DRUGS, NONSTEROIDAL (NSAIDs) 104
Saleto-600 - See ANTI-INFLAMMATORY
   DRUGS, NONSTEROIDAL (NSAIDs) 104
Saleto-800 - See ANTI-INFLAMMATORY
   DRUGS, NONSTEROIDAL (NSAIDs) 104
Saleto-CF - See
   ACETAMINOPHEN 4
   DEXTROMETHORPHAN 296
   PHENYLPROPANOLAMINE 668
Saleto-D - See
   ACETAMINOPHEN 4
   CAFFEINE 186
   PHENYLPROPANOLAMINE 668
   SALICYLATES 744
Salflex - See SALICYLATES 744
Salgesic - See SALICYLATES 744
SALICYLAMIDE - See SALICYLATES 744
SALICYLATES 744
Salicylazosulfapyridine - See
   SULFASALAZINE 766
SALICYLIC ACID - See KERATOLYTICS 464
SALICYLIC ACID & SULFUR - See
   KERATOLYTICS 464
SALICYLIC ACID, SULFUR & COAL TAR - See
   ANTISEBORRHEICS (Topical) 118
Saligel - See KERATOLYTICS 464
Sal-Infant - See ASPIRIN 132
SALMETEROL - See BRONCHODILATORS,
   ADRENERGIC 174
Salocol - See
   ASPIRIN 132
   CAFFEINE 186
Salofalk - See MESALAMINE 524
Salonil - See KERATOLYTICS 464
Salphenyl - See
   ACETAMINOPHEN & SALICYLATES 6
   ANTIHISTAMINES 98
   PHENYLEPHRINE 664

INDEX

Sal-Plant Gel Topical Solution - See
  KERATOLYTICS 464
SALSALATE - See SALICYLATES 744
Salsitab - See SALICYLATES 744
Saluron - See DIURETICS, THIAZIDE 324
Salutensin - See RAUWOLFIA & THIAZIDE
  DIURETICS 722
Salutensin-Demi - See RAUWOLFIA &
  THIAZIDE DIURETICS 722
Sandimmune - See CYCLOSPORINE 282
Sanorex - See APPETITE SUPPRESSANTS 130
Sans-Acne - See ANTIBACTERIALS FOR
  ACNE (Topical) 66
Sansert - See METHYSERGIDE 540
SAQUINAVIR - See PROTEASE INHIBITORS 700
Sarisol No. 2 - See BARBITURATES 148
Sarna HC - See ADRENOCORTICOIDS
  (Topical) 16
Sarodant - See NITROFURANTOIN 604
S.A.S. Enteric-500 - See SULFASALAZINE 766
S.A.S.-500 - See SULFASALAZINE 766
Sastid (AL) Scrub - See KERATOLYTICS 464
Sastid Plain - See KERATOLYTICS 464
Sastid Plain Shampoo and Acne Wash - See
  KERATOLYTICS 464
Sastid Soap - See KERATOLYTICS 464
Satric - See METRONIDAZOLE 544
Scabicide - See PEDICULICIDES (Topical) 642
SCOPOLAMINE - See CYCLOPLEGIC,
  MYDRIATIC (Ophthalmic) 278
SCOPOLAMINE (Hyoscine) 746
Scot-Tussin - See
  GUAIFENESIN 398
  PHENYLEPHRINE 664
Scot-Tussin DM - See
  ANTIHISTAMINES 98
  DEXTROMETHORPHAN 296
Scot-Tussin Original 5-Action Cold Medicine -
  See
  ANTIHISTAMINES 98
  CAFFEINE 186
  PHENYLEPHRINE 664
  SALICYLATES 744
SD Deprenyl - See SELEGILINE 748
Seba-Nil - See ANTIACNE, CLEANSING
  (Topical) 60
Sebasorb Liquid - See KERATOLYTICS 464
Sebex - See KERATOLYTICS 464
Sebex-T Tar Shampoo - See
  ANTISEBORRHEICS (Topical) 118
Sebucare - See KERATOLYTICS 464
Sebulex Antiseborrheic Treatment and
  Conditioning Shampoo - See
  KERATOLYTICS 464
Sebulex Antiseborrheic Treatment Shampoo -
  See KERATOLYTICS 464
Sebulex Conditioning Shampoo - See
  KERATOLYTICS 464
Sebulex Conditioning Suspension Shampoo -
  See ANTISEBORRHEICS (Topical) 118

Sebulex Cream Medicated Shampoo - See
  KERATOLYTICS 464
Sebulex Lotion Shampoo - See
  ANTISEBORRHEICS (Topical) 118
Sebulex Medicated Dandruff Shampoo with
  Conditioners - See KERATOLYTICS 464
Sebulex Medicated Shampoo - See
  KERATOLYTICS 464
Sebulex Regular Medicated Dandruff
  Shampoo - See KERATOLYTICS 464
Sebulex Shampoo - See KERATOLYTICS 464
Sebulon - See ANTISEBORRHEICS (Topical) 118
Sebutone - See ANTISEBORRHEICS (Topical)
  118
SECOBARBITAL - See BARBITURATES 148
SECOBARBITAL & AMOBARBITAL - See
  BARBITURATES 148
Seconal - See BARBITURATES 148
Sectral - See BETA-ADRENERGIC BLOCKING
  AGENTS 162
Sedabamate - See MEPROBAMATE 518
Sedapap - See
  ACETAMINOPHEN 4
  BARBITURATES 148
Sedative - See
  BELLADONNA ALKALOIDS &
    BARBITURATES 154
  ISOMETHEPTENE,
    DICHLORALPHENAZONE &
    ACETAMINOPHEN 446
  PANCREATIN, PEPSIN, BILE SALTS,
    HYOSCYAMINE, ATROPINE,
    SCOPOLAMINE & PHENOBARBITAL 628
  THEOPHYLLINE, EPHEDRINE &
    BARBITURATES 786
  THEOPHYLLINE, EPHEDRINE,
    GUAIFENESIN & BARBITURATES 790
Sedative-hypnotic agent - See
  BARBITURATES 148
  CHLORAL HYDRATE 216
  TRIAZOLAM 818
  ZOLPIDEM 858
Sedatuss - See DEXTROMETHORPHAN 296
Seldane D - See PSEUDOEPHEDRINE 706
SELEGILINE 748
SELENIUM SULFIDE - See
  ANTISEBORRHEICS (Topical) 118
Selexid - See PENICILLINS 648
Selsun - See ANTISEBORRHEICS (Topical) 118
Selsun Blue - See ANTISEBORRHEICS
  (Topical) 118
Selsun Blue Dry Formula - See
  ANTISEBORRHEICS (Topical) 118
Selsun Blue Extra Conditioning Formula - See
  ANTISEBORRHEICS (Topical) 118
Selsun Blue Extra Medicated Formula - See
  ANTISEBORRHEICS (Topical) 118
Selsun Blue Oily Formula - See
  ANTISEBORRHEICS (Topical) 118
Selsun Blue Regular Formula - See
  ANTISEBORRHEICS (Topical) 118

Sine-Aid Maximum Strength Gelcaps - See
  ACETAMINOPHEN 4
  PSEUDOEPHEDRINE 706
Sinemet - See CARBIDOPA & LEVODOPA 202
Sinemet CR - See CARBIDOPA & LEVODOPA
  202
Sine-Off Maximum Strength Allergy/Sinus
  Formula Caplets - See
  ACETAMINOPHEN 4
  ANTIHISTAMINES 98
  PSEUDOEPHEDRINE 706
Sine-Off Maximum Strength No Drowsiness
  Formula Caplets - See
  ACETAMINOPHEN 4
  PSEUDOEPHEDRINE 706
Sine-Off Sinus Medicine - See
  ANTIHISTAMINES 98
  ASPIRIN 132
  PHENYLPROPANOLAMINE 668
Sinequan - See ANTIDEPRESSANTS,
  TRICYCLIC 82
Singlet - See
  ACETAMINOPHEN 4
  ANTIHISTAMINES 98
  PSEUDOEPHEDRINE 706
Singulair - See LEUKOTRIENE MODIFIERS 480
Sinubid - See ACETAMINOPHEN 4
Sinucon Pediatric Drops - See
  ANTIHISTAMINES 98
  PHENYLEPHRINE 664
  PHENYLPROPANOLAMINE 668
Sinufed Timecelles - See
  GUAIFENESIN 398
  PSEUDOEPHEDRINE 706
Sinulin - See
  ACETAMINOPHEN 4
  ANTIHISTAMINES 98
  PHENYLPROPANOLAMINE 668
Sinumist-SR - See GUAIFENESIN 398
Sinupan - See
  GUAIFENESIN 398
  PHENYLEPHRINE 664
Sinus Excedrin Extra Strength - See
  ACETAMINOPHEN 4
  PSEUDOEPHEDRINE 706
Sinus Excedrin Extra Strength Caplets - See
  ACETAMINOPHEN 4
  PSEUDOEPHEDRINE 706
Sinus Excedrin No Drowsiness - See
  ACETAMINOPHEN 4
  PSEUDOEPHEDRINE 706
Sinus Excedrin No Drowsiness Caplets - See
  ACETAMINOPHEN 4
  PSEUDOEPHEDRINE 706
Sinus Relief - See
  ACETAMINOPHEN 4
  PSEUDOEPHEDRINE 706
SinuStat - See PSEUDOEPHEDRINE 706
Sinutab - See
  ACETAMINOPHEN 4
  ANTIHISTAMINES 98

PSEUDOEPHEDRINE 706
Sinutab Extra Strength - See
  ACETAMINOPHEN 4
  ANTIHISTAMINES 98
  PSEUDOEPHEDRINE 706
Sinutab II Maximum Strength - See
  ACETAMINOPHEN 4
  PSEUDOEPHEDRINE 706
Sinutab Maximum Strength Sinus Allergy -
  See ACETAMINOPHEN 4
Sinutab Maximum Strength Sinus Allergy
  Caplets - See ACETAMINOPHEN 4
Sinutab Maximum Strength without
  Drowsiness - See
  ACETAMINOPHEN 4
  PSEUDOEPHEDRINE 706
Sinutab Maximum Strength without
  Drowsiness Caplets - See
  ACETAMINOPHEN 4
  PSEUDOEPHEDRINE 706
Sinutab No Drowsiness - See
  ACETAMINOPHEN 4
  PSEUDOEPHEDRINE 706
Sinutab No Drowsiness Extra Strength - See
  ACETAMINOPHEN 4
  PSEUDOEPHEDRINE 706
Sinutab Regular - See
  ACETAMINOPHEN 4
  ANTIHISTAMINES 98
  PSEUDOEPHEDRINE 706
Sinutab SA - See
  ACETAMINOPHEN 4
  ANTIHISTAMINES 98
  PHENYLPROPANOLAMINE 668
Sinutrex Extra Strength - See
  ACETAMINOPHEN 4
  ANTIHISTAMINES 98
  PSEUDOEPHEDRINE 706
SINUvent - See
  GUAIFENESIN 398
  PHENYLPROPANOLAMINE 668
Skalaxin - See MUSCLE RELAXANTS,
  SKELETAL 570
Skelex - See MUSCLE RELAXANTS,
  SKELETAL 570
Sleep inducer (hypnotic) - See
  ETHCHLORVYNOL 352
Sleep-Eze 3 - See ANTIHISTAMINES 98
Slo-Bid - See BRONCHODILATORS,
  XANTHINE 176
Slo-bid Gyrocaps - See BRONCHODILATORS,
  XANTHINE 176
Slo-Niacin - See NIACIN (Vitamin B-3, Nicotinic
  Acid, Nicotinamide) 596
Slo-Phyllin - See BRONCHODILATORS,
  XANTHINE 176
Slo-Phyllin GG - See THEOPHYLLINE &
  GUAIFENESIN 784
Slo-Phyllin Gyrocaps - See
  BRONCHODILATORS, XANTHINE 176
Slow Fe - See IRON SUPPLEMENTS 444

T

INDEX

Temazin Cold - See
  ANTIHISTAMINES 98
  PHENYLPROPANOLAMINE 668
Temgesic - See NARCOTIC ANALGESICS 580
Temovate - See ADRENOCORTICOIDS
  (Topical) 16
Temovate E - See ADRENOCORTICOIDS
  (Topical) 16
Temovate Emollient - See
  ADRENOCORTICOIDS (Topical) 16
Temovate Gel - See ADRENOCORTICOIDS
  (Topical) 16
Temovate Scalp Application - See
  ADRENOCORTICOIDS (Topical) 16
Tempo - See ANTACIDS 54
Tempra - See ACETAMINOPHEN 4
Tempra Caplets - See ACETAMINOPHEN 4
Tempra Chewable Tablets - See
  ACETAMINOPHEN 4
Tempra Double Strength - See
  ACETAMINOPHEN 4
Tempra Drops - See ACETAMINOPHEN 4
Tempra D.S. - See ACETAMINOPHEN 4
Tempra Infants - See ACETAMINOPHEN 4
Tempra Syrup - See ACETAMINOPHEN 4
Ten K - See POTASSIUM SUPPLEMENTS 678
Tencet - See
  ACETAMINOPHEN 4
  BARBITURATES 148
Tenex - See GUANFACINE 408
Tenol - See ACETAMINOPHEN 4
Tenol Plus - See ACETAMINOPHEN &
  SALICYLATES 6
Tenoretic - See BETA-ADRENERGIC
  BLOCKING AGENTS & THIAZIDE
  DIURETICS 164
Tenormin - See BETA-ADRENERGIC
  BLOCKING AGENTS 162
TENOXICAM - See ANTI-INFLAMMATORY
  DRUGS, NONSTEROIDAL (NSAIDs) 104
Tenuate - See APPETITE SUPPRESSANTS 130
Tenuate Dospan - See APPETITE
  SUPPRESSANTS 130
T.E.P. - See THEOPHYLLINE, EPHEDRINE &
  BARBITURATES 786
Tepanil - See APPETITE SUPPRESSANTS 130
Tepanil Ten-Tab - See APPETITE
  SUPPRESSANTS 130
Teramin - See APPETITE SUPPRESSANTS 130
Terazol 3 - See ANTIFUNGALS (Vaginal) 92
Terazol 7 - See ANTIFUNGALS (Vaginal) 92
TERAZOSIN - See ALPHA ADRENERGIC
  RECEPTOR BLOCKERS 22
TERBINAFINE - See ANTIFUNGALS (Topical) 90
TERBUTALINE - See BRONCHODILATORS,
  ADRENERGIC 174
TERCONAZOLE - See ANTIFUNGALS (Vaginal)
  92
Terfluzine - See PHENOTHIAZINES 662
Terfluzine Concentrate - See
  PHENOTHIAZINES 662

Terphan - See DEXTROMETHORPHAN 296
TERPIN HYDRATE 778
Terpin Hydrate and Codeine Syrup - See
  NARCOTIC ANALGESICS 580
  TERPIN HYDRATE 778
Terpin-Dex - See
  DEXTROMETHORPHAN 296
  TERPIN HYDRATE 778
Terramycin - See TETRACYCLINES 782
Tersac Cleansing Gel - See KERATOLYTICS
  464
**Tersa-Tar Mild Therapeutic Shampoo with
  Protein and Conditioner** - See COAL TAR
  (Topical) 254
Tersa-Tar Soapless Tar Shampoo - See COAL
  TAR (Topical) 254
Tersa-Tar Therapeutic Shampoo - See COAL
  TAR (Topical) 254
Tes Est Cyp - See ANDROGENS &
  ESTROGENS 40
Teslac - See TESTOLACTONE 780
Testa-C - See ANDROGENS 38
Testamone 100 - See ANDROGENS 38
Testaqua - See ANDROGENS 38
Test-Estro Cypionate - See ANDROGENS &
  ESTROGENS 40
Testex - See ANDROGENS 38
Testoderm with Adhesive - See ANDROGENS
  38
Testoject-50 - See ANDROGENS 38
Testoject-LA - See ANDROGENS 38
TESTOLACTONE 780
Testone L.A. - See ANDROGENS 38
TESTOSTERONE - See ANDROGENS 38
TESTOSTERONE & ESTRADIOL - See
  ANDROGENS & ESTROGENS 40
Testred - See ANDROGENS 38
Testred-Cypionate 200 - See ANDROGENS 38
Testrin P.A. - See ANDROGENS 38
TETRACAINE - See
  ANESTHETICS (Mucosal-Local) 42
  ANESTHETICS (Rectal) 44
  ANESTHETICS (Topical) 46
TETRACAINE & MENTHOL - See
  ANESTHETICS (Rectal) 44
  ANESTHETICS (Topical) 46
TETRACYCLINE - See TETRACYCLINES 782
TETRACYCLINE (Ophthalmic) - See
  ANTIBACTERIALS (Ophthalmic) 68
TETRACYCLINE (topical) - See
  ANTIBACTERIALS FOR ACNE (Topical) 66
TETRACYCLINES 782
Tetracyn - See TETRACYCLINES 782
TETRAHYDROZILINE - See
  DECONGESTANTS (Ophthalmic) 290
Teveten - See ANGIOTENSIN II RECEPTOR
  ANTAGONISTS 48
Texacort - See ADRENOCORTICOIDS
  (Topical) 16
T-Gel - See COAL TAR (Topical) 254

INDEX

INDEX

Triminol Cough - See
  ANTIHISTAMINES 98
  DEXTROMETHORPHAN 296
  PSEUDOEPHEDRINE 706
TRIMIPRAMINE - See ANTIDEPRESSANTS,
  TRICYCLIC 82
Trimox - See PENICILLINS 648
Trimpex - See TRIMETHOPRIM 824
Trimstat - See APPETITE SUPPRESSANTS 130
Trimtabs - See APPETITE SUPPRESSANTS
  130
Trinalin Repetabs - See
  ANTIHISTAMINES 98
  PSEUDOEPHEDRINE 706
Trind - See
  ANTIHISTAMINES 98
  PHENYLPROPANOLAMINE 668
Trind DM Liquid - See
  ANTIHISTAMINES 98
  DEXTROMETHORPHAN 296
  PHENYLPROPANOLAMINE 668
Tri-Nefrin Extra Strength - See
  ANTIHISTAMINES 98
  PHENYLPROPANOLAMINE 668
Trinex - See
  ANTIHISTAMINES 98
  GUAIFENESIN 398
  PSEUDOEPHEDRINE 706
Tri-Norinyl - See CONTRACEPTIVES, ORAL
  262
Triofed - See
  ANTIHISTAMINES 98
  PSEUDOEPHEDRINE 706
Tri-Ophthalmic - See ANTIBACTERIALS
  (Ophthalmic) 68
Triotann - See
  ANTIHISTAMINES 98
  PHENYLEPHRINE 664
Triotann Pediatric - See
  ANTIHISTAMINES 98
  PHENYLEPHRINE 664
TRIOXSALEN - See PSORALENS 708
Tri-Pain - See ACETAMINOPHEN &
  SALICYLATES 6
Tripalgen Cold - See
  ANTIHISTAMINES 98
  PHENYLPROPANOLAMINE 668
TRIPELENNAMINE - See ANTIHISTAMINES 98
Triphasil - See CONTRACEPTIVES, ORAL 262
Tri-Phen-Chlor - See
  ANTIHISTAMINES 98
  PHENYLEPHRINE 664
  PHENYLPROPANOLAMINE 668
Tri-Phen-Chlor Pediatric - See
  ANTIHISTAMINES 98
  PHENYLEPHRINE 664
  PHENYLPROPANOLAMINE 668
Tri-Phen-Chlor T.R. - See
  ANTIHISTAMINES 98
  PHENYLEPHRINE 664

PHENYLPROPANOLAMINE 668
Triphenyl - See
  ANTIHISTAMINES 98
  PHENYLPROPANOLAMINE 668
Triphenyl Expectorant - See
  GUAIFENESIN 398
  PHENYLPROPANOLAMINE 668
Triphenyl T.D. - See
  ANTIHISTAMINES 98
  PHENYLPROPANOLAMINE 668
Triple Antibiotic - See
  ANTIBACTERIALS (Ophthalmic) 68
  ANTIBACTERIALS (Topical) 72
Triple X - See PEDICULICIDES (Topical) 642
Tripodrine - See
  ANTIHISTAMINES 98
  PSEUDOEPHEDRINE 706
Triposed - See
  ANTIHISTAMINES 98
  PSEUDOEPHEDRINE 706
TRIPROLIDINE - See ANTIHISTAMINES 98
TRIPTANS 826
Triptil - See ANTIDEPRESSANTS, TRICYCLIC
  82
Trip-Tone - See ANTIHISTAMINES 98
Triquilar - See CONTRACEPTIVES, ORAL 262
Trisoralen - See PSORALENS 708
Tristatin II - See NYSTATIN 610
Trisulfam - See
  SULFONAMIDES 770
  TRIMETHOPRIM 824
Tritann Pediatric - See
  ANTIHISTAMINES 98
  PHENYLEPHRINE 664
Tri-Tannate - See
  ANTIHISTAMINES 98
  PHENYLEPHRINE 664
Tri-Tannate Plus Pediatric - See
  ANTIHISTAMINES 98
  PHENYLEPHRINE 664
Tri-Thalmic - See ANTIBACTERIALS
  (Ophthalmic) 68
Tri-Vi-Flor - See VITAMINS & FLUORIDE 850
Trivora - See CONTRACEPTIVES, ORAL 262
Trocal - See DEXTROMETHORPHAN 296
TROGLITAZONE 828
Tronolane - See ANESTHETICS (Rectal) 44
Tronothane - See
  ANESTHETICS (Rectal) 44
  ANESTHETICS (Topical) 46
TROVAFLOXACIN - See
  FLUOROQUINOLONES 372
Trovan - See
  ANGIOTENSIN II RECEPTOR
    ANTAGONISTS 48
  FLUOROQUINOLONES 372
Truphylline - See BRONCHODILATORS,
  XANTHINE 176
Trusopt - See DORZOLAMIDE 330

INDEX

Ty-Cold Cold Formula - See
ACETAMINOPHEN 4
ANTIHISTAMINES 98
DEXTROMETHORPHAN 296
PSEUDOEPHEDRINE 706
Tylaprin with Codeine - See NARCOTIC
ANALGESICS & ACETAMINOPHEN 582
Tylenol - See ACETAMINOPHEN 4
Tylenol Allergy Sinus Gelcaps - See
ACETAMINOPHEN 4
ANTIHISTAMINES 98
PSEUDOEPHEDRINE 706
**Tylenol Allergy Sinus NightTime Maximum
Strength Caplets** - See
ACETAMINOPHEN 4
ANTIHISTAMINES 98
PSEUDOEPHEDRINE 706
Tylenol Arthritis Extended Relief - See
ACETAMINOPHEN 4
Tylenol Caplets - See ACETAMINOPHEN 4
Tylenol Children's Chewable Tablets - See
ACETAMINOPHEN 4
Tylenol Children's Elixir - See
ACETAMINOPHEN 4
Tylenol Children's Suspension Liquid - See
ACETAMINOPHEN 4
Tylenol Cold and Flu - See
ACETAMINOPHEN 4
ANTIHISTAMINES 98
DEXTROMETHORPHAN 296
PSEUDOEPHEDRINE 706
Tylenol Cold and Flu No Drowsiness Powder
- See
ACETAMINOPHEN 4
DEXTROMETHORPHAN 296
PSEUDOEPHEDRINE 706
Tylenol Cold Medication - See
ACETAMINOPHEN 4
ANTIHISTAMINES 98
DEXTROMETHORPHAN 296
PSEUDOEPHEDRINE 706
Tylenol Cold Medication, Non-Drowsy - See
ACETAMINOPHEN 4
DEXTROMETHORPHAN 296
PSEUDOEPHEDRINE 706
Tylenol Cold Night Time - See
ACETAMINOPHEN 4
ANTIHISTAMINES 98
DEXTROMETHORPHAN 296
PSEUDOEPHEDRINE 706
**Tylenol Cold No Drowsiness Formula
Gelcaps** - See
ACETAMINOPHEN 4
DEXTROMETHORPHAN 296
PSEUDOEPHEDRINE 706
Tylenol Cough - See
ACETAMINOPHEN 4
DEXTROMETHORPHAN 296
PSEUDOEPHEDRINE 706

Tylenol Cough with Decongestant - See
ACETAMINOPHEN 4
DEXTROMETHORPHAN 296
PSEUDOEPHEDRINE 706
Tylenol Extra Strength - See
ACETAMINOPHEN 4
Tylenol Infants' Drops - See
ACETAMINOPHEN 4
Tylenol Junior Strength - See
ACETAMINOPHEN 4
Tylenol Junior Strength Chewable Tablets -
See ACETAMINOPHEN 4
Tylenol Maximum Strength Cough - See
ACETAMINOPHEN 4
DEXTROMETHORPHAN 296
Tylenol Maximum Strength Flu Gelcaps - See
ACETAMINOPHEN 4
DEXTROMETHORPHAN 296
PSEUDOEPHEDRINE 706
Tylenol Maximum Strength Gelcaps - See
ACETAMINOPHEN 4
Tylenol No.1 - See NARCOTIC ANALGESICS &
ACETAMINOPHEN 582
Tylenol No.1 Forte - See NARCOTIC
ANALGESICS & ACETAMINOPHEN 582
Tylenol Regular Strength Caplets - See
ACETAMINOPHEN 4
Tylenol Regular Strength Tablets - See
ACETAMINOPHEN 4
Tylenol Sinus Maximum Strength - See
ACETAMINOPHEN 4
PSEUDOEPHEDRINE 706
Tylenol Sinus Maximum Strength Caplets - See
ACETAMINOPHEN 4
PSEUDOEPHEDRINE 706
Tylenol Sinus Maximum Strength Gelcaps -
See PSEUDOEPHEDRINE 706
Tylenol Sinus Medication - See
ACETAMINOPHEN 4
PSEUDOEPHEDRINE 706
Tylenol Sinus Medication Extra Strength - See
ACETAMINOPHEN 4
PSEUDOEPHEDRINE 706
Tylenol with Codeine - See NARCOTIC
ANALGESICS & ACETAMINOPHEN 582
Tylenol with Codeine No. 1 - See NARCOTIC
ANALGESICS & ACETAMINOPHEN 582
Tylenol with Codeine No. 2 - See NARCOTIC
ANALGESICS & ACETAMINOPHEN 582
Tylenol with Codeine No. 3 - See NARCOTIC
ANALGESICS & ACETAMINOPHEN 582
Tylenol with Codeine No. 4 - See NARCOTIC
ANALGESICS & ACETAMINOPHEN 582
Tylosterone - See ANDROGENS &
ESTROGENS 40
Tylox - See NARCOTIC ANALGESICS &
ACETAMINOPHEN 582
Ty-Pap - See ACETAMINOPHEN 4
Tyrodone - See
NARCOTIC ANALGESICS 580
PSEUDOEPHEDRINE 706

U

UAA - See ATROPINE, HYOSCYAMINE, METHENAMINE, METHYLENE BLUE, PHENYLSALICYLATE & BENZOIC ACID 136

Ugesic - See NARCOTIC ANALGESICS & ACETAMINOPHEN 582

Ulcidine - See HISTAMINE H₂ RECEPTOR ANTAGONISTS 412

Ulone - See CHLOPHEDIANOL 214

ULR-LA - See
GUAIFENESIN 398
PHENYLPROPANOLAMINE 668

Ultra Pred - See ANTI-INFLAMMATORY DRUGS, STEROIDAL (Ophthalmic) 108

Ultra Tears - See PROTECTANT (Ophthalmic) 702

ULTRAbrom PD - See
ANTIHISTAMINES 90
PSEUDOEPHEDRINE 706

Ultracef - See CEPHALOSPORINS 210

Ultragesic - See NARCOTIC ANALGESICS & ACETAMINOPHEN 582

Ultralente - See INSULIN 434

Ultralente Iletin I - See INSULIN 434

Ultram - See TRAMADOL 814

UltraMOP - See PSORALENS 708

Ultrase MT 12 - See PANCRELIPASE 630

Ultrase MT 20 - See PANCRELIPASE 630

Ultrase MT 24 - See PANCRELIPASE 630

Ultravate - See ADRENOCORTICOIDS (Topical) 16

Ultrazine-10 - See PHENOTHIAZINES 662

UNDECYLENIC ACID - See ANTIFUNGALS (Topical) 90

Unguentine - See ANESTHETICS (Topical) 46

Unguentine Plus - See ANESTHETICS (Topical) 46

Unguentine Spray - See ANESTHETICS (Topical) 46

Uni-Bent Cough - See ANTIHISTAMINES 98

Uni-Bronchial - See THEOPHYLLINE & GUAIFENESIN 784

Unicort - See ADRENOCORTICOIDS (Topical) 16

Uni-DeCon - See
ANTIHISTAMINES 98
PHENYLEPHRINE 664
PHENYLPROPANOLAMINE 668

Unilax - See
LAXATIVES, SOFTENER/LUBRICANT 474
LAXATIVES, STIMULANT 476

Unipen - See PENICILLINS 648

Uniphyl - See BRONCHODILATORS, XANTHINE 176

Unipres - See RESERPINE, HYDRALAZINE & HYDROCHLOROTHIAZIDE 726

Uniretic - See
ANGIOTENSIN-CONVERTING ENZYME (ACE) INHIBITORS 50
DIURETICS, THIAZIDE 324

Unisom Nighttime Sleep Aid - See ANTIHISTAMINES 98

Unisom SleepGels Maximum Strength - See ANTIHISTAMINES 98

Uni-Tussin - See GUAIFENESIN 398

Uni-Tussin DM - See
DEXTROMETHORPHAN 296
GUAIFENESIN 398

Univasc - See ANGIOTENSIN-CONVERTING ENZYME (ACE) INHIBITORS 50

Univol - See ANTACIDS 54

Unproco - See
DEXTROMETHORPHAN 296
GUAIFENESIN 398

Urabeth - See BETHANECHOL 168

Uracel - See SALICYLATES 744

Urecholine - See BETHANECHOL 168

Urex - See METHENAMINE 528

Uridon - See DIURETICS, THIAZIDE 324

Uridon Modified - See ATROPINE, HYOSCYAMINE, METHENAMINE, METHYLENE BLUE, PHENYLSALICYLATE & BENZOIC ACID 136

Urimed - See ATROPINE, HYOSCYAMINE, METHENAMINE, METHYLENE BLUE, PHENYLSALICYLATE & BENZOIC ACID 136

Urinary Antiseptic No. 2 - See ATROPINE, HYOSCYAMINE, METHENAMINE, METHYLENE BLUE, PHENYLSALICYLATE & BENZOIC ACID 136

Urised - See ATROPINE, HYOSCYAMINE, METHENAMINE, METHYLENE BLUE, PHENYLSALICYLATE & BENZOIC ACID 136

Uriseptic - See ATROPINE, HYOSCYAMINE, METHENAMINE, METHYLENE BLUE, PHENYLSALICYLATE & BENZOIC ACID 136

Urispas - See FLAVOXATE 366

Uritab - See ATROPINE, HYOSCYAMINE, METHENAMINE, METHYLENE BLUE, PHENYLSALICYLATE & BENZOIC ACID 136

Uritin - See ATROPINE, HYOSCYAMINE, METHENAMINE, METHYLENE BLUE, PHENYLSALICYLATE & BENZOIC ACID 136

Uritol - See DIURETICS, LOOP 318

Urobak - See SULFONAMIDES 770

Urocit-K - See CITRATES 238

Urodine - See PHENAZOPYRIDINE 660

Urogesic - See PHENAZOPYRIDINE 660

Uro-KP-Neutral - See POTASSIUM & SODIUM PHOSPHATES 672

Uro-Mag - See ANTACIDS 54

Uroplus DS - See
SULFONAMIDES 770
TRIMETHOPRIM 824

Uroplus SS - See
SULFONAMIDES 770
TRIMETHOPRIM 824

Urotoin - See NITROFURANTOIN 604

Uro-Ves - See ATROPINE, HYOSCYAMINE, METHENAMINE, METHYLENE BLUE, PHENYLSALICYLATE & BENZOIC ACID 136
Urozide - See DIURETICS, THIAZIDE 324
Ursinus Inlay - See
ASPIRIN 132
PSEUDOEPHEDRINE 706
URSODIOL 830
Ursofalk - See URSODIOL 830
Utex-S.R. - See
GUAIFENESIN 398
PHENYLPROPANOLAMINE 668
Uticort - See ADRENOCORTICOIDS (Topical) 16
U-Tract - See ATROPINE, HYOSCYAMINE, METHENAMINE, METHYLENE BLUE, PHENYLSALICYLATE & BENZOIC ACID 136

V

Vagistat - See ANTIFUNGALS (Vaginal) 92
Vagistat-1 - See ANTIFUNGALS (Vaginal) 92
VALACYCLOVIR - See ANTIVIRALS FOR HERPES VIRUS 122
Valadol - See ACETAMINOPHEN 4
Valadol Liquid - See ACETAMINOPHEN 4
Valergen-10 - See ESTROGENS 350
Valergen-20 - See ESTROGENS 350
Valergen-40 - See ESTROGENS 350
Valertest No. 1 - See ANDROGENS & ESTROGENS 40
Valertest No. 2 - See ANDROGENS & ESTROGENS 40
Valisone - See ADRENOCORTICOIDS (Topical) 16
Valisone Reduced Strength - See ADRENOCORTICOIDS (Topical) 16
Valisone Scalp Lotion - See ADRENOCORTICOIDS (Topical) 16
Valium - See BENZODIAZEPINES 156
Valnac - See ADRENOCORTICOIDS (Topical) 16
Valorin - See ACETAMINOPHEN 4
Valorin Extra - See ACETAMINOPHEN 4
Valpin 50 - See ANTICHOLINERGICS 74
VALPROIC ACID 832
Valrelease - See BENZODIAZEPINES 156
VALSARTAN - See ANGIOTENSIN II RECEPTOR ANTAGONISTS 48
Valtrex - See - See ANTIVIRALS FOR HERPES VIRUS 122
Vanacet - See NARCOTIC ANALGESICS & ACETAMINOPHEN 582
Vancenase - See ADRENOCORTICOIDS (Nasal Inhalation) 10
Vancenase AQ - See ADRENOCORTICOIDS (Nasal Inhalation) 10
Vanceril - See ADRENOCORTICOIDS (Oral Inhalation) 12
Vancocin - See VANCOMYCIN 834
VANCOMYCIN 834
Vanex Expectorant - See
GUAIFENESIN 398

NARCOTIC ANALGESICS 580
PSEUDOEPHEDRINE 706
Vanex Forte Caplets - See
ANTIHISTAMINES 98
PHENYLEPHRINE 664
PHENYLPROPANOLAMINE 668
Vanex Forte R - See ANTIHISTAMINES 98
Vanex LA - See
GUAIFENESIN 398
PHENYLPROPANOLAMINE 668
Vanex-HD - See
ANTIHISTAMINES 98
NARCOTIC ANALGESICS 580
PHENYLEPHRINE 664
Vanoxide 5 Lotion - See BENZOYL PEROXIDE 158
Vanquin - See ANTHELMINTICS 56
Vanquis - See ACETAMINOPHEN & SALICYLATES 6
Vanquish - See CAFFEINE 186
Vanseb Cream Dandruff Shampoo - See
ANTISEBORRHEICS (Topical) 118
KERATOLYTICS 464
Vanseb Lotion Dandruff Shampoo - See
ANTISEBORRHEICS (Topical) 118
KERATOLYTICS 464
Vanseb-T - See ANTISEBORRHEICS (Topical) 118
Vantin - See CEPHALOSPORINS 210
Vapocet - See NARCOTIC ANALGESICS & ACETAMINOPHEN 582
Vapo-Iso - See BRONCHODILATORS, ADRENERGIC 174
Vaponefrin - See BRONCHODILATORS, ADRENERGIC 174
Vascor - See CALCIUM CHANNEL BLOCKERS 192
Vascular headache suppressant - See
ISOMETHEPTENE, DICHLORALPHENAZONE & ACETAMINOPHEN 446
Vaseretic - See ANGIOTENSIN-CONVERTING ENZYME (ACE) INHIBITORS & HYDROCHLOROTHIAZIDE 52
Vasoclear - See DECONGESTANTS (Ophthalmic) 290
Vasoclear A - See DECONGESTANTS (Ophthalmic) 290
Vasocon - See DECONGESTANTS (Ophthalmic) 290
Vasocon Regular - See DECONGESTANTS (Ophthalmic) 290
Vasocon-A - See DECONGESTANTS (Ophthalmic) 290
Vasoconstrictor - See
CAFFEINE 186
ERGOTAMINE 342
ERGOTAMINE, BELLADONNA & PHENOBARBITAL 344
METHYSERGIDE 540
ORPHENADRINE, ASPIRIN & CAFFEINE 618

INDEX

Vicks NyQuil Multi-Symptom LiquiCaps - See
 ACETAMINOPHEN 4
 ANTIHISTAMINES 98
 DEXTROMETHORPHAN 296
 PSEUDOEPHEDRINE 706
**Vicks Pediatric Formula 44D Cough and
 Decongestant** - See
 DEXTROMETHORPHAN 296
 PSEUDOEPHEDRINE 706
Vicks Pediatric Formula 44E - See
 DEXTROMETHORPHAN 296
 GUAIFENESIN 398
**Vicks Pediatric Formula 44M Multi-Symptom
 Cough & Cold** - See
 ANTIHISTAMINES 98
 DEXTROMETHORPHAN 296
 PSEUDOEPHEDRINE 706
Vicks Sinex - See PHENYLEPHRINE 664
**Vicks Sinex 12-Hour Formula Decongestant
 Nasal Spray** - See OXYMETAZOLINE
 (Nasal) 624
**Vicks Sinex 12-Hour Formula Decongestant
 Ultra Fine Mist** - See OXYMETAZOLINE
 (Nasal) 624
**Vicks Sinex Long-Acting 12 Hour Nasal
 Spray** - See OXYMETAZOLINE (Nasal) 624
Vicodin - See NARCOTIC ANALGESICS &
 ACETAMINOPHEN 582
Vicodin ES - See NARCOTIC ANALGESICS &
 ACETAMINOPHEN 582
Vicodin-Tuss - See
 GUAIFENESIN 398
 NARCOTIC ANALGESICS 580
Vicoprofen - See
 ANTI-INFLAMMATORY DRUGS,
 NONSTEROIDAL (NSAIDs) 104
 NARCOTIC ANALGESICS 580
Vi-Daylin/F - See VITAMINS & FLUORIDE 850
Videx - See NUCLEOSIDE REVERSE
 TRANSCRIPTASE INHIBITORS 608
Vincol - See TIOPRONIN 802
Vioform Hydrocortisone Cream - See
 ANTIBACTERIALS, ANTIFUNGALS
 (Topical) 64
Vioform Hydrocortisone Lotion - See
 ADRENOCORTICOIDS (Topical) 16
 ANTIBACTERIALS, ANTIFUNGALS (Topical)
 64
Vioform Hydrocortisone Mild Cream - See
 ANTIBACTERIALS, ANTIFUNGALS
 (Topical) 64
Vioform Hydrocortisone Mild Ointment - See
 ANTIBACTERIALS, ANTIFUNGALS
 (Topical) 64
Vioform Hydrocortisone Ointment - See
 ANTIBACTERIALS, ANTIFUNGALS
 (Topical) 64
Viokase - See PANCRELIPASE 630
Vi-Penta F - See VITAMINS & FLUORIDE 850
Viprynium - See ANTHELMINTICS 56

Viracept - See PROTEASE INHIBITORS 700
Viramune - See NON-NUCLEOSIDE REVERSE
 TRANSCRIPTASE INHIBITORS 606
Viranol - See KERATOLYTICS 464
Viranol Ultra - See KERATOLYTICS 464
Virazid - See RIBAVIRIN 732
Virazole - See RIBAVIRIN 732
Viridium - See PHENAZOPYRIDINE 660
Virilon - See ANDROGENS 38
Virolon IM - See ANDROGENS 38
Viro-Med - See
 ANTIHISTAMINES 98
 ASPIRIN 132
 DEXTROMETHORPHAN 296
 GUAIFENESIN 398
 PSEUDOEPHEDRINE 706
Viroptic - See ANTIVIRALS (Ophthalmic) 126
Viscerol - See DICYCLOMINE 300
Visine - See DECONGESTANTS (Ophthalmic)
 290
Visine L.R. - See DECONGESTANTS
 (Ophthalmic) 290
Viskazide - See BETA-ADRENERGIC
 BLOCKING AGENTS & THIAZIDE
 DIURETICS 164
Visken - See BETA-ADRENERGIC BLOCKING
 AGENTS 162
Vistacrom - See CROMOLYN 266
Vistaril - See HYDROXYZINE 426
Vitabec 6 - See PYRIDOXINE (Vitamin B-6) 710
VitaCarn - See LEVOCARNITINE 484
**Vitalax Super Smooth Sugar Free Orange
 Flavor** - See LAXATIVES, BULK-FORMING
 470
Vitalax Unflavored - See LAXATIVES, BULK-
 FORMING 470
VITAMIN A 838
Vitamin A Acid Cream - See RETINOIDS
 (Topical) 730
Vitamin A Acid Gel - See RETINOIDS (Topical)
 730
Vitamin B-1 - See THIAMINE (Vitamin B-1) 792
Vitamin B-2 - See RIBOFLAVIN (Vitamin B-2) 734
Vitamin B-3 - See NIACIN (Vitamin B-3, Nicotinic
 Acid, Nicotinamide) 596
Vitamin B-5 - See PANTOTHENIC ACID
 (Vitamin B-5) 632
Vitamin B-6 - See PYRIDOXINE (Vitamin B-6) 710
Vitamin B-9 - See FOLIC ACID (Vitamin B-9) 382
VITAMIN B-12 (Cyanocobalamin) 840
VITAMIN C (Ascorbic Acid) 842
VITAMIN D 844
VITAMIN E 846
VITAMIN K 848
Vitamin supplement - See
 FOLIC ACID (Vitamin B-9) 382
 NIACIN (Vitamin B-3, Nicotinic Acid,
 Nicotinamide) 596
 PANTOTHENIC ACID (Vitamin B-5) 632
 PYRIDOXINE (Vitamin B-6) 710

Zanaflex - See TIZANIDINE 804
Zantac - See HISTAMINE H$_2$ RECEPTOR ANTAGONISTS 412
Zantac 75 - See HISTAMINE H$_2$ RECEPTOR ANTAGONISTS 412
Zantac Efferdose - See HISTAMINE H$_2$ RECEPTOR ANTAGONISTS 412
Zantac Geldose - See HISTAMINE H$_2$ RECEPTOR ANTAGONISTS 412
Zantac-C - See HISTAMINE H$_2$ RECEPTOR ANTAGONISTS 412
Zantryl - See APPETITE SUPPRESSANTS 130
Zapex - See BENZODIAZEPINES 156
Zarontin - See ANTICONVULSANTS, SUCCINIMIDE 80
Zaroxolyn - See DIURETICS, THIAZIDE 324
Zeasorb-AF Powder - See ANTIFUNGALS (Topical) 90
Zebeta - See BETA-ADRENERGIC BLOCKING AGENTS 162
Zebrax - See
   BENZODIAZEPINES 156
   CLIDINIUM 240
Zephrex - See
   GUAIFENESIN 398
   PSEUDOEPHEDRINE 706
Zephrex-LA - See
   GUAIFENESIN 398
   PSEUDOEPHEDRINE 706
Zerit - See NUCLEOSIDE REVERSE TRANSCRIPTASE INHIBITORS 608
Zeroxin-5 Gel - See BENZOYL PEROXIDE 158
Zeroxin-10 Gel - See BENZOYL PEROXIDE 158
Zestoretic - See ANGIOTENSIN-CONVERTING ENZYME (ACE) INHIBITORS & HYDROCHLOROTHIAZIDE 52
Zestril - See ANGIOTENSIN-CONVERTING ENZYME (ACE) INHIBITORS 50
Zetar - See COAL TAR (Topical) 254
Zetar Emulsion - See COAL TAR (Topical) 254
Zetar Medicated Antiseborrheic Shampoo - See COAL TAR (Topical) 254
Zetran - See BENZODIAZEPINES 156
Ziac - See BETA-ADRENERGIC BLOCKING AGENTS & THIAZIDE DIURETICS 164
Ziagen - See NUCLEOSIDE REVERSE TRANSCRIPTASE INHIBITORS 608
ZIDOVUDINE - See NUCLEOSIDE REVERSE TRANSCRIPTASE INHIBITORS 608
Zilactin-L - See ANESTHETICS (Mucosal-Local) 42
ZILEUTON - See LEUKOTRIENE MODIFIERS 480
ZINC ACETATE - See ZINC SUPPLEMENTS 856
ZINC GLUCONATE - See ZINC SUPPLEMENTS 856
ZINC SULFATE - See ZINC SUPPLEMENTS 856
ZINC SUPPLEMENTS 856

Zinc-220 - See ZINC SUPPLEMENTS 856
Zincate - See ZINC SUPPLEMENTS 856
Zincon - See ANTISEBORRHEICS (Topical) 118
Zithromax - See MACROLIDE ANTIBIOTICS 502
ZNP - See ANTISEBORRHEICS (Topical) 118
Zocor - See HMG-CoA REDUCTASE INHIBITORS 414
ZOLMITRIPTAN - See TRIPTANS 826
Zoloft - See SERTRALINE 750
ZOLPIDEM 858
Zomig - See TRIPTANS 826
Zonalon - See DOXEPIN (Topical) 332
Zorprin - See ASPIRIN 132
Zotrix - See CAPSAICIN 198
Zotrix-HP - See CAPSAICIN 198
Zovia 1/35E - See CONTRACEPTIVES, ORAL 262
Zovia 1/50E - See CONTRACEPTIVES, ORAL 262
Zovirax - See ANTIVIRALS FOR HERPES VIRUS 122
Zovirax Ointment - See ANTIVIRALS (Topical) 128
Zyban - See BUPROPION 178
Zydone - See NARCOTIC ANALGESICS & ACETAMINOPHEN 582
Zyflo - See LEUKOTRIENE MODIFIERS 480
Zyloprim - See ALLOPURINOL 20
Zymase - See PANCRELIPASE 630
Zymenol - See LAXATIVES, SOFTENER/LUBRICANT 474
Zyprexa - See OLANZAPINE 612
Zyrtec - See ANTIHISTAMINES, NONSEDATING 100